Lung and Pleural
Pathology

Lung and Pleural Pathology

Editor

Philip T. Cagle, MD
Medical Director, Pulmonary Pathology
Department of Pathology and Genomic Medicine
Houston Methodist Hospital
Houston, Texas

Professor of Pathology
Department of Pathology and Laboratory Medicine
Weill Cornell Medical College
New York, New York

Timothy Craig Allen, MD, JD
Professor, Department of Pathology
Director of Anatomic Pathology
The University of Texas Medical Branch
Galveston, Texas

New York   Chicago   San Francisco   Athens   London   Madrid   Mexico City
Milan   New Delhi   Singapore   Sydney   Toronto

1 2 3 4 5 6 7 8 9 0 CTP/CTP 19 18 17 16 15

ISBN 978-0-07-180955-9
MHID 0-07-180955-4

This book was set in Utopia Std 10/12 by MPS Limited.
The editors were Andrew Moyer and Regina Y. Brown.
The production supervisor was Catherine H. Saggese.
Production management was provided by Asheesh Ratra, MPS Limited.
China Translation & Printing Services, Ltd. was printer and binder.

This book is printed on acid-free paper.

Cataloging-in-publication data for this book is on file at the Library of Congress.

McGraw-Hill books are available at special quantity discounts to use as premiums and sales promotions, or for use in corporate training programs. To contact a representative, please visit the Contact Us pages at www.mhprofessional.com.

Dedication

Philip T. Cagle: Dedicated to my three friends with whom I have worked in the same department since we began together as trainees: Mary R. Schwartz, Dina R. Mody, and Luan D. Truong; and to our departmental administrator, Will H. Kyle, whose support and friendship has seen me through many tough times over the years.

Timothy Craig Allen: To my mentors, S. Donald Greenberg and Philip T. Cagle.

Contents

Contributors

Roberto Barrios, MD
Professor of Pathology and Genomic Medicine, Institute for
    Academic Medicine
Full Clinical Member, Houston Methodist Research Institute
Department of Pathology & Genomic Medicine
J.C. Walter Jr. Transplant Center
Houston Methodist Hospital
Houston, Texas
    Chapter 23, 24

Mary Beth Beasley, MD
Associate Professor of Pathology
Mount Sinai Medical Center
New York, New York
    Chapter 5

Melanie C. Bois, MD
Resident Physician
Mayo Clinic
Rochester, Minnesota
    Chapter 21

Alain C. Borczuk, MD
Columbia University Medical Center
Professor of Pathology at CUMC
New York, New York
    Chapter 11

Nahal Boroumand, MD
Assistant Professor of Pathology
Department of Pathology
University of Texas Medical Branch
Galveston, Texas
    Chapter 19, 25

Yasmeen Butt, MD
Pathology Resident
Department of Pathology
UT Southwestern Medical Center
Dallas, Texas
    Chapter 6, 7

Eunice K. Choi, MD
Department of Pathology and Genomic Medicine
Houston Methodist Hospital
Houston, Texas
    Chapter 17

Sanja Dacic, MD, PhD
Professor of Pathology
University of Pittsburgh
Pittsburgh, Pennsylvania
    Chapter 30

Subba Digumarthy, MD
Assistant Professor of Radiology, Harvard Medical School
Thoracic Radiologist, Massachusetts General Hospital
Boston, Massachusetts
    Chapter 4

Alexander G. Duarte, MD
Division of Pulmonary, Critical Care and Sleep Medicine
Professor, University of Texas Medical Branch
Galveston, Texas
    Chapter 15

Junya Fukuoka, MD, PhD
Professor, Department of Pathology
Nagasaki University Graduate School of Biomedical
    Sciences
Nagasaki, Japan
    Chapter 18

William K. Funkhouser Jr, MD, PhD
Professor, Pathology and Lab Medicine
UNC School of Medicine
Director, Anatomic and Surgical Pathology
UNC Hospitals
Chapel Hill, North Carolina
    Chapter 1

Miguel O. Gaxiola, MD
Pathologist, Head of Laboratory of Morfology
Instituto Nacional de Enfermedades Respiratorias(INER)
México City, México
    Chapter 23

Yimin Ge, MD
Department of Pathology and Genomic Medicine
Houston Methodist Hospital
Weill Medical College of Cornell University
Houston, Texas
    Chapter 17, 19, 25

Kimberly Golden, MD
Resident Physician, Department of Pathology
Northwestern University, Feinberg School of Medicine
Chicago, Illinois
Chapter 9

Alfredo Valero Gómez, MD
Fellow 2nd Year Pediatric Pathology, National Autonomous
    University of Mexico
Department of Pathology, National Medical Center "La
    Raza", Mexican Social Security Institute
México City, México
Chapter 24

Blythe K. Gorman, MD
Staff Pathologist
Department of Pathology and Genomic Medicine
Houston Methodist Hospital
Assistant Professor
Weill Cornell Medical College of Cornell University
Houston, Texas
Chapter 14

Abida K. Haque, MD
Department of Pathology and Genomic Medicine
Houston Methodist Hospital
Professor, Weill Medical School of Cornell University
New York, New York
Chapter 15

Aliya Husain, MD
Department of Pathology
The University of Chicago
Chicago, Illinois
Chapter 2

Jaishree Jagirdar, MD
Director of Anatomic Pathology and Professor of Pathology
Department of Pathology
University of Texas Health Science Center at San Antonio
San Antonio, Texas
Chapter 16

Kirk D. Jones, MD
Professor of Pathology
University of California San Francisco
San Francisco, California
Chapter 22

Fumi Kawakami, MD
Department of Diagnostic Pathology
Kobe University Hospital
Hyogo, Japan
Chapter 27, 28

Jason T. Koshy, MD
Resident
University of Texas Medical Branch
Galveston, Texas
Chapter 29

William B. Laskin, MD
Surgical Pathologist
Northwestern Memorial Hospital, Feinberg School Of
    Medicine
Northwestern University
Chicago, Illinois
Chapter 9

Rodolfo Laucirica, MD
Professor of Pathology and Immunology
Baylor College of Medicine
Director of Cytopathology
Ben Taub General Hospital
Houston, Texas
Chapter 13

Leslie A. Litzky, MD
Perelman School of Medicine at the University of
    Pennsylvania
Professor of Pathology and Laboratory Medicine
Director, Section of Medical Pathology at the Hospital of the
    University of Pennsylvania
Philadelphia, Pennsylvania
Chapter 10

Alberto M. Marchevsky, MD
Director, Pathology and Mediastinal Pathology
Department of Pathology and Laboratory Medicine
Cedars-Sinai
Los Angeles, California
Chapter 26

Mari Mino-Kenudson, MD
Associate Professor of Pathology, Harvard Medical School
Staff Pathologist, Massachusetts General Hospital
Boston, Massachusetts
Chapter 4

Mizuki Nishino, MD
Assistant Professor, Harvard Medical School
Staff Radiologist, Dana Farber Cancer Institute
Boston, Massachusetts
Chapter 3

Michiya Nishino, MD, PhD
Instructor of Pathology, Harvard Medical School
Staff pathologist/Cytopathologist, Beth Israel Deaconess
    Medical Center
Department of Pathology, Beth Israel Deaconess Medical
    Center
Boston, Massachusetts
Chapter 4

Andrew Paul Norgan, MD, PhD
Resident, Clinical Pathology
Department of Laboratory Medicine and Pathology
Mayo Clinic
Rochester, Minnesota
Chapter 12

Sergio Piña-Oviedo, MD
Resident
Department of Pathology and Genomic Medicine
Houston Methodist Hospital
Houston, Texas
Chapter 14

Jennifer Pogoriler, MD, PhD
Boston Children's Hospital
Boston, Massachusetts
Chapter 2

Kirtee Raparia, MD
Assistant Professor of Pathology
Northwestern University, Feinberg School of Medicine
Chicago, Illinois
Chapter 8

Michael P. Sedrak, MD
Surgical Pathology Fellow
University of Texas Medical Branch
Galveston, Texas
Chapter 29

Umar Nisar Sheikh, MD
Cytopathology Fellow
Department of Pathology and Laboratory Medicine
Emory University Hospital
Atlanta, Georgia
Chapter 20

Lynette M. Sholl, MD
Assistant Professor, Harvard Medical School
Associate Pathologist, Brigham and Women's Hospital
Boston, Massachusetts
Chapter 3

Arlene Sirajuddin, MD
Assistant Professor of Radiology
Department of Medical Imaging
College of Medicine
University of Arizona
Tucson, Arizona
Chapter 8

Deepika Sirohi, MD
Resident
Department of Pathology
University of Texas Health Science Center at San Antonio
San Antonio, Texas
Chapter 16

Charles E. Stager, PhD
Associate Professor of Pathology and Immunology
Baylor College of Medicine
Director of Microbiology
Ben Taub General Hospital
Houston, Texas
Chapter 13

Hidehiro Takei, MD
Department of Pathology and Genomic Medicine
Houston Methodist Hospital
Houston, Texas
Chapter 27, 28

Tomonori Tanaka, MD
Fellow, Department of Pathology
Nagasaki University Graduate School of Biomedical Sciences
Nagasaki, Japan
Chapter 18

Anatoly Urisman, MD, PhD
Clinical Instructor
Department of Pathology
University of California San Francisco
San Francisco, California
Chapter 22

Hironori Uruga, MD, PhD
Attending Physician
Department of Respiratory Medicine
Respiratory Center, Toranomon Hospital
Tokyo, Japan
Chapter 4

Celina Villa, MD
Resident Physician, Department of Pathology
Northwestern University, Feinberg School of Medicine
Chicago, Illinois
Chapter 9

Anjana Yeldandi, MD
Associate Professor in Pathology
Department of Pathology
Northwestern University, Feinberg School of Medicine
Chicago, Illinois
Chapter 9

Haijun Zhou, MD, PhD
Department of Pathology and Genomic Medicine
Houston Methodist Hospital
Houston, Texas
Chapter 17

Preface

There has been revolution in pulmonary pathology.

Lung cancer diagnoses now routinely utilize tumors' molecular characteristics to inform individual patient-centered precision treatment. The classification scheme of adenocarcinoma, the most common lung cancer, has evolved to reflect a new understanding of treatment and prognosis. Interstitial lung diseases are being increasingly better understood, with implications for newer treatments. Pulmonary infections with global implications such as SARS and avian flu have caught the public's attention. Authored by leaders in pulmonary pathology, *Lung and Pleural Pathology* was written to incorporate the most up-to-date information and fully embrace the very recent revolutionary advances in pulmonary disease.

Further, *Lung and Pleural Pathology* was written with a careful eye toward ease of use. Exhaustive pulmonary pathology treatises exist, but for general pathologists or pathologists with subspecialty expertise in areas other than pulmonary pathology—pathologists who routinely diagnose the vast majority of lung and pleural diseases—the very nature of those books makes them too unwieldy for everyday use. *Lung and Pleural Pathology*, utilizing a large number of images and charts in each chapter, is an up-to-date, exhaustive treatise that is nonetheless easy and quick for a pathologist to use on a daily basis, either in print or electronically. Its ease of use makes *Lung and Pleural Pathology* an excellent tool for the fast provision of pertinent, up-to-date information about lung and pleural diseases that can assist with diagnosis, consultation with clinicians, tumor boards, and discussions with patients and families.

Many thanks to the dedication and hard work of the authors in sharing their knowledge and understanding of the many pulmonary diseases for the betterment of patient care and diagnostic accuracy.

Philip T. Cagle
Timothy Craig Allen

Overview of Lung Diseases

William K. Funkhouser

TAKE HOME PEARLS

- The lung is a sophisticated machine that facilitates countercurrent diffusion of oxygen and carbon dioxide across a living semipermeable alveolar membrane between (liquid) blood and (gaseous) inhaled air.
- The lung functions automatically, is position independent, adapts to changes in demand and gas concentration, autoregulates perfusion to match ventilation, automatically responds to injury and infection, and is self-cleaning.
- It must be emphasized that individual signs and symptoms are rarely specific for a particular lung disease, and should be considered along with radiographic and morphologic findings to narrow the differential diagnosis.
- A major challenge for the current generation of surgical pathologists and cytopathologists is determining the appropriate allocation of scarce tissue for morphologic diagnosis, flow cytometric study, cytogenetics, prognostic/predictive variable subtyping, and biorepository placement for future research.

INTRODUCTION

The lung is an amazing organ. It is a sophisticated machine that facilitates countercurrent diffusion of oxygen and carbon dioxide across a living semipermeable alveolar membrane between (liquid) blood and (gaseous) inhaled air. It functions automatically, is position independent, adapts to changes in demand and gas concentration, autoregulates perfusion to match

ventilation, automatically responds to injury and infection, and is self-cleaning.

Lung diseases are etiologically heterogeneous and encompass developmental anomalies, infections, dust inhalation, ischemia, neoplasm, degeneration, and autoimmunity. The pathogenesis of lung disease may involve inflammation, fibrosis, excesses/deficits, necrosis, and hemorrhage; with resulting distortion of normal function, including abnormalities of ventilation, perfusion, and gas exchange.

HISTORY OF RELEVANT DISCOVERIES

Our current understanding of lung disease was many centuries in the making, and is worthy of a brief overview. The pre-Renaissance understanding of human anatomy and physiology was limited by Aristotle's and Galen's fixed concepts of nature, with its four elements, four humors, four temperaments, and four causes, and with the concept of lung function as a bellows for the heart via the pulmonary vein. Vesalius (1543) corrected Galenic misunderstanding of human cardiac anatomy, noting that there is no normal interventricular septal blood flow.[1,2] His contemporary Colombo (1559) correctly modeled pulmonary blood flow, identifying pulmonary veins as carrying blood, not air, to the left atrium.[3] Harvey (1628) corrected Galenic misunderstanding of blood production, consumption, and flow, including the identification of parallel pulmonary and systemic circulation of a stable blood volume.[3] Malpighi (1661) identified microscopically the capillaries that

Harvey had assumed must exist to connect arteries to veins in the lung.[4] Carbon dioxide was described by van Helmant (ca 1630), and oxygen by Scheele and Priestley (1774).[5] The concept of partial pressures of different molecules in a mixture was defined by Dalton (1801), and the concept of predictable equilibrium of a molecule between gas and liquid phases, based on partial pressures, by Henry (1803).[6] Hemoglobin was discovered by Hunefeld in 1840, and oxygen binding to hemoglobin by Hoppe-Seyler in the mid-19th century. The mathematics of molecular diffusion was described by Fick (1855). The development, approximately 1905-1915, of a closed system pulmonary function test device that could measure ventilatory volumes and vary the mixtures of oxygen and carbon dioxide allowed measurement of the effect of their binding to hemoglobin (the Haldane effect), and the effects of carbon dioxide and hydrogen on oxygen binding to hemoglobin (the Bohr effect).[7] Improved microscopic image quality resulted from French and German development of the substage condenser and apochromatic lenses in the late 19th century. Radiographic discoveries, predominantly in the last century, have significantly enhanced the understanding of lung disease. These include plain film radiographs (Roentgen, 1895) and tomographic technologies starting in the 1970s for humans, based on physical chemistry and radionuclide chemistry (CT scan, Hounsfield), MRI (Damadian, Lauterbur), and PET (Brownell, Kuhl).[8-11] Radionuclide estimates of pulmonary ventilation and perfusion were developed by Knipping (1957) and Wagner (1963), allowing estimates of ventilation:perfusion matching.[12]

NORMAL LUNG DEVELOPMENT

The normal adult lung is a complex system of conducting airways, gas exchange surfaces, and paired arterio-capillary-venous vascular networks. The embryonic lung develops as a ventral foregut derivative that progressively bifurcates to create branchpoints ("carinas") for conducting airways (bronchi, then bronchioles, then alveolar ducts). Conducting airways form during the "pseudoglandular" phase by 15 weeks' gestational age, and protoalveoli are evident in loose mesenchyme during the "canalicular" phase by 24 weeks' gestational age. The mesenchyme is progressively excluded or flattened between developing alveoli, such that an adult lung has back-to-back alveolar airspaces separated by elastin-rich, capillary-rich interstitial stroma.[13,14]

The rate-limiting steps for postpartum lung function appear to be diffusion distance and water surface tension. Human beings have thin alveolar type 1 epithelial cells and a fused basement membrane that minimizes gas diffusion distance between alveoli and capillaries, but also with type 2 cells that secrete sufficient surfactant by 36 weeks' gestational age to break the surface tension of the water lining the alveolar surface. Together, thin alveolar type 1 cells and functional type 2 cells ensure mechanical opening and ventilation of alveoli, with effective gas exchange, in 95% of newborns by 36 weeks' gestational age.[14,15]

NORMAL ADULT LUNG

The trachea and bronchi are encircled by near-circumferential cartilage rings which prevent collapse of these large-caliber airways during the positive intrathoracic pressure expiratory phase of the ventilatory cycle. These airways show lush surface cilia and submucosal glands that secrete mucin. Moving distally past the bronchus are bronchioles that retain the surface cilia, but definitionally do not have cartilage rings or submucosal glands. Bronchi and bronchioles are paired with pulmonary artery branches of similar caliber. More distally/peripherally, alveolar ducts have a simple nonciliated epithelium, and move gas to and from lobules of alveoli. Incomplete ridges subdivide the alveolar surface area into intersecting spheres which in tissue sections look like incomplete circles separated by thin, delicate, capillary-rich alveolar septa. The capillaries within the alveolar septa are surrounded by abundant elastin, and together comprise the interstitium. Overall, it is estimated that there are 300 million alveoli in the adult lung, together comprising 80 m² of alveolar surface for gas exchange.[15,16]

Normal lung mechanics and normal conducting airways facilitate compliant ventilation of clean, dry alveoli, and that thin delicate elastic alveolar septa facilitate countercurrent gas exchange between alveolar gas oxygen and RBC hemoglobin-bound carbon dioxide. Oxygen and carbon dioxide diffuse according to their relative concentration gradients, the unique diffusion characteristics for each molecule, and the diffusion distance, according to Fick law.[17] Ideally, there is physiologic autoregulation of ventilation and perfusion, such that there is minimal dead space (ventilated but not perfused) and minimal shunting (perfused but not ventilated). Pulmonary function testing allows estimation of capacities (total, residual, expiratory reserve), usual function (tidal volume, respiratory rate, minute ventilation), and maximal function (forced expiratory volume within 1 second and between 25% and 75% of expired volume).

HOST RESPONSES TO LUNG INJURIES AND INFECTIONS

The lung has a limited set of architectural and cytologic responses to injury and infection. These include accumulation of cells, accumulation of fluids, architectural remodeling, and altered flow in airways and vessels.

Inflammation and Specific Immune Responses

In immunocompetent patients, inflammatory cells traffic into the lung in response to infections and allergens, and immune cells traffic into the lung in response to infections and allografts. Neutrophils accumulate in response to bacterial infection. Eosinophils accumulate in association with type 1 hypersensitivity (allergic) responses. Lymphocytes accumulate in response to viral infections and allografts. Histiocytes accumulate in response to dusts, aspirated foodstuffs, or myco-bacterial/fungal infections, and can accumulate as epithelioid histiocytes into granulomata, or as multinucleated giant cells in foreign body responses. Lymphohistiocytic infiltrates and nodules can be seen in autoimmune diseases such as rheumatoid arthritis, systemic lupus erythematosus, and Sjögren syndrome.[18-20] Pericapillary cuffing by lymphocytes is seen in acute cellular rejection of lung allografts, unfortunately mimicking host response to virus.

Most bacteria trigger an acute inflammatory response which may evolve into bronchopneumonia with sheets of neutrophils accumulating within affected alveolar airspaces (bronchopneumonia. Some bacteria, such as *Staphylococcus* and *Klebsiella*, can trigger associated parenchymal necrosis. Viruses trigger a chronic inflammatory response, with accumulation of lymphocytes in the interstitium at the site of viral proliferation. Some viruses, such as cytomegalovirus, adenovirus, herpes, and measles, show a recognizable viral cytopathic effect. Most fungi and mycobacteria trigger focal stromal accumulation of epithelioid histiocytes, forming granulomas.[21]

In immunosuppressed patients, whether iatrogenic due to chemotherapy, allograft, or chronic corticosteroids, or secondary to HIV infection, the usual stigmata of host response to infection may be muted or absent, and a high index of suspicion must be maintained for infection in immunosuppressed patients. Reflex screening for common infectious agents like viruses and fungi may be helpful in these patients. Epstein-Barr virus can show a polyclonal blast response but can transform B lymphocytes, with clonal proliferation into recognizable lymphoma.

Fibroblastic/Fibrocytic Proliferation

Fibroblastic proliferation in alveoli can be seen as a late phase of infections (organizing pneumonia) and after the fibrin-rich first week of diffuse alveolar damage (organizing phase diffuse alveolar damage). Fibroblastic proliferation in the interstitium can be seen after the fibrin-rich first week of diffuse alveolar damage, and in usual interstitial pneumonitis. Mature fibrosis from fibrocytic synthesis of collagen can be seen in

remodeled lung. Survived diffuse alveolar damage, obliterative bronchiolitis, fibrogenic dust pneumoconiosis, autoimmune diseases, fibrous nonspecific interstitial pneumonia, usual interstitial pneumonia, and honeycomb lung are good examples.[22-24]

Intra-alveolar Macrophage Accumulation

Pulmonary alveolar macrophages are infrequent (approximately one per alveolar cross section) in normal lung. These marrow-derived cells function as phagocytes. Accumulation of alveolar macrophages can be seen following dust inhalation (cigarette smoke, silicates), distal to airway obstruction (postobstructive pneumonia/endogenous lipoid pneumonia), following mineral oil aspiration (exogenous/extrinsic lipoid pneumonia), and as foreign body giant cells following foodstuff aspiration.[25,26]

Type 2 Cell Proliferation After Necrosis of Type 1 Cells

Type 2 cell hyperplasia is seen in association with exudative phase diffuse alveolar damage, and is presumed to represent the local stem cell hyperplasia that repopulates the denuded type 1 cells of the alveolar surface.[27]

Mucocyte Hyperplasia

Surface and submucosal glandular hyperplasia of mucocytes can be seen in association with chronic dust inhalation, for example, cigarette smoking, asthma, cystic fibrosis, and primary ciliary dyskinesia.

Conducting Airway Smooth Muscle

Smooth muscle hyperplasia can be seen in the hyperreactive airway disease, asthma, and as a metaplastic proliferation in honeycomb lung.[27]

Mesothelial Hyperplasia

Mesothelial hyperplasia can be seen in association with adjacent infections, fibrinous pleuritis, granulomatous inflammation, and pleural metastasis. Mesothelial hyperplasia can be cytologically extremely atypical, and may easily mimic pleural diffuse malignant mesothelioma.

Neoplastic Transformation

Normal cells in the lung can become transformed into clonal neoplasms, with accumulation in the lung related to loss of growth control. Chronic exposure to aromatic mutagens in smoke can lead to neoplastic transformation of normal and metaplastic epithelium. The working hypothesis for pathogenesis of approximately 90% of the common lung primary carcinomas (essentially all small cell carcinomas and squamous cell carcinomas, and most adenocarcinomas) is that mutagens form adducts with DNA, with subsequent mutation of DNA during S phase of the cell cycle, with clonal transformation via loss of control over proliferation and programmed cell death/apoptosis.[20] Many primary pleural diffuse malignant mesotheliomas are associated with increased exposure to asbestos, of unclear pathogenesis. The lung and pleura can host involvement by metastasis from nonpulmonary primary carcinoma, sarcoma, and melanoma, and these metastases are thought to be more common than lung primaries. Rare lymphomas can develop within the lung and pleura, but are more likely to involve lymph nodes or thymus.

Accumulation of Fluid or Fibrin

Fluids normally present in the lung can be present in excess, leading to clinical disease. Transudate free water can accumulate in the interstitium +/− the alveolar airspaces when capillary hydrostatic pressure exceeds the limit for the capillary basement membrane. Congestive left heart failure, mitral stenosis, and pulmonary venoocclusive disease are examples. Surfactant can accumulate in alveolar airspaces due to dust inhalation, overproduction, or underclearance (pulmonary alveolar proteinosis). Hemorrhage into the lung parenchyma can occur with vasculitis (Wegener granulomatosis, Churg-Strauss syndrome, Goodpasture syndrome, systemic lupus erythematosus), necrotizing granulomatous inflammation in response to fungus or mycobacteria, vasoinvasive *Aspergillus*, or ischemic infarction.[28,29] Mucin can accumulate in individuals with chronic dust exposure (chronic bronchitis), chronic asthma, chronic infection (cystic fibrosis, primary ciliary dyskinesia, allergic bronchopulmonary aspergillosis), and can lead to mucous plugs that cannot be cleared with normal pulmonary toilet. Ischemic necrosis or inflammation can lead to increased permeability of the capillary basement membrane, with resultant serum leakage into the interstitium and/or alveolar airspaces, with coagulation cascade activation and fibrin accumulation (exudative phase of diffuse alveolar damage).

Necrosis

Central coagulative necrosis is typical for the granulomatous host response to fungal or mycobacterial infections, and geographic coagulative necrosis can be seen in association with the granulomatous vasculitis of Wegener granulomatosis, and Churg-Strauss syndrome.[30] Necrosis and granuloma formation are

not expected in association with lupus or Goodpasture syndrome. Also, ischemic infarction occurs roughly in 10% of patients with survivable pulmonary emboli, and classically presents with a pleural-based triangle with the obstructed pulmonary artery at its apex.

Architectural Destruction or Remodeling

Architectural destruction and remodeling encompasses alveolar septal destruction; parenchymal fibrosis with remodeling; conducting airway dilation, constriction, and obstruction; and vascular hypertrophy and stenosis due to high pressure or high flow. Destruction of elastase by cigarette smoking or via α1-antitrypsin deficiency leads to rupture and destruction of alveolar septa, with evolution of progressively larger-diameter alveolar airspaces, with commensurate loss of gas exchange surface area.[31,32] Alveolar parenchyma and adjacent subpleural stroma can be remodeled by fibrosing diseases such as usual interstitial pneumonia, pneumoconiosis (environmental fibrosing silicate dusts), autoimmune diseases (systemic lupus erythematosus, rheumatoid arthritis), and following spontaneous pneumothorax.

Altered Flow

Both bronchi and bronchioles can be progressively dilated by chronic inflammation and scarring associated with congenital mutations (cystic fibrosis, primary ciliary dyskinesia), chronic infections, or proximal airway obstruction. Acute constriction of conducting airways (asthma) is due to airway hyperreactivity to a variety of triggers, and is usually reversible. Subacute obstruction of bronchioles by fibroblastic plugs can be seen in bronchiolitis obliterans. Chronic constriction of bronchioles by either submucosal or luminal fibrosis (obliterative bronchiolitis) can be due to a drug side effect, or to chronic allograft rejection following lung transplantation.[33,34] Chronic elevation of pulmonary arterial pressure or flow (typically due to left to right shunts) can lead to secondary muscular arterial medial and intimal hypertrophy/fibrosis (pulmonary arterial hypertension).

DIFFERENT CLASSIFICATION SCHEMES FOR LUNG DISEASES

Pathologists generally consider disease entities in terms of etiology, pathogenesis, natural history, and effects on normal anatomy/physiology with their clinical and radiographic correlates. Recently, demand for molecular subtyping of neoplasms to identify cases with treatable mutations has taught us that we are guiding the hands of the medical oncologist as well as the surgeon. Classifications of lung diseases vary depending on these different perspectives on diseases.

Etiology and Pathogenesis

Etiologic categories include germline mutations (cystic fibrosis, primary ciliary dyskinesia), infections (bacteria, mycoplasma, mycobacteria, fungus, virus), mutagens (lung cancers), allergens (hypersensitivity pneumonitis, asthma), autoimmunity (rheumatoid arthritis, systemic lupus erythematosus, Goodpasture syndrome, Sjögren syndrome, Wegener granulomatosis), dusts/smoke (silicosis, asbestosis, chronic obstructive pulmonary disease), aspiration, degenerative (emphysema), and idiopathic. Pathogenetic categories include dilation (bronchiectasis), constriction (asthma), obstruction (pulmonary embolism, mucus plug), rupture (emphysema), necrosis (pulmonary embolism with infarct), inflammation (pneumonia, autoimmunity), fibrosis (usual interstitial pneumonia, autoimmunity, fibrosing dust response), and clonal neoplastic proliferation (lung cancers).

Clinical Presentation

Onset

Lung diseases vary in their onset and progression of signs and symptoms, ranging from acute to chronic. For example, diffuse alveolar damage develops abruptly, usually following shock of any cause, such that the patient or their family can usually identify the exact clinical event that triggered the start of diffuse alveolar damage. Subacute diseases develop over a period of weeks to months, and may be seasonal in nature, as with hypersensitivity pneumonitis. Chronic diseases such as usual interstitial pneumonia develop over a period of months to years, with insidious progression of signs and symptoms. Some diseases, such as hypersensitivity pneumonitis or eosinophilic pneumonia, can have a variety of presentations ranging from acute to chronic.[35]

Duration

Lung diseases vary widely in duration. Some are self-limited, such as treated bronchopneumonia and resolving diffuse alveolar damage. Some are seasonal, such as allergy-triggered asthma. Others, such as usual interstitial pneumonia, are chronic and progressive.

Signs and symptoms

Many of the clinical presenting signs of patients with lung diseases are nonspecific for a particular lung disease or class of diseases. Cough can be seen in diseases ranging from infections (mycoplasmal or bacterial bronchopneumonia) to reactive mucocyte hyperplasia (chronic bronchitis), to fibrosing remodeling diseases (usual interstitial pneumonia). Sputum production can be seen in lung diseases ranging from germline mutations affecting epithelial water balance and/or ciliary torque (cystic fibrosis, primary ciliary dyskinesia) to reactive mucocyte hyperplasia (chronic bronchitis), to hyper-reactive airways (asthma). Fever can be seen in lung diseases ranging from infections, such as bacterial bronchopneumonia, to autoimmune diseases such as systemic lupus erythematosus, to B symptoms in some lymphomas. Arthritis can be the presenting symptom for autoimmune diseases (rheumatoid arthritis, systemic lupus erythematosus) or bacterial sepsis leading to multiorgan failure (diffuse alveolar damage). The lung can be involved primarily by autoimmune diseases, or secondarily as a consequence of therapeutic immunosuppression of autoimmune diseases. A history of seasonal allergy may guide the diagnosis of a particular trigger for asthma, and can be used to guide the removal of allergens from the home and workplace in patients with asthma and extrinsic allergic alveolitis. Unintentional weight loss can be seen in association with inflammatory bowel diseases and with neoplastic cachexia.

Likewise, many of the clinical presenting symptoms of patients with lung diseases are nonspecific. Dyspnea can be seen in lung diseases ranging from vascular diseases (pulmonary emboli, congestive heart failure) to shock (diffuse alveolar damage), to hyperreactive airways (asthma), to smoke-associated chronic obstructive pulmonary disease. Malaise and loss of appetite are similarly nonspecific for narrowing the differential to even a class of lung diseases. It must be emphasized that individual signs and symptoms are rarely specific for a particular lung disease, and should be considered along with radiographic and morphologic findings to narrow the differential diagnosis.

Relevant medical history

Medications can damage the lung directly, or can be associated with increased risk for diseases that involve the lung secondarily. Salicylates taken for inflammatory bowel disease can trigger organizing pneumonia, and chemotherapeutic agents can directly damage the delicate airspace epithelium. Inhaled recreational drugs can contain particular dusts that trigger foreign body responses. Cigarettes can cause direct carcinogen-adduct damage to exposed epithelium, leading to metaplasia, dysplasia, and invasive carcinoma. Also, immunosuppressive agents, including systemic cytotoxic drugs and systemic corticosteroids, can predispose the individual to lung infections, and to diffuse alveolar damage following systemic sepsis.

Concurrent illnesses can predispose to immunosuppression and secondary lung infection, based on the inherent pathogenesis of the disease, such as HIV infection, or the immunosuppressive medications used to treat the disease, for example, autoimmune diseases and allografts. Travel history may be relevant to the workup of eosinophilic pneumonia, infectious pneumonia, and parasitic infestation, particularly if to known endemic areas.

Radiographic Findings

X-ray, CT scan, and MRI make use of the relative density differences between air and water/water-containing tissues, and bone. However, water density in alveolar parenchyma is nonspecific for water, and may be mimicked by blood, pus, infection, or postobstructive changes. Water density in large conducting airways can be mimicked by mucus plugs, carcinoid tumors, or carcinomas. CT scan may be able to distinguish mucin density from water density. Likewise, air densities are nonspecific for emphysema-associated septal destruction, and can be seen in hyperinflation, such as in asthma, or in subtotal proximal airway obstruction, as may occur, for example, with carcinoid tumor. The caliber of airways and their peribronchovascular stroma may narrow the differential diagnosis. For example, high-resolution CT scan may allow diagnosis of bronchiectatic airway dilation, and may allow diagnosis of the peribronchovascular stromal expansion seen with sarcoidosis, extrinsic allergic alveolitis, or pulmonary Langerhans cell histiocytosis.[36]

Pathologic Findings

Anatomic pathology

Many of the lung diseases affect particular anatomic compartments within the lung. These compartments include the tracheobronchus, bronchioles, peribronchovascular stroma, alveoli, alveolar septa/ interstitium, blood vessels, lymphatics, and pleura. The tracheobronchial airway is uniquely held open by cartilage rings and supplied with mucin by abundant submucosal glands, so is affected by certain diseases, such as salivary gland–type neoplasms, chronic bronchitis, and scleroderma, which do not affect the more distal bronchiolar conducting airways.

The bronchiolar airways are involved by certain diseases that are uncommon in the more proximal tracheobronchial tree, such as respiratory bronchiolitis/ interstitial lung disease, obliterative bronchiolitis. Peribronchovascular stroma can be involved by sarcoidosis, hypersensitivity pneumonia, and pulmonary Langerhans cell histiocytosis. Alveolar air spaces can be involved by infectious agents, including bacteria and fungi, and their host inflammatory responses, aspirated material, blood, pus, and free water. The alveolar septa/ interstitium of lung can be expanded by inflammatory cells, fibroblasts, fibrin, and free water, and can be destroyed and remodeled by fibrosis. Blood vessels can be obstructed by thromboemboli, can hypertrophy in

response to elevated pulmonary artery pressure or flow (pulmonary artery hypertension), can become inflamed and necrotic (Wegener granulomatosis, Churg-Strauss syndrome). Lymphatics can become dilated in children (lymphangiectasia), and lymphatic-distribution nonnecrotizing granulomatous inflammation can be seen in sarcoidosis. Pleural mesothelium can proliferate and become cytologically extremely atypical, can leak serum and develop fibrinous pleuritis, and can be involved by metastases.

Clinical and molecular pathology

Ancillary tests such as serologies, cultures, viral load polymerase chain reaction, and molecular/cytogenetic tests can provide additional support for putative morphologic diagnoses, including serologic testing for autoimmune diseases (Wegener granulomatosis, Churg-Strauss syndrome, rheumatoid arthritis, systemic lupus erythematosus), cultures/sensitivities (bacteria, fungi, and mycobacteria), qualitative polymerase chain reaction (influenza), and cytogenetic screens for pathognomonic translocations (synovial sarcoma, primitive neuroectodermal tumor). They may also be able to identify molecular therapeutic targets, such as quantitative polymerase chain reaction for Epstein-Barr virus viral load in posttransplant lymphoproliferative disease, cytogenetic screen for ALK translocation, and nucleic acid resequencing for activating mutations in EGFR exons 18-21 in lung adenocarcinoma, or to exclude certain therapies based on nucleic acid resequencing involving activating mutations in KRAS in lung adenocarcinoma.

Integration of Clinical, Radiographic, and Pathologic Findings

Accurate lung disease diagnosis frequently requires an integrated approach involving clinical presentation, radiographic findings, gross features, microscopic morphologic findings, and clinical lab data. Clinical presentation generates an initial differential diagnosis, and drives ordering of radiographs and radiology-guided or surgical tissue sampling. X-ray, CT scan, MRI, and PET scan are performed in order to narrow the differential diagnosis. Tissue sampling is performed with the anticipation that it will provide sufficient lesional tissue to allow both morphologic diagnosis and, when necessary, molecular subtyping, which in turn will drive clinical management. A major challenge for the current generation surgical pathologists and cytopathologists is determining the appropriate allocation of scarce tissue for morphologic diagnosis, flow cytometric study, cytogenetics, prognostic/predictive variable subtyping, and biorepository placement for future research.

REFERENCES

1. West JB. Galen and the beginnings of Western physiology. *Am J Physiol Lung Cell Mol Physiol*. 2014;307(2):L121-L128.

2. West JB. History of respiratory mechanics prior to World War II. *Compr Physiol*. 2012;2(1):609-619.

3. Castaneda AR. From Glenn to Fontan. A continuing evolution. *Circulation*. 1992;86(5 suppl):II80-II84.

4. Pearce JM. Malpighi and the discovery of capillaries. *Eur Neurol*. 2007;58(4):253-255.

5. Sternbach GL, Varon J. The discovery and rediscovery of oxygen. *J Emerg Med*. 2005;28(2):221-224.

6. Fishman GA. John dalton: though in error, he still influenced our understanding of congenital color deficiency. *Ophthalmic Genet*. 2008;29(4):162-165.

7. Tyuma I. The Bohr effect and the Haldane effect in human hemoglobin. *Jpn J Physiol*. 1984;34(2):205-216.

8. Scatliff JH, Morris PJ. From Roentgen to magnetic resonance imaging: the history of medical imaging. *N C Med J*. 2014;75(2):111-113.

9. Reed AB. The history of radiation use in medicine. *J Vasc Surg*. 2011;53(1 suppl):3S-5S.

10. Bautz W, Kalender W. [Godfrey N. Hounsfield and his influence on radiology]. *Radiologe*. 2005;45(4):350-355.

11. Prasad A. The (amorphous) anatomy of an invention: the case of magnetic resonance imaging (MRI). *Soc Stud Sci*. 2007;37(4):533-560.

12. Isawa T. [Pulmonary nuclear medicine]. *Kaku Igaku*. 1995;32(11):1281-1288.

13. Boyden EA. Observations on the anatomy and development of the lungs. *J Lancet*. 1953;73(12):509-512.

14. Wells LJ, Boyden EA. The development of the bronchopulmonary segments in human embryos of horizons XVII to XIX. *Am J Anat*. 1954;95(2):163-201.

15. Pump KK. The morphology of the finer branches of the bronchial tree of the human lung. *Dis Chest*. 1964;46:379-398.

16. Godwin JD, Tarver RD. Accessory fissures of the lung. *AJR Am J Roentgenol*. 1985;144(1):39-47.

17. Roetman EL, Barr RE. The mechanical basis for Fick's law and its generalizations. *Adv Exp Med Biol*. 1976;75:261-265.

18. Kitaichi M. Pathology of pulmonary sarcoidosis. *Clin Dermatol*. 1986;4(4):108-115.

19. Nagai A. Pathology and pathophysiology of chronic obstructive pulmonary disease. *Intern Med*. 2002;41(4):265-269.

20. Allen TC, Cagle PT, Popper HH. Basic concepts of molecular pathology. *Arch Pathol Lab Med*. 2008;132(10):1551-1556.

21. Bals R, Hiemstra PS. Innate immunity in the lung: how epithelial cells fight against respiratory pathogens. *Eur Respir J*. 2004;23(2):327-333.

22. Lynch JP 3rd, Wurfel M, Flaherty K, et al. Usual interstitial pneumonia. *Semin Respir Crit Care Med*. 2001;22(4):357-386.

23. Flaherty KR, Travis WD, Colby TV, et al. Histopathologic variability in usual and nonspecific interstitial pneumonias. *Am J Respir Crit Care Med*. 2001;164(9):1722-1727.

24. Harrison NK, Myers AR, Corrin B, et al. Structural features of interstitial lung disease in systemic sclerosis. *Am Rev Respir Dis*. 1991;144(3 pt 1):706-713.

25. Lotem J, Shabo Y, Sachs L. The network of hemopoietic regulatory proteins in myeloid cell differentiation. *Cell Growth Differ*. 1991;2(9):421-427.

26. Warner AE. Pulmonary intravascular macrophages. Role in acute lung injury. *Clin Chest Med*. 1996;17(1):125-135.

27. Tomashefski JF Jr. Pulmonary pathology of acute respiratory distress syndrome. *Clin Chest Med*. 2000;21(3):435-466.

28. Schwarz MI, Fontenot AP. Drug-induced diffuse alveolar hemorrhage syndromes and vasculitis. *Clin Chest Med*. 2004;25(1):133-140.

29. Collard HR, Schwarz MI. Diffuse alveolar hemorrhage. *Clin Chest Med*. 2004;25(3):583-592, vii.

30. Travis WD, Hoffman GS, Leavitt RY, Pass HI, Fauci AS. Surgical pathology of the lung in Wegener's granulomatosis. Review of 87 open lung biopsies from 67 patients. *Am J Surg Pathol*. 1991;15(4):315-333.

31. Cuvelier A, Muir JF, Hellot MF, et al. Distribution of alpha(1)-antitrypsin alleles in patients with bronchiectasis. *Chest*. 2000;117(2):415-419.

32. Shin MS, Ho KJ. Bronchiectasis in patients with alpha 1-antitrypsin deficiency. A rare occurrence? *Chest*. 1993;104(5):1384-1386.

33. Cordier JF. Bronchiolitis obliterans organizing pneumonia. *Semin Respir Crit Care Med*. 2000;21(2):135-146.

34. Lazor R, Vandevenne A, Pelletier A, Leclerc P, Court-Fortune I, Cordier JF. Cryptogenic organizing pneumonia. Characteristics of relapses in a series of 48 patients. The Groupe d'Etudes et de Recherche sur les Maladies "Orphelines" Pulmonaires (GERM"O"P). *Am J Respir Crit Care Med*. 2000;162(2 pt 1):571-577.

35. Sharma OP, Fujimura N. Hypersensitivity pneumonitis: a non-infectious granulomatosis. *Semin Respir Infect*. 1995;10(2):96-106.

36. Barker AF. Bronchiectasis. *N Engl J Med*. 2002;346(18):1383-1393.

2 Pediatric Pulmonary Diseases

Jennifer Pogoriler and Aliya Husain

TAKE HOME PEARLS

- The spectrum of pediatric lung disease in children is different from that seen in the adult.
- Lung development, age of the patient, and clinical features are key elements in forming the differential diagnosis.
- Comparison with normal lung of the appropriate gestation is helpful in evaluating lung biopsy in infants.
- Electron microscopy is helpful in evaluating surfactant dysfunction disorders.
- Histochemical and immunohistochemical stains are important in confirming infections.
- The majority of tumors in the lung are metastases from elsewhere; primary lung tumors are rare in children.

APPROACH TO PEDIATRIC LUNG DISEASE

Although children, particularly older adolescents, may rarely develop diffuse lung diseases similar to those seen in adults, there is a separate spectrum of developmental and/or genetic diseases specific to childhood. These diseases typically present in infancy. Recently established European registries[1,2] confirm the early presentation of most diffuse lung diseases and have found that the most common forms include surfactant disorders, hemosiderosis, sarcoidosis, and hypersensitivity pneumonitis. However, these registries included both those diagnoses made on biopsy and those made

on clinical and radiological evidence and may not represent the same spectrum of diseases seen in biopsy specimens.

The recent American Thoracic Society guidelines for evaluation of pediatric diffuse lung disease[3] endorse separating interstitial conditions from other causes of diffuse lung disease including cystic fibrosis, immunodeficiency, congenital heart disease, bronchopulmonary dysplasia, infection, primary ciliary dyskinesia, and recurrent aspiration. If these are excluded clinically and other testing is not diagnostic or an urgent diagnosis is required, surgical lung biopsy is strongly recommended to further classify the disease. Classification incorporating clinical and radiological features should be based on a recent scheme (originally designed for children under 2 years of age) that separates disorders into those more common in infancy (diffuse developmental disorders, growth abnormalities, surfactant dysfunction diseases, pulmonary interstitial glycogenosis, and neuroendocrine cell hyperplasia of infancy) and those without specific age of onset (disorders of normal or immunocompromised hosts, systemic disease processes, and vascular diseases).[4] However, others have argued that, particularly in older children, the spectrum of disease may need to be broadened.[5] Despite clinical, imaging, and surgical lung biopsy, a fraction of cases may remain unclassifiable.[1,6,7]

Lung development is traditionally divided into the histologic stages of pseudoglandular, canalicular, saccular, and alveologenesis, but the disorders associated with abnormal lung development can be more simply understood as disorders in airway development (usually localized as in bronchial atresia with congenital pulmonary airway malformations) or disorders in alveologenesis (usually diffuse, including diffuse developmental disorders and lung disease of prematurity). Localized pediatric lung lesions, either solid or cystic, are also distinct from the typical masses seen in adults. Common benign localized lesions in pediatrics include malformations, many of which are variations of bronchial obstruction with associated cystic lesions (sequestrations and congenital pulmonary airway malformations). Most pediatric lung tumors are metastatic; primary lung tumors are rare and are most commonly carcinoid tumors, inflammatory myofibroblastic tumors, or pleuropulmonary blastoma. Salivary-gland type tumors are also more common in children than in adults.[8-10]

SPECIAL CONSIDERATIONS OF SPECIMEN HANDLING

Consensus guidelines for the handling of fresh tissue for pediatric pulmonary biopsies advocate dividing the wedge resection for special testing including culture, electron microscopy, and potential special studies requiring frozen tissue (molecular, immunofluorescence, or genetic testing). Specific protocols are available,[11] although tissue sterility may be better preserved when cultures are sent as separate specimens directly from the operating room. Electron microscopy should be considered in all diffuse lung diseases. In addition to surfactant deficiency, electron microscopy may be helpful to identify glycogen in pulmonary interstitial glycogenosis, since glycogen can be lost in paraffin processing.

DISORDERS OF LUNG DEVELOPMENT

Diffuse developmental disorders mimicking an arrest in early lung development present in term infants. A clinical differential diagnosis for acute respiratory distress at birth in a term infant with diffuse lung disease includes diffuse developmental defects, surfactant abnormalities, and meconium aspiration.

They are extremely rare and have nearly 100% mortality without transplant. They are occasionally seen in biopsy but are more frequent at autopsy. Given the rarity of the diffuse developmental disorders, there may be some overlap in features between subtypes, and diagnostic criteria are not well defined. Later defects in alveologenesis are commonly seen in association with lung disease of prematurity, congenital heart disease, and chromosomal syndromes.

Although the exact period during which alveologenesis takes place is a matter of debate, much of it occurs during the first several years of life. Lung growth

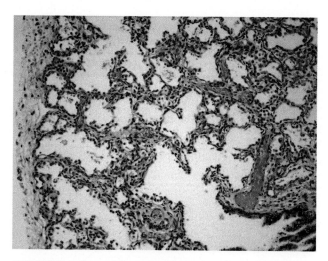

FIGURE 2-1 Normal lung. Normal alveolar architecture is seen in this section of the lung from a term infant.

in older children is more dependent on the increasing size of the alveoli. Evaluation of all infant lung biopsies for diffuse lung disease should begin with assessment of normal development. The alveoli of infants should be small and polygonal (*Figure 2-1*). Secondary crests, where new alveolar walls are projecting from the saccules, may be seen in infants and have a double row of capillaries before fusion creates a single capillary layer. Comparison with normal lung of the same age is helpful when evaluating the size and shape of alveoli.

Acinar Dysplasia

Clinical features of acinar dysplasia

Acinar dysplasia has also been referred to as Type 0 congenital pulmonary airway malformation (see below) and presents at birth with severe respiratory failure and pulmonary hypertension. Patients typically survive for only hours to days. The small number of reported cases suggests a female predominance, and there are reports of familial disease; however, a specific genetic defect has not been identified. The lungs are usually small relative to the size/weight expected for the infant's size.

Imaging features of acinar dysplasia

Imaging demonstrates bilateral small lung volumes which may be hazy on chest x-ray, but the findings on both chest x-ray and fetal ultrasound are nonspecific.

Histologic features of acinar dysplasia

The features of acinar dysplasia have been described in case reports or very small series.[12-15] The lungs resemble late pseudoglandular lung development with primitive airways widely spaced by abundant mesenchyme. Increased cartilage is associated with the abnormal

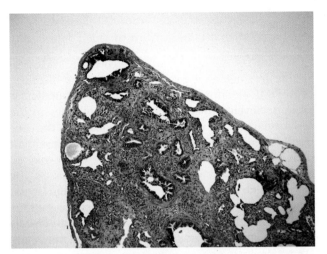

FIGURE 2-2 Acinar dysplasia. This is a lung biopsy from a full-term, 1-week-old infant who died several days later. The architecture is notable for bronchioles that extend to the pleural surface with extremely limited alveolar development. This marked lack of lung development is most likely a variant of acinar dysplasia, although even this degree of alveolar development is unusual in this condition.

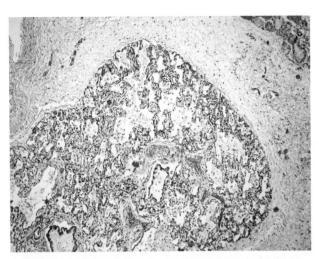

FIGURE 2-3 Alveolar dysplasia. This autopsy specimen from a term infant who developed respiratory distress at birth and died at 2 weeks of age shows slightly enlarged airspaces and thickened alveolar septa. These findings have been suggested to represent alveolar dysplasia, but the contribution of ventilation to this morphology cannot be excluded.

proximal airways. There is differentiation to cuboidal or columnar ciliated epithelium. Alveoli are virtually entirely absent, resulting in bronchioles that extend to the pleura or to the interlobular septa, although there may be some variation in severity even within a single patient (*Figure 2-2*). Other reported abnormalities include absent arteries accompanying terminal bronchioles.

Congenital Alveolar Dysplasia

Clinical features of alveolar dysplasia

Congenital alveolar dysplasia (CAD) also typically presents in the full-term neonate with respiratory failure and may have associated pulmonary hypertension. Only extremely rare cases of this entity have been reported, and the diagnostic criteria are not well defined, but rare patients with this form of abnormal development have survived to childhood.

Imaging features of alveolar dysplasia

The imaging features are not well defined and are not specific.

Histologic features of alveolar dysplasia

Extremely rare case reports of this entity exist.[16-19] CAD is characterized by an arrest in lung development superficially resembling the late canalicular or saccular stage; however, there is normal epithelial differentiation of the airways, and the small airspaces are lined by mature epithelium rather than the cuboidal epithelium of early development. In addition, there are numerous

capillaries in the septa. Importantly, normal numbers and location of capillaries are present, and there is no misalignment of pulmonary veins. Medial hypertrophy of pulmonary arteries may be present. Additional reported features include prominent connective tissue associated with bronchovascular bundles, interlobular septa, and the pleura.

For several reasons, the diagnosis of CAD is problematic.[20] The original historic descriptions included patients with what is now recognized as hyaline membrane disease. Currently, criteria distinguishing mesenchymal changes specific to this disorder from those due to therapy are undefined, and it is uncommon to see a biopsy or autopsy from an infant who has not been aggressively treated (*Figure 2-3*). Moreover, some patients with CAD have cells with clear cytoplasm in the mesenchyme. The degree of overlap with PIG (see below) is unknown. Finally, some cases reportedly have features that overlap with alveolar capillary dysplasia with misalignment of the pulmonary veins.

Alveolar Capillary Dysplasia With Misalignment of Pulmonary Veins

Clinical features of alveolar capillary dysplasia with misalignment of pulmonary veins

Similar to acinar dysplasia and CAD, alveolar capillary dysplasia with misalignment of pulmonary veins (ACDMPV) also presents with respiratory distress usually within days of birth. Severe pulmonary hypertension is always present. It is the most common of the diffuse developmental disorders, and recent reports of presentations later in infancy suggest the possibility of a broader spectrum of both clinical and pathological disease than was initially appreciated. Patients with ACDMPV often have other associated developmental defects, particularly in the gastrointestinal tract, but cardiac or genitourinary anomalies have also been reported. ACDMPV should be suspected in term neonates with idiopathic persistent pulmonary hypertension of the newborn.[21] Mutations in the transcription factor FOXF1 have been identified in a subset of patients with this disorder.

Imaging features of alveolar capillary dysplasia with misalignment of pulmonary veins

The imaging features of ACDMPV are nonspecific and range from a normal chest x-ray to diffuse ground glass opacities.[22]

Histologic features of alveolar capillary dysplasia with misalignment of pulmonary veins

Similar to congenital alveolar dysplasia, the histology of ACDMPV[23] superficially resembles the canalicular stage of development. Importantly, capillaries in the septa are markedly reduced and are located in the center of the septa (*Figure 2-4*), away from the basement membrane. Immunohistochemistry for CD34 may be useful to highlight the location and number of vessels. The veins, which normally run in the interlobular septa, are aberrantly located in the bronchovascular bundle. The differential diagnosis for these thin-walled vessels in the septa includes dilated lymphatics (which are D2-40 positive and usually have thinner walls and an absence of blood in the lumen) or thin-walled arteriolar branches. However, while an occasional

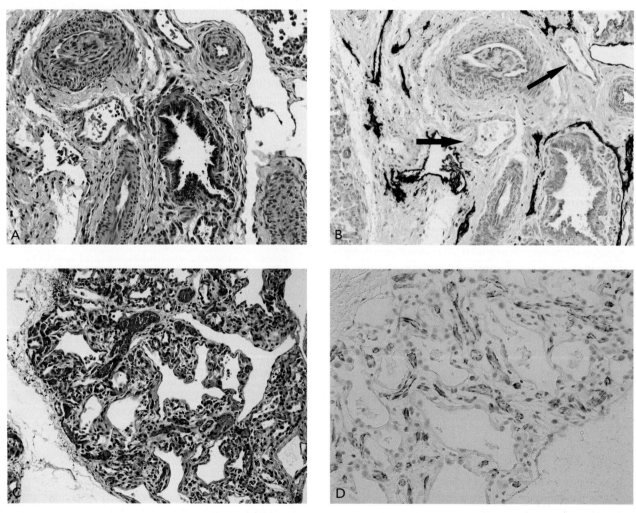

FIGURE 2-4 Alveolar capillary dysplasia with misalignment of the pulmonary veins. This biopsy from a 12-day-old infant with persistent pulmonary hypertension shows muscularized, thin-walled veins (a) in the bronchovascular bundles. Unlike the lymphatics, the veins are negative on by immunohistochemistry for D2-40 (b, arrow). The architecture is simplified with insufficient alveolar development and decreased, central alveolar wall capillaries (c) that do not form appropriate air-blood barriers. Immunohistochemistry for CD31 (d) highlights the scant capillaries and their abnormal location.

thin-walled arteriole might be seen, thin-walled vessels in most bronchovascular bundles are not typical. Similar mislocalization of vein-like structures into the bronchovascular bundles has recently been reported in bronchopulmonary dysplasia,[24] but the prevalence of this finding is unclear. In addition to the abnormal development of capillaries and veins, pulmonary arteries show marked hypertensive changes, similar to that seen in idiopathic persistent pulmonary hypertension of the newborn. Lymphangiectasia may also be present. In patients with less severe disease, the airspace developmental arrest and capillary abnormalities may be patchy and overall less severe. Cases with well-developed capillaries opposed to the alveolar basement membrane with misplacement of the veins have been described as an overlap of CAD/ACD.[19,20] The best classification of these cases is unclear.

Lung Disease of Prematurity

Clinical features of lung disease of prematurity

Given improved care of preterm infants including prenatal steroids, surfactant, and altered ventilation strategies, both respiratory distress syndrome (RDS, hyaline membrane disease) and chronic lung disease of prematurity are much less frequent than in the past. RDS, presenting shortly after birth with tachypnea and cyanosis, is due to a deficiency in surfactant either due to immaturity of the lung or rarely to genetic defects in surfactant (see below). Patients without acute RDS may still develop chronic lung disease of prematurity.

Chronic lung disease of prematurity (bronchopulmonary dysplasia, BPD) is found in preterm infants who require mechanical ventilation. Severity-based classifications of BPD are now defined based on the need for supplemental oxygen at different gestational ages. With improvements in prenatal care, BPD is now found predominantly in neonates at the earliest ages of gestation and at very low birth weights. Other factors including infection and poorly understood genetic changes also likely underlie the predisposition of some infants for both RDS and BPD. Outcomes for BPD are variable and depend on severity of the disease. Respiratory symptoms may persist into adulthood, but other patients show marked improvement. Infants are at increased risk of poor neurological outcomes.

Imaging features of lung disease of prematurity

In RDS, imaging shows small lung volumes, diffuse ground glass opacities, and air bronchograms. In BPD, chest x-ray may appear near normal while high resolution CT can show areas of hypertransradiancy due to decreased vascularity, patchy hyperinflation, and other nonspecific abnormalities.[25]

Histologic features of lung disease of prematurity

Typical findings of RDS are seen at autopsy and consist of eosinophilic hyaline membranes (*Figure 2-5*) similar to diffuse alveolar damage (see Chapter 20) in adults, although in patients who die within hours of birth the membranes may not yet have accumulated. Similar findings are seen in other causes of diffuse lung damage, including infection, and are not specific for RDS. Mortality from RDS is usually seen in only the most premature infants or those with other complications, and it follows aggressive treatment. Superimposed changes relating to treatment or other conditions may be difficult or impossible to separate from those due to RDS itself.

Historically, BPD developed in infants who were born at later preterm dates and treated with higher oxygen concentrations and higher pressures. The combination of oxygen and mechanical trauma resulted in damage to the airway epithelium with resulting epithelial necrosis, squamous metaplasia, fibrosis, and smooth muscle hypertrophy. There was marked but variable fibrosis and extension of muscle into the alveolar septa. These features of "old BPD" are no longer seen in their original severity, although chronic airway changes may be present.

Instead, a "new BPD" is seen in infants treated with prenatal corticosteroids, surfactant, and improved ventilation strategies who are born at gestational ages prior to the stage of alveologenesis. "New BPD" is predominantly characterized by an arrest in alveologenesis. This deficient alveolarization (alveolar growth abnormality) is one of the more common diagnoses in biopsies of infants[1,7] as well as one of the more commonly overlooked abnormalities. It is associated not only with lung disease of prematurity, but also with pulmonary hypoplasia, congenital heart disease, and chromosomal

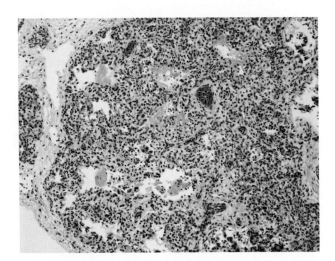

FIGURE 2-5 **Respiratory distress syndrome. This autopsy specimen from a 1-day-old infant born at 27 weeks' gestation shows hyaline membrane formation.**

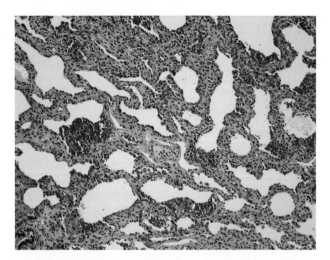

FIGURE 2-6 Bronchopulmonary dysplasia. This biopsy from a 3-month-old, former premature infant shows simplified, round airspaces with thickened alveolar septa.

disorders. In these cases, it is rarely biopsied except to rule out other superimposed etiologies when the patient's symptoms are out of proportion to those that are expected.

Depending on the severity of the changes, disorders in alveolar growth may be more or less difficult to recognize. Identification is facilitated by comparison to normal lung of the same age. In alveolar growth abnormalities, the lobules have fewer alveoli, with each airspace being larger in size and round (in comparison to the normal polygonal shape). Mild interstitial fibrosis may be present (*Figure 2-6*). Assessment of radial alveolar count (see below) can be helpful but lacks reproducibility.[26,27] In addition to these diffuse changes, focal changes of pulmonary interstitial glycogenosis (see below) as well as pulmonary hypertensive changes are often found.[1,4,7]

Pulmonary Hyperplasia

Clinical features of pulmonary hyperplasia

During early lung development, airway fluid promotes airway branching and development, and obstructions that prevent fluid from leaving the lung are associated with hyperplasia. This may rarely be seen diffusely but is more commonly focal. Congenital high airway obstruction such as laryngeal atresia in Fraser syndrome is extremely rare and presents with diffuse pulmonary hyperplasia and massive ascites. In contrast, local hyperplasia is secondary to permanent or transient bronchial obstruction. The underlying etiologies include bronchial atresia, bronchomalacia, mucous plugging, or external compression (such as by abnormal pulmonary vessels). Localized hyperplasia may be asymptomatic or may present with respiratory distress, depending on

the extent of involvement. Common forms of localized hyperplasia include CPAM type 3 (identified in neonates as involving most or all of one lung with high rates of respiratory distress due to the extent of involvement), and polyalveolar lobe, usually seen in isolation in the left upper lobe.

Imaging features of pulmonary hyperplasia

Pulmonary hyperplasia appears as a localized increase in lung transparency due to increased airspaces, sometimes with a shift of the mediastinum due to mass effect. Imaging demonstrating this local "congenital lobar emphysema" may correspond to either polyalveolar lobe with increased numbers of alveoli or to lung with hyperinflated but normal numbers of alveoli.

Histologic features of pulmonary hyperplasia

Polyalveolar lung is a localized lesion recognized to have increased numbers of alveoli based on an increased radial alveolar count (*Figure 2-7A*). It is often seen in association with bronchial atresia (see below). These cases of congenital lobar emphysema may or may not be accompanied by actual architectural enlargement of airspaces (*Figure 2-7B*).[28] The radial alveolar count can be determined by drawing a line drawn perpendicularly from the center of a respiratory bronchiole to the closest pleural surface or interlobular septum and counting the number of alveoli crossed by the line. This should be averaged over at least 10 fields.[29] Age-related normal values (with large standard deviations) are available, but the reproducibility of this measurement has been questioned[30,31] due to interobserver variability, state of lung inflation, and the location of the lung sections. Identification of sufficient numbers of appropriate airways may be impossible in surgical lung biopsies. CPAM type 3 (see below), is typically seen in neonates or fetuses and demonstrates immature lung with increased numbers of alveoli, increasing the total tissue between interlobular septa.

Pulmonary Hypoplasia

Clinical features of pulmonary hypoplasia

Pulmonary hypoplasia is almost always secondary to other developmental defects including oligohydramnios (due to premature rupture of membranes or genitourinary malformation), congenital diaphragmatic hernia or other space-occupying lesions of the thorax, decreased perfusion due to cardiovascular anomalies, or musculoskeletal disorders with an abnormally shaped thorax or impaired fetal breathing. Patients present with respiratory distress and outcomes

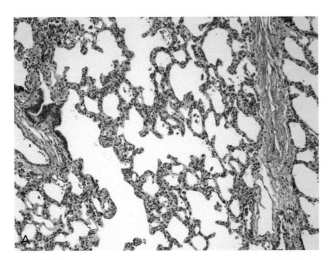
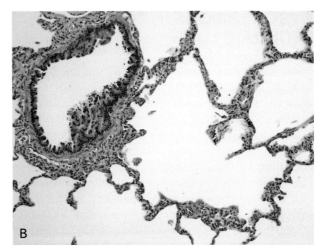

FIGURE 2-7 Congenital lobar emphysema. This infant with hyperlucency and presumed CPAM had no airway malforma-tion but did show increased radial alveolar count, consistent with polyalveolar lobe (a). In another infant with localized hyperlucency, normal numbers of enlarged alveoli were present consistent with congenital lobar emphysema (b).

are typically related to the severity of the hypoplasia and associated underlying condition.

Imaging features of pulmonary hypoplasia

Prenatal ultrasound may show a decreased thorax: abdomen circumference or alterations in other ratios of lung volumes, and fetal MRI may be used to calculate relative lung volumes, but the ability of these techniques to predict mortality due to postnatal pulmonary hypo-plasia is poor.[32] Postnatally, various imaging modalities show a shifted mediastinum (with unilateral hypoplasia), abnormally shaped thorax, or bell-shaped diaphragm.

Histologic features of pulmonary hypoplasia

Pulmonary hypoplasia is most commonly defined as a decreased lung weight:body weight ratio (<1.2% at 28 weeks' gestation or <1.5% at earlier gestation), although other measures including lung volumes and radial alveolar counts have been used, and based on strict weight standards alone more subtle degrees of pulmonary hypoplasia may be missed.[33,34] Postmortem lung weights may be unreliable if markedly increased due to edema, inflammation, or hemorrhage. Reported histologic findings have been variable and may depend on the timing and type of underlying condi-tion. Findings may include abnormalities in branching morphogenesis and/or alveologenesis. Although some lungs may appear histologically normal, maturation is typically delayed[35,36] (*Figure 2-8*), resulting in simpli-fied airspaces, increased mesenchyme, and decreased radial alveolar counts.

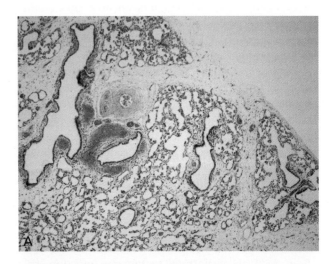
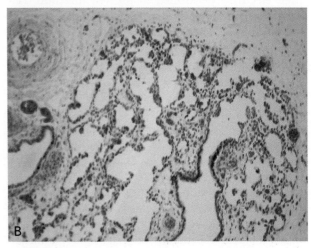

FIGURE 2-8 **Pulmonary hypoplasia. In this full-term infant with congenital renal aplasia, there is marked simpli-fication of the airways (a) with respiratory bronchioles approaching the pleura (b).**

CYSTIC LESIONS IN THE PEDIATRIC LUNG

Localized benign developmental lesions of the lung include congenital pulmonary adenomatoid malformations/congenital cystic adenomatoid malformations (CPAM, CCAM), bronchogenic cysts, intra- and extralobar sequestrations, bronchial atresia, and congenital lobar emphysema. Some lesions may be classified according to these traditional categories (described below), but there is often marked histologic overlap, and the underlying pathophysiology is likely similar. During early lung development, airway fluid promotes airway branching and development, and local obstructions that prevent fluid from leaving the lung are associated with focal hyperplasia with either relatively normal histology or cystically abnormal airways. Bronchial atresia may be identified as a component of many or even most of these cystic entities[37,38] which are often characterized by abnormal development of the airways and/or parenchyma. It has been suggested that the particular appearance of a cystic lesion may be the result of the timing, location, or degree of obstruction during development.[39]

Although previously considered to be rare and associated with marked morbidity, the incidence of these lesions is increasing due to widespread prenatal imaging. Many lesions are identified in utero, and serial imaging during pregnancy may show improvement or resolution over time as the lesion stops growing while the surrounding lung continues to grow. Relatively small residual lesions are often identified on postnatal imaging. Intrauterine therapy is reserved for large lesions with associated fetal hydrops, while in asymptomatic neonates surgery is typically deferred for several months. Lobectomy or segmentectomy is often electively performed to prevent infection, rule out associated malignancy, and improve growth of the remaining lung.[40] Less commonly, these lesions may be identified in older children and adolescents either incidentally or due to superimposed infection.

The features used to categorize these lesions include the vascular supply (pulmonary or systemic), location (intra- or extrapleural), relationship to the bronchial tree (normal connection, bronchial atresia, connection to gastrointestinal tract), macroscopic cyst size, and microscopic type of cyst lining. Specimens received from thoracoscopic procedures are often fragmented, and correlation with surgical or radiographic information may be required for diagnosis. In practice, precise classification may be difficult. Since the prognosis is predominantly dependent on associated malformations, the relative size of the lesion, and any associated pulmonary hypoplasia of the uninvolved lobes, a descriptive diagnosis is often sufficient.

Bronchogenic Cysts

Clinical features of bronchogenic cysts

Bronchogenic cysts are most commonly detected in the mediastinum but may also be found as intrapulmonary masses or rarely in other locations inside or even out of the thorax. They are often discovered incidentally but may present with respiratory distress due to compression of airways or with infection. They are through to arise due to aberrant outpouching in the foregut early in development.

Imaging features of bronchogenic cysts

Imaging demonstrates well-circumscribed, rounded, fluid-filled masses, sometimes with compression effects on surrounding structures. Importantly, there is no communication with the spinal cord as in neuroenteric cysts.

Histologic features of bronchogenic cysts

These unilocular single cysts do not connect to the tracheobronchial tree and are lined by ciliated columnar epithelium with submucosal glands, focal cartilage, and smooth muscle. The epithelium may undergo various types of metaplasia, but the presence of submucosal glands and cartilage is a helpful feature (*Figure 2-9*). The differential diagnosis includes duplication cysts of the gastrointestinal tract, which may also be lined by respiratory-type epithelium but have two layers of muscularis and lack cartilage. Different authors have applied different criteria to the exact wall components required to define these cysts, but in the absence of definitive features, a specimen may safely be called a foregut cyst.

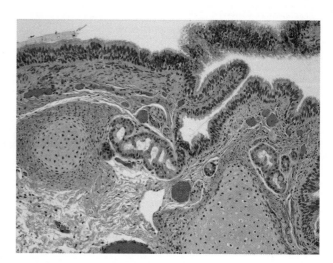

FIGURE 2-9 Bronchogenic cyst. This cyst is lined by respiratory-type epithelium and has both cartilage and submucosal glands in the wall.

Bronchial Atresia

Clinical features of bronchial atresia

Bronchial atresia is classically asymptomatic and detected incidentally in older children. In isolated bronchial atresia the left upper lobe is most commonly involved. Obstruction of airflow can lead to congenital lobar emphysema (CLE) due to air trapping and overdistension of the distal lung, or to polyalveolar lobe, a localized form of pulmonary hyperplasia (see above). Bronchial atresia is often a component of CPAMs and sequestrations (see below).

Imaging features of bronchial atresia

Imaging findings include the combination of radiodense opacity (mucocele) and distal hyperlucency of the overexpanded distal lung.[41] In neonatal cases, the distal lung may instead show features of fluid trapping as the amniotic fluid fails to be cleared through the obstructed airway.

Histologic features of bronchial atresia

Classic forms of bronchial atresia are associated with a large mucocele (*Figure 2-10*) just distal to the point of obstruction with mucous and foamy macrophages in the distal airways. Air trapping leads to hyperexpanded parenchyma, sometimes with emphysematous changes, similar to other causes of congenital lobar emphysema. Parenchymal changes are variable but include polyalveolar lobe, a form of localized pulmonary hyperplasia (see above), and focal changes similar to those seen in CPAM, especially type 2, as well as less well-characterized subtle maldevelopment.[39]

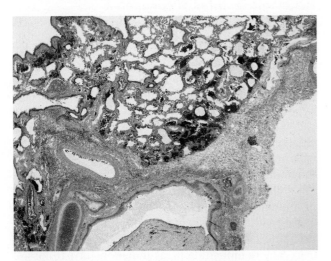

FIGURE 2-10 Bronchial atresia. This localized cystic lesion resected from a 7-month-old infant shows a mucocele (bottom center) in the large airway at the edge of the resection with associated abnormal, large airspaces distally.

Pulmonary Sequestration

Clinical features of pulmonary sequestration

Pulmonary sequestrations are portions of lung with a systemic vascular supply without connection to the main tracheobronchial tree, either with bronchial atresia or rarely with connection to the gastrointestinal tract. Extralobar sequestrations are invested in their own pleura and occur most commonly in the thorax, although they can be subdiaphragmatic. They are thought to be due to an early developmental defect with development of separate lung tissue outside the normal lungs, similar to bronchogenic cysts. However, unlike bronchogenic cysts they are often associated with other congenital anomalies. Intralobar sequestrations are within the lung proper and less commonly associated with other malformations. They are most often detected in the lower lobe. They previously presented at older ages due to infection and were hypothesized to be secondary to recurrent inflammation, but they are now commonly detected prenatally and understood to be developmental malformations. Although the pulmonary parenchyma in sequestrations may occasionally be morphologically unremarkable, it often shows at least focal abnormalities similar to CPAM, particularly type 2. Bronchial atresia is often identified on imaging or microdissection.

Imaging features of pulmonary sequestration

If they are large, feeding vessels may be identified on ultrasound, but typically imaging findings do not distinguish between intrapulmonary sequestration and CPAM (see below).

Histologic features of pulmonary sequestration

Although pulmonary sequestrations may demonstrate normal lung development, they often have at least focal parenchymal maldevelopment similar to type 2 CPAM (*Figure 2-11A*) (see below).[42] In older children, superimposed chronic inflammation may be present (*Figure 2-11B*). Features of bronchial atresia including mucous plugging and foamy histiocytes can often be seen, and abnormally large arteries should be seen entering the pleura (*Figure 2-11C*), consistent with the systemic blood supply.

Congenital Pulmonary Airway Malformations

Clinical features of congenital pulmonary airway malformations

CPAMs, also known as cystic adenomatoid malformations, are located within the lung and receive their blood supply from the pulmonary circulation. CPAMs

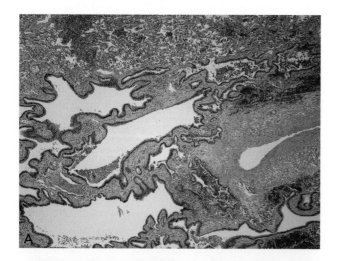

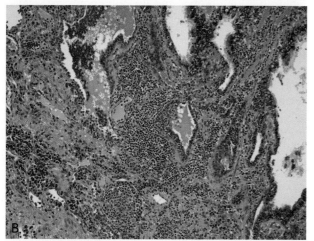

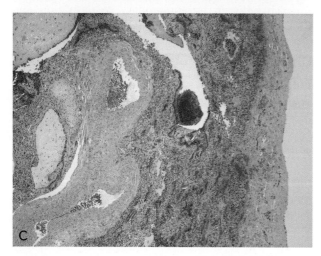

FIGURE 2-11 Sequestrations. This intralobar sequestration (a) shows focally increased bronchioles (bottom), similar to changes seen in type 2 CPAM but was supplied by systemic vessels. Other parts of the sequestration show relatively normal lung development (top). Lesions identified in older children as in this 7 year old (b) may show marked chronic inflammation secondary to repeated infection. This extralobar sequestration (c) has a large muscular artery near the peripheral pleura. The mucostasis in adjacent bronchi is consistent with its lack of connection to the tracheobronchial tree.

comprise malformed lung components with a wide range of morphologies ranging from predominantly cartilaginous, mimicking proximal bronchial components, to predominantly cystic with lining similar to alveolar walls. This spectrum of lesions has been classified into types 0-4 based on proximal to distal morphology (*Table 2-1*).[43] Both size of cyst and the microscopic components of the wall are important to classification, and the type of CPAM may correlate with other malformations and prognosis. Clinical features vary with the subtype of lesion but predominantly depend on the size of the lesion and its effect on surrounding structures or on associated malformations. Presentation may therefore vary from an incidental finding to marked respiratory distress. Mucinous adenocarcinoma has been reported to develop in association with type 1 CPAM, although the absolute risk is likely to be low and these patients classically do well. Types 2 and 3 CPAMs are more likely to do poorly due to associated malformations or to the size of the lesion. Most type 4 CPAMs probably represent pleuropulmonary blastoma (see below).

Imaging features of congenital pulmonary airway malformations

Imaging features depend on the subtype of CPAM and may vary from a large unilocular cyst to numerous small, multilocular cysts, to solid appearing (microcystic) lesions.[44] Imaging cannot reliably distinguish CPAM from sequestrations, which often have CPAM-type features. CPAMs detected in prenatal ultrasound may grow over the course of development but typically stabilize and then regress in later intrauterine life.

Histologic features of congenital pulmonary airway malformations

Type 0 CPAM is not a localized lesion but is instead the diffuse lung developmental defect now more commonly called acinar dysplasia (discussed above), and is essentially an absence of the development of alveoli. Type I CPAM is reportedly the most common subtype of CPAM and is characterized by large cysts lined by bronchial type airway epithelium occasionally with mucous cells or cartilage in the wall (*Figure 2-12*). Bland tufts of mucinous cells may be demarcated from the surrounding epithelium, and there are numerous case reports of mucinous "bronchioloalveolar" adenocarcinoma arising within or adjacent to type 1 CPAMs in both children and adults.[45-47] Even small clusters of mucinous cells may demonstrate K-ras mutations or p16 loss of heterozygosity, suggesting that they are potentially preneoplastic lesions.[48] Generous sampling should be performed to exclude areas of carcinoma. Type 2 CPAM (*Figure 2-13*) has smaller cysts with increased bronchioles described as "back-to-back"; however

Table 2-1 Classification of Cystic Pulmonary Adenomatoid Malformation

	Type 0	Type 1	Type 2	Type 3	Type 4
Clinical	Rare diffuse developmental defect also known as acinar dysplasia	Most common	Features often seen in bronchopulmonary sequestration	Rare	Rare, controversial entity
		Rarely associated with mucinous adenocarcinoma		Corresponds to localized hyperplasia (usually affecting most of the lung)	Most are Type 1 PPB
Normal counterpart	Trachea/bronchi	Distal bronchus	Bronchioles	Terminal bronchioles/acini	Acini
Macroscopic	No cysts	Up to 10 cm cysts	Cystic (up to 2 cm) and solid areas	Predominantly solid	Large cysts
	Relatively solid				
Microscopic appearance	Extensive loose mesenchymal tissue with small spaces lined by pseudostratified epithelium	Cuboidal to ciliated pseudostratified +/− mucous cells +/− cartilage	"Back-to-back" bronchioles	Resembles canalicular stage of development	Thin-walled cysts lined by mature pneumonocytes
			+/− skeletal muscle		

variable numbers of alveoli are seen in the background. Mature or immature skeletal muscle may be present in the walls, but a cambium layer or immature smooth muscle should not be present. Similar abnormal development is often seen focally in sequestrations, and the diagnosis requires clinical correlation. Type 3 CPAM (*Figure 2-14*), which is essentially a form of pulmonary hyperplasia secondary to bronchial obstruction, resembles immature lung with increased airspaces. It is typically a large lesion involving the entire lobe of a lung and presents early in life with respiratory distress due to mass effect. It was originally described as "adenomatoid" or mimicking the canalicular stage of lung development; however, the normal interlobular

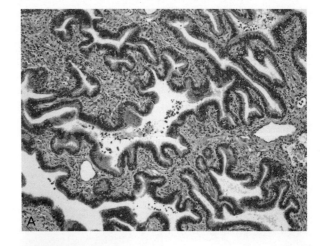

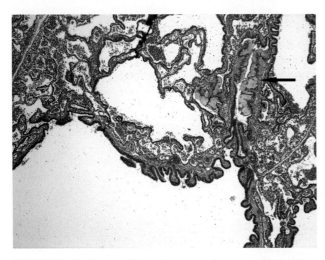

FIGURE 2-12 Congenital pulmonary airway malformation type 1. This **CPAM** has large cysts. The walls are lined by respiratory type epithelium, and there is focal proliferation of mucogenic cells (arrow).

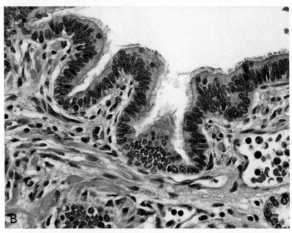

FIGURE 2-13 Congenital pulmonary airway malformation type 2. This mass removed from a 4-week-old infant is a small cyst **CPAM** characterized by "back-to-back" bronchioles without cartilage or mucous cells. At high power (b), striated skeletal muscle can be seen in the interstitium.

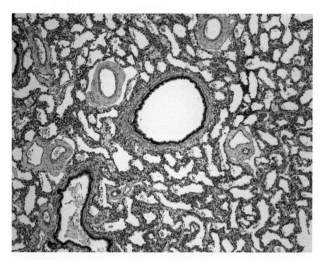

FIGURE 2-14 Congenital pulmonary airway malformation type 3. This CPAM has elongated, immature airspaces lined by cuboidal epithelium, resembling the canalicular stage of lung development.

septa are widely spaced apart due to the increased intervening airspaces which are often immature in appearance since the lesion is often seen in fetal or neonatal lung. The existence of type 4 CPAM (*Figure 2-15*) is controversial, with many or all cases in fact representing the cystic variant of pleuropulmonary blastoma.[49,50] Although embryonal rhabdomyosarcomas have been described as arising from CPAM, it is now generally accepted that these represent type I pleuropulmonary blastomas (see below). Any immature smooth muscle, cartilage, or focally increased mesenchyme in a cystic lesion should prompt a consideration of pleuropulmonary blastoma.

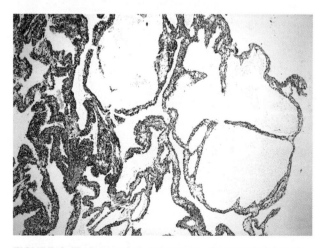

FIGURE 2-15 Congenital pulmonary airway malformation type 4. This CPAM (Used with permission of Dr J T Stocker, Bethesda, MD) has large, uniform, thin-walled cysts. No cambium layer is present; however, the presence of any immature mesenchymal component or cytogenetic abnormality would be suspicious for type 1 pleuropulmonary blastoma.

Pulmonary Interstitial Emphysema

Clinical features of pulmonary interstitial emphysema

Pulmonary interstitial emphysema (PIE) is the result of dissection of air out of the airspaces and into the interstitial tissue. PIE is predominantly seen in ventilated preterm infants, particularly those with respiratory distress syndrome. The incidence of PIE has markedly decreased due to gentler ventilation methods. It is speculated that the increased immature mesenchyme is more prone to rupture at higher pressures. Complications include rupture of air into the pleural space resulting in pneumothorax, or rupture of air centrally resulting in pneumomediastinum. Although PIE is typically transient, rare localized persistence of interstitial air results in persistent pulmonary interstitial emphysema (PPIE). Surgery is not typically a treatment for PIE, but PPIE may be resected to rule out other cystic lung masses.

Imaging features of pulmonary interstitial emphysema

The bronchovascular bundles appear as solid linear or dot-like structures within an air-filled cyst.[51]

Histologic features of pulmonary interstitial emphysema

Because PIE is typically seen in premature infants with other underlying conditions requiring ventilation, the changes are superimposed on underlying lung disease of prematurity. Air frequently dissects into the lymphatics, and if it is contained within lymphatics, the findings cannot be histologically distinguished from pulmonary lymphangiectasia; however, the air filled subpleural cystic spaces should be identified on gross examination. Rupture of the air into the connective tissue of the bronchovascular bundles or below the pleural surface results in unlined "cystic" spaces (*Figure 2-16*). Immunohistochemistry for D2-40 or cytokeratins demonstrates the absence of a cystic lining. Severe cases may be accompanied by hemorrhage into the connective tissue. PPIE is associated with a foreign-body giant cell response to the air (*Figure 2-16B and C*).

DISORDERS OF SURFACTANT METABOLISM

Genetic Disorders of Surfactant Metabolism

Clinical features of dysfunctional surfactant metabolism

Genetic disorders of surfactant metabolism include disorders of production (surfactant deficiency disorders) and disorders of clearance. Surfactant deficiency

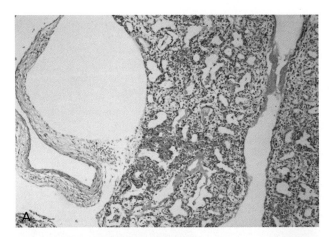

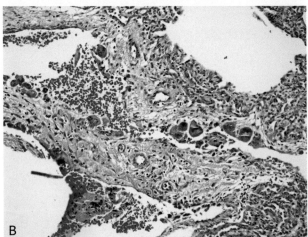

FIGURE 2-16 Pulmonary interstitial emphysema. In this premature infant with respiratory distress syndrome, in addition to hyaline membrane disease there are air-filled spaces in the interstitium without either epithelial or endothelial lining (a). Persistent interstitial emphysema, as seen in this 2-week-old premature infant shows cystic spaces lined by multinucleated giant cells as a reaction to interstitial air (b).

disorders include mutations in surfactant proteins (SPB,[52-54] SPC[55-57]), transport proteins (ABCA3[58]), and transcription factors (Nkx2.1/TTF1[59,60]), while defects in surfactant clearance are due to defective macrophage function (granulocyte macrophage colony-stimulating factor receptors GM-CSF2RA[61,62] and GM-CSF2RB).[63] In cases with typical clinical and imaging findings, genetic testing may make surgical lung biopsy unnecessary[3]; however, the sensitivity of genetic testing is not known, and the absence of a detected mutation does not rule out the diagnosis of a surfactant deficiency disorder.

Although surfactant deficiency was initially described in full-term infants with SPB mutation and refractory respiratory distress similar to lung disease of prematurity, it is now recognized that some mutations (SPC and ABCA3) may also present later in childhood or even in adults as interstitial lung disease. SPB and ABCA3 are both autosomal recessive disorders. Classically, SPB mutations present in the neonate, although mutations that result in decreased expression rather than complete loss of the protein have milder symptoms. The more common ABCA3 mutation may present in neonates, later in childhood or in adults. SPC mutations are inherited in an autosomal dominant manner with presentation in older infants, children, or even adults with usual interstitial pneumonia. Genotype-phenotype correlations are not well established due to the large number of described mutations. Case reports of successful treatment of surfactant deficiency disorders[64] with immunomodulatory agents have recently been published, but given the variable clinical presentations of different patients, it is unknown if the outcome simply reflected the natural history of the disease in those patients. The only current treatment is otherwise lung transplant.

Mutations in the transcription factor Nkx2.1 (TTF1) are associated with congenital hypothyroidism and neurologic abnormalities in addition to pulmonary hypoplasia and abnormal surfactant metabolism; however, the presentation in any given case is highly variable and the lungs are not uniformly involved.

Mutations in genes coding for the GM-CSF receptor (CSF2RA and CSF2RB) are extremely rare x-linked/autosomal recessive disorders that present in childhood with accumulation of surfactant protein similar to pulmonary alveolar proteinosis. Successful treatment with bronchoalveolar lavage has been reported.[65] Penetrance also appears to be variable.

Imaging features of dysfunctional surfactant metabolism

CT features of surfactant deficiency disorders include ground glass opacities and prominent interlobular septa, peripheral cysts, and patchy or severe fibrosis. The findings depend on the age of the patient and the type of deficiency.

Histologic features of dysfunctional surfactant metabolism

Although some histologic patterns are suggestive of particular surfactant mutations, there is marked variability in clinical and histologic patterns even with mutations in the same gene. Molecular testing is required to make a specific diagnosis. As more and more cases are reported, the spectrum of histologic patterns reported for each genotype is increasing. On the other hand, even in the absence of a detected mutation, certain histologic patterns are highly suggestive of an as-yet undetected surfactant gene mutation.[3,4] In infants, histologic patterns associated with surfactant dysfunction include both an intra-alveolar component (varying from predominantly PAS-positive, diastase-resistant eosinophilic material with cholesterol clefts to predominantly foamy macrophages) and an interstitial component with septal widening due to both type 2 pneumocyte hyperplasia as well as increased interstitial cells.

Among the classic patterns of surfactant deficiency disorders are congenital alveolar proteinosis (CAP), desquamative interstitial pneumonia (DIP), and chronic pneumonitis of infancy (CNI), while older infants and adolescents may demonstrate nonspecific interstitial pneumonitis. In adults, SPC and ABCA3 deficiencies are associated with usual interstitial pneumonia. CAP, classically associated with SPB mutation but also reported with other genes, demonstrates alveolar filling with PAS-positive surfactant material, foamy macrophages, and cholesterol clefts (*Figure 2-17*). In contrast to secondary PAP (see below), in which the underlying lung architecture is generally preserved, CAP is characterized by interstitial fibrosis and type 2 pneumocyte hyperplasia. In CNI,[66] the accumulation of intra-alveolar material is patchy, and the more dominant finding is widening of the interstitium with bland mesenchymal cells accompanied by type 2 pneumocyte hyperplasia. In DIP there is diffuse filling of the airspaces with macrophages, type 2 pneumocyte hyperplasia, and variable thickening of the alveolar walls (*Figure 2-18*). Despite the unfortunate fact that this pattern shares its name with the unrelated adult smoking–associated interstitial lung disease, in infants DIP is considered likely to represent surfactant deficiency even in the absence of a documented mutation.

Pathology findings in Nkx2.1/TTF1 disease are variable and may include deficient alveolarization in

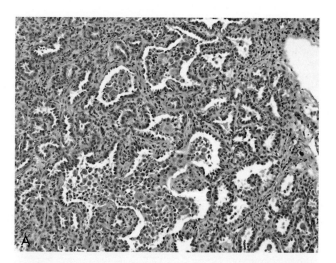

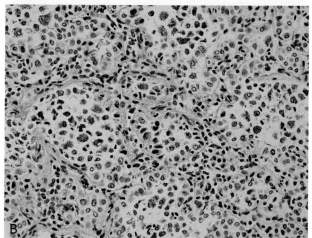

FIGURE 2-18 **Surfactant deficiency. This biopsy is from a 4-month-old infant with SFPC mutation and DIP-pattern shows numerous macrophages filling the alveolar spaces with reactive type 2 pneumocyte hyperplasia and mild widening of the alveolar septa. PAS with diastase (b) shows scant accumulation of PAS-positive material both in the macrophages and free in the airspaces.**

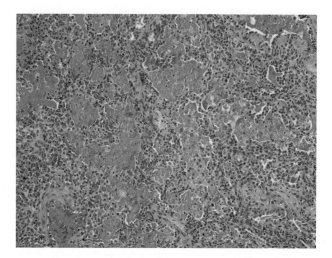

FIGURE 2-17 **Surfactant deficiency. This 4-week-old male with respiratory distress (a) shows the pattern of congenital alveolar proteinosis with marked accumulation of eosinophilic globular material in the airspaces. The alveoli are lined by hyperplastic type 2 pneumocytes with slight thickening of the alveolar walls due to chronic inflammatory cells.**

addition to typical findings of surfactant deficiency. However, these patients may even have normal-appearing lung. The CSF2RA and CSF2RB mutations present with histology similar to secondary PAP (see below).

Special techniques including immunohistochemistry and electron microscopy may contribute to the diagnosis in some cases. The accumulation of abnormal but immunoreactive protein in many SPC and ABCA3 mutations limits the utility of these antibodies; however, most, but not all mutations in SPB result in loss of SPB protein expression. With the clinical availability of genetic testing, the role of immunohistochemistry is decreasing. Electron microscopy may demonstrate absent surfactant or abnormal lamellar bodies. Classically, surfactant B mutations result in the absence of normal lamellar bodies with the accumulation of complex lamellar and vesicular bodies while ABCA3 mutations result in dense inclusions within concentric membranes.[67] SPC mutations have no abnormalities by electron microscopy. The full spectrum of EM findings in all the varieties of surfactant deficiencies has yet to be described, and the absence of EM findings does not exclude a diagnosis of surfactant deficiency.

The differential diagnosis for surfactant deficiency disorders depends on the age of the patient and histologic associated patterns. For DIP the differential includes metabolic diseases with accumulation of histiocytes, such as Gaucher's disease. Type 2 pneumocyte hyperplasia and interstitial inflammation can be seen in various infections, although there is usually a greater inflammatory cell component. In older children with NSIP, the differential diagnosis includes rheumatologic diseases, hypersensitivity, and infection.

Pulmonary Alveolar Proteinosis

Clinical features of pulmonary alveolar proteinosis

In contrast to surfactant deficiency disorders, pulmonary alveolar proteinosis (PAP) is due to deficient alveolar macrophage function leading to accumulation of surfactant material. It may be secondary to inhalation of toxins, autoimmunity, marrow suppression, or congenital disorders. In adults the most common form of PAP is autoimmune with antibodies to GM-CSF; however, this disorder is rare in children. PAP may also be seen in patients with marked immunodeficiencies, particularly in patients (including children), with myeloid leukemias.[68] This form of PAP is often associated with infections including fungus and nocardia.[69]

Imaging features of pulmonary alveolar proteinosis

The classic imaging feature of PAP is described as "crazy paving," a geographic or diffuse pattern of patchy ground glass opacities and septal thickening.[70]

Histologic features of pulmonary alveolar proteinosis

PAP is characterized by airspace accumulation of grungy eosinophilic material, cholesterol clefts, and foamy macrophages (*Figure 2-19*). The intraalveolar material is PAS positive and diastase resistant. This material is typically much more abundant than in surfactant deficiency disorders. More importantly, the underlying architecture of the lung is preserved without widening of the alveolar septa or type 2 pneumocyte hyperplasia. The differential diagnosis for eosinophilic material

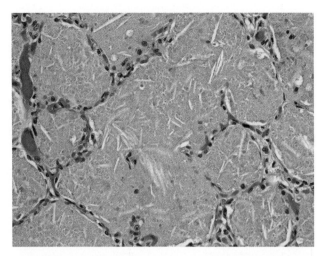

FIGURE 2-19 **Secondary pulmonary alveolar proteinosis. This autopsy specimen from an 8-year-old with secondary PAP associated with immune dysregulation due to juvenile rheumatoid arthritis and methotrexate treatment shows granular eosinophilic material with cholesterol clefts but good preservation of the alveolar architecture.**

filling the airspaces includes pulmonary edema (PAS negative) and pneumocystis (GMS positive). In immunosuppressed patients with PAP an infectious organism should be carefully sought.

OTHER DISORDERS SPECIFIC TO INFANCY

Pulmonary Interstitial Glycogenosis

Clinical features of pulmonary interstitial glycogenosis

PIG is a recently described[71] poorly defined entity presenting within days to weeks after birth. It may be the sole anomaly in a term infant but is often present in association with other features including deficient alveolarization in association with prematurity, congenital heart defects, chromosomal anomalies, or vascular disorders. Some patients have been treated with corticosteroids, but the significance of the finding and appropriate treatment are unknown.[72] It is generally believed to have a good prognosis and to resolve spontaneously.[73]

Imaging features of pulmonary interstitial glycogenosis

CT findings are nonspecific and may include septal widening, ground glass and reticular opacities, hyperinflation, and architectural distortion. The findings may be the result of the associated lung disorders rather than PIG alone.

Histologic features of pulmonary interstitial glycogenosis

The findings of PIG may be diffuse or patchy and may be seen in isolation or in association with other chronic lung disease. The alveolar septa are widened with an influx of spindle cells with pale or bubbly glycogen-laden cytoplasm (*Figure 2-20A*). PAS-positive (*Figure 2-20B*), diastase sensitive (*Figure 2-20C*) material may be present, but glycogen may be washed out by processing and may be better demonstrated by electron microscopy. There is an absence of type 2 pneumocyte hyperplasia or marked filling of the alveolar spaces with cells or debris.[71]

Neuroendocrine Cell Hyperplasia of Infancy

Clinical features of neuroendocrine cell hyperplasia of infancy

Infants with neuroendocrine cell hyperplasia of infancy present with tachypnea, retractions, crackles, and hypoxia, usually within the first few months of life. Familial cases have been reported,[74] and one family with mutation of NKX2.1/TTF1 mutation has been described,[75] but the genetic basis is otherwise undefined. An environmental trigger has been suggested but not identified. Infants often show failure to thrive, and treatment is supportive. Gradual improvement into early childhood is typical with no reported deaths,[76] but long-term follow-up studies are unavailable.

Imaging features of neuroendocrine cell hyperplasia of infancy

The CT features of NEHI are well described and include geographic ground glass opacities in the right middle and lingual lobes as well as mosaic air trapping in other lobes.[77] The findings may be specific enough to avoid a surgical lung biopsy with consistent clinical features.

Histologic features of neuroendocrine cell hyperplasia of infancy

Lung biopsy shows "normal" or near normal architectural findings, although focal airway inflammation or fibrosis may be present and does not exclude the diagnosis; indeed, a recent retrospective review found that cases of NEHI were missed and given a descriptive diagnosis of chronic bronchiolitis.[6] Immunohistochemistry for bombesin or serotonin demonstrates an increase in neuroendocrine cells in the terminal airways and alveolar ducts.[78] Other neuroendocrine markers are significantly less sensitive. Neuroendocrine cells are normally found as single cells or small clusters in

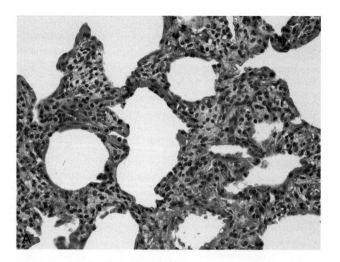

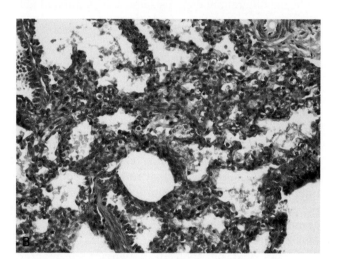

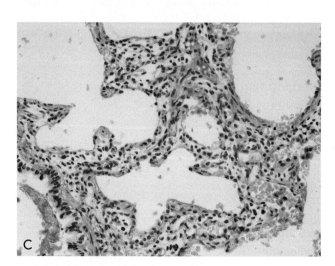

FIGURE 2-20 Pulmonary interstitial glycogenosis. This biopsy from an infant with respiratory distress shows thickened alveolar septa with scattered round to ovoid cells with clear cytoplasm (a). PAS stain (b) shows some of the cells have glycogen in their cytoplasm, which is absent in following digestion with diastase (c).

control lungs, and they are increased in other forms of pediatric lung disease including bronchopulmonary dysplasia, cystic fibrosis, prematurity, and mechanical ventilation.[79] Suggested values for increased neuroendocrine cells include neuroendocrine cells in >70% of airways or comprising >10% of a single area; however, these values may be seen in other chronic lung diseases and even in control lungs. Morphometric analysis also shows a significant increase in neuroendocrine cells, but given the extensive variability between patients the diagnosis requires correlation with clinical and radiographic findings.[79]

PEDIATRIC PULMONARY VASCULAR DISORDERS

Congenital Heart Disease

Clinical features of congenital heart disease

Patients with congenital heart disease are known to be at risk for developmental alveolar abnormalities and pulmonary hypertension. Most biopsies are performed to rule out other causes of imaging or functional abnormalities. Although pulmonary arterial hypertensive changes were previously graded to evaluate reversibility after surgical correction of cardiac defects, catheterization-based measurements are more appropriate, and biopsy is no longer performed for this purpose.

Histologic features of congenital heart disease

Children with congenital heart disease may have alveolar developmental abnormalities with simplified lobules including a reduction in alveolar number and an enlargement and simplification of alveolar shape (*Figure 2-21*). Pulmonary hypertensive changes (see Chapter 14) are frequent, and in patients with left-to-right shunts these may be graded according to the Heath-Edwards classification, but grading is not used for surgical prognosis. Grades 1 to 3 of the classification include muscularization of arterioles, medial hypertrophy of arteries, and intimal fibrosis. Grades 4 to 6 encompass complex lesion including plexiform lesions, dilatation lesions, and fibrinoid necrosis. Plexiform lesions should be distinguished from recanalizing thromboemboli which can be seen in other conditions. Plexiform lesions comprise a cellular proliferation of modified endothelial cells creating slit-like channels that may be enclosed within the artery or may extend through the wall. In contrast, recanalized thromboemboli have rounder, patent lumen with more fibrotic stroma and are completely enclosed within the vessel.

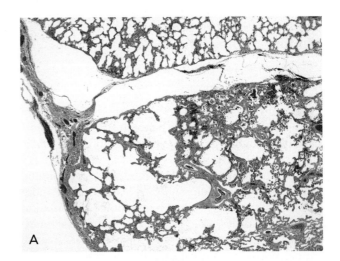

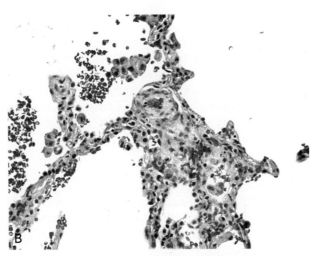

FIGURE 2-21 **Congenital heart disease. In this biopsy from a 7-month-old infant with trisomy 21 and complete atrioventricular canal defect, the airspaces are markedly variably in size with relatively normal alveoli at the top and simplified, enlarged airspaces at the bottom (a). These alveolar growth abnormalities might be due to congenital heart disease or chromosomal anomalies. There is associated lymphangiectasis in the interlobular septum. High power (b) shows thickening of the alveolar arterioles and scattered hemosiderin-laden macrophages.**

In infants, both intimal fibrosis and complex lesions are extremely rare. Instead, extension of muscle into the more distal arterioles and a reduction in the number of arterioles are common. However, quantification of these changes is not practical in a diagnostic setting. In addition to arterial changes, other vascular changes such as lymphangiectasias are common in patients with all types of heart failure. Heart disease with left heart failure or other causes of venous hypertension may have hemosiderin-laden macrophages in the airspaces and marked congestion of the alveolar capillaries.

Pulmonary Arteriovenous Malformations

Clinical features of pulmonary arteriovenous malformations

Pulmonary arteriovenous malformations (AVMs) are rare anomalous connections between arteries and veins most commonly seen in hereditary hemorrhagic telangiectasia (HHT, Osler-Weber-Rendu syndrome). HHT is due to autosomal dominant mutations in endoglin, ALK1, or SMAD4. Pulmonary AVMs are much more commonly seen with endoglin mutations. Presentation of HHT is usually with epistaxis due to mucosal telangiectasias; the pulmonary AVMs themselves may cause hypoxemia or paradoxical emboli to the systemic circulation, depending on size. Up to 35% of children with HHT have pulmonary AVMs on screening, although they are rarely symptomatic until adult life.[80] More rarely pulmonary AVMs are acquired abnormalities following congenital heart surgery or hepatopulmonary syndrome. Treatment is usually by embolization,[81] but rarely cases of diffuse lung disease require surgical treatment.

Imaging features of pulmonary arteriovenous malformations

Patients with HHT usually have screening for AVMs including contrast echocardiography and contrast CT.

Histologic features of pulmonary arteriovenous malformations

Pulmonary AVMs, similar to those elsewhere, are typically formed of thick-walled arteries draining directly into thin-walled veins (*Figure 2-22*). Aneurysmal dilations may be present. Evidence of prior bleeding including hemosiderin-laden macrophages and hemosiderin within connective tissue may be present. Elastic tissue stain may be used to highlight the abnormal vessels but in practice is rarely necessary. In addition to typical large AVMs, a subset of HHT patients has classic diffuse pulmonary arterial hypertensive changes including plexiform lesions.

Diffuse Pulmonary Lymphangiomatosis

Clinical features of diffuse pulmonary lymphangiomatosis

Pulmonary lymphangiomatosis is a rare disorder due to a proliferation of lymphatic vessels. Involvement may be limited to the chest or can be widespread. Although the proliferation of vessels is presumed to have been present since birth, presentation with wheezing or dyspnea is often later in childhood or more rarely in adults. Involvement may be limited to the lungs or occur more diffusely.

Imaging features of diffuse pulmonary lymphangiomatosis

CT shows increased thickening of the compartments normally containing lymphatics—bronchovascular bundles, interlobular septa, and the pleura. With involvement of the lymph nodes there is increased soft tissue at the hilum and in the mediastinum.

Histologic features of diffuse pulmonary lymphangiomatosis

In contrast to lymphangiectasis (see below) lymphangiomatosis is distinguished by increased numbers of lymphatic spaces which are usually not

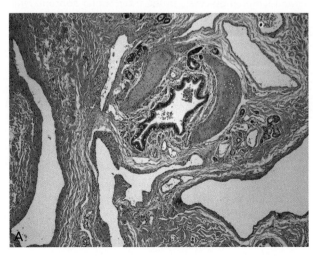
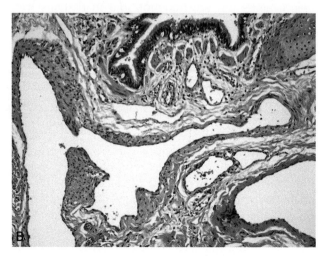

FIGURE 2-22 Arteriovenous malformation (a and b). This 5-year old presented with recurrent pneumonia. There are multiple vascular channels with transition from arterial to venous wall (40× and 100×).

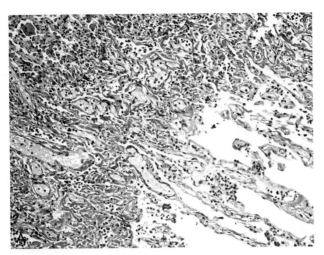 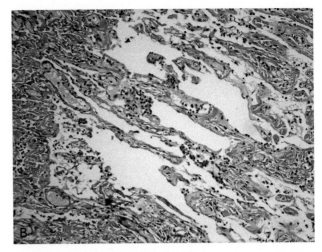

FIGURE 2-23 Pulmonary lymphangiomatosis. This 17-year old with pulmonary lymphangiomatosis has increased, small, anastomosing, thin-walled lymphatics in the interlobular septum (a). At higher power, scattered inflammatory cells are seen in the septum (b).

markedly enlarged but show complex anastomoses (*Figure 2-23*). These follow the normal lymphatic distribution. There is often an associated spindle-cell proliferative component which may be "kaposiform."[82] More recently, this lymphangiomatosis with a prominent spindle cell component has been termed "kaposiform lymphangiomatosis" and may be a more aggressive variant.[83]

The differential diagnosis for lymphatic lesion or cystic lesions with a spindle cell component includes predominantly parenchymal lesions such as lymphangioma and arteriovenous malformations, lymphangioleiomyomatosis (LAM), and lymphangiectasis. In LAM, the lesions form larger cystic spaces, involve the parenchyma, and are positive for estrogen and progesterone receptors and HMB-45. In lymphangiectasis, the thin-walled lymphatics are not increased in number but are markedly dilated. In both lymphangiomatosis and lymphangiectasis D2-40 immunohistochemistry can be used to stain lymphatic endothelium.

Congenital Pulmonary Lymphangiectasis

Clinical features of congenital pulmonary lymphangiectasis

In contrast to lymphangiomatosis, there is no proliferation of lymphatic vessels; instead, there is diffuse dilation. It typically presents in neonates with respiratory distress.[84] Rarely lymphangiectasis is a primary disorder with a high rate of mortality; however, it is more commonly secondary to cardiovascular disease. Diffuse lymphangiectasia may be frequently found in congenital heart disease patients, particularly those with impaired venous return. In these cases the prognosis is dependent on the underlying heart defect. Similar features may be found as lesions localized to a single lobe or the mediastinum and present in older children or adults.[85]

Imaging features of congenital pulmonary lymphangiectasis

Chest x-ray shows hyperlucent lung with increased interstitial markings. CT may show septal and peribronchiolar thickening with focal ground glass attenuation and pleural effusions.

Histologic features of congenital pulmonary lymphangiectasis

Widely ectatic lymphatic spaces are seen around the bronchovascular bundles, in the interlobular septa and the pleura (*Figure 2-24*). In autopsy specimens, some degree of lymphangiectasia may be seen secondary to inflation of the lungs. The lymphatic spaces follow the normal distribution (pleura, interlobular septa, bronchovascular bundles). There is no increase in the number or complexity of lymphatics, but the walls may be abnormally muscularized and thickened. Associated fibrosis has been reported in long-standing adult cases. Immunohistochemistry for D2-40 can confirm that they are lymphatics rather than abnormal veins.

The lymphatics may also be widely dilated (due to filling with air) in cases of pulmonary interstitial emphysema (see above); however, in these cases gross examination should show large pockets of air trapping under the pleura and along the septa. Dissection of air into the interstitium without any type of cystic lining may also be present.

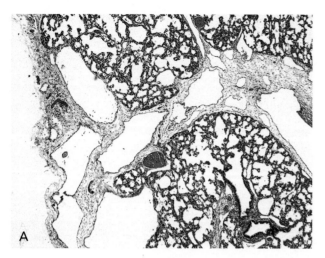
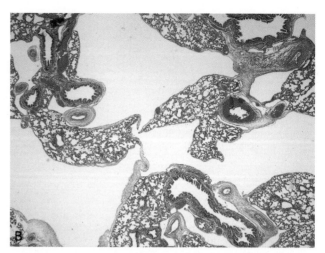

FIGURE 2-24 **Pulmonary lymphangiectasia. In this infant with congenital pulmonary lymphangiectasia, the lymphatics of the interlobular septa and pleura (a) and bronchovascular bundle (b) are markedly dilated.**

OTHER DIFFUSE LUNG DISEASES COMMON TO INFANTS AND CHILDREN

Lymphocytic Interstitial Pneumonia

Clinical features of lymphocytic interstitial pneumonia

Lymphocytic interstitial pneumonia (LIP) is a diffuse interstitial lung disease due to a benign, polyclonal proliferation of lymphocytes and plasma cells. It is virtually always seen in immunodeficient children, particularly those with perinatally acquired HIV infection. In these patients, it is considered an AIDS defining illness.

Imaging features of lymphocytic interstitial pneumonia

Findings are variable and nonspecific but may include ground glass opacities and septal thickening.

Histologic features of lymphocytic interstitial pneumonia

The alveolar septa are marked distended by an inflammatory infiltrate including lymphocytes, plasma cells, and histiocytes (*Figure 2-25*). Occasional poorly formed granulomas may be seen. The pattern is similar to the nonspecific interstitial pneumonia seen in adults but with denser infiltrates and more marked expansion of the interstitium. However, no specific criteria exist to differentiate these two entities. The differential diagnosis includes lymphoid hyperplasia, CMV, pneumocystis, chronic hypersensitivity, and connective tissue disease. Other forms of lymphoid hyperplasia including

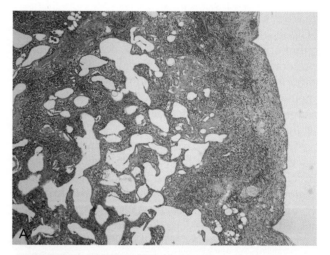
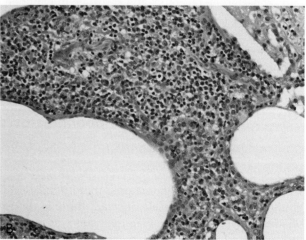

FIGURE 2-25 **Lymphocytic interstitial pneumonia. In this 5-year-old patient with AIDS and LIP, the alveolar walls are markedly distended with a mixed inflammatory infiltrate (a), consisting predominantly of lymphocytes, histiocytes, and plasma cells (b).**

follicular bronchiolitis may also be seen in patients with HIV. Special stains should always be performed to rule out infection.

Hemorrhagic Syndromes

Clinical features of hemorrhagic syndromes

The presentation of pulmonary hemorrhage includes hypoxemia, diffuse alveolar infiltrates, hemoptysis, and anemia. Alveolar hemorrhage syndromes are grouped into those with and without capillaritis.[86] Causes of hemorrhage without capillaritis include cardiac diseases, Heiner syndrome (reaction to cow's milk in infants), and idiopathic pulmonary hemosiderosis (IPS). Disorders associated with capillaritis include connective tissue diseases and vasculitides. A history of autoantibodies including c- or p-ANCA or anti-GBM antibodies should raise the suspicion of a vasculitic disease (Chapter 15); however, the vasculitic diseases with pulmonary capillary involvement are rare in children. IPS is sometimes associated with celiac disease and IgA deficiency, but the pathogenesis is not known.

Although idiopathic pulmonary hemosiderosis (IPS) may be diagnosed based on clinical features and a BAL with hemosiderin-laden macrophages,[87] biopsy is often undertaken to rule out capillaritis. Identification of capillaritis is important because these diseases often require more aggressive immunosuppressive treatment. Despite the absence of inflammation or known immune-mediated etiology, IPS often responds to steroids. Studies examining long-term outcome of IPS are limited due to the variable and sometimes uninvestigated underlying etiology. Patients may die of massive pulmonary hemorrhage or survive with normal lung function or restrictive lung disease. A subset develops rheumatologic disorders.[88]

Imaging features of hemorrhagic syndromes

Imaging shows a nonspecific diffuse alveolar infiltrate which may eventually progress to fibrosis. MRI findings may suggest the presence of hemosiderin based on its magnetic properties.

Histologic features of hemorrhagic syndromes

Biopsy demonstrates hemosiderin-laden macrophages filling alveolar spaces and in the interstitium (*Figure 2-26*). Acute pulmonary hemorrhage without hemosiderin may be an artifact of the procedure or could reflect extremely early disease. Prussian blue stain demonstrates iron not only in macrophages but also in pneumocytes, encrusting elastic fibers and free in the interstitium. Nonspecific reactive changes seen in addition to the hemosiderin include interstitial fibrosis, reactive pneumocytes, and peribronchiolar inflammation in long-standing cases. Capillaritis, defined as fibrinoid necrosis of the capillary wall with a neutrophilic infiltrate, should be carefully searched for (see Chapter 15). Increased neutrophils, apoptotic debris, and fibrinoid changes are described, but the threshold level of these findings and reproducibility of a diagnosis of capillaritis have not been defined.

Obliterative Bronchiolitis

Clinical features of obliterative bronchiolitis

Obliterative bronchiolitis may be seen in children, as in adults, in many forms of lower airway injury including infection, transplant rejection, graft-versus-host

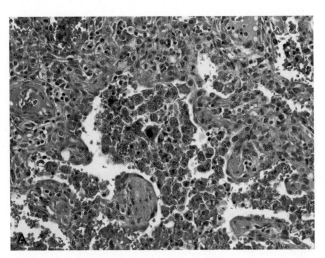 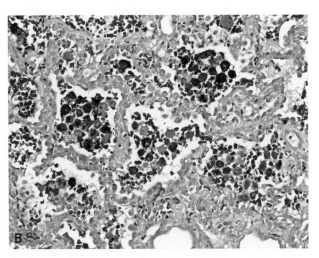

FIGURE 2-26 Idiopathic pulmonary hemosiderosis. This biopsy from a 2-year old who presented with hemoptysis shows both hemosiderin and more recent blood within alveolar macrophages (a). Prussian blue stain (b) shows iron within the macrophages and in the interstitium.

disease, chronic aspiration, autoimmunity, inhalation, hypersensitivity, or drug reaction (see Chapter 22); however, postinfectious obliterative bronchiolitis is primarily a pediatric disease and occurs most commonly following adenovirus infection, particularly in patients with a severe clinical presentation. Postinfectious obliterative bronchiolitis tends to have a better outcome than the types typically seen in adults.[89-91]

Imaging features of obliterative bronchiolitis

Chest x-ray shows prominent interstitium and hyperinflation. CT findings are highly specific and include mosaic perfusion, vascular attenuation, and central bronchiectasis.

Histologic features of obliterative bronchiolitis

In obliterative bronchiolitis the lesions vary from complete obliteration of the bronchiole lumen to a subtle increase in fibrous tissue below the epithelium, causing only partial obstruction of the airway (*Figure 2-27*).[92] This may be accompanied by variable degrees of chronic inflammation. Complete replacement of the bronchiole by fibrous tissue may results in an apparently unpaired pulmonary artery. Biopsy diagnosis is complicated by the patchy nature of the disease, which may show only subtle findings despite severe clinical presentation. The presence of mucostasis with foamy macrophages secondary to obstruction helps support the diagnosis. Although associated with adenovirus infection, obliterative bronchiolitis is a chronic change and adenoviral inclusions are not identified. Obliterative bronchiolitis should be differentiated from the airway obstruction due to intraluminal Masson bodies that are a feature of organizing pneumonia (previously termed bronchiolitis obliterans organizing pneumonia or BOOP).

Aspiration Injury

Clinical features of aspiration injury

Aspiration occurs in many or most normal patients. Pathological aspiration is dependent on the quantity or type of material aspirated or abnormal macrophage clearance. Significant aspiration is commonly seen in children with neurologic compromise or severe reflux. Symptoms and presentation depend on the type and quantity of material aspirated and may range from diffuse alveolar damage to localized foreign-body reaction and obliterative bronchiolitis. Meconium aspiration, specific to the neonate, is a cause of persistent pulmonary hypertension and respiratory distress in the full-term infant.

Imaging features of aspiration injury

Imaging features are nonspecific and reflect the pattern of lung response ranging from diffuse opacities to patchy atelectasis and hyperlucency due to airtrapping, or chronic changes including those of obliterative bronchiolitis.

Histologic features of aspiration injury

In most cases aspiration is difficult to definitively identify due to the nonspecific changes. Depending on the material, quantity, and timing histologic changes may vary from diffuse alveolar damage to foreign body granulomas to obliterative bronchiolitis. Identification of foreign material including meat, starches (often polarizable and sometimes PAS positive), or seeds is rare. Large oil droplets may be identified either by oil red O on frozen section or as empty spaces with associated giant cell reaction (*Figure 2-28*). In the absence of giant cells, the presence of round, empty spaces may simply correspond to entrapped air. Oil or lipid may also be associated with

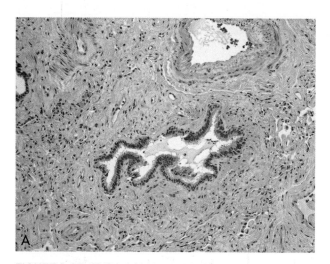
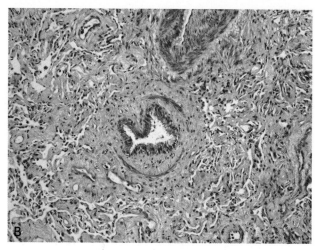

FIGURE 2-27 Obliterative bronchiolitis. In this patient, the airway epithelium is lifted away from the underlying smooth muscle (a). The fibrosis is highlighted in blue by this trichrome stain (b).

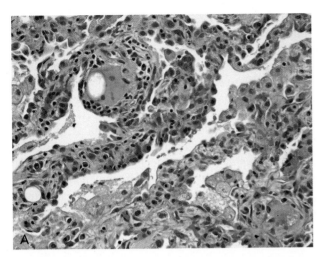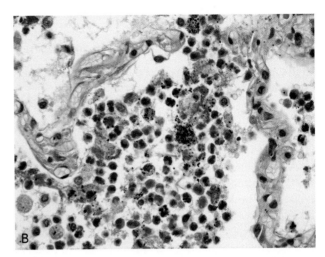

FIGURE 2-28 Microaspiration. Microaspiration due to gastroesophageal reflux (a) shows a multinucleated giant cell and foamy macrophages associated with mild chronic inflammation and interstitial fibrosis. Massive acute aspiration pneumonia (b) shows aspirated bile pigment and intra-alveolar neutrophils.

foamy macrophages, but these are a nonspecific finding also seen in obstruction, storage diseases, or resolving hemorrhage. In meconium aspiration, yellow-brown meconium may be identified, but more often there is a nonspecific acute inflammatory response that must be correlated with the clinical history.

Chronic Granulomatous Disease

Clinical features of granulomatous disease

Chronic granulomatous disease (CGD) is due to x-linked (most common) or autosomal recessive mutations in subunits of the NADPH oxidase complex resulting in defective leukocyte function and susceptibility to infection, particularly with catalase-positive organisms requiring the respiratory burst of phagocyte function for effective killing. Diagnosis requires specialized functional testing for NADPH oxidase activity or genetic testing. Although the lungs are the most prevalent site of disease and pneumonia is the most common cause of death[93] lung biopsies are rarely performed.

Imaging features of granulomatous disease

Imaging features of CGD are nonspecific and depend on the type of organism and may include abscesses, bronchiectasis, and diffuse infiltrates.

Histologic features of granulomatous disease

The classic feature of CGD is the presence of granulomas, and in one case series of surgical open lung biopsies found that all patients demonstrated at least some form of granuloma, most classically neutrophilic microabscesses with palisading granulomas[94] (*Figure 2-29*). Culture demonstrated fungal, bacterial,

and mycobacterial organisms associated with granulomas. In other reports of pediatric patients with lung biopsies, only a subset of cases demonstrated granulomas, and nonspecific changes including fibrosis and acute or chronic inflammation or even minimal abnormalities were also be seen.[95] These differences may reflect sampling. In both series histologic identification of organisms was low. The differential diagnosis includes other immunodeficiencies or infection in an immunocompetent patient as well as sarcoidosis. Although sarcoidosis is typically nonnecrotizing, necrotizing granulomas may be present. Moreover, in a small biopsy, the typical lymphatic distribution of the granulomas may not be apparent. Clinical correlation is required for the diagnosis of CGD.

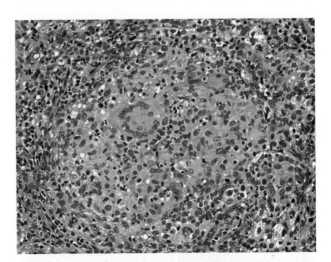

FIGURE 2-29 Chronic granulomatous disease. This 6-week-old infant presented with diffuse lung disease. Biopsy demonstrated granulomas with marked neutrophilic infiltrates, and follow-up testing demonstrated chronic granulomatous disease.

Respiratory Viral Infections

Clinical features of respiratory viral infections

In the nonimmunocompromised child, viral infection is commonly acquired through transplacental (cytomegalovirus [CMV], human immunodeficiency virus [HIV]), or intrapartum (herpes simplex virus [HSV]) or airborne (respiratory syncytial virus [RSV], human metapneumovirus [MPV], and adenovirus) transmission.[96,97] Of these, CMV is usually asymptomatic and often does not involve the lung. In this day and age, HIV infection of the mother is likely to be known and transmission to the baby is diagnosed by HIV nucleic acid detection in two separate specimens. Neonatal HSV infection manifests in the first week of life and may be relatively benign or result in disseminated disease with skin and mucous membrane lesions, meningoencephalitis, hepatitis, and, less commonly, pneumonia. RSV is the most important pathogen in childhood and causes regularly recurring epidemics in winter and early spring. The patient presents with fever, cough, rhinitis, pharyngitis, and dyspnea. MPV accounts for about 10% of community-acquired pneumonia and the presenting features are similar to those of RSV. The diagnosis depends on serologic tests. Adenoviral infections are commonly seen in children younger than 5 years who are in day care centers or other closed environments and in school going children. These present as bronchitis, bronchiolitis, or pneumonia.

In the immunocompromised child (such as transplant recipient, or congenital or acquired immunodeficiency) the most significant viral pneumonias are due to CMV or adenovirus. These patients have extensive disease and may die if not treated aggressively.

Imaging features of respiratory viral infections

Radiologic features vary depending on the extent of infection from patchy to extensive alveolar infiltrates. The causative organism can be suggested based on the clinical setting and imaging findings.

Histologic features of respiratory viral infections

The diagnosis of viral pneumonia is based on clinical and laboratory findings and the lung is rarely biopsied. The main indication for a biopsy, often a wedge, is the immunocompromised host since these patients are very sick and may have more than one organism causing infections. Also, the differential diagnosis is broader (such as rejection, malignancy) than in the normal child. CMV is easily and reliably identified by its characteristic cytopathic effect of enlarged cell with single intranuclear and multiple cytoplasmic inclusions (as in the adult). HSV pneumonia is patchy, with areas of necrosis within which normal sized cells contain intranuclear inclusions

(homogenous and glassy, occupying the entire nucleus and pushing the chromatin to the periphery of the nucleus or smaller, deeply eosinophilic, round or polygonal, separated from the nuclear membrane by a clear halo). In RSV pneumonia there are syncytial giant cells within inflammation in airways and alveoli. Multiple cytoplasmic eosinophilic inclusions can be seen within the giant cells. Adenovirus pneumonia is characterized by severe necrotizing bronchitis, bronchiolitis, and alveolitis (*Figure 2-30*). Within areas of necrosis infected cells are identified by the somewhat enlarged smudged nuclei due to the viral inclusions. The above infections can be confirmed immunohistochemically by using specific commercially available antibodies.

PRIMARY PEDIATRIC LUNG NEOPLASMS

Primary lung tumors of children are rare, with carcinoid tumors, pleuropulmonary blastoma, and inflammatory myofibroblastic tumor being the most common primary tumors. The differential diagnosis of a mass lesion includes the infectious/inflammatory lesions as well as primary tumors.

Carcinoid Tumor

Clinical features of carcinoid tumor

Carcinoid tumors are the most common malignancy of the lung in children, although all tumors are rare in this age group.[8,10,98] There is no external predisposing factor. Carcinoids occur in adolescents (mean age 12 years) with no sex predilection. Being endobronchial masses, the presenting symptoms include persistent cough, wheezing, pneumonia, and hemoptysis. Carcinoid syndrome is rare. They may arise from the lobar bronchi (75%), mainstem bronchi (10%), or within the lung parenchyma (15%). Carcinoids are low-grade tumors but local invasion and distant metastasis have been reported in about a quarter of children with overall survival of 90%.[10]

Imaging features of carcinoid tumor

Chest radiographic finding is that of a round or ovoid well-circumscribed opacity. Computed tomography (CT) shows a soft tissue attenuation mass with well-defined or lobulated margins. Focal internal calcification is more likely to be seen in centrally located tumors than in peripheral ones. There is intense enhancement within the tumor on postcontrast CT.[99]

Histologic features of carcinoid tumor

Histologic features of carcinoid tumors are similar to those seen in adults. The tumor cells form nests, cords, trabeculae, and ribbons. In general, the cells are uniform with moderate pale eosinophilic cytoplasm, round to oval nuclei, and only focal nuclear enlargement and atypia (*Figure 2-31*). Occasionally, spindle cells may predominate. The chromatin pattern is "salt and pepper" and nucleoli are inconspicuous. The tumors are subclassified into typical and atypical based on necrosis and mitosis (nuclear atypia does not affect the classification). Typical carcinoids have no necrosis (surface ulceration of tumor protruding into the airway does not count) and only one or less mitosis per 10 high power fields (HPFs). Atypical carcinoids have focal necrosis and/or 2 to 10 mitoses per 10 HPFs. This subclassification requires adequate sampling of the tumor, which is possible only on resection.

Carcinoid tumors are strongly positive for keratins and neuroendocrine markers (synaptophysin and chromogranin) which are helpful in interpreting small biopsies (*Figure 2-31B*). Proliferative index using Ki-67 staining has only a limited role in predicting short-term survival.[100]

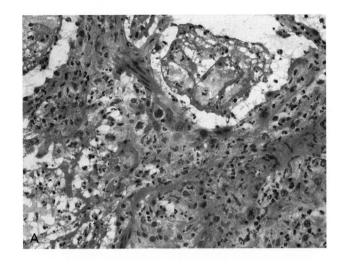
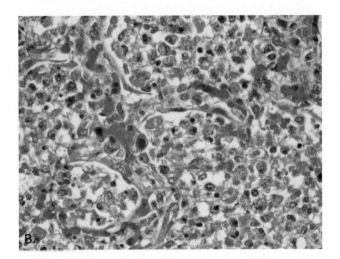
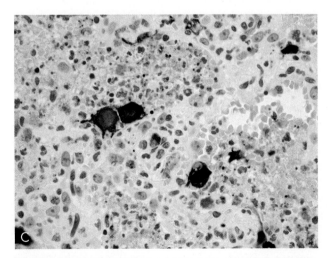

FIGURE 2-30 **Adenovirus pneumonia. Frozen section in immunocompromised host such as transplant recipient can be very helpful in diagnosis. This patient had bilateral infiltrates and infection was suggested on frozen section (a). Smudgy purple adenovirus intranuclear inclusion is seen in a pneumocyte (b). Antibody to adenovirus is commercially available for IHC stain which shows both nuclear and cytoplasmic positivity in infected cells (c).**

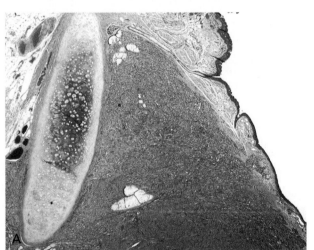
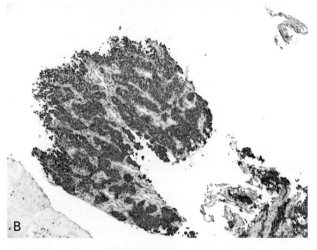

FIGURE 2-31 **Carcinoid. Endobronchial typical carcinoid growing between respiratory mucosa and cartilage island (a). Carcinoid tumor, staining for chromogranin in an endobronchial biopsy (b).**

Pleuropulmonary Blastoma

Clinical features of pleuropulmonary blastoma

Pleuropulmonary blastoma (PPB) is a rare primary pulmonary sarcoma presenting in infants and young children. It is associated with germline mutations in DICER1, an RNase III endonuclease required for miRNA and siRNA processing.[101] The mechanism underlying tumorigenesis is not understood, but transformation does not appear to involve loss of the wild-type gene. Associated tumors in these patients and their families include cystic nephroma, Sertoli-Leydig cell tumors and other ovarian nongerm cell tumors, multinodular goiter, embryonal rhabdomyosarcoma, primitive neuroectodermal tumor, Wilms tumor, medulloblastoma, and hamartomatous polyps. Importantly, penetrance is variable and most mutational carriers do not develop disease.[102,103]

Imaging features of pleuropulmonary blastoma

PPBs may be discovered on incidental imaging with features similar to CPAM (see above), or they may present with pneumothorax. Although not specific, pneumothorax is considered a feature suspicious for PPB. Type 3 PPBs form solid masses.

Histologic features of pleuropulmonary blastoma

PPB is divided into three subtypes: type I is purely cystic, type III is solid, and type II has intermediate features. The lesions are believed to progress from type I to III as the malignant mesenchymal cells overgrow the benign epithelium of the cystic component. Correspondingly, type I presents in younger children and has a much more favorable prognosis. Type I PPB is a circumscribed mass with cystic components lined by benign flat to cuboidal epithelial cells (*Figure 2-32*). The septa are typically variable in thickness and composition, although in young children they may be more uniform. The key feature is identification of at least focally immature mesenchymal cells. The most common immature feature (90% of cases) is a cambium layer, although this may be very focal. Areas of both immature cartilage and rhabdomyoblasts are also identified, while nodules of blastema are infrequent. Histologically suggestive features include cartilage and even focal thickening and increased cellularity of the septa. In difficult cases, clinical features favoring PPB include presentation with pneumothorax, presence of cystic nephromas or other tumors, or a family history. Chromosomal abnormalities have been reported in many PPBs including Trisomy 8.[104]

The differential diagnosis for type I PPB is other cystic lung lesions, particularly type 4 CPAM. The existence of a benign type 4 CPAM is very controversial, and virtually the entire lesion should be submitted to exclude a primitive mesenchymal component in a type

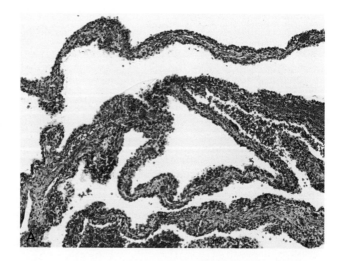

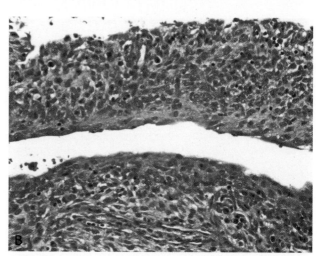

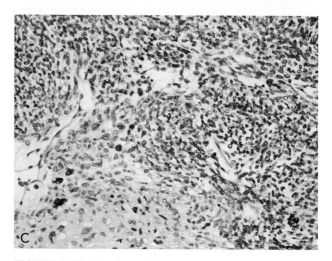

FIGURE 2-32 Pleuropulmonary blastoma. In this type 1 pleuropulmonary blastoma the cyst is thin-walled and lined by benign epithelium (a). There is only focal condensation of spindle cells below the epithelium. Other areas are more easily as malignant (b) as identified by this cellular mesenchyme in the cyst wall (Used with permission of Dr J Hicks, Texas Children's Hospital). Type 3 (solid) and type 2 (mixed) are more easily identified by solid malignant mesenchymal components (c).

4 CPAM. Other cystic lung lesions containing cartilage such as bronchogenic cyst and type 1 CPAM might be considered. Chromosomal abnormalities that support a diagnosis of PPB in these cases include trisomy for chromosome 2 or 8.[105,106]

Recurrences often present with more solid features. The solid areas of PPB types II and III may be blastematous or sarcomatoid.[107-109] Lesions formerly diagnosed as primary pulmonary rhabdomyosarcomas are now classified as type 3 PPB. For type II PPB the differential diagnosis includes primary or metastatic biphasic lesions including synovial sarcoma, Wilms tumor, or salivary gland–type tumors.

Inflammatory Myofibroblastic Tumor

Clinical features of inflammatory myofibroblastic tumor

Inflammatory myofibroblastic tumor (IMT) is among the most common lung tumors in children and adolescents. In a small number of patients it may be accompanied by nonspecific signs and symptoms including fever, malaise, anemia, and erythrocytosis, but it generally presents due to mass effect. Although it most often behaves in a benign fashion, it has the potential to recur and to metastasize.[110]

Imaging features of inflammatory myofibroblastic tumor

Imaging demonstrates a mass lesion. The findings are not specific.

Histologic features of inflammatory myofibroblastic tumors

The mass most often comprises of bland spindled cell with a prominent mixed inflammatory infiltrate usually including lymphocytes, plasma cells, and eosinophils (*Figure 2-33*). Atypical features may include hypercellularity, fascicular or herringbone pattern, necrosis, or

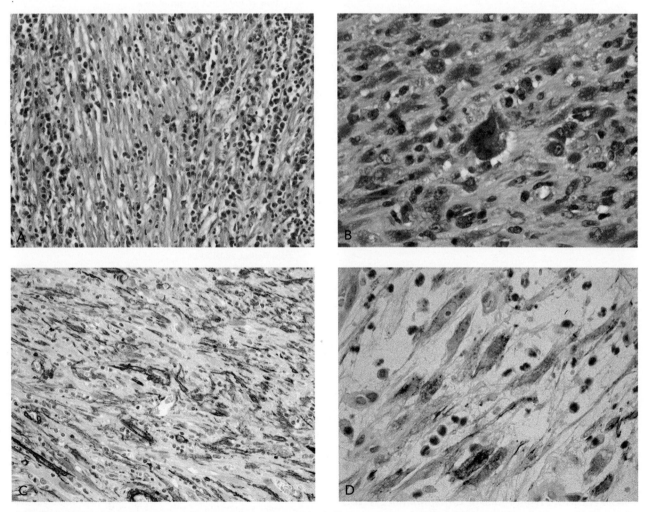

FIGURE 2-33 Inflammatory myofibroblastic tumor. This inflammatory myofibroblastic tumor shows spindled cells intermixed with a lymphoplasmacytic infiltrate (a). Occasional atypical cells (b) do not affect the prognosis. Immunohistochemistry for SMA (c) shows a "tram-trak" appearance typical of myofibroblastic cells. Immunohistochemistry for ALK (d) is helpful when positive.

cellular atypia including pleomorphism, ganglion-like cells, giant cells, or anaplasia. A round or polygonal cell component may be present, and these features do not relate to clinical outcome.[111] In some areas, the inflammation may be scant and the spindle cells variable cellular. Given the morphologic spectrum, particularly on a small biopsy the differential diagnosis includes other lesions with a mixed inflammatory infiltrate including hematopoietic neoplasms and infections as well as other spindle-cell predominant lesions including leiomyosarcoma and fibromatosis.

Immunohistochemistry for ALK may be helpful in identifying the subset of cases that are positive for ALK translocation; however, the absence of ALK staining does not exclude the possibility of ALK translocation.[88] Conflicting reports regarding the prognostic impact of ALK translocation have been published, which may be due to the rarity of the tumor or the variety of methods used to detect the translocation,[112] but the rare tumors with distant metastases and poor outcomes have been ALK negative.

Fetal Lung Interstitial Tumor (FLIT)

This recently described tumor[106,113] presents in neonates as a solid mass with features similar to the canalicular stage of development. This mass is sharply circumscribed, sometimes partially encapsulated, and shows abnormal airspaces spaces lined by cuboidal cells with interstitial bland cells without atypia or mitosis. The interstitial cells may have clear cytoplasm with PAS-positive glycogen. There is overlap between these described cases and the microscopic descriptions of type 3 CPAM, which usually involves an entire lobe rather than a circumscribed mass. The adjacent lung was unremarkable, and no recurrence was documented on follow-up.

Congenital Peribronchial Myofibroblastic Tumor

This is an extremely rare benign tumor found in fetuses and neonates.[114-116] It classically presents with hydrops in the fetus or neonatal respiratory distress due to mass effect; however, recurrence has never been reported, even with positive margins. Imaging demonstrates a solid mass. Although predominantly comprised of bland fascicles of spindle cells, areas of hemangiopericytoma-like vessels and round cells may be present. Both mitosis and necrosis as well as infiltration into the surrounding lung are common. There may be partial SMA expression, and electron microscopy findings are consistent with myofibroblastic differentiation. A cartilaginous component has been reported in some cases, although more frequently this seems to correspond to entrapped airway cartilage. It has been speculated

that the cartilaginous component may increase as the infant ages. Cytogenetics may show complex karyotypic rearrangements. Despite these features the behavior is benign.

REFERENCES

1. Griese M, Haug M, Brasch F, et al. Incidence and classification of pediatric diffuse parenchymal lung diseases in Germany. *Orphanet J Rare Dis.* 2009;4:26.
2. Nathan N, Taam RA, Epaud R, et al. A national internet-linked based database for pediatric interstitial lung diseases: the French network. *Orphanet J Rare Dis.* 2012;7:40.
3. Kurland G, Deterding RR, Hagood JS, et al. An official American Thoracic Society clinical practice guideline: classification, evaluation, and management of childhood interstitial lung disease in infancy. *Am J Respir Crit Care Med.* 2013;188:376.
4. Deutsch GH, Young LR, Deterding RR, et al. Diffuse lung disease in young children: application of a novel classification scheme. *Am J Respir Crit Care Med.* 2007;176:1120.
5. Rice A, Tran-Dang MA, Bush A, Nicholson AG. Diffuse lung disease in infancy and childhood: expanding the chILD classification. *Histopathology.* 2013;63:743.
6. Soares JJ, Deutsch GH, Moore PE, et al. Childhood interstitial lung diseases: an 18-year retrospective analysis. *Pediatrics.* 2013;132:684.
7. Langston C, Dishop MK. Diffuse lung disease in infancy: a proposed classification applied to 259 diagnostic biopsies. *Pediatr Dev Pathol.* 2009;12:421.
8. Yu DC, Grabowski MJ, Kozakewich HP, et al. Primary lung tumors in children and adolescents: a 90-year experience. *J Pediatr Surg.* 2010;45:1090.
9. Lal DR, Clark I, Shalkow J, et al. Primary epithelial lung malignancies in the pediatric population. *Pediatr Blood Cancer.* 2005;45:683.
10. Dishop MK, Kuruvilla S. Primary and metastatic lung tumors in the pediatric population: a review and 25-year experience at a large children's hospital. *Arch Pathol Lab Med.* 2008;132:1079.
11. Langston C, Patterson K, Dishop MK, et al. A protocol for the handling of tissue obtained by operative lung biopsy: recommendations of the chILD pathology co-operative group. *Pediatr Dev Pathol.* 2006;9:173.
12. Rutledge JC, Jensen P. Acinar dysplasia: a new form of pulmonary maldevelopment. *Hum Pathol.* 1986;17:1290.
13. Chow CW, Massie J, Ng J, et al. Acinar dysplasia of the lungs: variation in the extent of involvement and clinical features. *Pathology.* 2013;45:38.
14. DeBoer EM, Keene S, Winkler AM, Shehata BM. Identical twins with lethal congenital pulmonary airway malformation type 0 (acinar dysplasia): further evidence of familial tendency. *Fetal Pediatr Pathol.* 2012;31:217.
15. Langenstroer M, Carlan SJ, Fanaian N, Attia S. Congenital acinar dysplasia: report of a case and review of literature. *AJP Rep.* 2013;3:9.
16. Hegde S, Pomplun S, Hannam S, Greenough A. Nonfatal congenital alveolar dysplasia due to abnormalities of NO synthase isoforms. *Acta Paediatr.* 2007;96:1248.
17. Mac MH. Congenital alveolar dysplasia; a developmental anomaly involving pulmonary alveoli. *Pediatrics.* 1948;2:43.
18. Mac MH. Congenital alveolar dysplasia of the lungs. *Am J Pathol.* 1948;24:919.
19. Melly L, Sebire NJ, Malone M, Nicholson AG. Capillary apposition and density in the diagnosis of alveolar capillary dysplasia. *Histopathology.* 2008;53:450.

20. Drut R. Capillary apposition and density in the diagnosis of alveolar capillary dysplasia. *Histopathology.* 2010;56:401.

21. Sen P, Thakur N, Stockton DW, et al. Expanding the phenotype of alveolar capillary dysplasia (ACD). *J Pediatr.* 2004;145:646.

22. Bishop NB, Stankiewicz P, Steinhorn RH. Alveolar capillary dysplasia. *Am J Respir Crit Care Med.* 2011;184:172.

23. Wagenvoort CA. Misalignment of lung vessels: a syndrome causing persistent neonatal pulmonary hypertension. *Hum Pathol.* 1986;17:727.

24. Galambos C, Sims-Lucas S, Abman SH. Histologic evidence of intrapulmonary anastomoses by three-dimensional reconstruction in severe bronchopulmonary dysplasia. *Ann Am Thorac Soc.* 2013;10:474.

25. Rossi UG, Owens CM. The radiology of chronic lung disease in children. *Arch Dis Child.* 2005;90:601.

26. Husain AN, Siddiqui NH, Stocker JT. Pathology of arrested acinar development in postsurfactant bronchopulmonary dysplasia. *Hum Pathol.* 1998;29:710.

27. Margraf LR, Tomashefski JF Jr, Bruce MC, Dahms BB. Morphometric analysis of the lung in bronchopulmonary dysplasia. *Am Rev Respir Dis.* 1991;143:391.

28. Tapper D, Schuster S, McBride J, et al. Polyalveolar lobe: anatomic and physiologic parameters and their relationship to congenital lobar emphysema. *J Pediatr Surg.* 1980;15:931.

29. Emery JL, Mithal A. The number of alveoli in the terminal respiratory unit of man during late intrauterine life and childhood. *Arch Dis Child.* 1960;35:544.

30. Cooney TP, Thurlbeck WM. The radial alveolar count method of Emery and Mithal: a reappraisal 2—intrauterine and early postnatal lung growth. *Thorax.* 1982;37:580.

31. Cooney TP, Thurlbeck WM. The radial alveolar count method of Emery and Mithal: a reappraisal 1—postnatal lung growth. *Thorax.* 1982;37:572.

32. van Teeffelen AS, Van Der Heijden J, Oei SG, et al. Accuracy of imaging parameters in the prediction of lethal pulmonary hypoplasia secondary to mid-trimester prelabor rupture of fetal membranes: a systematic review and meta-analysis. *Ultrasound Obstet Gynecol.* 2012;39:495.

33. Husain AN, Hessel RG. Neonatal pulmonary hypoplasia: an autopsy study of 25 cases. *Pediatr Pathol.* 1993;13:475.

34. De Paepe ME, Friedman RM, Gundogan F, Pinar H. Postmortem lung weight/body weight standards for term and preterm infants. *Pediatr Pulmonol.* 2005;40:445.

35. Wigglesworth JS, Desai R, Guerrini P. Fetal lung hypoplasia: biochemical and structural variations and their possible significance. *Arch Dis Child.* 1981;56:606.

36. Reale FR, Esterly JR. Pulmonary hypoplasia: a morphometric study of the lungs of infants with diaphragmatic hernia, anencephaly, and renal malformations. *Pediatrics.* 1973;51:91.

37. Riedlinger WF, Vargas SO, Jennings RW, et al. Bronchial atresia is common to extralobar sequestration, intralobar sequestration, congenital cystic adenomatoid malformation, and lobar emphysema. *Pediatr Dev Pathol.* 2006;9:361.

38. Kunisaki SM, Fauza DO, Nemes LP, et al. Bronchial atresia: the hidden pathology within a spectrum of prenatally diagnosed lung masses. *J Pediatr Surg.* 2006;41:61.

39. Langston C. New concepts in the pathology of congenital lung malformations. *Semin Pediatr Surg.* 2003;12:17.

40. Stanton M, Njere I, Ade-Ajayi N, et al. Systematic review and meta-analysis of the postnatal management of congenital cystic lung lesions. *J Pediatr Surg.* 2009;44:1027.

41. Schuster SR, Harris GB, Williams A, et al. Bronchial atresia: a recognizable entity in the pediatric age group. *J Pediatr Surg.* 1978;13:682.

42. Conran RM, Stocker JT. Extralobar sequestration with frequently associated congenital cystic adenomatoid malformation, type 2: report of 50 cases. *Pediatr Dev Pathol.* 1999;2:454.

43. Stocker JT, Madewell JE, Drake RM. Congenital cystic adenomatoid malformation of the lung. Classification and morphologic spectrum. *Hum Pathol.* 1977;8:155.

44. Epelman M, Kreiger PA, Servaes S, et al. Current imaging of prenatally diagnosed congenital lung lesions. *Semin Ultrasound CT MR.* 2010;31:141.

45. Korol E. The correlation of carcinoma and congenital cystic emphysema of the lungs; report of ten cases. *Dis Chest.* 1953;23:403.

46. Summers RJ, Shehata BM, Bleacher JC, et al. Mucinous adenocarcinoma of the lung in association with congenital pulmonary airway malformation. *J Pediatr Surg.* 2010;45:2256.

47. Ramos SG, Barbosa GH, Tavora FR, et al. Bronchioloalveolar carcinoma arising in a congenital pulmonary airway malformation in a child: case report with an update of this association. *J Pediatr Surg.* 2007;42:E1.

48. Lantuejoul S, Nicholson AG, Sartori G, et al. Mucinous cells in type 1 pulmonary congenital cystic adenomatoid malformation as mucinous bronchioloalveolar carcinoma precursors. *Am J Surg Pathol.* 2007;31:961.

49. Hill DA, Dehner LP. A cautionary note about congenital cystic adenomatoid malformation (CCAM) type 4. *Am J Surg Pathol.* 2004;28:554.

50. MacSweeney F, Papagiannopoulos K, Goldstraw P, et al. An assessment of the expanded classification of congenital cystic adenomatoid malformations and their relationship to malignant transformation. *Am J Surg Pathol.* 2003;27:1139.

51. Donnelly LF, Lucaya J, Ozelame V, et al. CT findings and temporal course of persistent pulmonary interstitial emphysema in neonates: a multiinstitutional study. *AJR Am J Roentgenol.* 2003;180:1129.

52. deMello DE, Nogee LM, Heyman S, et al. Molecular and phenotypic variability in the congenital alveolar proteinosis syndrome associated with inherited surfactant protein B deficiency. *J Pediatr.* 1994;125:43.

53. deMello DE, Heyman S, Phelps DS, et al. Ultrastructure of lung in surfactant protein B deficiency. *Am J Respir Cell Mol Biol.* 1994;11:230.

54. Nogee LM, Garnier G, Dietz HC, et al. A mutation in the surfactant protein B gene responsible for fatal neonatal respiratory disease in multiple kindreds. *J Clin Invest.* 1994;93:1860.

55. Nogee LM, Dunbar AE 3rd, Wert SE, et al. A mutation in the surfactant protein C gene associated with familial interstitial lung disease. *N Engl J Med.* 2001;344:573.

56. Nogee LM, Dunbar AE 3rd, Wert S, et al. Mutations in the surfactant protein C gene associated with interstitial lung disease. *Chest.* 2002;121:20S.

57. Thomas AQ, Lane K, Phillips J 3rd, et al. Heterozygosity for a surfactant protein C gene mutation associated with usual interstitial pneumonitis and cellular nonspecific interstitial pneumonitis in one kindred. *Am J Respir Crit Care Med.* 2002;165:1322.

58. Shulenin S, Nogee LM, Annilo T, et al. ABCA3 gene mutations in newborns with fatal surfactant deficiency. *N Engl J Med.* 2004;350:1296.

59. Galambos C, Levy H, Cannon CL, et al. Pulmonary pathology in thyroid transcription factor-1 deficiency syndrome. *Am J Respir Crit Care Med.* 2010;182:549.

60. Hamvas A, Deterding RR, Wert SE, et al. Heterogeneous pulmonary phenotypes associated with mutations in the thyroid transcription factor gene NKX2-1. *Chest.* 2013;144:794.

61. Martinez-Moczygemba M, Doan ML, Elidemir O, et al. Pulmonary alveolar proteinosis caused by deletion of the GM-CSFRalpha gene in the X chromosome pseudoautosomal region 1. *J Exp Med.* 2008;205:2711.

62. Suzuki T, Sakagami T, Rubin BK, et al. Familial pulmonary alveolar proteinosis caused by mutations in CSF2RA. *J Exp Med.* 2008;205:2703.

63. Tanaka T, Motoi N, Tsuchihashi Y, et al. Adult-onset hereditary pulmonary alveolar proteinosis caused by a single-base deletion in CSF2RB. *J Med Genet.* 2011;48:205.

64. Rosen DM, Waltz DA. Hydroxychloroquine and surfactant protein C deficiency. *N Engl J Med.* 2005;352:207.

65. Suzuki T, Maranda B, Sakagami T, et al. Hereditary pulmonary alveolar proteinosis caused by recessive CSF2RB mutations. *Eur Respir J.* 2011;37:201.

66. Katzenstein AL, Gordon LP, Oliphant M, Swender PT. Chronic pneumonitis of infancy. A unique form of interstitial lung disease occurring in early childhood. *Am J Surg Pathol.* 1995; 19:439.

67. Edwards V, Cutz E, Viero S, et al. Ultrastructure of lamellar bodies in congenital surfactant deficiency. *Ultrastruct Pathol.* 2005;29:503.

68. Dirksen U, Hattenhorst U, Schneider P, et al. Defective expression of granulocyte-macrophage colony-stimulating factor/interleukin-3/interleukin-5 receptor common beta chain in children with acute myeloid leukemia associated with respiratory failure. *Blood.* 1998;92:1097.

69. Punatar AD, Kusne S, Blair JE, et al. Opportunistic infections in patients with pulmonary alveolar proteinosis. *J Infect.* 2012;65:173.

70. Holbert JM, Costello P, Li W, et al. CT features of pulmonary alveolar proteinosis. *AJR Am J Roentgenol.* 2001;176:1287.

71. Canakis AM, Cutz E, Manson D, O'Brodovich H. Pulmonary interstitial glycogenosis: a new variant of neonatal interstitial lung disease. *Am J Respir Crit Care Med.* 2002;165:1557.

72. Deutsch GH, Young LR. Pulmonary interstitial glycogenosis: words of caution. *Pediatr Radiol.* 2010;40:1471.

73. Deutsch GH, Young LR. Histologic resolution of pulmonary interstitial glycogenosis. *Pediatr Dev Pathol.* 2009;12:475.

74. Popler J, Gower WA, Mogayzel PJ Jr, et al. Familial neuroendocrine cell hyperplasia of infancy. *Pediatr Pulmonol.* 2010;45:749.

75. Young LR, Deutsch GH, Bokulic RE, et al. A Mutation in TTF1/NKX2.1 Is Associated With Familial Neuroendocrine Cell Hyperplasia of Infancy. *Chest.* 2013;144:1199.

76. Lukkarinen H, Pelkonen A, Lohi J, et al. Neuroendocrine cell hyperplasia of infancy: a prospective follow-up of nine children. *Arch Dis Child.* 2013;98:141.

77. Brody AS, Guillerman RP, Hay TC, et al. Neuroendocrine cell hyperplasia of infancy: diagnosis with high-resolution CT. *AJR Am J Roentgenol.* 2010;194:238.

78. Deterding RR, Pye C, Fan LL, Langston C. Persistent tachypnea of infancy is associated with neuroendocrine cell hyperplasia. *Pediatr Pulmonol.* 2005;40:157.

79. Young LR, Brody AS, Inge TH, et al. Neuroendocrine cell distribution and frequency distinguish neuroendocrine cell hyperplasia of infancy from other pulmonary disorders. *Chest.* 2011;139:1060.

80. Latino GA, Al-Saleh S, Alharbi N, et al. Prevalence of pulmonary arteriovenous malformations in children versus adults with hereditary hemorrhagic telangiectasia. *J Pediatr.* 2013;163:282.

81. Meek ME, Meek JC, Beheshti MV. Management of pulmonary arteriovenous malformations. *Semin Intervent Radiol.* 2011; 28:24.

82. Tazelaar HD, Kerr D, Yousem SA, et al. Diffuse pulmonary lymphangiomatosis. *Hum Pathol.* 1993;24:1313.

83. Croteau SE, Kozakewich HP, Perez-Atayde AR, et al. Kaposiform lymphangiomatosis: a distinct aggressive lymphatic anomaly. *J Pediatr.* 2014;164(2):383-388.

84. Bellini C, Boccardo F, Campisi C, Bonioli E. Congenital pulmonary lymphangiectasia. *Orphanet J Rare Dis.* 2006;1:43.

85. Brown M, Pysher T, Coffin CM. Lymphangioma and congenital pulmonary lymphangiectasis: a histologic, immunohistochemical, and clinicopathologic comparison. *Mod Pathol.* 1999; 12:569.

86. Susarla SC, Fan LL. Diffuse alveolar hemorrhage syndromes in children. *Curr Opin Pediatr.* 2007;19:314.

87. Salih ZN, Akhter A, Akhter J. Specificity and sensitivity of hemosiderin-laden macrophages in routine bronchoalveolar lavage in children. *Arch Pathol Lab Med.* 2006;130:1684.

88. Saeed MM, Woo MS, MacLaughlin EF, et al. Prognosis in pediatric idiopathic pulmonary hemosiderosis. *Chest.* 1999;116:721.

89. Colom AJ, Teper AM, Vollmer WM, Diette GB. Risk factors for the development of bronchiolitis obliterans in children with bronchiolitis. *Thorax.* 2006;61:503.

90. Smith KJ, Fan LL. Insights into post-infectious bronchiolitis obliterans in children. *Thorax.* 2006;61:462.

91. Moonnumakal SP, Fan LL. Bronchiolitis obliterans in children. *Curr Opin Pediatr.* 2008;20:272.

92. Mauad T, Dolhnikoff M. Histology of childhood bronchiolitis obliterans. *Pediatr Pulmonol.* 2002;33:466.

93. van den Berg JM, van Koppen E, Ahlin A, et al. Chronic granulomatous disease: the European experience. *PLoS One.* 2009;4:e5234.

94. Moskaluk CA, Pogrebniak HW, Pass HI, et al. Surgical pathology of the lung in chronic granulomatous disease. *Am J Clin Pathol.* 1994;102:684.

95. Levine S, Smith VV, Malone M, Sebire NJ. Histopathological features of chronic granulomatous disease (CGD) in childhood. *Histopathology.* 2005;47:508.

96. Mani H, Stocker J. Congenital and acquired systemic infectious diseases. In: Stocker JT, Dehner LP, Husain AN, eds. *Stocker & Dehner's Pediatric Pathology.* 3rd ed. Philadelphia, PA: Lippincott Williams & Wilkins; 2011:186.

97. Stocker JT, Mani H, Husain AN. The respiratory tract. In: Stocker JT, Dehner LP, Husain AN, eds. *Stocker & Dehner's Pediatric Pathology.* 3rd ed. Philadelphia, PA: Lippincott Williams & Wilkins; 2011:441.

98. Roby BB, Drehner D, Sidman JD. Pediatric tracheal and endobronchial tumors: an institutional experience. *Arch Otolaryngol Head Neck Surg.* 2011;137:925.

99. Amini B, Huang SY, Tsai J, et al. Primary lung and large airway neoplasms in children: current imaging evaluation with multidetector computed tomography. *Radiol Clin North Am.* 2013;51:637.

100. Walts AE, Ines D, Marchevsky AM. Limited role of Ki-67 proliferative index in predicting overall short-term survival in patients with typical and atypical pulmonary carcinoid tumors. *Mod Pathol.* 2012;25:1258.

101. Hill DA, Ivanovich J, Priest JR, et al. DICER1 mutations in familial pleuropulmonary blastoma. *Science.* 2009;325:965.

102. Foulkes WD, Bahubeshi A, Hamel N, et al. Extending the phenotypes associated with DICER1 mutations. *Hum Mutat.* 2011;32:1381.

103. Slade I, Bacchelli C, Davies H, et al. DICER1 syndrome: clarifying the diagnosis, clinical features and management implications of a pleiotropic tumour predisposition syndrome. *J Med Genet.* 2011;8:273.

104. Vargas SO, Nose V, Fletcher JA, Perez-Atayde AR. Gains of chromosome 8 are confined to mesenchymal components in pleuropulmonary blastoma. *Pediatr Dev Pathol.* 2001;4:434.

105. Novak R, Dasu S, Agamanolis D, et al. Trisomy 8 is a characteristic finding in pleuropulmonary blastoma. *Pediatr Pathol Lab Med.* 1997;17:99.

106. de Chadarevian JP, Liu J, Pezanowski D, et al. Diagnosis of "fetal lung interstitial tumor" requires a FISH negative for trisomies 8 and 2. *Am J Surg Pathol.* 2011;35:1085; author reply 1086.

107. Priest JR, McDermott MB, Bhatia S, et al. Pleuropulmonary blastoma: a clinicopathologic study of 50 cases. *Cancer.* 1997;80:147.

108. Priest JR, Hill DA, Williams GM, et al. Type I pleuropulmonary blastoma: a report from the International Pleuropulmonary Blastoma Registry. *J Clin Oncol.* 2006;24:4492.

CHAPTER 2

109. Hill DA, Jarzembowski JA, Priest JR, et al. Type I pleuropulmonary blastoma: pathology and biology study of 51 cases from the international pleuropulmonary blastoma registry. *Am J Surg Pathol.* 2008;32:282.

110. Siminovich M, Galluzzo L, Lopez J, et al. Inflammatory myofibroblastic tumor of the lung in children: anaplastic lymphoma kinase (ALK) expression and clinico-pathological correlation. *Pediatr Dev Pathol.* 2012;15:179.

111. Coffin CM, Hornick JL, Fletcher CD. Inflammatory myofibroblastic tumor: comparison of clinicopathologic, histologic, and immunohistochemical features including ALK expression in atypical and aggressive cases. *Am J Surg Pathol.* 2007;31:509.

112. Alaggio R, Cecchetto G, Bisogno G, et al. Inflammatory myofibroblastic tumors in childhood: a report from the Italian Cooperative Group studies. *Cancer.* 2010;116:216.

113. Dishop MK, McKay EM, Kreiger PA, et al. Fetal lung interstitial tumor (FLIT): A proposed newly recognized lung tumor of infancy to be differentiated from cystic pleuropulmonary blastoma and other developmental pulmonary lesions. *Am J Surg Pathol.* 2010;34:1762.

114. Kim Y, Park HY, Cho J, et al. Congenital peribronchial myofibroblastic tumor: a case study and literature review. *Korean J Pathol.* 2013;47:172.

115. Alobeid B, Beneck D, Sreekantaiah C, et al. Congenital pulmonary myofibroblastic tumor: a case report with cytogenetic analysis and review of the literature. *Am J Surg Pathol.* 1997; 21:610.

116. Huppmann AR, Coffin CM, Hoot AC, et al. Congenital peribronchial myofibroblastic tumor: comparison of fetal and postnatal morphology. *Pediatr Dev Pathol.* 2011;14:124.

CHAPTER 2

3 Adenocarcinoma

Lynette M. Sholl and Mizuki Nishino

TAKE HOME PEARLS

- Adenocarcinoma is the most common type of lung cancer diagnosed today. Outcomes are strongly related to stage at the time of diagnosis. Over half of patients have metastatic disease at presentation; patients with advanced (stage IV) disease have a mean five-year survival of less than 5%.
- Lung adenocarcinoma is more common in patients with a history of smoking; however, of all the lung cancer subtypes, adenocarcinoma is the most common diagnosed in nonsmokers. The risk factors for development of lung adenocarcinoma in nonsmokers are not well understood; however, this population is significantly more likely to have activating mutations in oncogenes that predict response to tyrosine kinase inhibitor therapies.
- The identification of genetic subgroups of lung adenocarcinoma has driven the evolution of a more granular histologic classification system. "Adenocarcinoma, mixed subtype" is replaced by "Adenocarcinoma, [designate subtype]-predominant." The diagnostic entity bronchioloalveolar carcinoma, a clinically heterogeneous diagnosis that in practice included in situ tumors with excellent prognosis and aggressive invasive tumors, has been eliminated. In its place, adenocarcinoma in situ designates small tumors with pure lepidic growth and no invasion, minimally invasive adenocarcinoma designates tumors with predominant lepidic growth and less than 5 mm of nonlepidic and/or invasive histology,

and adenocarcinoma, lepidic-predominant, designates tumors with greater than 5 mm of invasion, this final group being associated with relatively more aggressive behavior in most studies. The term "mucinous BAC" is replaced by invasive mucinous adenocarcinoma.
- EGFR or ALK alterations occur in 20% to 25% of lung adenocarcinomas and are associated with response to targeted inhibitors. Clinical practice guidelines now recommend testing for EGFR and ALK alterations in all advanced lung adenocarcinomas for selection of first-line therapy in patients whose tumors harbor EGFR-activating mutations or ALK rearrangements, respectively.
- Most advanced lung adenocarcinomas are diagnosed on small biopsy or cytology specimens. In 30% of these specimen types, morphologic features distinguishing adenocarcinoma and squamous cell carcinoma are lacking, and the term *nonsmall cell lung carcinoma* is no longer sufficient for guiding therapy. Therefore, immunohistochemistry studies may be used judiciously to make a definitive diagnosis, while conserving as much tissue as possible for downstream molecular profiling.

WHO CLASSIFICATION OF PULMONARY ADENOCARCINOMA

In the 2004 edition of the World Health Organization's classification of lung tumors, adenocarcinomas were

41

Table 3-1 2004 WHO Classification and 2011 IASLC/ATS/ERS/2015 WHO Classification: A Comparison of Published Lung Adenocarcinoma Classification Systems

2004 WHO Classification of Lung Adenocarcinomas	2011 IASLC/ATS/ERS/ 2015 WHO Classification of Lung Adenocarcinomas
Adenocarcinoma, mixed subtype	Preinvasive lesions
Acinar adenocarcinoma	Atypical adenomatous hyperplasia
Papillary adenocarcinoma	Adenocarcinoma in situ
Bronchioloalveolar carcinoma	Nonmucinous
Nonmucinous	Mucinous
Mucinous	Mixed mucinous/nonmucinous
Mixed mucinous/nonmucinous or indeterminate	Minimally invasive adenocarcinoma
Solid adenocarcinoma with mucin production	Nonmucinous
Fetal adenocarcinoma	Mucinous
Mucinous "colloid" carcinoma	Mixed mucinous/nonmucinous
Mucinous cystadenocarcinoma	Invasive adenocarcinoma
Signet ring adenocarcinoma	Lepidic predominant
Clear cell adenocarcinoma	Acinar predominant
	Papillary predominant
	Micropapillary predominant
	Solid predominant with mucin
	Variants of invasive adenocarcinoma
	Invasive mucinous adenocarcinoma
	Colloid
	Fetal
	Enteric

divided according to their histology into five major subtypes, including mixed, acinar, papillary, bronchioloalveolar, and solid with mucin production.[1] These classifiers have served as the backbone of the histologic diagnosis of adenocarcinoma for the last decade; however, extensive study of the utility of this classification system as well as major advances in the field of lung cancer biology have triggered the need for an updated system.

The mixed subtype category accounts for the vast majority of lung adenocarcinomas, which are broadly recognized to have wide intratumoral morphologic heterogeneity but may frequently show a predominant growth pattern. With our improved understanding of the genetics of lung adenocarcinoma, it has become clear that certain growth patterns are associated with underlying molecular alterations with important predictive and prognostic implications.[2-4] Thus, the mixed subtype categorization is considered insufficiently specific for today's practice.

The bronchioloalveolar (BAC) category, which was further subdivided into mucinous, nonmucinous, and mixed or indeterminate types, has likewise proven problematic. While BAC was strictly defined as a tumor growing along preexisting septal structures and lacking evidence of invasion, this term has been used broadly in clinical practice, encompassing a genetically and clinically diverse spectrum of tumors.[5-8]

Thus, a new classification scheme representing the combined recommendations of the International Society for the Study of Lung Cancers (IASLC), the American Thoracic Society (ATS), and the European Respiratory Society (ERS) was published in 2011 and served as the template for the revised 2015 WHO classification system (*Table 3-1*).[9] These newer recommendations eliminate the term "mixed subtype" and advise the pathologist to define a predominant subtype and semiquantitatively document other minor but distinctive patterns. In addition, this scheme replaces the term *BAC* with *adenocarcinoma in situ* and provides a mechanism to more accurately classify predominantly in situ lesions with minimal invasion (both defined in detail below).

EPIDEMIOLOGY OF ADENOCARCINOMA

In the United States, an estimated 230,000 people will be diagnosed with and 160,000 will die from lung cancer in 2013.[10] Worldwide, there are an estimated

1.6 million new diagnoses per year, with the highest incidences in North America and Central and Eastern Europe.[11] Historically, many epidemiologic databases have categorized lung cancers as either small cell carcinoma or nonsmall cell carcinoma, therefore the incidence of lung adenocarcinoma in particular is difficult to estimate; however, the National Cancer Institute estimates that 40% of lung cancers are adenocarcinomas, making it the most common type of lung cancer diagnosed today.[12]

Over half of patients have advanced (distantly metastatic) disease at the time of a lung cancer diagnosis, whereas only 15% of patients have disease confined to the lung at the time of diagnosis.[10] Survival is strongly dependent on stage of disease at diagnosis, with a 5-year survival ranging from 73% for patients with pathologic stage IA nonsmall cell lung carcinoma to 2% for patients with clinical stage IV disease.[13] Adenocarcinoma has a favorable prognosis when compared with other histologic subtypes of lung cancer for localized and regional disease[14]; however, this advantage is lost for patients with distant disease.[15]

DEMOGRAPHICS OF ADENOCARCINOMA

The incidence of lung cancer is 1.5- to 2-fold higher in men than in women, across all races. This incidence ranges from a low of 40.6 per 100,000 Hispanic men to 95.8 per 100,000 Black men and 26.3 per 100,000 Hispanic women to 54.6 per 100,000 White women. Based on data from the last decade, the median age of diagnosis of lung cancer was 70, and the median age of death due to lung cancer was 72. Lung cancer incidence and mortality has declined in men since the early 1990s, whereas in women both incidence and mortality increased significantly from the 1970s to the early 2000s; only in the last decade has this trend reversed in women.[10] Smokers have a 10-fold increased incidence of lung cancer; however, adenocarcinoma is significantly associated with lower median pack years of smoking (41.5 vs 61.8 pack years for other histologies) and when diagnosed in former smokers tends to present at a later time since quitting than other lung cancer types.[16] Indeed, adenocarcinoma histology is more common among nonsmokers than smokers (62% vs 19%).[17] While general trends in tobacco use can be correlated with lung cancer epidemiology, the National Cancer Institute's Surveillance, Epidemiology, and End Results (SEER) database and other population-based registries do not collect patient smoking data, therefore it is difficult to estimate the incidence of lung cancer in never smokers (defined as individuals who have smoker fewer than 100 cigarettes in their lifetime).[18] Over 50% of women with lung cancer are never smokers, as compared to 15% to 20% of men.[19] The rate of lung cancer in never smokers varies significantly based on race/ethnicity. Several large California-based studies reported that 46% to 71% of Asian/Pacific Islanders with lung cancer were never smokers, as compared to 10% to 40% of non-Hispanic Whites.[20,21]

ETIOLOGIES OF ADENOCARCINOMA

Smoking-Related Adenocarcinoma

The first large-scale epidemiologic studies to link cigarette smoking with lung cancer were published in 1950, when squamous cell carcinoma outnumbered adenocarcinoma by a ratio of 18:1.[22] By the mid-1990s, this ratio dropped dramatically to close to 1:1, and in women the diagnosis of adenocarcinoma is 1.5-fold more common than squamous cell carcinoma.[23] This shift in lung tumor type has been associated with the widespread adoption of filtered cigarettes; this type of cigarette generally reduces the yield of tar delivered to the lung and is associated with a reduced risk for lung cancer in long-term smokers as compared to unfiltered cigarettes. However, smokers tend to draw larger "puff volumes" when smoking filtered, as compared to unfiltered, cigarettes, leading to exposure of the peripheral lung to higher doses of the toxic compounds within smoke, including systemic carcinogens such as 4-(methylnitrosamino)-1-(3-pyridyl)-1-butanone (NNK), a nitrosamine. In addition, changes in the manufacturing of tobacco of the last half century have led to increases in the nitrate content, leading to higher concentrations of NNK in the inhaled cigarette smoke.[24] In the absence of the protective epithelial defenses of the proximal airways (ie, the mucociliary elevator), the peripheral lung compartments are thought to be relatively more susceptible to the toxic effects of the inhaled carcinogens.[22] The tumor mutation frequency is significantly higher in adenocarcinomas from smokers than from never smokers; lung adenocarcinoma in smokers ranks behind only melanoma and lung squamous carcinoma in terms of somatic mutation rate.[25] Mutations in lung adenocarcinoma most commonly take the form of transversions (purine to pyrimidine substitution, or vice versa)[25,26]; *KRAS*, *STK11/LKB1*, and *KEAP* are among the most commonly mutated genes in adenocarcinomas arising in smokers[25] (*Table 3-2*).

Table 3-2 Distinctive Molecular Profiles of Adenocarcinomas Arising in Smokers and Never-Smokers

	Smokers	Never Smokers	References
Median mutation frequency	9.8 per Mb	1.7 per Mb	Imielinski et al, 2012
Commonly mutated genes			Ding et al, 2008
	KRAS	EGFR	Imielinski et al, 2012
	STK11	ALK fusions	Takeuchi et al, 2012
	KEAP	ROS1 fusions	Kwak et al, 2010
	SMARCA4	RET fusions	Bergethon et al, 2012
Mutation types	C>A and C>G transversions	C>T transitions	Riely et al, 2008
		within CpG islands	Imielinski et al, 2012

Nonsmoking-Related Adenocarcinoma

While the association between cigarette smoking and lung cancer development is well established, 25% of lung cancer cases worldwide develop in patients with no history of smoking, ranging from 10% to 15% of lung cancers in Europe and North America to 30% to 40% of lung cancers in Asian countries.[17] Second-hand smoke is an established risk factor in this population, and other potential risk factors include environmental exposures such as cooking fumes, asbestos, and heavy metals, as well as viral infections such as human papillomavirus.[27] Genome-wide association studies have identified genetic polymorphisms that may contribute to an increased risk of lung cancer in never smokers, including *TERT* and the glypican *GPC5*.[28,29] To some extent, never smokers have phenotypically and genetically distinct lung carcinomas; these are most commonly adenocarcinomas with mutation rates that are 5- to 10-fold less than those seen in smokers.[30] In addition, adenocarcinomas arising in never smokers are more likely to harbor activating mutations in *EGFR* or oncogenic fusions involving *ALK*, *ROS*, and *RET* genes, findings of significance for selecting first-line therapies in these patients[31,32] (*Table 3-2*).

DIAGNOSTIC CRITERIA OF ADENOCARCINOMA

Clinical Features of Adenocarcinoma

The clinical features of adenocarcinoma depend on its location of origin within the lung and its stage at the time of diagnosis. Many patients with advanced disease present with symptoms attributable to their metastatic tumor. Most adenocarcinomas arise in the lung periphery, where they may present incidentally on lung imaging or may be asymptomatic and only recognized after the tumor has metastasized. According to data collected over the last 30 years of the 20th century, common presenting symptoms include cough in up to 75% of patients, particularly if the tumor arises centrally and involves a central airway; chest pain in 20% as a result of pleural, chest wall, or mediastinal invasion; hemoptysis in up to 50% as a result of tumor eroding into an adjacent bronchovascular bundle; and dyspnea in 25% as a result of airway obstruction, extensive parenchymal or lymphatic infiltration by tumor, or pleural effusion.[33-35] Patients with advanced invasive mucinous adenocarcinoma (formerly "mucinous BAC") may present with bronchorrhea, characterized by cough productive of abundant, thin, mucus.

In contrast to this older literature, recent studies of early stage lung cancer suggest that only half of patients come to clinical attention due to one or more of these thoracic symptoms; tumors in the remaining half of patients are detected incidentally as a result of imaging for other indications or in lung cancer screening programs.[36] In fact, large national studies have shown that low-dose CT-based screening in smokers leads to an increase in the diagnosis of lung cancer and reduced lung cancer mortality,[37,38] which will likely lead to an adoption of more routine imaging-based lung cancer screening programs and, if effective, a continuing reduction in the number of patients presenting symptomatically.

Imaging Features of Adenocarcinoma

Chest Radiograph and Computed Tomography Characteristics of Adenocarcinoma

Imaging plays a critical role in the evaluation of lung adenocarcinoma as well as other types of lung cancer, and is essential for detection, diagnosis, staging, as well as for assessment of surgical resectability and tumor response to therapy. While chest radiograph remains a practical imaging tool for initial evaluation, the technical advances and increased availability of multidetector row CT has markedly increased the role of CT in the assessment of lung cancer. Notably, the results of

National Lung Screening Trial (NLST) involving 53,454 persons at high risk for lung cancer demonstrated a relative reduction in mortality from lung cancer with low-dose CT screening of 20.0%, comparing to the screening by chest radiograph.[37] On the other hand, in the prostate, lung, colorectal, and ovarian (PLCO) screening involving 154,901 participants, annual radiograph screening did not reduce lung cancer mortality compared to the usual medical care.[39] In July 2013, the US Preventive Services Task Force issued a draft recommendation for annual screening for lung cancer with low-dose CT in persons at high risk for lung cancer based on age and smoking history,[40] further increasing the role of CT in detection and diagnosis of lung cancer.

Peripheral tumors

Adenocarcinoma of the lung commonly presents as a peripheral tumor. When the tumor is below 1 cm in diameter, it is rarely visible on chest radiograph.[41] The appearance on CT has been well described and studied in correlation with pathological classifications of adenocarcinoma and its spectrum.

Atypical adenomatous hyperplasia (AAH) and adenocarcinoma in situ (AIS) represent the precursor lesions of invasive adenocarcinoma, which are discussed in detail later in the chapter. On CT, AAH demonstrates a well-defined pure ground glass nodule, typically measuring 5 mm or less, and remains unchanged over years.[42-45] AIS also most commonly presents as a ground glass nodule that measures 3 cm or less on CT, and can be accompanied with a bubble-like lucency. Solid or part solid nodules are an unusual manifestation of AIS.[42,43,46] Minimally invasive adenocarcinoma (MIA), on the other hand, is seen as a part-solid nodule with predominant ground glass component with a small solid component which is 5 mm or less. The solid component correlates with areas of invasion, while ground glass component correlates with lepidic growth on pathology.[47] As precursor lesions and early adenocarcinomas often present as small ground glass nodules or part solid nodules (*Figure 3-1*), an appropriate radiological follow-up strategy is needed to assess change over time and detect any signs of transformation into more invasive tumor. For this purpose, a statement from the Fleischner Society has recently been published, describing the recommendations for the management of subsolid pulmonary nodules detected on CT.[48]

In terms of invasive adenocarcinoma, nonmucinous tumors usually present as a solid or part solid lesion, with the solid component measuring greater than 5 mm on CT (*Figure 3-2*). The size of the solid component provides important staging and prognostic information. Less commonly, the lesion can present as a consolidative opacity or lobar distribution of ground glass opacity.[45] Invasive mucinous adenocarcinomas are seen on CT as a solid nodule (*Figure 3-3*), part solid

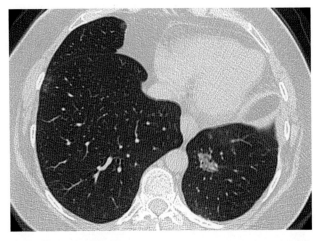

FIGURE 3-1 CT scan of the chest demonstrates a ground-glass nodule in the left base. Pathology reveals a lepidic-predominant adenocarcinoma with a minor component of acinar pattern.

nodules or a lobar or sublobar dense consolidation with air bronchograms. "CT angiogram sign" is noted on contrast-enhanced CT when pulmonary arteries are seen transversing the consolidated lesion, which is often seen in mucinous adenocarcinoma, however, is not a specific sign.[45,49]

Several imaging studies investigated the association between CT findings and clinical outcome and prognosis in small lung adenocarcinomas. Kodama et al performed a semiquantitative analysis of ground glass opacities in 104 small lung adenocarcinomas (<2 cm), and demonstrated better prognosis in tumors with >50% ground glass opacities.[50] A study by Aoki et al investigated the CT features of 127 patients with lung

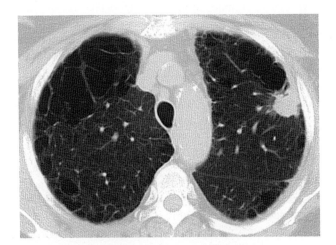

FIGURE 3-2 Coronal reformatted CT image of the chest demonstrates a bilobed nodule with spiculated margin. Note centrilobular and paraseptal emphysema in the upper lungs and interstitial lung disease in the peripheral portions of lower lungs. Pathology revealed a solid-predominant adenocarcinoma.

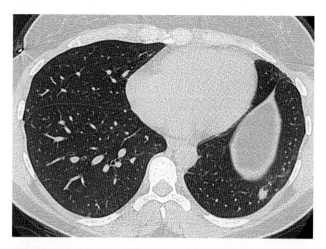

FIGURE 3-3 CT scan of the chest shows an irregular nodule in the periphery of the left base. Pathology reveals a mucinous adenocarcinoma with predominant lepidic pattern.

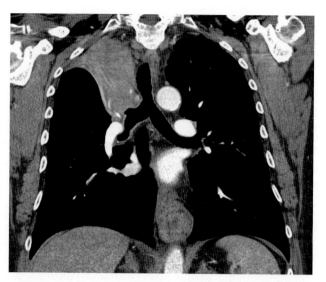

FIGURE 3-4 CT scan of the chest demonstrates an enhancing mass obstructing the right upper lobe bronchus, surrounded by the collapsed right upper lobe.

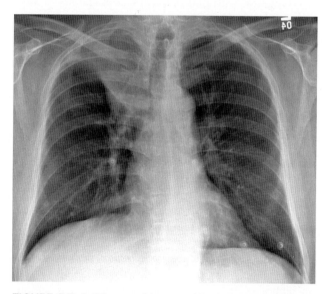

FIGURE 3-5 A 69-year-old man with shortness of breath and hemoptysis. Frontal chest radiograph demonstrates a right upper lobe collapse with the "Golden S sign" with the reverse S-shaped minor fissure, indicative of underlying central obstructive mass.

adenocarcinomas less than 3 cm, and demonstrated that adenocarcinomas with >50% ground glass components had significantly lower frequencies of lymph node metastasis and vascular invasion, and had significantly better prognosis compared to adenocarcinomas with ground glass components <50%. Coarse speculation and thickening of bronchovascular bundles around the tumors on CT were significantly associated with lymph node metastasis and vascular invasion on pathology.[51]

Central tumors

Although less common than peripheral tumors, lung adenocarcinoma can present as a central tumor, which can be associated with secondary signs on imaging including atelectasis, lobar collapse, and air trapping, due to the obstruction of major bronchus (*Figure 3-4*). These findings are noted on chest radiographs, and represent the classic patterns of radiographic manifestation of lung cancer. For example, right upper lobe collapse due to tumoral obstruction of right upper lobe bronchus presents as "Golden S sign" (*Figure 3-5*), in which the opacity due to collapsed right upper lobe is seen over the reverse S-shaped minor fissure with downward convexity of the medial portion of the fissure by a large central mass.[41,52] In case of left upper lobe collapse, hazy opacity extending from the left hilum and loss of cardiac and mediastinal silhouette are noted on the frontal radiograph, because the collapsed upper lobe moves forward and pulls the expanded lower lobe behind it.[41] These secondary signs of central tumors should prompt further evaluation.

Local invasion and intrathoracic spread

Assessment of invasion into adjacent structures, such as mediastinum, heart and great vessels, chest wall, and pleura, is an important component of T staging and evaluation of surgical resectability. CT is often useful as a noninvasive tool for this purpose. The utility of CT in assessing hilar and mediastinal invasion has been well studied, and the sensitivity of determining mediastinal invasion by single-detector or electron beam CT with or without the use of helical scanning ranges from 40% to 84% and specificity from 57% to 94%.[53-55] The assessment of chest wall and pleural invasion can be challenging. Of note, visceral pleural invasion increases the T staging from T1 to T2 and the tumor from stage IA to stage IB, even for tumors less than 3 cm. The seventh edition of the Union Internationale Contre le Cancer

TNM staging system recommends the use of elastic stains for determination of visceral pleural invasion.[56,57] On imaging, the conventional CT criteria include >3 cm tumoral contact with the pleura, an obtuse angle, and associated pleural thickening, which are very sensitive but nonspecific in determining chest wall invasion.[58] A recent study by Imai et al proposed the use of a ratio between the interface length between tumor and neighboring structures (arch distance) and the maximum tumor diameter. The arch distance-to-maximum tumor diameter ratio was correlated with pleural status (pl1, pl2, and pl3) after Elastica-Masson staining in 169 NSCLC patients.[59] The arch distance to maximum tumor diameter ratio becomes higher as pleural status advances. The cutoff ratio of 0.9 best distinguished between pl3 tumors and pl1 and pl2 tumors, with the sensitivity of 89.7%, specificity of 96.0%, PPV of 83.9%, NPV of 97.6%, accuracy of 94.8%, and area-under-the-curve for diagnosis of invasion of 0.976, an improvement compared to the conventional CT criteria.[59]

Patterns of intrathoracic spread can be either lymphangitic or hematogenous. In cases of lymphangitic spread of the tumor, the involvement of the lymphatic system of the lungs is noted on CT, including irregular thickening of the interlobular septa and the bronchovascular bundles, typically with lower lung distribution and asymmetric involvement (*Figure 3-6*). In cases of hematogenous metastasis, military nodules are distributed at random in relation to secondary pulmonary lobules.

PET/CT Features of Adenocarcinoma

PET/CT using Fluorine-18 (^{18}F)-fluorodeoxyglucose (FDG) is a useful modality for the diagnosis of lung cancer including lung adenocarcinoma, with its ability to differentiate malignant versus benign lung nodules

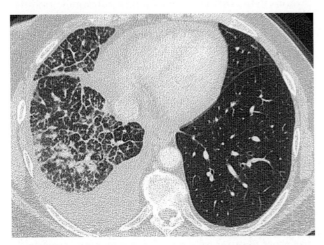

FIGURE 3-6 A 60-year-old woman with metastatic adenocarcinoma of the lung. CT scan of the chest demonstrates irregular thickening of the interlobular septa and bronchovascular bundles in the right lung, associated with pleural effusion, demonstrating lymphangitic spread of the tumor.

based on the FDG uptake that reflects the degree of glucose metabolism. Standard uptake value (SUV) is commonly used as a quantitative parameter on PET studies. In a study by Patz et al in 1993, FDG-PET was shown to be useful in differentiating benign from malignant solitary pulmonary nodules, with 100% specificity for benign nodules with a cutoff SUV of 2.5.[60] In a meta-analysis of 22 studies using FDG-PET for diagnosis of solitary pulmonary nodules, pooled sensitivity was 0.95, pooled specificity was 0.82, and the area under the ROC curve was 0.94.[61] FDG-PET/CT also has an established role in staging of lung cancer, as demonstrated by a recent randomized trial of 189 patients, demonstrating the improved sensitivity in preoperative staging by adding a PET/CT examination.[62]

Multiple prior studies have documented the association between FDG uptake and histologic subtypes of lung cancer, including lower FDG uptake in better-differentiated lung carcinomas, lower uptake in adenocarcinomas than in squamous cell carcinomas, and lower uptake in BAC than in non-BAC adenocarcinomas.[63-67] A prospective study of 178 patients with potentially resectable NSCLC demonstrated that adenocarcinoma (excluding BAC) had lower FDG uptake and Ki-67 scores than squamous cell carcinoma or large cell undifferentiated carcinomas, BAC had lower FDG uptake and Ki-67 scores compared to any other histologic subtype, and FDG uptake significantly correlated with Ki-67 scores, indicating the close relationship between tumor proliferation and tumor glucose metabolism in NSCLC.[68]

MRI Findings of Adenocarcinoma

MRI is used less frequently as a first-line modality for the assessment of lung adenocarcinoma, but it provides clinically useful information without ionizing radiation. It is especially useful when findings on CT are inconclusive, and better tissue contrast resolution on MRI may resolve ambiguous clinical findings. One such example includes the evaluation of chest wall and pleural invasion. In cases with chest wall invasion, MRI shows infiltration or disruption of the normal extrapleural fat plane on T1-weighted images or parietal pleural signal hyperintensity on T2-weighted images.[53] Short-tau inversion recovery (STIR) technique can demonstrate tumor with high signal intensity within the suppressed signal intensities of chest wall structures, enabling the determination of tumor extent within the chest wall.[53] In addition to the static MRI technique, the breathing dynamic cine MR has been studied in the assessment of chest wall invasion in a study of 14 patients by Sakai et al.[69] Tumors invading the chest wall are fixed, while tumors without invasion move freely along the parietal pleura on cine MRI. The sensitivity, specificity, and accuracy of dynamic cine MRI for detecting chest wall invasion were 100%, 70%, and 76%, respectively, improved over conventional CT and MR techniques. Dynamic MRI, in conjunction with CT and static MRI, can be a useful tool to further improve the assessment of invasion.

In addition to the high tissue contrast and multiplanar capability of conventional MRI, recent advancements in MR imaging technology also allow for the evaluation of lung adenocarcinoma using dynamic-contrast-enhanced MRI and diffusion-weighted imaging, which will be discussed subsequently.

Features of Adenocarcinoma by Advanced Imaging Techniques

Advanced CT techniques

MDCT with thin-section images provide volumetric data for the assessment of tumor volumes that were shown to be highly reproducible in lung nodules and cancers.[70,71] The volumetric analysis has been applied to differentiate lung cancer from benign nodules, assess biologic behaviors of lung cancers of different pathological subtypes, and monitor tumor response to therapy.[72] In a study by Wilson et al, volumetric measurement of lung cancer was used to characterize the growth rate of lung cancer according to histologic subtypes.[73] Volumetric doubling time was analyzed in 63 NSCLC detected in the Pittsburgh Lung Screening Study, and was classified as rapid (<183 days), typical (183-365 days), and slow (>365 days). Adenocarcinoma/BAC comprised 86.7% of the slow doubling time group compared with 20% of the rapid doubling time group, while squamous cell cancer comprised 60% of the rapid doubling time group compared with 3.3% of the slow doubling time group. Adenocarcinoma/BACs had longer doubling time than squamous cell carcinoma (median doubling time of 387 vs 160 days, $P = 0.0031$), indicating the slower growth of adenocarcinoma compared to squamous cell carcinoma.[73]

Further application of MDCT technology has given rise to the quantitative evaluation of vascularity and perfusion of lung nodules and cancers by dynamic-contrast-enhanced (DCE) CT. The ability of DCE-CT to differentiate malignant versus benign solitary pulmonary nodules has been extensively tested over the past 15 years. In the meta-analysis by Cronin et al in 2008, which included 10 DCE-CT studies, the pooled sensitivity was 0.93, the pooled specificity was 0.76, and the area under the receiver operating characteristics curve was 0.93 for DCE-CT, similar to other modalities including MR, FDG-PET, and ^{99m}Tc-depreotide SPECT.[61] Several studies demonstrated correlation between tumoral vascularity and perfusion parameters on DCE-CT with the extent of microvessel density on histology.[74,75]

Advanced PET techniques

While ^{18}F-FDG is by far the most commonly used PET tracer in clinical practice, a variety of newer PET tracers that can visualize different biological activities of the tumor other than glucose metabolism have been developed and studied. One such tracer is ^{18}F-fluorothymidine (FLT), a thymidine analogue that can be used to noninvasively assess tumor proliferation on imaging. In a study of 30 solitary pulmonary nodules by Buck et al, the ^{18}F-FLT uptake was specific to malignant lesions that were predominantly NSCLC, and was highly correlated with proliferative activity determined by Ki-67 immunostaining.[76] Further development and clinical application of novel PET tracers that are specific to biological activities of tumors will aid in our understanding of lung cancer biology, including adenocarcinoma.

Advanced MRI techniques

Dynamic-contrast-enhanced (DCE) MRI using gadolinium chelates has enabled detailed, noninvasive assessment of tumor perfusion and vascularity. DCE-MRI has been extensively studied in differentiating benign and malignant solitary pulmonary nodules.[77-79] A meta-analysis including six DCE-MRI studies reported between 1990 and 2005 showed a pooled sensitivity of 0.94, a pooled specificity of 0.79, and an area under the ROC curve of 0.94 for DCE-MRI in diagnosing malignant nodule, which was comparable to other methods such as DCE-CT, FDG-PET, and ^{99m}Tc-depreotide SPECT.[61] A recent study of 30 patients with solitary pulmonary nodule found that the tracer transport rate constant (k_{ep}) between plasma and the extravascular extracellular space was the most significant perfusion index for differentiating malignant from benign nodules, with 76% sensitivity, 100% specificity, and 80% accuracy, when a cutoff of k_{ep} 1.0 min^{-1} was used.[80]

Diffusion-weighted imaging (DWI) provides different tissue contrast compared to that on conventional MR sequences, and reflects the diffusion motion of water protons in the tissues.[81] A study of 54 pulmonary nodules using DWI reported that the signal intensity of malignant nodules was significantly higher than that of benign nodules.[81] In a study of 140 pulmonary nodules and masses by Mori et al, the minimum apparent coefficient (ADC) showed a significantly higher specificity than PET (0.97 vs 0.79) in differentiating malignant versus benign nodules.[82] In patients with proven lung cancer, ADCs of well-differentiated adenocarcinoma are higher than those of other lung carcinoma histologies.[83] DCE-MRI and DWI are also currently under active investigation as methods to assess tumor response to therapy.

Gross Features of Adenocarcinoma

The gross features of lung adenocarcinoma are variable and depend in large part on the histologic subtype and pattern of growth and spread. As these tumors most commonly arise in a peripheral location, examination of external lung may reveal puckering or dimpling of

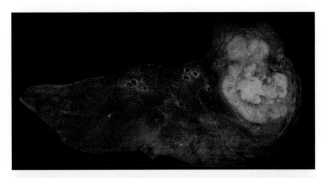

FIGURE 3-7 This peripherally located tumor is grossly well circumscribed with central necrosis and some surrounding parenchymal hemorrhage. Histologic review showed adenocarcinoma, solid predominant, with minor acinar pattern.

the pleura overlying the tumor. Tumors with pleural invasion may be associated with focal pleuritis with associated roughening of the pleural surface by fibrous adhesions. WHO categorizes lung adenocarcinomas into six patterns of macroscopic growth: (1) peripheral, (2) central or endobronchial, (3) diffuse consolidative, (4) disseminated disease that can mimic interstitial pneumonia, (5) disseminated disease involving visceral pleura, and (6) tumor arising in established fibrosis.[1]

Peripheral tumors containing predominantly invasive histology typically appear grossly tan to white with a fleshy consistency and relatively well-defined borders. Focal scarring or necrosis may be present (*Figure 3-7*). Tumors with a predominant lepidic component tend to have a more subtle gross appearance, with less distinct borders and less contrast with the surrounding lung parenchyma. On close examination, the fine septations of the involved lung appear thickened and pale as a result of the tumor growing along the preexisting alveoli. Areas of consolidation or scarring within these lepidic-predominant tumors often correspond with invasive patterns histologically (*Figure 3-8*).

The cut surface of centrally located tumors will have a similar appearance to those arising in the periphery, however, are more likely to have adjacent organizing pneumonia due to involvement of central airways with postobstructive complications (*Figure 3-9*). When present, organizing pneumonia can be grossly difficult to distinguish from neoplastic tissue and can lead to an overestimation of tumor size both radiographically and macroscopically.

Tumors with a predilection for extensive aerogenous spread, such as mucinous or nonmucinous adenocarcinomas with a predominance of lepidic or papillary growth (including tumors formerly known as "mucinous BAC") are frequently associated with more extensive disease and may not be amenable to surgical resection. Grossly, these tumors may have a dominant mass with smaller surrounding tumor nodules of similar coloration and consistency (*Figure 3-10*). Invasive mucinous adenocarcinomas can grow diffusely in the lung without significant disruption of the underlying architecture; this fact, along with abundant intra-alveolar mucin deposition, leads to a grossly consolidative appearance that mimics a lobar or sublobar pneumonia (*Figure 3-11*).

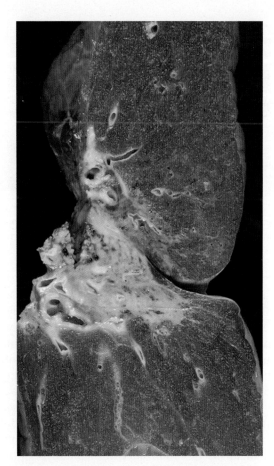

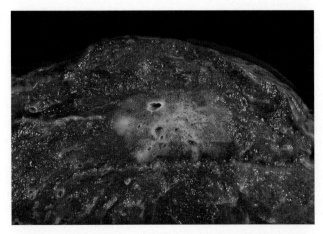

FIGURE 3-8 A small, peripheral nodule corresponding to a ground glass opacity on CT scan. Histologic review revealed a lepidic-predominant adenocarcinoma.

FIGURE 3-9 A central tumor with associated scar. Histologic review revealed an adenosquamous carcinoma.

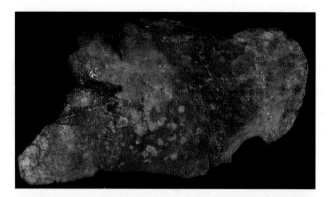

FIGURE 3-10 A pale, peripherally located dominant mass is surrounded by numerous smaller but similar-appearing nodules. Pathology review revealed a papillary-predominant tumor with minor lepidic pattern with aerogenous and lymphatic spread.

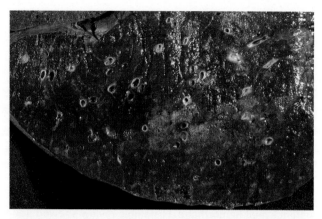

FIGURE 3-12 An autopsy specimen from a patient with relapsed *EGFR*-mutated lung adenocarcinoma with bilateral lymphangitic spread of disease and widespread distant metastases. The cut surface of the lung reveals multiple tan, ill-defined nodules.

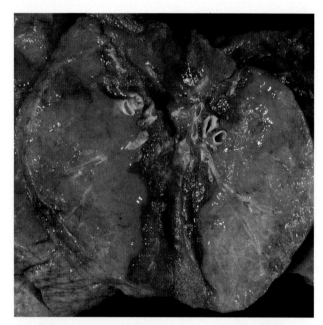

FIGURE 3-11 The lung has been serially sectioned and opened like a book, revealing sublobar consolidation due to invasive mucinous adenocarcinoma (formerly "mucinous BAC").

Lung adenocarcinoma can present with disseminated pulmonary disease either in the form of innumerable bilateral tumor nodules secondary to hematogenous spread or as a mimic of interstitial pneumonia as a result of extensive lymphangitic involvement; this pattern is also seen in forms of local relapse following systemic therapy. A dominant mass may or may not be readily identified. In the form of disease mimicking interstitial pneumonia, the tumor nodules may be ill-defined, appearing as multifocal to diffuse areas of tan discoloration and consolidation; peripheral infarcts may be present due to plugging of the vasculature by tumor (*Figure 3-12*). When disseminated disease

preferentially involves the pleural lymphatics, the lung may become encased by tumor, in a pattern mimicking malignant mesothelioma.

Tumor arising in a localized scar or on the background of a chronic fibrosing lung disease may be difficult to detect radiographically and thus may be found incidentally at autopsy or, for patients undergoing lung transplantation, at the time that the native lung is examined by pathology.[84] The tumor will typically have poorly defined margins in this context, particularly when arising on a background of significant fibrosis and architectural distortion. However, a dense, mass-like consolidation is typically identifiable, and the presence of softened or friable tissue, necrosis, and pronounced pleural puckering (in the case of peripheral lesions) may aid in distinguishing the tumor (*Figure 3-13*).

Histologic Features of Adenocarcinoma

Acinar Pattern

The acinar pattern is commonly reported as a predominant growth pattern (40%-50% of lung adenocarcinomas in some studies),[85] although this observation may vary in different populations.[86] This pattern is characterized by glandular structures lined by neoplastic cells. These glands may appear as simplified acini or as complex branching structures with varying amounts of intervening stromal mesenchymal and inflammatory cells. Tumor cell shape can be cuboidal, hobnail, or columnar (*Figures 3-14* and *3-15*). The cytoplasm may range from scant to voluminous and appear eosinophilic, clear, or palely basophilic depending on the relative amount of acidophilic proteins, glycogen, or mucin present. The architectural and cytologic features vary widely from one patient's tumor to the next, and even within an individual tumor.

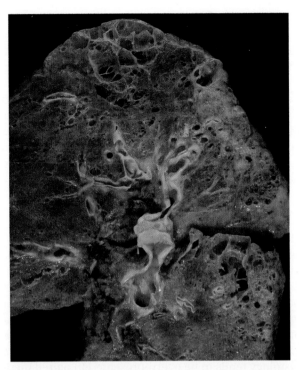

FIGURE 3-13 A peripheral lung adenocarcinoma diagnosed incidentally in an explanted lung following transplantation for end-stage emphysema and fibrosis. The contours of the tumor are difficult to define due to significant background architectural distortion.

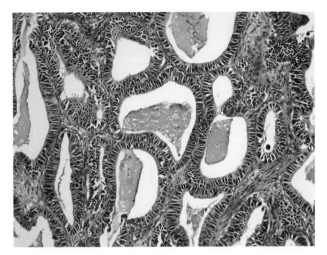

FIGURE 3-15 **Acinar pattern with columnar tumor cells (400×).**

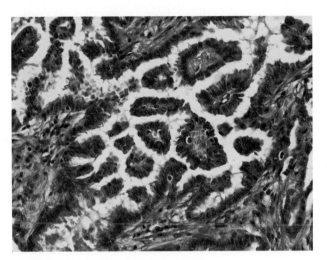

FIGURE 3-16 **Papillary pattern (400×).**

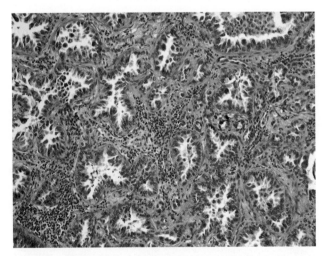

FIGURE 3-14 **Acinar pattern with cuboidal tumor cells and irregular gland contours (400×).**

Papillary Pattern

Identification of the papillary pattern of growth is subject to significant interobserver variability and in some cases may be difficult to distinguish from lepidic, acinar, and micropapillary patterns.[87] In contrast to the lepidic pattern, which largely conforms to the shape of the underlying lung architecture, the papillary pattern

shows complex secondary and tertiary structures comprised of tumor cells lining fibrovascular cores. This pattern may be seen in close continuity with acinar and papillary patterns, thus contributing to difficulty in distinguishing them. As with acinar pattern, the tumor cell shape, nuclear to cytoplasmic ratio, and cytoplasmic qualities vary widely (*Figure 3-16*).

Solid Pattern

Pathologist interobserver agreement studies have shown that the solid pattern is the most reproducibly identified of all adenocarcinoma patterns.[87] A predominance of solid-pattern architecture is associated with aggressive tumor behavior.[88] Solid growth is marked by nests and sheets of round to ovoid to polygonal tumor cells commonly growing in an interlocking "paving stone" fashion (*Figure 3-17*). Less

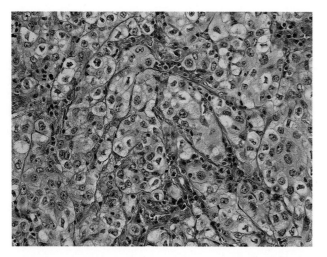

FIGURE 3-17 Solid pattern with clear cell change (400×).

commonly, the tumor cells grow in highly infiltrative nests with poorly defined cell-cell borders and cellular overlapping or in tumor nests that have distinctive peripheral palisading and can mimic large cell neuroendocrine carcinoma. Tumor nests can occasionally have central necrosis. The cytoplasm is frequently abundant and clear cell change is common in this pattern. Solid pattern growth with prominent signet ring cell differentiation has been associated with *ALK* gene rearrangements.[89,90]

Lepidic Pattern

Lepidic pattern is defined as the presence of tumor cells growing along preexisting alveolar structures, often with associated septal widening by fibroblasts and inflammatory cell infiltrates (*Figure 3-18*). By definition, lepidic pattern shows no evidence of invasion into stroma, pleura, or lymphovascular spaces.[9] Tumors with a pure lepidic pattern lacking evidence of invasion should be categorized as adenocarcinoma in situ (discussed below). Tumor cells may be nonmucinous, mucinous, or a combination of both. The lepidic growth pattern can be identified with relatively little interobserver variability[87]; however, as stated earlier it can be difficult to discriminate from papillary pattern, particularly when involved septa are truncated and fail to form a complete alveolar unit, mimicking the appearance of papillary structures.

Micropapillary Pattern

This pattern was introduced in the 2004 WHO classification but was not treated as a separate subtype at that time.[1] The 2011 IASLC/ATS/ERS and 2015 WHO classifications recommend identification of the micropapillary pattern in patients with early stage disease, as it has been associated with poor prognosis in several studies of early-stage adenocarcinoma.[9] Even when present as a minor subtype in the primary tumor, micropapillary histology tends to be overrepresented in paired metastatic samples, suggesting that this pattern correlates with increased capacity for vascular invasion and distant spread.[91] However, pathologists are least likely to arrive at concordance when assessing micropapillary pattern, with substantial disagreement when it comes to discriminating between papillary and micropapillary categories.[87] Micropapillary pattern is defined as the presence of papillae lacking a fibrovascular core; the tumor cells may be clustered in groups as small as three or four cells resembling florets floating freely in airspaces, and will have a very similar appearance whether present in the alveolated lung spaces or within lymphatics or vessels (*Figure 3-19*).

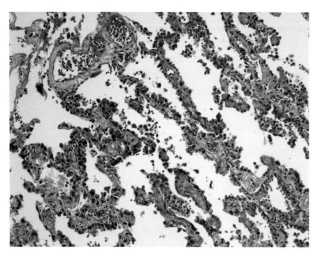

FIGURE 3-18 Lepidic pattern (400×).

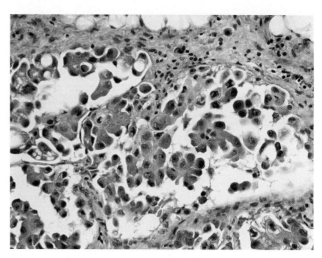

FIGURE 3-19 Micropapillary pattern. Note small papillary clusters of tumor cells lacking evident fibrovascular cores (400×).

CYTOLOGIC FEATURES OF ADENOCARCINOMA

Cytologic features, when taken together with the histologic patterns and stromal features, closely reflect the molecular relatedness of different tumor nodules in one patient and can predict if these tumors represent metastatic disease or distinct primaries.[92] The cytomorphology of lung adenocarcinoma is variable, depending on grade and, to some extent, the subtype. In cytologic preparations, a definitive morphologic distinction between adenocarcinoma and squamous cell carcinoma can be made in close to 70% of cases, a figure that improves to over 80% when a paired biopsy specimen is reviewed simultaneously.[93] Adenocarcinoma cytomorphology is characterized by cohesive sheets and three-dimensional clusters of tumor cells with irregular nuclei, chromatin consistency ranging from finely to coarsely granular, prominent nucleoli, and foamy cytoplasm with vacuolization.[94]

It is frequently not possible to predict the histologic subtype of adenocarcinoma with confidence on cytologic preparations; however, some cytomorphologic features can be correlated with the histology pattern as determined by surgical pathology review. Acinar spaces may be prominent in tumors with acinar pattern histology (*Figure 3-20*). Mucinous adenocarcinomas have flat, honeycomb-like sheets of tumor cells with relatively uniform, low-grade nuclei with distinctive grooves and abundant intracellular and extracellular mucin (*Figure 3-21*). The pattern of growth of lepidic-predominant nonmucinous adenocarcinomas is typically not discernable in cytologic preparations. Papillary pattern can be

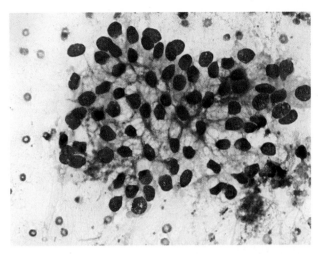

FIGURE 3-21 Lung adenocarcinoma with mucinous histology. This smear shows the characteristic flat, honeycomb sheets of this tumor type. (Romanowsky stain.) (Used with permission of Dr Christopher French, Brigham and Women's Hospital.)

distinguished based on the presence of malignant cells growing in a crowded manner along fibrovascular cores (*Figure 3-22*). In contrast, the tumor cells of micropapillary pattern adenocarcinoma are present as small, tight clusters lacking a fibrovascular core (*Figure 3-23*). Solid pattern is associated with large, solid clusters of tumor cells typically with high-grade nuclear features including marked nuclear enlargement, irregular contours, and large nucleoli. Cytoplasmic vacuolation may be prominent (*Figure 3-24*).

Distinctive cytomorphologic features of fetal adenocarcinoma include cohesive aggregates comprised of cells containing uniform, ovoid nuclei, subnuclear vacuoles, finely granular chromatin and the presence

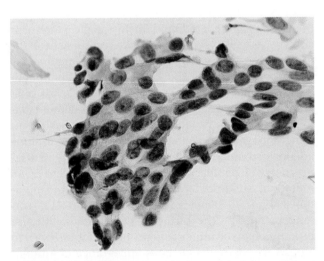

FIGURE 3-20 Lung adenocarcinoma with acinar pattern histology. Tumor cells are uniform in size with two prominent acinar spaces visible. Chromatin is finely granular. (Smear, Papanicolaou stain.) (Used with permission of Dr Christopher French, Brigham and Women's Hospital.)

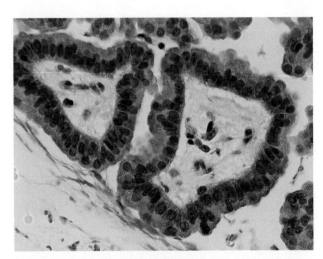

FIGURE 3-22 Lung adenocarcinoma with papillary pattern histology. Crowded tumor cells line a fibrovascular stalk. (Cell block, H&E stain.) (Used with permission of Dr Christopher French, Brigham and Women's Hospital.)

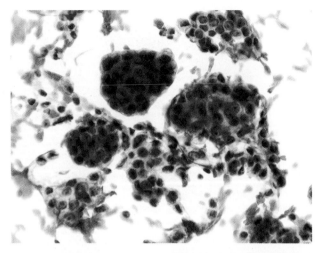

FIGURE 3-23 Lung adenocarcinoma with micropapillary pattern histology. Tumor cells are arranged in compact balls without a fibrovascular stalk. (Smear, Romanowsky stain.) (Used with permission of Dr Christopher French, Brigham and Women's Hospital.)

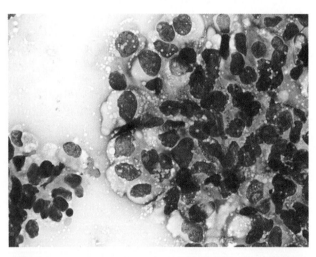

FIGURE 3-24 Lung adenocarcinoma with solid pattern histology. Smear reveals large clusters of densely packed tumor cells with large nuclei with irregular nuclear contours and prominent nucleoli. Tumor cell cytoplasm shows clearing, a common finding in this histologic subtype. (Romanowsky stain.) (Used with permission of Dr Christopher French, Brigham and Women's Hospital.)

of admixed squamous morules.[95] The rare category of colloid adenocarcinoma (including tumors formerly classified as mucinous cystadenocarcinoma) can be difficult to identify on cytology preparations due to the scant cellularity of this tumor type; however, clues to the diagnosis may include the presence of abundant mucin, few, low-grade neoplastic cells, and a radiographic correlate of a cystic lung lesion.[96]

HISTOLOGIC SUBTYPES OF ADENOCARCINOMA

Invasive lung adenocarcinomas demonstrate marked inter- and intratumoral morphologic heterogeneity,[1] an observation that likely reflects the presence of several functionally distinct cell populations in the lung. Debate surrounds the identity of the cell of origin of human lung adenocarcinomas, although in vitro and mouse model studies have identified several putative adenocarcinoma precursor cells including the bronchioloalveolar stem cell (BASC)[97] and type 2 alveolar epithelial cells.[98,99] Microarray expression studies and massively parallel sequencing efforts also support the concept that lung adenocarcinomas comprise a diverse group of tumors with distinctive biologic and clinical characteristics that tend to cluster with specific histologic subtypes.[2,25,100]

Invasive Adenocarcinomas With a Predominant Subtype

In recognition of frequent intratumoral morphologic heterogeneity, the 1999 and 2004 WHO classification systems recommended use of the term *adenocarcinoma, mixed subtype.*[1] However, this term failed to reflect the underlying genetic diversity of these tumors, which may contain one of several mutually exclusive genetic alterations that (1) correlate with specific clinical features and (2) may predict response to available targeted therapies. Thus, the field saw a shift in diagnostic terminology, with an evolving emphasis on the predominant tumor features, in an effort to better correlate histologic features with these unique genetic alterations. The 2011 IASLC/ATS/ERS lung adenocarcinoma classification recommended consistent documentation of the predominant histologic pattern or subtype, as well as semiquantitative recording of all the minor patterns or subtypes present in 5% increments.[9] As described in detail above, the predominant pattern does correlate significantly with prognosis, with solid and micropapillary predominant tumors demonstrating more aggressive biologic behavior. Studies examining the genotype-phenotype correlations in lung adenocarcinoma have demonstrated a strong association between papillary-predominant pattern and *EGFR* mutations, solid-predominant pattern and *KRAS* mutations, and solid-signet ring cell features and *ALK* rearrangement.[4,89,101] The inclusion of a semiquantitative description of the minor patterns present is intended to emphasize the heterogeneous appearance of a tumor and to permit more detailed comparison to other pulmonary tumors when attempting to make a distinction between metastatic disease and multiple synchronous primaries.[9]

Mucinous Adenocarcinoma

Mucinous adenocarcinomas, previously classified as "mucinous BAC," is a variant of adenocarcinoma that represents a clinical entity distinct from nonmucinous adenocarcinomas. These tumors, which often present with multifocal disease, lobar or multilobar consolidation, and bronchorrhea, are highly correlated with oncogenic *KRAS* mutations and anticorrelated with *EGFR* mutations.[3] Despite the predominance of lepidic pattern, these tumors are now recognized to contain invasive growth in most cases, and thus rarely are purely in situ lesions.

Histologically, mucinous adenocarcinoma has a very characteristic appearance of clustered well-differentiated neoplastic epithelium with abundant intracellular mucin. The tumor clusters will often appear abruptly and in a discontinuous fashion on otherwise unremarkable alveolar walls and often lack associated septal thickening. Areas of invasion will exhibit increased fibrosis with neoplastic gland formation. These tumors are highly productive of mucin, leading to filling of the surrounding airspaces by extracellular mucin and abundant muciphages (*Figure 3-25*). The predilection for aerogenous spread frequently leads to a lobar pattern of involvement with multiple foci of invasive and in situ tumor bathed in mucin and associated inflammatory cells.

Minimally Invasive Adenocarcinoma

The concept of minimally invasive adenocarcinoma (MIA) was introduced in the 2011 IASLC/ATS/ERS classification recommendations. This tumor type is defined as a solitary, lepidic-predominant adenocarcinoma measuring ≤3 cm and containing areas of invasion that measure no more than 5 mm in any one focus.[9] The invasive component is defined as any nonlepidic pattern of tumor growth or any area showing evidence of stromal invasion, recognizing that distinguishing stromal invasion from focal architectural collapse and scar is not always possible. Tumors with lymphovascular invasion or necrosis should be categorized as adenocarcinoma, lepidic predominant, rather than MIA. Retrospective reclassification studies of early stage adenocarcinomas suggest that MIA has a 100% 5-year disease-free survival, identical to that of adenocarcinoma in situ.[102-105] The distinction between MIA and adenocarcinoma in situ is discussed in greater detail below.

Fetal Adenocarcinoma

Fetal adenocarcinoma is a variant of adenocarcinoma that can be divided into low-grade and high-grade forms. Low-grade, well-differentiated fetal adenocarcinoma is a clinically, morphologically, and genetically distinctive category of lung adenocarcinoma notable for presentation in younger adults (at a mean age in the fourth decade), slight female predilection, strong nuclear and cytoplasmic expression of β-catenin protein indicative of activation of the WNT signaling pathway, and a high frequency of β-catenin mutations.[106] This low-grade tumor is associated with an indolent disease course.[107] Histologically, this tumor is characterized by organized glands and trabeculae comprised of monomorphic columnar cells containing abundant intracellular glycogen that tends to aggregate in the subnuclear cytoplasm (*Figure 3-26*). Squamous morules may be a prominent feature. The overall histology

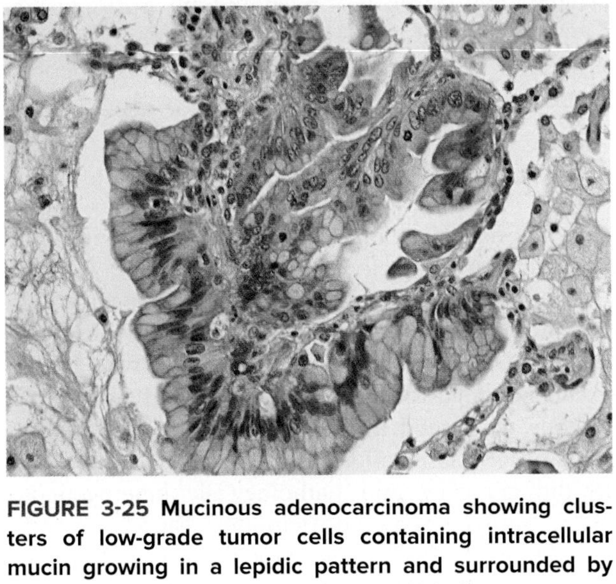

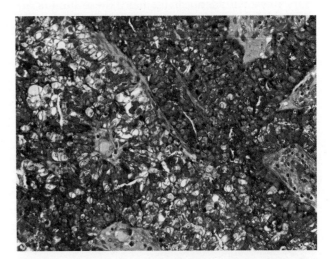

FIGURE 3-25 Mucinous adenocarcinoma showing clusters of low-grade tumor cells containing intracellular mucin growing in a lepidic pattern and surrounded by extracellular mucin and muciphages (400×).

FIGURE 3-26 Well-differentiated fetal adenocarcinoma. Monomorphic columnar tumor cells form crowded acini and trabeculae. Tumor cells contain abundant glycogen (PAS stain, 400×).

is reminiscent of endometrioid adenocarcinoma; however, fibroblastic and myofibroblastic stromal proliferation may also be prominent.[108]

High-grade lung adenocarcinoma with fetal lung-like morphology, in contrast, appears to represent a more heterogeneous group of tumors. These tumors contain a fetal-like pattern with high-grade nuclear features, disorganized architecture, necrosis, and admixed adenocarcinoma of conventional histology.[107] Morita et al identified *EGFR* and *KRAS* mutations in this tumor type at the expected frequency, leading these authors to conclude that high-grade lung adenocarcinoma with fetal-like morphology represents a pattern of lung adenocarcinoma, rather than a distinct clinical entity.[109]

Colloid Adenocarcinoma

Colloid adenocarcinoma of the lung, including the rare tumors formerly classified as "mucinous cystadenocarcinoma," are a variant of pulmonary adenocarcinoma that are morphologically identical to colloid adenocarcinomas of the gastrointestinal tract.[9] These tumors may appear radiographically as cystic masses; on histologic examination they comprise circumscribed pools of mucin containing floating neoplastic epithelium (*Figure 3-27*) and may be partially encapsulated. The tumor cells are typically well differentiated.

Enteric Adenocarcinoma

The 2011 IASLC/ATS/ERS guidelines recommend including this variant of adenocarcinoma in the classification schema, in order to bring attention to the existence of primary lung tumors that share morphologic and immunophenotypic characteristics with primary intestinal adenocarcinomas.[9] These tumors are heterogeneous, like most conventional lung adenocarcinomas, but are characterized by tall-columnar neoplastic epithelium with eosinophilic cytoplasm, vesicular nuclei, and some nuclear palisading. Morphologic features resembling colorectal carcinoma can predominate in some cases, leading to diagnostic confusion. Immunohistochemistry studies also support a gastrointestinal phenotype; these tumors will show CDX2 and CK20 expression, while also retaining CK7 and, in a minority of cases, TTF-1 and SP-A expression[110] (*Figure 3-28*). It is not clear if these relatively rare tumors have any distinct clinical features; however, it is important to clinically and radiographically exclude a gastrointestinal tract primary.

PRECURSOR LESIONS OF INVASIVE ADENOCARCINOMA

Atypical Adenomatous Hyperplasia

Atypical adenomatous hyperplasia (AAH) is now widely accepted as an early neoplastic precursor to invasive adenocarcinoma. AAH is frequently detected incidentally in lung tissues resected for lung cancer and for other indications, may be multifocal, and can be found in both smokers and nonsmokers.[111] High-sensitivity molecular studies have detected oncogenic *EGFR* and *KRAS* mutations in AAH lesions,[112,113] suggesting that these events occur early in lung tumorigenesis. AAH can be difficult to distinguish from adenocarcinoma in situ; however, AAH is typically ≤5 mm and can be discriminated from surrounding lung tissue by the presence of increased epithelial cell density with some cellular overlapping, hyperchromatic nuclei, and hobnail cytomorphology (*Figure 3-29*). This lesion should be distinguished from reactive bronchiolar metaplasia and reactive pneumocyte atypia, particularly in the context of prior chemoradiotherapy or other lung injury.

Adenocarcinoma In Situ

In a seminal report in 1995, Noguchi et al proposed a classification system that highlighted the 100% disease-free survival of surgically resected small adenocarcinomas with in situ growth only (type A) or those with in situ growth and focal stromal collapse (type B). The excellent prognosis of these tumor types was subsequently confirmed in Western populations.[114] In the 2004 WHO classification, these tumors were included in the clinically and pathologically heterogeneous "BAC" subtype of adenocarcinoma.[1] The 2011 recommendations reclassify tumors with pure in situ (lepidic) growth as adenocarcinoma in situ, and multiple subsequent retrospective reclassification studies have

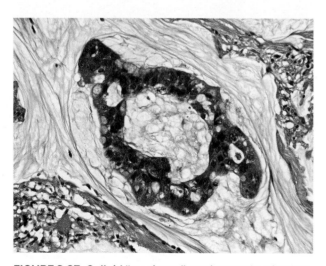

FIGURE 3-27 Colloid "mucinous" carcinoma showing low-grade neoplastic cell clusters floating in abundant mucin (400×).

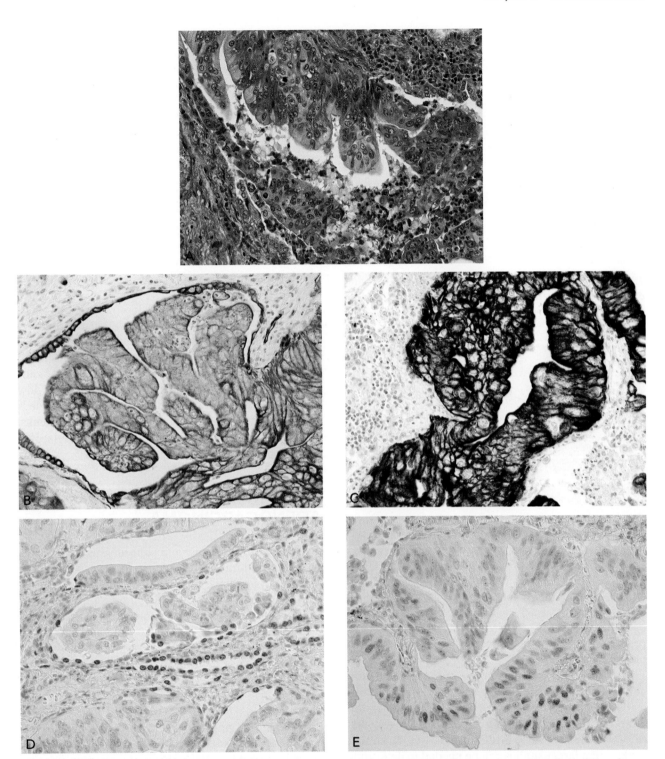

FIGURE 3-28 Enteric adenocarcinoma. **(A)** Hematoxylin and eosin stain shows columnar cell morphology with abundant eosinophilic cytoplasm and some nuclear palisading; **(B)** CK7 immunostain; **(C)** CK20 immunostain; **(D)** TTF-1 immunostain is negative in the tumor cells and positive in entrapped nonneoplastic pneumocytes; **(E)** CDX2 immunostain is weakly positive in the tumor cells. (All panels at 400×.)

confirmed the association with 100% 5-year disease-free survival.[101,102,104]

AIS is defined as an adenocarcinoma measuring ≤3 cm with lepidic growth only and lacking evidence for stromal, lymphovascular, and pleural invasion. Most

AIS has nonmucinous cytomorphology; while AIS and AAH can be difficult to distinguish, AIS typically has more striking atypia than AAH, including more pronounced cellular crowding with nuclear overlap and columnar cell change.[1] Interstitial widening may be

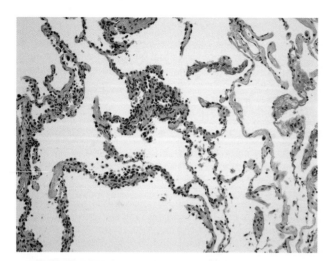

FIGURE 3-29 Atypical adenomatous hyperplasia. Note discrete transition from normal on the right to neoplastic on the left (200×).

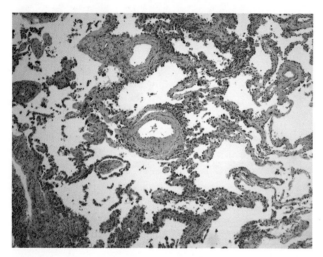

FIGURE 3-30 Adenocarcinoma in situ.

prominent in the septal structures underlying the neoplastic cells[9] (*Figure 3-30*).

Identification of small areas of invasion can be difficult and prone to significant interobserver variability,[87] leading to overlap between the AIS and MIA categories. However, most available outcomes data suggest that MIA, like AIS, has 100% 5-year disease-free survival; it is likely that larger studies will be needed to determine the significance, if any, of this distinction in clinical practice.[102-105]

IMMUNOHISTOCHEMICAL FEATURES OF ADENOCARCINOMA

Lung adenocarcinoma is characteristically thyroid transcription factor-1 (TTF1, or NKX2.1) positive. This lineage-specific transcription factor is 70% to 80%

sensitive for detection of lung adenocarcinomas and is highly specific in the differential with squamous cell carcinoma (discussed further below). TTF-1 is also expressed in thyroid neoplasms; therefore, care must be taken to exclude metastatic tumors of primary thyroid origin in the appropriate clinical context. Concern regarding the suboptimal sensitivity of this marker for lung adenocarcinoma has led to the clinical implementation of other markers, including surfactant proteins and napsin. Napsin is an aspartic proteinase involved in surfactant B processing with an equivalent to 10% to 15% improved sensitivity over TTF-1 in detection of lung adenocarcinoma.[115,116] Napsin is equivalent to TTF-1 in terms of specificity relative to the differential with squamous cell carcinoma; however, it is also expressed in renal neoplasms, and with greatest frequency in those of papillary subtype.[116]

Over 80% of lung adenocarcinomas are CK7 positive and CK20 negative. Enteric adenocarcinomas of the lung are typically strongly positive for both CK7 and CK20, and mucinous adenocarcinomas are CK7 negative and CK20 positive.[117] Poorly differentiated adenocarcinomas frequently lose expression of these low molecular weight keratins. The CK7+/CK20− profile is shared with breast carcinoma, Müllerian carcinomas, and malignant mesothelioma, therefore, is a relatively nonspecific in a broader differential.[118]

MOLECULAR FEATURES OF ADENOCARCINOMA

Just as it is histologically and clinically heterogeneous, lung adenocarcinoma is now recognized to be molecularly heterogeneous. Importantly, many of the oncogenic alterations that have been identified in lung adenocarcinomas predict response to targeted therapies. The discovery of molecular subtypes predicting response to targeted inhibitors has triggered a revolution in biomarker identification and companion diagnostic development in tumors arising in the lung and other organs. Many of these oncogenic driving alterations occur in a mutually exclusive manner, leading to the recognition of relatively distinct clinicopathologic subtypes of lung adenocarcinoma, many of which have been discussed in detail earlier in this chapter. This section will focus on alterations for which established targeted therapies are now available in clinical practice.

Approximately 60% of lung adenocarcinomas harbor a well-characterized oncogenic alteration. In most populations, *KRAS* is the most commonly mutated oncogene in lung adenocarcinoma, occurring in an estimated 20% to 30% of these tumors; at this time, there are no targeted therapies that have been proven effective at inhibiting oncogenic KRAS signaling. *EGFR* is mutated in 15% to 30% of lung adenocarcinomas, with a higher frequency among Asian populations. Other mutations (*Figure 3-31*) generally occur in 5% or less of lung adenocarcinomas; the significance of these less common mutations in terms of prognosis and response to targeted therapies is the subject of intense clinical investigation. A variety of oncogenic fusion genes have been identified in lung cancer since 2007, leading to a surge in cytogenetics (namely fluorescence in situ hybridization or FISH)–based diagnostics and to the development of several novel immunohistochemical tools for detection of aberrantly expressed fusion proteins such as ALK and ROS1. With the increasing use of next generation sequencing, identification of novel gene-level and chromosome-level alterations will likely lead to new therapeutic targets in lung adenocarcinoma.

Targeted EGFR Therapy in Lung Cancer

The epidermal growth factor receptor (*EGFR*) is an ErbB transmembrane growth factor receptor that shares homology with *ERBB2* (*HER2/neu*). Upon ligand binding to the extracellular ligand-binding domain, ErbB family receptors form homodimers or heterodimers leading to activation of the cytoplasmic tyrosine kinase with downstream activation of the PI3K/AKT/mTOR and RAS/RAF/MAPK pathways. The effects of EGFR signaling include growth, proliferation, and cell motility. In light of these properties and the recognition that EGFR is overexpressed in 60% of lung cancers,[119] it has long been implicated as an oncogene in this tumor type and is an attractive target for anticancer therapies. Attempts to inhibit EGFR signaling using monoclonal antibody-based approaches to blocking ligand binding have yielded disappointing results. In contrast, small molecule inhibitors that block the ATP-binding groove in the tyrosine kinase domain were very promising in preclinical and early clinical studies. However, when tested in larger clinical phase III trials of unselected patients with advanced stage nonsmall cell lung carcinoma, the tyrosine kinase inhibitors (TKIs) gefitinib and erlotinib showed little to no benefit as compared to conventional chemotherapy.[120] However, a subset of patients demonstrated a remarkable and sustained response to these TKIs; these patients tended to be female nonsmokers. Early reports also suggested "bronchoalveolar carcinoma" and Asian ethnicity predicted response.[121]

Several groups identified, nearly simultaneously, the molecular underpinnings for this dramatic response in selected patients: somatic gain-of-function *EGFR* mutations occurring in "hot spots" in the tyrosine kinase domain (exons 18 through 21).[122-124] These studies reported, and extensive international effort confirmed, that approximately 90% of EGFR-activating mutations occur as short in-frame deletions involving the conserved Leu Arg Glu Ala (LREA) motif in exon 19 or as a missense point mutation (Leu858Arg) in exon 21.[125] Less frequent mutations occur in exon 18 at Gly719 and in exon 21 at Leu861Gln. Multiple large clinical trials subsequently confirmed the association between *EGFR* mutation status and response to TKI therapy.[126,127]

In contrast to the wild type (nonmutated) state, the presence of an activating kinase domain mutation leads to EGFR tyrosine kinase activation independent of ligand binding, with downstream proliferative and anti-apoptotic signaling. This is thought to form the basis of EGFR dependency, or "oncogene addiction," and subsequently to tumor cell sensitivity to EGFR inhibition. As compared to wild-type *EGFR*, these activating mutations also stabilize the interaction between tyrosine kinase inhibitor and the kinase. Therefore, EGFR-TKIs preferentially inhibit mutant as compared to wild-type *EGFR*, leading to enhanced efficacy and reduced toxicity.[128]

EGFR Mutation and Tumor Histology

In the early clinical trials of EGFR TKIs, the only histologic criteria for enrollment was *nonsmall cell lung carcinoma*. However, it soon became evident that this was insufficiently specific, as *EGFR* mutations occur almost exclusively in adenocarcinomas, or in the unusual mixed tumors that contain at least a component of

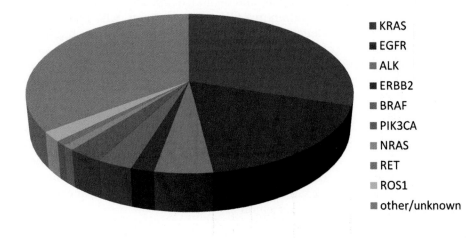

- ■ KRAS
- ■ EGFR
- ▨ ALK
- ■ ERBB2
- ■ BRAF
- ▨ PIK3CA
- ▨ NRAS
- ■ RET
- ▨ ROS1
- ■ other/unknown

FIGURE 3-31 Oncogenes that are altered in lung adenocarcinoma. The size of the pie sliver reflects their documented frequency in this tumor type. Most occur in a mutually exclusive fashion; however, PIK3CA and some BRAF mutations occur in tandem with other driving alterations. (Data derived from the Cosmic Sanger somatic mutation database [http://cancer.sanger.ac.uk/cancergenome/projects/cosmic/].)

adenocarcinoma.[125] Squamous cell carcinomas virtually never harbor *EGFR* mutations, and those that reportedly do most likely represent undersampled adenosquamous carcinoma or mischaracterized poorly differentiated solid subtype adenocarcinoma.[129] The range of histologic appearances of *EGFR*-mutated lung adenocarcinoma is broad; however, several large genotype-phenotype studies suggest a strong correlation with papillary pattern; in some cases histologic heterogeneity in *EGFR* mutated tumors can be attributed at least in part to progressive genomic alterations at the EGFR locus, with lower grade lepidic or papillary components harboring copy number neutral EGFR locus and high-grade solid components containing high-level EGFR amplification.[130]

EGFR Copy Number and Protein Expression

In the mid-2000s, several groups suggested there was an association between *EGFR* copy number gain as detected using FISH techniques and response to EGFR-TKIs. However, in most phase III trials, response rates in patients whose tumors had *EGFR* copy number gain failed to match those of patients whose tumors harbored an activating mutation (approximately 30% vs 70% response rates, respectively).[125] Retrospective studies of tumors from patients who received EGFR TKIs shed some light on why some of the tumors with *EGFR* copy number gain showed response. Focused, high-level amplification of the *EGFR* gene is a relatively rare event in *EGFR*-mutated tumors (as compared to copy number gain due to polysomy of chromosome 7, which is quite common in lung adenocarcinoma irrespective of mutation status), but when it does occur, it preferentially involves an allele with an underlying *EGFR* activating mutation.[130] These observations comport with the concept of oncogene dependency, as the presence of high-level amplification correlates with more advanced stage and higher grade disease (suggesting a role in promoting tumorigenesis) and has been associated with dramatic response to TKI therapy. *EGFR* copy number gain is also associated with increased EGFR protein expression. However, this protein expression is not specific to tumors with underlying activating mutations and is a poor surrogate for mutation status in predicting response to EGFR TKIs.[131] As a result, current clinical practice guidelines for EGFR testing in lung adenocarcinoma strongly recommend use of mutation analysis, but not *EGFR* copy number or protein expression for selection of patients for targeted therapy.[125]

Mechanisms of Resistance to EGFR Inhibitors

Patients with sensitizing *EGFR* mutations almost inevitably relapse while receiving targeted therapy, typically after a 1-year interval. When tissue is taken at the time of relapse, approximately 50% of tumors undergoing mutation analysis will show the Thr790Met resistance mutation in *EGFR* exon 20, in addition to their original activating mutation.[132,133] Gene amplification of *MET*, a receptor tyrosine kinase with protean effects on cellular growth and proliferation, occurs in up to 20% of relapsed tumors and may or may not be independent of the *EGFR* resistance mutation.[134] Less common forms of resistance include ERBB2 (HER2/neu) amplification, PIK3CA pathway activation, and evolution to small cell carcinoma. Trials of second-generation EGFR inhibitors have thus far failed to demonstrate efficacy in relapsed disease. Other strategies under consideration include chemotherapy, combined EGFR inhibition and chemotherapy, MET inhibition, or inhibition of other activated parallel or downstream pathways.[135] Primary resistance to EGFR inhibitors also exists in the form of other exon 20 mutations in the *EGFR* gene. These are relatively uncommon insertion/duplication mutations that actually trigger EGFR activation but in most cases also confer resistance to erlotinib and gefitinib.[128]

ALK Rearrangement in Lung Adenocarcinoma

Soda et al first identified anaplastic lymphoma kinase (*ALK*) gene rearrangements in lung carcinomas in 2007, at which time they described the fusion of *ALK* to *EML4* via a small intrachromosomal inversion event on chromosome 2.[136] ALK is a tyrosine kinase, the overactivation of which is well described in the pathogenesis of other tumor types including anaplastic large cell lymphoma and inflammatory myofibroblastic tumor.[89] Preclinical data suggested that tumor cells harboring *ALK* gene rearrangements were sensitive to treatment with the multitargeted tyrosine kinase inhibitor, crizotinib. Clinical trials were rapidly developed utilizing FISH for detection of *ALK* rearrangements in order to select candidates for therapy with crizotinib. These trials led to identification *ALK* rearrangements in ~5% of lung adenocarcinomas and demonstrated a 57% response rate to crizotinib in *ALK*-positive patients, with many experiencing dramatic shrinkage of their tumor burden[137] (*Figure 3-32*). Less than a year after these trials were published, the US Food and Drug Administration approved crizotinib for treatment of advanced stage ALK-positive nonsmall cell lung cancer.[138] Follow-up phase III trials also demonstrated the superiority of crizotinib as compared to chemotherapy in ALK-positive lung cancer, with response rates of 65% vs 20%, respectively.[139] Current clinical and pathology clinical practice guidelines recommend testing for *ALK* rearrangements in patients with advanced lung adenocarcinoma.[125]

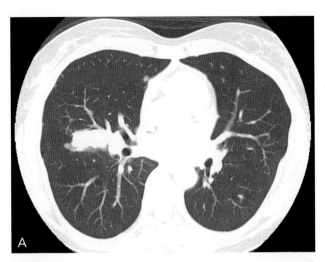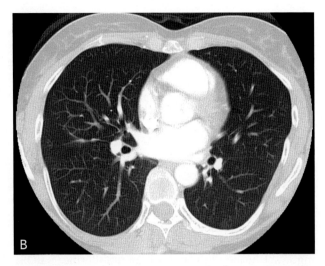

FIGURE 3-32 A 52-year-old woman with ALK-positive lung adenocarcinoma. Computed tomography images from pre-treatment (October 2011) show a solid mass in the central right lung with surround ground glass opacities. Following treatment with crizotinib, CT images (February 2013) show near complete response. (Used with permission of Bruce Johnson, MD, Dana Farber Cancer Institute, Boston, MA.)

Testing for *ALK* Rearrangement in Lung Adenocarcinoma

FISH for *ALK* rearrangements was used to select patients for therapy in the clinical trials reporting the efficacy of crizotinib; subsequently, the *ALK* Break Apart FISH Probe Kit (Abbott Molecular, Des Plaines, IL) was approved by the FDA as a companion diagnostic for use of this drug in lung cancers.[140] The *ALK* FISH assay has presented challenges, however, because the small intrachromosomal inversion that represents the most common alteration leads to a subtle (>2 probe diameter) separation in the 5′ and 3′ signals.[137] In addition, cells without a rearrangement can have nonspecific signal separation not dissimilar to that seen in truly rearranged tumor cells. These interpretive difficulties lead to both false-negative and false-positive results and contribute to significant interobserver variability.

Notably, *EML4-ALK* fusions upregulate ALK transcription and protein expression. Preceding the discoveries in lung cancer, immunohistochemistry for ALK protein expression was widely available for use in the diagnosis of anaplastic large cell lymphoma (ALCL); however, the antibodies that were sensitive to ALK over-expression in ALCL were insufficiently sensitive for its detection in *ALK*-rearranged lung cancers.[141] Efforts to develop more sensitive antibodies led to the commercial availability of clones 5A4 and D5F3, both of which have a sensitivity and specificity of 95% to 100% for the detection of *ALK*-rearranged lung tumors, when compared to FISH.[141,142] However, robust outcomes data using immunohistochemistry as selection criteria for treating *ALK*-rearranged patients with crizotinib is lacking. As a result, the clinical practice guidelines strongly recommend use of FISH for selection of patients for

therapy with crizotinib; however, labs may consider using carefully validated immunohistochemistry to screen out negative cases[125] (*Figure 3-33*).

Unique Clinicopathologic Features of *ALK* Rearranged Lung Tumors

ALK rearrangement in lung adenocarcinoma is associated with relatively distinctive clinical and pathologic characteristics. Patients whose tumors harbor *ALK* rearrangements tend to be young, never smokers who present with a high stage of disease, and appear to have a poorer prognosis as compared to ALK-negative tumors.[89,143] Aside from rare case reports, most literature indicates that *ALK* rearrangements and *EGFR* and *KRAS*

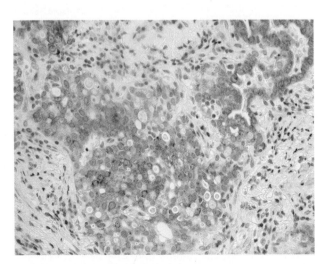

FIGURE 3-33 ALK protein overexpression in a tumor with an *ALK* gene rearrangement (clone 5A4, 400×).

mutations occur in a mutually exclusive fashion.[144] Published studies report various morphologic associations; however, most describe a correlation with solid pattern histology and frequent signet ring cells.[89] One published scoring system reports that identification of solid, papillary, or micropapillary histology paired with the presence of signet ring or hepatoid cytomorphology has a sensitivity of 88% for predicting *ALK* rearrangements[90] (*Figure 3-34*).

ROS1 *and* RET *Rearrangements in Lung Carcinoma*

ROS1 has been recognized as an oncogene for over two decades, following the identification of activating *ROS1* fusions in glioblastoma multiforme.[145] ROS1 fusions were first discovered in nonsmall cell lung carcinomas using a phosphoproteomic screen and were subsequently described in approximately 1% to 2% of NSCLC.[146,147] *CD74*, *SLC34A2*, *SDC4*, and *FIG1* are among several fusion partners that drive ROS1 overexpression and trigger oncogenic transformation in in vitro and in vivo studies.[146,147] Importantly, preclinical and early clinical reports have demonstrated that *ROS1*-translocated lung adenocarcinomas can be inhibited by crizotinib, the same multitargeted inhibitor that has shown efficacy in *ALK*-rearranged tumors.[148]

ROS1 translocations can be detected using FISH or immunohistochemistry approaches. Published FISH assays describe a break-apart probe design spanning the common break point region (including exons 32, 34, and 35) in the *ROS1* gene.[32,148] The presence of an *ROS1* rearrangement leads to a split signal in the majority of cases; *ROS1* translocations most commonly result from interchromosomal events, thus the distance between the probes in a rearranged case is typically greater than that seen in *ALK*-rearranged lung tumors, lending itself to more straightforward interpretation. Immunohistochemistry using the commercially available D4D6 clone has a published sensitivity of up to 100% and specificity of 92% for detection of *ROS1*-rearranged lung adenocarcinomas, and thus may also be a useful screening tool[149] (*Figure 3-35*).

The clinical characteristics of patients with ROS1 rearranged lung tumors are similar to those with ALK-rearranged tumors, and include never-smoking status, younger age, and adenocarcinoma histology. *ROS1* rearrangements have been described almost exclusively in tumors that lack other driving molecular alterations in genes such as *EGFR*, *KRAS*, and *ALK*. Overall, *ROS1*-rearranged tumors are rare, accounting for 1% to 2% of lung adenocarcinomas overall; however, they appear to account for over 10% of adenocarcinomas arising in never smokers with otherwise "pan wild-type" mutational status.[32,148,149]

Interestingly, *ROS1*-rearranged lung adenocarcinomas have histologic features that overlap with those described in *ALK*-rearranged tumors, including solid and papillary-pattern growth with cribriforming, prominent mucin production, and frequent psammomatous calcifications (*Figure 3-36*). *ALK* and *ROS1* are in fact phylogenetically related, suggesting these two genes may have similar oncogenic function when overexpressed.[89,90,149]

RET gene rearrangements in lung cancer are uncommon, thought to occur at a frequency similar to that of *ROS1* rearrangements in the lung. Approaches to detection of *RET* rearrangement include FISH and reverse-transcriptase polymerase chain reaction (RT-PCR); however, to date, screening for *RET* rearrangements has not been widely implemented in clinical practice. The most commonly described fusion product is *KIF5B-RET*, resulting from a small intrachromosomal inversion on

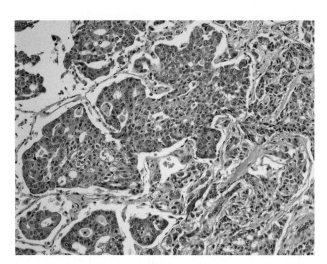

FIGURE 3-34 An *ALK*-rearranged lung adenocarcinoma growing in solid nests with cribriform spaces containing mucin (400×).

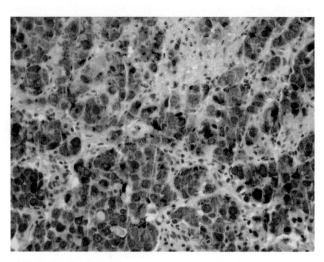

FIGURE 3-35 *ROS1* protein overexpression in a tumor with *ROS1* gene rearrangement. Staining pattern is cytoplasmic and variably granular (Clone D4D6).

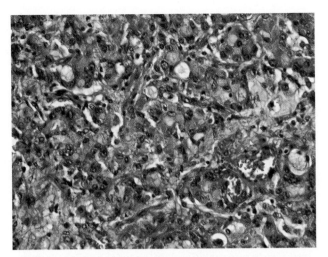

FIGURE 3-36 *ROS1*-rearranged lung adenocarcinoma growing in solid nests with frequent signet ring cells and cribriform spaces containing mucin (400×).

chromosome 10.[32] Similar to *ALK*, this inversion leads to a subtle split in the 5' and 3' probes when applying a break-apart FISH strategy, leading to significant difficulties in assay validation and practical interpretation. Difficulties associated with obtaining sufficiently high-quality RNA from archival, fixed tissues has generally precluded adoption of RT-PCR as a screening tool in clinical practice.[125] Thus, the clinical and pathologic features of RET-rearranged tumors have not been firmly established across different populations. That said, early evidence suggests that *RET*-rearranged tumors are more common in never smokers and occur preferentially in adenocarcinoma[150]; however, there is one report of RET rearrangement occurring in a carcinoid tumor.[151] Early evidence suggests that *RET*-rearranged lung tumors will respond to therapy with the MET and VEGFR2 inhibitor cabozantanib.[152]

HEREDITARY SYNDROMES ASSOCIATED WITH ADENOCARCINOMA

Lung adenocarcinomas are reported in families with a variety of hereditary cancer syndromes; however, there are few hereditary syndromes in which lung adenocarcinoma is a dominant feature. For instance, lung adenocarcinomas are reported in families with Li Fraumeni syndrome, an autosomal recessive disorder characterized by germline TP53 mutations. However, in contrast to breast carcinoma, soft tissue sarcomas, and adrenocortical carcinoma, lung cancers do not appear to occur in excess in these individuals relative to the general population.[153] Ataxia-telangiectasia is an autosomal recessive disorder characterized by neurodegeneration, immune deficiency and hematologic malignancies, and results from mutations in the DNA repair gene, ataxia

telangiectasia mutated (ATM). Some investigators have reported an association between polymorphisms in the gene and risk of nonsmall cell lung cancer[154-156]; however, population-based studies have failed to identify ATM risk alleles in lung cancer patients.[157] Similarly, individuals who are heterozygous for ATM mutations have an increased risk of female breast cancer but not for other cancer types, including lung cancer.[158] Other well-characterized hereditary cancer syndromes such as breast ovarian cancer syndrome, Lynch syndrome, and familial adenomatous polyposis (FAP) are not associated with an excess risk of primary lung tumors. That said, low-grade fetal adenocarcinoma, a rare and unique tumor subtype characterized by aberrant Wnt pathway signaling, has been reported in a patient with FAP.[106]

Within the last decade, however, several putative hereditary cancer syndromes have emerged that appear to have a more significant association with lung adenocarcinoma. Mutations in Brca1-associated protein-1 (*BAP-1*), a tumor suppressor gene in the BRCA1 growth control pathway, were originally described in families with high rates of mesothelioma and uveal melanoma, and are thought to increase the risk of developing malignant mesothelioma following exposure to asbestos.[159,160] Biallelic inactivation of BAP-1 has been identified in lung adenocarcinomas arising in families with *BAP-1* germline mutations.[161]

Routine testing of lung tumors for *EGFR* gene mutations for treatment selection led to identification of a family with multiple nonsmall cell lung carcinomas containing de novo (pretreatment) Thr790Met resistance mutations. Further studies confirmed this alteration was present in the germline, a finding that suggests a form of heritable genetic susceptibility to lung adenocarcinoma.[162] These alterations appear to be rare; one institutional report identified germline Thr790Met variants in 1% of all patients with lung adenocarcinoma tested for *EGFR* mutations. These tumors typically harbor a second activating mutation in *EGFR* in *cis* (on the same allele) with the germline Thr790Met alteration.[163]

APPROACH TO THE DIAGNOSIS OF POORLY-DIFFERENTIATED ADENOCARCINOMA ON SMALL BIOPSIES

With the discovery of specific, targetable oncogenic alterations in lung tumors, and the recognition that the best characterized of these alterations (ie, EGFR and ALK) occur almost exclusively in adenocarcinomas, it has become imperative for the practicing pathologist to accurately diagnose this tumor type, even on limited material. The previous practice of diagnosing "nonsmall cell lung carcinoma" on small biopsies and/or in morphologically indeterminate tumors must be minimized to ensure that patients are properly triaged for molecular testing to guide selection of therapy. In addition, tumor type is associated with differential response to some chemotherapies, with adenocarcinoma demonstrating an improved response rate to pemetrexed and bevacizumab as compared to squamous cell carcinoma, and may predict adverse outcomes, with a risk of life-threatening pulmonary hemorrhage in patients with lung squamous cell carcinoma receiving bevicuzimab.[9,164]

In practice, many patients for whom molecular testing and adjuvant therapy are indicated have advanced disease and do not undergo tumor resection. Instead, less morbid procedures including small biopsies or fine needle aspirations are performed for diagnosis and staging purposes. On average, the pathologist is able to make a definitive morphologic diagnosis of adenocarcinoma or squamous cell carcinoma in only about 70% of small biopsies and cytology specimens.[165] As a result, ancillary immunohistochemistry studies have become critical for accurate and complete characterization of lung tumor tissues. Of course, no single immunohistochemical marker can distinguish between adenocarcinoma and squamous cell carcinoma in 100% of cases; therefore, a small panel of markers may be employed to make this distinction with confidence. Stains must be chosen judiciously, however, to conserve adequate tissue for molecular testing, particularly for small biopsies.

Much effort has gone into examining the best panel of immunohistochemistry markers for distinguishing between adenocarcinoma and squamous cell carcinoma. The original 2011 classification recommended combined use of TTF-1 to stain adenocarcinoma and p63 to stain squamous cell carcinoma.[9] These markers have their limitations, however. P63 in particular, while highly sensitive for squamous cell carcinoma, is notoriously nonspecific, staining up to a third of adenocarcinomas. This can lead to diagnostic confusion, particularly in TTF-1 weak or negative adenocarcinomas. Fortunately, a more specific isoform of p63, ΔNp63 or p40, is significantly more specific, reportedly expressed in only 3% of lung adenocarcinomas and even then present in fewer than 5% of tumor cells.[166] Therefore,

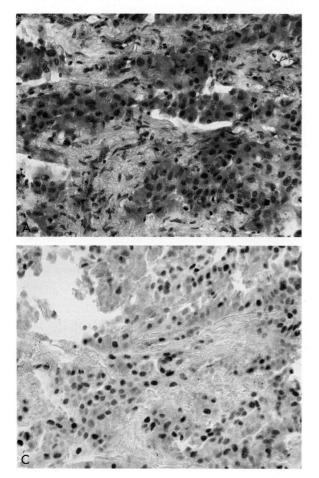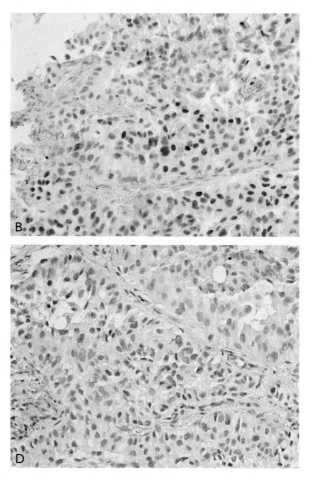

FIGURE 3-37 Immunohistochemistry in a small lung cancer biopsy with ambiguous morphologic features. (A) Tumor was called nonsmall cell lung carcinoma, NOS, based on the H&E appearance; (B) TTF-1 is strongly positive; (C) p63 is positive in most tumor cells; (D) p40 is negative, confirming nonspecific reactivity of the p63 antibody. Final diagnosis was nonsmall cell lung carcinoma, favor adenocarcinoma. (All images at 400×.)

Table 3-3 Use of Immunohistochemistry to Guide Diagnosis of Lung Adenocarcinomas on Small Biopsies

Scenario	TTF-1	P63/p40	Diagnosis	Frequency	Next Steps
1	+	−/−	NSCLC, favor ACA	~80% ACA	
2	+	+/+[a] (in same cells)	NSCLC, favor ACA	0% SQC	
3	−	+/+	NSCLC, favor SQC	0% ACA 95% SQC	
4	+	+/+ (in different cells)	NSCLC, NOS, favor adenosquamous carcinoma	Rare (~1% of NSCLC)	Final diagnosis deferred to resection specimen
5	−	−/−	NSCLC, NOS[b]	10%-15% of ACA 0% SQC	Napsin, mucin
6	−	+/−	NSCLC, NOS[b]	Rare	Napsin, mucin

ACA, adenocarcinoma; NOS, not otherwise specified; NSCLC, nonsmall cell lung carcinoma; SQC, squamous cell carcinoma.
[a]Nonspecific p63 expression in lung ACA can range from focal to diffuse. When p40 expression is seen, it is typically present in 5% or fewer tumor cells.
[b]Exclude metastatic disease.

updated recommendations incorporate use of this antibody into the diagnosis on small biopsies[167] (*Figure 3-37*). TTF-1 is highly specific for adenocarcinoma in the differential with squamous cell carcinoma; however, it is only about 70% to 80% sensitive, leaving the possibility of metastatic disease to the lung in the differential for any tumor with combined TTF-1 and p63 or p40 negativity. Napsin may improve upon the sensitivity of TTF-1 (although there is conflicting literature on this point), and may be incorporated into the diagnostic panel.[116] Optimally, because napsin is a cytoplasmic marker and TTF-1 a nuclear marker, the two antibodies can be combined for simultaneous detection, thus increasing diagnostic sensitivity while conserving tumor tissue. Other immunohistochemistry markers, such as low and high molecular weight cytokeratins, have limited sensitivity and specificity in this differential and should be used only as second- or third-line tools. In a small number of cases, further classification of a tumor simply is not possible, in which case the diagnosis should be rendered as nonsmall cell lung carcinoma, not otherwise specified (NOS). In these cases, the clinical scenario, including patient risk factors and imaging findings, may be used to guide the decision to undergo molecular profiling or select chemotherapy.[9] *Table 3-3* summarizes the existing recommendations for use of immunohistochemistry in small biopsy diagnoses.

ADENOSQUAMOUS CARCINOMA

Clinical Features of Adenosquamous Carcinoma

Adenosquamous carcinomas are rare, representing on the order of 1% of lung carcinomas. Strictly speaking, the diagnosis of these tumors is limited to resection specimens, where the two components can be accurately quantified (see histologic features section below). Although this tumor type is more commonly seen in smokers, their clinical behavior is otherwise indistinguishable from adenocarcinomas,[1] and molecular profiling suggests that adenosquamous carcinomas and adenocarcinomas have shared genetic features.[168] Microdissection studies of *EGFR*- and *KRAS*-mutated adenosquamous carcinomas show that the tumor mutation profile is shared by both adeno- and squamous cell carcinoma components, arguing that these do not represent the collision of two separate tumors, but instead one distinct entity.[168,169] Studies comprehensively reviewing the pathologies of patients with "squamous cell carcinomas" containing *EGFR* activating mutations reclassify many of these as adenosquamous carcinomas that were initially undersampled.[129]

Imaging Features of Adenosquamous Carcinoma

Studies examining the computed tomography features of adenosquamous carcinoma show that 80% of these tumors arise in the periphery with a mean diameter of 3.8 cm (±1.9), with central tumors tending to be larger. 80% or more of adenosquamous tumors have margins that are lobulated, spiculated, and/or ill defined (*Figure 3-38*). On PET studies, the mean SUVmax is 8.3 (±3.9) with a higher SUVmax correlating with poor outcomes.[170]

Gross Features of Adenosquamous Carcinoma

Adenosquamous carcinomas are grossly similar to adenocarcinomas. Consistent with radiographic findings, these tumors are more commonly peripheral than central. Some studies indicate that these tumors are associated with more aggressive features, including

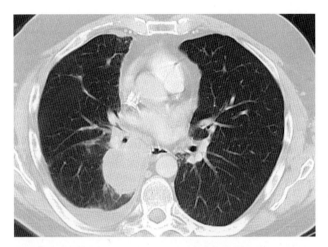

FIGURE 3-38 CT scan of the chest demonstrates a mass in the right lower lobe abutting the right lower lobe bronchus. Pathology review reveals adenosquamous carcinoma.

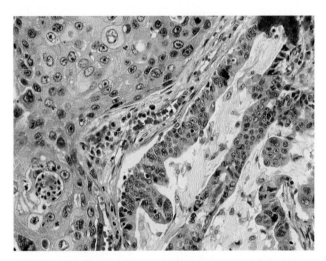

FIGURE 3-39 Closely intermixed neoplastic mucin-producing glands and keratinizing nests of squamous cells in an adenosquamous carcinoma.

larger size, pleural invasion, and multiple ipsilateral tumors, necessitating larger resections on average than adenocarcinomas.[171]

Histologic Features of Adenosquamous Carcinoma

Adenosquamous carcinomas are defined as nonsmall cell carcinomas containing at least 10% each of morphologically evident adenocarcinoma and squamous cell carcinoma. Components of glandular, papillary, or lepidic growth may be adjacent to or admixed with tumor nests showing features of squamous differentiation including keratinization or intercellular bridges (*Figure 3-39*). Tumors with predominantly solid pattern adenocarcinoma may be distinguished with the help of mucin stains; however, in light of the fact that mucin

droplets can be found in squamous cell carcinoma, immunohistochemistry for TTF-1 and p63 or p40 are more likely to clearly define the two components.[172]

REFERENCES

1. Travis W, Brambilla E, Muller-Hermelink HK, Harris CC, eds. *Pathology and Genetics of Tumours of the Lung, Pleura, Thymus, and Heart.* Lyon, France: IARCPress; 2004.
2. Motoi N, Szoke J, Riely GJ, et al. Lung adenocarcinoma: modification of the 2004 WHO mixed subtype to include the major histologic subtype suggests correlations between papillary and micropapillary adenocarcinoma subtypes, EGFR mutations and gene expression analysis. *Am J Surg Pathol.* 2008;32(6):810-827.
3. Finberg KE, Sequist LV, Joshi VA, et al. Mucinous differentiation correlates with absence of EGFR mutation and presence of KRAS mutation in lung adenocarcinomas with bronchioloalveolar features. *J Mol Diagn.* 2007;9(3):320-326.
4. Hwang DH, Szeto DP, Perry AS, Bruce JL, Sholl LM. Pulmonary large cell carcinoma lacking squamous differentiation is clinicopathologically indistinguishable from solid-subtype adenocarcinoma. *Arch Pathol Lab Med.* 2014;138(5):626-635.
5. Sakuma Y, Matsukuma S, Yoshihara M, et al. Distinctive evaluation of nonmucinous and mucinous subtypes of bronchioloalveolar carcinomas in EGFR and K-ras gene-mutation analyses for japanese lung adenocarcinomas: confirmation of the correlations with histologic subtypes and gene mutations. *Am J Clin Pathol.* 2007;128(1):100-108.
6. Garfield DH, Cadranel J, West HL. Bronchioloalveolar carcinoma: the case for two diseases. *Clin Lung Cancer.* 2008;9(1):24-29.
7. Travis WD, Garg K, Franklin WA, et al. Evolving concepts in the pathology and computed tomography imaging of lung adenocarcinoma and bronchioloalveolar carcinoma. *J Clin Oncol.* 2005;23(14):3279-3287.
8. Varlotto JM, Flickinger JC, Recht A, Nikolov MC, DeCamp MM. A comparison of survival and disease-specific survival in surgically resected, lymph node-positive bronchioloalveolar carcinoma versus nonsmall cell lung cancer: implications for adjuvant therapy. *Cancer.* 2008;112(7):1547-1554.
9. Travis WD, Brambilla E, Noguchi M, et al. International Association for the Study of Lung Cancer/American Thoracic Society/European Respiratory Society: international multidisciplinary classification of lung adenocarcinoma. *J Thorac Oncol.* 2011;6(2):244-285.
10. Howlader N, Noone AM, Krapcho M, et al. SEER cancer statistics review, 1975-2010. National Cancer Institute. Bethesda, MD. http://seer.cancer.gov/csr/1975_2010.
11. Jemal A, Bray F, Center MM, Ferlay J, Ward E, Forman D. Global cancer statistics. *CA Cancer J Clin.* 2011;61(2):69-90.
12. Non-small cell lung cancer treatment (PDQ). National Cancer Institute. http://www.cancer.gov/cancertopics/pdq/treatment/non-small-cell-lung. Updated 20132013.
13. Goldstraw P, Crowley J, Chansky K, et al. The IASLC lung cancer staging project: proposals for the revision of the TNM stage groupings in the forthcoming (seventh) edition of the TNM classification of malignant tumours. *J Thorac Oncol.* 2007;2(8):706-714.
14. Strauss GM, Jemal A, McKenna MB, Strauss JA, Cummings KM. Lung cancer survival in relation to histologic subtype: an analysis based upon surveillance epidemiology and end results (SEER) data: B4-06 [abstract]. *J Thorac Oncol.* 2007;2(8):345-346.
15. Cetin K, Ettinger DS, Hei YJ, O'Malley CD. Survival by histologic subtype in stage IV nonsmall cell lung cancer based on data

from the surveillance, epidemiology and end results program. *Clin Epidemiol.* 2011;3:139-148.

16. Lee BW, Wain JC, Kelsey KT, Wiencke JK, Christiani DC. Association of cigarette smoking and asbestos exposure with location and histology of lung cancer. *Am J Respir Crit Care Med.* 1998;157(3 Pt 1):748-755.

17. Sun S, Schiller JH, Gazdar AF. Lung cancer in never smokers—a different disease. *Nat Rev Cancer.* 2007;7(10):778-790.

18. Jemal A, Thun MJ, Ries LA, et al. Annual report to the nation on the status of cancer, 1975-2005, featuring trends in lung cancer, tobacco use, and tobacco control. *J Natl Cancer Inst.* 2008;100(23):1672-1694.

19. Parkin DM, Bray F, Ferlay J, Pisani P. Global cancer statistics, 2002. *CA Cancer J Clin.* 2005;55(2):74-108.

20. Ou SH, Ziogas A, Zell JA. Asian ethnicity is a favorable prognostic factor for overall survival in non-small cell lung cancer (NSCLC) and is independent of smoking status. *J Thorac Oncol.* 2009;4(9):1083-1093.

21. Gomez SL, Chang ET, Shema SJ, et al. Survival following non-small cell lung cancer among Asian/Pacific Islander, Latina, and non-Hispanic white women who have never smoked. *Cancer Epidemiol Biomarkers Prev.* 2011;20(3):545-554.

22. Wynder EL, Muscat JE. The changing epidemiology of smoking and lung cancer histology. *Environ Health Perspect.* 1995;103(suppl 8):143-148.

23. Parkin DM, Whelan SL, Ferlay J, Teppo L, Thomas DB. *Cancer Incidence in Five Continents.* Vol VIII, no 155. Lyon, France: IARCPress; 2002.

24. Hoffmann D, Rivenson A, Hecht SS. The biological significance of tobacco-specific N-nitrosamines: smoking and adenocarcinoma of the lung. *Crit Rev Toxicol.* 1996;26(2):199-211.

25. Imielinski M, Berger AH, Hammerman PS, et al. Mapping the hallmarks of lung adenocarcinoma with massively parallel sequencing. *Cell.* 2012;150(6):1107-1120.

26. Riely GJ, Kris MG, Rosenbaum D, et al. Frequency and distinctive spectrum of KRAS mutations in never smokers with lung adenocarcinoma. *Clin Cancer Res.* 2008;14(18):5731-5734.

27. Subramanian J, Govindan R. Lung cancer in never smokers: a review. *J Clin Oncol.* 2007;25(5):561-570.

28. Wang Y, Broderick P, Webb E, et al. Common 5p15.33 and 6p21.33 variants influence lung cancer risk. *Nat Genet.* 2008;40(12):1407-1409.

29. Li Y, Sheu CC, Ye Y, et al. Genetic variants and risk of lung cancer in never smokers: a genome-wide association study. *Lancet Oncol.* 2010;11(4):321-330.

30. Ding L, Getz G, Wheeler DA, et al. Somatic mutations affect key pathways in lung adenocarcinoma. *Nature.* 2008;455(7216):1069-1075.

31. Shigematsu H, Lin L, Takahashi T, et al. Clinical and biological features associated with epidermal growth factor receptor gene mutations in lung cancers. *J Natl Cancer Inst.* 2005;97(5):339-346.

32. Takeuchi K, Soda M, Togashi Y, et al. RET, ROS1 and ALK fusions in lung cancer. *Nat Med.* 2012;18(3):378-381.

33. Hyde L, Hyde CI. Clinical manifestations of lung cancer. *Chest.* 1974;65(3):299-306.

34. Chute CG, Greenberg ER, Baron J, Korson R, Baker J, Yates J. Presenting conditions of 1539 population-based lung cancer patients by cell type and stage in New Hampshire and Vermont. *Cancer.* 1985;56(8):2107-2111.

35. Kuo CW, Chen YM, Chao JY, Tsai CM, Perng RP. Non-small cell lung cancer in very young and very old patients. *Chest.* 2000;117(2):354-357.

36. Taiwo EO, Yorio JT, Yan J, Gerber DE. How have we diagnosed early-stage lung cancer without radiographic screening? A contemporary single-center experience. *PLoS One.* 2012;7(12):e52313.

37. National Lung Screening Trial Research Team, Aberle DR, Adams AM, et al. Reduced lung-cancer mortality with low-dose computed tomographic screening. *N Engl J Med.* 2011;365(5):395-409.

38. National Lung Screening Trial Research Team, Church TR, Black WC, et al. Results of initial low-dose computed tomographic screening for lung cancer. *N Engl J Med.* 2013;368(21):1980-1991.

39. Oken MM, Hocking WG, Kvale PA, et al. Screening by chest radiograph and lung cancer mortality: the prostate, lung, colorectal, and ovarian (PLCO) randomized trial. *JAMA.* 2011;306(17):1865-1873.

40. Screening for lung cancer: U.S. preventive services task force recommendation statement DRAFT. http://www.uspreventiveservicestaskforce.org/. Updated 2013. Accessed August 28, 2013.

41. Armstrong P. Neoplasms of the lung, airway and pleura. In: Armstrong P, Wilson AG, Dee P, Hansell DM, eds. *Imaging of the Diseases of the Chest.* 3rd ed. London, United Kingdom: Mosby; 2000:305-404.

42. Hansell DM, Bankier AA, MacMahon H, McLoud TC, Muller NL, Remy J. Fleischner society: glossary of terms for thoracic imaging. *Radiology.* 2008;246(3):697-722.

43. Suzuki K, Asamura H, Kusumoto M, Kondo H, Tsuchiya R. "Early" peripheral lung cancer: prognostic significance of ground glass opacity on thin-section computed tomographic scan. *Ann Thorac Surg.* 2002;74(5):1635-1639.

44. Takashima S, Sone S, Li F, Maruyama Y, Hasegawa M, Kadoya M. Indeterminate solitary pulmonary nodules revealed at population-based CT screening of the lung: using first follow-up diagnostic CT to differentiate benign and malignant lesions. *AJR Am J Roentgenol.* 2003;180(5):1255-1263.

45. Gaikwad A, Gupta A, Hare S, et al. Primary adenocarcinoma of lung: a pictorial review of recent updates. *Eur J Radiol.* 2012;81(12):4146-4155.

46. Kim TJ, Goo JM, Lee KW, Park CM, Lee HJ. Clinical, pathological and thin-section CT features of persistent multiple ground-glass opacity nodules: comparison with solitary ground-glass opacity nodule. *Lung Cancer.* 2009;64(2):171-178.

47. Godoy MC, Naidich DP. Subsolid pulmonary nodules and the spectrum of peripheral adenocarcinomas of the lung: recommended interim guidelines for assessment and management. *Radiology.* 2009;253(3):606-622.

48. Naidich DP, Bankier AA, MacMahon H, et al. Recommendations for the management of subsolid pulmonary nodules detected at CT: a statement from the Fleischner Society. *Radiology.* 2013;266(1):304-317.

49. Im JG, Han MC, Yu EJ, et al. Lobar bronchioloalveolar carcinoma: "angiogram sign" on CT scans. *Radiology.* 1990;176(3):749-753.

50. Kodama K, Higashiyama M, Yokouchi H, et al. Prognostic value of ground-glass opacity found in small lung adenocarcinoma on high-resolution CT scanning. *Lung Cancer.* 2001;33(1):17-25.

51. Aoki T, Tomoda Y, Watanabe H, et al. Peripheral lung adenocarcinoma: correlation of thin-section CT findings with histologic prognostic factors and survival. *Radiology.* 2001;220(3):803-809.

52. Golden R. The effect of bronchostenosis upon the roentgen ray shadow in carcinoma of the bronchus. *AJR Am J Roentgenol.* 1925;13:21.

53. Koyama H, Ohno Y, Seki S, et al. Magnetic resonance imaging for lung cancer. *J Thorac Imaging.* 2013;28(3):138-150.

54. Glazer HS, Kaiser LR, Anderson DJ, et al. Indeterminate mediastinal invasion in bronchogenic carcinoma: CT evaluation. *Radiology.* 1989;173(1):37-42.

55. White PG, Adams H, Crane MD, Butchart EG. Preoperative staging of carcinoma of the bronchus: can computed tomographic scanning reliably identify stage III tumours? *Thorax.* 1994;49(10):951-957.

56. Sobin LH, Gospodarowicz MK, Wittekind C, eds. *UICC TNM Classification of Malignant Tumors.* 7th ed. New York: Wiley-Blackwell; 2009.

57. Travis WD, Brambilla E, Rami-Porta R, et al. Visceral pleural invasion: pathologic criteria and use of elastic stains: proposal for the 7th edition of the TNM classification for lung cancer. *J Thorac Oncol*. 2008;3(12):1384-1390.

58. Grenier P, Dubary B, Carette MF, Frija G, Musset D, Chastang C. Preoperative thoracic staging of lung cancer: CT and MR evaluation. *Diagn Interv Radiol*. 1989;1:23-28.

59. Imai K, Minamiya Y, Ishiyama K, et al. Use of CT to evaluate pleural invasion in non-small cell lung cancer: measurement of the ratio of the interface between tumor and neighboring structures to maximum tumor diameter. *Radiology*. 2013;267(2):619-626.

60. Patz EF Jr, Lowe VJ, Hoffman JM, et al. Focal pulmonary abnormalities: evaluation with F-18 fluorodeoxyglucose PET scanning. *Radiology*. 1993;188(2):487-490.

61. Cronin P, Dwamena BA, Kelly AM, Carlos RC. Solitary pulmonary nodules: meta-analytic comparison of cross-sectional imaging modalities for diagnosis of malignancy. *Radiology*. 2008;246(3):772-782.

62. Fischer B, Lassen U, Mortensen J, et al. Preoperative staging of lung cancer with combined PET-CT. *N Engl J Med*. 2009;361(1):32-39.

63. Jeong HJ, Min JJ, Park JM, et al. Determination of the prognostic value of [(18)F]fluorodeoxyglucose uptake by using positron emission tomography in patients with non-small cell lung cancer. *Nucl Med Commun*. 2002;23(9):865-870.

64. Higashi K, Ueda Y, Seki H, et al. Fluorine-18-FDG PET imaging is negative in bronchioloalveolar lung carcinoma. *J Nucl Med*. 1998;39(6):1016-1020.

65. Kim BT, Kim Y, Lee KS, et al. Localized form of bronchioloalveolar carcinoma: FDG PET findings. *AJR Am J Roentgenol*. 1998;170(4):935-939.

66. Port JL, Andrade RS, Levin MA, et al. Positron emission tomographic scanning in the diagnosis and staging of non-small cell lung cancer 2 cm in size or less. *J Thorac Cardiovasc Surg*. 2005;130(6):1611-1615.

67. Eschmann SM, Friedel G, Paulsen F, et al. Is standardised (18)F-FDG uptake value an outcome predictor in patients with stage III non-small cell lung cancer? *Eur J Nucl Med Mol Imaging*. 2006;33(3):263-269.

68. Vesselle H, Salskov A, Turcotte E, et al. Relationship between non-small cell lung cancer FDG uptake at PET, tumor histology, and ki-67 proliferation index. *J Thorac Oncol*. 2008;3(9):971-978.

69. Sakai S, Murayama S, Murakami J, Hashiguchi N, Masuda K. Bronchogenic carcinoma invasion of the chest wall: evaluation with dynamic cine MRI during breathing. *J Comput Assist Tomogr*. 1997;21(4):595-600.

70. Zhao B, James LP, Moskowitz CS, et al. Evaluating variability in tumor measurements from same-day repeat CT scans of patients with non-small cell lung cancer. *Radiology*. 2009;252(1):263-272.

71. Nishino M, Guo M, Jackman DM, et al. CT tumor volume measurement in advanced non-small-cell lung cancer: performance characteristics of an emerging clinical tool. *Acad Radiol*. 2011;18(1):54-62.

72. Nishino M, Jackman DM, Hatabu H, Janne PA, Johnson BE, Van den Abbeele AD. Imaging of lung cancer in the era of molecular medicine. *Acad Radiol*. 2011;18(4):424-436.

73. Wilson DO, Ryan A, Fuhrman C, et al. Doubling times and CT screen-detected lung cancers in the Pittsburgh Lung Screening Study. *Am J Respir Crit Care Med*. 2012;185(1):85-89.

74. Yi CA, Lee KS, Kim EA, et al. Solitary pulmonary nodules: dynamic enhanced multi-detector row CT study and comparison with vascular endothelial growth factor and microvessel density. *Radiology*. 2004;233(1):191-199.

75. Tacelli N, Remy-Jardin M, Copin MC, et al. Assessment of non-small cell lung cancer perfusion: pathologic-CT correlation in 15 patients. *Radiology*. 2010;257(3):863-871.

76. Buck AK, Schirrmeister H, Hetzel M, et al. 3-deoxy-3-[(18)F]fluorothymidine-positron emission tomography for noninvasive assessment of proliferation in pulmonary nodules. *Cancer Res*. 2002;62(12):3331-3334.

77. Ohno Y, Hatabu H, Takenaka D, Adachi S, Kono M, Sugimura K. Solitary pulmonary nodules: potential role of dynamic MR imaging in management initial experience. *Radiology*. 2002;224(2):503-511.

78. Schaefer JF, Vollmar J, Schick F, et al. Solitary pulmonary nodules: dynamic contrast-enhanced MR imaging--perfusion differences in malignant and benign lesions. *Radiology*. 2004;232(2):544-553.

79. Tozaki M, Ichiba N, Fukuda K. Dynamic magnetic resonance imaging of solitary pulmonary nodules: utility of kinetic patterns in differential diagnosis. *J Comput Assist Tomogr*. 2005;29(1):13-19.

80. Mamata H, Tokuda J, Gill RR, et al. Clinical application of pharmacokinetic analysis as a biomarker of solitary pulmonary nodules: dynamic contrast-enhanced MR imaging. *Magn Reson Med*. 2012;68(5):1614-1622.

81. Satoh S, Kitazume Y, Ohdama S, Kimula Y, Taura S, Endo Y. Can malignant and benign pulmonary nodules be differentiated with diffusion-weighted MRI? *AJR Am J Roentgenol*. 2008;191(2):464-470.

82. Mori T, Nomori H, Ikeda K, et al. Diffusion-weighted magnetic resonance imaging for diagnosing malignant pulmonary nodules/masses: comparison with positron emission tomography. *J Thorac Oncol*. 2008;3(4):358-364.

83. Matoba M, Tonami H, Kondou T, et al. Lung carcinoma: diffusion-weighted mr imaging--preliminary evaluation with apparent diffusion coefficient. *Radiology*. 2007;243(2):570-577.

84. Arcasoy SM, Hersh C, Christie JD, et al. Bronchogenic carcinoma complicating lung transplantation. *J Heart Lung Transplant*. 2001;20(10):1044-1053.

85. von der Thusen JH, Tham YS, Pattenden H, et al. Prognostic significance of predominant histologic pattern and nuclear grade in resected adenocarcinoma of the lung: potential parameters for a grading system. *J Thorac Oncol*. 2013;8(1):37-44.

86. Yoshizawa A, Sumiyoshi S, Sonobe M, et al. Validation of the IASLC/ATS/ERS lung adenocarcinoma classification for prognosis and association with EGFR and KRAS gene mutations: analysis of 440 japanese patients. *J Thorac Oncol*. 2013;8(1):52-61.

87. Thunnissen E, Beasley MB, Borczuk AC, et al. Reproducibility of histopathological subtypes and invasion in pulmonary adenocarcinoma. an international interobserver study. *Mod Pathol*. 2012;25(12):1574-1583.

88. Barletta JA, Yeap BY, Chirieac LR. Prognostic significance of grading in lung adenocarcinoma. *Cancer*. 2010;116(3):659-669.

89. Rodig SJ, Mino-Kenudson M, Dacic S, et al. Unique clinicopathologic features characterize ALK-rearranged lung adenocarcinoma in the western population. *Clin Cancer Res*. 2009;15(16):5216-5223.

90. Nishino M, Klepeis VE, Yeap BY, et al. Histologic and cytomorphologic features of ALK-rearranged lung adenocarcinomas. *Mod Pathol*. 2012;25(11):1462-1472.

91. Sica G, Yoshizawa A, Sima CS, et al. A grading system of lung adenocarcinomas based on histologic pattern is predictive of disease recurrence in stage I tumors. *Am J Surg Pathol*. 2010;34(8):1155-1162.

92. Girard N, Deshpande C, Lau C, et al. Comprehensive histologic assessment helps to differentiate multiple lung primary nonsmall cell carcinomas from metastases. *Am J Surg Pathol*. 2009;33(12):1752-1764.

93. Sigel CS, Moreira AL, Travis WD, et al. Subtyping of non-small cell lung carcinoma: a comparison of small biopsy and cytology specimens. *J Thorac Oncol*. 2011;6(11):1849-1856.

94. Cibas ES, Ducatman BS, eds. *Cytology: Diagnostic Principles and Clinical Correlates*. 2nd ed. London, United Kingdom: Saunders; 2003.

95. Geisinger KR, Travis WD, Perkins LA, Zakowski MF. Aspiration cytomorphology of fetal adenocarcinoma of the lung. *Am J Clin Pathol.* 2010;134(6):894-902.

96. Butnor KJ, Sporn TA, Dodd LG. Fine needle aspiration cytology of mucinous cystadenocarcinoma of the lung: report of a case with radiographic and histologic correlation. *Acta Cytol.* 2001;45(5):779-783.

97. Kim CF, Jackson EL, Woolfenden AE, et al. Identification of bronchioalveolar stem cells in normal lung and lung cancer. *Cell.* 2005;121(6):823-835.

98. Barkauskas CE, Cronce MJ, Rackley CR, et al. Type 2 alveolar cells are stem cells in adult lung. *J Clin Invest.* 2013;123(7):3025-3036.

99. Lin C, Song H, Huang C, et al. Alveolar type II cells possess the capability of initiating lung tumor development. *PLoS One.* 2012;7(12):e53817.

100. Director's Challenge Consortium for the Molecular Classification of Lung Adenocarcinoma, Shedden K, Taylor JM, et al. Gene expression-based survival prediction in lung adenocarcinoma: a multi-site, blinded validation study. *Nat Med.* 2008;14(8):822-827.

101. Tsuta K, Kawago M, Inoue E, et al. The utility of the proposed IASLC/ATS/ERS lung adenocarcinoma subtypes for disease prognosis and correlation of driver gene alterations. *Lung Cancer.* 2013;81(3):371-376.

102. Yanagawa N, Shiono S, Abiko M, Ogata SY, Sato T, Tamura G. New IASLC/ATS/ERS classification and invasive tumor size are predictive of disease recurrence in stage I lung adenocarcinoma. *J Thorac Oncol.* 2013;8(5):612-618.

103. Yoshizawa A, Motoi N, Riely GJ, et al. Impact of proposed IASLC/ATS/ERS classification of lung adenocarcinoma: prognostic subgroups and implications for further revision of staging based on analysis of 514 stage I cases. *Mod Pathol.* 2011;24(5):653-664.

104. Woo T, Okudela K, Mitsui H, et al. Prognostic value of the IASLC/ATS/ERS classification of lung adenocarcinoma in stage I disease of japanese cases. *Pathol Int.* 2012;62(12):785-791.

105. Russell PA, Wainer Z, Wright GM, Daniels M, Conron M, Williams RA. Does lung adenocarcinoma subtype predict patient survival?: a clinicopathologic study based on the new international association for the study of lung Cancer/American thoracic Society/European respiratory society international multidisciplinary lung adenocarcinoma classification. *J Thorac Oncol.* 2011;6(9):1496-1504.

106. Nakatani Y, Masudo K, Miyagi Y, et al. Aberrant nuclear localization and gene mutation of beta-catenin in low-grade adenocarcinoma of fetal lung type: up-regulation of the Wnt signaling pathway may be a common denominator for the development of tumors that form morules. *Mod Pathol.* 2002;15(6):617-624.

107. Nakatani Y, Kitamura H, Inayama Y, et al. Pulmonary adenocarcinomas of the fetal lung type: a clinicopathologic study indicating differences in histology, epidemiology, and natural history of low-grade and high-grade forms. *Am J Surg Pathol.* 1998;22(4):399-411.

108. Nakatani Y, Dickersin GR, Mark EJ. Pulmonary endodermal tumor resembling fetal lung: a clinicopathologic study of five cases with immunohistochemical and ultrastructural characterization. *Hum Pathol.* 1990;21(11):1097-1107.

109. Morita S, Yoshida A, Goto A, et al. High-grade lung adenocarcinoma with fetal lung-like morphology: clinicopathologic, immunohistochemical, and molecular analyses of 17 cases. *Am J Surg Pathol.* 2013;37(6):924-932.

110. Inamura K, Satoh Y, Okumura S, et al. Pulmonary adenocarcinomas with enteric differentiation: histologic and immunohistochemical characteristics compared with metastatic colorectal cancers and usual pulmonary adenocarcinomas. *Am J Surg Pathol.* 2005;29(5):660-665.

111. Kitagawa H, Goto A, Niki T, Hironaka M, Nakajima J, Fukayama M. Lung adenocarcinoma associated with atypical adenomatous hyperplasia. A clinicopathological study with special reference to smoking and cancer multiplicity. *Pathol Int.* 2003;53(12):823-827.

112. Ikeda K, Nomori H, Ohba Y, et al. Epidermal growth factor receptor mutations in multicentric lung adenocarcinomas and atypical adenomatous hyperplasias. *J Thorac Oncol.* 2008;3(5):467-471.

113. Sakamoto H, Shimizu J, Horio Y, et al. Disproportionate representation of KRAS gene mutation in atypical adenomatous hyperplasia, but even distribution of EGFR gene mutation from preinvasive to invasive adenocarcinomas. *J Pathol.* 2007;212(3):287-294.

114. Yim J, Zhu LC, Chiriboga L, Watson HN, Goldberg JD, Moreira AL. Histologic features are important prognostic indicators in early stages lung adenocarcinomas. *Mod Pathol.* 2007;20(2):233-241.

115. Mukhopadhyay S, Katzenstein AL. Subclassification of non-small cell lung carcinomas lacking morphologic differentiation on biopsy specimens: utility of an immunohistochemical panel containing TTF-1, napsin A, p63, and CK5/6. *Am J Surg Pathol.* 2011;35(1):15-25.

116. Bishop JA, Sharma R, Illei PB. Napsin A and thyroid transcription factor-1 expression in carcinomas of the lung, breast, pancreas, colon, kidney, thyroid, and malignant mesothelioma. *Hum Pathol.* 2010;41(1):20-25.

117. Shah RN, Badve S, Papreddy K, Schindler S, Laskin WB, Yeldandi AV. Expression of cytokeratin 20 in mucinous bronchioloalveolar carcinoma. *Hum Pathol.* 2002;33(9):915-920.

118. Gyure KA, Morrison AL. Cytokeratin 7 and 20 expression in choroid plexus tumors: utility in differentiating these neoplasms from metastatic carcinomas. *Mod Pathol.* 2000;13(6):638-643.

119. Tateishi M, Ishida T, Mitsudomi T, Kaneko S, Sugimachi K. Immunohistochemical evidence of autocrine growth factors in adenocarcinoma of the human lung. *Cancer Res.* 1990;50(21):7077-7080.

120. Thatcher N, Chang A, Parikh P, et al. Gefitinib plus best supportive care in previously treated patients with refractory advanced non-small-cell lung cancer: results from a randomised, placebo-controlled, multicentre study (Iressa Survival Evaluation in Lung Cancer). *Lancet.* 2005;366(9496):1527-1537.

121. Miller VA, Kris MG, Shah N, et al. Bronchioloalveolar pathologic subtype and smoking history predict sensitivity to gefitinib in advanced non-small-cell lung cancer. *J Clin Oncol.* 2004;22(6):1103-1109.

122. Paez JG, Janne PA, Lee JC, et al. EGFR mutations in lung cancer: correlation with clinical response to gefitinib therapy. *Science.* 2004;304(5676):1497-1500.

123. Lynch TJ, Bell DW, Sordella R, et al. Activating mutations in the epidermal growth factor receptor underlying responsiveness of non-small-cell lung cancer to gefitinib. *N Engl J Med.* 2004;350(21):2129-2139.

124. Pao W, Miller V, Zakowski M, et al. EGF receptor gene mutations are common in lung cancers from "never smokers" and are associated with sensitivity of tumors to gefitinib and erlotinib. *Proc Natl Acad Sci U S A.* 2004;101(36):13306-13311.

125. Lindeman NI, Cagle PT, Beasley MB, et al. Molecular testing guideline for selection of lung cancer patients for EGFR and ALK tyrosine kinase inhibitors: guideline from the college of American pathologists, international association for the study of lung cancer, and association for molecular pathology. *J Mol Diagn.* 2013;15(4):415-453.

126. Maemondo M, Inoue A, Kobayashi K, et al. Gefitinib or chemotherapy for non-small-cell lung cancer with mutated EGFR. *N Engl J Med.* 2010;362(25):2380-2388.

127. Mok TS, Wu YL, Thongprasert S, et al. Gefitinib or carboplatin-paclitaxel in pulmonary adenocarcinoma. *N Engl J Med.* 2009;361(10):947-957.

128. Sharma SV, Bell DW, Settleman J, Haber DA. Epidermal growth factor receptor mutations in lung cancer. *Nat Rev Cancer.* 2007;7(3):169-181.

129. Rekhtman N, Paik PK, Arcila ME, et al. Clarifying the spectrum of driver oncogene mutations in biomarker-verified squamous carcinoma of lung: lack of EGFR/KRAS and presence of PIK3CA/AKT1 mutations. *Clin Cancer Res.* 2012;18(4):1167-1176.

130. Sholl LM, Yeap BY, Iafrate AJ, et al. Lung adenocarcinoma with EGFR amplification has distinct clinicopathologic and molecular features in never-smokers. *Cancer Res.* 2009;69(21):8341-8348.

131. Sholl LM, Xiao Y, Joshi V, et al. EGFR mutation is a better predictor of response to tyrosine kinase inhibitors in non-small cell lung carcinoma than FISH, CISH, and immunohistochemistry. *Am J Clin Pathol.* 2010;133(6):922-934.

132. Pao W, Miller VA, Politi KA, et al. Acquired resistance of lung adenocarcinomas to gefitinib or erlotinib is associated with a second mutation in the EGFR kinase domain. *PLoS Med.* 2005;2(3):e73.

133. Hammerman PS, Janne PA, Johnson BE. Resistance to epidermal growth factor receptor tyrosine kinase inhibitors in non-small cell lung cancer. *Clin Cancer Res.* 2009;15(24):7502-7509.

134. Turke AB, Zejnullahu K, Wu YL, et al. Preexistence and clonal selection of MET amplification in EGFR mutant NSCLC. *Cancer Cell.* 2010;17(1):77-88.

135. Cadranel J, Ruppert AM, Beau-Faller M, Wislez M. Therapeutic strategy for advanced EGFR mutant non-small-cell lung carcinoma. *Crit Rev Oncol Hematol.* 2013;88(3):477-493.

136. Soda M, Choi YL, Enomoto M, et al. Identification of the transforming EML4-ALK fusion gene in non-small-cell lung cancer. *Nature.* 2007;448(7153):561-566.

137. Kwak EL, Bang YJ, Camidge DR, et al. Anaplastic lymphoma kinase inhibition in non-small-cell lung cancer. *N Engl J Med.* 2010;363(18):1693-1703.

138. FDA approval for crizotinib. National Cancer Institute. http://www.cancer.gov/cancertopics/druginfo/fda-crizotinib. Updated 2013. Accessed August 30, 2013.

139. Shaw AT, Kim DW, Nakagawa K, et al. Crizotinib versus chemotherapy in advanced ALK-positive lung cancer. *N Engl J Med.* 2013;368(25):2385-2394.

140. Vysis ALK break apart FISH probe kit, with the vysis paraffin pretreatment IV and post hybridization wash buffer kit, ProbeChek ALK negative control slides, and ProbeChek ALK positive control slides - P110012. U.S. Food and Drug Administration. http://www.fda.gov/MedicalDevices/ProductsandMedicalProcedures/DeviceApprovalsandClearances/Recently-ApprovedDevices/ucm270832.htm. Updated 2012. Accessed August 30, 2013.

141. Mino-Kenudson M, Chirieac LR, Law K, et al. A novel, highly sensitive antibody allows for the routine detection of ALK-rearranged lung adenocarcinomas by standard immunohistochemistry. *Clin Cancer Res.* 2010;16(5):1561-1571.

142. Sholl LM, Weremowicz S, Gray SW, et al. Combined use of ALK immunohistochemistry and FISH for optimal detection of ALK-rearranged lung adenocarcinomas. *J Thorac.Oncol.* 2013;8(3):322-328.

143. Yang P, Kulig K, Boland JM, et al. Worse disease-free survival in never-smokers with ALK+ lung adenocarcinoma. *J Thorac Oncol.* 2012;7(1):90-97.

144. Gainor JF, Varghese AM, Ou SH, et al. ALK rearrangements are mutually exclusive with mutations in EGFR or KRAS: an analysis of 1,683 patients with non-small cell lung cancer. *Clin Cancer Res.* 2013;19(15):4273-4281.

145. Birchmeier C, O'Neill K, Riggs M, Wigler M. Characterization of ROS1 cDNA from a human glioblastoma cell line. *Proc Natl Acad Sci U S A.* 1990;87(12):4799-4803.

146. Rikova K, Guo A, Zeng Q, et al. Global survey of phosphotyrosine signaling identifies oncogenic kinases in lung cancer. *Cell.* 2007;131(6):1190-1203.

147. Rimkunas VM, Crosby KE, Li D, et al. Analysis of receptor tyrosine kinase ROS1-positive tumors in non-small cell lung cancer: identification of a FIG-ROS1 fusion. *Clin Cancer Res.* 2012;18(16):4449-4457.

148. Bergethon K, Shaw AT, Ou SH, et al. ROS1 rearrangements define a unique molecular class of lung cancers. *J Clin Oncol.* 2012;30(8):863-870.

149. Sholl LM, Sun H, Butaney M, et al. ROS1 immunohistochemistry for detection of ROS1-rearranged lung adenocarcinomas. *Am J Surg Pathol.* 2013;37(9):1441-1449.

150. Wang R, Hu H, Pan Y, et al. RET fusions define a unique molecular and clinicopathologic subtype of non-small-cell lung cancer. *J Clin Oncol.* 2012;30(35):4352-4359.

151. Cai W, Su C, Li X, et al. KIF5B-RET fusions in chinese patients with non-small cell lung cancer. *Cancer.* 2013;119(8):1486-1494.

152. Drilon A, Wang L, Hasanovic A, et al. Response to cabozantinib in patients with RET fusion-positive lung adenocarcinomas. *Cancer Discov.* 2013;3(6):630-635.

153. Ruijs MW, Verhoef S, Rookus MA, et al. TP53 germline mutation testing in 180 families suspected of Li-Fraumeni syndrome: mutation detection rate and relative frequency of cancers in different familial phenotypes. *J Med Genet.* 2010;47(6):421-428.

154. Shen L, Yin ZH, Wan Y, Zhang Y, Li K, Zhou BS. Association between ATM polymorphisms and cancer risk: a meta-analysis. *Mol Biol Rep.* 2012;39(5):5719-5725.

155. Yang H, Spitz MR, Stewart DJ, Lu C, Gorlov IP, Wu X. ATM sequence variants associate with susceptibility to non-small cell lung cancer. *Int J Cancer.* 2007;121(10):2254-2259.

156. Lo YL, Hsiao CF, Jou YS, et al. ATM polymorphisms and risk of lung cancer among never smokers. *Lung Cancer.* 2010;69(2):148-154.

157. Schneider J, Illig T, Rosenberger A, Bickeboller H, Wichmann HE. Detection of ATM gene mutations in young lung cancer patients: a population-based control study. *Arch Med Res.* 2008;39(2):226-231.

158. Thompson D, Duedal S, Kirner J, et al. Cancer risks and mortality in heterozygous ATM mutation carriers. *J Natl Cancer Inst.* 2005;97(11):813-822.

159. Bott M, Brevet M, Taylor BS, et al. The nuclear deubiquitinase BAP1 is commonly inactivated by somatic mutations and 3p21.1 losses in malignant pleural mesothelioma. *Nat Genet.* 2011;43(7):668-672.

160. Testa JR, Cheung M, Pei J, et al. Germline BAP1 mutations predispose to malignant mesothelioma. *Nat Genet.* 2011;43(10):1022-1025.

161. Abdel-Rahman MH, Pilarski R, Cebulla CM, et al. Germline BAP1 mutation predisposes to uveal melanoma, lung adenocarcinoma, meningioma, and other cancers. *J Med Genet.* 2011;48(12):856-859.

162. Bell DW, Gore I, Okimoto RA, et al. Inherited susceptibility to lung cancer may be associated with the T790M drug resistance mutation in EGFR. *Nat Genet.* 2005;37(12):1315-1316.

163. Oxnard GR, Miller VA, Robson ME, et al. Screening for germline EGFR T790M mutations through lung cancer genotyping. *J Thorac Oncol.* 2012;7(6):1049-1052.

164. FDA approval for bevicuzimab. National Cancer Institute. http://www.cancer.gov/cancertopics/druginfo/fda-bevacizumab#Anchor-NSCLC. Updated 2013. Accessed August 31, 2013.

165. Rekhtman N, Ang DC, Sima CS, Travis WD, Moreira AL. Immunohistochemical algorithm for differentiation of lung adenocarcinoma and squamous cell carcinoma based on large series of whole-tissue sections with validation in small specimens. *Mod Pathol.* 2011;24(10):1348-1359.

166. Bishop JA, Teruya-Feldstein J, Westra WH, Pelosi G, Travis WD, Rekhtman N. p40 (DeltaNp63) is superior to p63 for the diagnosis of pulmonary squamous cell carcinoma. *Mod Pathol.* 2012;25(3):405-415.

167. Travis WD, Brambilla E, Noguchi M, et al. Diagnosis of lung cancer in small biopsies and cytology: implications of the 2011 international association for the study of lung Cancer/American thoracic Society/European respiratory society classification. *Arch Pathol Lab Med.* 2013;137(5):668-684.

168. Shu C, Cheng H, Wang A, et al. Thymidylate synthase expression and molecular alterations in adenosquamous carcinoma of the lung. *Mod Pathol.* 2013;26(2):239-246.

169. Tochigi N, Dacic S, Nikiforova M, Cieply KM, Yousem SA. Adenosquamous carcinoma of the lung: a microdissection study of KRAS and EGFR mutational and amplification status in a western patient population. *Am J Clin Pathol.* 2011; 135(5):783-789.

170. Lee Y, Chung JH, Kim SE, Kim TJ, Lee KW. Adenosquamous carcinoma of the lung: CT, FDG PET, and clinicopathologic findings. *Clin Nucl Med.* 2014;39(2):107-112.

171. Mordant P, Grand B, Cazes A, et al. Adenosquamous carcinoma of the lung: surgical management, pathologic characteristics, and prognostic implications. *Ann Thorac Surg.* 2013;95(4):1189-1195.

172. Shimoji M, Nakajima T, Yamatani C, et al. A clinicopathological and immunohistological re-evaluation of adenosquamous carcinoma of the lung. *Pathol Int.* 2011;61(12):717-722.

4 Squamous Cell Carcinoma

Mari Mino-Kenudson, Michiya Nishino, Subba Digumarthy, and Hironori Uruga

TAKE HOME PEARLS

- Squamous cell carcinomas comprise 25% to 30% of all lung cancers and are strongly associated with tobacco smoking, male gender, and central location of the tumor. However, their prevalence and male:female ratio have recently been decreasing and tumors arising in the periphery of the lung have been increasingly identified due in part to the changes in smoking habits.
- Squamous cell carcinoma is defined as a malignant epithelial tumor of the lung exhibiting keratinization and/or intercellular bridges, and was classified into a classic form and four variants (papillary carcinoma, clear cell carcinoma, small cell carcinoma, and basaloid carcinoma). In the fifth edition of WHO classification, however, it is simplified as keratinizing and nonkeratinizing squamous cell carcinoma and basaloid carcinoma reflecting the differences in biology.
- Given the recent advances in treatment for lung cancer patients, the distinction of squamous cell carcinoma from nonsquamous cell carcinoma has become of paramount importance. It is recommended to subtype undifferentiated nonsmall cell carcinomas into squamous cell carcinoma or nonsquamous cell carcinoma applying a panel of immunomarkers even in small biopsy or cytology samples.
- Genetically a selective amplification of chromosome 3q, which includes oncogene *SOX2*, is the most prevalent alteration in lung squamous cell carcinomas, although *SOX2* does not appear to be a "driver" of neoplastic transformation. While no

targeted agents are clinically available for (conventional) squamous cell carcinoma to date, agents targeted to several molecular alterations such as *FGFR* amplification and PI3K-AKT pathway activation are being evaluated in clinical trials Thus, it is anticipated that molecular targeted therapy will play a role in treatment for squamous cell carcinoma in the near future.

WHO CLASSIFICATION OF PULMONARY SQUAMOUS CELL CARCINOMA

Squamous cell carcinoma is traditionally defined as a malignant epithelial tumor showing keratinization and/or intercellular bridges that arises from bronchial epithelium. In the 2004 WHO classification, invasive squamous cell carcinoma consisted of a classic form and variants—papillary carcinoma, clear cell carcinoma, small cell carcinoma, and basaloid carcinoma[1]; however, it has been simplified as keratinizing and nonkeratinizing squamous cell carcinoma and basaloid carcinoma in the fifth edition of WHO classification. It is important to note that nonkeratinizing squamous cell carcinoma includes "undifferentiated nonsmall cell carcinoma" with an immunophenotype of squamous cell carcinoma that has been historically classified into the large cell carcinoma category. Nonkeratinizing squamous cell carcinoma is confirmed by its immunostaining pattern, immunopositive for p40, and immunonegative for TTF-1.

EPIDEMIOLOGY OF SQUAMOUS CELL CARCINOMA

Squamous cell carcinomas account for 25% to 30% of all lung cancers. Of the major histologic nonsmall cell lung cancer (NSCLC) subtypes, squamous cell carcinomas are associated most strongly with cigarette smoking, with over 90% of these tumors occurring in cigarette smokers. Squamous cell carcinomas comprise 53% of lung cancers from smokers, compared to 18% of those from never smokers.[2] The risk for lung cancer among smokers shows a sex predilection, with women having much higher risk than men. The relative risk for squamous cell carcinoma and small cell carcinoma is 17.5 in women compared with 12.7 in men, although for adenocarcinoma it is 2.0 and 2.8, respectively.[3]

Squamous cell carcinoma used to be the most common subtype of NSCLC, but the proportion of squamous cell carcinomas relative to adenocarcinomas has been decreasing since the 1960s.[4] This shift in prevalence has been attributed to several factors including improved imaging modalities leading to the detection of small peripheral tumors, recent smoking cessation rates, changes in cigarette design and composition, and a change in cigarette smoke inhalation patterns.[5-7] Currently, adenocarcinoma is the most common subtype of lung cancer in many countries, but substantial regional differences remain in the proportion of squamous cell carcinomas relative to adenocarcinomas.[8]

Squamous cell carcinomas of the lung are typically central airway tumors involving the main stem and lobar and segmental bronchi; however, recent series have revealed an increasing prevalence of peripheral squamous cell carcinomas, which are becoming as common as central squamous cell carcinomas.[9]

ETIOLOGY OF SQUAMOUS CELL CARCINOMA

Squamous cell carcinomas arise from basal cells or metaplastic goblet cells, which sequentially develop into squamous metaplasia, squamous dysplasia, carcinoma in situ, and invasive carcinoma. Exposure to tobacco products, inflammation, or irritation could trigger this sequential process. Smoking is the most notable cause of inflammation and irritation, although exposure to secondhand smoke, ambient fine particulate matter ($PM_{2.5}$) air pollution, cooking oil vapors, indoor coal burning, and viral infections (eg, human papilloma virus) are candidate triggers.[2,10] Arsenic exposure is also strongly associated with squamous cell carcinoma.[11] Interestingly, whole genome sequencing analysis performed in a single arsenic-related lung squamous cell carcinoma has shown a lower number of point mutations, a remarkably high fraction of T>G/A>C transversions and low fraction of C>A/G>T transversions, which is uncharacteristic of lung squamous cell carcinomas. Furthermore, the analysis identified a unique TP53 point mutation (G>C), which is extremely rare (<0.2%) in lung cancers but has been observed in other arsenic-related malignancies. The results support the notion that arsenic induces lung cancers through mechanisms distinct from tobacco and other nonarsenic carcinogens.[12]

DEMOGRAPHICS AND CLINICAL FEATURES OF SQUAMOUS CELL CARCINOMA

Lung cancer is typically a disease of later life. In the elderly, cigarette smoking is the most notable cause, and this age group therefore has a higher proportion of squamous cell carcinomas compared to the younger group (under 40 years of age) in which the proportion of adenocarcinomas is higher.[13] Squamous cell carcinoma used to be predominantly a disease seen in men due to the differences in smoking habits between the genders. For instance, the male: female ratio for squamous cell carcinoma was more than 20:1 in France, Italy, the Netherlands, Slovenia, and Spain up until around 1990. Along with the recent changes in smoking habits, the male: female ratio fell to less than 3:1 in Canada, Iceland, and Sweden and among Caucasians in the United States by the late 1990s.[8]

Clinically, patients with central tumors can present with cough, shortness of breath, and fever secondary to obstructive pneumonia and atelectasis. Hemoptysis is an important feature that can be related to both central and peripheral locations and an increased propensity for cavitation. In general, squamous cell carcinomas tend to be locally aggressive and sometimes extend along the bronchus so that the assessment of the bronchial resection margin, in particular at the time of intraoperative consultation, is extremely important. Conversely, they develop metastasis to distant organs less frequently than adenocarcinomas. Squamous cell carcinomas that involve the superior sulcus (apical pleuropulmonary groove) are the predominant tumor type associated with Pancoast syndrome. The condition is characterized by pain (usually in the shoulder and less commonly in the forearm, scapula, and fingers), Horner syndrome, bony destruction, and hand muscle atrophy.[14] Multiple paraneoplastic syndromes have been reported in association with lung cancer. Of these, hypercalcemia is most commonly seen in patients with squamous cell carcinoma. Cancer-associated hypercalcemia is usually due to bone metastases, but occasionally occurs in the absence of metastatic disease, where it is typically mediated by parathyroid-related protein that increases both bone reabsorption and renal tubular reabsorption of calcium. Serum parathyroid hormone levels are characteristically low or unmeasurable in these cases.[15] Tumor-related leukocytosis due to the autonomous production of granulocyte and granulocyte-macrophage colony-stimulating factors is another paraneoplastic syndrome associated with lung cancer; 60 of 227 lung cancers with tumor-related leukocytosis were reported as squamous cell carcinomas.[16]

SQUAMOUS CELL CARCINOMA AND INTERSTITIAL PNEUMONIA

Smoking is strongly associated with both lung cancer and interstitial pneumonia, in particular idiopathic pulmonary fibrosis (IPF). Therefore, some patients have both diseases, with 9.8% to 38% of IPF patients also having lung cancer.[17] Squamous cell carcinoma is typically the most common histology in lung cancers arising in patients with IPF.[18,19] The lung cancer development in the background of IPF is attributed not only to tobacco exposure as a mutual cause but also to fibrosis since the tumors typically develop in the peripheral lung parenchyma exhibiting fibrosis and epithelial dysplasia.[17] Interestingly, computed tomography often shows a nodule or mass in the transitional zone between fibrotic and normal lung tissue in patients with IPF and lung cancer.[20] It is clinically important to identify and confirm the diagnosis of interstitial pneumonia in the background of lung cancer since treatments for lung cancer such as surgical resection, radiation therapy, and chemotherapy can trigger acute exacerbation of interstitial pneumonia.

The syndrome of combined pulmonary fibrosis and emphysema (CPFE) is a recently described entity, and is characterized by the coexistence of centrilobular and/or paraseptal emphysema and pulmonary fibrosis depicted by imaging study.[21] It is associated with high prevalence of pulmonary hypertension and poor prognosis. Virtually all patients are smokers and thus at high risk of developing lung cancer. About half of those patients

reportedly develop lung cancer,[22] and squamous cell carcinoma is more prevalent than adenocarcinoma.[23] It remains unclear whether the risk of developing lung cancer is higher in CPFE than in IPF, however.[19,24]

TREATMENT FOR SQUAMOUS CELL CARCINOMA

Similar to the other NSCLCs, surgical resection is the standard therapy for patients with stage IA squamous cell carcinoma, while surgical resection with adjuvant chemotherapy is commonly indicated for patients with stage IB, IIA, and IIB disease. The management of stage IIIA and IIIB squamous cell carcinoma is still open to debate and the combination of all three or any combinations of two modalities among surgical resection, platinum-based chemotherapy, and radiation therapy can be applied. For stage IV disease and recurrent disease, chemotherapy is essentially the treatment for squamous cell carcinoma.[25] The first-line chemotherapy for squamous cell carcinoma is usually platinum based, and a non-platinum monotherapy is typically used as the second or third line. Chemotherapy for NSCLCs has recently been split into that for squamous cell carcinoma and that for nonsquamous cell carcinoma. Pemetrexed, a multitargeted folate antimetabolite, showed higher efficacy for adenocarcinoma than squamous cell carcinoma,[26] while bevacizumab, an antivascular endothelial growth factor monoclonal antibody, is not approved for squamous cell carcinoma due to the possibility of fatal hemoptysis in those patients.[26] Molecular targeted therapies (eg, epidermal growth factor receptor inhibitors and anaplastic lymphoma kinase inhibitors) are playing an increasingly important role in the treatment of lung cancer, but the corresponding mutations are typically identified in nonsquamous NSCLCs, and no therapy targeted to molecular alterations commonly seen in squamous cell carcinoma is currently available outside of clinical trials (*Table 4-1*). Consequently, the histologic distinction of squamous cell carcinoma from nonsquamous cell

Table 4-1 Histology (and Cytology) Matters in NSCLC

Drug	Class	Why Histology (and Cytology) Matters
Pemetrexed (Alimta)	Folate antimetabolite	Better activity against NSCLC with nonsquamous histology[30]
Bevacizumab (Avastin)	Anti-VEGF-A monoclonal antibody	Use only in NSCLC with nonsquamous histology (risk of severe pulmonary hemorrhage in squamous cell carcinoma)[26]
Gefitinib (Iressa)	EGFR tyrosine kinase inhibitors	Activity against NSCLC with *EGFR*-activating mutations (almost exclusively adenocarcinomas)[31,32,33]
Erlotinib (Tarceva)		
Afatinib (Gilotrif)		
Crizotinib (Xalkori)	ALK tyrosine kinase inhibitor	Activity against NSCLC with *ALK* rearrangements (almost exclusively adenocarcinomas)[34,35]
Ceritinib (Zykadia)		

carcinoma has become extremely important for treatment decision making. Unfortunately, the development of novel chemotherapeutic agents and/or new regimens for squamous cell carcinoma is not as progressive as that for adenocarcinoma. However, immunotherapies such as antiprogrammed death 1 (PD-1) antibody and anticytotoxic T-lymphocyte antigen-4 (CTLA-4) antibody have shown better response in patients with squamous cell carcinoma than those with adenocarcinoma in phase I and II trials.[27-29] While the findings need to be confirmed by additional studies, the immunotherapies are expected as new therapeutic modalities for patients with squamous cell carcinoma.

IMAGING FEATURES OF SQUAMOUS CELL CARCINOMA

Imaging plays an important role in detection, diagnosis, and staging of squamous cell lung cancer. The modalities that are commonly used are conventional radiography, computed tomography (CT), magnetic resonance imaging (MRI), and positron emission tomography (PET). The recent advances in such as imaging CT texture analysis, dual energy CT, and MRI-PET enable better tissue characterization and treatment planning.

Radiography

In asymptomatic patients, the radiographic diagnosis of lung cancer frequently occurs in the context of screening and detection of lung nodules on routine chest radiographs that are performed for preoperative and treatment workup of other diseases and preemployment screening. A nodule has to reach the size of at least 9 mm before it is reliably detected on radiograph.[36] The density of the nodule is also very important. Nodules that are dense and of solid morphology are more readily detected on radiographs. In general, detection of small lung nodules is difficult on radiograph due to overlying and overlapping vessels and bones, factors that may obscure significant portion of lung parenchyma (*Figure 4-1*). The concept of "doubling time" is very important in radiology. A malignant nodule has a doubling time of 7 to 465 days.[37] A doubling time outside this range is unusual for squamous cell carcinoma of lung. Nodules that are greater than 2 cm in size are more likely to be malignant.

Squamous cell carcinoma of the lung is overwhelmingly found in the inner third of the lung and around the hila. Only a third of these cancers are found in the periphery of the lung,[38] although an increasing number of squamous cell carcinomas are being detected in the periphery.[9] As the central cancers arise from lining cells of major bronchi, the tumors occlude the lumen and cause atelectasis of the distal lung and postobstructive

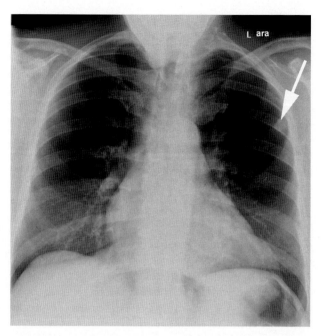

FIGURE 4-1 Chest radiograph shows 2-cm squamous cell carcinoma in the left upper lobe that is obscured by the overlying the rib an (arrow).

pneumonia.[39] The lung collapse is characterized by increased density of lung with associated volume loss and absence of air bronchograms within the lung opacity. A segmental or lobar collapse results in an opacity that reaches up to the hilum of the lung. A combination of central hilar mass with associated distal collapse of the lung is characteristic of a central squamous cell lung cancer (*Figure 4-2*). A right hilar mass causing collapse of right upper lobe produces characteristic "reverse S sign of Golden," where the right minor fissure is concave superiorly and laterally and convex inferiorly and medially. If there is postobstructive pneumonia, loss of volume may not be apparent and air bronchogram can be seen.

Cavitation is an important and common feature of squamous cell carcinoma. A cavity is defined as abnormal hollow space in lung parenchyma that may be empty or filled with fluid. Cavitation is also a prominent feature of several infections such as lung abscess and tuberculosis. The cavity in malignancy is usually thick walled (>5 mm) and has nodularity along the inner wall.[40] The cavitary squamous cell carcinoma is thought to have poorer prognosis compared to solid squamous cell carcinoma, presumably due to delay in diagnosis from overlapping features with infection and also differences in tumor biology.[41,42] Pancoast tumor is nonsmall cell lung cancer that arises in the lung apex and can invade adjacent chest wall and mediastinal structures. Historically, squamous cell carcinoma accounted for the majority of Pancoast tumors. The radiographic features are characterized by a mass in

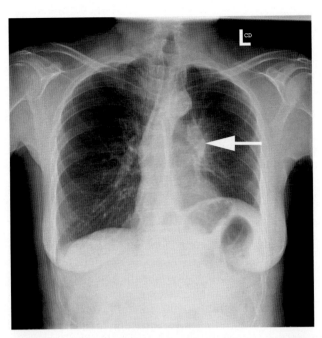

FIGURE 4-2 Chest radiograph shows central squamous cell carcinoma in the left upper lobe bronchus causing left upper lobe collapse (arrow).

the lung apex that extends into the mediastinum, and may cause destruction of adjacent ribs and vertebrae (*Figure 4-3*). The radiographic features in early stages can be very subtle and can easily be missed.[43,44]

Mediastinal widening is suggestive of metastatic lymphadenopathy; however, plain radiography is not sensitive to detect mediastinal nodal disease. Pleural effusions cause blunting of costophrenic angles and opacification of hemithorax, depending on the amount of fluid.

Computed Tomography

Computed tomography (CT) is the modality of choice for screening patients for lung cancer and for characterization of lung nodules detected on chest radiography.[45]

There is significant overlap in morphology of tumors on CT between squamous cell carcinoma and adenocarcinoma of the lung, but there are some useful pointers: (1) Squamous cell carcinoma is solid in CT attenuation, and ground glass and mixed solid and ground glass morphology is rare and uncommon. (2) Cavitation is significantly more common in squamous cell carcinoma (*Figure 4-4*). (3) Internal air bronchogram is rare in squamous cell cancer. (4) Pleural tags and spiculated margins are less common in squamous cell carcinoma.[46]

The assessment of lymph nodes on CT is primarily based on size and enhancement pattern. In the setting of malignancy, a lymph node that is greater than 1 cm in short axis is considered metastatic. In a meta-analysis of lymph nodes detected on CT, which is performed as part of preoperative staging of NSCLC, the sensitivity, specificity, and accuracy of CT compared to the final pathology are 33% to 75%, 66% to 90%, 64% to 79%, respectively.[47] Several modifications such as increasing the size threshold above 1 cm and measuring volume or circumference of lymph nodes are suggested, to increase the accuracy of CT interpretation.[48] Heterogeneous enhancement of lymph nodes with necrosis is a feature of pathological lymph nodes and is more commonly seen in squamous cell cancer (*Figure 4-5*).[49]

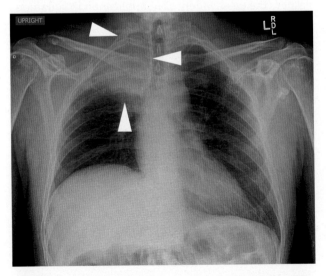

FIGURE 4-3 Chest radiograph shows right apical squamous cell carcinoma (Pancoast tumor) extending into mediastinum and causing osteolysis of right first rib (arrows).

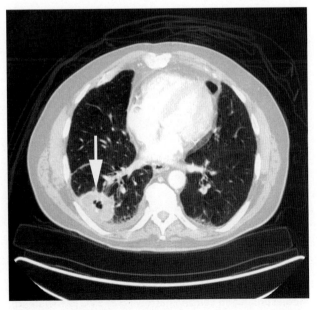

FIGURE 4-4 Chest CT shows 4-cm peripheral cavitary squamous cell carcinoma in the right lower lobe (arrow).

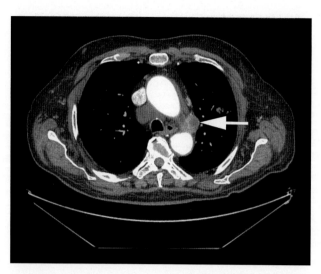

FIGURE 4-5 Chest CT in mediastinal window shows a metastatic necrotic lymph node in the AP window (arrow) from squamous cell carcinoma of the left upper lobe.

CT is widely used to identify patients with resectable lung cancer. Invasion into mediastinum by central squamous cell cancer is considered surgically inoperable in most situations. The CT findings are often divided into "definite" and "indeterminate" categories to assess mediastinal invasion. The findings such as gross involvement of mediastinal fat, encasement of mediastinal vessels and structures, and destruction of vertebra, by tumor are considered definite signs of mediastinal invasion (*Figure 4-6*). Only contact between the mediastinum and lung mass with loss of fat plane is considered an indeterminate sign. These patients may have resectable tumor on surgical exploration.[50,51]

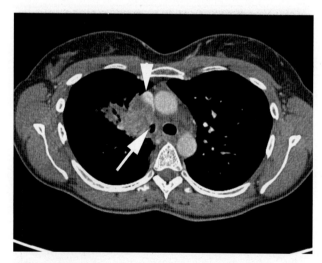

FIGURE 4-6 Chest CT in mediastinal window shows squamous cell carcinoma of the right upper lobe invading the mediastinum and causing narrowing of SVC (arrow head). Notice also the occlusion of right upper lobe bronchus (arrow).

Assessment of chest wall and parietal pleural invasion, in peripheral squamous cell cancer, is important for planning surgery and can adversely affect the prognosis. There are several signs that suggest chest wall and pleural invasion such as: (1) greater than 3 cm contact between the mass and pleura; (2) pleural thickening and obliteration of extra pleural fat; (3) presence of pleural tags; (4) presence of extrapleural mass; and (5) destruction of adjacent bone. Among these signs presence of extrapleural mass with bone destruction is the only sign that has high accuracy in predicting invasion. In the absence of this sign the sensitivity and specificity range from 38% to 87% and 40% to 90%, respectively.[52] The presence of large pleural effusion is suggestive of metastases to the pleura. Pleural thickening and pleural nodules on CT increase the accuracy of diagnosis. Even in the absence of effusion, pleural nodularity and fissural thickening are suggestive of pleural metastases.[53]

Pulmonary lymphangitic carcinomatosis is defined as diffuse infiltration and obstruction of the pulmonary lymphatic vessels by malignant cells. This is more common in adenocarcinoma of the lung. In squamous cell cancer this is usually seen around the primary tumor.[54]

Magnetic Resonance Imaging

Magnetic resonance imaging (MRI) does not involve ionizing radiation, has superior tissue contrast resolution to CT, and has the ability to characterize tissues. However, imaging time is significantly longer and has lower spatial resolution compared to CT. MRI is also limited due to cardiac and respiratory motion artifacts and low proton density in the normal lungs. Therefore, MRI is typically used in special situations for its superior contrast resolution and ability to characterize tissues. The most widely used application in squamous cell lung cancer is in the evaluation of Pancoast tumor and assessment of mediastinal and chest wall invasion.

When compared to contrast-enhanced single helical CT, cardiac-gated contrast-enhanced MR is superior for detection of hilar and mediastinal invasion. The sensitivity, specificity, and accuracy were 78% to 90%, 73% to 87%, and 75% to 88%, respectively.[55] Similarly MRI is more sensitive in demonstrating chest wall invasion, by showing abnormal signal and loss of fat in extrapleural fat on T1-weighted images and high signal in parietal pleura on T2-weighted images. The sensitivity is further increased by using intravenous gadolinium. The fixity of chest wall to pleura and therefore tumor invasion can be demonstrated on dynamic cine MRI. During respiration, normal parietal pleura slide freely against the chest wall, whereas they move in unison if there is invasion.[56,57]

The assessment of mediastinal and hilar nodes ideally requires cardiac and/or respiratory triggered image acquisition to reduce image artifacts. Metastatic

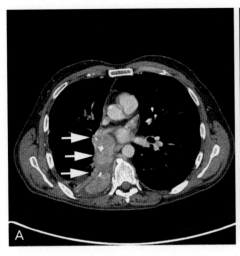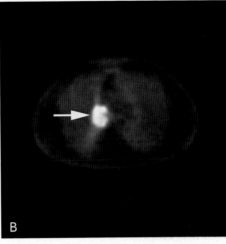

FIGURE 4-7 Chest CT (A) in mediastinal window shows a right lower lobe central mass causing collapse of the right lower lobe (arrows), the mass and collapse are indistinguishable on CT. PET image (B) shows central mass has intense 18-FDG uptake (arrow) whereas distal collapsed lung is not 18-FDG avid.

lymph nodes have high signal intensity on T2-weighted imaging and show abnormal enhancement after administration of intravenous gadolinium. STIR turbo SE imaging and diffusion-weighted imaging improve the sensitivity and accuracy.[58] Studies have shown similar accuracy in detection of metastatic lymph nodes, between CT-PET and whole body MRI.[59]

MRI is superior to CT or PET for evaluation of brain parenchyma and detection of brain metastasis. MRI is also sensitive to detection of early marrow changes and can detect bone metastasis earlier than CT.[60]

Positron Emission Tomography

Positron emission tomography (PET) is considered the best imaging tool in staging of lung cancer and is superior to anatomical imaging such as CT and MRI.[61] The radiotracer used in imaging is 18-fluorodeoxyglucose (18-FDG) and is analogous to glucose. 18-FDG accumulates in sites of increased glucose uptake such as cancerous lesions. PET imaging has lower spatial resolution compared to CT and is most useful when used in conjunction with CT.

Although the determination of T stage is mostly based on anatomical imaging, PET is useful in selected situations. For instance, it is useful in separating the 18-FDG avid central tumor from distal atelectasis and allows accurate measurement of tumor for planning radiotherapy (*Figure 4-7*).[62] Similarly PET can be useful in diagnosing early chest wall invasion.

In patients with resectable lung cancer, nodal disease is the most important prognostic factor. PET imaging is superior to CT imaging in assessment of nodal metastases and has sensitivity and specificity of 83 % and 92% compared to 59 % and 78% of CT.[63] The combination of PET with CT further improves the accuracy.

The most important contribution of whole body PET imaging is in determining the "M" stage and is the most

cost-effective method. In patients selected for resection, PET imaging may detect occult metastasis in 5% to 29% of patients.[64] The incidence of distant metastases increases with increased T and N stage of cancer. The commonest sites of metastases are adrenal glands, liver, brain, bones, and distant lymph nodes (*Figure 4-8*). Malignant pleural disease from metastasis can be seen up to 15% of patients with NSCLC. Increased FDG uptake is suggestive of metastasis, and has a negative predictive value of 100% and positive predictive value of 63% to 79%.[65] However, pleural infections and inflammatory conditions can also have increased FDG uptake, thus the increased FDG uptake of pleura needs to be interpreted with caution.

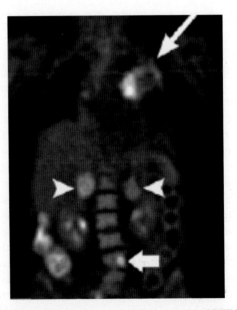

FIGURE 4-8 Whole body attenuation corrected PET image shows FDG avid left upper lobe mass (arrow), bilateral adrenal metastases (arrow head), and L4 vertebral body metastasis (short arrow).

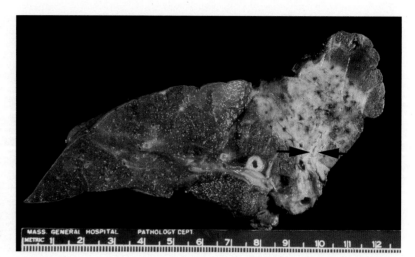

FIGURE 4-9 Gross photograph of a central squamous cell carcinoma partially occluding the bronchial lumen (arrows). The tumor exhibits a white, relatively firm cut surface with scattered anthracosis.

Recent Advances

CT texture histogram analysis is a technique that can characterize tissue based on pixel intensity values. It has been shown that this technique may be able to differentiate histologic subtypes of lung nodules[66] and may be useful in identifying squamous cell carcinoma. The tissue heterogeneity in NSCLC was found to be an independent prognostic factor in predicting survival.[67]

Dual energy CT and functional MR imaging of lungs can assess and quantify lung perfusion and ventilation and are helpful in planning surgery and radiation therapy to minimize injury of normal lung parenchyma.[68,69]

GROSS FEATURES OF SQUAMOUS CELL CARCINOMA

Squamous cell carcinoma has traditionally been considered as a tumor of the central airway (*Figure 4-9*), but an increasing number of peripheral tumors (*Figure 4-10*) are being reported and they now comprise up to half of all squamous cell carcinomas.[9] The cut surface is usually white or gray and frequently soft and friable, but depending on the severity of fibrosis, they may become firm. Focal carbon pigment deposits may be present in the center and star-like retractions on the periphery. The tumor may grow to a large size and may cavitate due to central necrosis. Central tumors form intraluminal polypoid masses and/or infiltrate through the bronchial wall into the surrounding tissues and may occlude the bronchial lumen, resulting in atelectasis, bronchiectasis, obstructive pneumonia, and bronchopneumonia.[1] Hilar lymph nodes are often enlarged due to direct invasion and/or metastasis by tumor and/or reactive lymphadenopathy secondary to obstructive or infective pneumonia.

HISTOLOGIC FEATURES OF SQUAMOUS CELL CARCINOMA— DIAGNOSTIC CRITERIA OF SQUAMOUS CELL CARCINOMA

Squamous cell carcinoma has been traditionally defined as a malignant epithelial tumor showing keratinization (*Figure 4-11A*) and/or intercellular bridges (*Figure 4-11B*) that arises from bronchial epithelium.[1] The keratinization includes layered keratin and cytoplasmic keratin of individual tumor cells. Keratin pearl formation may also be seen. The 2015 WHO classification recognizes nonkeratinizing squamous cell carcinomas that can be identified by their immunostaining pattern (immunopositive for squamous markers, immunonegative for TTF-1). Traditionally, squamous cell carcinomas of the lung have been graded into well, moderately, and poorly differentiated tumors based on a degree of squamous differentiation. In the well-differentiated tumors, there are tumor nests exhibiting prominent keratinization and intercellular bridges, while those features are found only in a small area of the tumor in the poorly differentiated tumors. The moderately differentiated tumors show an intermediate degree of squamous differentiation that is between well and poorly differentiated tumors (*Figure 4-12*).[70] Similar to squamous cell carcinomas of the nasopharynx, the lung counterpart can be classified into keratinizing and nonkeratinizing tumors. In the nonkeratinizing tumors, there is typically a lack of maturation in the epithelial nests. As the name implies, the tumors do not generally exhibit histologic evidence of keratinization, although some degree may be seen.[71] Thus, nonkeratinizing squamous cell carcinomas are essentially graded as poorly differentiated tumors. As noted above, nonkeratinizing squamous cell carcinoma, diagnosed as squamous marker immunopositive and TTF-1 immunonegative, is recognized in the 2015 WHO classification.

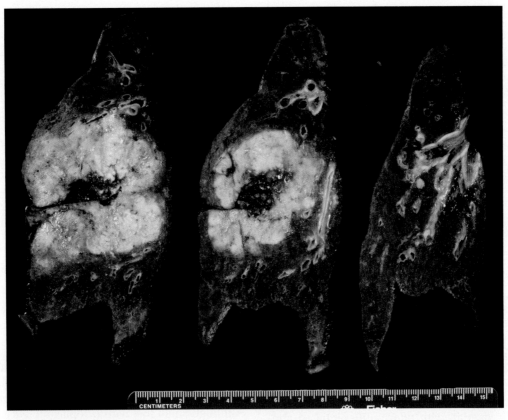

FIGURE 4-10 Gross photograph of peripheral squamous cell carcinoma with central necrosis and hemorrhage.

An issue associated with the grading and subtyping is that there is no standardized cutoff for distribution (%) of tumor cells with keratinization in each category (well, moderately, and poorly differentiated or keratinizing vs nonkeratinizing).[72] The assessment of keratinization is also subject to tissue sampling. In any event, most squamous cell carcinomas are

moderately differentiated,[70] and the degree of keratinization does not appear to be associated with patient outcomes.[72-74] For instance, a recent study with a large cohort of lung squamous cell carcinomas, that applied a cutoff of 5% for keratinizing pattern (including layered and cytoplasmic keratinization) to differentiating keratinizing versus nonkeratinizing tumors,

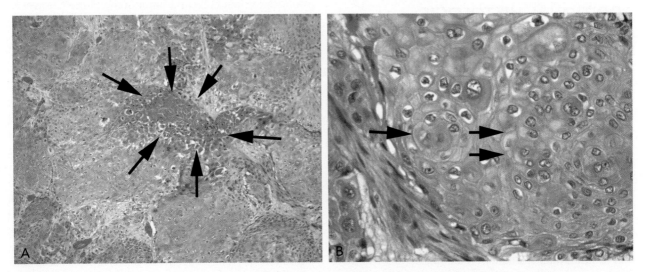

FIGURE 4-11 An example of squamous cell carcinoma with keratinization (arrow heads) (A) and intercellular bridges (arrows) (B).

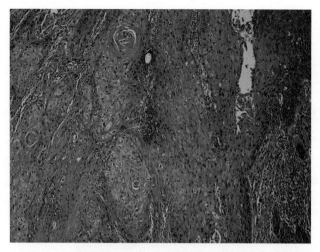

FIGURE 4-12 An example of moderately differentiated squamous cell carcinoma.

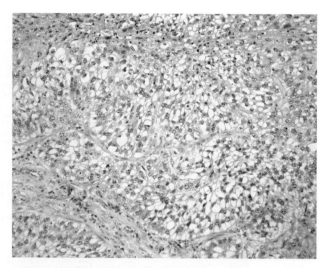

FIGURE 4-13 Squamous cell carcinoma with prominent clear cell features.

failed to demonstrate the prognostic significance of the subtyping.[72] Despite the lack of clear prognostic significance, recognizing a nonkeratinizing subtype of squamous cell carcinoma in the lung has become clinically important since these tumors can have morphologic overlap with poorly differentiated adenocarcinomas with pseudosquamous features.[72] As previously mentioned, the differentiation between the two entities has molecular and therapeutic implications, and thus, it is of paramount importance to achieve accurate diagnosis using immunohistochemistry for adenocarcinoma and squamous markers (refer to the Approach to the Diagnosis of Poorly Differentiated Squamous Cell Carcinoma on Small Biopsy Specimens section).

ADDITIONAL HISTOLOGIC FEATURES AND PATTERNS OF SQUAMOUS CELL CARCINOMA

The fourth WHO classification published in 2004 recognized four histologic variants of squamous cell carcinoma based on their cytomorphologic characteristics. Three variants (clear cell, small cell, and papillary) do not appear to have distinct clinicopathological features.[72] Therefore, these variants have been removed from the 2015 WHO classification. However, these histologic features remain of value as differential diagnoses of other types of lung cancer, including small cell carcinoma and metastases from other organs. Basaloid carcinoma remains part of the 2015 WHO classification of squamous cell carcinoma and also incorporates those cancers previously classified as basaloid under large cell carcinomas.

Clear Cell Features

Some squamous cell carcinomas consist predominantly or almost entirely of cells with clear cytoplasm that is secondary to glycogen accumulation (*Figure 4-13*).[75] Although small foci with cytoplasmic clearing are not infrequently seen not only in squamous cell carcinomas but also in other types of lung cancer, and have been reported in approximately a third of resected lung cancers (except for small cell carcinoma), the foci usually involve only 10% to 20% of the entire tumor in most cases. Conversely, tumors consisting predominantly (more than 50%) of malignant cells with abundant clear cytoplasm are rare and have been reported in less than 6% of squamous cell carcinomas.[76] In those cases, it is important to differentiate from large cell carcinoma and adenocarcinoma of the lung with clear cell changes and metastatic clear cell carcinoma of the kidney; however, they do not appear to have a prognostic significance compared to those without clear cell changes.[76]

Small Cell Features

Some poorly differentiated squamous cell carcinomas histologically and/or cytologically resemble small cell carcinoma, but retain immunohistochemical and/or characteristics of squamous differentiation (*Figure 4-14A-D*).[77] It is important to distinguish squamous cell carcinoma with small cell features from true small cell carcinoma and combined small cell carcinoma with squamous cell carcinoma, given the difference in treatment between small cell carcinoma and nonsmall cell carcinoma. Small cell features consist of small tumor cells arranged in sheets, nests, and/or cords with abundant mitoses and necrosis. Nuclear molding and/ or Azzopardi effect (crush artifact with encrustation

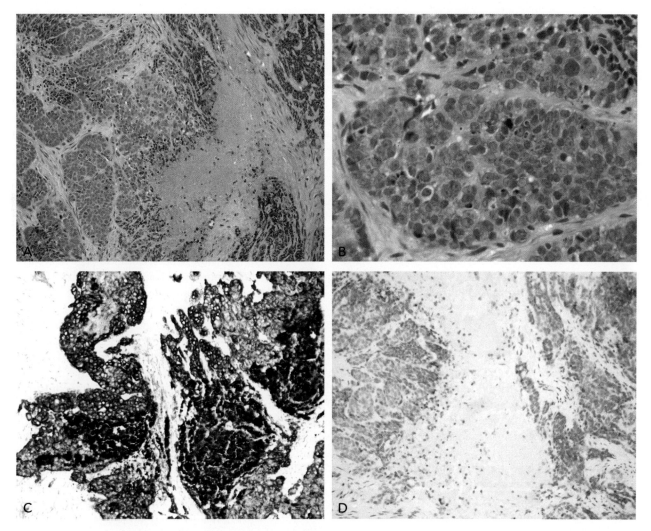

FIGURE 4-14 An example of squamous cell carcinoma with small cell features. The tumor exhibits nests and/or cords of small-sized cells with a high N/C ratio. Whereas the presence of nuclear molding (on the right side) is suggestive of small cell carcinoma (A), the tumor cells exhibit conspicuous nucleoli (B). Immunohistochemistry shows the tumor cells to be positive for cytokeratin 5/6 (C) and p40, and negative for synaptophysin (D) and other neuroendocrine markers consistent with squamous cell carcinoma.

of basophilic nuclear DNA around blood vessels) may be seen in some cases (*Figure 4-14A*). However, these tumors usually lack the characteristic nuclear features of small cell carcinoma having coarse or vesicular chromatin, more prominent nucleoli, more cytoplasm, and more distinct cell borders (*Figure 4-14B*). Focal intercellular bridges or keratinization may be seen. Importantly, immunohistochemical study confirms squamous differentiation (diffuse expression of squamous cell markers such as p40, p63, and CK5/6) (*Figure 4-14C*) and the lack of neuroendocrine differentiation (negative expression of neuroendocrine markers such as chromogranin A and synaptophysin) (*Figure 4-14D*). Electromicroscopy also shows the absence of neurosecretory granules.[78,79]

Papillary Architectural Features

Some squamous cell carcinomas may show exophytic and endobronchial papillary growth or superficial papillary spreading. In the latter case, there may be a very limited amount of intraepithelial spread without invasion, but invasion is seen in most cases. The tumor cells exhibit squamous differentiation with numerous nuclear abnormalities, but unequivocal keratinization is typically absent, and the tumor cells may resemble transitional cell carcinoma (*Figure 4-15*).[80] Given the exophytic and endobronchial growth resulting in symptoms and signs secondary to airway obstruction in the majority of the tumors, they are often diagnosed and treated at their early stage. Although the prognosis of

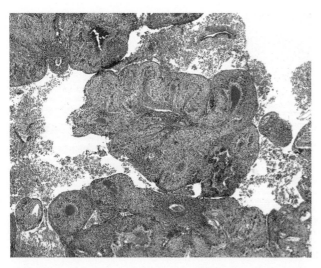

FIGURE 4-15 Papillary architectural features with an exophytic growth. The tumor cells do not exhibit unequivocal keratinization and somewhat resemble transitional cell carcinoma.

squamous cell carcinomas with papillary architecture appears to be better than all resected lung cancers, it is no better than that of stage I tumors.[80-82] The differential diagnosis includes papilloma and metastatic carcinomas with an endobronchial growth, such as papillary thyroid carcinoma. The former is usually benign and rarely solitary, and often develops as part of laryngotracheal papillomatosis in young patients.[80]

Basaloid Carcinoma

Basaloid carcinoma is a rare subtype of lung cancer with a reported incidence of 5% to 6% of nonsmall cell lung cancers.[83,84] Basaloid tumors were previously classified as a variant of squamous cell carcinoma or that of large cell carcinoma based on the presence or absence of squamous differentiation on morphology, respectively, in accordance with the 2004 *WHO Classification of Tumours: Tumours of the Lung, Pleura, Thymus and Heart*.[1,85] All of these tumors are now classified under squamous cell carcinoma in the 2015 WHO classification. Basaloid squamous cell carcinomas exhibit a proliferation of small cells with lobular architecture or anastomotic trabecular growth and prominent peripheral palisading of tumor nuclei, along with obvious squamous differentiation in a minor component (*Figure 4-16*). The basaloid features consist of scanty cytoplasm, consequently, high nuclear/cytoplasmic ratio, a greater amount of hyperchromatic nuclei that lack prominent nucleoli, and high mitotic activity (15-50 per 2 mm²). Proliferative index as indicated by Ki-67 ranges from 50% to 80%. Comedo-type necrosis is common and rosette may be seen in one-third of cases, but nuclear molding is essentially absent. Poorly differentiated lung carcinomas with an extensive basaloid pattern but lacking morphologic squamous differentiation (keratinization and/or intercellular bridges) were previously regarded as the basaloid variant of large cell carcinoma.[85,86] However, growing evidence indicates that the latter is also of a squamous lineage confirmed by immunohistochemical expression of squamous markers.[87,88] Thus, it appears more practical to classify all lung carcinomas with prominent basaloid features as squamous cell carcinomas. Indeed, the 2015 WHO classification categorizes all of these tumors as squamous cell carcinomas, including those that were previously categorized as large cell carcinomas.

There have been conflicting reports on the prognosis of patients with basaloid carcinoma.[72,83,89-91] Although the largest series to date has reported that basaloid carcinomas had a shorter patient survival than nonbasaloid squamous cell carcinoma,[83] studies from East Asian countries have failed to show the prognostic significance of basaloid carcinomas compared

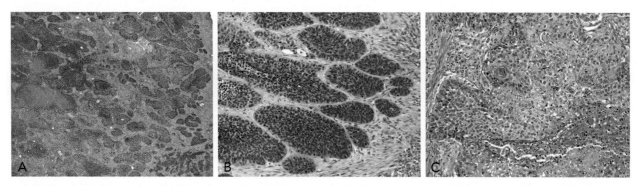

FIGURE 4-16 A basaloid squamous cell carcinoma consists mostly of small cells with lobular architecture or anastomotic trabecular growth (**A**), and prominent peripheral palisading of tumor nuclei that exhibit high nuclear/cytoplasmic ratio and a greater amount of hyperchromasia, but lack prominent nucleoli (**B**). Obvious squamous differentiation is seen in a minor component (**C**).

to poorly differentiated, nonbasaloid squamous cell carcinomas,[90,91] and the recent study from the United States has reported that patients with basaloid squamous cell carcinomas had a trend for better prognosis than those with nonbasaloid tumors.[72] Interestingly, squamous cell carcinomas with basaloid differentiation and severe nuclear atypia exhibited more intense SOX2 protein expression than other tumors, while SOX2 expression was associated with better overall survival in squamous cell carcinomas in one study.[92] The differences in the prognosis of basaloid squamous cell carcinomas between the studies may be due to variations in several factors including the histologic type of basaloid tumors (the degree of basaloid differentiation) disease stage and treatment, ethnic differences, and/or interobserver agreement on basaloid features. While the prognostic significance and reproducibility of the basaloid features in lung squamous cell carcinoma warrant further investigation, the basaloid variant is important as a differential diagnosis of other types of lung cancer including large cell neuroendocrine carcinoma, small cell carcinoma, adenoid cystic carcinoma, NUT carcinoma, and poorly differentiated (nonbasaloid) squamous cell or adenocarcinoma (refer to the Differential Diagnosis of Squamous Cell Carcinoma of the Lung section).

Alveolar Space-Filling Pattern

An alveolar space-filling growth pattern appears to correspond to favorable prognosis in squamous cell carcinomas.[9,93] This pattern is seen predominantly in peripheral squamous cell carcinomas and displays cohesive aggregates of malignant squamous cells filling airspaces with intact nondisrupted alveolar septa as if

the tumor cells could grow and penetrate the pores of Kohn (*Figure 4-17A*). The preserved alveolar framework can be confirmed by an elastic stain and benign alveolar pneumocytes that form an intact flattened continuous layer of lining cells can be highlighted by TTF1, Napsin A, and/or cytokeratin 7 stains (*Figure 4-17B*).[9,93,94] Peripheral squamous cell carcinomas consisting solely of this pattern are rare (0%-4.6%), but as a prominent feature, the pattern has been identified in approximately one-fourth of peripheral squamous cell carcinomas.[9,93,94] The two studies from Japan reported the 5-year disease free survival rate of 100% in five cases with a pure alveolar space-filling growth pattern and 19 (of 82) cases with an alveolar space-filling ratio of 70% or more.[9,93] Given the nondestructive growth and favorable prognosis, this pattern is likely equivalent to lepidic pattern of lung adenocarcinoma.

CYTOLOGIC FEATURES OF SQUAMOUS CELL CARCINOMA

As discussed previously, due to recent advances in the treatment and molecular diagnostics of nonsmall cell lung cancer (NSCLC), the ability to distinguish its two principal subtypes—squamous cell carcinoma and adenocarcinoma—is increasing in importance. However, because approximately 70% of patients with lung cancer present at an advanced stage with unresectable disease, the only pathologic material available for analysis may be cytology specimens procured from minimally invasive procedures such as transthoracic and endobronchial fine needle aspiration (FNA) biopsies, bronchial brushings/washings, sputum collection, and thoracentesis in the setting of malignant pleural effusions. Pathologists

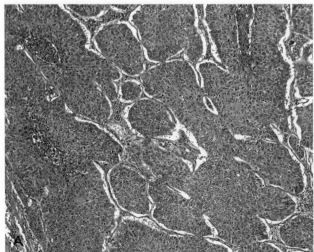
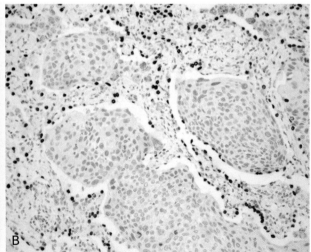

FIGURE 4-17 A peripheral squamous cell carcinoma with cohesive aggregates of malignant squamous cells filling airspaces with intact nondisrupted alveolar septa (A) that are confirmed by a TTF-1 immunostain highlighting a flat, continuous layer of benign alveolar pneumocytes (B).

must not only be able to establish a diagnosis of malignancy on these cytology specimens, but also to subtype NSCLC into squamous cell carcinoma versus adenocarcinoma (vs others) and to triage cytologic specimens appropriately for molecular testing.[95,96]

The International Association for the Study of Lung Cancer/American Thoracic Society/European Respiratory Society (IASCLS/ATS/ERS) recommends the following terminology for squamous cell carcinomas in cytology and small biopsy specimens: "squamous cell carcinoma" for cases that show characteristic cytomorphology of squamous cell differentiation, and "NSCLC, favor squamous cell carcinoma" for morphologically poorly differentiated cases that show immunohistochemical evidence (eg, ΔNp63/p40 expression) of squamous differentiation.[96,97]

Cytologic Features of Well-Differentiated Squamous Cell Carcinoma

The cytologic features of squamous cell carcinoma depend on the extent of squamous differentiation. Aspirates of well-differentiated squamous cell carcinoma characteristically show single dispersed cells in a necrotic background, frequently with many anucleate cells (*Figure 4-18*). Tumor cells range from polygonal to elongated, tadpole-like shapes (*Figures 4-19 to 4-21*). The cytoplasm of keratinizing cells often appears densely eosinophilic (hematoxylin and eosin stain), orangeophilic (Papanicolaou stain), or pale "robin's-egg blue" (air-dried Romanowsky-stained preparations). Keratin pearls may be present. The nuclei are hyperchromatic and may be range from small, pyknotic forms to those that are large with markedly irregular contours.

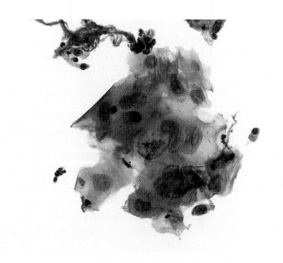

FIGURE 4-19 Transbronchial fine needle aspiration of a well-differentiated squamous cell carcinoma shows a cluster of cells with abundant, dense, orangeophilic cytoplasm and large, irregular nuclei (Papanicolaou stain, 40×).

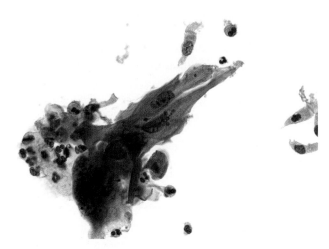

FIGURE 4-20 The same tumor from *Figure 4-22* is shown. These tumor cells show the elongated and densely orangeophilic cytoplasm characteristic of well-differentiated squamous cell carcinoma. The benign bronchial columnar cells in the background serve as a size reference (Papanicolaou stain, 40×).

Nucleoli are typically inconspicuous due to the coarseness of the chromatin.

Cytologic Features of Moderately to Poorly Differentiated Squamous Cell Carcinoma

In contrast, moderately and poorly differentiated squamous cell carcinomas are often aspirated as cohesive tissue fragments (*Figures 4-22 to 4-24*). Tumor cells have moderate to scant amounts of cytoplasm and large nuclei, bringing about higher nuclear/cytoplasmic ratios compared to their well-differentiated counterparts.

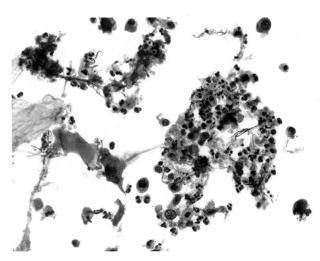

FIGURE 4-18 Transbronchial fine needle aspiration of a well-differentiated squamous cell carcinoma showing necroinflammatory debris, anucleated squamous cells, and singly dispersed tumor cells (Papanicolaou stain, 20×).

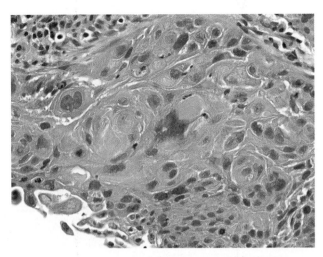

FIGURE 4-21 Endobronchial biopsy of the well-differentiated portion of the squamous cell carcinoma shown in *Figures 4-22 and 4-23* (hematoxylin and eosin, 40×).

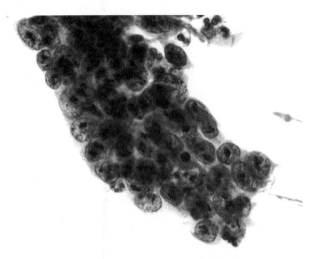

FIGURE 4-23 Transbronchial fine needle aspiration of a poorly differentiated squamous cell carcinoma. No keratinization or cytomorphologic evidence of squamous differentiation is seen. Tumor cells have scant cytoplasm, large nuclei, finely granular chromatin, and prominent nucleoli (Papanicolaou stain, 40×).

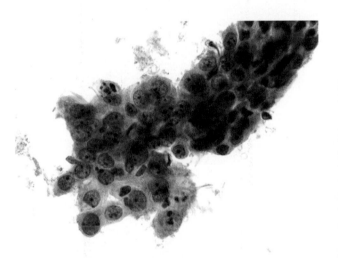

FIGURE 4-22 Transbronchial fine needle aspiration of a moderately to poorly differentiated squamous cell carcinoma. The tumor cells are cohesive, have ill-defined cell borders, high nuclear-to-cytoplasmic ratios, finely granular chromatin, and prominent nucleoli (Papanicolaou stain, 40×).

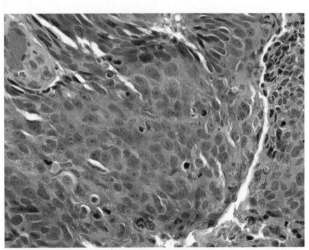

FIGURE 4-24 Endobronchial biopsy of the poorly differentiated portion of the squamous cell carcinoma shown in *Figure 4-25* (hematoxylin and eosin, 40×).

Keratinization is focal or may be completely absent. The chromatin tends to be granular rather than hyperchromatic, and nucleoli may be prominent. In aspirates of poorly differentiated carcinomas, immunohistochemistry on cell block preparations may be essential for accurately classifying tumors.

Differential Diagnosis

The cytomorphologic distinction between the well-differentiated forms of pulmonary squamous cell carcinoma and adenocarcinoma is usually straightforward (*Tables 4-2* and *4-3*). Whereas well-differentiated

Table 4-2 Cytologic Differential Diagnosis of Pulmonary Squamous Cell Carcinoma

Malignant
- Adenocarcinoma
- Squamous cell carcinoma from the upper aerodigestive tract
- Small cell carcinoma

Benign
- Mesothelial cells
- Squamous metaplasia/reactive or reparative changes
- Radiation/chemotherapy effect
- Vegetable matter

Table 4-3 Comparison of Cytologic Features of Well-Differentiated and Moderately to Poorly Differentiated Pulmonary Squamous Cell Carcinoma With Common Differential Diagnoses

Cytologic Feature	Squamous Cell Carcinoma, Well-Differentiated	Squamous Cell Carcinoma, Moderately to Poorly Differentiated	Adenocarcinoma	Mesothelial Cells	Reactive Squamous Cells
Low-power appearance	Single, dispersed cells ± necrosis	Cohesive tissue fragments ± single cells and necrosis	Variable depending on subtype: loosely cohesive three-dimensional clusters, papillae, disorganized honeycomb-like sheets, single cells	Flat, loosely cohesive sheets with slit-like spaces between cells ("windows")	Clusters with few single cells ± necrosis; adjacent injury and/or inflammation may be present
Cytoplasm	Keratinized, dense, glassy cytoplasm that can stain eosinophilic (H&E), orangeophilic (Papanicolaou stain), or robin's-egg blue (Romanowsky stain) Polygonal to elongated spindle and tadpole shapes Keratin pearls	Usually more uniform cytology than keratinizing, well-differentiated forms Focal to absent keratinization Dense and smooth cytoplasm	Vacuolated, foamy, translucent ± cytoplasmic mucin	Abundant, dense cytoplasm with lighter/paler periphery	Keratinization can be variable
Cell borders	Well-defined with intercellular bridges	Poorly defined			
N/C ratio	Lower	Higher	Variable	Lower	Low to normal
Nuclear placement	Usually central	Usually central	Can be eccentric	Usually central	
Nuclear shape	Small and pyknotic to large, often angular and irregular contours	Large, variably irregular	Ovoid, may be variably grooved and irregular	Round/oval, variably grooved	Ovoid, typically smooth contoured
Chromatin	Dense, hyperchromatic	Finely granular, pale	Finely granular, pale (can be coarse in poorly differentiated tumors)	Finely granular	Finely granular, pale
Nucleoli	Not prominent	Often prominent	Often prominent	Small, can be prominent	Often prominent

squamous cell carcinomas typically appear as single cells dispersed in a necrotic background on cytology specimens, adenocarcinomas are characteristically aspirated as loosely cohesive three-dimensional clusters, disorganized honeycomb-like sheets, and papillae with a variable amount of singly dispersed cells. Adenocarcinomas also tend to have foamy, variably vacuolated cytoplasm, occasional cytoplasmic mucin, and ovoid nuclei with prominent nucleoli. Of note, a subset of adenocarcinomas may demonstrate abundant, densely eosinophilic cytoplasm, mimicking the cytomorphology of squamous cell carcinoma.[98,99] Small cell carcinoma may also overlap in cytomorphology with poorly differentiated squamous cell carcinoma, particularly in cases in which the squamous cells adopt a basaloid appearance. In cases where the cytomorphology does not indicate a specific line of differentiation, a minimal panel of immunohistochemical stains (discussed below) may help establish the diagnosis.

For sputum samples and specimens obtained endoscopically, squamous dysplasias and squamous cell carcinomas of the upper aerodigestive tract (UADT) may be sampled unintentionally. Attempts to distinguish squamous cell carcinomas arising in the lung versus those arising from a head/neck primary site have been described, but there are no specific markers to date that separate these two entities.[100,101] Ultimately, this distinction rests on clinical history and imaging findings; a history of UADT dysplasia or carcinoma and the absence of a dominant lung mass on imaging would favor UADT contamination.

With their large polygonal shapes and abundant eosinophilic cytoplasm, benign and malignant mesothelial cells can also mimic squamous cell carcinomas, particularly in transthoracic FNA specimens in which incidental sampling of the mesothelium may occur. In contrast to squamous cell carcinomas, mesothelial cells are often aspirated as loosely cohesive sheets with intercellular spaces ("windows"). Mesothelial cells also have fine chromatin, grooved nuclei, and a characteristic "two-tone" cytoplasm with dense perinuclear and lighter peripheral zones, the latter of which may have a "frilled skirt" appearance due to the presence of long microvilli.

Airway epithelium can undergo squamous metaplasia and reactive changes in the setting of acute lung injury and necrotizing/cavitary lesions (such as tuberculosis, fungal infections, abscess, and bronchiectasis with pneumonia). Compared to squamous cell carcinoma, reactive/reparative squamous epithelium tend to be more cohesive, be smaller in size, show less nuclear pleomorphism, and have smudgier chromatin.[102] However, in some cytologic specimens, the presence of necroinflammatory debris and keratinizing cells with degenerative atypia may be difficult to distinguish from squamous cell carcinoma; in these cases, an indeterminate (ie, atypical or suspicious) cytologic diagnosis may be appropriate to avoid a false-positive interpretation, particularly when the clinical history and/or radiographic findings suggests an inflammatory or infectious process.

Radiation and chemotherapy-induced atypia is characterized by cytomegaly (resulting in low or normal nuclear-to-cytoplasmic ratios), cytoplasmic and nuclear vacuolation, multinucleation, pale to finely granular chromatin, and prominent nucleoli.

Vegetable matter—either from oral contaminant or aspirated into the lungs—may also mimic squamous cells due to their distinct cell borders and pyknotic nuclei. However, the rigidity and regularity of the cell walls should help distinguish plant cells from squamous epithelium.

IMMUNOHISTOCHEMICAL FEATURES OF SQUAMOUS CELL CARCINOMA

A variety of markers have been reported in pulmonary squamous cell carcinomas. While many of these antibodies are sensitive for squamous differentiation, most suffer from only moderate specificity, particularly in their ability to distinguish squamous cell carcinoma from adenocarcinoma. Therefore, a limited panel of antibodies—preferably used in a stepwise algorithmic approach—is recommended to permit specific subtyping of poorly differentiated NSCLC (discussed in next section). Evolving markers with greater specificity for squamous differentiation (eg, ΔNp63/p40) and the combination of antibody panels into cocktails that can be applied to single slides may allow better specificity while conserving tissue for molecular analysis.[103-105] A brief description of antibodies supporting squamous differentiation is provided here.

Cytokeratins (Cytoplasmic Staining)

Lung squamous cell carcinomas typically show diffuse and strong cytoplasmic staining with antibody cocktails against pan-cytokeratin (eg, AE1/AE3) and high molecular weight cytokeratins such as CK903 (34βE12) and cytokeratin 5/6. However, the utility of these markers for NSCLC subtyping is limited by variable staining in lung adenocarcinomas as well.[106-108] Most pulmonary squamous cell carcinomas also express low molecular weight cytokeratins such as those detected by Cam5.2. In contrast to lung adenocarcinomas, which generally show a CK7+/CK20− immunophenotype, the majority of pulmonary squamous cell carcinomas are negative for both CK7 and CK20.[109,110]

p63 (Nuclear Staining)

P63 is a p53-related transcription factor that is important for epithelial development. As such, p63 is expressed in squamous epithelia of various tissues, basal/myoepithelial cells of glandular structures such as breast and prostate, and reserve cells of the respiratory tract. Squamous cell carcinoma consistently shows nuclear expression of p63, but variable levels of p63 staining can also be seen in lung adenocarcinomas well as lung small cell carcinomas, lymphomas, and other tumor types.[107,108,111-119] The *p63* gene encodes multiple isoforms, including those with a functional transactivation domain at the N-terminus of the protein (TA-p63) and those lacking the N-terminal transactivation domain (ΔNp63). TA-p63 is thought to function as a tumor suppressor gene, much like p53; in contrast, ΔNp63 (discussed below) may operate as an oncogene based on its role in stem/progenitor-cell maintenance.[120-122] Most immunohistochemistry laboratories currently use anti-p63 monoclonal antibody clone 4A4, which recognizes both TA-p63 and ΔNp63 isoforms.

ΔNp63 (p40) (Nuclear Staining)

The p40 antibody specifically recognizes p63 isoforms that lack the N-terminal transactivation domain (ΔNp63). Several studies have demonstrated that p40 shows superior specificity and equivalent sensitivity for detecting squamous cell carcinoma, compared to the p63 4A4 antibody.[123-125] In the rare lung adenocarcinomas that have been reported to show ΔNp63/p40 immunoreactivity, positive staining was limited to 5% or less of the tumor cells.[123,124] In contrast to p63, ΔNp63/p40 has not been detected in small cell lung carcinomas or large cell lymphomas.[114,123]

Desmosomal Proteins (Membranous/Cytoplasmic Staining)

Recent studies have reported increased expression of some desmosomal cell adhesion proteins (desmocollin-3, desmoglein-3, and plakophilin-1) in squamous cell carcinomas compared to adenocarcinomas. Additionally, desmocollin-3 appears to have high specificity in distinguishing squamous cell carcinoma from neuroendocrine carcinomas.[126] While these markers appear specific for squamous cell carcinoma, their utility is limited by their relatively low sensitivity, particularly in poorly differentiated squamous cell carcinomas.[108,127,128] Therefore, while staining for desmocollin-3 supports squamous differentiation, its absence is not helpful for subtyping NSCLC.

Miscellaneous Squamous Markers

Additional markers that have recently been investigated for recognizing squamous cell carcinomas include glypican-3, S100A2, S100A7, and SOX2.[108,126,129]

The sensitivity and specificity of these markers vary between reports, and their utility in NSCLC subtyping remains to be established.

Issues in Differentiating Pulmonary Squamous Cell Carcinoma From Other Tumors by Immunohistochemistry

Thyroid transcription factor 1 (TTF-1/NKX2-1) and the aspartic proteinase Napsin A are markers with high specificity for lung adenocarcinoma.[106-108,124,130-137] However, focal or weak nuclear staining of squamous cell carcinomas for TTF-1 has been described in rare cases; this aberrant staining pattern appears to be more common using the SPT24 clone compared to the 8G7G3/1 clone of TTF-1 monoclonal antibodies.[107,138] Similarly, a few studies have reported the detection of Napsin A staining in pulmonary squamous cell carcinomas.[104,136,139,140] In addition, pulmonary macrophages and type 2 pneumocytes are also immunoreactive for Napsin A; when entrapped within a tumor or present in small biopsy or cellblock specimens, these cells may be a source of false-positive Napsin A immunoreactivity in some squamous cell carcinomas that may be misinterpreted as adenocarcinoma.[141]

To date, there is no marker that reliably distinguishes primary squamous cell carcinoma of the lung from squamous cell carcinomas arising from other sites. As a surrogate marker for high-risk HPV infection, strong p16 staining in squamous cell carcinomas has been suggested to indicate origin from the uterine cervix (or, by extension, a subset of oropharyngeal squamous cell carcinomas) instead of the lung. However, p16 immunoreactivity has been shown in 21% to 35% of pulmonary squamous cell carcinomas, so its effectiveness in excluding pulmonary origin is limited.[142,143]

MOLECULAR FEATURES OF SQUAMOUS CELL CARCINOMA

Recent advances in the field of cancer biology and therapeutics have led to the discovery of oncogenic driver mutations and the development of targeted agents that have shown substantial efficacy in clinical trials.[31,34] Unfortunately, however, the effective targeted therapies have disproportionally impacted adenocarcinomas compared to squamous cell carcinomas.[144] It is likely attributed to a high overall mutation rate and marked genomic complexity of lung squamous cell carcinoma[145] that makes the identification of driver mutations difficult. Nevertheless, alterations of multiple genes and pathways have been examined in squamous cell carcinoma by means of somatic copy number alterations, whole genome/exome sequencing, gene expression, and DNA methylation, and histologic subtype specific alterations (compared to those of lung adenocarcinoma) have been reported.[146] Selected alterations that appear to have clinical implications are discussed here.

Somatic Copy Number Alteration

At the level of whole chromosome arm somatic copy number alterations (SCNAs), the most significant difference between squamous cell carcinoma and adenocarcinoma is a selective amplification of chromosome 3q in lung squamous cell carcinoma[145-147]; Amplification of 8q is also more specific for squamous cell carcinoma.[146,147] Candidate oncogenes located in those regions include *SOX2* and *PIK3CA* (3q) and *FGFR1* and *BRF2* (8q).[146] Of those, high-level amplification of *SOX2* (located on chromosome 3q26) has been reported in approximately 20% of lung squamous cell carcinomas.[148,149]

SOX2 is a transcription factor and is a critical regulator of normal stem cell function in embryonic and neural stem cells.[150-152] It is thought to play a crucial role in the development of airway epithelium.[153] The recent study by Bass et al has demonstrated SOX2 expression is required for proliferation and independent growth of lung cell lines; however, ectopic expression of SOX2 alone was not able to transform immortalized tracheobronchial epithelial cells.[149] Thus, *SOX2* amplification is not qualified as a "driver" event, and may represent a "priming" event that requires additional downstream events to be fully transforming.[144]

Similarly, amplification of *FGFR1* (located on chromosome 8p12) is enriched in squamous cell carcinomas compared to adenocarcinomas, and has been reported in approximately 20% of lung squamous cell carcinomas.[154] FGFR1 is a member of the FGFR family of receptor tyrosine kinase and its activation results in downstream signaling via PI3K/AKT and/or RAS/MAPK pathways that, in turn, promote cell growth, survival migration, and angiogenesis in various cancers.[155] Dysregulation of the FGFR1-4 signaling has been demonstrated in multiple cancers, but *FGFR1* mutations are rare in lung cancer.[145] Currently, multiple multitargeted tyrosine kinase inhibitors that have activity against FGFR1 are in development, and some are being evaluated specifically for lung cancers harboring *FGFR1* amplification (https://clinicaltrials.gov/). Thus *FGFR1* florescence in situ hybridization (FISH) to detect amplification is being implemented as part of clinical molecular testing (*Figure 4-25*).

Gene Mutations

The most comprehensive sequencing analyses of lung squamous cell carcinomas (n = 178), performed by the Cancer Genome Atlas (TCGA) research network, has identified a number of frequently mutated genes. They are *TP53, CDKN2A, PTEN, PIK3CA, KEAP1, MLL2, HLA-A, NFE2L2, NOTCH1,* and *RB1*.[145] In addition,

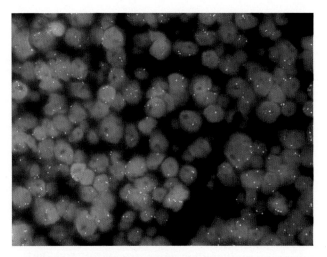

FIGURE 4-25 FGFR amplification: Fluorescence in situ hybridization (FISH) of fibroblast growth factor receptor 1 (FGFR1) demonstrates FGFR1 gene amplification in this tumor. Amplified FGFR1 is seen as an isolated cluster of red signals. Of note, the amplification is present in some and not all tumor cells.

individual sequencing studies of lung squamous cell carcinomas have reported recurrent mutations in several additional genes, including *BAI3, FBXW7, GRN8, MUC16, RUNX1T1, STK11, ERBB4, AKT1,* and *DDR2*.[145,156-158] Notably, *KRAS* and *EGFR* mutations that are frequently seen in lung adenocarcinomas, as well as gene rearrangements, are (vanishingly) rare in squamous cell carcinomas.[146]

Among the aforementioned mutations, those in *TP53* (located on chromosome 17p13) are a frequent event in lung cancer, present in the majority of NSCLCs including 65% of squamous cell carcinomas,[159] while mutations of *NFE2L2* (*NRF2*), *AKT1,* and *DDR2* are predominantly seen in squamous cell carcinomas.[146] Of those, *NFE2L2* (*NRF2*) mutations are identified in 10% to 15% of lung squamous cell carcinomas (as opposed to 1%-2% of adenocarcinomas).[145,158,160-162] *NRF2* (located on chromosome 2q31) is a redox-sensitive transcription factor that regulates the expression of antioxidant enzymes and several antiapoptotic proteins, which confer cytoprotection against endogenous and oxidative stress. *KEAP1* (located on chromosome 19p13) negatively regulates *NRF2* activity by targeting it for degradation. Mutations in *NRF2* interfere with proper *NRF2-KEAP1* binding and inhibit KEAP1-mediated degradation of NRF2.[158] *KEAP1* mutations and LOH have been reported in lung cancer and result in NFR2 activation, but *KEAP1* mutations have been predominantly identified in adenocarcinomas.[160] In addition, aberrant expressions of *NRF2* and *KEAP1* are more prevalent than mutations in lung cancer, suggesting the involvement of other mechanisms for NRF2/KEAP1 pathway dysregulation.[163]

CHAPTER 4

A somatic mutation in *AKT* (located on 14q32), *E17K*, that involves the pleckstrin homology domain, constitutively activates the protein kinase. The *AKT1 E17K* mutation has been found in 5.5% of 36 squamous cell lung cancers along with 2% to 6% of other cancers, but not in lung adenocarcinoma (0/53).[164,165] The *AKT1* mutation is mutually exclusive with those in *PIK3CA* and complete loss of PTEN protein expression, indicating that the *AKT1* mutation is sufficient for pathologic activation of PI3K/AKT pathway.[164] Several AKT inhibitors are in clinical development, it remains unknown whether cancers with these mutations will be sensitive to single-agent AKT inhibitors.[144]

DDR2 (located on 1q23) is a receptor tyrosine kinase that binds collagen and has been shown to promote cell migration, proliferation, and survival.[166,167] A study has shown *DDR2* kinase gene mutations in 3.2% (9/277) of primary lung squamous cell cancers and 15% (2/13) of cell lines.[156] Knockdown of *DDR2* by RNA interference or by the multitargeted kinase inhibitor, dasatinib, in cell lines with *DDR2* mutations led to inhibition of proliferation, and ectopic expression of mutated *DDR2* led to cellular transformation. Furthermore, a patient with lung squamous cell carcinoma that responded to dasatinib and erlotinib treatment harbored a *DDR2* kinase domain mutation.[156] Although preliminary, these results suggest that these mutations may be oncogenic, and tumors harboring *DDR2* mutations may be sensitive to drugs that inhibit its kinase activity.

DNA Methylation

Although the data are limited, integration of global DNA methylation and the corresponding gene expression profiles indicate that aberrant DNA methylation may play a role in DNA replication, recombination, and repair functions. In addition, methylation of *HOXA2* and *HOXA10* genes may have prognostic significance.[168,169]

miRNA

miRNA signatures may be able to classify lung cancers into histologic subtypes more accurately than global mRNA expression profiles.[170] Of those, miR-205 appears to be highly specific for squamous cell carcinoma.[171]

Somatically Altered Pathways

The integration of data obtained by the various types of molecular assays provides a more comprehensive understanding of tumor biology. The inclusion of pathway or network analysis can aid in interpreting how a set of alterations work in conjunction to promote tumors. Several affected pathways have been identified in lung squamous cell carcinoma. In the TCGA study, genes involved in oxidative stress response and squamous differentiation were frequently altered. The former consisted of mutations and SCNAs of *NFR2* and *KEAP1* and/or deletion or mutation of *CUL3*. Mutations in *KEAP1* and *CUL3* showed a pattern consistent with loss of function, and were mutually exclusive with mutations in *NFR2*. They were collectively found in 34% of cases. The latter consisted of overexpression and amplification of *SOX2* and *TP63*, loss-of-function mutations in *NONTCH1*, *NOTCH2*, and *ASCL4* and focal deletions in *FOXP1*, and were collectively identified in 44% of samples. Similar to the oxidative stress response pathway, alterations in *NOTCH1*, *NOTCH2*, and *ASCL4* were mutually exclusive and exhibited minimal overlap with amplification of *TP63* and/or *SOX2*, indicating that alterations in individual genes within the pathway have overlapping functional consequences. In addition, there were frequent alterations in *CDKN2A*/RB1 and PI3K/AKT pathways. Of therapeutic relevance, approximately 70% of lung squamous cell carcinomas had alterations in one of the PI3K/AKT, receptor tyrosine kinase, or RAS/MAPK pathways in which multiple inhibitors are available or in development.[145]

mRNA Expression Profiling and Subtype Classification

Lung squamous cell carcinoma can be classified into subtypes not only by histology, but also by molecular profiling. A study using five published discovery cohorts and one validation cohort has identified four subtypes of lung squamous cell carcinoma based on the difference in mRNA expressions.[172] They are primitive, classical, basal, and secretory subtypes, and appear to have different survival outcomes, patient populations, and biological processes.

The primitive subtype is characterized by overexpression of genes associated with cellular proliferation (MCM10, E2F3, TS, and POLA1), and is associated with the highest female ratio, poorly differentiated histology, and worst recurrence free and overall survivals compared to the other subtypes. The classical subtype exhibits genes associated with xenobiotic metabolism, which detoxifies foreign chemicals, and is enriched with a gene signature derived from lung cell lines exposed to cigarette smoke, including genes such as *AKR1C3*. This subtype has the greatest concentration of smokers and the heavy smoking history, the highest male ratio, and overexpression of *TP63*, *SOX2*, and *PIK3CA*, recapitulating conventional squamous cell carcinoma of the lung.[145] Genes associated with immune response including *NF-κB* targeted genes are overexpressed in the secretory subtype. This type also overexpresses the lung secretory cell markers including *MUC1* and pulmonary surfactant proteins. Interestingly, genes, are commonly expressed in normal submucosal glands, as well as *TTF-1* are overexpressed in the secretory subtype compared to the other types. The basal subtype expression profile reveals overexpression of genes associated with cell adhesion, epidermal development, including *keratin 5*, and several *S100* family genes, including *S100A2* that is a marker specific for the basal layer of the lung epithelium and squamous cell carcinoma.[173] In addition, the basal subtype is enriched with genes whose products are localized in the basement membrane. Interestingly, this subtype is associated with well-differentiated histology and the least extrapulmonary recurrence compared to the other subtypes, and thus, it appears to be distinct from the morphologic basaloid variant (despite the similarity in the terminology).

The aforementioned TCGA study confirmed the four subtypes, and also found considerable correlations between the expression subtypes and genomic alterations in copy number, mutation, and methylation. For instance, the classical subtype is characterized by alterations in *KEAP1*, *NFR2*, and *PTEN*, as well as pronounced hypermethylation and chromosomal instability, but is negatively associated with amplification of *FGFR1* and *WHSC1L1*. By contrast, the primitive expression subtype more commonly exhibited *RB1* and *PTEN* alterations, and the basal subtype harbors *NF1* alterations.[145]

DIFFERENTIAL DIAGNOSIS OF SQUAMOUS CELL CARCINOMA OF THE LUNG

The differential diagnoses of pulmonary squamous cell carcinoma are broad and include other types of lung cancer, squamous cell carcinoma metastatic or extension from other organs, and benign diseases (*Table 4-4*). Of those, the one that we most frequently encounter in daily practice is poorly differentiated NSCLCs; in particular, adenocarcinoma with solid pattern since a pseudosquamous appearance may be seen in a decent

minority of lung adenocarcinomas.[72] Keratinization is a pathognomonic feature of squamous cell carcinoma, thus differential diagnosis arises mainly in poorly differentiated tumors or small biopsy specimens showing no morphological features of squamous cell differentiation. In these cases, a limited panel of immunomarkers (p40 or p63/TTF-1) and a mucin stain are necessary to differentiate the two entities (refer to the Approach to the Diagnosis of Poorly Differentiated Squamous Cell Carcinoma on Small Biopsy Specimens section). Of note, focal intracellular mucin can occasionally be present in tumors that are clearly squamous cell carcinoma.[1] The other differential diagnoses are discussed individually.

Neuroendocrine Carcinoma

Both large cell neuroendocrine carcinoma and small cell carcinoma are differential diagnoses of squamous cell carcinoma, in particular, the basaloid variant. Palisading and rosette-like structures can be seen in the latter, thus mimicking large cell neuroendocrine carcinoma (*Figure 4-26*). Cytologic features useful in differentiating the basaloid variant from large cell neuroendocrine carcinoma include smaller cell size, higher N/Cs, and lack of nucleoli.[87,90,174] The small cell variant of squamous cell carcinoma (or basaloid variant with a small cell size) has tumor cells of very small size that can closely resemble small cell carcinoma. In cytology, features helpful in distinguishing the two entities include greater intercellular cohesion, less apoptotic bodies, more vesicular chromatin and visible nucleoli, a lack of pyknotic-like chromatin, focal squamous

Table 4-4 Histologic Differential Diagnosis of Pulmonary Squamous Cell Carcinoma

Malignant
- Adenocarcinoma with solid pattern
- Large cell carcinoma
- Large cell neuroendocrine carcinoma
- Small cell carcinoma
- Thymic carcinoma
- Metastasis from other organs (eg, head and neck, esophagus, cervix)
- Adenoid cystic carcinoma
- NUT carcinoma

Benign
- Squamous papilloma
- Diffuse alveolar damage with squamous metaplasia

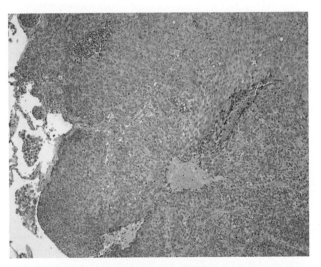

FIGURE 4-26 Large cell neuroendocrine carcinoma demonstrating a lobular growth of polygonal tumor cells with peripheral palisading and comedo necrosis mimicking the basaloid variant of squamous cell carcinoma.

differentiation, and less conspicuous rosettes and molding, favoring the squamous cell carcinoma variant over small cell carcinoma.[87,90,174] Unfortunately, however, distinguishing the two entities in biopsy samples, especially in poorly preserved or crushed specimens, can be extremely difficult, since peripheral palisading that facilitates separation of basaloid from nonbasaloid tumors may be obscured, as may the nuclear features that aid in the distinction in those samples.

Immunohistochemistry may be of value in assessing the differential diagnosis. Diffuse, strong keratin p40, p63, or CK5/6 that characterizes squamous cell carcinomas is absent in the neuroendocrine carcinomas. Conversely, diffuse staining of multiple neuroendocrine markers and TTF-1, characteristic of most neuroendocrine carcinomas, are not seen in squamous cell carcinomas, although CD56 can be infrequently positive in the latter.[87,114,174,175]

Thymic Carcinoma

A primary pulmonary squamous cell carcinoma with massive involvement of the anterior mediastinal tissue can be difficult to differentiate from thymic squamous cell carcinoma. The differentiation requires careful correlation with operative and radiologic findings. Immunohistochemistry may aid in differentiating the two entities since immunoreactivity to Pax8 and FOXN1 has been reported in the majority of thymic carcinomas, while these markers are usually negative in primary lung carcinomas.[176]

Metastasis From Other Organs

Distinguishing primary lung squamous cell carcinoma from metastasis in patients with prior history of squamous cell carcinoma of other sites, such as head and neck, esophagus, or cervix can be challenging and often requires genotypic fingerprinting, such as p53 mutation and/or LOH involving microsatellite markers[100,101,177,178] or HPV genotyping.[179-181] Of note, p16 immunostaining that is used as a surrogate marker for the presence of HPV in the cervix or head and neck may not be useful in this setting since p16 is overexpressed in 40% of primary lung cancers that do not harbor HPV.[180]

Adenoid Cystic Carcinoma

Adenoid cystic carcinoma of the solid or basaloid type can resemble the basaloid variant.[182,183] Ancillary tests that help to separate the two entities include immunohistochemistry for CD117 and myoepithelial markers such as smooth muscle actin and demonstration of MYB gene rearrangements by FISH.[184,185]

NUT Carcinoma

NUT carcinoma is a primitive tumor of a squamous lineage that portends a poor prognosis. It is defined by the presence of a t(15;19) chromosomal translocation, driven by the resultant *BRD4-NUT* fusion oncogene. The distinction of NUT carcinoma from poorly differentiated squamous cell carcinoma is challenging as they share squamous differentiation and immunophenotype (*Figure 4-27*), and can only be made using *NUT* FISH and/or a highly specific monoclonal NUT antibody.[186]

Squamous Papilloma

Differentiation of very well-differentiated central airway squamous carcinoma of the papillary variant from squamous papilloma can be difficult, requiring demonstration of invasion.[80]

Benign Conditions

Squamous metaplasia with cytologic atypia in diffuse alveolar damage (DAD) may also be confused with squamous cell carcinoma. The presence of characteristic features of DAD such as hyaline membranes, diffuse alveolar septal connective tissue proliferation, pneumocyte hyperplasia along with bronchiolocentricity of the squamous changes would favor a metaplastic process. In the lung parenchyma, squamous cell carcinoma not infrequently entraps alveolar pneumocytes. The latter may exhibit reactive atypia (*Figure 4-28*), leading to histological misinterpretation as adenosquamous carcinoma.

Adenosquamous Carcinoma Versus Squamous Cell Carcinoma With a Minor Component of Adenocarcinoma

Adenosquamous carcinoma is defined as a tumor showing components of squamous cell carcinoma and adenocarcinoma, each component comprising at least 10% of the tumor.[187] Growing evidence, however, supports the importance of reporting a minor component of the histologic subtypes comprising <10%, since tumors with mixed features can reflect the genetic status of either component regardless of the proportion. Tumors with a minor (<10%) component of (unequivocal) adenocarcinoma in otherwise classic squamous cell carcinoma may harbor oncogenic mutations, which are typically seen in adenocarcinomas such as *KRAS* and *EGFR* mutations, much more frequently than pure squamous cell carcinomas.[188,189]

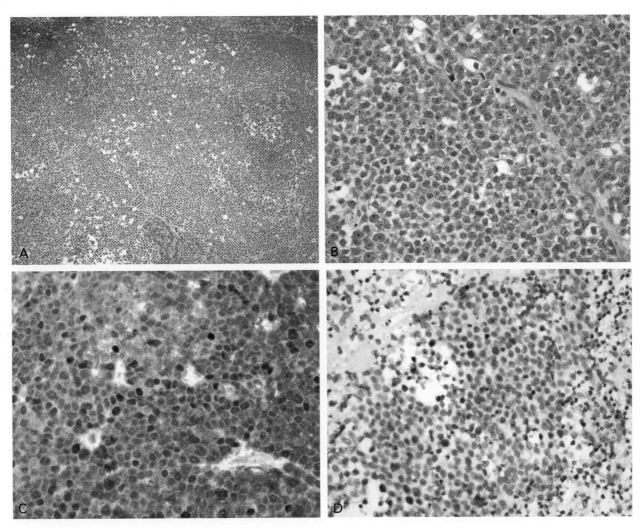

FIGURE 4-27 An example of NUT carcinoma consists of diffuse and monotonous sheets (A) of undifferentiated tumor cells (B). Immunohistochemistry reveals the expressions of p63 (C) and NUT (D) in the tumor cells, confirming the diagnosis.

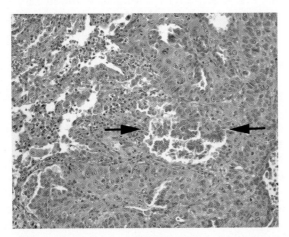

FIGURE 4-28 Squamous cell carcinoma extending into alveolar spaces and adjacent, reactive pneumocytes with a micropapillary pattern of proliferation mimicking adenocarcinoma. This combination may lead to a misinterpretation of adenosquamous cell carcinoma.

HEREDITARY SYNDROMES ASSOCIATED WITH SQUAMOUS CELL CARCINOMA

There have been no hereditary syndromes identified in association with lung squamous cell carcinoma. Genome-wide studies of patients with lung cancer, however, have revealed the association between squamous cell carcinoma and polymorphic variation in the 9p21 (*CDKN2A/CDKN2B*), and 12q13.33 (*RAD52*) loci,[190-193] as well as 6p21-22.[193,194] Recently, Wang et al also showed the association of rare variants 13q13.1 (*BRCA2*) and 22q12.1 (*CHEK2*) with squamous cell carcinoma.[195] Given the recent implementation of next generation sequencing in clinical molecular testing, additional susceptibility genes/factors may be discovered in lung squamous cell carcinoma in the future.

CHAPTER 4

PRECURSOR LESIONS OF SQUAMOUS CELL CARCINOMA

Squamous Metaplasia

Squamous metaplasia is characterized by focal or diffuse replacement of the normal ciliated columnar epithelial cells by stratified squamous epithelial cells (*Figure 4-29*). Squamous metaplasia is a common finding in tobacco smokers, and its incidence and extent increases in proportion to smoking history.[196,197] It is thought that the rugged stratified squamous epithelium may be more resistant to the noxious chemicals in cigarette smoke that the ciliated columnar epithelium would not tolerate, and the phenotypic change likely arises by reprogramming of stem cells to differentiate along a new pathway rather than transdifferentiation of the columnar epithelium to squamous epithelium.[198] Given the frequent association with chronic inflammation and lack of evidence that links to increased risk for developing lung cancer, squamous metaplasia represents reactive changes as opposed to true neoplastic (preinvasive) lesions.[197,199-201]

Squamous Dysplasia and Squamous Cell Carcinoma In Situ

Squamous dysplasia and carcinoma in situ (CIS) constitute preinvasive lesions of lung squamous cell carcinoma. The preinvasive lesion occurs in individuals with significant tobacco smoking history (more than 30 pack years of cigarette smoking) and with obstructive airway disease, but the lesion itself seldom leads to symptoms.[202,203] Dysplastic foci may persist in the airway for many years but progression of individual lesions to malignancy is rare.[204,205] A chance of developing into invasive squamous cell carcinoma, however, increases as dysplasia progresses, and 19% to as many as 50% of

patients with severe dysplasia and the majority of those with CIS develop invasive lesions.[206,207] Since the entire central airway is exposed to tobacco smoking, squamous dysplasia and CIS may develop anywhere in the airway, typically as multiple lesions, the phenomenon is well-known as "field cancerization,"[204,207,208] although they may occur at a single site. Of those, foci of CIS usually arise near bifurcations of segmental bronchi, subsequently extending proximally into the adjacent lobar bronchus and distally into segmental branches. The lesions are less frequently seen in the trachea.[209]

Given the high rate of severe dysplasia developing into invasive squamous cell carcinoma,[206] early diagnosis and treatment of preinvasive lesions are important. Unfortunately, however, routine white-light bronchoscopy is not useful to diagnose these lesions, since it can detect only one-quarter of moderate to severe dysplasia and CIS lesions.[210] In order to improve the detection of high-grade dysplastic lesions, image-enhanced endoscopies including autofluorescence bronchoscopy (AFB) and narrow band imaging (NBI), endobronchial ultrasonography (EBUS), and optical coherence tomography (OCT) are warranted. AFB uses different wavelengths of light to enhance a contrast between normal bronchial tissue and malignant lesion.[211] A meta-analysis has shown the high sensitivity and moderate specificity of AFB, 90% and 56%, respectively.[212] The clinician can evaluate microvascular structures of tissue by NBI, irradiating special blue light and green light.[213] The sensitivity of NBI for preinvasive lesions has been reported to be from 90% to 100 %.[206] OCT, which is similar to an ultrasound imaging using an infrared light instead of sound, is also expected to be useful in the diagnosis of preinvasive lesions.

Morphologically, preinvasive lesions of lung squamous cell carcinoma encompass a broad range of cytoarchitectural atypia. Grading of preinvasive lesions is similar to that in other sites such as the cervix and esophagus. Some prefer a four-tiered grading system consisting of mild, moderate, and severe dysplasia, as well as CIS, while others tend to lump the grades together into low-grade (*Figure 4-30*) and high-grade preinvasive lesions, the latter category including CIS (*Figure 4-31*). With increasing grades of dysplasia, neoplastic cells involve and replace more of the epithelium, but the lesion remains confined to the basement membrane. Mild dysplasia is characterized by minimal cytological and architectural abnormalities with basal zone expansion with increased cellularity and vertically oriented nuclei limited to the lower third of the epithelial layer. Mitoses are absent or very rare. Importantly, there is continuous progression of maturation from base to luminal surface. Moderate dysplasia exhibits more cytologic abnormalities, but still has finely granular cytoplasm. Progression of maturation from base to luminal surface is only partially present,

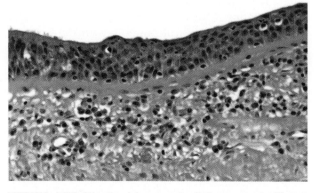

FIGURE 4-29 Focal replacement of the normal ciliated columnar epithelial cells by stratified squamous epithelial cells (squamous metaplasia).

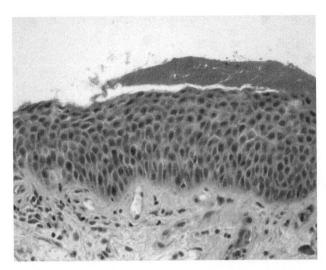

FIGURE 4-30 An example of low-grade squamous dysplasia.

and Basal zone expansion with cellular crowding and vertically oriented nuclei occupy the lower two-thirds of the epithelium. Mitotic figures are present, but are limited in the lower third. Severe dysplasia is characterized by prominent cellular pleomorphism, coarse and uneven chromatin, and frequent and conspicuous nucleoli. Basal zone expansion reached the upper third, but superficial cell flattening is still identified, and vertically oriented nuclei and mitotic figures are confined to the lower two-thirds. In contrast to dysplasia, maturation is essentially absent in CIS, and thus, the epithelium could be inverted with little change in appearance. CIS exhibits significant cytologic abnormalities with coarse and uneven chromatin. There is no consistent orientation of nuclei in relation to epithelial surface and mitotic figures are present through full thickness of the epithelium. Both squamous

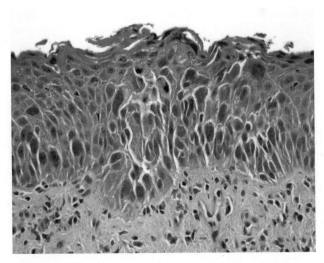

FIGURE 4-31 An example of high-grade squamous dysplasia.

dysplasia and CIS typically show a flat morphology, and the thickness of epithelial cell layer increases along with the progression of dysplasia, while CIS may or may not appear thickened. However, a more unusual form exists where the CIS exhibits an exophytic, polypoid, or papillary growth without mucosal invasion (*Figure 4-32A*).[209,214]

In a subset of squamous dysplastic changes, the basal membrane thickens and there are capillary loops projecting into the dysplastic bronchial lining that results in papillary protrusions of the epithelium. These lesions are termed angiogenic squamous dysplasia. LOH at chromosome 3p has been reported in about half of such lesions, but no confirmed *TP53* mutations have been identified. Thus, angiogenic squamous dysplasia may reflect aberrant patterns of microvascularization at an early stage of bronchial carcinogenesis.[215,216]

Given that the cytoarchitectural abnormalities are on the spectrum, there can be considerable overlap between the four categories, and a range of dysplasia may be seen within any particular case. As such, there are problems of reproducibility in the dysplasia grading, although one study involving pathologists with different levels of experience has shown that interobserver and intraobserver concordance on grading of preinvasive lesions of the lung squamous cell carcinoma was similar to that in other grading systems in histopathology, with no significant decrease in variability by abridging the system.[217] Another issue associated with grading of dysplasia is its partial involvement of the epithelial layer. Squamous metaplasia (and subsequent squamous dysplasia) is believed to develop the preexisting basal cell hyperplasia. Squamous differentiation may occur in the basal cell layer undermining differentiated respiratory epithelium (immature squamous metaplasia). If the neoplastic process starts before the squamous metaplasia replaces the full thickness of respiratory epithelium, marked cytologic atypia may be seen underneath ciliated and/or mucus secreting columnar cells. It is difficult to apply the grading system that is made for a full-thickness squamous epithelium to the partially transformed epithelium. In this setting, the assessment only on the epithelium with squamous differentiation using a two-tiered grading system (low grade vs high grade) appears to be more practical.[214] In any case, grading of preinvasive squamous lesions may not be clinically relevant since they are not visible under conventional bronchoscopy, and thus, the surgical pathologist infrequently encounters these lesions in endoscopic biopsy material. Whereas squamous dysplasia and/or CIS are relatively frequent in lung resection specimens for lung cancer from cigarette smokers, classification of the preinvasive lesions is less important in this context, outside of any academic considerations. However, given the advancement of

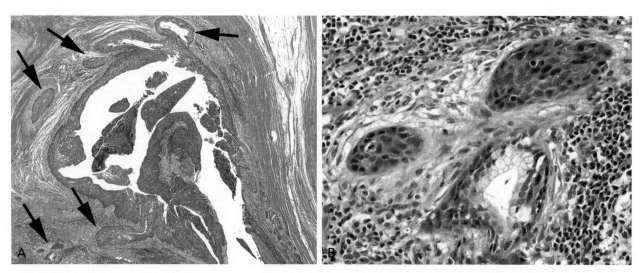

FIGURE 4-32 A squamous cell carcinoma in situ with an exophytic growth involving bronchial gland ducts (arrows) but no invasion (A). The bronchial gland involvement by dysplastic epithelium mimics invasive carcinoma (B).

bronchoscopic techniques, grading of the preinvasive lesions in biopsy specimens may become important for treatment decision making in the near future.

Differential Diagnosis of Squamous Dysplasia and Squamous Cell Carcinoma In Situ

There are several benign and malignant lesions that resemble squamous dysplasia and/or CIS morphologically. These include basal cell hyperplasia, regenerative/reactive atypia secondary to severe inflammation, erosion or ulcer, and chemotherapy and/or radiation effects. Squamous papilloma is also a differential diagnosis of CIS with an exophytic growth. Malignancies that mimic dysplasia include lateral spread or extension onto the overriding surface epithelium of invasive squamous cell carcinoma. Of those, basal cell hyperplasia that is defined as thickening of the basal epithelial cell layer (more than three cells thick) and is likely a precursor to squamous metaplasia needs to be differentiated from mild dysplasia.[214] Squamous papilloma lacks cytologic atypia and shows orderly maturation from the basal layer toward the surface. It is rarely solitary, and often develops as part of laryngotracheal papillomatosis in young patients.[80] Distinction of squamous dysplasia from regenerative/reactive atypia may be difficult, especially in biopsy specimens. Regenerative epithelium lacks significant nuclear pleomorphism, crowding or stratification, and does not show abnormal mitoses. It is commonly associated with prominent inflammation and/or fibrinopurulent exudates indicative of erosion/ulcer. In addition, surface maturation is usually present. After Radiation and/or chemotherapy may induce reactive atypia in metaplastic squamous epithelium

(*Figure 4-33*). Atypical squamous cells secondary to the therapy do not exhibit an increased nuclear/cytoplasmic ratio, although the cells can be significantly enlarged, but instead reveal cytoplasmic vacuolation. Similar therapeutic effects may be seen in the background stromal cells. Lateral spread or surface extension of invasive squamous cell carcinoma needs to be distinguished from dysplasia or CIS since the distinction may have implications for staging and assessing resection margins. In these cases, nuclear pleomorphism is usually more pronounced than high-grade dysplasia, and there is a sharp demarcation between the carcinomatous and noncarcinomatous components.[218] Conversely, extension of CIS into the bronchial gland ducts may mimic invasion (*Figure 4-32B*). The presence of necrosis and the knowledge of an endoscopic mass favor invasive carcinoma.[219]

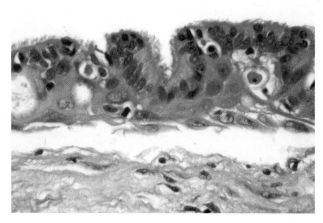

FIGURE 4-33 Atypical squamous cells secondary to radiation therapy undermining ciliated columnar epithelium.

Stepwise Molecular Alterations in Squamous Carcinogenesis of the Lung

The development of lung squamous cell carcinoma follows sequential accumulation of genetic and epigenetic alterations in the bronchial epithelial cells that accompany the severity of histologic changes.[216,220] Progressive allelic losses at multiple 3p chromosome sites (including SOX2 and PI3K) and 9p21 (p16[INK4a]) are the earliest detectable changes that can be identified in the morphologically normal-appearing bronchial epithelium. Later changes occur at 8p21–23, 13q14 (RB), and 17p13 (TP53). Of those, LOH at chromosome 8p21-23 can be seen in dysplasia while *TP53* inactivation is commonly associated with CIS and invasive carcinoma. PI3K pathway activation as well as p16[INK4a] methylation has also been detected at an early stage of squamous carcinogenesis. PI3K pathway activation has been observed in the cytologically normal bronchial epithelium of smokers with lung cancer and those with dysplastic lesions[221] while the frequency of p16[INK4a] methylation increases during histologic progression from 24% in squamous metaplasia to 50% in CIS.[220]

APPROACH TO THE DIAGNOSIS OF POORLY DIFFERENTIATED SQUAMOUS CELL CARCINOMA ON SMALL BIOPSY SPECIMENS

Morphologic distinction between squamous cell carcinoma, lung adenocarcinoma, and other neoplasms may not be possible for poorly differentiated tumors. In these cases, a limited panel of immunohistochemical stains can help pathologists distinguish between these therapeutically relevant tumor subtypes.[95,106,108,136,222-225] When using stains on cytology and small biopsy specimens, a minimal panel is advised to conserve cellular material for molecular studies.[96]

A minimal panel consisting of one lung adenocarcinoma marker (eg, TTF-1 or Napsin A) and one squamous marker (eg, p40, p63, or cytokeratin 5/6) may be sufficient for distinguishing adenocarcinoma from squamous cell carcinoma in most cytology and small biopsy specimens, with the stepwise addition of more markers in immunophenotypically equivocal cases. In addition to their utility in supporting classification as an adenocarcinoma, TTF-1 and Napsin A each offers the advantage of corroborating a lung origin for the tumor.

Poorly differentiated lung tumors that show diffuse positivity for a squamous marker and no expression of an adenocarcinoma marker should be diagnosed as "NSCLC, favor squamous cell carcinoma" (*Figure 4-34*). Conversely, poorly differentiated tumors with diffuse expression of an adenocarcinoma marker and no expression of squamous markers should be classified as "NSCLC, favor adenocarcinoma". In each of these cases, a note in the report should indicate that the favored subtype was based on immunophenotype rather than morphology.

Due to the relatively low specificity of cytokeratin 5/6 and p63 (4A4) for squamous cell carcinoma (compared to the specificity of TTF-1 and Napsin A for lung adenocarcinoma), we recommend that small samples of tumor that show unequivocal positivity for TTF-1 or Napsin A should be classified as "NSCLC, favor adenocarcinoma" even in the presence of cytokeratin 5/6 and/or p63 (4A4) positivity.[96,105,107,113,123] With the emergence of ΔNp63 (p40) as a squamous marker with superior specificity to p63 (4A4), overlapping adenocarcinoma/squamous immunophenotypes may become less common.[123] In cases where a small biopsy or cellblock specimen shows distinct populations of tumor cells that stain for adenocarcinoma versus squamous markers, a note suggesting the possibility of adenosquamous carcinoma may be raised. However, the definitive diagnosis of adenosquamous carcinoma should be reserved for resection specimens in which examination of the

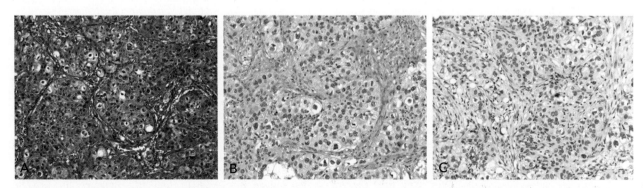

FIGURE 4-34 **A biopsy shows poorly differentiated nonsmall cell carcinoma with a nesting pattern of growth and no obvious squamous or glandular differentiation (A). A two-marker immunohistochemistry panel reveals positive nuclear staining of p40 in the majority of tumor cells (B) and completely negative TTF-1 expression (C) consistent with nonsmall cell carcinoma favor squamous cell carcinoma.**

CHAPTER 4

tumor shows adenocarcinoma and squamous cell carcinoma, each comprising at least 10% of the tumor volume.

In cases of poorly differentiated tumors that show no staining for adenocarcinoma or squamous markers, an expanded antibody panel may be necessary. Positivity for cytokeratin can confirm the diagnosis of carcinoma, while negativity for S100, CD45, and CD34 can exclude other epithelioid neoplasms such as melanoma, hematolymphoid tumors, and vascular tumors, respectively. For poorly differentiated carcinomas, additional antibody panels or molecular studies that are guided by clinical and radiographic findings may be helpful to identify an extrapulmonary primary site.[226-228] Ultimately, a diagnosis of "nonsmall cell carcinoma, not otherwise specified," may be most appropriate.

Of note, poorly differentiated mediastinal or intrathoracic epithelioid malignancies should also alert the pathologist to the possibility of the highly aggressive NUT carcinoma.[229-234] These tumors are defined by the presence of a t(15;19) chromosomal translocation, driven by the resultant *BRD4-NUT* fusion oncogene, and sometimes show focal morphologic and/or immunophenotypic evidence of squamous differentiation.[186] A NUT-specific antibody has been reported to show a speckled nuclear staining pattern in NUT carcinomas and may be useful for identifying this malignancy.[235]

REFERENCES

1. Hammar SP, Brambilla C, Pugatch B, et al. Squamous cell carcinoma. In: Travis WD, Brambilla C, Muller-Hermelink HK, Harris CC, eds. *WHO Classification of Tumours: Tumours of the Lung, Pleura, Thymus and Heart.* Lyon, France: IARC press; 2004:26-30.
2. Sun S, Schiller JH, Gazdar AF. Lung cancer in never smokers—a different disease. *Nat Rev Cancer.* 2007;7(10):778-790.
3. Sobue T, Yamamoto S, Hara M, Sasazuki S, Sasaki S, Tsugane S. Cigarette smoking and subsequent risk of lung cancer by histologic type in middle-aged Japanese men and women: the JPHC study. *Int J Cancer.* 2002;99(2):245-251.
4. Sagerup CM, Smastuen M, Johannesen TB, Helland A, Brustugun OT. Sex-specific trends in lung cancer incidence and survival: a population study of 40,118 cases. *Thorax.* 2011;66(4):301-307.
5. Levi F, Franceschi S, La Vecchia C, Randimbison L, Te VC. Lung carcinoma trends by histologic type in Vaud and Neuchatel, Switzerland, 1974-1994. *Cancer.* 1997;79(5):906-914.
6. Stellman SD, Muscat JE, Hoffmann D, Wynder EL. Impact of filter cigarette smoking on lung cancer histology. *Prev Med.* 1997;26(4):451-456.
7. Forey BA, Lee PN, Fry JS. Updating UK estimates of age, sex and period specific cumulative constant tar cigarette consumption per adult. *Thorax.* 1998;53(10):875-878.
8. Devesa SS, Bray F, Vizcaino AP, Parkin DM. International lung cancer trends by histologic type: male:female differences diminishing and adenocarcinoma rates rising. *Int J Cancer.* 2005;117(2):294-299.
9. Funai K, Yokose T, Ishii G, et al. Clinicopathologic characteristics of peripheral squamous cell carcinoma of the lung. *Am J Surg Pathol.* 2003;27(7):978-984.
10. Turner MC, Krewski D, Pope CA 3rd, Chen Y, Gapstur SM, Thun MJ. Long-term ambient fine particulate matter air pollution and lung cancer in a large cohort of never-smokers. *Am J Respir Crit Care Med.* 2011;184(12):1374-1381.
11. Taeger D, Johnen G, Wiethege T, et al. Major histopathological patterns of lung cancer related to arsenic exposure in German uranium miners. *Int Arch Occup Environ Health.* 2009;82(7):867-875.
12. Martinez VD, Thu KL, Vucic EA, et al. Whole-genome sequencing analysis identifies a distinctive mutational spectrum in an arsenic-related lung tumor. *J Thorac Oncol.* 2013;8(11):1451-1455.
13. Girones Sarrio R, Torregrosa MD, Lopez P, Gomez-Codina J, Rosell R. Smoking habits in elderly lung cancer patients: still no changes in epidemiology? A single-center experience. *Clin Transl Oncol.* 2010;12(10):686-691.
14. Rusch VW. Management of Pancoast tumours. *Lancet Oncol.* 2006;7(12):997-1005.
15. Davidson LA, Black M, Carey FA, Logue F, McNicol AM. Lung tumours immunoreactive for parathyroid hormone related peptide: analysis of serum calcium levels and tumour type. *J Pathol.* 1996;178(4):398-401.
16. Kasuga I, Makino S, Kiyokawa H, Katoh H, Ebihara Y, Ohyashiki K. Tumor-related leukocytosis is linked with poor prognosis in patients with lung carcinoma. *Cancer.* 2001;92(9):2399-2405.
17. King TE Jr, Pardo A, Selman M. Idiopathic pulmonary fibrosis. *Lancet.* 2011;378(9807):1949-1961.
18. Saito Y, Kawai Y, Takahashi N, et al. Survival after surgery for pathologic stage IA non-small cell lung cancer associated with idiopathic pulmonary fibrosis. *Ann Thorac Surg.* 2011;92(5):1812-1817.
19. Kwak N, Park CM, Lee J, et al. Lung cancer risk among patients with combined pulmonary fibrosis and emphysema. *Respir Med.* 2014;108(3):524-530.
20. Kishi K, Homma S, Kurosaki A, Motoi N, Yoshimura K. High-resolution computed tomography findings of lung cancer associated with idiopathic pulmonary fibrosis. *J Comput Assist Tomogr.* 2006;30(1):95-99.
21. Cottin V, Cordier JF. The syndrome of combined pulmonary fibrosis and emphysema. *Chest.* 2009;136(1):1-2.
22. Kitaguchi Y, Fujimoto K, Hanaoka M, Kawakami S, Honda T, Kubo K. Clinical characteristics of combined pulmonary fibrosis and emphysema. *Respirology.* 2010;15(2):265-271.
23. Girard N, Marchand-Adam S, Naccache J-M, et al. Lung cancer in combined pulmonary fibrosis and emphysema - a series of 47 Western patients. *J Thorac Oncol.* 2014;9(8):1162-1170.
24. Usui K, Tanai C, Tanaka Y, Noda H, Ishihara T. The prevalence of pulmonary fibrosis combined with emphysema in patients with lung cancer. *Respirology.* 2011;16(2):326-331.
25. Ettinger DS, Wood DE, Akerkey W, et al. Non-small cell lung cancer, version 4. 2014. *J Natl Compr Canc Netw.* 2014.
26. Scagliotti GV, Parikh P, von Pawel J, et al. Phase III study comparing cisplatin plus gemcitabine with cisplatin plus pemetrexed in chemotherapy-naive patients with advanced-stage non-small-cell lung cancer. *J Clin Oncol.* 2008;26(21):3543-3551.
27. Lynch TJ, Bondarenko I, Luft A, et al. Ipilimumab in combination with paclitaxel and carboplatin as first-line treatment in stage IIIB/IV non-small-cell lung cancer: results from a randomized, double-blind, multicenter phase II study. *J Clin Oncol.* 2012;30(17):2046-2054.
28. Topalian SL, Hodi FS, Brahmer JR, et al. Safety, activity, and immune correlates of anti-PD-1 antibody in cancer. *N Engl J Med.* 2012;366(26):2443-2454.
29. Sundar R, Soong R, Cho BC, Brahmer JR, Soo RA. Immunotherapy in the treatment of non-small cell lung cancer. *Lung Cancer.* 2014;85(2):101-109.
30. Johnson DH, Fehrenbacher L, Novotny WF, et al. Randomized phase II trial comparing bevacizumab plus carboplatin and

paclitaxel with carboplatin and paclitaxel alone in previously untreated locally advanced or metastatic non-small-cell lung cancer. *J Clin Oncol.* 2004;22(11):2184-2191.

31. Mok TS, Wu YL, Thongprasert S, et al. Gefitinib or carboplatin-paclitaxel in pulmonary adenocarcinoma. *New Engl J Med.* 2009;361(10):947-957.

32. Janne PA, Wang X, Socinski MA, et al. Randomized phase II trial of erlotinib alone or with carboplatin and paclitaxel in patients who were never or light former smokers with advanced lung adenocarcinoma: CALGB 30406 trial. *J Clin Oncol.* 2012; 30(17):2063-2069.

33. Sequist LV, Yang JC, Yamamoto N, et al. Phase III study of afatinib or cisplatin plus pemetrexed in patients with metastatic lung adenocarcinoma with EGFR mutations. *J Clin Oncol.* 2013;31(27):3327-3334.

34. Kwak EL, Bang YJ, Camidge DR, et al. Anaplastic lymphoma kinase inhibition in non-small-cell lung cancer. *New Engl J Med.* 2010;363(18):1693-1703.

35. Shaw AT, Kim DW, Mehra R, et al. Ceritinib in ALK-rearranged non-small-cell lung cancer. *New Engl J Med.* 2014; 370(13):1189-1197.

36. Kundel HL. Predictive value and threshold detectability of lung tumors. *Radiology.* 1981;139(1):25-29.

37. Geddes DM. The natural history of lung cancer: a review based on rates of tumour growth. *Br J Dis Chest.* 1979;73(1):1-17.

38. Colby TV, Koss MN, Travis WD. *Tumors of the Lower Respiratory Tract, Fascicle 13.* Washington, DC: Armed Forces Institute of Pathology; 1995.

39. Chaudhuri MR. Primary pulmonary cavitating carcinomas. *Thorax.* 1973;28(3):354-366.

40. Woodring JH, Fried AM, Chuang VP. Solitary cavities of the lung: diagnostic implications of cavity wall thickness. *AJR Am J Roentgenol.* 1980;135(6):1269-1271.

41. Gasinska A, Kolodziejski L, Niemiec J, Dyczek S. Clinical significance of biological differences between cavitated and solid form of squamous cell lung cancer. *Lung Cancer.* 2005;49(2):171-179.

42. Pentheroudakis G, Kostadima L, Fountzilas G, et al. Cavitating squamous cell lung carcinoma-distinct entity or not? Analysis of radiologic, histologic, and clinical features. *Lung Cancer.* 2004;45(3):349-355.

43. Arcasoy SM, Jett JR. Superior pulmonary sulcus tumors and Pancoast's syndrome. *New Engl J Med.* 1997;337(19): 1370-1376.

44. Bruzzi JF, Komaki R, Walsh GL, et al. Imaging of non-small cell lung cancer of the superior sulcus: part 2: initial staging and assessment of resectability and therapeutic response. *Radiographics.* 2008;28(2):561-572.

45. Aberle DR, Adams AM, Berg CD, et al. Reduced lung-cancer mortality with low-dose computed tomographic screening. *New Engl J Med.* 2011;365(5):395-409.

46. Koenigkam Santos M, Muley T, Warth A, et al. Morphological computed tomography features of surgically resectable pulmonary squamous cell carcinomas: impact on prognosis and comparison with adenocarcinomas. *Eur J Radiol.* 2014;83(7):1275-1281.

47. Kramer H, Groen HJ. Current concepts in the mediastinal lymph node staging of nonsmall cell lung cancer. *Ann Surg.* 2003;238(2):180-188.

48. Kudo S, Imai K, Ishiyama K, et al. New CT criteria for nodal staging in non-small cell lung cancer. *Clin Imaging.* 2014; 38(4):448-453.

49. Wong CY, Nunez R, Bohdiewicz P, et al. Patterns of abnormal FDG uptake by various histological types of non-small cell lung cancer at initial staging by PET. *Eur J Nucl Med.* 2001;28(11):1702-1705.

50. Verschakelen JA, Bogaert J, De Wever W. Computed tomography in staging for lung cancer. *Eur Respir J Suppl.* 2002;35:40s-48s.

51. Bonomo L, Ciccotosto C, Guidotti A, Storto ML. Lung cancer staging: the role of computed tomography and magnetic resonance imaging. *Eur J Radiol.* 1996;23(1):35-45.

52. Pennes DR, Glazer GM, Wimbish KJ, Gross BH, Long RW, Orringer MB. Chest wall invasion by lung cancer: limitations of CT evaluation. *AJR Am J Roentgenol.* 1985;144(3):507-511.

53. Hwang JH, Song KS, Park SI, Lim TH, Kwon KH, Goo DE. Subtle pleural metastasis without large effusion in lung cancer patients: preoperative detection on CT. *Korean J Radiol.* 2005; 6(2):94-101.

54. Prakash P, Kalra MK, Sharma A, Shepard JA, Digumarthy SR. FDG PET/CT in assessment of pulmonary lymphangitic carcinomatosis. *AJR Am J Roentgenol.* 2010;194(1):231-236.

55. Ohno Y, Adachi S, Motoyama A, et al. Multiphase ECG-triggered 3D contrast-enhanced MR angiography: utility for evaluation of hilar and mediastinal invasion of bronchogenic carcinoma. *J Magn Reson Imaging.* 2001;13(2):215-224.

56. Freundlich IM, Chasen MH, Varma DG. Magnetic resonance imaging of pulmonary apical tumors. *J Thorac Imaging.* 1996;11(3):210-222.

57. Sakai S, Murayama S, Murakami J, Hashiguchi N, Masuda K. Bronchogenic carcinoma invasion of the chest wall: evaluation with dynamic cine MRI during breathing. *J Comput Assist Tomogr.* 1997;21(4):595-600.

58. Nomori H, Mori T, Ikeda K, et al. Diffusion-weighted magnetic resonance imaging can be used in place of positron emission tomography for N staging of non-small cell lung cancer with fewer false-positive results. *J Thorac Cardiovasc Surg.* 2008;135(4):816-822.

59. Yi CA, Shin KM, Lee KS, et al. Non-small cell lung cancer staging: efficacy comparison of integrated PET/CT versus 3.0-T whole-body MR imaging. *Radiology.* 2008;248(2):632-642.

60. Ohno Y, Koyama H, Onishi Y, et al. Non-small cell lung cancer: whole-body MR examination for M-stage assessment–utility for whole-body diffusion-weighted imaging compared with integrated FDG PET/CT. *Radiology.* 2008;248(2):643-654.

61. Kalff V, Hicks RJ, MacManus MP, et al. Clinical impact of (18)F fluorodeoxyglucose positron emission tomography in patients with non-small-cell lung cancer: a prospective study. *J Clin Oncol.* 2001;19(1):111-118.

62. van Baardwijk A, Baumert BG, Bosmans G, et al. The current status of FDG-PET in tumour volume definition in radiotherapy treatment planning. *Cancer Treat Rev.* 2006;32(4):245-260.

63. Birim O, Kappetein AP, Stijnen T, Bogers AJ. Meta-analysis of positron emission tomographic and computed tomographic imaging in detecting mediastinal lymph node metastases in nonsmall cell lung cancer. *Ann Thorac Surg.* 2005;79(1):375-382.

64. Schrevens L, Lorent N, Dooms C, Vansteenkiste J. The role of PET scan in diagnosis, staging, and management of non-small cell lung cancer. *Oncologist.* 2004;9(6):633-643.

65. Schaffler GJ, Wolf G, Schoellnast H, et al. Non-small cell lung cancer: evaluation of pleural abnormalities on CT scans with 18F FDG PET. *Radiology.* 2004;231(3):858-865.

66. Ganeshan B, Miles KA. Quantifying tumour heterogeneity with CT. *Cancer Imaging.* 2013;13:140-149.

67. Ganeshan B, Panayiotou E, Burnand K, Dizdarevic S, Miles K. Tumour heterogeneity in non-small cell lung carcinoma assessed by CT texture analysis: a potential marker of survival. *Eur Radiol.* 2012;22(4):796-802.

68. Zhang LJ, Yang GF, Wu SY, Xu J, Lu GM, Schoepf UJ. Dual-energy CT imaging of thoracic malignancies. *Cancer Imaging.* 2013;13:81-91.

69. Sommer G, Bauman G, Koenigkam-Santos M, et al. Non-contrast-enhanced preoperative assessment of lung perfusion in patients with non-small-cell lung cancer using Fourier decomposition magnetic resonance imaging. *Eur J Radiol.* 2013;82(12):e879-887.

70. Cardesa A, Gal A, Nadal A, Zidar N. Squamous cell carcinoma. In: Barnes L, Eveson JW, Reichart P, Sidransky D, eds. *WHO Classification of Tumours: Head and Neck Tumours.* Lyon, France: TARC press; 2005:118-121.

71. Chan JKC, Bray F, McCarron PF, W., et al. Nasopharyngeal carcinoma. In: Barnes L, Eveson JW, Reichart P, Sidransky D, eds. *WHO Classification of Tumours: Head and Neck Tumours.* Lyon, France: IARC press; 2005:85-97.

72. Kadota K, Nitadori J, Woo KM, et al. Comprehensive pathological analyses in lung squamous cell carcinoma: single cell invasion, nuclear diameter, and tumor budding are independent prognostic factors for worse outcomes. *J Thorac Oncol.* 2014 Aug;9(8):1126-39.

73. Takahashi Y, Ishii G, Taira T, et al. Fibrous stroma is associated with poorer prognosis in lung squamous cell carcinoma patients. *J Thorac Oncol.* 2011;6(9):1460-1467.

74. Maeshima AM, Maeshima A, Asamura H, Matsuno Y. Histologic prognostic factors for small-sized squamous cell carcinomas of the peripheral lung. *Lung Cancer.* 2006;52(1):53-58.

75. Edwards C, Carlile A. Clear cell carcinoma of the lung. *J Clin Pathol.* 1985;38(8):880-885.

76. Katzenstein AL, Prioleau PG, Askin FB. The histologic spectrum and significance of clear-cell change in lung carcinoma. *Cancer.* 1980;45(5):943-947.

77. Travis WD. Pathology of lung cancer. *Clin Chest Med.* 2011; 32(4):669-692.

78. Hammar S. The use of electron microscopy and immunohistochemistry in the diagnosis and understanding of lung neoplasms. *Clin Lab Med.* 1987;7(1):1-30.

79. Churg A, Johnston WH, Stulbarg M. Small cell squamous and mixed small cell squamous--small cell anaplastic carcinomas of the lung. *Am J Surg Pathol.* 1980;4(3):255-263.

80. Dulmet-Brender E, Jaubert F, Huchon G. Exophytic endobronchial epidermoid carcinoma. *Cancer.* 1986;57(7):1358-1364.

81. Sherwin RP, Laforet EG, Strieder JW. Exophytic endobronchial carcinoma. *J Thorac Cardiovasc Surg.* 1962;43:716-730.

82. Woolner LB, Andersen HA, Bernatz PE. "Occult" carcinoma of the bronchus: a study of 15 cases of in situ or early invasive bronchogenic carcinoma. *Diseases of the Chest.* 1960;37:278-288.

83. Moro-Sibilot D, Lantuejoul S, Diab S, et al. Lung carcinomas with a basaloid pattern: a study of 90 cases focusing on their poor prognosis. *Eur Respir J.* 2008;31(4):854-859.

84. Kim DJ, Kim KD, Shin DH, Ro JY, Chung KY. Basaloid carcinoma of the lung: a really dismal histologic variant? *Ann Thorac Surg.* 2003;76(6):1833-1837.

85. Brambilla E, Pugatch B, Geisinger K, et al. Large cell carcinoma. In: Travis WD, Brambilla C, Muller-Hermelink HK, Harris CC, eds. *WHO Classification of Tumours: Tumours of the Lung, Pleura, Thymus and Heart.* Lyon, France: IARC press; 2004:45-50.

86. Brambilla E, Moro D, Veale D, et al. Basal cell (basaloid) carcinoma of the lung: a new morphologic and phenotypic entity with separate prognostic significance. *Hum Pathol.* 1992;23(9):993-1003.

87. Crapanzano JP, Loukeris K, Borczuk AC, Saqi A. Cytological, histological, and immunohistochemical findings of pulmonary carcinomas with basaloid features. *Diagn Cytopathol.* 2011;39(2):92-100.

88. Rossi G, Mengoli MC, Cavazza A, et al. Large cell carcinoma of the lung: clinically oriented classification integrating immunohistochemistry and molecular biology. *Virchows Arch.* 2014;464(1):61-68.

89. Moro D, Brichon PY, Brambilla E, Veale D, Labat F, Brambilla C. Basaloid bronchial carcinoma. A histologic group with a poor prognosis. *Cancer.* 1994;73(11):2734-2739.

90. Kim MJ, Ha SY, Kim NR, Cho HY, Chung DH, Kim GY. Aspiration cytology features of pulmonary basaloid carcinoma. *Cytopathology.* 2009;20(5):336-339.

91. Wang LC, Wang L, Kwauk S, et al. Analysis on the clinical features of 22 basaloid squamous cell carcinoma of the lung. *J Cardiothorac Surg.* 2011;6:10.

92. Brcic L, Sherer CK, Shuai Y, Hornick JL, Chirieac LR, Dacic S. Morphologic and clinicopathologic features of lung squamous cell carcinomas expressing Sox2. *Am J Clin Pathol.* 2012;138(5):712-718.

93. Watanabe Y, Yokose T, Sakuma Y, et al. Alveolar space filling ratio as a favorable prognostic factor in small peripheral squamous cell carcinoma of the lung. *Lung Cancer.* 2011;73(2):217-221.

94. Yousem SA. Peripheral squamous cell carcinoma of lung: patterns of growth with particular focus on airspace filling. *Hum Pathol.* 2009;40(6):861-867.

95. Rekhtman N, Brandt SM, Sigel CS, et al. Suitability of thoracic cytology for new therapeutic paradigms in non-small cell lung carcinoma: high accuracy of tumor subtyping and feasibility of EGFR and KRAS molecular testing. *J Thorac Oncol.* 2011;6(3):451-458.

96. Travis WD, Brambilla E, Noguchi M, et al. Diagnosis of lung cancer in small biopsies and cytology: implications of the 2011 International Association for the Study of Lung Cancer/American Thoracic Society/European Respiratory Society classification. *Arch Pathol Lab Med.* 2013;137(5):668-684.

97. Travis WD, Brambilla E, Noguchi M, et al. International association for the study of lung cancer/american thoracic society/european respiratory society international multidisciplinary classification of lung adenocarcinoma. *J Thorac Oncol.* 2011; 6(2):244-285.

98. Nishino M, Klepeis VE, Yeap BY, et al. Histologic and cytomorphologic features of ALK-rearranged lung adenocarcinomas. *Mod Pathol.* 2012;25(11):1462-1472.

99. Solis LM, Raso MG, Kalhor N, Behrens C, Wistuba II, Moran CA. Primary oncocytic adenocarcinomas of the lung: a clinicopathologic, immunohistochemical, and molecular biologic analysis of 16 cases. *Am J Clin Pathol.* 2010;133(1):133-140.

100. Geurts TW, van Velthuysen ML, Broekman F, et al. Differential diagnosis of pulmonary carcinoma following head and neck cancer by genetic analysis. *Clin Cancer Res.* 2009;15(3):980-985.

101. Leong PP, Rezai B, Koch WM, et al. Distinguishing second primary tumors from lung metastases in patients with head and neck squamous cell carcinoma. *J Natl Cancer Inst.* 1998;90(13):972-977.

102. Crapanzano JP, Zakowski MF. Diagnostic dilemmas in pulmonary cytology. *Cancer.* 2001;93(6):364-375.

103. Brown AF, Sirohi D, Fukuoka J, et al. Tissue-preserving antibody cocktails to differentiate primary squamous cell carcinoma, adenocarcinoma, and small cell carcinoma of lung. *Arch Pathol Lab Med.* 2013;137(9):1274-1281.

104. Fatima N, Cohen C, Lawson D, Siddiqui MT. TTF-1 and Napsin A double stain: a useful marker for diagnosing lung adenocarcinoma on fine-needle aspiration cell blocks. *Cancer Cytopathol.* 2011;119(2):127-133.

105. Rossi G, Pelosi G, Graziano P, Barbareschi M, Papotti M. A reevaluation of the clinical significance of histological subtyping of non–small-cell lung carcinoma: diagnostic algorithms in the era of personalized treatments. *Int J Surg Pathol.* 2009; 17(3):206-218.

106. Mukhopadhyay S, Katzenstein AL. Subclassification of non-small cell lung carcinomas lacking morphologic differentiation on biopsy specimens: utility of an immunohistochemical panel containing TTF-1, napsin A, p63, and CK5/6. *Am J Surg Pathol.* 2011;35(1):15-25.

107. Rekhtman N, Ang DC, Sima CS, Travis WD, Moreira AL. Immunohistochemical algorithm for differentiation of lung adenocarcinoma and squamous cell carcinoma based on large series of whole-tissue sections with validation in small specimens. *Mod Pathol.* 2011;24(10):1348-1359.

CHAPTER 4

108. Tsuta K, Tanabe Y, Yoshida A, et al. Utility of 10 immunohistochemical markers including novel markers (desmocollin-3, glypican 3, S100A2, S100A7, and Sox-2) for differential diagnosis of squamous cell carcinoma from adenocarcinoma of the Lung. *J Thorac Oncol.* 2011;6(7):1190-1199.

109. Chu P, Wu E, Weiss LM. Cytokeratin 7 and cytokeratin 20 expression in epithelial neoplasms: a survey of 435 cases. *Mod Pathol.* 2000;13(9):962-972.

110. Gruver AM, Amin MB, Luthringer DJ, et al. Selective immunohistochemical markers to distinguish between metastatic high-grade urothelial carcinoma and primary poorly differentiated invasive squamous cell carcinoma of the lung. *Arch Pathol Lab Med.* 2012;136(11):1339-1346.

111. Bishop JA, Benjamin H, Cholakh H, Chajut A, Clark DP, Westra WH. Accurate classification of non-small cell lung carcinoma using a novel microRNA-based approach. *Clin Cancer Res.* 2010;16(2):610-619.

112. Pelosi G, Pasini F, Olsen Stenholm C, et al. p63 immunoreactivity in lung cancer: yet another player in the development of squamous cell carcinomas? *J Pathol.* 2002;198(1):100-109.

113. Yoshida A, Tsuta K, Watanabe S, et al. Frequent ALK rearrangement and TTF-1/p63 co-expression in lung adenocarcinoma with signet-ring cell component. *Lung Cancer.* 2011;72(3):309-315.

114. Butnor KJ, Burchette JL. p40 (DeltaNp63) and keratin 34betaE12 provide greater diagnostic accuracy than p63 in the evaluation of small cell lung carcinoma in small biopsy samples. *Hum Pathol.* 2013;44(8):1479-1486.

115. Chilosi M, Zamo A, Brighenti A, et al. Constitutive expression of DeltaN-p63alpha isoform in human thymus and thymic epithelial tumours. *Virchows Arch.* 2003;443(2):175-183.

116. Di Como CJ, Urist MJ, Babayan I, et al. p63 expression profiles in human normal and tumor tissues. *Clin Cancer Res.* 2002;8(2):494-501.

117. Hallack Neto AE, Siqueira SA, Dulley FL, Ruiz MA, Chamone DA, Pereira J. p63 protein expression in high risk diffuse large B-cell lymphoma. *J Clin Pathol.* 2009;62(1):77-79.

118. Hedvat CV, Teruya-Feldstein J, Puig P, et al. Expression of p63 in diffuse large B-cell lymphoma. *Appl Immunohistochem Mol Morphol.* 2005;13(3):237-242.

119. Nylander K, Vojtesek B, Nenutil R, et al. Differential expression of p63 isoforms in normal tissues and neoplastic cells. *J Pathol.* 2002;198(4):417-427.

120. Candi E, Dinsdale D, Rufini A, et al. TAp63 and DeltaNp63 in cancer and epidermal development. *Cell Cycle.* 2007;6(3):274-285.

121. Gressner O, Schilling T, Lorenz K, et al. TAp63alpha induces apoptosis by activating signaling via death receptors and mitochondria. *EMBO J.* 2005;24(13):2458-2471.

122. Hibi K, Trink B, Patturajan M, et al. AIS is an oncogene amplified in squamous cell carcinoma. *Proc Natl Acad Sci U S A.* 2000;97(10):5462-5467.

123. Bishop JA, Teruya-Feldstein J, Westra WH, Pelosi G, Travis WD, Rekhtman N. p40 (DeltaNp63) is superior to p63 for the diagnosis of pulmonary squamous cell carcinoma. *Mod Pathol.* 2012;25(3):405-415.

124. Pelosi G, Fabbri A, Bianchi F, et al. DeltaNp63 (p40) and thyroid transcription factor-1 immunoreactivity on small biopsies or cellblocks for typing non-small cell lung cancer: a novel two-hit, sparing-material approach. *J Thorac Oncol.* 2012;7(2):281-290.

125. Pelosi G, Rossi G, Cavazza A, et al. DeltaNp63 (p40) distribution inside lung cancer: a driver biomarker approach to tumor characterization. *Int J Surg Pathol.* 2013;21(3):229-239.

126. Masai K, Tsuta K, Kawago M, et al. Expression of squamous cell carcinoma markers and adenocarcinoma markers in primary pulmonary neuroendocrine carcinomas. *Appl Immunohistochem Mol Morphol.* 2013;21(4):292-297.

127. Cui T, Chen Y, Yang L, et al. Diagnostic and prognostic impact of desmocollins in human lung cancer. *J Clin Pathol.* 2012;65(12):1100-1106.

128. Gomez-Morales M, Camara-Pulido M, Miranda-Leon MT, et al. Differential immunohistochemical localization of desmosomal plaque-related proteins in non-small-cell lung cancer. *Histopathology.* 2013;63(1):103-113.

129. Sholl LM, Long KB, Hornick JL. Sox2 expression in pulmonary non-small cell and neuroendocrine carcinomas. *Appl Immunohistochem Mol Morphol.* 2010;18(1):55-61.

130. Bishop JA, Sharma R, Illei PB. Napsin A and thyroid transcription factor-1 expression in carcinomas of the lung, breast, pancreas, colon, kidney, thyroid, and malignant mesothelioma. *Hum Pathol.* 2010;41(1):20-25.

131. Hirano T, Auer G, Maeda M, et al. Human tissue distribution of TA02, which is homologous with a new type of aspartic proteinase, napsin A. *Jpn J Cancer Res.* 2000;91(10):1015-1021.

132. Hirano T, Gong Y, Yoshida K, et al. Usefulness of TA02 (napsin A) to distinguish primary lung adenocarcinoma from metastatic lung adenocarcinoma. *Lung Cancer.* 2003;41(2):155-162.

133. Stoll LM, Johnson MW, Burroughs F, Li QK. Cytologic diagnosis and differential diagnosis of lung carcinoid tumors a retrospective study of 63 cases with histologic correlation. *Cancer Cytopathol.* 2010;118(6):457-467.

134. Suzuki A, Shijubo N, Yamada G, et al. Napsin A is useful to distinguish primary lung adenocarcinoma from adenocarcinomas of other organs. *Pathol Res Pract.* 2005;201(8-9):579-586.

135. Ueno T, Linder S, Elmberger G. Aspartic proteinase napsin is a useful marker for diagnosis of primary lung adenocarcinoma. *Br J Cancer.* 2003;88(8):1229-1233.

136. Whithaus K, Fukuoka J, Prihoda TJ, Jagirdar J. Evaluation of napsin A, cytokeratin 5/6, p63, and thyroid transcription factor 1 in adenocarcinoma versus squamous cell carcinoma of the lung. *Arch Pathol Lab Med.* 2012;136(2):155-162.

137. Yang M, Nonaka D. A study of immunohistochemical differential expression in pulmonary and mammary carcinomas. *Mod Pathol.* 2010;23(5):654-661.

138. Matoso A, Singh K, Jacob R, et al. Comparison of thyroid transcription factor-1 expression by 2 monoclonal antibodies in pulmonary and nonpulmonary primary tumors. *Appl Immunohistochem Mol Morphol.* 2010;18(2):142-149.

139. Turner BM, Cagle PT, Sainz IM, Fukuoka J, Shen SS, Jagirdar J. Napsin A, a new marker for lung adenocarcinoma, is complementary and more sensitive and specific than thyroid transcription factor 1 in the differential diagnosis of primary pulmonary carcinoma: evaluation of 1674 cases by tissue microarray. *Arch Pathol Lab Med.* 2012;136(2):163-171.

140. Pereira TC, Share SM, Magalhaes AV, Silverman JF. Can we tell the site of origin of metastatic squamous cell carcinoma? An immunohistochemical tissue microarray study of 194 cases. *Appl Immunohistochem Mol Morphol.* 2011;19(1):10-14.

141. Ordonez NG. A word of caution regarding napsin A expression in squamous cell carcinomas of the lung. *Am J Surg Pathol.* 2012;36(3):396-401.

142. Doxtader EE, Katzenstein AL. The relationship between p16 expression and high-risk human papillomavirus infection in squamous cell carcinomas from sites other than uterine cervix: a study of 137 cases. *Hum Pathol.* 2012;43(3):327-332.

143. Wang CW, Wu TI, Yu CT, et al. Usefulness of p16 for differentiating primary pulmonary squamous cell carcinoma from cervical squamous cell carcinoma metastatic to the lung. *Am J Clin Pathol.* 2009;131(5):715-722.

144. Heist RS, Sequist LV, Engelman JA. Genetic changes in squamous cell lung cancer: a review. *J Thorac Oncol.* 2012;7(5):924-933.

145. Cancer Genome Atlas Research N. Comprehensive genomic characterization of squamous cell lung cancers. *Nature.* 2012;489(7417):519-525.

146. Pikor LA, Ramnarine VR, Lam S, Lam WL. Genetic alterations defining NSCLC subtypes and their therapeutic implications. *Lung Cancer*. 2013;82(2):179-189.

147. Staaf J, Isaksson S, Karlsson A, et al. Landscape of somatic allelic imbalances and copy number alterations in human lung carcinoma. *Int J Cancer*. 2013;132(9):2020-2031.

148. Hussenet T, Dali S, Exinger J, et al. SOX2 is an oncogene activated by recurrent 3q26.3 amplifications in human lung squamous cell carcinomas. *PLoS One*. 2010;5(1):e8960.

149. Bass AJ, Watanabe H, Mermel CH, et al. SOX2 is an amplified lineage-survival oncogene in lung and esophageal squamous cell carcinomas. *Nat Genet*. 2009;41(11):1238-1242.

150. Wernig M, Meissner A, Foreman R, et al. In vitro reprogramming of fibroblasts into a pluripotent ES-cell-like state. *Nature*. 2007;448(7151):318-324.

151. Yu J, Vodyanik MA, Smuga-Otto K, et al. Induced pluripotent stem cell lines derived from human somatic cells. *Science*. 2007;318(5858):1917-1920.

152. Takahashi K, Yamanaka S. Induction of pluripotent stem cells from mouse embryonic and adult fibroblast cultures by defined factors. *Cell*. 2006;126(4):663-676.

153. Que J, Luo X, Schwartz RJ, Hogan BL. Multiple roles for Sox2 in the developing and adult mouse trachea. *Development*. 2009;136(11):1899-1907.

154. Weiss J, Sos ML, Seidel D, et al. Frequent and focal FGFR1 amplification associates with therapeutically tractable FGFR1 dependency in squamous cell lung cancer. *Sci Transl Med*. 2010;2(62):62ra93.

155. Mason I. Initiation to end point: the multiple roles of fibroblast growth factors in neural development. *Nat Rev Neurosci*. 2007;8(8):583-596.

156. Hammerman PS, Sos ML, Ramos AH, et al. Mutations in the DDR2 kinase gene identify a novel therapeutic target in squamous cell lung cancer. *Cancer Discov*. 2011;1(1):78-89.

157. Kan Z, Jaiswal BS, Stinson J, et al. Diverse somatic mutation patterns and pathway alterations in human cancers. *Nature*. 2010;466(7308):869-873.

158. Shibata T, Ohta T, Tong KI, et al. Cancer related mutations in NRF2 impair its recognition by Keap1-Cul3 E3 ligase and promote malignancy. *Proc Natl Acad Sci U S A*. 2008;105(36):13568-13573.

159. Kishimoto Y, Murakami Y, Shiraishi M, Hayashi K, Sekiya T. Aberrations of the p53 tumor suppressor gene in human non-small cell carcinomas of the lung. *Cancer Res*. 1992;52(17):4799-4804.

160. Singh A, Bodas M, Wakabayashi N, Bunz F, Biswal S. Gain of Nrf2 function in non-small-cell lung cancer cells confers radioresistance. *Antioxid Redox Signal*. 2010;13(11):1627-1637.

161. Singh A, Misra V, Thimmulappa RK, et al. Dysfunctional KEAP1-NRF2 interaction in non-small-cell lung cancer. *PLoS Med*. 2006;3(10):e420.

162. Kim YR, Oh JE, Kim MS, et al. Oncogenic NRF2 mutations in squamous cell carcinomas of oesophagus and skin. *J Pathol*. 2010;220(4):446-451.

163. Solis LM, Behrens C, Dong W, et al. Nrf2 and Keap1 abnormalities in non-small cell lung carcinoma and association with clinicopathologic features. *Clin Cancer Res*. 2010;16(14):3743-3753.

164. Carpten JD, Faber AL, Horn C, et al. A transforming mutation in the pleckstrin homology domain of AKT1 in cancer. *Nature*. 2007;448(7152):439-444.

165. Malanga D, Scrima M, De Marco C, et al. Activating E17K mutation in the gene encoding the protein kinase AKT1 in a subset of squamous cell carcinoma of the lung. *Cell Cycle*. 2008;7(5):665-669.

166. Olaso E, Labrador JP, Wang L, et al. Discoidin domain receptor 2 regulates fibroblast proliferation and migration through the extracellular matrix in association with transcriptional activation of matrix metalloproteinase-2. *J Biol Chem*. 2002;277(5):3606-3613.

167. Ikeda K, Wang LH, Torres R, et al. Discoidin domain receptor 2 interacts with Src and Shc following its activation by type I collagen. *J Biol Chem*. 2002;277(21):19206-19212.

168. Heller G, Babinsky VN, Ziegler B, et al. Genome-wide CpG island methylation analyses in non-small cell lung cancer patients. *Carcinogenesis*. 2013;34(3):513-521.

169. Lockwood WW, Wilson IM, Coe BP, et al. Divergent genomic and epigenomic landscapes of lung cancer subtypes underscore the selection of different oncogenic pathways during tumor development. *PLoS One*. 2012;7(5):e37775.

170. Calin GA, Croce CM. MicroRNA signatures in human cancers. *Nat Rev Cancer*. 2006;6(11):857-866.

171. Lebanony D, Benjamin H, Gilad S, et al. Diagnostic assay based on hsa-miR-205 expression distinguishes squamous from nonsquamous non-small-cell lung carcinoma. *J Clin Oncol*. 2009;27(12):2030-2037.

172. Wilkerson MD, Yin X, Hoadley KA, et al. Lung squamous cell carcinoma mRNA expression subtypes are reproducible, clinically important, and correspond to normal cell types. *Clin Cancer Res*. 2010;16(19):4864-4875.

173. Smith SL, Gugger M, Hoban P, et al. S100A2 is strongly expressed in airway basal cells, preneoplastic bronchial lesions and primary non-small cell lung carcinomas. *Br J Cancer*. 2004;91(8):1515-1524.

174. Maleki Z. Diagnostic issues with cytopathologic interpretation of lung neoplasms displaying high-grade basaloid or neuroendocrine morphology. *Diagn Cytopathol*. 2011;39(3):159-167.

175. Sturm N, Lantuejoul S, Laverriere MH, et al. Thyroid transcription factor 1 and cytokeratins 1, 5, 10, 14 (34betaE12) expression in basaloid and large-cell neuroendocrine carcinomas of the lung. *Hum Pathol*. 2001;32(9):918-925.

176. Weissferdt A, Moran CA. Immunohistochemistry in the diagnosis of thymic epithelial neoplasms. *Appl Immunohistochem Mol Morphol*. 2014;22(7):479-487.

177. van der Sijp JR, van Meerbeeck JP, Maat AP, et al. Determination of the molecular relationship between multiple tumors within one patient is of clinical importance. *J Clin Oncol*. 2002;20(4):1105-1114.

178. Geurts TW, Nederlof PM, van den Brekel MW, et al. Pulmonary squamous cell carcinoma following head and neck squamous cell carcinoma: metastasis or second primary? *Clin Cancer Res*. 2005;11(18):6608-6614.

179. Weichert W, Schewe C, Denkert C, Morawietz L, Dietel M, Petersen I. Molecular HPV typing as a diagnostic tool to discriminate primary from metastatic squamous cell carcinoma of the lung. *Am J Surg Pathol*. 2009;33(4):513-520.

180. Yanagawa N, Wang A, Kohler D, et al. Human papilloma virus genome is rare in North American non-small cell lung carcinoma patients. *Lung Cancer*. 2013;79(3):215-220.

181. Bishop JA, Ogawa T, Chang X, et al. HPV analysis in distinguishing second primary tumors from lung metastases in patients with head and neck squamous cell carcinoma. *Am J Surg Pathol*. 2012;36(1):142-148.

182. Emanuel P, Wang B, Wu M, Burstein DE. p63 Immunohistochemistry in the distinction of adenoid cystic carcinoma from basaloid squamous cell carcinoma. *Mod Pathol*. 2005;18(5):645-650.

183. Morice WG, Ferreiro JA. Distinction of basaloid squamous cell carcinoma from adenoid cystic and small cell undifferentiated carcinoma by immunohistochemistry. *Hum Pathol*. 1998;29(6):609-612.

184. Persson M, Andren Y, Mark J, Horlings HM, Persson F, Stenman G. Recurrent fusion of MYB and NFIB transcription factor genes in carcinomas of the breast and head and neck. *Proc Natl Acad Sci U S A*. 2009;106(44):18740-18744.

185. Mitani Y, Rao PH, Futreal PA, et al. Novel chromosomal rearrangements and break points at the t(6;9) in salivary adenoid cystic carcinoma: association with MYB-NFIB chimeric fusion,

MYB expression, and clinical outcome. *Clin Cancer Res.* 2011;17(22):7003-7014.

186. French CA. Pathogenesis of NUT midline carcinoma. *Annu Rev Pathol.* 2012;7:247-265.

187. Brambrilla E, Travis WD. Adenosquamous carcinoma. In: Travis WD, Brambrilla C, Muller-Hermelink HK, Harris CC, eds. *WHO Classification of Tumours: Tumours of the Lung, Pleura, Thymus and Heart.* Lyon, France: IARC press; 2004:51-52.

188. Pan Y, Wang R, Ye T, et al. Comprehensive analysis of oncogenic mutations in lung squamous cell carcinoma with minor glandular component. *Chest.* 2014;145(3):473-479.

189. Chi A, Johnstone S, Nishino M, Mark E, Mio-Kenudson M. The prevalence and implication of adenocarcinoma component in lung cancer with morphological diagnosis of squamous cell carcinoma. *Mod Pathol.* 2014;27.

190. Broderick P, Wang Y, Vijayakrishnan J, et al. Deciphering the impact of common genetic variation on lung cancer risk: a genome-wide association study. *Cancer Res.* 2009;69(16):6633-6641.

191. Landi MT, Chatterjee N, Yu K, et al. A genome-wide association study of lung cancer identifies a region of chromosome 5p15 associated with risk for adenocarcinoma. *Am. J. Hum. Genet.* 2009;85(5):679-691.

192. Shi J, Chatterjee N, Rotunno M, et al. Inherited variation at chromosome 12p13.33, including RAD52, influences the risk of squamous cell lung carcinoma. *Cancer Discov.* 2012;2(2):131-139.

193. Timofeeva MN, Hung RJ, Rafnar T, et al. Influence of common genetic variation on lung cancer risk: meta-analysis of 14 900 cases and 29 485 controls. *Hum Mol Genet.* 2012;21(22): 4980-4995.

194. Walsh KM, Gorlov IP, Hansen HM, et al. Fine-mapping of the 5p15.33, 6p22.1-p21.31, and 15q25.1 regions identifies functional and histology-specific lung cancer susceptibility loci in African-Americans. *Cancer Epidemiol Biomarkers Prev.* 2013;22(2):251-260.

195. Wang Y, McKay JD, Rafnar T, et al. Rare variants of large effect in BRCA2 and CHEK2 affect risk of lung cancer. *Nat Genet.* 2014;46(7):736-741.

196. Peters EJ, Morice R, Benner SE, et al. Squamous metaplasia of the bronchial mucosa and its relationship to smoking. *Chest.* 1993;103(5):1429-1432.

197. Auerbach O, Forman JB, Gere JB, et al. Changes in the bronchial epithelium in relation to smoking and cancer of the lung; a report of progress. *New Engl J Med.* 1957;256(3):97-104.

198. Kumar V. *Cellular responses to stress and toxic insults: adaptation, injury and death.* Kumar V, Abbas AK, Fausto N, Aster JC, eds. Pathologic Basis of Disease. Elsevier, New York; 2010:3-42.

199. Wistuba II, Behrens C, Milchgrub S, et al. Sequential molecular abnormalities are involved in the multistage development of squamous cell lung carcinoma. *Oncogene.* 1999;18(3):643-650.

200. Lam S, leRiche JC, Zheng Y, et al. Sex-related differences in bronchial epithelial changes associated with tobacco smoking. *J Natl Cancer Inst.* 1999;91(8):691-696.

201. Hirsch FR, Franklin WA, Gazdar AF, Bunn PA Jr. Early detection of lung cancer: clinical perspectives of recent advances in biology and radiology. *Clin Cancer Res.* 2001;7(1):5-22.

202. Moro-Sibilot D, Jeanmart M, Lantuejoul S, et al. Cigarette smoking, preinvasive bronchial lesions, and autofluorescence bronchoscopy. *Chest.* 2002;122(6):1902-1908.

203. Hirsch FR, Prindiville SA, Miller YE, et al. Fluorescence versus white-light bronchoscopy for detection of preneoplastic lesions: a randomized study. *J Natl Cancer Inst.* 2001; 93(18):1385-1391.

204. Jeremy George P, Banerjee AK, Read CA, et al. Surveillance for the detection of early lung cancer in patients with bronchial dysplasia. *Thorax.* 2007;62(1):43-50.

205. Hoshino H, Shibuya K, Chiyo M, et al. Biological features of bronchial squamous dysplasia followed up by autofluorescence bronchoscopy. *Lung Cancer.* 2004;46(2):187-196.

206. Nakajima T, Yasufuku K. Early lung cancer: methods for detection. *Clin Chest Med.* 2013;34(3):373-383.

207. Ishizumi T, McWilliams A, MacAulay C, Gazdar A, Lam S. Natural history of bronchial preinvasive lesions. *Cancer Metastasis Rev.* 2010;29(1):5-14.

208. Jeanmart M, Lantuejoul S, Fievet F, et al. Value of immunohistochemical markers in preinvasive bronchial lesions in risk assessment of lung cancer. *Clin Cancer Res.* 2003;9(6):2195-2203.

209. Franklin WA, Wistuba II, Geisinger K, et al. Squamous dysplasia and carcinoma in-situ. In: Travis WD, Brambilla C, Muller-Hermelink HK, Harris CC, eds. *WHO Classification of Tumours: Tumours of the Lung, Pleura, Thymus and Heart.* Lyon, France: IARC press; 2004:85-97.

210. Lam S, Kennedy T, Unger M, et al. Localization of bronchial intraepithelial neoplastic lesions by fluorescence bronchoscopy. *Chest.* 1998;113(3):696-702.

211. Ikeda N, Hayashi A, Iwasaki K, et al. Comprehensive diagnostic bronchoscopy of central type early stage lung cancer. *Lung Cancer.* 2007;56(3):295-302.

212. Chen W, Gao X, Tian Q, Chen L. A comparison of autofluorescence bronchoscopy and white light bronchoscopy in detection of lung cancer and preneoplastic lesions: a meta-analysis. *Lung Cancer.* 2011;73(2):183-188.

213. Yasufuku K. Early diagnosis of lung cancer. *Clin Chest Med.* 2010;31(1):39-47, Table of Contents.

214. Kerr KM. Pulmonary preinvasive neoplasia. *J Clin Pathol.* 2001;54(4):257-271.

215. Keith RL, Miller YE, Gemmill RM, et al. Angiogenic squamous dysplasia in bronchi of individuals at high risk for lung cancer. *Clin Cancer Res.* 2000;6(5):1616-1625.

216. Hirsch FR, Merrick DT, Franklin WA. Role of biomarkers for early detection of lung cancer and chemoprevention. *Eur Respir J.* 2002;19(6):1151-1158.

217. Nicholson AG, Perry LJ, Cury PM, et al. Reproducibility of the WHO/IASLC grading system for pre-invasive squamous lesions of the bronchus: a study of inter-observer and intra-observer variation. *Histopathology.* 2001;38(3):202-208.

218. Shimizu M, Ban S, Odze RD. Squamous dysplasia and other precursor lesions related to esophageal squamous cell carcinoma. *Gastroenterol Clin North.* 2007;36(4):797-811, v-vi.

219. Kerr K, Popper H. The differential diagnosis of pulmonary preinvasive lesions. In: Timens W, Popper H, eds. *Pathology of the Lung.* Vol 39. European Respiratory Monograph: European Respiratory Society; Wakefield, UK. 2007:37-62.

220. Wistuba II, Gazdar AF. Lung cancer preneoplasia. *Annu Rev Pathol.* 2006;1:331-348.

221. Gustafson AM, Soldi R, Anderlind C, et al. Airway PI3K pathway activation is an early and reversible event in lung cancer development. *Sci Transl Med.* 2010;2(26):26ra25.

222. Khayyata S, Yun S, Pasha T, et al. Value of P63 and CK5/6 in distinguishing squamous cell carcinoma from adenocarcinoma in lung fine-needle aspiration specimens. *Diagn Cytopathol.* 2009;37(3):178-183.

223. Loo PS, Thomas SC, Nicolson MC, Fyfe MN, Kerr KM. Subtyping of undifferentiated non-small cell carcinomas in bronchial biopsy specimens. *J Thorac Oncol.* 2010;5(4):442-447.

224. Sigel CS, Moreira AL, Travis WD, et al. Subtyping of non-small cell lung carcinoma: a comparison of small biopsy and cytology specimens. *J Thorac Oncol.* 2011;6(11):1849-1856.

225. Pelosi G, Rossi G, Bianchi F, et al. Immunohistochemistry by means of widely agreed-upon markers (cytokeratins 5/6 and 7, p63, thyroid transcription factor-1, and vimentin) on small biopsies of non-small cell lung cancer effectively parallels the corresponding profiling and eventual diagnoses on surgical specimens. *J Thorac Oncol.* 2011;6(6):1039-1049.

226. Bahrami A, Truong LD, Ro JY. Undifferentiated tumor: true identity by immunohistochemistry. *Arch Pathol Lab Med.* 2008;132(3):326-348.

CHAPTER 4

227. Monzon FA, Koen TJ. Diagnosis of metastatic neoplasms: molecular approaches for identification of tissue of origin. *Arch Pathol Lab Med.* 2010;134(2):216-224.

228. Oien KA, Dennis JL. Diagnostic work-up of carcinoma of unknown primary: from immunohistochemistry to molecular profiling. *An Oncol.* 2012;23(suppl 10):x271-277.

229. Bauer DE, Mitchell CM, Strait KM, et al. Clinicopathologic features and long-term outcomes of NUT midline carcinoma. *Clin Cancer Res.* 2012;18(20):5773-5779.

230. Evans AG, French CA, Cameron MJ, et al. Pathologic characteristics of NUT midline carcinoma arising in the mediastinum. *Am J Surg Pathol.* 2012;36(8):1222-1227.

231. Kees UR, Mulcahy MT, Willoughby ML. Intrathoracic carcinoma in an 11-year-old girl showing a translocation t(15;19). *Am J Pediatr Hematol Oncol.* 1991;13(4):459-464.

232. Kubonishi I, Takehara N, Iwata J, et al. Novel t(15;19)(q15;p13) chromosome abnormality in a thymic carcinoma. *Cancer Res.* 1991;51(12):3327-3328.

233. Lee AC, Kwong YI, Fu KH, Chan GC, Ma L, Lau YL. Disseminated mediastinal carcinoma with chromosomal translocation (15;19). A distinctive clinicopathologic syndrome. *Cancer.* 1993;72(7):2273-2276.

234. Tanaka M, Kato K, Gomi K, et al. NUT midline carcinoma: report of 2 cases suggestive of pulmonary origin. *Am J Surg Pathol.* 2012;36(3):381-388.

235. Haack H, Johnson LA, Fry CJ, et al. Diagnosis of NUT midline carcinoma using a NUT-specific monoclonal antibody. *Am J Surg Pathol.* 2009;33(7):984-991.

Neuroendocrine Carcinomas

Mary Beth Beasley

TAKE HOME PEARLS

- Ki-67 (mib-1) may be useful in separating high-grade NE carcinomas from carcinoids, but is not currently useful in reliably distinguishing TC from AC.
- Mitotic activity and necrosis which discriminate TC from AC may be present focally within a tumor. For this reason, subclassification should be done on a large/resected specimen and should generally not be done on a small biopsy specimen.
- A diagnosis of large cell neuroendocrine carcinoma requires the presence of both a neuroendocrine growth pattern and demonstration of neuroendocrine differentiation by ancillary markers.
- Small cell carcinoma may have more overt neuroendocrine growth patterns on resected specimens and the cell size may appear larger than in transbronchial biopsies.
- The nuclei of small cell carcinoma are oval/spindle in shape and have granular chromatin with absent or inconspicuous nucleoli; large cell neuroendocrine carcinoma in contrast has round nuclei with vesicular chromatin and prominent nucleoli may be present.
- Appropriately prepared sections are important for discriminating LCNEC from SCLC as too thick and/or overstained sections may obscure nuclear and cellular detail.

INTRODUCTION

Terminology of Neuroendocrine Carcinomas

Neuroendocrine carcinomas of the lung primarily include the low-grade typical carcinoid (TC), the intermediate-grade atypical carcinoid (AC), and the high-grade tumors, large cell neuroendocrine carcinoma (LCNEC) and small cell carcinoma (SCLC).[1] Carcinoid tumorlets, typically an incidental finding, and the putative preneoplastic lesion of diffuse idiopathic neuroendocrine cell hyperplasia (DIPNECH) are also included in this grouping.[1] The terminology of pulmonary neuroendocrine carcinomas differs somewhat from that used in other organ systems, primarily by the retention of the "carcinoid" nomenclature in the World Health Organization (WHO) classification of lung tumors. Other classification systems paralleling those of other locations such as Grades 1, 2, and 3 or well, moderately, and poorly differentiated neuroendocrine carcinomas have been proposed, as they are felt by some to better reflect the malignant nature of the carcinoids in particular.[2,3] Alternate nomenclature will be included where appropriate in the text below.

The 2004 WHO classification of neuroendocrine tumors is discussed below and summarized in *Tables 5-1* and *5-2*. An updated WHO classification has an anticipated publication date of late 2014/early 2015. The current nomenclature will be retained; however, large cell neuroendocrine carcinoma will be moved into a stand-alone category as opposed to being included as a subtype of large cell carcinoma as it was in the 2004 classification.

Other tumors with neuroendocrine differentiation occurring as primary lung neoplasms include primitive neuroectodermal tumor and, rarely, primary pulmonary neuroblastoma, discussed herein. Expression of neuroendocrine markers may also occur in pulmonary blastomas. Paragangliomas arise more commonly as

Table 5-1 WHO Classification of Pulmonary Neuroendocrine Tumors/Lesions

Carcinoid tumorlet
Diffuse idiopathic neuroendocrine cell hyperplasia
Carcinoid tumors
   Typical carcinoid
   Atypical carcinoid
Large cell neuroendocrine carcinoma
   Combined large cell neuroendocrine carcinoma
Small cell carcinoma
   Combined small cell carcinoma

posterior mediastinal tumors but may involve the lung secondarily. While case reports exist, their occurrence as primary lung parenchymal tumors is controversial.[1] Finally, it should be noted that a small subset of non-small cell lung carcinomas without overt neuroendocrine morphology may show positive staining with one or more neuroendocrine markers. Such tumors have been termed most commonly as *nonsmall cell carcinoma with neuroendocrine differentiation,* although alternative nomenclature such as *nonsmall cell carcinoma with occult neuroendocrine differentiation* has also been used. This subset of tumors has been the subject of much debate but the balance of literature suggests that this feature does not convey any particular significance in regard to prognosis or response to chemotherapy at the present time.[3]

Epidemiology of Neuroendocrine Carcinomas

Neuroendocrine carcinomas as a whole comprise roughly 20% of all pulmonary malignancies. Small cell carcinomas account for the majority of these while carcinoid tumors comprise 1% to 2%. Large cell neuroendocrine carcinomas are very rare and comprise 1% or less of all lung malignancies.[3,4] The frequency of SCLC appears to be decreasing.[5]

Etiologies of Neuroendocrine Carcinomas

Traditionally, the neuroendocrine carcinomas of the lung have been viewed as a continuum of tumors arising from neuroendocrine cells of the airways. However, it appears that TC and AC are related to each other on demographic and molecular grounds and are distinct from LCNEC and SCLC.[3,6-8] The cell of origin is currently a matter of debate and while the carcinoids may possibly arise from pulmonary neuroendocrine cells it is more likely that the high-grade tumors arise from a pluripotent stem cell.[9] The putative precursor lesion DIPNECH has been associated with TC and AC but not

Table 5-2 Diagnostic Criteria of Major Pulmonary Neuroendocrine Carcinomas

Typical carcinoid:
  Growth pattern: classically organoid with vascular background
    Other growth patterns: trabecular, papillary, prominent rosettes, "follicular," "pseudoglandular," pleomorphic cells
    Other background patterns: fibrotic, "amyloid like," ossified, mucinous (very rare)
  Cellular features: classically uniform round cells, granular "salt and pepper" chromatin, scant to moderately abundant cytoplasm
    Other cellular features: oncocytic cells, clear cells, pigmented cells
  Mitotic activity: less than 2 mitoses per 2 mm^2
  Necrosis: absent
Atypical carcinoid:
  Growth pattern: organoid with vascular background; range of patterns similar to typical carcinoid
  Cellular features: similar to typical carcinoid
  Mitotic activity: 2 to 10 mitoses per 2 mm^2 (Note: Tumors with necrosis but fewer than 2 mitoses per 2 mm^2 should still be classified as AC)
  Necrosis: Yes—usually punctate within center of cell nests; may have more extensive necrosis
Large cell neuroendocrine carcinoma:
  Growth pattern: organoid, usually with peripheral palisading of cells, rosette formation
  Cellular features: polygonal cell shape, round nuclei with vesicular chromatin, prominent nucleoli often present, moderately abundant cytoplasm, cell borders typically distinct.
  Mitotic activity: greater than 10 per 2 mm^2, most cases substantially higher
  Necrosis: Not a defining criterion but usually present, either in center of cell nests or in larger sheets
Small cell carcinoma:
  Growth pattern: typically solid sheets
    Other: organoid growth, rosette formation, papillary morphology—these patterns usually seen in large/resected specimens if present
  Cellular features: Oval to spindle cells, generally 3-4× the size of a lymphocytes, granular chromatin, scant cytoplasm, absent/inconspicuous nucleoli, cell borders typically indistinct
    Other: Cells may appear larger in resected specimens, cytoplasm may be more visible but N/C ratio still very high
  Mitoses: Greater than 10 per 2 mm^2, most cases substantially higher
  Necrosis: Not a defining features but usually present, ranging from individual cell necrosis to large sheets

with the high-grade tumors.[1,10-13] Conversely, the high-grade tumors may occur in combination with other types of lung carcinoma such as adenocarcinoma or squamous cell carcinoma, or they may be mixed with each other. Such combined morphology has not been reported in the carcinoids.[4,7] The high-grade neuroendocrine carcinomas, SCLC, and LCNEC are seen almost exclusively in cigarette smokers, whereas smoking is not as clearly associated with AC and appears unassociated with TC.[1,4,14]

CARCINOID TUMORLETS

Carcinoid tumorlets are defined as carcinoid tumors measuring 5 mm or less in diameter. By definition they lack mitotic activity and necrosis. They are located within airway walls, and the majority represent incidental findings in airways with prior injury (*Figure 5-1*). Carcinoid tumorlets may be encountered in the lung adjacent to peripheral carcinoids in particular, and do not appear to impact prognosis. Carcinoid tumorlets may also occur as a component of DIPNECH, which is discussed in this chapter.[1,14]

DIFFUSE IDIOPATHIC PULMONARY NEUROENDOCRINE CELL HYPERPLASIA

Diffuse idiopathic neuroendocrine cell hyperplasia (DIPNECH) is defined as a generalized proliferation of pulmonary neuroendocrine cells, which may occur as linear hyperplasia within airway epithelium (*Figure 5-2*), cellular clusters (neuroendocrine bodies) within the mucosa or extend beyond the basement membrane to form carcinoid tumorlets. The proliferating neuroendocrine cells are oval to spindle shaped and have finely granular chromatin. The extent of involvement may be highlighted by staining with neuroendocrine markers such as chromogranin, synaptophysin,

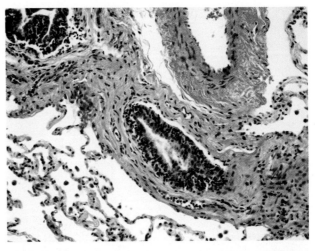

FIGURE 5-2 Neuroendocrine cell hyperplasia within an airway wall—note the expansion of uniform oval cells but the basement membrane remains intact (H&E 200×).

or CD56 (*Figure 5-3*). The involved airways may show inflammatory infiltrates or fibrotic features of constrictive bronchiolitis. DIPNECH is considered a precursor lesion and carcinoid tumor(s) may also be present. The majority of reported cases have been typical carcinoid but examples associated with atypical carcinoid have also been reported.[1,10-13]

DIPNECH should be discriminated from carcinoid tumorlets which not infrequently occur in the lung adjacent to peripherally located carcinoids. Such lesions are confined to the region of the tumor and do not involve the lung diffusely. Radiographic findings may be helpful in discriminating the two in small resections where the extent of disease is unclear.[1,10-13]

DIPNECH has been reported most frequently in the fifth and sixth decades and has been reported more

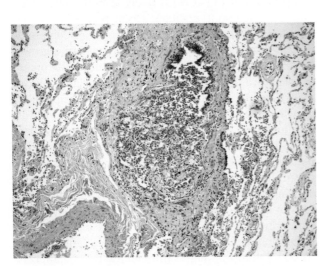

FIGURE 5-1 Carcinoid tumorlet. Carcinoid tumorlets are proliferations of neuroendocrine cells located within airway walls and measuring 5 mm or less (H&E 100×).

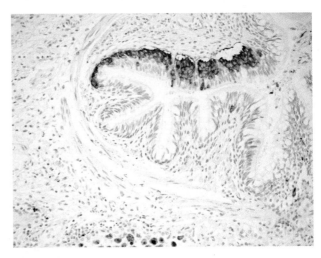

FIGURE 5-3 Neuroendocrine cell hyperplasia—A synaptophysin stains highlights subtle areas of hyperplasia (synaptophysin 200×).

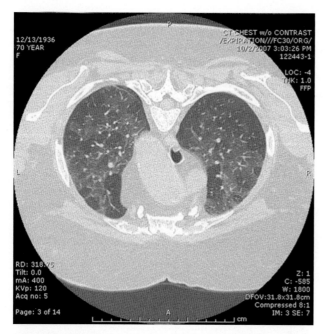

FIGURE 5-4 Expiratory CT scan of DIPNECH showing mosaic attenuation due to air trapping.

frequently in women. Most patients present with a history of shortness of breath and wheezing, which is frequently misdiagnosed as asthma, while other patients are identified incidentally.[12,13]

High-resolution CT scans show nodular bronchial wall thickening along with mosaic attenuation (*Figure 5-4*).[13]

DIPNECH is a chronic disease with the majority of patients experiencing slowly progressive disease which may stabilize over time. Occasional patients may develop more aggressive disease for unclear reasons. If DIPNECH is associated with a carcinoid tumor, the presence of the carcinoid governs the behavior of disease and the presence of DIPNECH does not appear to impact the overall survival related to the carcinoid alone.[1,10-13]

TYPICAL CARCINOID TUMOR (GRADE 1 NEUROENDOCRINE CARCINOMA)

Diagnostic Criteria of Typical Carcinoid Tumor

Typical carcinoid (TC) is defined by the WHO criteria as a carcinoid tumor greater than 5 mm in size with fewer than 2 mitoses per 2 mm^2 and lacking necrosis.[1]

Clinical Features of Typical Carcinoid Tumor

Carcinoids occur in a younger age group overall than conventional lung carcinomas and are generally seen in patients under 60 years of age. Carcinoids frequently arise in the central airways and may produce symptoms secondary to obstruction. Thirty to forty percent of tumors arise in a peripheral location and may be asymptomatic. Rarely, carcinoid syndrome, Cushing syndrome, and acromegaly may occur due to peptide production by the tumor. Lymph node metastases occur in 5% to 15% of TC. While TC generally behaves in a low-grade, indolent fashion, a small percentage or tumors will evolve into widespread fatal disease. The 5-year survival rate is approximately 90%.[3,6,15-17]

Imaging Features of Typical Carcinoid Tumor

Imaging typically shows an endobronchial tumor that may show associated calcification. Secondary atelectasis or bronchiectasis may be seen. PET studies generally show minimal to low avidity.[18,19]

Gross Features of Typical Carcinoid Tumor

Carcinoid tumors are typically tan-yellow and well circumscribed. Central tumors usually extend into the bronchial lumen. The amount of endobronchial tumor may be deceptive as the tumor may grow between the cartilaginous plates into the adjacent tissue. Peripheral tumors may not show an overt association with an airway.[1,3,18]

Histologic Features of Typical Carcinoid Tumor

TC are typically composed of uniform populations of polygonal cells with moderate to abundant eosinophilic cytoplasm and nuclei with finely granular chromatin and inconspicuous nucleoli. Occasional tumors may have clear or oncocytic cells, and tumors containing melanin have also been reported.[20] TC shows growth patterns typical of neuroendocrine tumors. The organoid (*Figure 5-5*) and trabecular patterns (*Figure 5-6*) are most frequent. Rosette formation (*Figure 5-7*), papillary growth (*Figure 5-8*), "pseudoglandular" (*Figure 5-9*), and follicular growth patterns (*Figures 5-10A* and *B*) may also be encountered, and occasionally a mixture of patterns may occur in the same tumor. The background stroma is typically highly vascular although fibrosis, amyloid like stroma, and, rarely, cartilage and bone formation may be encountered. Rare examples may have a prominent mucinous stroma (*Figures 5-11A* and *B*).[21] Peripheral tumors in particular have a tendency to show spindle cell morphology although the cells retain classic nuclear features and generally show a nested growth pattern (*Figure 5-12*).[3,7,18]

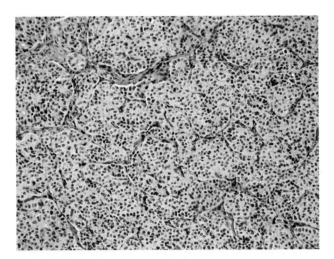

FIGURE 5-5 Typical carcinoid showing classic organoid growth with a finely vascular stroma. Nuclei are round, relatively uniform and have finely granular chromatin (H&E 200×).

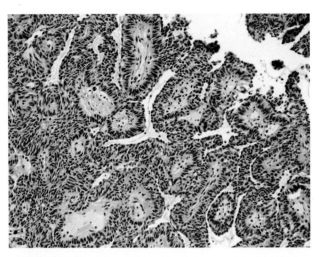

FIGURE 5-8 Typical carcinoid showing papillary growth with fibrovascular cores (H&E 200×).

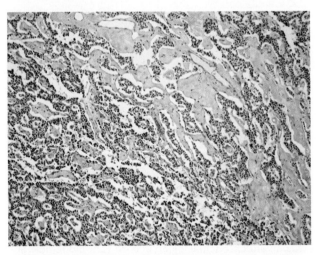

FIGURE 5-6 Typical carcinoid showing prominent trabecular growth and a fibrotic, hyalinized stroma (H&E 200×).

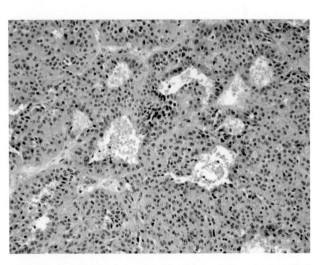

FIGURE 5-9 Typical carcinoid with solid and so-called "pseudoglandular growth." This tumor is also composed of cells with prominent oncocytic cytoplasm (H&E 200×).

Cytologic Features of Typical Carcinoid Tumor

Cytology specimens generally demonstrate dyscohesive cells, sometimes showing rosette formation, in a clean background. Fragments of capillaries may be seen. As in surgical specimens, the chromatin is finely granular and nucleoli are inconspicuous or absent.[1,3]

Immunohistochemical Features of Typical Carcinoid Tumor

TC are typically positive for cytokeratins AE1/AE3 and Cam 5.2. High molecular weight cytokeratins such as 34BE12 are usually negative. Neuroendocrine markers (chromogranin, synaptophysin, CD56) are positive.

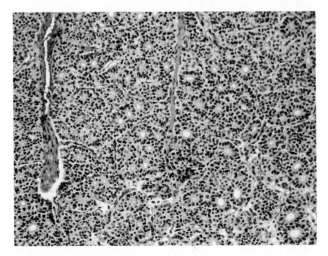

FIGURE 5-7 Typical carcinoid showing prominent rosette formation (H&E 200×).

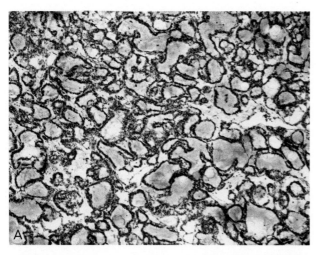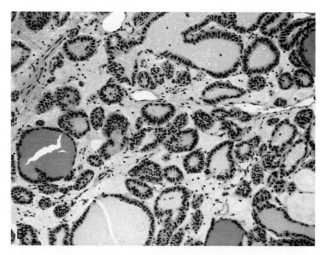

FIGURE 5-10 A: Frozen section of typical carcinoid showing striking follicular growth, greatly mimicking thyroid tissue (H&E 200×). B: Permanent section of 9A. Typical carcinoid showing a pattern of follicular growth with "colloid-like" material (H&E 200×).

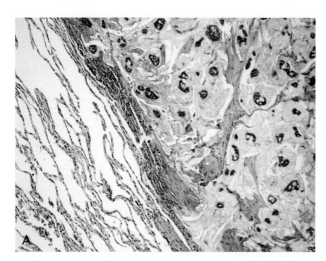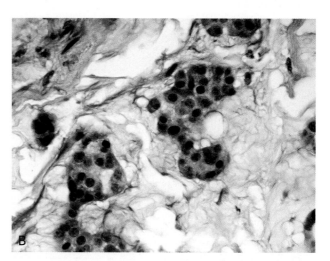

FIGURE 5-11 A: Typical carcinoid with mucinous stroma—This was an endobronchial lesion in a 40-year-old female and comprises tumor cells set in an extracellular mucinous matrix (H&E 100×). B: Typical carcinoid with mucinous stroma—Higher power demonstrated the tumor cells were uniform and had granular chromatin. Keratins and neuroendocrine markers were positive, BRST-2, mammaglobin, ER, PR, and CDX-2 were negative (H&E 600×).

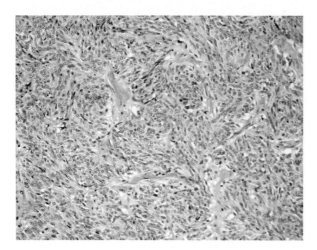

FIGURE 5-12 Typical carcinoid with spindle cell morphology and classic organoid growth (H&E 200×).

A panel is recommended as rarely an individual NE marker may be negative.[1,3]

Molecular Features of Typical Carcinoid Tumor

Carcinoid tumors in general show a very low somatic mutation rate. Mutations of MEN1 (chromosome 11p13 deletions) have been reported in up to 40% of sporadic carcinoids, which is a unique mutation that has not been reported in the high-grade neuroendocrine carcinomas.[22-25] Mutations in eukaryotic translation initiation factor 1A (EIF1AX) and trafficking and E3 ubiquitin ligase have also been reported.[6,24,26] Loss of Rb and abnormalities of E2F1 are only rarely seen in carcinoid tumors in contrast to high-grade neuroendocrine carcinomas.[27,28] Additionally, carcinoids have a lower rate of telomerase activity and have infrequent mutations in p53.[29,30] Overall, methylation with associated inactivation of tumor suppressor genes is rare in carcinoids compared to other lung cancers.[30] Carcinoid tumors have not been found to harbor mutations of epidermal grown factor receptor (EGFR) or other members of the ERB family of receptor kinases. Similarly, KRAS sequencing has demonstrated no mutations, with tumors studied found to be wild type. ALK mutations have not been reported but have not been extensively studied.[3,6,9,16,24,26,31,32] In regard to areas of potential interest for targeted therapy, agents directed toward the mammalian target of rapamycin (mTOR) pathway and vascular endothelial growth factor (VEGF) have shown some promise in trial settings but their utility is still under investigation.[32-35]

ATYPICAL CARCINOID TUMOR (GRADE 2 NEUROENDOCRINE CARCINOMA)

Diagnostic Criteria of Atypical Carcinoid Tumor

Atypical carcinoids (AC) are defined in the WHO classification as a carcinoid tumor with 2 to 10 mitoses per 2 mm² *or* necrosis. Most AC will have both features; however, occasional tumors will have necrosis and fewer than 2 mitoses per 2 mm² and such tumors should be classified as AC.[1] Of note, both TC and AC may show cellular pleomorphism and this by itself is not a discriminating feature between TC and AC.[1,17,36] AC is generally characterized by the same array of histologic growth patterns and cytologic features as TC. Most commonly, however, an organoid pattern is present (*Figure 5-13*).

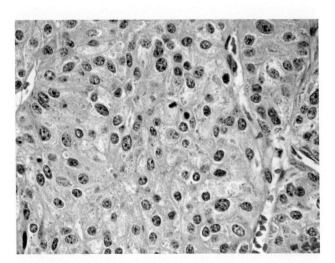

FIGURE 5-13 Atypical carcinoid—atypical carcinoid with organoid growth and a mitotic figure. This tumor also has oncocytic cytoplasm (H&E 400×).

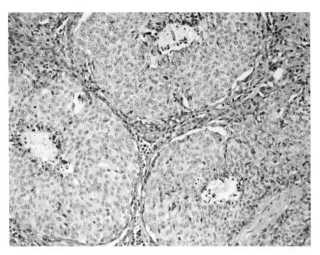

FIGURE 5-14 Atypical carcinoid—atypical carcinoid with organoid growth and central necrosis within cellular nests (H&E 200×).

Areas of necrosis are typically punctate and located centrally within tumor nests, although larger areas of necrosis may be encountered (*Figure 5-14*).[37] Mitotic activity may be focal and should be counted in the area of highest mitotic activity.[14,36] It should be noted that the definition of 2 to 10 mitoses per 2 mm² and while this corresponds to 10 high power fields on many microscope models, those with wide field objectives may need to adjust field counts accordingly.[38]

Clinical, Imaging, Gross, and Immunohistochemical Features

Clinical, imaging, gross, and immunohistochemical features of AC are essentially identical to those of TC (see above). AC, however, typically exhibits more aggressive behavior than TC, with lymph node metastases occurring in approximately 30% to 50% of cases.[3,4,14,18,36] Reported 5-year survival rates are somewhat variable, likely due to inclusion of some tumors in older literature, which would be more properly classified as LCNEC using the current criteria. Utilizing the current WHO criteria, the 5- and 10-year survival rates for AC are approximately 60% and 40%, respectively.[6,14,15,36]

A special note should be made in regard to Ki-67 staining. Proliferation markers have prognostic implications in neuroendocrine carcinomas of nonpulmonary sites, and have been extensively studied in pulmonary neuroendocrine tumors. Although on average AC has a higher proliferative index than TC and a variety of cutoff have been proposed to aid in discrimination between the two, it is generally felt that the role of Ki-67 in discriminating TC from AC has not been definitively established.[3,39,40]

Molecular Features of Atypical Carcinoid Tumor

Similar to TC, AC has been associated with mutations of the *MEN1* gene but at a higher frequency than TC.[22,24,26] Mutations generally follow a similar pattern to those found in TC but are typically found at a slightly higher frequency (see typical carcinoid section above). Both carcinoids show low rates of loss of heterozygosity at 3P, 13q, 9q21, and 17p, which are seen with a high rate of frequency in the high-grade neuroendocrine carcinomas.[6,9,16,24,26,32,41]

SMALL CELL CARCINOMA (GRADE 3 NEUROENDOCRINE CARCINOMA, SMALL CELL TYPE)

Diagnostic Criteria of Small Cell Carcinoma

Small cell carcinoma (SCLC) is defined by the WHO criteria as a malignant epithelial tumor consisting of small cells with scant cytoplasm, ill-defined cell borders, granular nuclear chromatin, and absent/inconspicuous nucleoli. The cells are characteristically oval or spindle shaped and nuclear molding may be present. Necrosis is usually present and is often extensive. The mitotic count is by definition greater than 10 mitoses per 2 mm^2 but is typically in excess of 60 to 70 mitoses per 10 HPF.[1,42]

Clinical Features of Small Cell Carcinoma

SCLC is classically located centrally and patients typically present with symptoms related to local tumor growth. Most patients present with extrapulmonary spread at the time of diagnosis. SCLC is associated with a variety of paraneoplastic syndromes such as SIAHD, Cushing syndrome, Eaton-Lambert syndrome, encephalopathy, and numerous others, which are not typically associated with other lung carcinomas. Approximately 5% to 10% of SCLC may present in a peripheral location.[18,43,44] SCLC is a high-grade malignancy with an exceedingly poor prognosis with a 5-year survival rate of 5% or less.[43] Traditionally, SCLC has been treated as distinct from other lung carcinomas as the primary treatment is chemotherapy as opposed to surgery. As most patients present with non-resectable disease, chemotherapy is still the primary treatment for most cases; however, surgical treatment is appropriate for peripheral and low-stage SCLC.[45,46]

Imaging Features of Small Cell Carcinoma

SCLC characteristically presents as a large hilar mass, usually with bulky hilar adenopathy. Peripheral SCLC appear as a solid mass which is often deceptively well circumscribed. SCLC is generally highly PET avid.[18]

Gross Features of Small Cell Carcinoma

SCLC is typically a large tan hilar mass with frequent involvement of lymph nodes. The tumor may spread along the bronchi in a subepithelial fashion.[1,8,14,47]

Histologic Features of Small Cell Carcinoma

SCLC is characterized by tumor cells that are classically described as being the size of three to four resting lymphocytes. The cells have very high nuclear to cytoplasmic ratios and cytoplasm is difficult to discern. Nuclei have hyperchromatic nuclei with granular chromatin and nucleoli are inconspicuous or absent. The cells are typically arranged in sheets; however, in larger specimens more overt neuroendocrine growth patterns may be observed, similar to those seen in carcinoid tumors (*Figure 5-15*). Similarly, cells may appear larger in resected specimens and more abundant cytoplasm may be seen (*Figures 5-16* and *5-17A* and *B*). SCLC may contain a range of cells sizes including occasional large cells and giant cells (*Figure 5-18*); however, unless these cells comprise greater than 10% of the tumor a diagnosis of combined SCLC should not be made. Mitotic activity is exceedingly high and necrosis is also generally present, particularly in larger samples. Blood vessels may become encrusted in nucleic acid material imparting a smudgy, basophilic appearance—so-called *Azzopardi effect*. "Crush artifact," often encountered in bronchial biopsy specimens of SCLC, is not pathognomonic and should not be taken as supportive evidence of

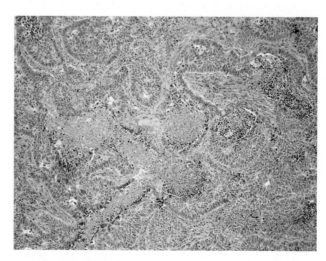

FIGURE 5-15 Small cell carcinoma—a resected small cell showing prominent organoid growth. From this power the tumor may potentially be mistaken for an atypical carcinoid (H&E 200×).

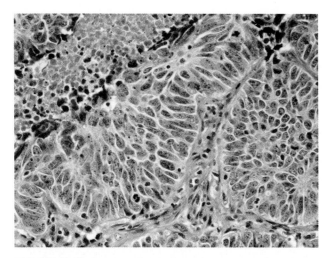

FIGURE 5-16 Small cell carcinoma—high power of the case in *Figure 5-15* showing typical cytologic features of small cell carcinoma with oval nuclei and finely granular chromatin, although the cells appear larger than in a typical bronchial biopsy (H&E 400×).

SCLC, as most any other tumor in the differential diagnosis of SCLC can also show crush artifact in a small biopsy.[4,6,7,18,44,48]

Cytologic Features of Small Cell Carcinoma

Cytology specimens typically show sheets of cells and individual bare nuclei. Apoptotic cells and necrosis are usually present.[3]

Immunohistochemical Features of Small Cell Carcinoma

The diagnosis of SCLC is generally made on light microscopy but immunohistochemistry may be necessary to separate SCLC from other tumors such as basaloid carcinoma or lymphoma. SCLC is typically positive for AE1/AE3 and Cam 5.2, often with a dot-like pattern, but paranuclear or diffuse cytoplasmic staining may also occur. Cytokeratin 34BE12 should be negative in pure SCLC. SCLC will generally express one or more NE markers (chromogranin, synaptophysin and CD56) but these markers must be interpreted in the morphologic context and up to 10% of SCLC may lack expression of NE markers due to low density of neuroendocrine granules.[42,49-51] TTF-1 is positive in up to 90% of SCLC depending on the clone utilized.[51,52] Napsin-A has thus far been consistently negative.[49] P63, often used as a marker of squamous differentiation, may be positive in SCLC although usually focally; however, p40 has thus far been negative.[53] C-kit is positive in over 60% of cases but has not shown any correlation with survival or with response to targeted therapy.[54,55]

Ki-67 is typically positive in close to 100% of tumor nuclei in SCLC. As state above, Ki-67 does not reliably discriminate between TC and AC nor does it discriminate between LCNEC and SCLC by itself, but it can aid in discriminating between high-grade and low-grade NE carcinomas with poor preservation in small biopsies. A partially crushed biopsy of a neuroendocrine tumor with 90% Ki-67 staining is not going to be TC or AC and, conversely, a negative or very low Ki-67 is not going to occur in a high-grade NE carcinoma.[3,39,40]

Molecular Features of Small Cell Carcinoma

SCLC is characterized by a wide range of genetic abnormalities, including inactivation of *TP53* and losses at chromosome 3p. Losses at 3p may involve several potential tumor suppressor genes such as *FHIT, RASSR1,*

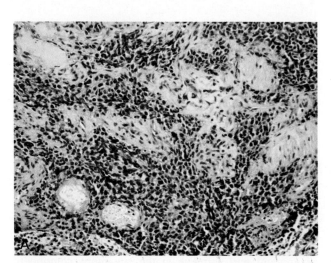
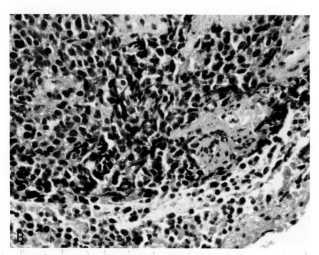

FIGURE 5-17 A: Small cell carcinoma—typical transbronchial biopsy of small cell carcinoma showing small cells, necrosis, and, while not pathognomonic, crush artifact (H&E 100×). B: Small cell carcinoma—high power of the case in 7-17A—at the same magnification, note how tumor cells appear smaller than those in the resected specimen in *Figure 5-16* (H&E 400×).

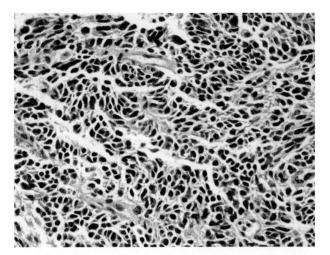

FIGURE 5-18 Small cell carcinoma—Small cell carcinoma may show a range of cell sizes. This case shows primarily classic cellular features but rare tumor giant cells are also present in the upper part of the picture. Unless a definitive secondary component comprises 10% or more of the total tumor, a diagnosis of a combined tumor should not be made (H&E 200×).

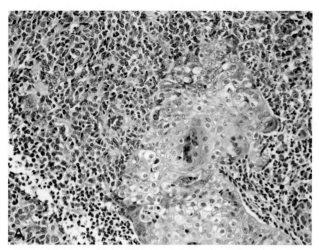

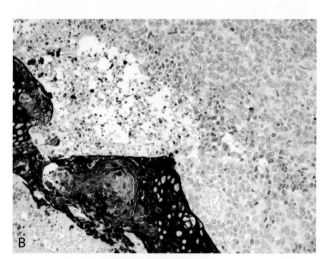

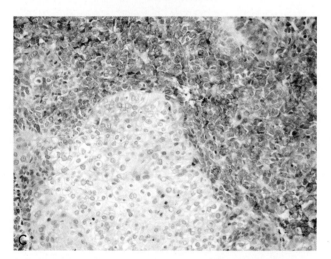

FIGURE 5-19 Combined small cell carcinoma. A: Small cell carcinoma combined with keratinizing squamous cell carcinoma (H&E 200×). B: The squamous cell carcinoma is positive for CK5/6 and the small cell component is negative (CK5/6 200×). C: CD56 is positive in the small cell component and negative in the squamous component (CD56 200×).

FUS1, VHL, DUTT1, and *FRA3B.* Losses on chromosomes 4q, 5q, 13q, and 15q have also been reported. Amplification of the *MYC* gene family and the *MAD1L1* gene has been reported.[9,26,31,41,43,52,56-63] Mutations of *Rb* are seen in almost all cases of SCLC, resulting in *Rb* loss and resulting *Rb* pathway disruption.[27] *PTEN* mutations, FGFR1 tyrosine kinase amplification, and SOX2 amplifications may also occur.[57,64] Both SCLC and LCNEC show high expression of hASH1, which is involved in neuroendocrine differentiation, with one reporting indicating higher expression in SCLC.[65,66] In spite of the myriad mutations present, therapeutic targets have been lacking. Recently *PARP1* and activation of the Hedgehog signaling pathway have been identified as potential targets of study. In general, SCLC lacks EGFR tyrosine kinase mutations and mutation testing is typically not recommended for pure SCLC.[67-70] However, adenocarcinomas harboring EGFR mutations have been reported to recur as SCLC, presumably as a resistance mechanism, yet retain the original EGFR mutation.[71,72]

COMBINED SMALL CELL CARCINOMA

Combined SCLC refers to SCLC combined with a component of nonsmall cell carcinoma, usually squamous cell, adenocarcinoma, or large cell carcinoma (*Figures 5-19A, B,* and *C*). SCLC may be combined with LCNEC and rarely with spindle or giant cell carcinoma. Because of the morphologic continuum between SCLC and LCNEC, at least 10% of the tumor should show clear evidence of LCNEC before being referred to as a combined tumor. Such tumors typically behave in a fashion similar to SCLC.[1,3,4]

LARGE CELL NEUROENDOCRINE CARCINOMA (GRADE 3 NEUROENDOCRINE CARCINOMA, LARGE CELL TYPE)

Diagnostic Criteria of Large Cell Neuroendocrine Carcinoma

Large cell neuroendocrine carcinoma (LCNEC) is defined by the WHO criteria as a tumor with histologic features of neuroendocrine morphology, large cell size, and expression of neuroendocrine markers by immunohistochemical methods. The mitotic rate is greater than 10 mitoses per 2 mm^2.[1,73]

Clinical Features of Large Cell Neuroendocrine Carcinoma

LCNEC has been reported most commonly as a peripheral lung tumor and may be asymptomatic at presentation. Twenty percent have been reported centrally. Clinical signs and symptoms are similar to other lung carcinomas. Paraneoplastic syndromes may be observed such as hypertrophic osteoarthropathy or hypercoagulable states.[3,4,18] The reported survival rates for LCNEC have been somewhat variable, likely due to the inclusion of tumors not meeting strict criteria. In spite of some reports indicating the prognosis for LCNEC is not substantially different from non-neuroendocrine lung carcinomas, most studies using strict criteria have demonstrated that the prognosis of LCNEC is poor and similar to that of SCLC.[2-4,8] Due to the rarity of LCNEC, optimal treatment has not been identified. Surgery is typically thought to be the treatment of choice although some studies have shown that chemotherapeutic regimens used for small cell may have some efficacy while other have not.[8,55]

Imaging Features of Large Cell Neuroendocrine Carcinoma

Imaging studies typically report a peripheral tumor, often with irregular margins and occasional calcification. Bulky mediastinal lymphadenopathy is usually absent. Cavitation is uncommon. Tumors are typically highly PET avid.[18]

Gross Features of Large Cell Neuroendocrine Carcinoma

LCNEC is typically a large mass in the lung periphery. Reports indicate a high frequency in the right upper lobe. Reported sizes range from 0.9 to 12 cm with an average of 3 to 4 cm. The tumor is typically tan-red with areas of necrosis and hemorrhage.[3,7,48,73]

Histologic Features of Large Cell Neuroendocrine Carcinoma

LCNEC is characterized by a neuroendocrine growth pattern similar to that seen in the carcinoid tumors. Organoid nests with peripheral palisading of tumor cells are most common and many cases show rosette formation. Necrosis is often present in the center of the nests but large areas of necrosis may be seen (*Figures 5-20* and *5-21*). The tumor cells are large with moderately abundant eosinophilic cytoplasm. Cell shape tends to be polygonal and cell borders are usually distinct. Nucleoli are frequently present and often large (*Figure 5-22*). The mitotic rate is by definition greater than 10 per 2 mm^2 but most cases have an excess of 30 mitoses per 2 mm^2 with an average of 75 per 2 mm^2.[1,3,7,14,18]

Cytologic Features of Large Cell Neuroendocrine Carcinoma

Diagnosis of LCNEC on cytology specimens or small biopsies in general is often difficult due to the lack of sufficient tissue to evaluate the growth pattern. The cytologic appearance is generally that of a high-grade nonsmall cell carcinoma.[3]

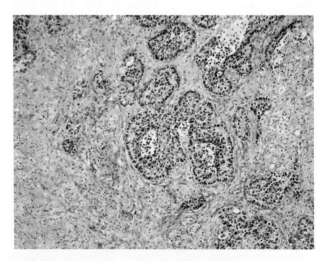

FIGURE 5-20 Large cell neuroendocrine carcinoma—low power demonstrating organoid growth pattern with peripheral palisading of tumor cells. Focal necrosis is present in the center of the nests (H&E 100×).

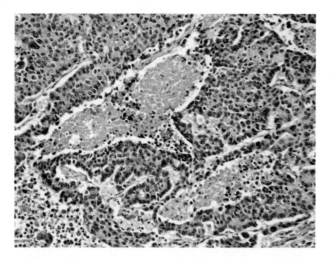

FIGURE 5-21 Large cell neuroendocrine carcinoma—organoid nest with larger area of necrosis. Focal rosette formation can be seen on the right (H&E 200×).

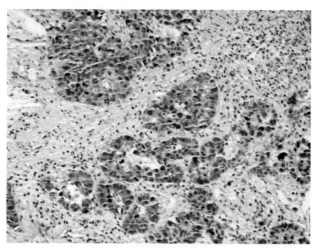

FIGURE 5-23 Large cell neuroendocrine carcinoma—By definition, neuroendocrine differentiation must be demonstrated by ancillary methods. This is an example of a positive synaptophysin stain in LCNEC (synaptophysin 200×).

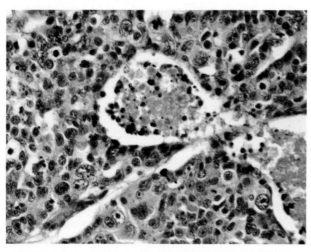

FIGURE 5-22 Large cell neuroendocrine carcinoma—Cells are polygonal in shape with vesicular chromatin and many cells have prominent nucleoli. Mitotic figures are present (H&E 400×).

Immunohistochemical Features of Large Cell Neuroendocrine Carcinoma

By definition LCNEC should have both neuroendocrine morphology and expression of neuroendocrine markers by immunohistochemistry (*Figure 5-23*). It should be noted that a marker with relative specificity for neuroendocrine differentiation should be utilized (ie, chromogranin, synaptophysin, CD56) as opposed to neuron-specific enolase (NSE), which also stains a high percentage of non-neuroendocrine lung carcinomas. Currently, there is no specific recommendation for a minimum required amount of staining although this is under review.[1,3,7,14,18]

Molecular Features of Large Cell Neuroendocrine Carcinoma

Molecular abnormalities in LCNEC share considerable overlap with those found in SCLC. Like SCLC, LCNEC shows a high level of expression of HASH1; however, expression of hairy enhancer split 1 (HES1), which is a negative regulator of neuroendocrine differentiation, is more highly expressed in LCNEC.[65,66,74] Other studies have shown statistically significant differences between LCNEC and SCLC, with LCNEC showing more frequent gains at 2q31, 2q32, and 2q33, more frequent loss at 6p21.3, and less frequent loss at 3p26, 4q21, 4q24, and 4q31 compared to SCLC.[16,23,26,31,41,55,58,60,61,75] Interestingly, a study by D'Adda et al studied genetic alterations in combined SCLC/LCNEC and found that both components showed common genetic alterations usually involved in early carcinogenesis and hypothesized a possible monoclonal carcinogenesis. While the authors did find some differences between the two components, they were found to have more commonality with each other than with known alterations in pure tumors, possibly suggesting that combined SCLC/LCNEC may represent a transition in the spectrum of high-grade neuroendocrine carcinomas.[76]

COMBINED LARGE CELL NEUROENDOCRINE CARCINOMA

Like SCLC, LCNEC may occur in combination with squamous cell carcinoma or adenocarcinoma, with each component comprising at least 10% of the tumor

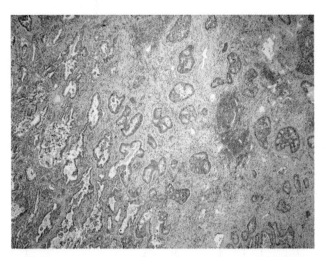

FIGURE 5-24 **Combined LCNEC—In this example LCNEC is present on the right and adenocarcinoma is present on the left (H&E 100×).**

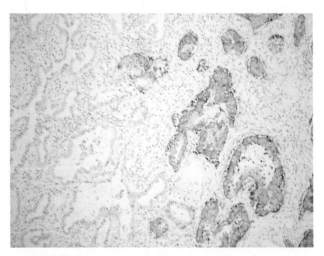

FIGURE 5-25 **Combined LCNEC—A CD56 stain highlights the LCNEC component while the adenocarcinoma component is negative (H&E 200×).**

(*Figures 5-24* and *5-25*). Such tumors are quite rare and the LCNEC component governs the behavior. LCNEC combined with SCLC should be termed *combined SCLC* and not *combined LCNEC* given that the LCNEC will generally drive treatment selection.[1,3,14]

OTHER NEUROENDOCRINE LESIONS OF THE LUNG

Primary Pulmonary Neuroblastoma

Neuroblastoma (NB) is the fourth most common childhood malignancy overall, with the majority of cases occurring in the abdomen, either in intra- or extraadrenal locations. Ganglioneuroblastoma (GNB) is a related tumor with a similar presentation but containing a

population of maturing ganglion cells. The vast majority of cases of NB and GNB are diagnosed prior to 5 years of age and only rare tumors have been reported in adults. Approximately 15% to 20% of cases occur in the thorax, where they typically arise from the sympathetic chain and present as posterior mediastinal masses. In this location symptoms are usually related to mass effect of the tumor but may be symptoms related to catecholamine release, such as diarrhea or myoclonus, may be present.[77-79]

Primary intrapulmonary NBs/GNBs are exceedingly rare, and, in spite of NB/GNB being largely a childhood tumor, the reported cases of intrapulmonary tumors have all been GNB and have been reported in a 47-year-old male,[77] a 38-year-old female, and a 20-year-old female.[79] Interestingly, a combined carcinoid/GNB has also been reported in a 69-year-old female.[78]

Of the pulmonary NBs/GNBs, two were solitary and one consisted of a dominant lesion and two smaller nodules. The main lesions either involved or were in the proximity of airways, were well circumscribed with a firm white cut surface and ranged from 3.0 to 5.0 cm. One patient was apparently asymptomatic and one presented with cough The third presented with protracted vomiting, nausea, diarrhea, abdominal pain, a 75-lb weight loss and hypercalcemia and was later discovered to have parathyroid hyperplasia, a pituitary adenoma, and an islet cell tumor, consistent with MEN1 syndrome.[77,79]

Histologically, neuroblastoma is characterized by a proliferation of small round blue cells with minimal identifiable stroma (*Figure 5-26*) although "differentiating" tumors may show fibrillary eosinophilic matrix. Homer-Wright rosettes may be encountered. GNBs contain identifiable ganglion cells. NBs/GNBs are usually negative for cytokeratins, actin, and desmin and positive for NSE, synaptophysin, and CD56. Chromogranin is typically negative. NB/GNB is negative for CD99 and β-2 microglobulin.[80]

Specific information regarding outcome and prognostic features of pulmonary neuroblastoma is lacking due to the rarity of these tumors. Features important in predicting outcome in general include the degree of gangliocytic differentiation and the so-called *mitotic karyorrhectic index* (number of mitotic and/or karyorrhectic cells in 5000 tumor cells in a *neuropil-free area*). Increased copy number of n-MYC is associated with a worse outcome.[80]

Primary Pulmonary Primitive Neuroectodermal Tumor

Primitive neuroectodermal tumor (PNET), a member of the Ewing sarcoma family of tumors, occurs most commonly as a soft tissue neoplasm. Roughly a third of PNET arise in the thorax, generally involving the chest

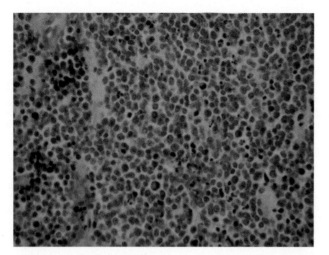

FIGURE 5-26 Neuroblastoma—an example of neuroblastoma showing diffuse sheets of small blue cells with minimal identifiable stroma (H&E 200×). (Used with permission of Dr Margret Magid.)

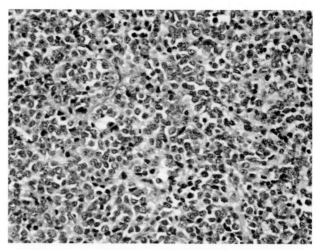

FIGURE 5-27 Primitive neuroectodermal tumor (PNET)— PNET is characterized by small blue cells with scant cytoplasm, dispersed chromatin, and inconspicuous nucleoli. This example shows sheet-like growth, but rosette formation may also be seen (H&E 400×).

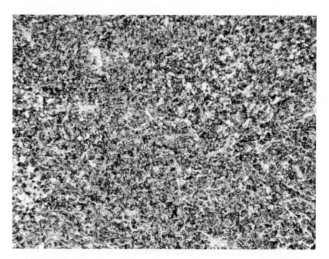

FIGURE 5-28 Primitive neuroectodermal tumor (PNET)— CD99, while not exclusively seen in PNET, is characteristically strongly positive (CD99 200×).

wall, where they have been historically known as *malignant small cell tumor of thoracopulmonary origin* or *Askin tumor*. While PNET may metastasize to the lung parenchyma, reported examples of primary intrapulmonary PNET are exceedingly rare. The source of origin is unclear but is thought to possibly arise from abnormal migration of neural crest cells. While PNET occurring in the soft tissues has experienced an improved survival with modern therapy, with reported 5-year survivals of up to 70%, PNET arising in the thorax tends to follow a more aggressive course, similar to PNET report in other visceral sites.[81-83] In the 2012 series of six patients, four patients had known follow-up and three were dead of disease.[84]

PNET involving the thorax generally occurs in children and teenagers but cases have been reported in older adults as well, with a slight male predominance. Presenting symptoms typically consist of chest pain, shortness of breath, and cough.[81,83] A 2012 series of six intrapulmonary PNET described the radiologic features in all cases as well-circumscribed parenchymal masses with contrast enhancement. The tumors were grossly described as ranging from 4 to 9.6 cm, well-circumscribed tumors with a friable yellow-white cut surface, soft consistency, and areas of necrosis and hemorrhage. Cystic degeneration was noted in one case and one case showed endobronchial involvement.[84]

Primary thoracic tumors are histologically the same as their soft tissue counterparts and consist of small closely packed small blue cells with high nuclear/cytoplasmic ratios, finely dispersed chromatin, and inconspicuous nucleoli (*Figure 5-27*). Cells are arranged in diffuse sheets of lobules with occasional rosette formation or prominent nuclear palisading. Necrosis and hemorrhage may be present. Mitotic activity is

usually present and may be high. The tumors may greatly resemble SCLC, and discrimination largely depends on immunohistochemical stains. PNET is typically positive for S-100, CD99, FLI-1, NSE, and synaptophysin, although positive staining for S-100 has not been as consistently reported in thoracopulmonary tumors in comparison to their soft tissue counterparts (*Figure 5-28*). Chromogranin and cytokeratin are typically negative, as is TTF-1. Conversely, SCLC is positive for cytokeratin, the majority of cases are positive for TTF-1, and most cases are negative for CD99. That being said, a small percentage of SCLC is positive for CD99 and PNET may occasionally be positive for keratin. The characteristic gene rearrangement found in PNET, t(11;22)(q24;q12), is helpful in problematic cases.[81-84]

REFERENCES

1. Travis WD, Brambilla E, Müller-Hermelink HK, Harris CC. *Pathology and Genetics: Tumours of the Lung, Pleura, Thymus and Heart.* In: Travis WD, Brambilla E, Harris CC, Muller-Hermelink HK, eds. Lyon, France: IARC; 2004.

2. Moran CA, Suster S, Coppola D, Wick MR. Neuroendocrine carcinomas of the lung: a critical analysis. *Am J Clin Pathol.* 2009;131(2):206-221.

3. Rekhtman N. Neuroendocrine tumors of the lung: an update. *Arch Pathol Lab Med.* 2010;134(11):1628-1638.

4. Lim E, Goldstraw P, Nicholson AG, et al. Proceedings of the IASLC International Workshop on Advances in Pulmonary Neuroendocrine Tumors 2007. *J Thorac Oncol.* 2008;3(10): 1194-1201.

5. Govindan R, Page N, Morgensztern D, et al. Changing epidemiology of small-cell lung cancer in the United States over the last 30 years: analysis of the surveillance, epidemiologic, and end results database. *J Clin Oncol.* 2006;24(28):4539-4544.

6. Bertino EM, Confer PD, Colonna JE, Ross P, Otterson GA. Pulmonary neuroendocrine/carcinoid tumors: a review article. *Cancer.* 2009;115(19):4434-4441.

7. Flieder DB. Neuroendocrine tumors of the lung: recent developments in histopathology. *Curr Opin Pulm Med.* 2002;8(4):275-280.

8. Travis WD. Lung tumours with neuroendocrine differentiation. *Eur J Cancer.* 2009;45(suppl 1):251-266.

9. Swarts DR, Ramaekers FC, Speel EJ. Molecular and cellular biology of neuroendocrine lung tumors: evidence for separate biological entities. *Biochim Biophys Acta.* 2012;1826(2):255-271.

10. Davies SJ, Gosney JR, Hansell DM, et al. Diffuse idiopathic pulmonary neuroendocrine cell hyperplasia: an under-recognised spectrum of disease. *Thorax.* 2007;62(3):248-252.

11. Falkenstern-Ge RF, Kimmich M, Friedel G, Tannapfel A, Neumann V, Kohlhaeufl M. Diffuse idiopathic pulmonary neuroendocrine cell hyperplasia: 7-year follow-up of a rare clinicopathologic syndrome. *J Cancer Res Clin Oncol.* 2011;137(10):1495-1498.

12. Gorshtein A, Gross DJ, Barak D, et al. Diffuse idiopathic pulmonary neuroendocrine cell hyperplasia and the associated lung neuroendocrine tumors: clinical experience with a rare entity. *Cancer.* 2012;118(3):612-619.

13. Nassar AA, Jaroszewski DE, Helmers RA, Colby TV, Patel BM, Mookadam F. Diffuse idiopathic pulmonary neuroendocrine cell hyperplasia: a systematic overview. *Am J Respir Crit Care Med.* 2011;184(1):8-16.

14. Travis WD. Advances in neuroendocrine lung tumors. *Ann Oncol.* 2010;21(suppl 7):vii65-vii71.

15. Mezzetti M, Raveglia F, Panigalli T, et al. Assessment of outcomes in typical and atypical carcinoids according to latest WHO classification. *Ann Thorac Surg.* 2003;76(6):1838-1842.

16. Righi L, Volante M, Rapa I, Scagliotti GV, Papotti M. Neuroendocrine tumours of the lung. A review of relevant pathological and molecular data. *Virchows Arch.* 2007;451(suppl 1):S51-S59.

17. Travis WD, Rush W, Flieder DB, et al. Survival analysis of 200 pulmonary neuroendocrine tumors with clarification of criteria for atypical carcinoid and its separation from typical carcinoid. *Am J Surg Pathol.* 1998;22(8):934-944.

18. Chong S, Lee KS, Chung MJ, Han J, Kwon OJ, Kim TS. Neuroendocrine tumors of the lung: clinical, pathologic, and imaging findings. *Radiographics.* 2006;26(1):41-57.

19. Erasmus JJ, Macapinlac HA. Low-sensitivity FDG-PET studies: less common lung neoplasms. *Semin Nucl Med.* 2012;42(4):255-260.

20. Gal AA, Koss MN, Hochholzer L, DeRose PB, Cohen C. Pigmented pulmonary carcinoid tumor. An immunohistochemical and ultrastructural study. *Arch Pathol Lab Med.* 1993;117(8):832-836.

21. Nannini N, Bertolini F, Cavazza A, Casali C, Mengoli MC, Rossi G. Atypical carcinoid with prominent mucinous stroma: a hitherto unreported variant of pulmonary neuroendocrine tumor. *Endocr Pathol.* 2010;21(2):120-124.

22. Debelenko LV, Swalwell JI, Kelley MJ, et al. MEN1 gene mutation analysis of high-grade neuroendocrine lung carcinoma. *Genes Chromosomes Cancer.* 2000;28(1):58-65.

23. Hofsli E. Genes involved in neuroendocrine tumor biology. *Pituitary.* 2006;9(3):165-178.

24. Leotlela PD, Jauch A, Holtgreve-Grez H, Thakker RV. Genetics of neuroendocrine and carcinoid tumours. *Endocr Relat Cancer.* 2003;10(4):437-450.

25. Walch AK, Zitzelsberger HF, Aubele MM, et al. Typical and atypical carcinoid tumors of the lung are characterized by 11q deletions as detected by comparative genomic hybridization. *Am J Pathol.* 1998;153(4):1089-1098.

26. Onuki N, Wistuba II, Travis WD, et al. Genetic changes in the spectrum of neuroendocrine lung tumors. *Cancer.* 1999;85(3):600-607.

27. Beasley MB, Lantuejoul S, Abbondanzo S, et al. The P16/cyclin D1/Rb pathway in neuroendocrine tumors of the lung. *Hum Pathol.* 2003;34(2):136-142.

28. Salon C, Merdzhanova G, Brambilla C, Brambilla E, Gazzeri S, Eymin B. E2F-1, Skp2 and cyclin E oncoproteins are upregulated and directly correlated in high-grade neuroendocrine lung tumors. *Oncogene.* 2007;26(48):6927-6936.

29. Nishio Y, Nakanishi K, Ozeki Y, et al. Telomere length, telomerase activity, and expressions of human telomerase mRNA component (hTERC) and human telomerase reverse transcriptase (hTERT) mRNA in pulmonary neuroendocrine tumors. *Jpn J Clin Oncol.* 2007;37(1):16-22.

30. Voortman J, Lee JH, Killian JK, et al. Array comparative genomic hybridization-based characterization of genetic alterations in pulmonary neuroendocrine tumors. *Proc Natl Acad Sci U S A.* 2010;107(29):13040-13045.

31. Kobayashi Y, Tokuchi Y, Hashimoto T, et al. Molecular markers for reinforcement of histological subclassification of neuroendocrine lung tumors. *Cancer Sci.* 2004;95(4):334-341.

32. Swarts DR, Van Neste L, Henfling ME, et al. An exploration of pathways involved in lung carcinoid progression using gene expression profiling. *Carcinogenesis.* 2013;34(12):2726-2737.

33. Dong M, Yao JC. mTOR inhibition, a potential novel approach for bronchial carcinoids. *Endocr Relat Cancer.* 2011;18(3):C15-C18.

34. Jafri N, Salgia R. Biology and novel therapeutics for neuroendocrine tumors of the lung. *J Biol Regul Homeost Agents.* 2004;18(3-4):275-290.

35. Kunnimalaiyaan M, Chen H. The Raf-1 pathway: a molecular target for treatment of select neuroendocrine tumors? *Anticancer Drugs.* 2006;17(2):139-142.

36. Beasley MB, Thunnissen FB, Brambilla E, et al. Pulmonary atypical carcinoid: predictors of survival in 106 cases. *Hum Pathol.* 2000;31(10):1255-1265.

37. Tsuta K, Raso MG, Kalhor N, Liu DD, Wistuba II, Moran CA. Histologic features of low- and intermediate-grade neuroendocrine carcinoma (typical and atypical carcinoid tumors) of the lung. *Lung Cancer.* 2011;71(1):34-41.

38. Thunnissen FB, Ambergen AW, Koss M, Travis WD, O'Leary TJ, Ellis IO. Mitotic counting in surgical pathology: sampling bias, heterogeneity and statistical uncertainty. *Histopathology.* 2001;39(1):1-8.

39. Erler BS, Presby MM, Finch M, et al. CD117, Ki-67, and p53 predict survival in neuroendocrine carcinomas, but not within the subgroup of small cell lung carcinoma. *Tumour Biol.* 2011;32(1):107-111.

40. Pelosi G, Rindi G, Travis WD, Papotti M. Ki-67 antigen in lung neuroendocrine tumors: unraveling a role in clinical practice. *J Thorac Oncol.* 2014;9(3):273-284.

41. Takeuchi T, Minami Y, Iijima T, Kameya T, Asamura H, Noguchi M. Characteristics of loss of heterozygosity in large cell

neuroendocrine carcinomas of the lung and small cell lung carcinomas. *Pathol Int.* 2006;56(8):434-439.

42. Beasley MB, Brambilla E, Travis WD. The 2004 World Health Organization classification of lung tumors. *Semin Roentgenol.* 2005;40(2):90-97.

43. Campbell AM, Campling BG, Algazy KM, el-Deiry WS. Clinical and molecular features of small cell lung cancer. *Cancer Biol Ther.* 2002;1(2):105-112.

44. Nicholson SA, Beasley MB, Brambilla E, et al. Small cell lung carcinoma (SCLC): a clinicopathologic study of 100 cases with surgical specimens. *Am J Surg Pathol.* 2002;26(9):1184-1197.

45. Badzio A, Kurowski K, Karnicka-Mlodkowska H, Jassem J. A retrospective comparative study of surgery followed by chemotherapy vs. non-surgical management in limited-disease small cell lung cancer. *Eur J Cardiothorac Surg.* 2004;26(1):183-188.

46. Koletsis EN, Prokakis C, Karanikolas M, Apostolakis E, Dougenis D. Current role of surgery in small cell lung carcinoma. *J Cardiothorac Surg.* 2009;4:30.

47. Butnor KJ, Beasley MB, Cagle PT, et al. Protocol for the examination of specimens from patients with primary non-small cell carcinoma, small cell carcinoma, or carcinoid tumor of the lung. *Arch Pathol Lab Med.* 2009;133(10):1552-1559.

48. den Bakker MA, Thunnissen FB. Neuroendocrine tumours—challenges in the diagnosis and classification of pulmonary neuroendocrine tumours. *J Clin Pathol.* 2013;66(10):862-869.

49. Bishop JA, Sharma R, Illei PB. Napsin A and thyroid transcription factor-1 expression in carcinomas of the lung, breast, pancreas, colon, kidney, thyroid, and malignant mesothelioma. *Hum Pathol.* 2010;41(1):20-25.

50. Guinee DG Jr, Fishback NF, Koss MN, Abbondanzo SL, Travis WD. The spectrum of immunohistochemical staining of small-cell lung carcinoma in specimens from transbronchial and open-lung biopsies. *Am J Clin Pathol.* 1994;102(4):406-414.

51. Wu M, Wang B, Gil J, et al. p63 and TTF-1 immunostaining. A useful marker panel for distinguishing small cell carcinoma of lung from poorly differentiated squamous cell carcinoma of lung. *Am J Clin Pathol.* 2003;119(5):696-702.

52. Kitamura H, Yazawa T, Sato H, Okudela K, Shimoyamada H. Small cell lung cancer: significance of RB alterations and TTF-1 expression in its carcinogenesis, phenotype, and biology. *Endocr Pathol.* 2009;20(2):101-107.

53. Au NH, Gown AM, Cheang M, et al. P63 expression in lung carcinoma: a tissue microarray study of 408 cases. *Appl Immunohistochem Mol Morphol.* 2004;12(3):240-247.

54. Pelosi G, Masullo M, Leon ME, et al. CD117 immunoreactivity in high-grade neuroendocrine tumors of the lung: a comparative study of 39 large-cell neuroendocrine carcinomas and 27 surgically resected small-cell carcinomas. *Virchows Arch.* 2004;445(5):449-455.

55. Rossi G, Cavazza A, Marchioni A, et al. Role of chemotherapy and the receptor tyrosine kinases KIT, PDGFRalpha, PDGFRbeta, and Met in large-cell neuroendocrine carcinoma of the lung. *J Clin Oncol.* 2005;23(34):8774-8785.

56. Anbazhagan R, Tihan T, Bornman DM, et al. Classification of small cell lung cancer and pulmonary carcinoid by gene expression profiles. *Cancer Res.* 1999;59(20):5119-5122.

57. Dacic S, Finkelstein SD, Baksh FK, Swalsky PA, Barnes LE, Yousem SA. Small-cell neuroendocrine carcinoma displays unique profiles of tumor-suppressor gene loss in relationship to the primary site of formation. *Hum Pathol.* 2002;33(9):927-932.

58. Hiroshima K, Iyoda A, Shida T, et al. Distinction of pulmonary large cell neuroendocrine carcinoma from small cell lung carcinoma: a morphological, immunohistochemical, and molecular analysis. *Mod Pathol.* 2006;19(10):1358-1368.

59. Kovatich A, Friedland DM, Druck T, et al. Molecular alterations to human chromosome 3p loci in neuroendocrine lung tumors. *Cancer.* 1998;83(6):1109-1117.

60. Nagashio R, Sato Y, Matsumoto T, et al. Significant high expression of cytokeratins 7, 8, 18, 19 in pulmonary large cell neuroendocrine carcinomas, compared to small cell lung carcinomas. *Pathol Int.* 2010;60(2):71-77.

61. Peng WX, Shibata T, Katoh H, et al. Array-based comparative genomic hybridization analysis of high-grade neuroendocrine tumors of the lung. *Cancer Sci.* 2005;96(10):661-667.

62. Taniwaki M, Daigo Y, Ishikawa N, et al. Gene expression profiles of small-cell lung cancers: molecular signatures of lung cancer. *Int J Oncol.* 2006;29(3):567-575.

63. Wistuba II, Gazdar AF, Minna JD. Molecular genetics of small cell lung carcinoma. *Semin Oncol.* 2001;28(2 suppl 4):3-13.

64. Sholl LM, Long KB, Hornick JL. Sox2 expression in pulmonary non-small cell and neuroendocrine carcinomas. *Appl Immunohistochem Mol Morphol.* 2010;18(1):55-61.

65. Jiang SX, Kameya T, Asamura H, et al. hASH1 expression is closely correlated with endocrine phenotype and differentiation extent in pulmonary neuroendocrine tumors. *Mod Pathol.* 2004;17(2):222-229.

66. Osada H, Tatematsu Y, Yatabe Y, Horio Y, Takahashi T. ASH1 gene is a specific therapeutic target for lung cancers with neuroendocrine features. *Cancer Res.* 2005;65(23):10680-10685.

67. Mountzios G, Dimopoulos MA, Soria JC, Sanoudou D, Papadimitriou CA. Histopathologic and genetic alterations as predictors of response to treatment and survival in lung cancer: a review of published data. *Crit Rev Oncol Hematol.* 2010;75(2):94-109.

68. Sartori G, Cavazza A, Sgambato A, et al. EGFR and K-ras mutations along the spectrum of pulmonary epithelial tumors of the lung and elaboration of a combined clinicopathologic and molecular scoring system to predict clinical responsiveness to EGFR inhibitors. *Am J Clin Pathol.* 2009;131(4):478-489.

69. Pirker R, Herth FJ, Kerr KM, et al. Consensus for EGFR mutation testing in non-small cell lung cancer: results from a European workshop. *J Thorac Oncol.* 2010;5(10):1706-1713.

70. Lindeman NI, Cagle PT, Beasley MB, et al. Molecular testing guideline for selection of lung cancer patients for EGFR and ALK tyrosine kinase inhibitors: guideline from the College of American Pathologists, International Association for the Study of Lung Cancer, and Association for Molecular Pathology. *J Thorac Oncol.* 2013;8(7):823-859.

71. Chang Y, Kim SY, Choi YJ, et al. Neuroendocrine differentiation in acquired resistance to epidermal growth factor receptor tyrosine kinase inhibitor. *Tuberc Respir Dis.* 2013;75(3):95-103.

72. Watanabe S, Sone T, Matsui T, et al. Transformation to small-cell lung cancer following treatment with EGFR tyrosine kinase inhibitors in a patient with lung adenocarcinoma. *Lung Cancer.* 2013;82(2):370-372.

73. Travis WD, Linnoila RI, Tsokos MG, et al. Neuroendocrine tumors of the lung with proposed criteria for large-cell neuroendocrine carcinoma. An ultrastructural, immunohistochemical, and flow cytometric study of 35 cases. *Am J Surg Pathol.* 1991;15(6):529-553.

74. Nasgashio R, Sato Y, Matsumoto T, et al. The balance between the expressions of hASH1 and HES1 differs between large cell neuroendocrine carcinoma and small cell carcinoma of the lung. *Lung Cancer.* 2011;74(3):405-410.

75. Peng WX, Sano T, Oyama T, Kawashima O, Nakajima T. Large cell neuroendocrine carcinoma of the lung: a comparison with large cell carcinoma with neuroendocrine morphology and small cell carcinoma. *Lung Cancer.* 2005;47(2):225-233.

76. D'Adda T, Pelosi G, Lagrasta C, et al. Genetic alterations in combined neuroendocrine neoplasms of the lung. *Mod Pathol.* 2008;21(4):414-422.

77. Cooney TP. Primary pulmonary ganglioneuroblastoma in an adult: maturation, involution and the immune response. *Histopathology.* 1981;5(4):451-463.

78. Freeman JK, Otis CN. Combined carcinoid tumor and ganglioneuroblastoma of the lung: a case report. *Int J Surg Pathol.* 2001;9(2):169-173.

79. Hochholzer L, Moran CA, Koss MN. Primary pulmonary ganglioneuroblastoma: a clinicopathologic and immunohistochemical study of two cases. *Ann Diagn Pathol.* 1998;2(3):154-158.

80. Lack EE. Neuroblastoma, ganglioneuroblastoma and other related tumors. In: Silverberg SG, ed. *Tumors of the Adrenal Glands and Extraadrenal Paraganglia. AFIP Atlas of Tumor Pathology.* 4th ed. Silver Spring, MD: ARP Press; 2007:435-476.

81. Choi EY, Gardner JM, Lucas DR, McHugh JB, Patel RM. Ewing sarcoma. *Semin Diagn Pathol.* 2014;31(1):39-47.

82. Murphey MD, Senchak LT, Mambalam PK, Logie CI, Klassen-Fischer MK, Kransdorf MJ. From the radiologic pathology archives: Ewing sarcoma family of tumors: radiologic-pathologic correlation. *Radiographics.* 2013;33(3):803-831.

83. Tsokos M, Alaggio RD, Dehner LP, Dickman PS. Ewing sarcoma/peripheral primitive neuroectodermal tumor and related tumors. *Pediatr Dev Pathol.* 2012;15(1 suppl):108-126.

84. Weissferdt A, Moran CA. Primary pulmonary primitive neuroectodermal tumor (PNET): a clinicopathological and immunohistochemical study of six cases. *Lung.* 2012;190(6):677-683.

CHAPTER 5

6 Large Cell and Other Carcinomas

Yasmeen Butt and Timothy Craig Allen

TAKE HOME PEARLS

- Large cell carcinoma, traditionally one of the mainstays of lung cancer diagnosis, is today an uncommonly rendered diagnosis.
- Marker-null large cell carcinomas are an uncommon subset of lung cancers that histologically show "large cell" features and are immunohistochemically negative for adenocarcinoma and squamous cell carcinoma markers.
- Mucoepidermoid carcinoma and adenoid cystic carcinoma are the most common salivary gland tumors arising within the lung.

LARGE CELL CARCINOMA

Large cell carcinoma, traditionally one of the mainstays of lung cancer diagnosis, is today an uncommonly rendered diagnosis because many lung cancers formerly termed large cell carcinoma are now being identified using immunohistochemical methods as poorly differentiated adenocarcinomas and poorly differentiated squamous cell carcinomas. The term large cell carcinoma is now dynamic and somewhat controversial; today the diagnosis pulmonary large cell carcinoma is essentially limited to lung cancers with "large cell" histology for which immunostaining for adenocarcinoma and squamous cell markers is unclear or unavailable, or for which immunostaining is negative (large cell carcinoma with null immunohistochemical features; "marker-null large cell carcinoma").[1-4] Importantly,

the diagnosis should be limited to resection specimens and not applied to biopsy or cytology samples that may represent an incomplete sampling of the different morphologies represented across any given tumor.[3]

Clinical Features of Marker-Null Large Cell Carcinoma

Marker-null large cell carcinomas, when compared with adenocarcinoma and squamous cell carcinomas of the lung, have a similar clinical presentation. Importantly, marker-null large cell carcinomas exhibit a worse overall and disease-free survival with a median disease-free survival of 0.6 years and a 5-year overall survival of only 12%.[4]

Imaging Features of Marker-Null Large Cell Carcinoma

Imaging of marker-null large cell carcinoma is also similar to pulmonary adenocarcinoma and pulmonary squamous cell carcinoma. They have been reported to present radiologically often as solid nodule that is greater than 5 cm in greatest dimension.[5,6]

Gross Features of Marker-Null Large Cell Carcinoma

Marker-null large cell carcinomas present grossly with features similar to other poorly differentiated pulmonary cancers. They are often larger than 5 cm and

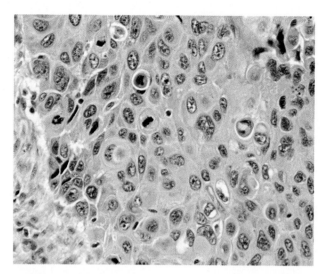

FIGURE 6-1 High-power image of pulmonary marker-null large cell carcinoma showing nonsmall cell neoplastic cells that lack squamous or adenocarcinomatous differentiation.

may have a sarcomatoid appearance—so-called "fish-flesh"—on cut surface, and can contain necrotic areas.[6]

Histologic Features of Marker-Null Large Cell Carcinoma

By their limiting diagnostic criteria, marker-null large cell carcinomas lack any squamous, glandular, or neuroendocrine differentiation (*Figure 6-1*). They are typically composed of solid sheets or large clusters of large polygonal cells, usually with prominent nuclei, vesicular chromatin, and obvious cytoplasmic membranes. And by definition, immunostains do not support squamous cell or adenocarcinomatous differentiation.

SALIVARY GLAND–TYPE CARCINOMAS OF THE LUNG

Mucoepidermoid Carcinoma

Of the salivary gland–type carcinomas, mucoepidermoid carcinomas are the most common, representing 0.1% to 0.2% of all primary lung tumors, and can present in any age group with no gender predilection.[7-17] The minor salivary glands that line the tracheobronchial tree are thought to be the origin of these tumors.[18]

Clinical features of mucoepidermoid carcinoma

Mucoepidermoid carcinomas usually involve large airways and present with associated respiratory symptoms

including hemoptysis, bronchitis, wheezing, cough, fever, and chest pain.[15] Rarely, they can involve the peripheral lung.[18]

Imaging features of mucoepidermoid carcinoma

Chest radiographs and computed tomography (CT) are generally not helpful in diagnosing mucoepidermoid carcinomas, in part because of the generally smaller size of these lesions, typically 9 to 40 mm; their endobronchial location; and potential interference from pneumonia or atelectasis.[9,18]

Gross features of mucoepidermoid carcinoma

Mucoepidermoid carcinomas are typically well circumscribed and present as an exophytic mass with a tan-white or gray-white or tan cut surface and can show areas of cystic degeneration or overtly mucoid features.[18,19]

Histologic features of mucoepidermoid carcinoma

Three components comprise mucoepidermoid carcinomas: mucus-secreting, squamous, and intermediate (or transitional) polygonal cells. These cells types range in frequency in any given tumor and serve as the primary basis for classification as low or high grade, with low grade lesions demonstrating tubulocystic pattern. High-grade lesions show more cytologic atypia and a higher mitotic activity. Calcification and prominent lymphoid proliferations can also assist with diagnosis[8,9,20] (*Figures 6-2 and 6-3*).

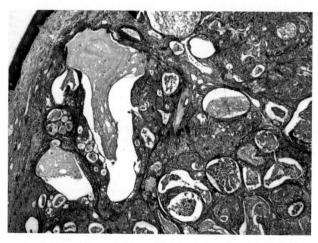

FIGURE 6-2 Low-power image of low-grade pulmonary mucoepidermoid carcinoma showing mucin-filled glands and surrounding nests of squamous and transitional epithelial cells.

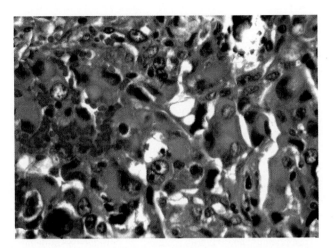

FIGURE 6-3 High-power image of high-grade pulmonary mucoepidermoid carcinoma showing increased cytologic atypia.

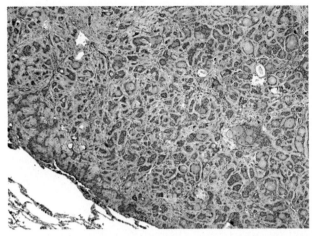

FIGURE 6-4 Lower power image of pulmonary adenoid cystic carcinoma showing islands and cords of neoplastic cells with interspersed extracellular basement membrane–like material.

ADENOID CYSTIC CARCINOMA

Although it is the second most common salivary gland–type pulmonary neoplasm, adenoid cystic carcinoma (ACC) is nonetheless rare, accounting for 0.09% to 0.2% of all primary lung neoplasms.[21,22]

Clinical Features of Adenoid Cystic Carcinoma

ACCs are characteristically centrally located with a minor asymptomatic subset, approximately 10%, forming in peripheral locations. The majority of ACCs present with dyspnea, wheezing, cough, pneumonia, and hemoptysis due to bronchial obstruction and/or erosion.[23,24] While slow growing in most patients, these tumors have been known to have multiple recurrences and eventual distant metastases.[25]

Imaging Features of Adenoid Cystic Carcinoma

ACCs appear as endobronchial masses typically measuring from 0.9 to 4.0 cm, averaging approximately 4 cm.[26]

Gross Features of Adenoid Cystic Carcinoma

Grossly, ACCs are deceptively well circumscribed, with a soft tan to yellow-white cut surface.

Histologic Features of Adenoid Cystic Carcinoma

ACCs have bland cytology and consist of compact polyhedral cells with amphophilic cytoplasm and round, hyperchromatic nucleoli. The cells are most often

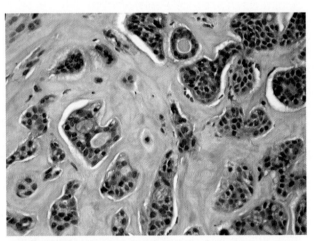

FIGURE 6-5 High-power image of pulmonary adenoid cystic carcinoma showing compact polyhedral cells with round, hyperchromatic nuclei.

arranged in a "jigsaw puzzle" pattern with islands and cords of cells with interspersed extracellular spaces containing basement membrane–like material or mucin (cribriform pattern). Less common patterns include the so-called "tubular pattern" with cells forming elongated cylinders and the "solid" pattern, which has minimal to no intercellular matric material[25] (*Figures 6-4* and *6-5*).

PULMONARY LYMPHOEPITHELIOMA–LIKE CARCINOMA

Pulmonary lymphoepithelioma–like carcinomas (LELCs) are relatively rare in the lung and were first reported in 1987.[27] LELC has also been reported in the bladder,[28] esophagus,[29] thymus,[30] salivary gland,[31] skin,[32] and the cervix.[33]

Clinical Features of Pulmonary Lymphoepithelioma–Like Carcinoma

In contrast to other non-small cell lung carcinomas, LELC affects younger nonsmoking patients, ranging from 42 to 80 years with a mean of 57 years in one study, with a higher predilection for Asians and a strong association with Epstein-Barr virus (EBV) infection.[34-37]

Imaging Features of Pulmonary Lymphoepithelioma–Like Carcinoma

LELCs commonly appear as peripheral nodules on CT scan, with direct pleural contact with a typically homogenous density and no lobe predilection.[38,39]

Gross Features of Pulmonary Lymphoepithelioma–Like Carcinoma

Grossly, tumors are solitary, well circumscribed, and range from 1 to 4.5 cm with a firm, tan-white cut surface.[39]

Histologic Features of Pulmonary Lymphoepithelioma–Like Carcinoma

These tumors are distinguished based on morphology, which consists of tumor cells with scanty eosinophilic cytoplasm, vesicular chromatin, variably shaped nuclei and 1 or 2 prominent nucleoli in solid nests surrounded by lymphocytic infiltrates.[39,40] Of note, LELCs must be differentiated from lymphomas, and are often distinguished based on immunohistochemistry for keratins and LCA[40,41] (*Figure 6-6*).

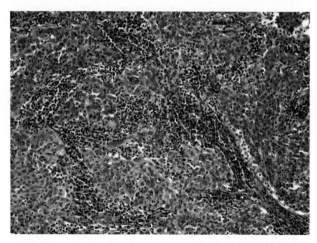

FIGURE 6-6 Medium-power image of pulmonary lymphoepithelioma–like carcinoma showing nests of large neoplastic cells with surrounding lymphocytic infiltrates.

REFERENCES

1. Brambilla E, Pugatch B, Geisinger KR. et al. Large cell carcinoma. In: Travis WD, Brambilla E, Müller-Hermelink HK, Harris CC, eds. *Pathology and Genetics of Tumours of the Lung, Pleura, Thymus and Heart.* Lyon, France: IARC Press; 2004:45-50.
2. Howlader N, Noone AM, Krapcho, M, et al. *SEER Cancer Statistics Review, 1975–2008.* Bethesda, MD: National Cancer Institute; 2011. http://seer.cancer.gov/csr/1975_2008/ Based on November 2010 SEER data submission, posted to the SEER Web site.
3. Travis WD, Brambilla E, Noguchi M, et al. International association for the study of lung cancer/american thoracic society/european respiratory society international multidisciplinary classification of lung adenocarcinoma. *J Thorac Oncol.* 2011;6:244-285.
4. Rekhtman N, Tafe LJ, Chaft JE, et al. Distinct profile of driver mutations and clinical features in immunomarker-defined subsets of pulmonary large-cell carcinoma. *Mod Pathol.* April 2013;26(4):511-522.
5. Gardiner N, Jogai S, Wallis A. The revised lung adenocarcinoma classification-an imaging guide. *J Thorac Dis.* October 2014;6(suppl 5):S537-S546.
6. Leslie KO, Wick MR. *Practical Pulmonary Pathology.* 2nd ed. Philadelphia, PA: Churchill Livingstone 2011:570.
7. Anton-Pacheco J, Jimenez MA, Rodriguez-Peralto JL, Cuadros J, Berchi FJ. Bronchial mucoepidermoid tumor in a 3-year-old child. *Pediatr Surg Int.* 1998;13:524-525.
8. Kim TS, Lee KS, Han J, et al. Mucoepidermoid carcinoma of the tracheobronchial tree: radiographic and CT findings in 12 patients. *Radiology.* 1999;212: 643-648.
9. Shilo K, Foss RD, Franks TJ, DePeralta-Venturina M, Travis WD. Pulmonary mucoepidermoid carcinoma with prominent tumor-associated lymphoid proliferation. *Am J Surg Pathol.* 2005;29:407-411.
10. Niggemann B, Gerstner B, Guschmann M, et al. An 11-yr-old male with pneumonia and persistent airway obstruction. *Eur Respir J.* 2002;19:582-584.
11. Martin-Ucar AE, Rocco G. Mucoepidermoid carcinoma in unilateral hypoplastic lung: a rare tumor in a rarer condition. *Ann Thorac Surg.* 2003;75:1020-1021.
12. Sanchez J, Serrano J, Gomez P, Roman J, Cosano A, Torres A. Bronchial mucoepidermoid carcinoma after allogeneic bone marrow transplantation. *J Clin Pathol.* 1997;50:969-970.
13. Stenman G, Petursdottir V, Mellgren G, Mark J. A child with a t(11;19)(q14-21;p12) in a pulmonary mucoepidermoid carcinoma. *Virchows Arch.* 1998;433:579-581.
14. Barrett W, Heaps LS, Diaz S, Sharma P, Arbuckle S, Smith A. Mucoepidermoid carcinoma of the bronchus in a 15-year-old girl with complex cytogenetic rearrangement involving 11q and over-expression of cyclin D1. *Med Pediatr Oncol.* 2002;39:49-51.
15. Dinopoulos A, Lagona E, Stinios I, Konstadinidou A, Kattamis C. Mucoepidermoid carcinoma of the bronchus. *Pediatr Hematol Oncol.* 2000;17:401-408.
16. Pandya H, Matthews S. Case report: mucoepidermoid carcinoma in a patient with congenital agenesis of the left upper lobe. *Br J Radiol.* 2003;76:339-342.
17. Colby T, Koss M, Travis W. Tumors of salivary gland type. In: IARC:Lyon *Tumors of the Lower Respiratory Tract.* Washington, DC: Armed Forces Institute of Pathology; 1995:65-89. *Atlas of Tumor Pathology;* 3rd series, fascicle 13.
18. Yousem SA, Hochholzer L. Mucoepidermoid tumors of the lung. *Cancer.* 1987;60:1346-1352.
19. Heitmiller RF, Mathisen DJ, Ferry JA, Mark EJ, Grillo HC. Mucoepidermoid lung tumors. *Ann Thorac Surg.* 1989;47:394-399.
20. Liu X, Adams AL. Mucoepidermoid carcinoma of the bronchus: a review. *Arch Pathol Lab Med.* September 2007;131(9):1400-1404.

21. Sweeney WB, Thomas JM. Adenoid cystic carcinoma of the lung. *Contemp Surg.* 1986;28:97-100.

22. Turnbull AD, Huvos AG, Goodner JT, Beattie EJ Jr. The malignant potential of bronchial adenoma. *Ann Thorac Surg.* 1972;14:453-464.

23. Youkouchi H, Otsuka Y, Otoguro Y, et al. Primary peripheral adenoid cystic carcinoma of the lung and literature comparison of features. *Intern Med.* 2007;46:1799-1803.

24. Inoue H, Iwashita A, Kanegae H, Higuchi K, Fujinaga Y, Matsumoto I. Peripheral pulmonary adenoid cystic carcinoma with substantial submucosal extension to the proximal bronchus. *Thorax.* 1991;46:147-148.

25. Bennett AK, Mills SE, Wick MR. Salivary-type neoplasms of the breast and lung. *Semin Diagn Pathol.* November 2003;20(4):279-304.

26. Moran CA, Suster S, Koss MN. Primary adenoid cystic carcinoma of the lung. A clinicopathologic and immunohistochemical study of 16 cases. *Cancer.* March 1994 1;73(5):1390-1397.

27. Begin LR, Eskandari J, Joncas J, et al. Epstein-Barr virus related lymphoepithelioma-like carcinoma of lung. *J Surg Oncol.* 1987;36:280-283.

28. Dinney CP, Ro JY, Babain RJ, et al. Lymphoepithelioma of the bladder: a clinicopathological study of three cases. *J Urol.* 1993;149:840-842.

29. Mori M, Matsuda H, Kuwano H, et al. Esophageal squamous cell carcinoma with lymphoid stroma: a case report. *Virchows Arch A Pathol Anat.* 1989;415:473-479.

30. Leyvraz S, Henle W, Chaminian AP, et al. Association of Epstein-Barr virus with thymic carcinoma. *N Engl J Med.* 1985;312:1296-1299.

31. Saemundsen AK, Albeck H, Hansen JPH, et al. Epstein-Barr virus in nasopharyngeal and salivary gland carcinomas of Greenland Eskimos. *Br J Cancer.* 1982;46:721-728.

32. Swanson SA, Cooper PH, Mills SE, et al. Lymphoepithelioma-like carcinoma of the skin. *Mod Pathol.* 1988;1:359-365.

33. Mills SE, Austin MB, Randall ME. Lymphoepithelioma-like carcinoma of the uterine cervix: a distinctive undifferentiated carcinoma with inflammatory stroma. *Am J Surg Pathol.* 1985;9:883-889.

34. Chan JKC, Hui PK, Tsang WYW, et al. Primary lymphoepithelioma-like carcinoma of the lung. *Cancer.* 1995;76:413-422.

35. Chen FF, Yan JJ, Lai WW, et al. Epstein-Barr virus-associated non-small cell lung carcinoma. *Cancer.* 1998;82:2334-2342.

36. Wong MP, Chung LP, Yuen ST, et al. In situ detection of Epstein-Barr virus in non-small cell lung carcinoma. *J Pathol.* 1995;177:233-240.

37. Chang YL, Wu CT, Shih JY, Lee YC. New aspects in clinicopathologic and oncogene studies of 23 pulmonary lymphoepithelioma-like carcinomas. *Am J Surg Pathol.* 2002 Jun;26(6):715-723.

38. Mo Y, Shen J, Zhang Y, et al. Primary lymphoepithelioma-like carcinoma of the lung: distinct computed tomography features and associated clinical outcomes. *J Thorac Imaging.* July 2014;29(4):246-251.

39. Castro CY, Ostrowski ML, Barrios R, et al. Relationship between Epstein-Barr virus and lymphoepithelioma like carcinoma of the lung: a clinicopathologic study of 6 cases and review of the literature. *Hum Pathol.* August 2001;32(8):863-872.

40. Liang Y, Wang L, Zhu Y, et al. Primary pulmonary lymphoepithelioma-like carcinoma: fifty-two patients with long-term follow-up. *Cancer.* October 1, 2012;118(19):4748-4758.

41. Thunnissen E, et al. Reproducibility of histopathological diagnosis in poorly differentiated NSCLC: an international multiobserver study. *J Thorac Oncol.* September 2014;9(9):1354-1362.

CHAPTER 6

Sarcomatoid Carcinoma and Sarcomas

Yasmeen Butt and Timothy Craig Allen

TAKE HOME POINTS

- Sarcomatoid carcinomas and primary pulmonary sarcomas are rare.
- Primary pulmonary sarcoma is a diagnosis of exclusion, and a thorough search for a nonpulmonary primary must be undertaken prior to diagnosis of a primary pulmonary sarcoma.
- The term *sarcomatoid carcinoma* encompasses four subtypes: pleomorphic (spindle/giant cell) carcinoma, pulmonary blastoma, pleuropulmonary blastoma, and pulmonary carcinosarcoma.
- The vast majority of synovial sarcomas contain a tumor-specific chromosome t(X;18)(p11.2;q11.2) translocation, the fusion genes of which often assist in the diagnosis of primary pulmonary synovial sarcoma.
- Pulmonary artery intimal sarcoma may be misdiagnosed clinically as pulmonary embolism.
- Kaposi sarcoma is the most common true sarcoma in the lung and traditionally has been associated with AIDS patients.
- Immunostaining patterns for primary pulmonary sarcomas generally mirror the patterns of their nonpulmonary counterparts.

SARCOMATOID CARCINOMA

Pulmonary sarcomatoid carcinomas are rare, comprising 0.3% of all lung malignancies, and primary pulmonary sarcomas are even rarer.[1-6] Over time the classification of lung malignancies has undergone significant changes. Currently, the term *sarcomatoid carcinoma* encompasses four subtypes: pleomorphic (spindle cell or giant cell) carcinoma, pulmonary blastoma, pleuropulmonary blastoma, and pulmonary carcinosarcoma.[7,8] (*Table 7-1*) There is a "continuum of differentiation" in morphology between these entities that is supported by molecular evidence that all of these entities originate from pluripotent stem cells in the lung.[9 15]

Clinical Features of Sarcomatoid Carcinoma

These tumors generally arise in older patients, ranging from approximately 30 to 85 years with median ages from 60 to 17 years. There is a male predominance. There is a strong association with smoking frequency and SCs.[5,11,16-24]

Imaging Features of Sarcomatoid Carcinoma

On CT scan, sarcomatoid carcinomas appear as any other lung neoplasm. The majority of SCs are centrally

Table 7-1 Pulmonary Sarcomatoid Carcinomas

Pleomorphic (spindle/giant cell) carcinoma
Pulmonary blastoma
Pleuropulmonary blastoma
Pulmonary carcinosarcoma

located with occasional endobronchial involvement and range in size from 1 to 28 cm with a mean size of 5 to 8 cm.[5,19,21,24-31]

Gross Features of Sarcomatoid Carcinoma

Grossly, SCs are unencapsulated and circumscribed with a variegated tan, white, or gray hemorrhagic cut surface and frequently have necrotic areas.[15]

Histologic Features of Sarcomatoid Carcinoma

Pleomorphic carcinomas are by definition poorly differentiated and lack features of squamous cell carcinoma, adenocarcinoma, or large cell carcinomas. They must have at least 10% giant or spindle cells. Rarely, a tumor will have pure giant or spindle cell morphology (giant cell carcinoma or spindle cell carcinoma, respectively), but typically an admixture is present[9,5,16,25,31] (*Figure 7-1*). Necrosis is a common feature and can be extensive. Epithelial markers can be used to identify carcinomatous differentiation in these tumors.[15]

Pulmonary blastomas are biphasic entities with a primitive mesenchymal stroma and a malignant epithelial component that approximates fetal lung in the pseudoglandular stage, consisting of tubules of nonciliated cells with subnuclear and supranuclear glycogen vacuoles.[32-35]

Pleuropulmonary blastomas consist of a heterogenous mixture of sarcomatous elements and primitive blastomatous features that are subtyped based on the mixture of solid and cystic components. Type I tumors are purely cystic, type II contain a mixture of solid and

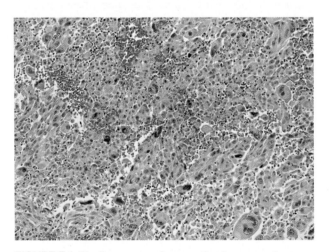

FIGURE 7-1 Medium-power image of pulmonary pleomorphic carcinoma showing a giant cell pattern with discohesive pleomorphic giant cells.

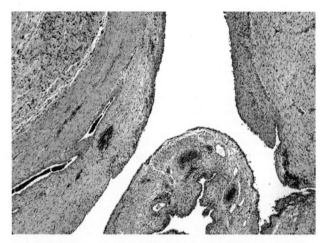

FIGURE 7-2 Low-power image of pleuropulmonary blastoma type I showing cystic spaces with associated wide septa and focal prominent blood vessels.

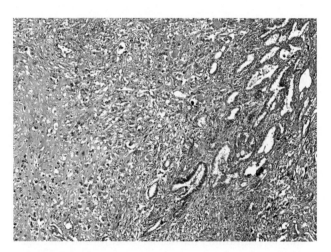

FIGURE 7-3 Medium-power image of pulmonary carcinosarcoma showing malignant cartilage adjacent to an adenocarcinomatous component of the tumor.

cystic components, and type III are purely solid[36-39] (*Figure 7-2*).

Pulmonary carcinosarcomas demonstrate a mixture of carcinomatous elements and identifiable sarcomatous elements such as skeletal muscle, cartilage, or bone[9] (*Figure 7-3*). The carcinoma component is most commonly squamous, followed by adenocarcinoma and adenosquamous carcinoma.[5,24]

PRIMARY PULMONARY SYNOVIAL SARCOMA

Pulmonary synovial sarcomas are most frequently metastatic tumors, typically from primary tumors in the lower limbs of older children and young adults. The vast majority of synovial sarcomas have a tumor-specific chromosome t(X;18)(p11.2;q11.2) translocation resulting in production of fusion genes. Fusion gene identification often assists in accurate diagnosis. All primary pulmonary sarcomas are rare, and primary pulmonary synovial sarcoma (SS) is no exception; however, they do rarely occur.

Clinical Features of Primary Pulmonary Synovial Sarcoma

Contrasted with pulmonary carcinomas, patients with SS are younger, with a mean age of 38.5 years on presentation. Symptoms are similar to other lung malignancies and include cough, hemoptysis, chest pain, and shortness of breath. However, if peripherally located, patients can be asymptomatic.

Imaging Features of Primary Pulmonary Synovial Sarcoma

Generally, imaging is nonspecific for SSs in the lung and there is no lobe predilection.[40] Some cases have shown flocculent or particular calcifications and cystic changes have been reported.[40-47]

Gross Features of Primary Pulmonary Synovial Sarcoma

Grossly, SSs are ill circumscribed with a fleshy tan-white cut surface and range in size from 0.6 to 17 cm.[48]

Histologic Features of Primary Pulmonary Synovial Sarcoma

Histologic features of pulmonary SSs are the same as in any other location and can be monophasic or biphasic. Sheets of spindle cells arranged in fascicles with indistinct cell borders and scant cytoplasm characterize monophasic SS, the more common histological variant in the lung. Biphasic types have an additional epithelial component consisting of cuboidal to low columnar cells lining clefts or gland-like spaces.[40]

As is the case with primary pulmonary sarcomas in general, the immunostaining pattern of primary pulmonary synovial sarcoma typically mirrors the pattern of its nonpulmonary counterpart. Immunostains therefore can be invaluable for the diagnosis of sarcoma, but unhelpful in determining whether the neoplasm is primary or metastatic to the lung.

PULMONARY ARTERY INTIMAL SARCOMA

Although not strictly a respiratory tract tumor, pulmonary artery intimal sarcoma is an intrathoracic sarcoma.

Clinical Features of Pulmonary Artery Intimal Sarcoma

Pulmonary artery intimal sarcoma is a rare and likely underdiagnosed tumor that is usually misdiagnosed clinically as a pulmonary embolism.[49] Patients are found to be nonresponsive to anticoagulant therapy. Presenting symptoms most commonly include dyspnea, back or chest pain, cough, and hemoptysis. Rarely, sudden death can occur.[50] Early diagnosis due to heightened clinicoradiologic suspicion provides the most likely opportunity for improved prognosis.

Imaging Features of Clinical Features of Pulmonary Artery Intimal Sarcoma

Imaging reveals a heterogeneous endoluminal mass that may be sessile or pedunculated.[51] CT and PET-CT are useful in evaluation of patients with severe dyspnea and a pulmonary artery filling defect, and often lead to the initial suspicion of pulmonary artery intimal sarcoma.

Gross Features of Clinical Features of Pulmonary Artery Intimal Sarcoma

Intimal sarcomas appear as gelatinous or mucoid clots in a vessel with variegated cut surfaces containing firm fibrotic areas that can be interspersed with bony or gritty areas in tumors with chondrosarcomatous or chondroid foci, respectively. Higher-grade lesions commonly demonstrate hemorrhage and necrosis.[52]

Histologic Features of Clinical Features of Pulmonary Artery Intimal Sarcoma

Multiple patterns can be seen in these lesions including undifferentiated pleomorphic sarcomas (most common) and myxofibrosarcomas with areas of bland spindle cells set in a dense fibrous background. About 17% of cases will demonstrate heterologous elements (chondrosarcoma or osteosarcoma).[53,54]

EPITHELIOID HEMANGIOENDOTHELIOMA

Clinical Features of Epithelioid Hemangioendothelioma

Epithelioid hemangioendotheliomas are seen predominantly in women (80%) younger than 40 years and are often asymptomatic incidental findings. Those with symptoms present with cough, dyspnea, and pleuritic chest pain.[55-59]

Imaging Features of Epithelioid Hemangioendothelioma

CT scan demonstrates bilateral multiple, small perivascular nodular lesions, each less than 2 cm that can have poorly or well-defined borders[60,61]

Gross Features of Epithelioid Hemangioendothelioma

Tumors are circumscribed with a chondroid appearing gray-white cut surface.[62]

Histologic Features of Epithelioid Hemangioendothelioma

The malignant cells are plump, epithelioid cells with abundant eosinophilic cytoplasm that are often embedded in a myxohyaline fibrous stroma surrounding the center of nodules which can demonstrate necrotic, sclerotic, or hypocellular centers. The lesion commonly extends through the pores of Kohn to give an intra-alveolar growth pattern. On cytology, the malignant cells have characteristic intracytoplasmic vacuoles.[9,63,64]

PRIMARY PULMONARY FIBROSARCOMA

Although most pulmonary sarcomas are of metastatic origin, rarely primary pulmonary fibrosarcomas occur. When identified, careful examination for a nonpulmonary primary is warranted before a diagnosis of primary pulmonary fibrosarcoma is rendered.

Clinical Features of Primary Pulmonary Fibrosarcoma

Clinically and pathologically, primary pulmonary fibrosarcomas can be divided into intrapulmonary and endobronchial types with the former occurring in middle age and elderly patients with a male predominance and the latter in young adults and children without a gender predilection. Symptoms include chest pain, cough, and hemoptysis in endobronchial cases and in a subset of the intrapulmonary cases.[65]

Imaging Features of Primary Pulmonary Fibrosarcoma

Primary pulmonary fibrosarcomas appear as discrete, homogenous masses on imaging with endobronchial lesion measuring less than 3 cm and intrapulmonary lesions ranging from 3.5 to 23 cm.[66]

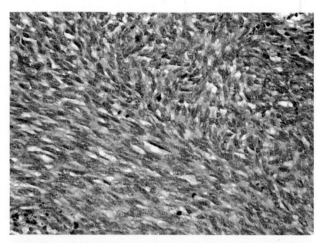

FIGURE 7-4 High-power image of primary pulmonary fibrosarcoma showing elongated spindle cells arranged in fascicles.

Gross Features of Primary Fibrosarcoma of the Lung

The masses are typically lobulated and the cut surfaces frequently show hemorrhage and necrosis.[66]

Histologic Features of Primary Fibrosarcoma of the Lung

As with its soft tissue locations, primary pulmonary fibrosarcomas are composed of elongated atypical spindled nuclei with indistinct cytoplasm, arranged in fascicles and sheets with a characteristic interdigitating growth pattern[65,67,68] (*Figure 7-4*). Mitoses may be prominent.

PRIMARY PULMONARY LEIOMYOSARCOMA

Leiomyosarcomas, sarcomas showing smooth muscle differentiation, typically arise within the soft tissues of the extremities. Metastatic tumor must be excluded before diagnosing primary pulmonary leiomyosarcoma.

Clinical Features of Primary Pulmonary Leiomyosarcoma

Primary pulmonary leiomyosarcomas are extremely rare as a primary lesion, with one large retrospective study citing them as representing only 0.03% of 10,000 malignancies.[65] These tumors are not related to smoking. They are typically endobronchial in location and present with chest pain, cough, and hemoptysis, although intraparenchymal lesions have been reported and are most often incidental findings and asymptomatic.[69,70]

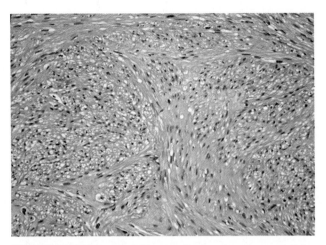

FIGURE 7-5 High-power image of primary pulmonary leiomyosarcoma showing bundles of elongated spindle cells, generally with rounded nuclear ends.

Imaging Features of Primary Pulmonary Leiomyosarcoma

Imaging demonstrates a sharply demarcated mass measuring from 3 to 15 cm that is often accompanied by hilar or mediastinal lymph node metastasis.[70,71]

Gross Features of Primary Pulmonary Leiomyosarcoma

Primary pulmonary leiomyosarcomas have a relatively firm, yellow to white cut surface and frequently have foci of hemorrhage and necrosis.[71]

Histologic Features of Primary Pulmonary Leiomyosarcoma

Histology mirrors that of leiomyosarcomas primary to other locations in the body, and consists of spindle cells haphazardly arranged in a whorled fashion with cells cut in cross sectioning demonstrating characteristic perinuclear lucencies.[69-71] Hemorrhage and necrosis may be present. Characteristically, elongated spindle cells with rounded nuclear ends are seen (*Figure 7-5*). Myxoid or hyalinized stroma may be present. Poorly differentiated tumors usually exhibit significant nuclear pleomorphism as well as atypical mitoses.

PRIMARY PULMONARY CHONDROSARCOMA

Chondrosarcomas most often occur in older adults and arise in the shoulders, ribs, or pelvis. Metastatic tumor to the lung must be excluded prior to diagnosis of primary pulmonary chondrosarcoma.

Clinical Features of Primary Pulmonary Chondrosarcoma

Primary pulmonary chondrosarcomas, as slow-growing tumors, have a slow onset of respiratory symptoms including cough, wheezing, chest pain, and hemoptysis.[72,73]

Imaging Features of Primary Pulmonary Chondrosarcoma

If intraluminal, imaging may not be able to detect these lesions. Detectable abnormalities include cystic changes or central calcifications in a sharply circumscribed, lobular mass.[73,74]

Gross Features of Primary Pulmonary Chondrosarcoma

Gross examination of a primary pulmonary chondrosarcoma reveals a lobulated mass with firm bluish foci corresponding to cartilaginous differentiation.[74]

Histologic Features of Primary Pulmonary Chondrosarcoma

Primary pulmonary chondrosarcomas are generally well-differentiated-appearing tumors. The lack of entrapped small airways, as seen in pulmonary chondroid hamartomas, even moderate nuclear pleomorphism, crowding, and binucleation along with an irregular microscopic interface with normal lung can all be clues to their diagnosis.[72,75] Of note, mesenchymal chondrosarcomas are a rare pediatric variant consisting of sheets of small round blue cells with interspersed embryonal cartilage. Hemangiopericytoid blood vessels can also be seen in this variant.[76]

PRIMARY PULMONARY RHABDOMYOSARCOMA

Metastatic disease, rather than primary, is significantly more common, and must be ruled out definitively before making a diagnosis of primary pulmonary rhabdomyosarcoma.

Clinical Features of Primary Pulmonary Rhabdomyosarcoma

Primary pulmonary rhabdomyosarcoma is an extremely rare pediatric malignancy with the majority occurring in children under 10 years of age.[77-80] Symptoms are similar to other lung-based malignancies and include dyspnea, wheezing, or cough. Patients can also present with a spontaneous pneumothorax if the RMSL is associated with a cystic lesion.[81,82]

Imaging Features of Primary Rhabdomyosarcoma of the Lung

Imaging typically reveals a nonspecific homogenous intraparenchymal mass or a mass within a cystic lesion.[82]

Gross Features of Primary Rhabdomyosarcoma of the Lung

Grossly, these lesions can be polypoid and located in a bronchial lumen or be seen as focal thickening of a cyst wall.[83]

Histologic Features of Primary Rhabdomyosarcoma of the Lung

The majority of these tumors exhibit either an alveolar or embryonal (solid) growth pattern[78,79] of small round blue cells with minimal amphophilic or eosinophilic cytoplasm, coarse clumped chromatin, and numerous mitotic and apoptotic cells.[83] Necrosis may be present. Primary pulmonary embryonal rhabdomyosarcoma typically shows sheets of small blue cells with interspersed fibrotic or myxoid stroma. Cells may be discohesive and frequently contain high-grade round to oval nuclei with a fine chromatin pattern (*Figures 7-6 and 7-7*). Primary pulmonary alveolar rhabdomyosarcoma typically exhibits pleomorphic large neoplastic cells with large eccentric nuclei, as well as multinucleated strap cells and tadpole cells with cytoplasmic tails.

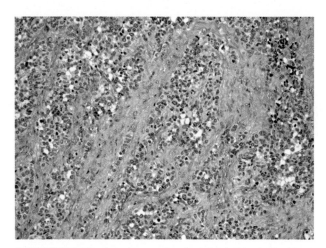

FIGURE 7-6 Medium-power image of primary pulmonary embryonal rhabdomyosarcoma showing sheets of small blue cells with associated fibrotic stroma.

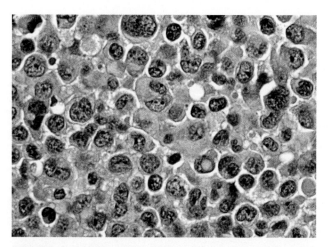

FIGURE 7-7 High-power image of primary pulmonary embryonal rhabdomyosarcoma showing somewhat discohesive high-grade neoplastic cells with round to oval nuclei and a fine chromatin pattern.

PRIMARY PULMONARY KAPOSI SARCOMA

Kaposi sarcoma is the most common true sarcoma in the lung and traditionally has been associated with in AIDS patients.[84-89]

Clinical Features of Primary Pulmonary Kaposi Sarcoma

In contrast with the cutaneous form, primary pulmonary Kaposi sarcoma tends to be detected later in the disease course after the mass has grown sufficiently to produce symptoms.[90] In addition to symptoms attributable to HIV/AIDS, patients will have stridor if an endobronchial lesion is present, cough, dyspnea, and hemoptysis.[91]

Imaging Features of Primary Pulmonary Kaposi Sarcoma

Findings are nonspecific and consist of ill-defined interstitial infiltrates.[92,93]

Gross Features of Primary Pulmonary Kaposi Sarcoma

Grossly, ill-defined areas of bruise-like discolorations are seen in the lung parenchyma.[94]

Histologic Features of Primary Pulmonary Kaposi Sarcoma

Microscopically, primary pulmonary Kaposi sarcoma consists of a combination disorganized fascicles of spindle cells with moderate cytologic atypia and ectatic thin-walled vessels that grow along and through pre-existing intrapulmonary fibrous septae. Additional features that can point to a KS diagnosis include hemosiderin and extravasated red blood cells.[91,95]

INFLAMMATORY MYOFIBROBLASTIC TUMOR

Inflammatory myofibroblastic tumors, considered by some to be a subset of inflammatory pseudotumors, remain controversial. Some authors consider IMTs to represent a reactive inflammatory condition, while others consider IMTs to represent a low-grade mesenchymal malignancy.

Clinical Features of Inflammatory Myofibroblastic Tumor

These tumors are most frequently found in the lung in children and young adults.[96] Up to 50% of patients present with systemic symptoms, including weight loss, fever, anemia, erythrocyte sedimentation rate elevation, leukothrombocytosis, and hyperglobulinemia in addition to any additional specific lung symptoms related to the tumor's physical location, which can include hemoptysis and chest pain.[97,98]

Imaging Features of Inflammatory Myofibroblastic Tumor

Inflammatory myofibroblastic tumors tend to be smaller than 5 cm but have been reported up to 10 cm and appear as a lobulated or globoid mass, commonly with internal calcifications.[99]

Gross Features of Inflammatory Myofibroblastic Tumor

These tumors appear deceptively well circumscribed and have yellow or gray-tan cut surfaces and can contain gritty calcified foci.[66]

Histologic Features of Inflammatory Myofibroblastic Tumor

Microscopically, they have irregular interfaces with surrounding normal lung tissues and consist of relatively bland appearing spindle cells with amphophilic or slightly eosinophilic cytoplasm arranged randomly or in poorly formed fascicles with variable amounts and types of admixed inflammatory cells.[96,97,100]

OTHER PRIMARY PULMONARY SARCOMAS

Additional rare sarcoma types have been reported in the literature as case studies including glomangiosarcoma,[101] angiosarcoma,[102,103] osteosarcoma,[102,104] liposarcoma,[105-107] malignant peripheral nerve sheath tumor,[108-111] and alveolar soft part sarcoma.[112-114] In all of these, it is important to rule out metastatic disease, which is much more likely, before diagnosing a primary pulmonary malignancy.

REFERENCES

1. Travis WD, Travis LB, Devesa SS. Lung cancer *Cancer*. 1995;75(1 suppl):191-202. Erratum in *Cancer*. June 15, 1995;75(12):2979.
2. Nascimento AG, Unni KK, Bernatz PE. Sarcomas of the lung. *Mayo Clin Proc*. June 1982;57(6):355-359.
3. Przygodzki RM, Moran CA, Suster S, Koss MN. Primary pulmonary rhabdomyosarcomas: a clinicopathologic and immunohistochemical study of three cases. *Mod Pathol*. August 1995;8(6):658-661.
4. Zeren H, Moran CA, Suster S, Fishback NF, Koss MN. Primary pulmonary sarcomas with features of monophasic synovial sarcoma: a clinicopathological, immunohistochemical, and ultrastructural study of 25 cases. *Hum Pathol*. May 1995;26(5):474-480.
5. Pelosi G, et al. Review article: pulmonary sarcomatoid carcinomas: a practical overview. *Int J Surg Pathol*. April 2010;18(2):103-120.
6. Wick MR, Ritter JH, Humphrey PA. Sarcomatoid carcinomas of the lung: a clinicopathologic review. *Am J Clin Pathol*. July 1997;108(1):40-53.
7. Huang IC, Ritter JH, Wick MR. Malignant nonepithelial neoplasms of the lungs and pleural surfaces. In: Aisner J, et al., eds. *Comprehensive Textbook of Thoracic Oncology*. Baltimore, MD: Williams & Wilkins; 1996:815-849.
8. Franks TJ, Galvin JR. Sarcomatoid carcinoma of the lung: histologic criteria and common lesions in the differential diagnosis. *Arch Pathol Lab Med*. January 2010;134(1):49-54.
9. Travis WD, Brambilla E, Müller-Hermelink HK, Harris CC, eds. *Pathology and Genetics of Tumours of the Lung, Pleura, Thymus and Heart*. Lyon, France: IARC Press; 2004. *World Health Organization Classification of Tumours*; vol 10.
10. Pelosi G, Sonzogni A, De Pas T, et al. Pulmonary sarcomatoid carcinomas: a practical overview. *Int J Surg Pathol*. 2010:18(2):103-120.
11. Rossi G, Cavazza A, Sturm N, et al. Pulmonary carcinomas with pleomorphic, sarcomatoid, or sarcomatous elements: a clinicopathologic and immunohistochemical study of 75 cases. *Am J Surg Pathol*. 2003;27(3):311-324.
12. Holst VA, Finkelstein S, Colby TV, Myers JL, Yousem SA. p53 and K-ras mutational genotyping in pulmonary carcinosarcoma, spindle cell carcinoma, and pulmonary blastoma: implications for histogenesis. *Am J Surg Pathol*. 1997;21(7):801-811.
13. Takahashi K, Kohno T, Matsumoto S, et al. Clonality and heterogeneity of pulmonary blastoma from the viewpoint of genetic alterations: a case report. *Lung Cancer*. 2007;57(1):103-108.
14. Dacic S, Finkelstein SD, Sasatomi E, Swalsky PA, Yousem SA. Molecular pathogenesis of pulmonary carcinosarcoma as determined by microdissection based allelotyping. *Am J Surg Pathol*. 2002;26(4):510-516.

15. Travis WD. Sarcomatoid neoplasms of the lung and pleura. *Arch Pathol Lab Med.* 2010 Nov;134(11):1645-1658.

16. Mochizuki T, Ishii G, Nagai K, et al. Pleomorphic carcinoma of the lung: clinicopathologic characteristics of 70 cases. *Am J Surg Pathol.* 2008;32(11): 1727-1735.

17. Nakajima M, Kasai T, Hashimoto H, Iwata Y, Manabe H. Sarcomatoid carcinoma of the lung: a clinicopathologic study of 37 cases. *Cancer.* 1999;15;86(4):608-616.

18. Addis BJ, Corrin B. Pulmonary blastoma, carcinosarcoma and spindle-cell carcinoma: an immunohistochemical study of keratin intermediate filaments. *J Pathol.* 1985;147(4):291-301.

19. Humphrey PA, Scroggs MW, Roggli VL, Shelburne JD. Pulmonary carcinomas with a sarcomatoid element: an immunocytochemical and ultrastructural analysis. *Hum Pathol.* 1988;19(2):155-165.

20. Ishida T, Tateishi M, Kaneko S, et al. Carcinosarcoma and spindle cell carcinoma of the lung: clinicopathologic and immunohistochemical studies. *J Thorac Cardiovasc Surg.* 1990;100(6):844-852.

21. Stackhouse EM, Harrison EG Jr, Ellis FH Jr. Primary mixed malignancies of lung: carcinosarcoma and blastoma. *J Thorac Cardiovasc Surg.* 1969;57(3):385-399.

22. Zimmerman KG, Sobonya RE, Payne CM. Histochemical and ultrastructural features of an unusual pulmonary carcinosarcoma. *Hum Pathol.* 1981;12(11):1046-1051.

23. Davis MP, Eagan RT, Weiland LH, Pairolero PC. Carcinosarcoma of the lung: Mayo Clinic experience and response to chemotherapy. *Mayo Clin Proc.* 1984;59(9):598-603.

24. Koss MN, Hochholzer L, Frommelt RA. Carcinosarcomas of the lung: a clinicopathologic study of 66 patients. *Am J Surg Pathol.* 1999;23(12):1514-1526.

25. Fishback NF, Travis WD, Moran CA, Guinee DG Jr, McCarthy WF, Koss MN. Pleomorphic (spindle/giant cell) carcinoma of the lung: a clinicopathologic correlation of 78 cases. *Cancer.* 1994;73(12):2936-2945.

26. Koss MN, Hochholzer L, O'Leary T. Pulmonary blastomas. *Cancer.* 1991;67(9):2368-2381.

27. Lee KG, Cho NH. Fine-needle aspiration cytology of pulmonary adenocarcinoma of fetal type: report of a case with immunohistochemical and ultrastructural studies. *Diagn Cytopathol.* 1991;7(4):408-414.

28. Nakatani Y, Dickersin GR, Mark EJ. Pulmonary endodermal tumor resembling fetal lung: a clinicopathologic study of five cases with immunohistochemical and ultrastructural characterization. *Hum Pathol.* 1990;21(11):1097-1107.

29. Yuki T, Sakuma T, Ohbayashi C, et al. Pleomorphic carcinoma of the lung: a surgical outcome. *J Thorac Cardiovasc Surg.* 2007;134(2):399-404.

30. Kim TH, Kim SJ, Ryu YH, et al. Pleomorphic carcinoma of lung: comparison of CT features and pathologic findings. *Radiology.* 2004;232(2): 554-549.

31. Francis D, Jacobsen M. Pulmonary blastoma. *Curr Top Pathol.* 1983;73:265-294.

32. Adluri RK, Boddu SR, Martin-Ucar A, Duffy JP, Beggs FD, Morgan WE. Pulmonary blastoma—a rare tumor with variable presentation. *Eur J Cardiothorac Surg.* 2006;29(2):236-239.

33. Robert J, Pache JC, Seium Y, de Perrot M, Spiliopoulos A. Pulmonary blastoma: report of five cases and identification of clinical features suggestive of the disease. *Eur J Cardiothorac Surg.* 2002;22(5):708-711.

34. Zaidi A, Zamvar V, Macbeth F, Gibbs AR, Kulatilake N, Butchart EG. Pulmonary blastoma: medium-term results from a regional center. *Ann Thorac Surg.* 2002;73(5):1572-1575.

35. Koss MN. Pulmonary blastomas. *Cancer Treat Res.* 1995;72:349-362.

36. Hill DA, Jarzembowski JA, Priest JR, Williams G, Schoettler P, Dehner LP. Type I pleuropulmonary blastoma: pathology and biology study of 51 cases from the international pleuropulmonary blastoma registry. *Am J Surg Pathol.* 2008;32(2):282-295.

37. Priest JR, McDermott MB, Bhatia S, Watterson J, Manivel JC, Dehner LP. Pleuropulmonary blastoma: a clinicopathologic study of 50 cases. *Cancer.* 1997;80(1):147-161.

38. Priest JR, Hill DA, Williams GM, et al. Type I pleuropulmonary blastoma: a report from the International Pleuropulmonary Blastoma Registry. *J Clin Oncol.* 2006;24(27):4492-4498.

39. Manivel JC, Priest JR, Watterson J, et al. Pleuropulmonary blastoma: the so-called pulmonary blastoma of childhood. *Cancer.* 1988;62(8):1516-1526.

40. Zeren H, Moran CA, Suster S, Fishback NF, Koss MN. Primary pulmonary sarcomas with features of monophasic synovial sarcoma: a clinicopathological, immunohistochemical, and ultrastructural study of 25 cases. *Hum Pathol.* 1995 May;26(5): 474-480.

41. Yoon GS, Park SY, Kang GH, Kim OJ. Primary pulmonary sarcoma with morphologic features of biphasic synovial sarcoma: a case report. *J Korean Med Sci.* February 1998;13(1):71-76.

42. Kaplan MA, Goodman MD, Satish J, Bhagavan BS, Travis WD. Primary pulmonary sarcoma with morphologic features of monophasic synovial sarcoma and chromosome translocation t(X; 18). *Am J Clin Pathol.* February 1996;105(2):195-199.

43. Roberts CA, Seemayer TA, Neff JR, Alonso A, Nelson M, Bridge JA. Translocation (X;18) in primary synovial sarcoma of the lung. *Cancer Genet Cytogenet.* May 1996;88(1):49-52.

44. Sekeres M, Vasconcelles MJ, McMenamin M, Rosenfeld-Darling M, Bueno R. Two patients with sarcoma. Case 1. Synovial cell sarcoma of the lung. *J Clin Oncol.* June 2000;18(11): 2341-2342.

45. Zaring RA, Roepke JE. Pathologic quiz case. Pulmonary mass in a patient presenting with a hemothorax. Diagnosis: primary pulmonary biphasic synovial sarcoma. *Arch Pathol Lab Med.* December 1999;123(12):1287-1289.

46. Bacha EA. Wright CD, Grillo HC, et al. Surgical treatment of primary pulmonary sarcomas. *Eur J Cardiothorac Surg.* April 1999;15(4):456-460.

47. Hisaoka M, Hashimoto H, Iwamasa T, Ishikawa K, Aoki T. Primary synovial sarcoma of the lung: report of two cases confirmed by molecular detection of SYT-SSX fusion gene transcripts. *Histopathology.* March 1999;34(3):205-210.

48. Begueret H, Galateau-Salle F, Guillou L, et al. Primary intrathoracic synovial sarcoma: a clinicopathologic study of 40 t(X;18)-positive cases from the French Sarcoma Group and the Mesopath Group. *Am J Surg Pathol.* 2005;29:339-346.

49. Mussot S, Ghigna MR, Mercier O, et al. Retrospective institutional study of 31 patients treated for pulmonary artery sarcoma. *Eur J Cardiothorac Surg.* 2013;43:787-93.

50. Parish JM, Rosenow ECI, Swensen SJ, et al. Pulmonary artery sarcoma. Clinical features. *Chest.* 1996;110:1480-1488.

51. Hynes JK, Smith HC, Holmes DR. Pulmonary artery sarcoma: preoperative diagnosis noninvasively by two-dimensional echocardiography. *Circulation.* 1983;67:459-477.

52. Travis WD. *Pathology and Genetics of Tumours of the Lung, Pleura, Thymus and Heart (IARC WHO Classification of Tumours).* IARC: Lyon: September 2004.

53. Huo L, Moran CA, Fuller GN, et al. Pulmonary artery sarcoma: a clinicopathologic and immunohistochemical study of 12 cases. *Am J Clin Pathol.* 2006;125:419-424.

54. Tavora F, Miettinen M, Fanburg-Smith J, et al. Pulmonary artery sarcoma: a histologic and follow-up study with emphasis on a subset of low-grade myofibroblastic sarcomas with a good long-term follow-up. *Am J Surg Pathol.* 2008;32:1751-1761.

55. Dail DH, Liebow AA, Gmelich JT, et al. Intravascular, bronchiolar, and alveolar tumor of the lung (IVBAT). An analysis of twenty cases of a peculiar sclerosing endothelial tumor. *Cancer.* February 1, 1983;51(3):452-464.

CHAPTER 7

56. Weiss SW, Ishak KG, Dail DH, Sweet DE, Enzinger FM. Epithelioid hemangioendothelioma and related lesions. *Semin Diagn Pathol.* November 1986;3(4):259-287.

57. Kitaichi M, Nagai S, Nishimura K, et al. Pulmonary epithelioid haemangioendothelioma in 21 patients, including three with partial spontaneous regression. *Eur Respir J.* July 1998;12(1):89-96.

58. Schattenberg T, Kam R, Klopp M, et al. Pulmonary epithelioid hemangioendothelioma: report of three cases. *Surg Today.* 2008;38(9):844-849.

59. Rock MJ, Kaufman RA, Lobe TE, Hensley SD, Moss ML. Epithelioid hemangioendothelioma of the lung (intravascular bronchioloalveolar tumor) in a young girl. *Pediatr Pulmonol.* 1991;11(2):181-186.

60. Ross GJ, Violi L, Friedman AC, Edmonds PR, Unger E. Intravascular bronchioloalveolar tumor: CT and pathologic correlation. *J Comput Assist Tomogr.* March-April 1989;13(2):240-243.

61. Ye B, Li W, Liu XY, et al. Multiple organ metastases of pulmonary epithelioid haemangioendothelioma and a review of the literature. *Med Oncol.* 2010. 27:49-54.

62. Zhang PJ, Livolsi VA, Brooks JJ. Malignant epithelioid vascular tumors of the pleura: report of a series and literature review. *Hum Pathol.* 2000. 31:29-34.

63. Dail DH, Liebow AA, Gmelich JT, et al. Intravascular, bronchiolar, and alveolar tumor of the lung (IVBAT). An analysis of twenty cases of a peculiar sclerosing endothelial tumor. *Cancer.* February 1, 1983;51(3):452-464.

64. Weiss SW, Ishak KG, Dail DH, Sweet DE, Enzinger FM. Epithelioid hemangioendothelioma and related lesions. *Semin Diagn Pathol.* November 1986;3(4):259-287.

65. Guccion JG, Rosen SH. Bronchopulmonary leiomyosarcoma and fibrosarcoma. A study of 32 cases and review of the literature. *Cancer.* September 1972;30(3):836-847.

66. Leslie KO, Wick MR. *Pulmonary Pathology.* 2nd ed. Philadelphia, PA; 2011.

67. Wick MR, Manivel JC. Primary sarcomas of the lung. In: Williams CJ, Krikorian JG, Green MR, Raghavan D, eds. *Textbook of Uncommon Cancer.* New York: John Wiley & Sons; 1988:335-381.

68. Logrono R, Filipowicz EA, Eyzaguirre EJ, Sawh RN. Diagnosis of primary fibrosarcoma of the lung by fine-needle aspiration and core biopsy. *Arch Pathol Lab Med.* August 1999;123(8):731-735.

69. Lillo-Gil R, Albrechtsson U, Jakobsson B. Pulmonary leiomyosarcoma appearing as a cyst. Report of one case and review of the literature. *Thorac Cardiovasc Surg.* August 1985;33(4):250-252.

70. Yu H, Ren H, Miao Q, Cui Q, Zhang Z, Xu L. Pulmonary leiomyosarcoma—report of three cases. *Chin Med Sci J.* September 1996;11(3):191-194.

71. Attanoos RL, Appleton MA, Gibbs AR. Primary sarcomas of the lung: a clinicopathological and immunohistochemical study of 14 cases. *Histopathology.* July 1996;29(1):29-36.

72. Hayashi T, Tsuda N, Iseki M, Kishikawa M, Shinozaki T, Hasumoto M. Primary chondrosarcoma of the lung. A clinicopathologic study. *Cancer.* July 1, 1993;72(1):69-

73. Fallahnejad M, Harrell D, Tucker J, Forest J, Blakemore WS. Chondrosarcoma of the trachea. Report of a case and five-year follow-up. *J Thorac Cardiovasc Surg.* February 1973;65(2):210-213.

74. Parker LA, Molina PL, Bignault AG, Fidler ME. Primary pulmonary chondrosarcoma mimicking bronchogenic cyst on CT and MRI. *Clin Imaging.* July-September 1996;20(3):181-183.

75. Sun CC, Kroll M, Miller JE. Primary chondrosarcoma of the lung. *Cancer.* November 1, 1982;50(9):1864-1866.

76. Kurotaki H, Tateoka H, Takeuchi M, Yagihashi S, Kamata Y, Nagai K. Primary mesenchymal chondrosarcoma of the lung. A case report with immunohistochemical and ultrastructural studies. *Acta Pathol Jpn.* May 1992;42(5):364-371.

77. McDermott VG, Mackenzie S, Hendry GM. Case report: primary intrathoracic rhabdomyosarcoma: a rare childhood malignancy. *Br J Radiol.* October 1993;66(790):937-941.

78. Schiavetti A, Dominici C, Matrunola M, Capocaccia P, Ceccamea A, Castello MA. Primary pulmonary rhabdomyosarcoma in childhood: clinico-biologic features in two cases with review of the literature. *Med Pediatr Oncol.* March 1996;26(3):201-207.

79. Noda T, Todani T, Watanabe Y, et al. Alveolar rhabdomyosarcoma of the lung in a child. *J Pediatr Surg.* November 1995;30(11):1607-1608.

80. Hancock BJ, Di Lorenzo M, Youssef S, Yazbeck S, Marcotte JE, Collin PP. Childhood primary pulmonary neoplasms. *J Pediatr Surg.* September 1993;28(9):1133-1136.

81. Allan BT, Day DL, Dehner LP. Primary pulmonary rhabdomyosarcoma of the lung in children. Report of two cases presenting with spontaneous pneumothorax. *Cancer.* March 1, 1987;59(5):1005-1011.

82. Murphy JJ, Blair GK, Fraser GC, et al. Rhabdomyosarcoma arising within congenital pulmonary cysts: report of three cases. *J Pediatr Surg.* October 1992;27(10):1364-1367.

83. Eriksson A, Thunell M, Lundqvist G. Pendulating endobronchial rhabdomyosarcoma with fatal asphyxia. *Thorax.* May 1982;37(5):390-391.

84. Meduri GU, Stover DE, Lee M, Myskowski PL, Caravelli JF, Zaman MB. Pulmonary Kaposi's sarcoma in the acquired immune deficiency syndrome. Clinical, radiographic, and pathologic manifestations. *Am J Med.* July 1986;81(1):11-18.

85. Purdy LJ, Colby TV, Yousem SA, Battifora H. Pulmonary Kaposi's sarcoma. Premortem histologic diagnosis. *Am J Surg Pathol.* May 1986;10(5):301-311.

86. Cadranel J, Naccache J, Wislez M, Mayaud C. Pulmonary malignancies in the immunocompromised patient. *Respiration.* 1999;66(4):289-309.

87. Katariya K, Thurer RJ. Malignancies associated with the immunocompromised state. *Chest Surg Clin N Am.* February 1999;9(1):63-77, viii.

88. Smith C, Lilly S, Mann KP, et al. AIDS-related malignancies. *Ann Med.* August 1998;30(4):323-344.

89. Hannon FB, Easterbrook PJ, Padley S, Boag F, Goodall R, Phillips RH. Bronchopulmonary Kaposi's sarcoma in 106 HIV-1 infected patients. *Int J STD AIDS.* September 1998;9(9):518-525.

90. Hanno R, Owen LG, Callen JP. Kaposi's sarcoma with extensive silent internal involvement. *Int J Dermatol.* November 1979;18(9):718-721.

91. Garay SM, Belenko M, Fazzini E, Schinella R. Pulmonary manifestations of Kaposi's sarcoma. *Chest.* January 1987;91(1):39-43.

92. O'Brien RF, Cohn DL. Serosanguineous pleural effusions in AIDS-associated Kaposi's sarcoma. *Chest.* September 1989;96(3):460-466.

93. Floris C, Sulis ML, Bernascani M, Turno R, Tedde A, Sulis E. Pneumothorax in pleuropulmonary Kaposi's sarcoma related to acquired immunodeficiency syndrome. *Am J Med.* July 1989;87(1):123-124.

94. Ognibene FP, Shelhamer JH. Kaposi's sarcoma. *Clin Chest Med.* September 1988;9(3):459-465.

95. Gal AA, Koss MN, Hartmann B, et al. A review of pulmonary pathology in the acquired immune deficiency syndrome. *Surg Pathol.* 1988;1:325-346.

96. Wick MR, Ritter JH, Nappi O. Inflammatory sarcomatoid carcinoma of the lung: report of three cases and clinicopathologic comparison with inflammatory pseudotumors in adult patients. *Hum Pathol.* September 1995;26(9):1014-1021.

97. Coffin CM, Dehner LP, Meis-Kindblom JM. Inflammatory myofibroblastic tumor, inflammatory fibrosarcoma, and related lesions: an historical review with differential diagnostic considerations. *Semin Diagn Pathol.* 1998;15:102-110.

98. Takeda S, Onishi Y, Kawamura T, Maeda H. Clinical spectrum of pulmonary inflammatory myofibroblastic tumor. *Interact Cardiovasc Thorac Surg.* August 2008;7(4):629-633.

99. Pettinato G, Manivel JC, De Rosa N, Dehner LP. Inflammatory myofibroblastic tumor (plasma cell granuloma). Clinicopathologic study of 20 cases with immunohistochemical and ultrastructural observations. *Am J Clin Pathol.* November 1990;94(5): 538-546.

100. Matsubara O, Tan-Liu NS, Kenney RM, Mark EJ. Inflammatory pseudotumors of the lung: progression from organizing pneumonia to fibrous histiocytoma or to plasma cell granuloma in 32 cases. *Hum Pathol.* July 1988;19(7):807-814.

101. Gaertner EM, et al. Pulmonary and mediastinal glomus tumors—report of five cases including a pulmonary glomangiosarcoma: a clinicopathologic study with literature review. *Am J Surg Pathol.* August 2000;24(8):1105-1114.

102. Corpa-Rodríguez ME, Mayoralas-Alises S, García-Sánchez J, Gil-Alonso JL, Díaz-Agero P, Casillas-Pajuelo M. [Postoperative course in 7 cases of primary sarcoma of the lung]. *Arch Bronconeumol.* November 2005;41(11):634-637.

103. Yousem SA. Angiosarcoma presenting in the lung. *Arch Pathol Lab Med.* February 1986;110(2):112-115.

104. Reingold IM, Amromin GD. Extraosseous osteosarcoma of the lung. *Cancer.* August 1971;28(2):491-498.

105. Sawamura K, Hashimoto T, Nanjo S, et al. Primary liposarcoma of the lung: report of a case. *J Surg Oncol.* 1982 Apr;19(4): 243-246.

106. Achir A, Ouadnouni Y, Smahi M, Bouchikh M, Msougar Y, Benosman A. Primary pulmonary liposarcoma—a case report. *Thorac Cardiovasc Surg.* March 2009;57(2):119-120.

107. Loddenkemper C, Pérez-Canto A, Leschber G, Stein H. Primary dedifferentiated liposarcoma of the lung. *Histopathology.* June 2005;46(6):710-712.

108. Attanoos RL, Appleton MA, Gibbs AR. Primary sarcomas of the lung: a clinicopathological and immunohistochemical study of 14 cases. *Histopathology.* July 1996;29(1):29-36.

109. Keel SB, Bacha E, Mark EJ, Nielsen GP, Rosenberg AE. Primary pulmonary sarcoma: a clinicopathologic study of 26 cases. *Mod Pathol.* December 1999;12(12):1124-1131.

110. Bartley TD, Arean VM. Intrapulmonary neurogenic tumors. *J Thorac Cardiovasc Surg.* July 1965;50:114-123.

111. Manabe H, Umemoto T, Takagi H, et al. [Primary neurogenous sarcoma of the lung; report of a case]. *Kyobu Geka.* April 2005;58(4):337-340.

112. Kim YD, Lee CH, Lee MK, et al. Primary alveolar soft part sarcoma of the lung. *J Korean Med Sci.* April 2007;22(2): 369-372.

113. Wakely PE Jr, McDermott JE, Ali SZ. Cytopathology of alveolar soft part sarcoma: a report of 10 cases. *Cancer.* December 25, 2009;117(6):500-507.

114. Ladanyi M, et al. The der(17)t(X;17)(p11;q25) of human alveolar soft part sarcoma fuses the TFE3 transcription factor gene to ASPL, a novel gene at 17q25. *Oncogene.* January 4, 2001;20(1):48-57.

Lymphomas

Kirtee Raparia and Arlene Sirajuddin

TAKE HOME PEARLS

- Pulmonary lymphoid system is composed of pulmonary lymphatics and the bronchus-associated lymphoid tissue (BALT).
- Primary lymphoid lesions encompass a wide range of benign and malignant lesions.
- Pulmonary lymphomas have become better-defined entities with the help of advanced technology such as multidetector chest CT, flow cytometric immunophenotyping, and molecular analysis.
- Primary lymphoid lesions of the lung are increasingly recognized as the number of posttransplant patients and patients on immunosuppressive therapies continue to rise.
- Marginal zone lymphoma of the lung is the most common type of pulmonary lymphoma (both primary and secondary) with an overall good prognosis.
- Lymphomatoid granulomatosis belongs in the group of lymphoproliferative neoplasms and is considered to be an EBV-driven B-cell neoplasm.
- Rare subtypes of lymphoma including T-cell, NK-cell, and ALK-positive lymphomas may also occur as primary neoplasms in the lung and a timely diagnosis and treatment is necessary in an attempt to improve patient survival rates.

CLASSIFICATION OF LYMPHOMAS AND LYMPHOMA-LIKE CONDITIONS IN THE LUNG

Primary lymphoid lesions of the lung includes nonneoplastic lymphocytic proliferations (follicular bronchiolitis, lymphoid interstitial pneumonia, and nodular lymphoid hyperplasia); neoplastic lymphocytic proliferations (low-grade B-cell lymphoma of MALT, other non-Hodgkin lymphomas, and Hodgkin lymphoma); and a miscellaneous group of lesions including lymphomatoid granulomatosis, posttransplant lymphoproliferative disorders, AIDS-related lymphoma, and intravascular lymphoma/lymphomatosis.

Primary pulmonary lymphoma (PPL) is defined as clonal lymphoid proliferation affecting one or both lungs (parenchyma and/or bronchi) in a patient with no previous extrapulmonary involvement at the time of diagnosis or during the subsequent 3 months. Primary lymphoma of the lung is a rare disorder and represents only 0.3% of all primary pulmonary malignancies: less than 1% of all the cases of non-Hodgkin lymphoma (NHL) and 3% to 4% of all the extranodal manifestations of NHL.[1] Lymphomatoid proliferation can also involve the lungs either by hematogenous dissemination of non-Hodgkin lymphoma or Hodgkin lymphoma (HL) or by contiguous invasion from a hilar or mediastinal site involved by lymphoma. These conditions are more frequent and are referred to as secondary involvement of the lung by lymphoma. Lymphomas in the lung are usually diagnosed by video-assisted thoracic surgery (VATS), open wedge biopsy, or lobectomy. However, more recently transbronchial biopsy or computed tomography (CT)–guided transthoracic needle biopsy can also yield promising results, if tissue is triaged carefully in clinically suspicious cases.[2]

DIAGNOSTIC METHODS FOR LYMPHOMA DIAGNOSIS AND EVALUATION

Diagnosis and classification of lymphomas is based on the morphologic, immunological, and genetic features that the lesional cells share with their normal B- and T-lymphocyte counterparts. Special studies such as immunohistochemistry, flow cytometric immunophenotyping, molecular genetics, and cytogenetics have recently evolved and can identify clonal populations in small samples and yield accurate and specific diagnoses. However, lack of clonality does not always prove that the lesion is benign and reactive. In such cases, the morphology and immunoarchitecture of the tissue sections is helpful in making the diagnosis and assessing the lineage of the infiltrate.

Immunohistochemistry

A panel of markers is decided based on morphologic differential diagnosis (no single marker is specific) which may include leukocyte common antigen (CD45/LCA), B-cell lineage markers (CD10, CD19, CD20, CD23, CD74, PAX-5, CD79a, CD13, IgD, kappa and lambda light chains), T-cell lineage markers (CD2, CD3, CD4, CD5, CD7, CD8, CD43, CD45RO, CD56, and CD57), monocyte cell markers (CD1a, CD15, CD21, CD68, and S100), and other miscellaneous markers like bcl-2, bcl-6, cyclinD1, CD15, CD30, ALK-1, TdT, and EMA, depending on the cytoarchitectural pattern of tumor.

Flow Cytometry

Flow cytometric immunophenotyping evaluates individual cells in fluid suspension for the presence and absence of specific antigens (phenotype). It allows the diagnosis of phenotypically abnormal cells belonging to the B-cell, T-cell, or NK-cell lineage, using three or four markers simultaneously in specific cell populations, and permitting evaluation even in a limited sample. The only caveat of flow cytometry is that immune architecture cannot be evaluated.

In Situ Hybridization

In situ hybridization (ISH) for kappa and lambda light chains aids in the diagnosis of B-cell lymphoid neoplasms. Additional, EBER (EBV ISH) is routinely used for prognostic purposes in certain types of lymphomas.

Fluorescence In Situ Hybridization

Many types of non-Hodgkin lymphomas have certain type of chromosomal translocations. Fluorescence in situ hybridization (FISH) can detect specific translocations associated with various lymphomas rapidly and with high specificity from fresh lesional tissue or from paraffin embedded tissue.

Polymerase Chain Reaction

Polymerase chain reaction (PCR) analysis can be performed on paraffin embedded tissue to document clonality, establish lineage, and evaluate for the presence of viruses. PCR is routinely used to analyze the immunoglobulin heavy and light chain rearrangements in B-cell neoplasms and T-cell receptor gene rearrangement in T-cell neoplasms.

NORMAL PULMONARY LYMPHATICS, LYMPHATIC ROUTES, BRONCHUS ASSOCIATED LYMPHOID TISSUE AND INTRAPULMONARY LYMPH NODES

The lung contains an extensive lymphatic network made up of lymphatic pathways that are located in the pleura and interlobular septa that channel lymphatic fluid toward parenchymal, septal, hilar, and mediastinal lymph nodes. This pulmonary lymphatic network consists of two subdivisions: the superficial lymphatic system and the deep lymphatic system (*Figure 8-1A*). The superficial lymphatic system, also known as the pleural lymphatics, arises in the pleural space and drains the outer portion of the lung toward the hilum. The deep lymphatic system, also known as the parenchymal lymphatics, arises at the level of the alveolar ducts and drains along the bronchovascular bundles toward the hilar nodes. The alveolar walls themselves contain no lymphatic spaces.

Organized lymphoid tissue in the periphery of the normal lung is limited to sparse submucosal aggregates of lymphocytes and intraparenchymal lymph nodes.[3] The lymphoid tissue is more substantial centrally along bronchioles and central airways. Various antigenic stimuli such as smoking, immunological disease, or

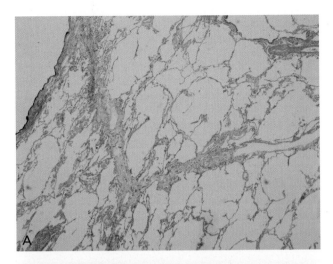

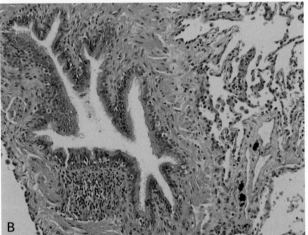

FIGURE 8-1 Pulmonary lymphatics and bronchial mucosa–associated lymphoid tissue (BALT): (A) Pulmonary lymphatics drain along the interlobular septa, pulmonary arteries and veins toward the hilum. (B) BALT accumulates adjacent to the airways after exposure to immunogenic material (200× magnification, hematoxylin-eosin stain).

chronic infection in the bronchi initiate the primary and secondary immune response, leading to lymphoid hyperplasia referred to as acquired *mucosa-associated lymphoid tissue* (MALT). In the lung, it is often referred to as bronchus-associated lymphoid tissue (BALT) (*Figure 8-1B*). Acquired MALT has a distinctive immune architecture with four compartments: B-cell-rich follicles, follicular mantle and marginal zones, and T-cell-rich interfollicular regions.

Intrapulmonary lymph nodes are encapsulated lymph nodes that usually occur at the bifurcations of large bronchi as well as in the lung periphery, located subpleurally or adjacent to interlobular septa. These are often seen in patients with dust exposure and cigarette smoking history. On imaging, they appear as single or multiple nodules.

FOLLICULAR BRONCHIOLITIS, LYMPHOID HYPERPLASIA, INFILTRATES, AND LYMPHOMA-LIKE CONDITIONS

Follicular Bronchiolitis

Demographics of follicular bronchiolitis

Patients usually present in middle age, although cases in children have been reported. It is slightly more common in males than females.[4]

Etiologies of follicular bronchiolitis

Follicular bronchiolitis is often associated with collagen vascular diseases, particularly rheumatoid arthritis, congenital or acquired immunodeficiency disorders such as IgA deficiency, AIDS, and common variable immunodeficiency, patients with hypersensitivity disorders associated with peripheral eosinophilia, and patients with chronic obstructive pulmonary diseases.[5,6]

Diagnostic criteria of follicular bronchiolitis

Follicular bronchiolitis is polyclonal hyperplasia and expansion of the BALT from chronic antigen stimulation around peribronchiolar regions and at bronchial bifurcations. These hyperplastic lymphoid follicles are primarily composed of polytypic B cells, with minimal lymphocytic infiltration into the adjacent alveolar interstitium and bronchiolar epithelium.[5,6]

Clinical features of follicular bronchiolitis

Symptoms include insidious onset of shortness of breath, dyspnea, cough, and weight loss. Surgical lung biopsy is usually necessary to establish a diagnosis, especially in the absence of suggestive clinical history.[7] These patients have overall good prognosis, but can be variable in younger patients. Treatment involves management of the underlying disease, steroids, and immunosuppressants.

Imaging features of follicular bronchiolitis

Follicular bronchiolitis involves the lung bilaterally and presents as centrilobular nodules and ground glass opacities on CT scan, which can range from 3 to 12 mm in size[8] (*Figure 8-2A*).

Gross and histologic features of follicular bronchiolitis

It is difficult to appreciate these lesions grossly since they are small. Histologically, follicular bronchiolitis

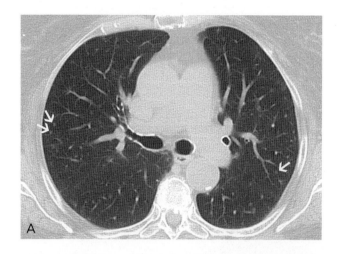

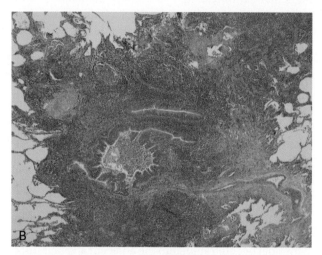

FIGURE 8-2 Follicular bronchiolitis. (A) Transverse CT image of the midlungs demonstrates multiple centrilobular nodules (arrows) in a patient with rheumatoid arthritis. (B) The bronchi and bronchioles are associated with hyperplastic polyclonal lymphoid follicles with reactive germinal centers compressing the lumens (hematoxylin-eosin, original magnifications ×40).

is characterized by eccentric peribronchiolar accumulation of hyperplastic lymphoid follicles primarily composed of polytypic B cells, distorting and narrowing the bronchiolar lumen. There is minimal interstitial involvement and the airspaces are not involved (*Figure 8-2B*).

Immunohistochemical features of follicular bronchiolitis

Follicular bronchiolitis is composed of mixture of B and T lymphocytes, which can be confirmed by CD3 and CD20 immunostains. The B cells in these lesions are polytypic, expressing both kappa and lambda light chains.

Nodular Lymphoid Hyperplasia (Pseudolymphoma)

Demographics of nodular lymphoid hyperplasia

Patients usually present in middle age, although cases in children have been reported.

Etiologies of nodular lymphoid hyperplasia

Nodular lymphoid hyperplasia (NLH) is associated with altered immune status (collagen vascular disease, acquired immune deficiency, dysgammaglobulinemia). It can be seen as an isolated finding in asymptomatic individuals.[9]

Diagnostic criteria of nodular lymphoid hyperplasia

NLH is a localized mass composed of polyclonal lymphoid hyperplasia in the pulmonary lung parenchyma along the course of the bronchovascular bundles.[10]

Clinical features of nodular lymphoid hyperplasia

NLH commonly occurs as an isolated finding in asymptomatic individuals. When symptoms are present, they include cough and dyspnea. Treatment is surgical resection.

Imaging features of nodular lymphoid hyperplasia

NLH can present as a nodule, mass, or focal area of mass-like consolidation within the lung on chest radiographs and CT.[5,9] Lesions are usually single, but can be multiple. Air bronchograms are often present within the lesion on CT. Mediastinal and hilar lymphadenopathy, as well as pleural effusion, is absent (*Figure 8-3A*).

Gross and histologic features of nodular lymphoid hyperplasia

NLH presents as a nodule or mass-like lesion with sharp demarcation from the surrounding normal lung parenchyma. NLH is composed of a polymorphous population of lymphoid cells (both B and T cells), lymphoid follicles with multiple germinal centers, as well as lymphoplasmacytosis in the interfollicular regions. Variable amounts of fibrosis may also be present in the lesion as well as occasional giant cells and macrophages. Lesions typically lack lymphoepithelial lesions, seen commonly in lymphoma (*Figure 8-3B*). Diagnosis requires surgical biopsy. NLH must be differentiated from MALT lymphoma (discussed later in the chapter), which is more common and other rare types of lymphomas such as follicular lymphoma and mantle cell lymphoma.

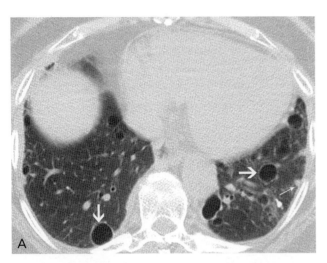 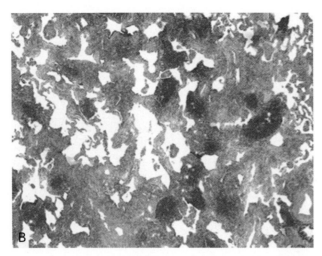

FIGURE 8-3 Nodular lymphoid hyperplasia. (A) Transverse CT image shows a nodule in the left lower lobe (arrow). **(B)** The nodules shows mixture of polyclonal B and T lymphocytes admixed with plasma cells and intervening fibrosis (hematoxylin-eosin, original magnifications ×40).

Immunohistochemical and molecular features of nodular lymphoid hyperplasia

Immunohistochemical studies are necessary to determine the polyclonal population of the lymphocytes and plasma cells as well as molecular genetic analysis to ensure that no rearrangements of the immunoglobulin light or heavy chains are present.

Lymphoid Interstitial Pneumonia

Demographics of lymphoid interstitial pneumonia

Lymphoid interstitial pneumonia (LIP) arises most commonly between the fourth and seventh decades of life, and is more common in women than men. It can be seen in children as well.

Etiologies of lymphoid interstitial pneumonia

LIP has been associated with multiple diseases such as autoimmune diseases, HIV in pediatric population, common variable immunodeficiency, collagen vascular diseases such as Sjögren syndrome, and Castleman disease.[5,9,11,12] It has been associated with chronic infections such as Ebstein-Barr virus, human herpes virus 8, and mycoplasma, and is also a known complication of graft-versus-host disease in bone marrow transplantation patients.

Diagnostic criteria of lymphoid interstitial pneumonia

LIP is a rare benign polyclonal lymphoproliferative disorder of the lung parenchyma, presenting as extensive and diffuse disease.

Clinical features of lymphoid interstitial pneumonia

Patients with LIP present with symptoms including insidious onset of cough, dyspnea, and weight loss. Approximately 60% of patients with LIP have dysproteinemia, which is usually some form of dysgammaglobulinemia, hypergammaglobulinemia being more common than hypogammaglobulinemia. Treatment involves corticosteroids as well as treatment of the underlying disease and outcomes are variable.

Imaging features of lymphoid interstitial pneumonia

Radiographic findings are nonspecific and range from nodular or reticular opacities in the lower lungs to no findings at all. CT shows ground glass opacity, centrilobular nodules, bronchovascular bundle thickening, and peribronchovascular cysts predominately in the lower lungs[13,14] (*Figure 8-4A*).

Gross and histologic features of lymphoid interstitial pneumonia

Grossly, it is difficult to define the lesion in most cases. Histologically, there is diffuse infiltration of lymphocytes (predominately T cells intermixed with some polytypic B cells) and plasma cells into the alveolar interstitium, resulting in expansion of the alveolar septa, with accentuation along bronchovascular bundles and lobular septae. Ill-defined granulomas and giant cells have been found in 20% to 50% of cases. Lymphoid follicles primarily composed of B cells are often present in LIP. Lymphoepithelial lesions and cellular infiltrates around the vessels can also be seen (*Figure 8-4B*).

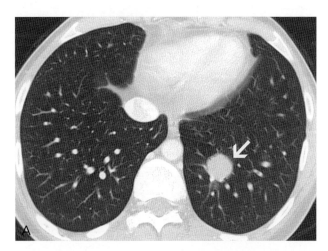
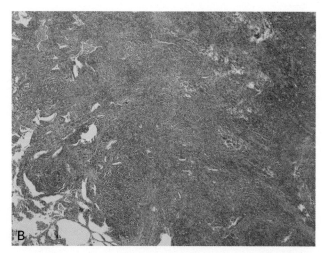

FIGURE 8-4 Lymphocytic interstitial pneumonia. (A) Transverse CT image shows cysts (big arrows) and nodules (small arrow) in a patient with Sjögren syndrome. (B) Lung parenchyma showing dominant interstitial pattern of distribution of primarily T cells intermixed with polytypic B cells and plasma cells, commonly seen in adults and children with altered immune status (hematoxylin-eosin, original magnifications ×40).

Immunohistochemical and molecular features of lymphoid interstitial pneumonia

Definitive pathologic diagnosis of LIP typically requires surgical biopsy, with immunohistochemical studies necessary to determine the polyclonal nature of the lymphocytes and distinguish LIP from lymphoma. AIDS-related lesions often show reactivity with p21 protein of human immunodeficiency virus.

LYMPHOMAS

Primary Pulmonary Non-Hodgkin Lymphomas

Primary pulmonary marginal zone lymphoma

Demographics of pulmonary marginal zone lymphoma

Marginal zone lymphoma (MZL) of MALT type arising from MALT of the bronchus is the most common primary lymphoma of the lung, accounting for approximately 70% cases of lung lymphomas. MZL almost exclusively affects adults, although rare cases in younger patients have been reported.[15,16]

Etiologies of pulmonary marginal zone lymphoma

MZL is acquired as secondary to long-term response to various antigenic stimuli such as smoking, immunological disease such as Sjögren syndrome, rheumatoid arthritis, Hashimoto thyroiditis, systemic lupus erythematosus, or infections such as hepatitis C and HIV.[17-19] Most patients who developed MZL as noted in few series were former or active smokers.[20-22]

Diagnostic criteria of pulmonary marginal zone lymphoma

MZL of the lung is composed of cells that morphologically and phenotypically resemble mature B cells, which have distinctive morphology and immunophenotype described below.

Clinical features of pulmonary marginal zone lymphoma

Patients with MZL may present with cough, fever, or unexplained weight loss, although many are entirely asymptomatic. These patients often present clinically with monoclonal gammopathy, most commonly reported paraprotein being IgM isotype.[19]

Patients with pulmonary MZL usually have limited disease and follow an indolent clinical course with a favorable outcome.[1,21,22] These patients do require long-term follow up and repeated biopsies and may develop relapses in the lung and in other MALT sites and some may undergo transformation to diffuse large B-cell lymphoma (DLBCL). The optimal management of pulmonary MZL with regard to surgical resection, chemotherapy or radiotherapy alone or in combination is not well established.

Imaging features of pulmonary marginal zone lymphoma

Most common radiologic findings are presence of solitary or multiple discrete nodules or areas of consolidation that may occupy one or both lungs in either a perihilar or peripheral distribution.[23-26] Air bronchograms are common[23,27,28] (Figure 8-5A).

Gross and histologic features of pulmonary marginal zone lymphoma

Grossly, the lesions are gray, tan, solid, poorly defined masses with a firm, fibrous, or granular cut surface. These lesions show a peculiar distribution of tumor cells accentuated along the bronchovascular bundles, interlobular septa, and visceral pleura. These lymphangitic infiltrates eventually coalesce into masses that can efface the lung parenchyma and form nodules or a more diffuse pattern. Invasion of bronchi, blood vessels, and pleura can also be seen. Most cases have interspersed intact or disrupted reactive lymphoid follicles (*Figure 8-5B*). Presence of lymphoepithelial lesions, defined by the infiltration and distortion of epithelial structures by aggregates of (usually three or more) neoplastic lymphoid cells, is an important diagnostic feature in MZL. Anticytokeratin antibody, along with CD20/CD19 and CD5 antibodies, can facilitate identification of the lymphoepithelial lesions, highlighting marginal zone B cells in these areas. The neoplastic cells are morphologically described as showing a spectrum of monocytoid, centrocyte-like or lymphoplasmacytic cytology and occasionally appearing as large transformed B lymphocytes. Plasma cells containing Dutcher bodies can also be seen.

Pulmonary MZL can be associated with prominent stromal deposition of amyloid in 1% to 6% of the pulmonary MZL cases.[19,29] Pulmonary MZL with light chain deposition disease has also been reported in an HIV-positive male.[30] Light chain deposition disease shows deposits similar to amyloid, but they are Congo red negative, while amyloid has characteristic Congo red positivity. However, light chain deposition disease has a granular appearance on electron microscopy compared to fibrils in amyloid.

Some cases of MZL may resemble pulmonary nodular lymphoid hyperplasia, but the latter shows polymorphous population of lymphoid cells (both B and T cells), confirmed by immunohistochemistry. In contrast, MZL shows a predominance of B cells with more distinct morphology of marginal zone cells in a diffuse pattern and in some cases coexpression of CD43 by B cells is present. If the lesion has many polytypic plasma cells, fibrosis, and vascular involvement by lymphoid infiltrate, IgG4-related sclerosing disease should be considered in the differential diagnosis. Staining for IgG4 and IgG should be performed and a higher ratio of IgG4-positive plasma cells to IgG-positive plasma cells (more than 40%) in combination with increased serum levels of IgG4 would support a diagnosis of IgG4 related sclerosing disease.

Immunohistochemical and molecular features of pulmonary marginal zone lymphoma

The immunophenotype of the neoplastic cells of MZL is positive for pan-B-cell antigens CD19, CD20, PAX-5,

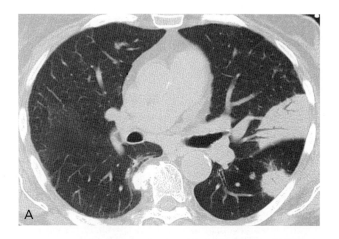

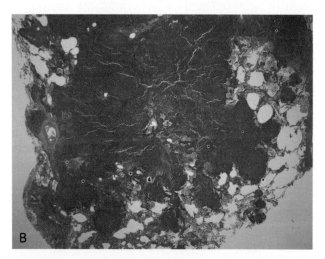

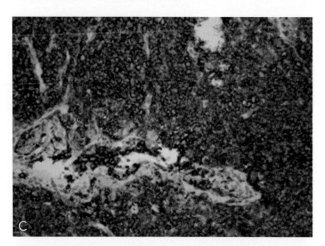

FIGURE 8-5 MALT lymphoma. (A) Transverse CT image shows mass-like consolidation containing air bronchograms in the lingua and left lower lobe. (B) Lung parenchyma with solid, dense nodules of lymphoid infiltrate spreading along the interstitium in the periphery and frequently invading the bronchi, blood vessels, and pleura (H&E, 20×). CD20 immunostaining (C) highlights the predominant B cells in the lymphoid infiltrate, which are monotypic (lambda restricted, not shown here) (hematoxylin-eosin, original magnifications ×20 [A] and CD20 immunostain ×200 [B]).

IgM (>IgA>IgG), occasionally CD43 and negative for IgD, CD5, CD10, CD23, terminal deoxynucleotidyltransferase (TdT), bcl-6, and cyclin D1 (*Figure 8-5C*). Plasma cells may be monotypic or polytypic. Flow cytometric immunophenotyping demonstrating the presence of monoclonal B-cell population aids in the diagnosis of clonality. Immunoglobulin gene rearrangement (IGH) studies may confirm the diagnosis.[31]

t(11;18)(q21;q21) chromosomal translocation resulting in the production of a fusion protein composed of the apoptosis inhibitor API2 on chromosome 11q21 and the paracaspase MALT1 on chromosome 18q21 is the most common structural abnormality identified in the primary pulmonary MZL.20 Other translocations [t(14;18) (q32;q21), t(1;14) (p22;q32), and t(3;14) (p14;q32)] as well as trisomy 18 and 3 have also been described in a subset of cases in other sites.[31]

Primary pulmonary diffuse large B-cell lymphoma

Demographics of primary large B-cell lymphoma
Primary pulmonary DLBCL is the second most common type of PPL accounting for approximately 12% to 20% of all the cases.[28,32-34] It commonly affects the adults in sixth and seventh decades of life.

Etiologies of primary large B-cell lymphoma
A subset of these lymphomas arises by transformation of preexisting or concurrent MZL, small lymphocytic lymphoma, and follicular lymphoma.[35]

Diagnostic criteria of primary large B-cell lymphoma
Primary large B-cell lymphoma is characterized by presence of atypical large B cells, causing destruction of the lung parenchyma.

Clinical features of primary large B-cell lymphoma
Patients usually present with cough or dyspnea and rarely hemoptysis. These neoplasms can be seen in both immunocompromised and immunocompetent patients. Diffuse large B-cell lymphomas are aggressive, but complete remission and long-term survival can be seen, with reported median survival time of approximately 8 to 10 years.[1]

Imaging features of primary large B-cell lymphoma
The radiologic appearance is similar to that of MZL except that pulmonary DLBCL may have areas of necrosis, giving rise to cavitation[32] (*Figure 8-6A*).

Gross and histologic features of primary large B-cell lymphoma
On gross examination, the tumor has a solid appearance with discrete borders and variable areas of necrosis. Primary diffuse large B-cell lymphoma in the lung forms confluent sheets of tumor cells and tends to destroy the normal lung parenchyma. The tumor is composed of large dyscohesive tumor cells with coarse chromatin, distinct nucleoli, and abundant amphophilic cytoplasm (*Figure 8-6B*). These are usually described as centroblastic or immunoblastic. An intravascular variant of large B-cell lymphoma, known as *intravascular lymphomatosis*, is also recognized by the World Health Organization (WHO) classification of lymphomas. These lymphomas have prominent pulmonary manifestations, but are an aggressive, systemic disease with worse prognosis for patients.[36]

Differential diagnosis based on morphology alone includes primary or metastatic carcinomas, metastatic

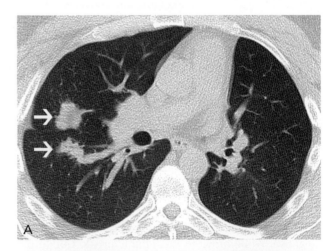

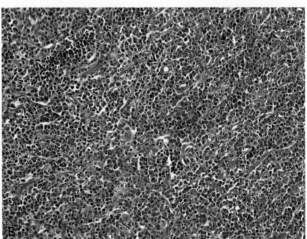

FIGURE 8-6 Diffuse large B-cell lymphoma. **(A)** Transverse CT image shows nodules within the right middle lobe and right lower lobe (arrows) in a patient with diffuse large B-cell lymphoma arising primarily in the lung. Note is made of a faint air bronchogram in the right lower lobe nodule. **(B)** Primary diffuse large B-cell lymphoma presenting as a mass with destruction of the lung parenchyma and showing atypical dyscohesive large cells with abundant cytoplasm, coarse chromatin, and prominent nucleoli (×400).

melanoma, and other epithelial malignancies. These are generally distinguishable by performing epithelial and hematopoietic immunohistochemical stains. Some cases of DLBCL may have an increased number of T cells and are diagnosed as T-cell-rich large B-cell lymphoma. However, lymphoepithelioma-like carcinoma or Hodgkin lymphoma should be excluded in these cases.

Immunohistochemical features of primary large B-cell lymphoma

The immunophenotype of the neoplastic cells are positive for CD19, CD20, CD79a and those of germinal center origin also express CD10 and bcl-6.

Lymphomatoid granulomatosis

Demographics of lymphomatoid granulomatosis

Lymphomatoid granulomatosis (LYG) is a disease that commonly affects adults in the fifth to sixth decade of life. It has a slight predisposition for males, with male-to-female ratio of 2:1.[37]

Etiologies of lymphomatoid granulomatosis

LYG has been shown to be associated with Ebstein-Barr virus (EBV) infection, many cases arising in the setting of immunodeficiency.

Diagnostic criteria of lymphomatoid granulomatosis

LYG is an angiocentric and angiodestructive process that commonly affects the lung as bilateral nodular infiltrates, mimicking granulomatosis with polyangiitis (formerly Wegener granulomatosis) both clinically and radiographically. Recent WHO classification has characterized lymphomatoid granulomatosis as a B-cell neoplasm.

Clinical features of lymphomatoid granulomatosis

The clinical features of LYG reflect systemic multiorgan disease. Pulmonary involvement usually is present, while the skin (50%), nervous system (25%), kidneys, and liver are affected less commonly, and late in the course of illness. The course of LYG patients has been described as usually progressive.[38] In the large studies, mortality rates range from 63% to 90% at 5 years. Treatment for LYG has varied according to grade; grade 3 is presently treated as diffuse large B-cell lymphoma, and shows a prognosis roughly similar to that of diffuse large B-cell lymphoma.[39]

Imaging features of lymphomatoid granulomatosis

CT shows nodules, masses, or an area of consolidation in a peribronchovascular distribution. Cavitation is sometimes present.[14,40] Lesions may contain air bronchograms or a peripheral ground glass halo.[41,42] Pleural effusion is sometimes present. Fluorodeoxyglucose positron emission tomography (FDG-PET) CT shows avid FDG uptake in these lesions[42] (*Figure 8-7A*).

Gross and histologic features of lymphomatoid granulomatosis

Grossly, lesions have homogenous white gray color on cut section with or without central areas of necrosis. Histologically, the tumor shows a nodular replacement of the lung parenchyma by a mixed mononuclear cell infiltrate with prominent vascular invasion and areas of necrosis surrounded by a rim of viable cells. The infiltrating cells show a varying number of small lymphocytes, histiocytes, plasma cells, and large transformed lymphocytes, which, at the high-grade end of the spectrum, occur in sheets, and are indistinguishable from diffuse large B-cell lymphoma (*Figure 8-7B*).

Grading of LYG according to WHO 2008 depends on proportion of large B cells stained with EBV by ISH, where grade 1 is composed of a polymorphous infiltrate with only a few large cells and less than five EBV-positive cells/HPF, and grade 3 shows numerous large B cells, necrosis, and EBV-positive cells (>50/HPF) . LYG of all grades is angiocentric, with accumulation of viable cells around the vessels, followed by angiodestruction, vascular invasion, luminal occlusion, and disruption of the vessels. Although the criteria of the 2008 WHO for classification of LYG are clear, there are some cases that do not fulfill all of the criteria. For practical purposes, Katzenstein et al have proposed the following criteria for LYG in a recent review: (1) Mixed mononuclear cell infiltrate containing large and small lymphoid cells, often along with plasma cells and histiocytes, which replaces the lung parenchyma and shows vascular infiltration. (2) Variable numbers of CD20-positive large B cells, often with atypia, present in a background of CD3-positive small lymphocytes. The other supportive findings include areas of necrosis, positive ISH for EBV-encoded RNA (EBER), and multiple lung nodules radiologically, as well as skin or nervous system involvement[43] (*Figure 8-7C*).

Although granulomatosis with polyangiitis (formerly Wegener granulomatosis) shows similarity to LYG clinically, radiologically, and somewhat histologically, it lacks the large CD20-positive B cells and contains large areas of basophilic necrosis with true granulomas and multinucleated giant cells. Other conditions in the differential diagnosis include viral pneumonia and bronchocentric granulomatosis, which lack the angiocentricity and lymphocyte rich population, and other lymphomas including Hodgkin lymphoma, T-cell-rich B-cell lymphoma, peripheral T-cell lymphoma, and NK/T-cell lymphoma. The lymphoid neoplasms in the differential diagnosis can be distinguished from LYG by the lack of atypical large CD20-positive cells and presence of immunophenotypes characteristic of each subtype.

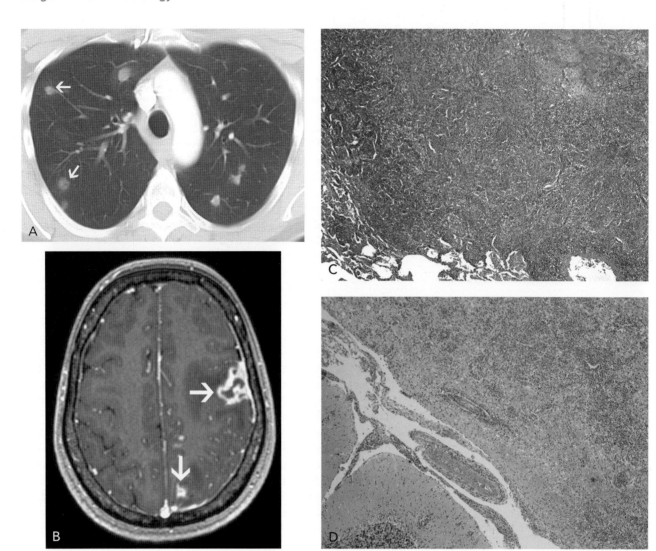

FIGURE 8-7 Lymphomatoid granulomatosis. (A) Transverse CT image shows multiple nodules (arrows) in both lungs. (B) Axial postcontrast MPRAGE image of the brain shows multiple peripherally enhancing lesions (arrows) in the same patient demonstrating CNS involvement by LYG. (C) Lung parenchyma shows nodular replacement of the lung parenchyma by a mixed mononuclear cell infiltrate with prominent vascular invasion and areas of necrosis surrounded by rim of viable cells. The patient also had brain lesions (D) showing tumor cells surrounding the vessels and areas of necrosis (hematoxylin-eosin, original magnifications ×40 [C] and ×40 [D]).

Immunohistochemical features of lymphomatoid granulomatosis

The large cells are CD20+, CD79a+, CD30+/−, CD15−, EBV+, while the small lymphocytes are mostly T cells, CD4>CD8.

Rare Non-Hodgkin lymphoma of B-cell lineage

A minority of patients with primary pulmonary lymphomas can also show the following subtypes including follicular lymphoma, Burkitt lymphoma, and mantle cell lymphoma, although these are rare neoplasms.[20,28,32,44]

Other Non-Hodgkin Lymphomas

Primary pulmonary plasmacytoma

Demographics of primary pulmonary plasmacytoma

Pulmonary plasmacytoma can be seen in both sexes with equal predilection.

Etiologies of primary pulmonary plasmacytoma

Primary plasmacytoma of the lung is exceedingly rare although pulmonary involvement with plasma cell myeloma is more common. Exact etiology of these lesions is unknown.

Diagnostic criteria of primary pulmonary plasmacytoma

Diagnosis is confirmed by the presence of diffuse sheets of monoclonal plasma cells.

Clinical features of primary pulmonary plasmacytoma

Most of the patients are asymptomatic at presentation; however, symptoms like dyspnea, fever, and hemoptysis have been reported. All patients with plasmacytoma of the lung should be worked up for complete evaluation of systemic plasma cell myeloma including serum and urine electrophoresis, skeletal survey, and bone marrow evaluation.

Unlike plasma cell myeloma, extramedullary plasmacytoma may not have serum M protein or Bence Jones light chains in the urine. However, up to 25% of patients with extramedullary plasmacytoma will show a monoclonal gammopathy.[45] Surgical resection is the best treatment for localized pulmonary plasmacytoma, which occasionally is combined with chemotherapy or radiotherapy.[46] The prognosis of these patients is generally better than that of patients with systematic plasma cell myeloma. Extramedullary plasmacytoma can develop into systemic myeloma in very few cases.[47]

Imaging features of primary pulmonary plasmacytoma

Imaging usually shows solitary or multiple nodules in the lung. Rare cases present with diffuse pleural involvement.[48]

Gross and histological findings of primary pulmonary plasmacytoma

Grossly the tumor presents as a discrete solitary mass or nodule in the lung or hilar areas with firm, fleshy, and dark-tan cut surface.[49] Amyloid deposition may be prominent grossly and microscopically.[50] Diagnosis is confirmed by the presence of diffuse sheets of plasma cells that show monoclonality.[51] Occasionally, the lesional cells are quite pleomorphic and would raise a differential diagnosis of bronchogenic carcinoma or metastatic melanoma. However, the amphophilic cytoplasm and paranuclear "hof" of plasma cells is quite helpful to make a correct diagnosis.

Immunohistochemical features of Primary pulmonary plasmacytoma

Plasma cells are negative for leukocyte common antigen (LCA) and B-cell markers. They will be positive for CD138 immunomarker and will show restrictive pattern of cytoplasmic immunoglobulin expression. Flow cytometry analysis also shows CD138 positivity in the plasma cells with restricted pattern of light chain expression. However, it is important to perform keratin, S-100, and other lineage markers to rule out lesions in differential diagnosis.

Plasma cell neoplasms, secondary involvement of the lung

Secondary involvement of the lung by disseminated plasma cell dyscrasia is more common than primary pulmonary plasmacytoma. These patients can develop nodular deposits of amyloid in the lung, which can be solitary or multiple.[29]

Primary Pulmonary Hodgkin Lymphoma

Hodgkin lymphoma in the lung

Demographics of Hodgkin lymphoma

Primary pulmonary Hodgkin lymphoma (HL) is a rare entity.[52-55] Hodgkin lymphoma is most commonly seen in the lung as secondary involvement. HL affects young adults with a mean age of 42 years and with slight female predisposition.

Etiologies of Hodgkin lymphoma

The exact etiology of HL is unknown.

Diagnostic criteria of Hodgkin lymphoma

Identification of large and pleomorphic "Reed-Sternberg" (RS) cells, when present, are quite diagnostic for HL.

Clinical features of Hodgkin lymphoma

Most patients present with concomitant cervical, mediastinal, or supraclavicular lymphadenopathy. Factors that correlate with a poor prognosis include age greater than 60 years, B symptoms, multiplicity and bilaterality of lung lesions, pleural effusion, and cavitation.[56] It is suggested that chemotherapy is recommended over radiotherapy in this disease because of the risk of radiation pneumonitis.

Imaging features of Hodgkin lymphoma

These patients present with single or multiple parenchymal masses, endobronchial lesions, or consolidation, which may be patchy (*Figure 8-8A*).

Gross and histologic features of Hodgkin lymphoma

The diagnosis of HL in the lung is based on the recognition of diagnostic Reed-Sternberg cells within the appropriate reactive cellular infiltrate in the background (*Figure 8-8B*). Nodular sclerosis and mixed cellularity are the common histologic types seen in the lung. Differential diagnoses for classic HL include solitary fibrous tumor with extensive inflammation and inflammatory myofibroblastic tumor.

Immunohistochemical features of Hodgkin lymphoma

Immunohistochemically, the tumor cells are positive for CD15+, CD30+, Pax5+, rarely CD20+, and negative for T-cell markers and CD45.[31,57]

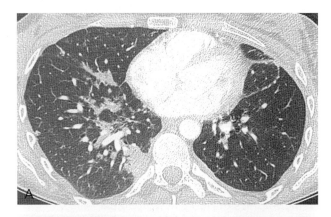

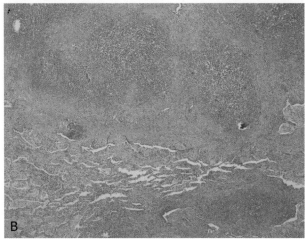

FIGURE 8-8 Hodgkin lymphoma. (A) Transverse CT image shows somewhat nodular consolidation along the right major fissure, subpleural nodules and nodular areas of density in the right lower lobe, as well as consolidation along the bronchovascular bundles in the right lower lobe (perilymphatic distribution) in this patient with primary Hodgkin lymphoma of the lung. **(B)** Primary Hodgkin lymphoma, a rare occurrence in the lung, showing a polymorphous lymphoid infiltrate with surrounding fibrosis and sharp interface with adjacent lung parenchyma (×40).

IMMUNODEFICIENCY-ASSOCIATED LYMPHOPROLIFERATIVE DISORDERS

Primary Effusion Lymphoma

Primary effusion lymphoma is a rare distinctive type of diffuse large B-cell lymphoma characterized by lymphomatous effusion of pleural, pericardial, or peritoneal cavities, without any solid mass.[58] Nearly all patients are HIV-positive young adults, males affected much more often than females. These neoplasms are human herpes virus 8 (HHV8) positive and can also be coinfected with EBV. The neoplastic cells are very large, uniform, and pleomorphic (immunoblast like), and some may resemble Reed-Sternberg cells. Neoplastic

cells express CD45 and are negative for B-cell antigens. However, immunoglobulin light and heavy chains are clonally rearranged supporting a B-cell lineage. It frequently is associated with mutations in the 5′ noncoding regions of BCL6 as well as the immunoglobulin gene variable regions. These patients carry a poor prognosis (*Figure 8-9A and B*).

Pyothorax-Associated Lymphoma

Pyothorax-associated lymphoma is a rare EBV-positive diffuse large B-cell lymphoma arising in patients with long-standing chronic pyothorax (treated with iatrogenic pneumothorax), secondary to tuberculosis. Patients present with a mass in the pleura, rarely accompanied by lung mass or pleural effusion. On

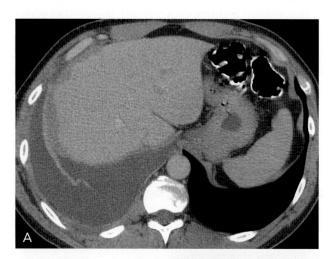

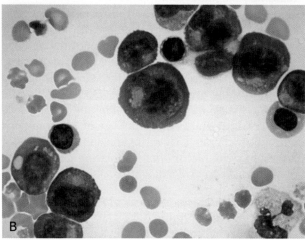

FIGURE 8-9 Primary effusion lymphoma. (A) Transverse CT image shows malignant right pleural effusion in this patient with primary effusion lymphoma. **(B)** Pleural fluid from a patient with primary effusion lymphoma shows pleomorphic large cells with irregular nuclear contours, prominent nucleoli, and moderately abundant cytoplasm (×1000).

microscopic examination, the tumor shows diffuse pro-liferation of large atypical cells, with centroblastic and/or immunoblastic or plasmacytoid features with areas of necrosis. Neoplastic cells express pan-B-cell anti-gens, MUM1, and rarely are CD138 positive, and are negative for CD10, bcl-6, and HHV-8. Patients carry a dismal prognosis.

Posttransplant Related Lymphoproliferative Disorders

Demographics of PTLD

Posttransplant-related lymphoproliferative disorder (PTLD) involves approximately 2% of transplant cases overall; however, incidence varies with each type of transplant. Children are more likely to develop PTLD than adults.

Etiology of PTLD

PTLD is a serious complication of solid organ and hematopoietic stem cell transplantation that is linked to immunosuppression, the Epstein-Barr virus (EBV), and cytomegalovirus (CMV). Although PTLD has been described after transplantation of all solid organs, its inci-dence varies depending on the organ transplanted. Lung transplant recipients show an incidence between 2.5% and 8%.[59] Most patients have systemic involvement at pre-sentation, but some patients may have disease confined to the allograft itself.[60] The etiologic factors that underlie different subtypes of PTLD, as well as the implications for differential therapy and survival, are unknown.[61]

Clinical features of PTLD

PTLD is a highly variable disease in its clinical presen-tation as well as in its pathologic characteristics. Most patients present with systemic disease at presentation.

Imaging features of PTLD

CT shows solitary or multiple nodules, masses, patchy airspace consolidation, and mediastinal and hilar lymphadenopathy. Multiple pulmonary nodules are the most common finding[14,62] (*Figure 8-10*).

Gross and histological features of PTLD

Grossly, it can be difficult to appreciate the lesion, unless nodules or masses are present. Microscopically, the lesions can vary from simple lymphoid hyper-plasia to aggressive lymphoproliferative neoplasm. Pathologically, there are two major subtypes of PTLD. Polymorphic PTLD is characterized morphologically by a plethora of monoclonal B cells in all stages of matu-ration as well as reactive T cells. Monomorphic PTLD

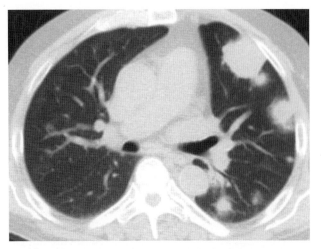

FIGURE 8-10 Posttransplant lymphoproliferative disorder. Transverse CT image shows multiple nodules in masses in both the lungs, left greater than right, in this renal trans-plant patient.

is a subtype of non-Hodgkin lymphoma that appears as homogeneous sheets of transformed, monoclonal B cells, often with cytogenetic abnormalities. Regardless of the histologic features, the lymphoid cells in most cases of PTLD contain EBV detected by immunohisto-chemistry or in situ hybridization. T-lineage PTLDs, spe-cifically of the gamma-delta-T-cell phenotype, although rare, can also occur after solid organ transplantation.[63] Classifying the PTLDs into morphologic and molecular categories plays an important role in initial treatment planning and prognosis and it is important to recog-nize that transplant patients can develop lymphomas of any subtype.[64] A systematic multidisciplinary (clinical, radiologic, virologic, and histologic) approach is man-datory for the diagnosis and management of PTLD in transplant recipients. In addition, staining for EBV anti-gens and quantification of EBV DNA in biopsy speci-mens should always be performed to understand the role of EBV infection in the pathogenesis of PTLD.[65]

LYMPHOMAS OF T-CELL LINEAGE

Peripheral T-Cell Lymphoma

Primary pulmonary peripheral T-cell lymphoma (PTCL) is an extremely rare and aggressive disease and is mostly found as case reports in the literature.[66] These patients are often clinically ill and may present with fever, cough, and dyspnea. The clinical course is usually aggressive, and relapses are more common for T-cell lymphoma than for the B-cell lymphomas. Patients with PTCL are usually adults with generalized disease; the lymph nodes, liver and spleen may be involved. It is more commonly seen in males.[67] Few case reports of primary pulmonary T-cell lymphoma in HTLV-1 carriers have also been reported.[66] The incidence of primary pulmonary T-cell lymphoma is higher in the Asian population than in the Western population, as is the case with T-cell lymphomas in general.[68]

The radiologic findings are similar to those associated with pulmonary MZL and consist mainly of ground glass attenuation and/or consolidation, centrilobular nodules, masses, thickening of bronchovascular bundles, and interlobular septal thickening in the peripheral lung. WHO has divided the mature T-cell neoplasms into specifically defined entities.[69] The cases that do not match one of the defined entities of PTCL are best categorized as "not otherwise specified," reflecting that we do not yet fully understand the underlying pathogenesis.

Histological examination of the lung shows diffuse infiltrates of large lymphoid cells with pleomorphic, vesicular nuclei, prominent nucleoli, and frequent mitoses. Rare cases also show predominance of small lymphoid cells with atypical, irregular nuclei. Angiocentricity is often seen in these neoplasms. Immunohistochemical staining demonstrates tumor cells with aberrant T-cell phenotype that are positive for CD3 with frequent downregulation of CD5 and CD7 and are negative for CD20, CD30 (Ki-1), and CD56. The Ki-67 proliferative index is usually high in these neoplasms, exceeding 70%. PTCL shows clonal T-cell receptor (TCR) gene rearrangements by PCR analysis in most cases. Most of the cases of primary pulmonary T-cell lymphoma reported in the literature were diagnosed by open lung biopsy. These patients receive chemotherapy, often with poor response.[67]

Anaplastic Large Cell Lymphoma

Anaplastic large cell lymphoma (ALCL) has a propensity to involve extranodal sites, particularly skin and rarely other extranodal sites such as lung. Primary pulmonary anaplastic large cell lymphoma has been reported in the literature as case reports only.[70,71] Patients with ALCL have a bimodal age distribution seen in children and adults, with male predominance.[72] ALCL has an aggressive clinical course and patients frequently present with systemic symptoms and advanced-stage disease. The tumor cells express a T-cell phenotype, and rarely may also have a null phenotype. ALCL is characterized by diffuse sheets of large cells with pleomorphic nuclei and abundant cytoplasm. The nuclear chromatin is usually finely clumped or dispersed with multiple small, basophilic nucleoli. The majority of these cells are positive for a pan-T-cell markers such as CD2, CD3, or CD45RO, although null phenotype may be negative for these markers. Consistent expression of CD30/Ki-1 is an important hallmark of this disease.

Most cases express cytotoxic granule-associated proteins such as TIA1, granzyme, and/or perforin. ALCL may mimic metastatic carcinoma or melanoma on morphology, thus performing a battery of hematopoietic and epithelial markers is obligatory as a diagnostic aid. A few studies from the literature suggest that the risk of progression to systemic disease and death is high in patients who present as primary pulmonary ALCL.[73]

ALCL should be distinguished from other T-cell large cell lymphomas by its reactivity with ALK immunostain or by presence of t(2;5) translocation involving the NPM and ALK genes. ALCL (ALK -negative) is included as a provisional entity in the recent WHO classification.

NK/T-Cell Lymphoma

NK/T-cell lymphoma is characterized by vascular destruction, prominent necrosis, and associated EBV infection. It is more prevalent in Asians and native American population of Mexico, Central and South America. The most frequent presentation of this tumor is extranodal, usually upper aerodigestive tract, but other sites of involvement are skin, soft tissue, gastrointestinal tract, testis, and the spleen. Rare cases with isolated lung involvement have been reported.[74] Patients often present with systemic symptoms and advanced stage, with involvement of multiple sites. The tumor cells show an angiocentric and angiodestructive pattern with broad cytologic spectrum. The major immunophenotype of these neoplasms include positivity for CD2, CD56, and cytoplasmic CD3 and negativity for surface CD3. NK/T-cell lymphoma occurring outside the nasal cavity is a highly aggressive neoplasm with poor response to therapy and short survival time.

PULMONARY INVOLVEMENT WITH SYSTEMIC HEMATOLOGIC MALIGNANCY

Secondary Pulmonary Non-Hodgkin and Hodgkin Lymphoma

Lung is a relatively frequent site of secondary involvement of lymphoma and is more common in patients with Hodgkin lymphoma (approximately 38% of cases) as compared to non-Hodgkin lymphoma (approximately 24%).[75,76] These patients have prior or concurrent nodal lesions of lymphoma or develop evidence of systemic lymphoma up to 6 months after presentation. Secondary involvement may result from direct mediastinal node extension or from lymphatic or hematogenous dissemination from distant sites. Nodules, masses, and consolidation are common radiologic pulmonary manifestations of secondary involvement

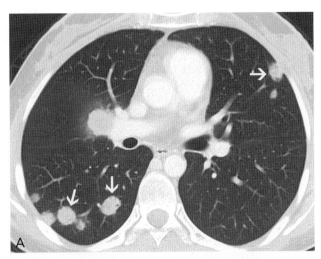
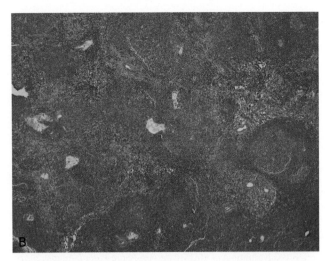

FIGURE 8-11 Pulmonary involvement with systemic hematologic malignancy. **(A)** Transverse CT shows multiple nodules (arrows) in this patient with diffuse systemic spread of non-Hodgkin lymphoma secondarily involving the lungs. **(B)** Patient with a history of marginal zone lymphoma of the stomach, now presenting with nodules in the lung, which shows dense nodules of lymphoid infiltrate spreading along the interstitium and invading the bronchi and the bronchioles (×40).

of the lung by lymphoma. Mediastinal lymphadenopathy and pleural effusion are also commonly present. Patients usually present with nonspecific pulmonary symptoms. A high suspicion of lung involvement by lymphoma should be considered in a patient with a prior history of lymphoma who develops lung lesions, necessitating further extensive workup where correlation of clinical, microbiologic, and histologic findings is necessary in these cases. Diagnosis of secondary pulmonary lymphomas is made using the same criteria as in the evaluation of lymph node biopsies (*Figure 8-11A and B*). These patients are staged using the Ann Arbor criteria, and their prognosis is determined by both stage and histologic subtype.

Follicular lymphoma, small lymphocytic lymphoma, and mantle cell lymphoma are the most common systemic B-cell lineage lymphomas to secondarily involve the lung. MZL frequently involves the lung secondarily after presentation in other mucosal sites. Clinical history, morphology, and immunohistochemical studies are necessary to provide an accurate diagnosis and classification for all of these cases. If the clinical history is known at the outset, sending tissue for flow cytometric analysis can provide accurate timely diagnosis and classification.

The vast majority of patients with T-cell lymphomas have systemic disease at presentation. Clinical history, histologic, immunophenotypic, viral, and cytogenetic analysis all contribute to diagnosing-specific subtypes of lymphoma, including T-cell prolymphocytic leukemia (T-PLL), angioimmunoblastic-type PTCL (AILD-PTCL), and T-cell ALCL. About 10% of patients with peripheral T-cell lymphoma have pulmonary involvement.[77]

REFERENCES

1. Cadranel J, Wislez M, Antoine M. Primary pulmonary lymphoma. *Eur Respir J.* September 2002;20(3):750-762.
2. William J, Variakojis D, Yeldandi A, Raparia K. Lymphoproliferative neoplasms of the lung: a review. *Arch Pathol Lab.* March 2013; 137(3):382-391.
3. Colby TV, Yousem SA. Pulmonary histology for the surgical pathologist. *Am J Surg Pathol.* March 1988;12(3):223-239.
4. Nicholson AG, Wotherspoon AC, Diss TC, et al. Reactive pulmonary lymphoid disorders. *Histopathology.* May 1995;26(5):405-412.
5. Gibson M, Hansell DM. Lymphocytic disorders of the chest: pathology and imaging. *Clinical Radiology.* July 1998;53(7): 469-480.
6. Travis WD, Galvin JR. Non-neoplastic pulmonary lymphoid lesions. *Thorax.* December 2001;56(12):964-971.
7. Aerni MR, Vassallo R, Myers JL, Lindell RM, Ryu JH. Follicular bronchiolitis in surgical lung biopsies: clinical implications in 12 patients. *Respir Med.* February 2008;102(2):307-312.
8. Howling SJ, Hansell DM, Wells AU, Nicholson AG, Flint JD, Muller NL. Follicular bronchiolitis: thin-section CT and histologic findings. *Radiology.* September 1999;212(3):637-642.
9. Kradin RL, Mark EJ. Benign lymphoid disorders of the lung, with a theory regarding their development. *Hum Pathol.* October 1983;14(10):857-867.
10. Bragg DG, Chor PJ, Murray KA, Kjeldsberg CR. Lymphoproliferative disorders of the lung: histopathology, clinical manifestations, and imaging features. *AJR Am J Roentgenol.* August 1994;163(2):273-281.
11. Tanaka N, Kim JS, Bates CA, et al. Lung diseases in patients with common variable immunodeficiency: chest radiographic, and computed tomographic findings. *J Comput Assist Tomogr.* September-October 2006;30(5):828-838.
12. Kaan PM, Hegele RG, Hayashi S, Hogg JC. Expression of bcl-2 and Epstein-Barr virus LMP1 in lymphocytic interstitial pneumonia. *Thorax.* January 1997;52(1):12-16.
13. Swigris JJ, Berry GJ, Raffin TA, Kuschner WG. Lymphoid interstitial pneumonia: a narrative review. *Chest.* December 2002;122(6): 2150-2164.

CHAPTER 8

14. Hare SS, Souza CA, Bain G, et al. The radiological spectrum of pulmonary lymphoproliferative disease. *Br J Radiol.* July 2012;85(1015):848-864.

15. Teruya-Feldstein J, Temeck BK, Sloas MM, et al. Pulmonary malignant lymphoma of mucosa-associated lymphoid tissue (MALT) arising in a pediatric HIV-positive patient. *Am J Surg Pathol.* March 1995;19(3):357-363.

16. Aghamohammadi A, Parvaneh N, Tirgari F, et al. Lymphoma of mucosa-associated lymphoid tissue in common variable immunodeficiency. *Leuk Lymphoma.* February 2006;47(2):343-346.

17. Hansen LA, Prakash UB, Colby TV. Pulmonary lymphoma in Sjogren's syndrome. *Mayo Clin Proc.* August 1989;64(8):920-931.

18. Luppi M, Longo G, Ferrari MG, et al. Additional neoplasms and HCV infection in low-grade lymphoma of MALT type. *Br J Haematol.* August 1996;94(2):373-375.

19. Kurtin PJ, Myers JL, Adlakha H, et al. Pathologic and clinical features of primary pulmonary extranodal marginal zone B-cell lymphoma of MALT type. *Am J Surg Pathol.* August 2001;25(8):997-1008.

20. Graham BB, Mathisen DJ, Mark EJ, Takvorian RW. Primary pulmonary lymphoma. *Ann Thorac Surg.* October 2005;80(4):1248-1253.

21. Stefanovic A, Morgensztern D, Fong T, Lossos IS. Pulmonary marginal zone lymphoma: a single centre experience and review of the SEER database. *Leuk Lymphoma.* July 2008;49(7):1311-1320.

22. Arkenau HT, Gordon C, Cunningham D, Norman A, Wotherspoon A, Chau I. Mucosa associated lymphoid tissue lymphoma of the lung: the Royal Marsden Hospital experience. *Leuk Lymphoma.* March 2007;48(3):547-550.

23. Wislez M, Cadranel J, Antoine M, et al. Lymphoma of pulmonary mucosa-associated lymphoid tissue: CT scan findings and pathological correlations. *Eur Respir J.* August 1999;14(2):423-429.

24. O'Donnell PG, Jackson SA, Tung KT, Hassan B, Wilkins B, Mead GM. Radiological appearances of lymphomas arising from mucosa-associated lymphoid tissue (MALT) in the lung. *Clin Radiol.* April 1998;53(4):258-263.

25. Imai H, Sunaga N, Kaira K, et al. Clinicopathological features of patients with bronchial-associated lymphoid tissue lymphoma. *Intern Med.* 2009;48(5):301-306.

26. Bae YA, Lee KS, Han J, et al. Marginal zone B-cell lymphoma of bronchus-associated lymphoid tissue: imaging findings in 21 patients. *Chest.* February 2008;133(2):433-440.

27. Habermann TM, Ryu JH, Inwards DJ, Kurtin PJ. Primary pulmonary lymphoma. *Semin Oncol.* June 1999;26(3):307-315.

28. Cordier JF, Chailleux E, Lauque D, et al. Primary pulmonary lymphomas. A clinical study of 70 cases in nonimmunocompromised patients. *Chest.* January 1993;103(1):201-208.

29. Dacic S, Colby TV, Yousem SA. Nodular amyloidoma and primary pulmonary lymphoma with amyloid production: a differential diagnostic problem. *Mod Pathol.* September 2000;13(9):934-940.

30. Bhargava P, Rushin JM, Rusnock EJ, et al. Pulmonary light chain deposition disease: report of five cases and review of the literature. *Am J Surg Pathol.* February 2007;31(2):267-276.

31. Ferry JA. *Extranodal Lymphomas.* Philadelphia, PA: Elsevier Saunders; 2011.

32. Li G, Hansmann ML, Zwingers T, Lennert K. Primary lymphomas of the lung: morphological, immunohistochemical and clinical features. *Histopathology.* June 1990;16(6):519-531.

33. Ferraro P, Trastek VF, Adlakha H, Deschamps C, Allen MS, Pairolero PC. Primary non-Hodgkin's lymphoma of the lung. *Ann Thorac Surg.* April 2000;69(4):993-997.

34. Kim JH, Lee SH, Park J, et al. Primary pulmonary non-Hodgkin's lymphoma. *Jpn J Clin Oncol.* September 2004;34(9):510-514.

35. Neri N, Jesus Nambo M, Aviles A. Diffuse large B-cell lymphoma primary of lung. *Hematology.* March 2011;16(2):110-112.

36. Kraus MD, Jones D, Bartlett NL. Intravascular lymphoma associated with endocrine dysfunction: a report of four cases and a review of the literature. *Am J Med.* August 1999;107(2):169-176.

37. Colby TV. Current histological diagnosis of lymphomatoid granulomatosis. *Mod Pathol.* January 2012;25(suppl 1):S39-S42.

38. Makol A, Kosuri K, Tamkus D, de MCW, Chang HT. Lymphomatoid granulomatosis masquerading as interstitial pneumonia in a 66-year-old man: a case report and review of literature. *J Hematol Oncol.* 2009;2:39.

39. Jung KH, Sung HJ, Lee JH, et al. A case of pulmonary lymphomatoid granulomatosis successfully treated by combination chemotherapy with rituximab. *Chemotherapy.* 2009;55(5):386-390.

40. Koss MN. Malignant and benign lymphoid lesions of the lung. *Ann Diagn Pathol.* June 2004;8(3):167-187.

41. Lee JS, Tuder R, Lynch DA. Lymphomatoid granulomatosis: radiologic features and pathologic correlations. *AJR Am J Roentgenol.* November 2000;175(5):1335-1339.

42. Chung JH, Wu CC, Gilman MD, Palmer EL, Hasserjian RP, Shepard JA. Lymphomatoid granulomatosis: CT and FDG-PET findings. *Korean J Radiol.* November-December 2011;12(6):671-678.

43. Katzenstein AL, Doxtader E, Narendra S. Lymphomatoid granulomatosis: insights gained over 4 decades. *Am J Surg Pathol.* December 2010;34(12):e35-e48.

44. Begueret H, Vergier B, Parrens M, et al. Primary lung small B-cell lymphoma versus lymphoid hyperplasia: evaluation of diagnostic criteria in 26 cases. *Am J Surg Pathol.* January 2002;26(1):76-81.

45. Shaikh G, Sehgal R, Mehrishi A, Karnik A. Primary pulmonary plasmacytoma. *J Clin Oncol.* June 20, 2008;26(18):3089-3091.

46. Ujiie H, Okada D, Nakajima Y, Yoshino N, Akiyama H. A case of primary solitary pulmonary plasmacytoma. *Ann Thorac Cardiovasc Surg.* 2012;18(3):239-242.

47. Mohammad Taheri Z, Mohammadi F, Karbasi M, et al. Primary pulmonary plasmacytoma with diffuse alveolar consolidation: a case report. *Patholog Res Int.* 2010;2010:463465.

48. Colonna A, Gualco G, Bacchi CE, et al. Plasma cell myeloma presenting with diffuse pleural involvement: a hitherto unreported pattern of a new mesothelioma mimicker. *Ann Diagn Pathol.* February 2010;14(1):30-35.

49. Kazzaz B, Dewar A, Corrin B. An unusual pulmonary plasmacytoma. *Histopathology.* September 1992;21(3):285-287.

50. Morinaga S, Watanabe H, Gemma A, et al. Plasmacytoma of the lung associated with nodular deposits of immunoglobulin. *Am J Surg Pathol.* December 1987;11(12):989-995.

51. Montero C, Souto A, Vidal I, Fernandez Mdel M, Blanco M, Verea H. [Three cases of primary pulmonary plasmacytoma]. *Arch Bronconeumol.* November 2009;45(11):564-566.

52. Nakachi S, Nagasaki A, Owan I, et al. [Primary pulmonary Hodgkin lymphoma—two case reports and a review of the literature]. *Gan To Kagaku Ryoho.* December 2007;34(13):2279-2282.

53. Kern WH, Crepeau AG, Jones JC. Primary Hodgkin's disease of the lung. Report of 4 cases and review of the literature. *Cancer.* November-December 1961;14:1151-1165.

54. Radin AI. Primary pulmonary Hodgkin's disease. *Cancer.* February 1, 1990;65(3):550-563.

55. Harper PG, Fisher C, McLennan K, Souhami RL. Presentation of Hodgkin's disease as an endobronchial lesion. *Cancer.* January 1, 1984;53(1):147-150.

56. Yousem SA, Weiss LM, Colby TV. Primary pulmonary Hodgkin's disease. A clinicopathologic study of 15 cases. *Cancer.* March 15, 1986;57(6):1217-1224.

57. Homma M, Yamochi-Onizuka T, Shiozawa E, et al. Primary pulmonary classical Hodgkin lymphoma with two recurrences in the mediastinum : a case report. *J Clin Exp Hematop.* 2010;50(2):151-157.

58. Nador RG, Cesarman E, Chadburn A, et al. Primary effusion lymphoma: a distinct clinicopathologic entity associated with

the Kaposi's sarcoma-associated herpes virus. *Blood.* July 15, 1996;88(2):645-656.

59. Paranjothi S, Yusen RD, Kraus MD, Lynch JP, Patterson GA, Trulock EP. Lymphoproliferative disease after lung transplantation: comparison of presentation and outcome of early and late cases. *J Heart Lung Transplant.* October 2001;20(10):1054-1063.

60. Randhawa PS, Yousem SA, Paradis IL, Dauber JA, Griffith BP, Locker J. The clinical spectrum, pathology, and clonal analysis of Epstein-Barr virus-associated lymphoproliferative disorders in heart-lung transplant recipients. *Am J Clin Pathol.* August 1989;92(2):177-185.

61. Kremer BE, Reshef R, Misleh JG, et al. Post-transplant lymphoproliferative disorder after lung transplantation: A review of 35 cases. *J Heart Lung Transplant.* March 2012;31(3):296-304.

62. Borhani AA, Hosseinzadeh K, Almusa O, Furlan A, Nalesnik M. Imaging of posttransplantation lymphoproliferative disorder after solid organ transplantation. *Radiographics.* July-August 2009;29(4):981-1000; discussion 1000-1002.

63. Steurer M, Stauder R, Grunewald K, et al. Hepatosplenic gammadelta-T-cell lymphoma with leukemic course after renal transplantation. *Hum Pathol.* February 2002;33(2):253-258.

64. Chadburn A, Chen JM, Hsu DT, et al. The morphologic and molecular genetic categories of posttransplantation lymphoproliferative disorders are clinically relevant. *Cancer.* May 15, 1998;82(10):1978-1987.

65. Baldanti F, Rognoni V, Cascina A, Oggionni T, Tinelli C, Meloni F. Post-transplant lymphoproliferative disorders and Epstein-Barr virus DNAemia in a cohort of lung transplant recipients. *Virol J.* 2011;8:421.

66. Minomo S, Takimoto T, Morimura O, et al. Primary pulmonary T-cell lymphoma in a human T-lymphotropic virus type-1 carrier showing atypical shadow. *J Thorac Oncol.* April 2010;5(4):558-559.

67. Bernabeu Mora R, Sanchez Nieto JM, Nieto Olivares A. Bilateral pulmonary nodules as a manifestation of primary pulmonary T-cell lymphoma. *Int J Hematol.* September 2009;90(2):153-156.

68. Shin CH, Paik SH, Park JS, et al. Primary pulmonary T-cell lymphoma: a case report. *Korean J Radiol.* March-April 2010;11(2):234-238.

69. Swerdlow SH, Campo E, Harris NL, et al. *WHO Classification of Tumours of Haematopoietic and Lymphoid Tissues.* Lyon, France: IARCPress; 2008.

70. Rush WL, Andriko JA, Taubenberger JK, et al. Primary anaplastic large cell lymphoma of the lung: a clinicopathologic study of five patients. *Mod Pathol.* December 2000;13(12):1285-1292.

71. Yang HB, Li J, Shen T. Primary anaplastic large cell lymphoma of the lung. Report of two cases and literature review. *Acta Haematol.* 2007;118(3):188-191.

72. Guerra J, Echevarria-Escudero M, Barrio N, Velez-Rosario R. Primary endobronchial anaplastic large cell lymphoma in a pediatric patient. *P R Health Sci J.* June 2006;25(2):159-161.

73. Chott A, Kaserer K, Augustin I, et al. Ki-1-positive large cell lymphoma. A clinicopathologic study of 41 cases. *Am J Surg Pathol.* May 1990;14(5):439-448.

74. Lee BH, Kim SY, Kim MY, et al. CT of nasal-type T/NK cell lymphoma in the lung. *J Thorac Imaging.* March 2006;21(1):37-39.

75. Berkman N, Breuer R. Pulmonary involvement in lymphoma. *Respir Med.* February 1993;87(2):85-92.

76. Berkman N, Breuer R, Kramer MR, Polliack A. Pulmonary involvement in lymphoma. *Leuk Lymphoma.* January 1996;20(3-4):229-237.

77. Fujisawa T, Suda T, Matsuura S, et al. Peripheral T-cell lymphoma with diffuse pulmonary infiltration and an increase in serum KL-6 level. *Respirology.* May 2007;12(3):452-454.

9 Benign Lung Neoplasms

William B. Laskin, Celina Villa, Kimberly Golden, and Anjana Yeldandi

TAKE HOME PEARLS

- Benign mesenchymal lung tumors other than hamartomas are exceedingly rare.
- Hamartomas are well-circumscribed, peripheral nodules incidentally found and associated with excellent prognosis following conservative resection.
- Cartilage predominant or monomorphic hamartomas need to be differentiated from the rare chondromas.
- Primary salivary gland–type neoplasms arising from the seromucinous glands are extremely rare and present as coin lesions or endobronchial lesions and treated with a conservative resection.
- Sclerosing hemangiomas are well-circumscribed, solitary lesions that can be mistaken for well-differentiated adenocarcinoma. Other cell types such as xanthomatous or foamy cells and hemosiderin pigment laden macrophages are often present. Histology is characterized by multiple architectural patterns with the vast majority of lesions (85%) demonstrating an admixture of hypocellular fibrosclerotic (scar-like) areas, foci exhibiting papillary growth, solid cell aggregates, and hemorrhagic ectatic spaces.
- A subset of inflammatory myofibroblastic tumors exhibit rearrangements involving the *ALK* gene on chromosome 2p23.
- Intrapulmonary solitary fibrous tumors are rare, compared with pleural based lesions, are firm, well-circumscribed, unencapsulated nodule. The tumor presents as a bland appearing spindle cells in a background of collagenized stroma. Characteristics of the lesion are hemangiopericytoma-like branching vessels and presence of pericellular collagen.
- Primary pulmonary desmoid tumors arising from the lung parenchyma or visceral pleura are exceedingly rare, but histologically identical to their soft tissue counterparts.
- Perivascular epithelioid cell tumors, or PEComas, are uncommon spindled and epithelioid cell mesenchymal neoplasms that coexpress smooth muscle and melanocytic immunomarkers and clear cell sugar tumors are the most common manifestation of the process in the lung. Metastatic clear cell renal cell carcinoma and metastatic melanoma have to be excluded before a diagnosis of clear cell sugar tumor is rendered. Lymphangioleiomyomatosis (LAM) is a rare condition that occurs almost exclusively in women of reproductive age. The classic triad of radiographic findings for LAM includes a reticular interstitial pattern, chylous pleural effusion, and pneumothorax.
- Solitary squamous papillomas and multifocal respiratory papillomas are associated with human papillomavirus (HPV) subtypes 6 and 11.

INTRODUCTION

Benign lung neoplasms include salivary gland–like neoplasms of the tracheobronchial seromucinous glands and a wide range of epithelial and mesenchymal tumors. These benign neoplasms are uncommon and often rare. A succinct review of these entities is presented here.

SALIVARY GLAND–TYPE TRACHEOBRONCHIAL NEOPLASMS

The submucosal glands of the tracheobronchial tree are composed of luminal (serous and mucinous) cells and myoepithelial cells morphologically and functionally identical to the cellular elements of the salivary gland. Albeit rare, benign and malignant lung tumors with morphological features identical to prototypic salivary gland tumors occur in the lung (salivary gland–type tumors). While most salivary gland–type tumors are malignant, this section will concentrate on potentially benign entities.

Pleomorphic Adenoma

Clinical features

Pleomorphic adenoma occurs over a wide age range from 11 to 75 years, but has a peak incidence in the sixth and seventh decades of life.[1] Pleomorphic adenoma is generally located centrally and less often in the peripheral lung where the lesion is commonly, but not always, attached to a distal (peripheral) bronchus.[2,3] Centrally located tumors come to clinical attention because of symptoms related to obstruction or hemoptysis.[2,3] As "benign metastasizing pleomorphic adenoma" of salivary gland infrequently metastasizes to the lung,[4] a primary salivary gland tumor should be excluded before rendering a diagnosis of primary pulmonary pleomorphic adenoma.

Imaging

Computerized tomography demonstrates a nondescript, well-circumscribed solid mass.

Gross features

The tumor ranges in size from 1 to 16 cm in greatest dimension.[5] Centrally located endobronchial tumors present as intraluminal polypoid or dome-shaped masses, whereas lesions arising within peripheral lung are well-circumscribed nodular masses. Macroscopically, pleomorphic adenoma typically is well circumscribed, but unencapsulated, with a soft to firm consistency. Cut surface has a glistening gray-white, myxoid appearance similar to its much more common salivary gland counterpart.

Histologic features

Pleomorphic adenomas consist of a variable admixture of spindled myoepithelial cells and epithelial structures within a myxoid or myxochondroid stromal matrix (*Figure 9-1*). The epithelial component is arranged in

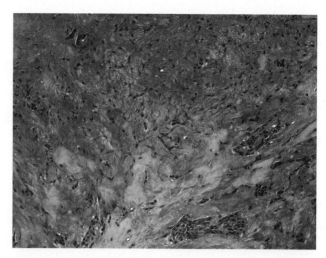

FIGURE 9-1 Pleomorphic adenoma: medium power of tumor with a variable admixture of spindle and epithelial structures within a myxochondroid stromal matrix.

cords, solid or cribriform nests, and oftentimes exhibits focal squamous or sebaceous differentiation. Spindled myoepithelial cells are mostly found in the stromal-rich matrix. Unlike its salivary gland counterpart, the epithelial component is less apt to demonstrate tubule formation and the stroma generally lacks well-formed cartilage.[2] Cellular variants are composed primarily of myoepithelial cells or epithelial elements with little intervening stroma.

Immunohistochemical profile

Tumor cells demonstrate an immunoprofile similar to their salivary gland counterparts with expression of broad-spectrum keratins, S-100 protein, smooth muscle actin, and glial fibrillary acidic protein.[2] Prostate specific antigen has also been detected in pulmonary pleomorphic adenomas.[6]

Clinical outcome

Outcome is generally good for conventional pleomorphic adenoma after complete excision. Incomplete excision leads to recurrence

Acinic Cell Tumor (Fechner Tumor)

First described in 1972 by Fechner and bearing his name (Fechner tumor),[7] the acinic cell tumor is an extremely rare neoplasm even among pulmonary salivary gland–like tumors. Electron microscopic studies confirm the presence of intracytoplasmic zymogen–type granules of varying electron density characteristic of acinar-type secretory cells. A primary salivary gland acinic cell tumor requires exclusion as these carcinomas have a propensity to metastasize years after surgical excision.

Clinical features

Most cases have been reported in middle-aged adults with a few tumors documented in children.[8,9] The lesion has a slight female predominance.[8] Patients with peripheral tumors are asymptomatic, while those with centrally located lesions oftentimes present with respiratory symptoms such as cough, dyspnea, or hemoptysis.[8,9]

Imaging

Imaging detects a nondescript, well-delineated solid pulmonary nodule.

Gross features

The tumor occurs anywhere throughout the lung from beneath the pleura to the central bronchi where the lesion grows as a submucosal mass.[7,8] Most tumors are between 1 and 4 cm in greatest dimension.[8] Gross examination reveals a well-circumscribed, subtly lobulated mass that may be encapsulated. The cut section is white to gray in color.

Histologic features

The process is usually well circumscribed with neoplastic cells arranged in glandular, solid, microcystic, papillary-cystic, follicular, or mixed patterns. In some tumors, fibroconnective tissue with an accompanying lymphoplasmacytic infiltrate partitions tumoral elements into organoid nests. The key lesional cell has a characteristic appearance with abundant basophilic granular cytoplasm, and a centrally placed, rounded nucleus with a variably sized nucleolus (*Figure 9-2*).

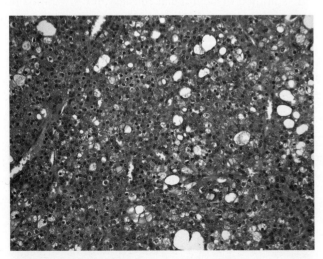

FIGURE 9-2 Acinic cell tumor: solid sheets of tumor cells with abundant basophilic granular cytoplasm, centrally placed rounded nucleus with a variably sized nucleolus.

Tumor cells occasionally have a "signet-ring" morphology, or clear, vacuolated, or oncocytic cytoplasm. Necrosis is absent, cytologic atypia is usually minimal, and mitotic figures are few in number. Histochemical staining with periodic acid-Schiff method (with and without diastase treatment) highlights the zymogen granules within tumor cell cytoplasm.[8]

Immunohistochemical profile

Like their salivary gland counterpart, tumor cells are immunoreactive for broad-spectrum keratins and epithelial membrane antigen, but do not express vimentin. Lysosomal proteins, α_1-antitrypsin and amylase, are occasionally identified.[8]

Clinical outcome

Acinic cell tumors are successfully treated with surgical excision.[8,10] Rare case reports documenting recurrence[11] or lymph node metastasis[10] serve as warnings that long-term patient surveillance is necessary.

Oncocytoma (Oxyphilic Adenoma)

Only a handful of pure pulmonary oncocytomas have been reported in the literature. As oncocytic metaplasia is a quite common phenomenon in the lung with an increasing age,[12] it is not surprising that lung tumors exhibiting oncocytic change exist. Indeed, oncocytic metaplasia is most commonly reported in carcinoid tumor, but myoepithelial tumors, mucoepidermoid carcinoma, mucous gland adenomas, and acinic cell tumors also have the potential for oncocytic change and must be excluded before the diagnosis of oncocytoma is rendered. Additionally, oncocytic carcinomas metastatic from other sites require exclusion.

Clinical features

Oncocytoma is a tumor that occurs primarily in adults and predilects to male smokers.[13] The process typically presents as a solitary lesion within the bronchus[13] but multiple pulmonary lesions has been described.[14]

Imaging

Imaging shows a nondescript, well-delineated solid mass.

Gross features

Tumors range from 1.0 to 3.5 cm in diameter.[13]

Gross examination reveals a well-circumscribed lesion with a solid, characteristically "mahogany-brown" cut surface which may show cystic change.

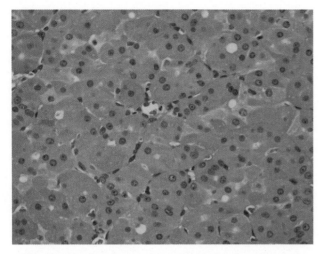

FIGURE 9-3 Oncocytoma: The lesion is composed of large polygonal cells with abundant, coarsely granular, eosinophilic cytoplasm and centrally placed, rounded nuclei with inconspicuous nucleoli.

Histologic features

Like oncocytomas of the kidney and salivary gland, the tumor is composed of large polygonal cells with abundant, coarsely granular, eosinophilic cytoplasm and a centrally placed, rounded nuclei with inconspicuous nucleoli (*Figure 9-3*). The tumor cells are usually arranged in sheets, but other architectural patterns including nested, acinar, cystic, or papillary-cystic growth may be observed. Importantly, the tumor should lack goblet and intermediate cells characteristic of mucoepidermoid carcinoma, cystic glandular structures with mucinous differentiation indicative of a mucous gland adenoma, histochemical evidence for acinic cell differentiation (periodic acid-Schiff-positive zymogen granules), and immunohistochemical expression of neuroendocrine markers.

Immunohistochemical profile

The cells express keratin and epithelial membrane antigen. Immunohistochemistry is important in excluding other primary and metastatic tumors exhibiting oncocytic change.

Clinical outcome

Pure oncocytomas are benign tumors cured by surgical excision.

Myoepithelioma

Myoepithelioma of the lung is an extremely rare form of monomorphic adenoma. As pleomorphic adenoma and epithelial-myoepithelial carcinoma may have a predominant myoepithelial component, both require exclusion before issuing a diagnosis of myoepithelioma. *EWSR1* translocations detected in visceral and soft tissue myoepithelial tumors have been identified in a primary pulmonary myoepithelial tumor as well.[15]

Clinical features

Benign myoepithelioma has been reported to arise in the endobronchus or peripheral lung in patients ranging in age from 18 to 77 years. One report details a case of a proximal endotracheal myoepithelioma.[16] Most patients present with respiratory symptoms related to bronchial obstruction.

Imaging

Imaging visualizes a nondescript, solid, well-delineated nodule. Cystic change was identified with magnetic resonance imaging in one case.[17] Positron emission tomography showed no increased uptake in the few patients.[18]

Gross features

Tumors range in size from 1.7 to 3.3 cm.[19] Grossly, myoepitheliomas are firm and well circumscribed with a gray-white and nodular cut surface. Cystic degeneration and hemorrhage infrequently occurs.

Histologic features

Microscopically, the neoplastic myoepithelial cell exhibits a broad morphological range including spindled, epithelioid (with eosinophilic or clear cytoplasm), and plasmacytoid morphotypes (*Figure 9-4*). These cell types are often mixed in any given lesion. Epithelioid myoepithelial cells are arranged in nodules and cord-like trabeculae, but no epithelial structures are allowed. The spindled myoepithelial cells assume a whorled or

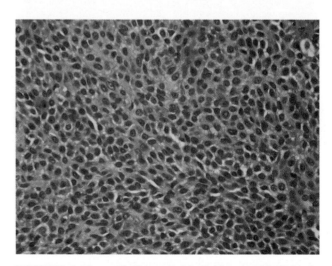

FIGURE 9-4 Myoepithelioma: Epithelioid myoepithelial cells are arranged in sheets without any epithelial structures.

fascicular growth pattern, sometimes with neural-like palisades. Focal myxochondroid stromal matrix is often identified. In contrast to malignant myoepitheliomas described in soft tissue, benign myoepitheliomas lack macronucleoli, nuclear hyperchromasia, and tumoral necrosis, and exhibit low mitotic activity.[20]

Immunohistochemical profile

Immunohistochemically, myoepitheliomas express muscle actins, S-100 protein, and less often keratin. Glial fibrillary acidic protein was found in one case of pulmonary myoepithelioma.[18]

Clinical outcome

Complete surgical excision is curative for benign myoepithelioma. Rare examples of pulmonary myoepithelioma exhibiting aggressive pathological features have resulted in distant metastasis and patient death.[21,22]

Mucus Gland Adenoma

Mucus gland adenoma morphologically and immunohistochemically recapitulates native bronchial glands and is found principally in bronchi with rare intrapulmonary examples documented without a bronchial association[23] and in the trachea.[24]

Clinical features

These tumors occur in adults with a peak incidence in the sixth decade of life and have no gender preference.[25] Most patients present with symptoms related to bronchial obstruction including cough, wheezing, hemoptysis, and obstructive pneumonia.[25]

Imaging

Plain radiograph and computerized tomography visualize a well-delineated nodule. An air meniscus sign on computerized tomography indicates the endobronchial location for the lesion (*Figure 9-5A*).[26]

Gross features

Mucinous gland adenomas range in size from less than 1 cm to approximately 7 cm in greatest dimension.[25] Grossly, they appear as well-defined, intraluminal bronchial masses having a firm consistency. The cut surface is shiny and gelatinous with mucous-filled cysts frequently observed.[25]

Histologic features

Microscopically, this lesion is an encapsulated, well-circumscribed aggregation of macro- and microcystic glands or papillary-cystic structures lined by cytologically bland flat, cuboidal, or columnar-shaped cells with abundant mucinous cytoplasm (*Figure 9-5B*). Clear or oncocytic cells are also identified in some examples (*Figure 9-5 C and D*). The process protrudes into the bronchial lumen but its bronchial wall component is delineated by bronchial cartilage. Fibrous septa possessing a variably cellular population of cytologically bland spindle cells emanate from the pseudocapsule and traverse the process.[25] A lymphoplasmacytic infiltrate is frequently present.[25]

Immunohistochemical profile

The tumor cells express keratins, including high-molecular-weight keratin, epithelial membrane antigen, and CEA, but not TTF-1.[25,27] Spindle cells within the stroma demonstrate a myoepithelial phenotype with keratin, muscle actin(s), and S-100 protein expression.[25]

Clinical outcome

Mucinous adenomas are cured by conservative surgical excision including "sleeve" resection of the bronchus.

Pneumocytic Adenomyoepithelioma

The pneumocytic adenomyoepithelioma is a recently described neoplasm exhibiting epithelial and myoepithelial differentiation and considered a subtype of salivary gland–type tumor of the lung.[28] Ultrastructural analysis confirms that type II pneumocytes and spindled myoepithelial cells are the two main cellular constituents of this neoplasm.[28]

Clinical features

The tumor presents primarily in women in the sixth and seventh decades of life[29] as solitary or less often multiple lesions.

Gross features

The tumor ranges in size from less than 1 to 2.6 cm in diameter. Lesions are solitary or multiple, well-circumscribed nodules with a solid, whorled, tan-white cut surface.[28]

Histological features

The tumor is well circumscribed but nonencapsulated. The epithelial component constitutes the bulk of the tumor and consists of mildly atypical cuboidal to low columnar cells and underlying basal cells. The epithelial component is arranged in tubular/glandular structures, and less frequently in nodular and trabecular arrays. Colloid-like material fills many of the glandular

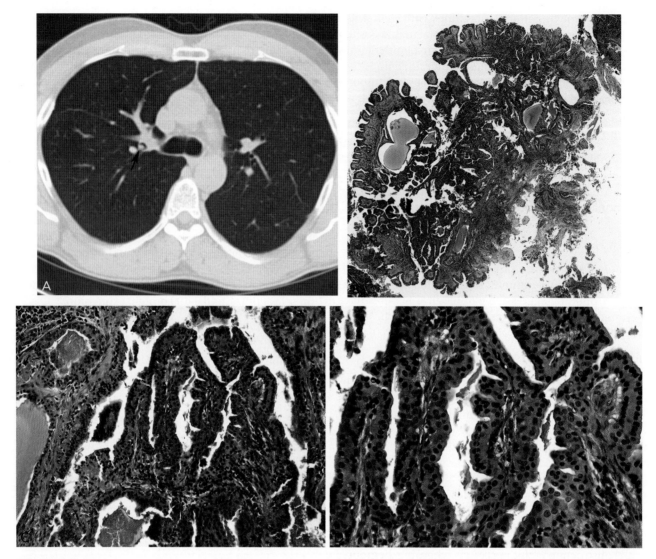

FIGURE 9-5 Mucous gland adenoma: A. CT scan demonstrating an endobronchial lesion. B. Lesion composed of glands, papillary-cystic structures lined by cytologically bland, flat, cuboidal cells. C, D. mucous gland adenoma: lesion with focal oncocytic morphology.

lumens (*Figure 9-6*). Intimately admixed with the glandular element, are bland spindle cells with eosinophilic cytoplasm arrayed in loose fascicles.

Immunohistochemical profile

Epithelial cells demonstrate type II pneumocyte differentiation by expressing keratins CAM5.2 and keratin 7, epithelial membrane antigen, CEA, surfactant apoprotein, and TTF-1. The underlying basal cells and the spindled element express myoepithelial markers, smooth muscle actin, high-molecular-weight keratin, S-100 protein, calponin, and p63.[28,29]

Clinical outcome

Short-term follow-up after surgical excision in a handful of cases revealed no recurrence of the tumor.[28]

HAMARTOMA

As classically defined, hamartomas are benign tumors composed of various mesenchymal elements appropriate to the organ, but which grow in a disorganized fashion. Accordingly, hamartoma is differentiated from monomorphic mesenchymal tumors such as leiomyoma, lipoma, and chondroma, by the presence of two or more different mesenchymal tissues in the former entity. In the past, the heterogeneous composition of pulmonary hamartoma, which characteristically includes cartilage, smooth muscle, fibromyxoid tissue, bone, and fat, resulted in a plethora of terms used to describe this process. Recent studies have demonstrated recombination of chromosomes 6p21 and 14q24 in examples of conventional pulmonary chondroid hamartoma supporting the notion that these are

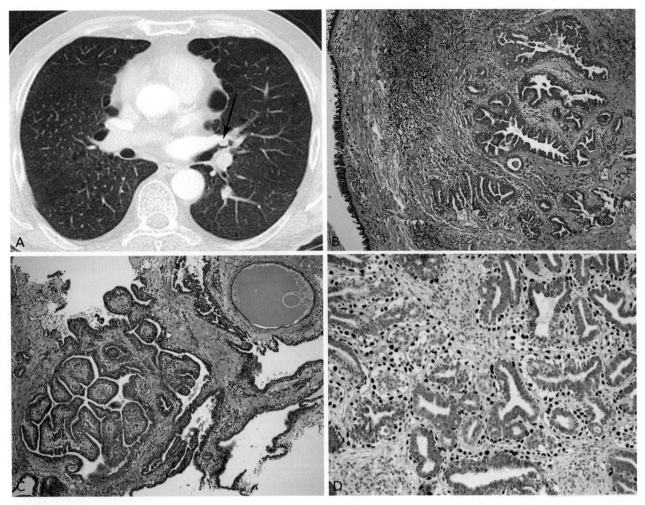

FIGURE 9-6 Adenomyoepithelioma: A. CT scan of lung with a well-defined endobronchial lesion. B, C. H&E section of the submucosal lesion with glandular structures and colloid-like material in a subtype of benign salivary gland tumor. D. P63 immunostain highlighting the basal cells.

neoplastic processes.[30] This section will focus on the most common manifestation of hamartomatous growth in the lung, the chondromatous hamartoma.

Clinical Features

Pulmonary hamartoma is the most common benign tumor of the lung representing 77% of all benign lung tumors in one study.[31] The tumor presents in adult patients with a peak incidence in the sixth and seventh decades of life and shows a strong male predominance.[32] Hamartomas are usually solitary with multiple lesions less commonly reported.[32] Peripherally located tumors account for approximately 90% of pulmonary hamartomas, are usually asymptomatic, and detected radiologically in over 60% of patients.[32] On the other hand, large endobronchial lesions may cause symptoms related to bronchial obstruction. In addition, synchronous primary or secondary lung neoplasms have

been reported in close to 30% of patients with pulmonary hamartoma.[32]

Imaging

Radiographically, pulmonary hamartoma appears as a well-circumscribed or lobulated nodule (*Figure 9-7*). Cartilage matrix calcifications, including "popcorn" calcifications, are identified in approximately 17% of cases.[32,33] Evidence of intralesional fat by computerized tomography also assists in the radiologic diagnosis.[34]

Gross Features

Pulmonary hamartomas usually range in size from millimeters to 6 cm in diameter.[32] Centrally located lesions are frequently intraluminal polypoid masses covered by intact bronchial mucosa. Macroscopically, hamartomas are well-circumscribed, unencapsulated,

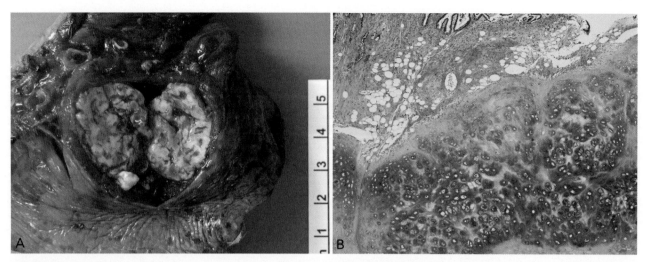

FIGURE 9-7 Hamartoma: A. Lung with a well-circumscribed, unencapsulated, lobulated mass with a firm to hard consistency and cut surface reflecting the presence of mature cartilaginous tissue. B. Cut section with mature cartilage, adipose tissue, and respiratory-type mucosa.

lobulated masses with a firm to hard consistency and a glistening cut surface reflecting the presence of mature cartilaginous tissue (*Figure 9-7*).

Histologic Features

In one large study, 71% of pulmonary hamartomas consist of ill-defined lobules of mature hyaline cartilage (predominant element in over 50% of cases) surrounded by fibromyxoid stroma (fibrochondromatous hamartoma).[32] Mature adipose tissue and loosely arranged fascicles of smooth muscle are additional elements commonly encountered.[32] The cartilaginous component can demonstrate matrix calcification and focal maturation to benign bone (enchondral ossification). Respiratory-type mucosa forms branching cleft-like spaces around islands of lesional tissue and has a propensity for undergoing metaplasia, or hyperplastic or papillary growth (*Figure 9-7*). Compared with peripheral lesions, endobronchial tumors tend to possess more of a fatty component (endobronchial lipomatous hamartoma) (*Figure 9-8A–D*).[35]

Immunohistochemical Profile

Immunohistochemistry is not useful in the diagnosis of this entity.

Clinical Outcome

Outcome is excellent with simple excision including wedge and "sleeve" resections. Large and symptomatic endobronchial lesions sometimes require lobectomy for cure.

SCLEROSING HEMANGIOMA (PNEUMOCYTOMA)

The term *sclerosing hemangioma* was used by Liebow and Hubbell because of the lesion's vague resemblance to cutaneous dermatofibroma (then also termed *sclerosing hemangioma*), and not as an acknowledgment to an alleged endothelial derivation.[36] Early studies claimed an endothelial, mesothelial, mesenchymal, or epithelial origin of the tumor, but subsequent, more sophisticated ultrastructural and immunohistochemical analyses finally demonstrated that the key lesional element of this enigmatic tumor showed varying degrees of epithelial (type II pneumocyte) differentiation.[37-39]

Clinical Features

Sclerosing hemangioma (pneumocytoma) is a tumor of the adult population with a peak incidence in the fifth decade of life and a strong female predominance.[39,40] Pneumocytoma typically presents as a solitary lesion located in the periphery of the lung and occasionally under the pleura. In approximately 4% of cases, the lesions are multiple.[39,40] Most tumors are asymptomatic and detected incidentally, but symptoms of cough, hemoptysis, or vague chest pain are reported in between 10% and 20% of cases.[39,40]

Imaging

Plain radiograph usually detects a well-delineated, round to oval mass that occasionally shows calcification. Computerized tomography visualizes a solid,

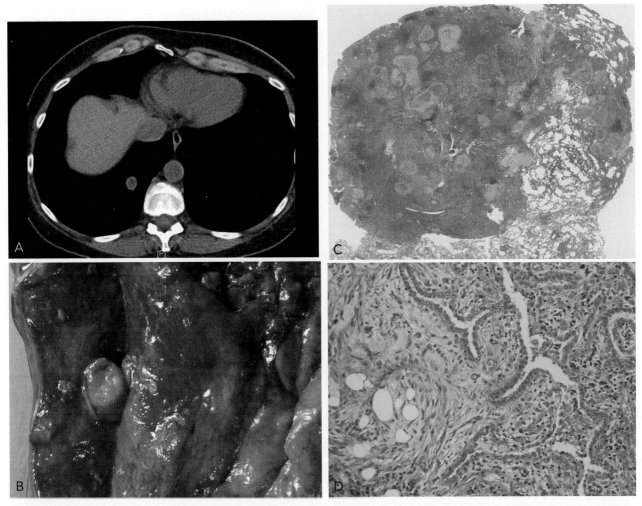

FIGURE 9-8 Hamartoma: A. CT scan with a well-defined parenchymal synchronous nodule from a patient with squamous cell carcinoma. **B.** Lung with a soft tan well-defined nodule, cut surface reflecting the presence of other noncartilaginous tissue. **C.** Low magnification of the H&E section with cartilaginous islands and predominant non cartilaginous tissue. **D.** Medium magnification of the mass with mature adipose tissue, spindle cells, and entrapped hyperplastic alveolar type epithelium.

homogenous high-density mass with low density foci representing cysts.

Gross Features

The lesion ranges in size from 0.4 to 8.0 cm with a mean size of about 3 cm. in maximum dimension.[39,40] Macroscopically, the peripheral pneumocytoma is usually a well-circumscribed, unencapsulated nodule (*Figure 9-9*), while the less often encountered pleural-based lesion is polypoid. The tumor has a firm to rubbery consistency with a tan-gray to yellow cut surface that exhibits foci of dark red hemorrhage. Cystic change is infrequently observed.

Histologic Features

The process is characterized by multiple architectural patterns with the vast majority of lesions (85%)

demonstrating an admixture of hypocellular fibrosclerotic (scar-like) areas, foci exhibiting papillary growth, solid cellular aggregates, and hemorrhagic ectatic spaces (*Figure 9-9*). Papillary, fibrosclerotic, and solid areas constituted the most frequently observed combination of architectural patterns (40% of tumors) in one large study.[39] Cytologically, pneumocytomas are composed of two cell types—mature surface respiratory epithelial cells and "round" cells. The surface cells that line luminal spaces are reminiscent of type II pneumocytes or Clara cells having a cuboidal or hobnail configuration with well-defined cytoplasmic borders and intranuclear cytoplasmic inclusions. The less mature "round" cells populate the core of papillary structures and comprise solid areas of the tumor. This component consists of ovoid to cuboidal cells with ill-defined cytoplasmic borders and lightly eosinophilic, vacuolated cytoplasm. Occasionally, "signet-ring"-like cytoplasmic inclusions of surfactant are identified within the

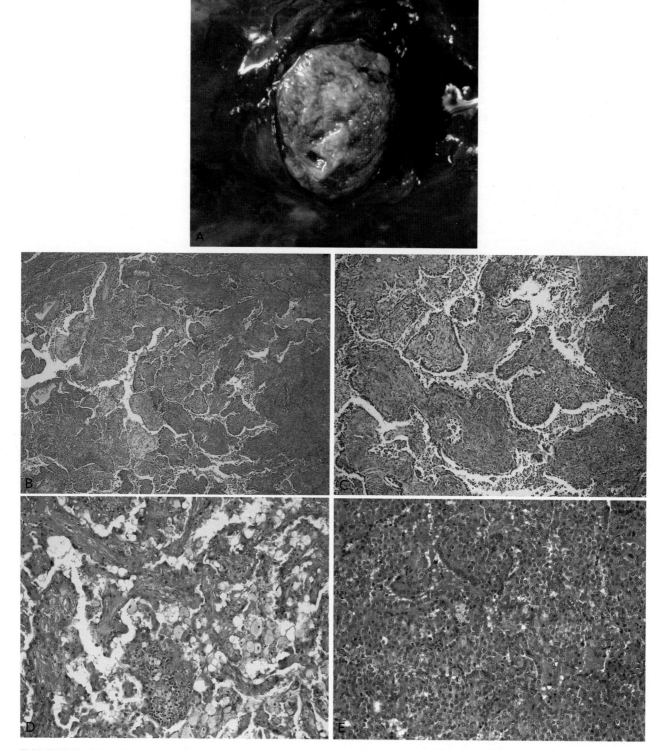

FIGURE 9-9 Sclerosing hemangioma: A. Lung with a well-defined fleshy tan mass. B-E. H&E sections with low to medium magnifications showing sclerotic papillary architecture, foamy macrophages, and solid with hemorrhagic areas.

"round" cell component. Hemosiderin deposition, cholesterol deposits, foci of dystrophic calcification, small areas of necrosis, and chronic inflammatory cell infiltrates are additional histological features identified within the lesion.[40]

Immunohistochemical Profile

The more mature appearing surface cells express keratins, TTF-1, epithelial membrane antigen, surfactant apoprotein, CEA, and neuroendocrine markers, neuron-specific enolase, synaptophysin, and chromogranin. The less mature, "round" cell element usually only shows epithelial membrane antigen and TTF-1 expression.[39]

Clinical Outcome

Prognosis for pneumocytoma is excellent after complete excision.[39,40] Metastatic spread of tumor to the subcapsular area of locoregional lymph nodes has been documented in the literature, but this event does not appear to result in an adverse outcome.[41]

LIPOMA

Lipoma of the lung is a rare lesion that can only be separated from the more common hamartoma by the absence of other mesenchymal elements after thorough pathologic examination.

Clinical Features

Lipomas arise primarily in the bronchus (*Figure 9-10*) as a submucosal, "dumbbell-shaped" or polypoid mass and less often in the peripheral lung.[42,43] The tumor presents in adults with a peak incidence in the fifth to seventh decades of life and shows a strong male bias and predilection to heavy smokers.[42-44] Patients with endobronchial tumors present with cough, shortness of breath, hemoptysis, or secondary pneumonia due to obstruction.[42,43]

Imaging

Computerized tomography is a sensitive technique for detecting a lipoma because the lesion characteristically has a density approximating that of pleural fat.[35]

Gross Features

Lipomas range in size from 1 to 7 cm[43] and consist of yellow to tan-yellow lobules of fat. A circumferential fibrous pseudocapsule, internal fibrous septation, or small foci of intralesional fibrosis may be observed.

Histologic Features

Lipomas consist of irregularly shaped lobules of mature adipocytes harboring small nuclei placated against the cell membrane. Foci of benign spindle cell growth reminiscent of spindle cell lipoma have been described.[43] Presence of osteocartilaginous metaplasia within the lipoma requires separation from cartilaginous elements of hamartoma.[44] Delicate fibrovascular stroma partitioning lobules of tumor and presence of atypical

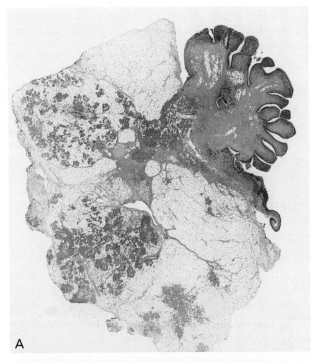

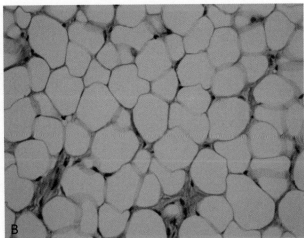

FIGURE 9-10 Lipomatous hamartoma: A. Endobronchial tumors tend to possess more of a fatty component (endobronchial lipomatous hamartoma). The overlying surface epithelium has pseudopapillomatous transformation with squamous metaplasia. **B.** High magnification of the lipomatous areas with benign appearing adipocytes consistent with lipoma/lipomatous hamartoma.

hyperchromatic cells and floret-like giant cells, which are hallmark features of atypical lipomatous tumor, have been reported in conventional endobronchial lipomas.[44]

Immunohistochemical and Molecular Profile

Immunohistochemistry is not useful in the diagnosis of this entity. One study failed to identify amplification of 12q13-15 region as in atypical lipomatous tumor, but did find *HMGA1* and *HMGA2* rearrangements like conventional lipoma.[44]

Clinical Outcome

Prognosis is excellent after complete surgical excision. Some bronchial-based lesions are curable with bronchoscopic resection including laser techniques and/or electrosurgical polypectomy.[42]

BENIGN VASCULAR TUMORS OF THE LUNG

Hemangioma and lymphangioma are rare, benign vascular tumors that clinically and radiologically have the potential to mimic other cystic, infectious, or neoplastic processes in the lung. Lymphangiomatosis, on the other hand, is a benign, but clinically aggressive intrapulmonary process with a poor prognosis.

Hemangioma

Clinical features

Intrapulmonary capillary and cavernous hemangiomas are extremely rare lesions that occur in patients of all ages, including children, and have no gender bias.[45,46] Hemangiomas are usually solitary lesions but can be multiple in some cases. The process shows no predilection for any particular area of the lower respiratory tract.[47] Most patients are asymptomatic, but symptoms including hemoptysis and cyanosis have been described.[46,47] Between 20% and 35% of patients with Rendu-Osler-Weber syndrome (hereditary telangiectasis) develop pulmonary arteriovenous malformations.[48]

Imaging features

Hemangiomas present as discrete, variably dense, and sometimes cystic masses (*Figure 9-11*). Calcifications within the mass indicate presence of phleboliths (calcifying thrombi within veins). Solitary capillary

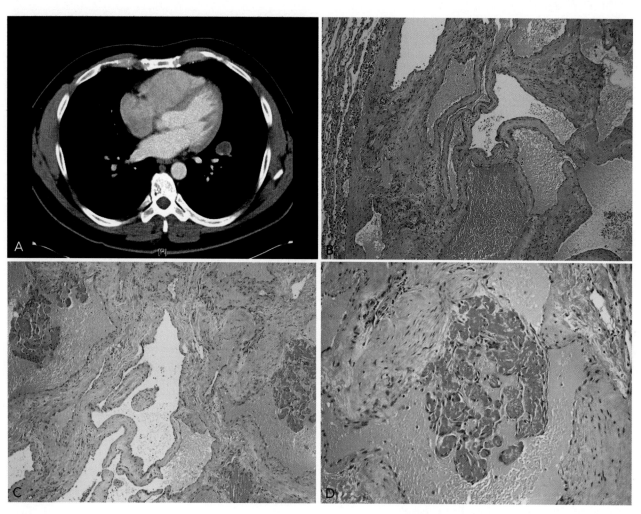

FIGURE 9-11 Hemangioma A: CT scan with a well-defined nodule. B: Low magnification of lung parenchyma with ectatic vascular spaces. C, D: Ectatic vascular spaces lined by bland endothelial cells and associated organizing thrombi.

hemangioma occasionally presents as "ground glass" opacities on computerized tomography.[45]

Gross features

Hemangiomas are hemorrhagic masses that frequently have a cystic or spongy cut surface with spaces filled with blood and thrombus.

Histologic features

Hemangiomas consist of a well-circumscribed, lobulated proliferation of capillary-sized (capillary hemangioma) or ectatic (cavernous hemangioma) vascular spaces lined by bland endothelial cells. Organizing thrombi (*Figure 9-11*) and phleboliths are oftentimes observed in cavernous hemangiomas. Both subtypes are typically solitary lesions, but multiple capillary hemangiomas, distinct from pulmonary capillary hemangiomatosis associated with veno-oclusive disease and pulmonary hypertension, have been reported in the pediatric population.[49]

Immunohistochemistry

Lesional cells of hemangiomas express endothelial-related markers, CD31, CD34, factor VIII–related antigen, Fli-1, and ERG.

Clinical outcome

Solitary hemangiomas are treated surgically. Embolization or α-interferon administration are modalities reserved for multifocal lesions that carry the potential for significant loss of pulmonary function and a poor outcome.[49]

Lymphangioma/Lymphangiomatosis

This category of vascular tumors includes circumscribed (lymphangioma) or diffuse (lymphangiomatosis) processes characterized by an increased number of benign, varying sized lymphatic channels. This contrasts lymphangiectasia in which native lymphatic vessels are dilated, but not increased in number. These disorders of lymphatic vessels are believed to result from congenital errors of lymphatic channel development.[50] This section will focus on lymphangioma and lymphangiomatosis.

Clinical features

Intrapulmonary lymphangioma presents in children and adults (peak incidence in the fourth decade of life) and shows no gender bias.[51] Intrapulmonary lymphangiomas are typically sporadic, but the process is associated with Klippel-Trenaunay-Weber and Maffucci

syndrome.[47] Lymphangiomatosis is a diffuse proliferation of benign lymphatic channels associated with multiorgan involvement in 75% of cases.[50] However, the diffuse pulmonary variant only affects the lung, mediastinum, and pleura. This process usually presents in late childhood with no gender predilection and manifests dyspnea, hemoptysis, asthmatic symptomatology, or chylous effusions.[50]

Imaging features

Computerized tomography of lymphangioma demonstrates a well-delineated, hypodense, cystic lesion not unlike other pulmonary cystic processes.[47] In lymphangiomatosis, imaging with computerized tomography reveals thickened interlobular septa, major fissures, airways, and pleura. Magnetic resonance imaging assists in determining the number of lesions and extent of the process within lung parenchyma.[50]

Gross features

Lymphangioma is an ill-defined mass composed of small, large, and cavernous spaces filled with serous or serosanguineous fluid.

Histologic features

Lymphangiomas consist of irregularly contoured spaces containing serous fluid and lined by attenuated, cytologically bland endothelial cell. The surrounding stroma oftentimes harbors bundles of smooth muscle and lymphoid aggregates or follicles. The numerous lymphatic channels in lymphangiomatosis course along the path of the preexisting lymphatic vessels in the lung.[52] A variably cellular proliferation of bland spindle cells accompanies the lymphatic proliferation in this disorder.

Immunohistochemistry

Along with consistent expression of CD31 and variable expression of CD34 lymphatic endothelial cells frequently express more specific lymphatic markers, D2-40 and PROX1.[53] The interstitial spindle cells in lymphangiomatosis are highlighted with desmin, muscle actins, and progesterone receptor protein[52] and do not express Melan-A or HMB-45 (like lymphangioleiomyomatosis).

Clinical outcome

Whereas some hemangiomas regress spontaneously, lymphangiomas require surgical excision as they have a tendency for recurrence if not completely removed. Sclerotherapy can be used alone or along with surgery for lymphangiomas and has shown good results.[54] The clinical course of lymphangiomatosis is characterized by relentless growth. Therapy revolves around decreasing symptoms related to the compressive effects of the lesions and includes drainage of chylous collections and sclerotherapy.[50]

PULMONARY CHONDROMA

Pulmonary chondroma is a benign tumor composed entirely of hyaline cartilage and occurs almost exclusively in young women as part of a syndrome described by Carney et al,[55] which includes extra-adrenal paragangliomas and epithelioid gastrointestinal stromal tumors of the stomach (Carney triad).

Clinical Features

Chondromas associated with Carney triad are asymptomatic and generally detected as part of the evaluation for manifestations of the syndrome.[56] Multiple chondromas are slightly more common than solitary lesions in Carney triad.[57] Sporadic chondromas occur more often in older adult males as a single endobronchial lesion and cause respiratory symptoms due to bronchial obstruction.[57]

Imaging

Plain radiographs show a solid, lobulated, well-circumscribed lesion that has a slight predilection for the lower lobes. Computerized tomography is a sensitive method for detecting cartilage matrix (central "popcorn"-like or peripheral) calcifications within the mass. This radiologic finding is observed in approximately 40% of Carney triad patients and assists in differentiating chondroma from metastatic gastrointestinal stromal tumor.[57]

Gross Features

Chondromas are distinctly lobulated masses with a firm, gritty consistency. The cut surface has a glistening cartilaginous appearance with a gray-white color.

Microscopic Features

The tumor is separated from lung parenchyma by a fibrous pseudocapsule and is composed exclusively of a cartilaginous matrix (*Figure 9-12*). The cartilage may be mature hyaline type or variably myxoid. Tumors generally exhibit mild to moderate hypercellularity, but cytological atypia is minimal. Cartilage matrix calcification or foci showing maturation to bone was observed in 14% of cases in one comprehensive study.[57] According to Rodriguez et al, pulmonary chondromas differ from cartilaginous hamartomas by their higher incidence of

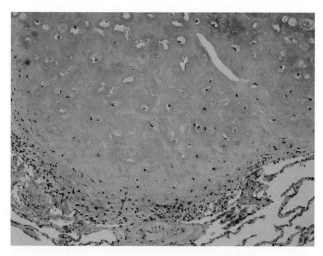

FIGURE 9-12 **Pulmonary chondroma: The tumor is composed exclusively of mature cartilaginous tissue.**

multiplicity, female predominance, and microscopic absence of respiratory epithelium surrounding islands of tumor and other mesenchymal elements.[57]

Clinical Outcome

Prognosis of chondroma is excellent after surgical excision. Patients with the Carney triad, whose prognosis is dependent on the clinical behavior of frequently coexisting paraganglioma and gastrointestinal stromal tumor,[56] have the potential to develop additional pulmonary chondromas.

LEIOMYOMA

Pulmonary leiomyomas arise from the muscular wall of the trachea, bronchus (*Figure 9-13*), or rarely from vascular structures within lung parenchyma.[58] Smooth muscle is frequently a component of pulmonary hamartoma, but the pulmonary leiomyoma should not possess additional mesenchymal elements after thorough pathological evaluation. As smooth muscle proliferations of the uterus, both benign ("benign metastasizing leiomyoma" and intravenous leiomyomatosis) and malignant (leiomyosarcoma), have the potential to metastasize to the lung, examination of the uterus and/or reviewing the patient's medical history for prior hysterectomy for uterine leiomyomas are recommended before rendering a diagnosis of primary pulmonary leiomyoma.

Clinical Features

Leiomyoma of the lung occurs in adults and has a peak incidence in the fourth and fifth decades of life. Tracheal lesions involve a slightly older population than

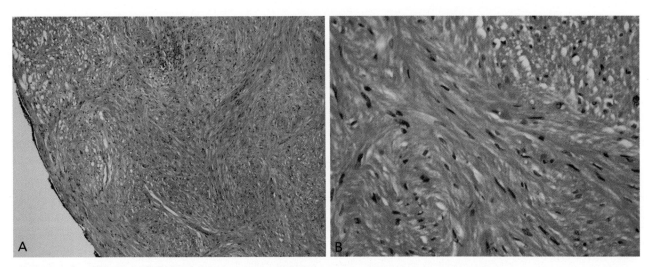

FIGURE 9-13 Pulmonary leiomyoma: A. Low magnification of benign spindle cell lesion beneath the flattened respiratory epithelium. **B.** Medium magnification of the tumor with fascicles of spindle cells consistent with smooth muscle origin.

intrapulmonary.[59] Tumors within lung parenchyma show a female bias whereas males more often develop tracheal leiomyomas.[59] Parenchymal lesions are usually asymptomatic and detected radiologically.

Imaging Features

Imaging detects a nondescript, well-delineated, oval, or round solid lesion.

Gross Features

Like the more commonly encountered leiomyoma in other locations, pulmonary leiomyoma is a well-circumscribed, firm lesion with a whorled and/or trabeculated cut surface.

Histologic Features

Leiomyomas are composed of elongated, intersecting fascicles of cytologically bland spindle cells with well-defined cell borders and eosinophilic, vaguely fibrillated cytoplasm. Presence of tumoral necrosis and conspicuous mitotic activity should raise the possibility of a primary or metastatic leiomyosarcoma. *Benign metastasizing leiomyoma* is a smooth muscle tumor arising from the myometrium of the uterus that "metastasizes" hematogenously to the lung (*Figure 9-14*). Features favoring this diagnosis are multiple lung tumors, the presence of the tumor within a vessel, entrapped respiratory mucosa within the mass, histological features compatible with uterine leiomyoma including stromal fibrosis, and a micro- or macrotrabecular growth

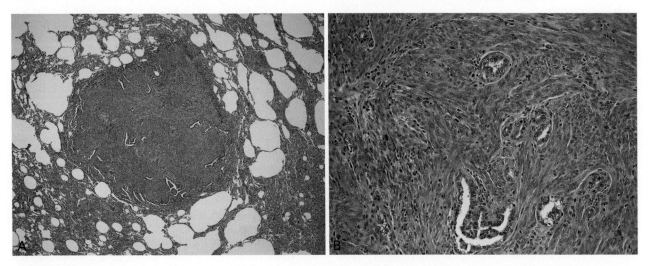

FIGURE 9-14 Benign metastasizing leiomyoma: A. Well-defined parenchymal spindle cell nodule with entrapped alveolar epithelium. **B.** Medium magnification demonstrating spindle cells consistent with smooth muscle and entrapped alveolar epithelium.

pattern of cells. Also, the smooth muscle cells of both uterine leiomyoma and intravenous leiomyomatosis immunohistochemically express Müllerian-related markers, estrogen receptor and progesterone receptor proteins, and/or Wilms tumor antigen-1 (WT-1).[60,61]

Immunohistochemical Profile

Leiomyomas demonstrate strong expression of myogenic markers, smooth muscle actin, muscle specific actin, calponin, caldesmon, and more variably, desmin. At least two immunomarkers are typically expressed in a bona fide smooth muscle tumor.

Clinical Outcome

Prognosis is excellent after complete surgical excision.

PULMONARY ADENOMA

In contrast to tracheobronchial-based salivary gland–type adenomas, alveolar and papillary adenomas are almost exclusively located in the peripheral lung. While some investigators consider these mature respiratory epithelial cell proliferations examples of monomorphic sclerosing hemangioma,[62] others categorize them as separate entities. The squamous, glandular, and mixed squamous cells and glandular adenomas are bronchial-based papillary lesions. Within this latter subset of adenomas, tumors with a squamous component possess a risk for malignant transformation.

Alveolar Adenoma

Benign proliferation of respiratory epithelial cells that ultrastructurally exhibit features of type II pneumocytes.[63]

Clinical features

These extremely rare tumors arise in the periphery of the lung of adults (peak incidence in the sixth decade of life) and show a female.[63-65] The lesion is typically asymptomatic and detected incidentally on imaging.

Imaging

Plain radiographs reveal a single, nondescript, well-delineated, noncalcified nodule in the periphery of the lung.

Gross features

The tumors are small with a mean size between 1.8 and 2.2 cm.[63-65] Alveolar adenomas are soft, lobulated lesions with a gray-white and oftentimes cystic cut surface.

Histologic features

Microscopically, alveolar adenomas are circumscribed but not encapsulated nodules. The lesions are composed of variably sized cysts containing eosinophilic material and lined by cytologically bland flattened, cuboidal, and hobnail cells. The stroma between the cysts is populated by a variably cellular proliferation of bland spindle cells and contains a modest chronic inflammatory component.

Immunohistochemical profile

The epithelial tumor cells express markers of type II pneumocytes including broad-spectrum and low-molecular-weight keratins, epithelial membrane antigen, TTF-1, surfactant B and C, and CEA.[63,65] The fibroblast-like spindle cells within the stromal express vimentin and CD34.[65]

Clinical outcome

Prognosis after surgical excision is excellent for this benign tumor.[63,64]

Papillary (Type II Pneumocyte/ Clara Cell) Adenoma

A benign papillary epithelial proliferation composed of cells ultrastructurally exhibiting differentiation along type II pneumocyte, Clara cell, and ciliated bronchial cell.[13]

Clinical features

This rare papillary neoplasm occurs in patients of all ages (peak incidence in the third decade of life) and shows no gender bias.[66] Patients are asymptomatic and the lesion is detected incidentally on imaging.

Imaging

Plain radiograph detects a small, well-marginated, nondescript, opacity nodule located in the peripheral lung.

Gross features

Tumors range from 1 to 4 cm in dimension.[13] Grossly, the tumor is a well-circumscribed, unencapsulated nodule with a gray-white, somewhat granular, cut surface.

Microscopic features

The tumor is usually well circumscribed, but may demonstrate modest invasion into parenchyma, pleura, endobronchial lumen, and also may invade veins.[66] The lesion consists of variably inflamed fibrovascular cores lined by cytologically bland cuboidal to low columnar cells. Ciliated[67] and oncocytic cells[68] are also identified. The rounded nuclei of the lesional cells frequently possess intranuclear inclusions. Rare examples of the papillary adenoma with extensively sclerotic stroma show histological overlap with sclerosing hemangioma (pneumocytoma).[69]

Immunohistochemical profile

The lesional cells exhibit type II pneumocyte differentiation by their expression of broad-spectrum keratin, TTF-1, CEA, and surfactant apoproteins.

Clinical outcome

This benign entity is cured with complete surgical excision.[66]

SOLITARY SQUAMOUS, GLANDULAR, AND MIXED SQUAMOUS AND GLANDULAR PAPILLOMAS

Clinical Features

Solitary papillomas, like the lesions of multifocal respiratory papillomatosis, are located in the major bronchi and less often in the trachea. In contrast to multifocal respiratory papillomatosis that presents in the pediatric age group, solitary lesions occur mostly in adults (peak incidence in the sixth decade of life and arise predominantly in males.[70,71] Most patients present with obstructive symptoms including cough, dyspnea, hemoptysis, or pneumonia.[70,71] The majority of patients with papillomas having a squamous component report a smoking history.[70,71] Conventional solitary squamous papillomas and especially multifocal respiratory papillomas are associated with human papillomavirus (HPV) subtypes 6 and 11.[70,72] Squamous papillomas with dysplasia (and a potential for malignant transformation) commonly harbor high-risk HPV subtypes 16 and 18.[72]

Imaging

Computerized tomographic studies demonstrate a small, nondescript intraluminal protuberance or nodule.

Gross Features

Papillomas are endobronchial cauliflower-like exophytic lesions that range from less than 1 to 2.5 cm.[70] The surface of the proliferation is smooth or verruciform.

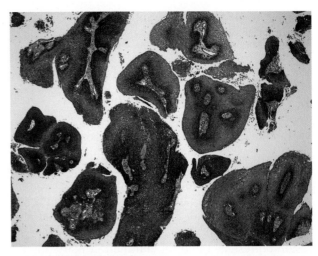

FIGURE 9-15 Multiple recurrent squamous papillomas in a young patient with laryngeal, upper and lower respiratory tract involvement.

Histologic Features

The squamous papilloma has a fibrovascular core covered by a keratinized stratified squamous epithelial lining (*Figure 9-15*). Rarely, the tumor will exhibit inverted growth with bulbous nests of squamous epithelium extend into the underlying stroma. In one large study, 14% of cases exhibited HPV viral cytopathic effect manifesting as squamous cells with irregularly contoured, hyperchromatic nuclei with perinuclear halos and binucleated cells, and 29% showed cytological dysplasia.[70] Glandular papillomas have arborizing fibrovascular stalks lined by cytologically bland columnar, cuboidal, and ciliated cells arranged in a flat or pseudostratified architecture. Mixed squamous and glandular papillomas are lined primarily by glandular mucosa (similar to that observed in pure glandular papillomas) but harbor scattered foci of keratinized squamous epithelium. The squamous component occasionally demonstrates varying degrees of dysplasia, but not HPV cytopathic effect.[70]

Immunohistochemical Profile

Immunohistochemistry is not valuable in the diagnosis of these lesions.

Clinical Outcome

Complete resection is curative for all three lesions. As studies claim that solitary papillomas with a squamous component can develop squamous cell carcinoma (and exhibit a 14% rate of malignant transformation),[71] patients who report tobacco use or have polyps showing the presence of squamous dysplasia[71] warrant close follow-up after surgical excision.

INFLAMMATORY MYOFIBROBLASTIC TUMOR

Within the spectrum of pulmonary fibroinflammatory tumefactions or inflammatory "pseudotumors," the inflammatory myofibroblastic tumor is a distinct clonal proliferation of myofibroblasts and fibroblasts accompanied by an inflammatory component. Inflammatory myofibroblastic tumor arises in a variety of anatomic sites with 25% to 40% occurring in the lung, where the lesion represents the most common primary pulmonary neoplasm in the pediatric population[73]). Over 30% of pulmonary inflammatory pseudotumors, most of which occur in children, demonstrate cytogenetic aberrations involving the *ALK* gene on 2p23 and/or overexpression of ALK protein, which indicates that a subset of these tumors are clonal neoplasms deserving of the name inflammatory myofibroblastic tumor.[74-76]

Clinical Features

Inflammatory myofibroblastic tumor of the lung occurs in patients of all ages, but mostly affects children and young adults, and shows an equal gender distribution. Patients are frequently asymptomatic with the remainder experiencing cough, dyspnea, hemoptysis, or chest pain.[77] Systemic signs and symptoms such as fever, leukocytosis, hyperglobulinemia, and anemia are reported in up to 30% of extrapulmonary cases[78,79] and result from interleukin secretion by the tumor.[80] A prior history of respiratory infection is documented in a significant minority of pediatric and adult patients with pulmonary tumors.

Imaging

Plain radiographs visualize a solitary, peripherally located, well-delineated mass in the majority of cases.[73] Multiple lesions are infrequently detected.[81] Computerized tomography reveals a well-delineated lobulated or spherical solid mass. Calcifications are commonly detected within the lesion.

Gross Features

Grossly, the inflammatory myofibroblastic tumor exhibits a broad size range, but most lesions measure between 1 and 6 cm in greatest dimension. The tumor is typically well demarcated from the surrounding parenchyma (*Figure 9-16*). The mass has a firm consistency and a yellow to tan, occasionally gritty cut surface. Focal calcification and hemorrhage may be present, but necrosis is exceptional.

Histologic Features

Histologically, the tumor is composed of spindled myofibroblasts with lightly eosinophilic, subtly fibrillar cytoplasm and a fusiform nucleus with a small but conspicuous nucleolus. Three growth patterns exist and oftentimes are mixed in any given lesion.[79] Short fascicular or whorled pattern of spindle cells with scanty collagenous or myxoid stroma is common in cellular areas of the tumor (compact spindle cell pattern), whereas an overly abundant myxoid stroma with granulation tissue–like vessels results in a more haphazard proliferation of cells reminiscent of nodular fasciitis (myxoid vascular pattern). Paucicellular areas with an abundance of collagen have a scar-like appearance (hypocellular fibrous pattern). Large, ganglion-like cells are typically identified within the lesion. The mitotic activity in most cases is low (<3 mitoses per 50 high-powered fields) with no atypical mitotic figures observed.[76] Lymphocytes, plasma cells, eosinophils, and neutrophils are found in varying proportions throughout the tumor, while xanthomatous histiocytes, multinucleated giant cells, and mast cells are less commonly identified. Foci of calcification or ossification are also observed in rare cases.

Immunohistochemical Profile

The spindle cells of inflammatory myofibroblastic tumor demonstrate smooth muscle or muscle-specific actin expression characteristically in a perimembranous or "tram-track" pattern, calponin, and focally, desmin.[79] Keratin expression is noted in one-third of cases.[79] Cytoplasmic ALK immunoexpression serves as a surrogate for *ALK* gene rearrangement (*Figure 9-16*) and was found in 46% of pulmonary cases in one study.[82] Two studies report immunohistochemical findings that correlate with an aggressive clinical course. In one study, all metastatic inflammatory myofibroblastic tumors (including three from the lung) lacked ALK immunoexpression[79] and in another report, expression of p53 was associated with recurrence and malignant transformation of the tumor.[83]

Clinical Outcome

Complete excision of the tumor is the mainstay of therapy. Difficulty in excising the tumor because of multifocality or location results in the potential for recurrence (approximately 25% of cases). Less than 5% of tumors

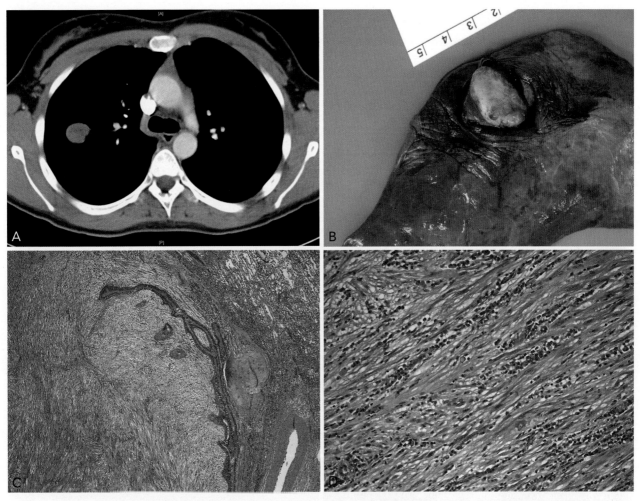

FIGURE 9-16 Inflammatory myofibroblastic tumor: A. CT scan of the chest with a solitary, peripherally located, well-delineated mass in the right lung. B. Well-defined tan to yellow nodule. C. Compact spindle cells in an abundant myxoid stroma. D. High magnification of the spindle cells associated with plasma cells and other inflammatory cells of varying proportion.

show documented extrapulmonary recurrence or metastasis[79,84]

INTRAPULMONARY SOLITARY FIBROUS TUMOR

Although first described as a pleural-based tumor, solitary fibrous tumor, initially classified as a localized subtype of fibrous mesothelioma, is a ubiquitous mesenchymal neoplasm. The inclusion of hemangiopericytoma and its variants into the solitary fibrous tumor category has no doubt resulted in a wider range of sites for this tumor. In the thorax, the vast majority of these tumors have a visceral pleural origin. Regarding intraparenchymal examples of solitary fibrous tumor, these lesions possibly arise from the subpleural mesenchyme in continuity with interlobular septa or from fibroblastic cells indigenous to the lung parenchyma.[85,86] The following discussion focuses on intraparenchymal tumors.

Clinical Features

Intrapulmonary solitary fibrous tumor (SFT) occurs principally in adults (peak incidence in the sixth decade)[87] with only rare case reports described in children.[88] The process has no gender bias.[87] Clinical signs and symptoms associated with intrapulmonary lesions have only been reported in few cases, and most were discovered incidentally on imaging.[85] Two rare phenomena associated with pleural-based solitary fibrous tumor include tumor-induced hypoglycemia due to secretion of insulin-like growth factor-II by tumor cells and pulmonary osteoarthropathy.[89]

Imaging

Computerized tomography visualizes a well-circumscribed, intraparenchymal mass.[87] Cystification, calcification, and foci of necrosis are infrequently identified.

Gross Features

Grossly, the tumors range in size from a few centimeters to over 20 cm with a mean size of about 8 cm.[87] The tumors are firm, well-circumscribed, lobulated, unencapsulated masses (*Figure 9-17*). By definition, no attachment to the visceral pleura is identified, although most lesions are peripherally located lesions.[87] Less than 5% of cases have multiple lesions in the same lobe.[87] Cut surface of the mass is tan to pale yellow in color, with foci of hemorrhage, cystification, and necrosis sometimes evident.

Histologic Features

Microscopically, the key mesenchymal element is a spindle cell with an oval, cytologically bland nucleus, and scanty, lightly eosinophilic cytoplasm. The spindle cells proliferate in a collagenous and less frequently, myxoid stroma, with ropy bands of eosinophilic collagen and pericellular collagen deposition common histologic findings (*Figure 9-17*). Spindle cells are arranged in herringbone or storiform arrays, around vessels (perivascular orientation), or in fascicles with nuclear palisading sometimes evident.[90] Areas of hypo- and hypercellularity within the lesion result in a multipatterned architecture. The characteristic of the process is the presence of irregularly contoured and branching, hemangiopericytoma-like vessels oftentimes with perivascular hyalinized collagen deposition. Cellular examples composed of fusiform cells with ill-defined cell borders and demonstrating a more haphazard ("patternless") growth pattern around "staghorn" vessels are reminiscent of classic hemangiopericytoma. A unique growth pattern observed in intrapulmonary solitary fibrous tumors is the presence of distorted runs of respiratory epithelium entrapped within the mass (*Figure 9-17*) imparting an adenofibromatous architecture to the process.[87]

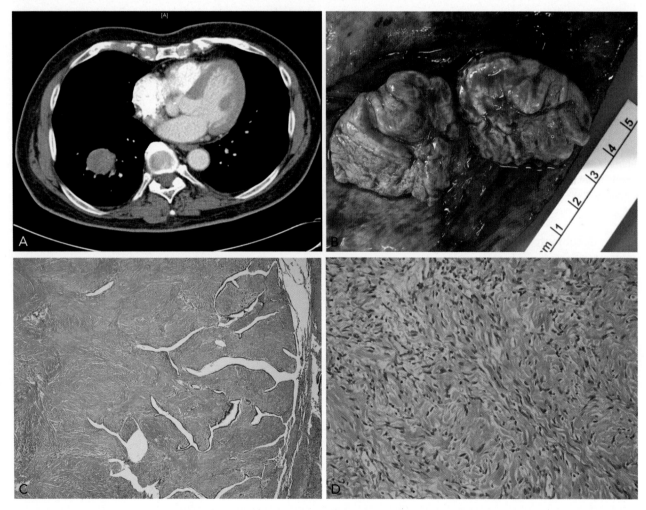

FIGURE 9-17 Intrapulmonary solitary fibrous tumor: **A.** CT scan of the chest with a solitary mass. **B.** Lobectomy with a lobulated tan, soft to firm mass. **C.** Spindle cells in a dense collagenous stroma and entrapped respiratory epithelium. **d.** The spindle cell proliferation in a collagenous and myxoid stroma, associated with ropy bands of eosinophilic collagen.

Immunohistochemical Profile

Tumor cells typically show strong and diffuse expression of CD34, bcl-2, and CD99; variable expression of epithelial membrane antigen, smooth muscle actin, and calponin; and focal expression of broad-spectrum keratin.[87] Tumors exhibiting high-grade malignant features typically show diminished expression of CD34.

Clinical Outcome

In one study, there was no statistical difference in survival between pleural and intraparenchymal lesions.[91] Tumors exhibiting increased cellularity, enlarged and hyperchromatic nuclei, mitotic activity of five or more mitoses per 10 high-powered fields, and tumoral necrosis have the potential for aggressive clinical behavior. Conversely, the presence of typical histologic features in a solitary fibrous tumor does not guarantee a favorable outcome.[87] Due to absence of reliable morphologic parameters for predicting clinical behavior of intrapulmonary as well as pleural-based solitary fibrous tumor, a complete surgical excision of the mass with long-term follow-up is recommended management for this tumor[87,92]

INTRATHORACIC FIBROMATOSIS (DESMOID-TYPE FIBROMATOSIS)

Clinical Features

The chest wall is the second most common location for deep fibromatosis (desmoid-type fibromatosis). At this site, the tumor originates from fascial or musculoaponeurotic tissue and grows into the overlying musculature of the chest wall. In contrast to the latter scenario, true intrathoracic desmoid tumors arising from the visceral pleura or lung parenchyma and extending into the pleura cavity without chest wall involvement are extremely rare lesions with only a handful of cases reported to date.[93-95] These tumors occur in middle-aged adults and show no gender bias. Lesions arise from the visceral pleura[93,96] or are associated with a bronchus.[95] A significant minority of patients report prior episodes of trauma prior to diagnosis.[93]

Imaging

Imaging visualizes a poorly defined, solid mass, which is indistinguishable from the solitary fibrous tumor.

Gross Features

Tumors reported in the literature range in size from 3.5 to 19 cm with a mean size of 9 cm.[93] The large size achieved by some examples of intrapulmonary

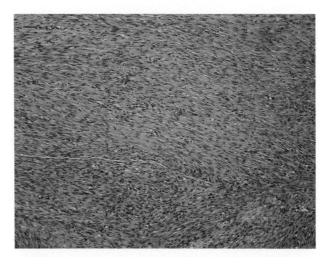

FIGURE 9-18 Desmoid tumor: Spindle cells distributed in fascicles and whorled arrays within a dense collagenous stroma, associated with a cytologically bland nucleus, small but conspicuous nucleolus, and scant eosinophilic cytoplasm.

desmoid-type fibromatosis is due to its covert intrathoracic location. Grossly, desmoids tumors are tan, firm, often polypoid masses arising from the visceral pleura and extending into the thoracic cavity. They have a pale, fibrous cut surface, and subtly infiltrative borders.

Histologic Features

Microscopically, intrathoracic desmoid–type fibromatosis, like their soft tissue counterparts, is composed of spindle cells with a cytologically bland nucleus possessing a small but conspicuous nucleolus and scant eosinophilic cytoplasm (*Figure 9-18*). The cells are evenly distributed in fascicles and whorled arrays within a dense, collagenous stroma. Small open and elongated, nonbranched vessels are uniformly distributed throughout the process.

Immunohistochemical Profile

Nuclear expression of β-catenin was observed in at least one-quarter of desmoid-type fibromatosis cells in over 70% of cases in one comprehensive study.[97] Cytoplasmic smooth muscle actin, oftentimes in a perimembranous ("tram-track") pattern, and calponin are muscle markers typically expressed by lesional cells.[98] The tumors also express cyclin D1 (downstream target of β-catenin), but are negative for CD34 (in contrast to solitary fibrous tumor).[95]

Clinical Outcome

Desmoid tumor is a benign entity usually treated with a complete surgical excision. However, adequate surgical excision does not guarantee a recurrence-free clinical course. One small study of intrathoracic desmoid tumors found recurrence in 25% of patients with negative surgical margins,[93] which is comparable to a 5-year recurrence rate of 29% reported for the more common chest wall tumorss.[99]

BENIGN PERIPHERAL NERVE SHEATH TUMORS

Benign intrathoracic neurogenic tumors are typically found in the posterior mediastinum (*Figure 9-19*). Primary neurogenic tumors of the lung are extremely rare lesions. In a 50-year survey of intrathoracic neurogenic tumors conducted in Japan, only 0.01% were intrapulmonary.[100] Neurogenic tumors are purported to arise from nerve segments located beneath bronchial mucosa. Clinically, benign peripheral nerve sheath tumors are usually asymptomatic, but endobronchial lesions may obstruct the bronchus causing cough, dyspnea, or obstructive pneumonia.

Neurofibroma

Clinical features

In general, this tumor occurs over a wide age range, but neurofibromas arising in the setting of neurofibromatosis type 1 affect a younger aged population.[101] The lesion shows a slight male predilection.

Imaging

Imaging reveals a well-delineated, nondescript nodule or fusiform mass within lung parenchyma.

Gross features

Grossly, neurofibromas are usually unencapsulated, but well-circumscribed, fusiform lesions. The process is associated with a bronchus and protrudes into the lumen. Plexiform neurofibromas are pathognomonic of neurofibromatosis type 1 and present as entangled masses of enlarged nerve bundles. Neurofibromas have a rubbery consistency and a glistening, myxoid cut surface.

Microscopic features

Microscopically, neurofibromas are expanded nerve segments containing elongated spindle cells with wavy, dark-stained nuclei attached to ropy strands of collagen within a myxocollagenous stroma. Mast cells are commonly found in the stroma. In contrast to malignant peripheral nerve sheath tumors, the cells of neurofibroma are spaced apart, small and uniform in size (although focal nuclear enlargement is allowed),

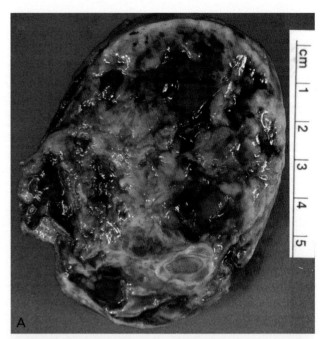

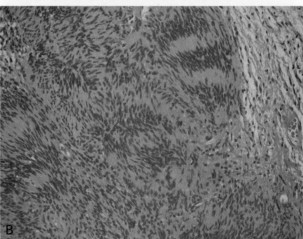

FIGURE 9-19 Schwannoma: A. Posterior mediastinal mass with well-circumscribed, encapsulated ovoid nodule, having a heterogenous cut surface with foci of hemorrhage and cystic degeneration. B. Characteristic hypercellular Antoni A areas with cells exhibiting nuclear palisading (Verocay bodies).

mitotically inactive, and not arranged in long fascicles (*Figure 9-20*).

Immunohistochemical profile

The immunohistochemical profile of neurofibroma is identical to extrapulmonary counterparts. Neurofibromas variably express S-100 protein (Schwann cells) and CD34 (endoneural fibroblasts). Residual axonal segments within the tumor express neurofilament protein. If encapsulated, spindled perineural cells within the fibrous sheath variably express epithelial membrane antigen.

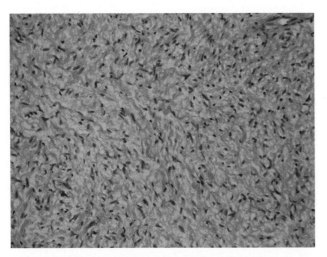

FIGURE 9-20 Neurofibroma: elongated spindle cells with wavy, dark-stained nuclei attached to ropy strands of collagen within a myxocollagenous stroma

Clinical outcome

Benign neurofibroma is treated with complete surgical excision.

Schwannoma

Clinical features

Intrapulmonary schwannomas are sporadic and solitary lesions that present at any age, but have a peak incidence in the fifth decade of life, and show a slight female predominance.[102] Nearly one-half of tumors are located near a bronchus while the other reported tumors were located in the peripheral lung and less often in the trachea.[102] Tumors located near proximal airways cause obstructive symptoms.[102]

Imaging

Imaging detects a nondescript well-delineated nodule usually associated with a bronchus or within the periphery of the lung.[102]

Gross feature

Schwannomas are well circumscribed, encapsulated round to ovoid nodules having a pale tan to white cut surface with foci of hemorrhage and cystic degeneration (*Figure 9-19*).

Microscopic features

Microscopically, schwannomas are composed spindled Schwann cells with serpentine-shaped, hyperchromatic nuclei having wavy and buckled contours and ill-defined, lightly eosinophilic cytoplasm. The cells are embedded in a fine, fibrillary collagenous stroma. Characteristic hypercellular Antoni A areas with cells exhibiting nuclear palisading (Verocay bodies) are found adjacent to hypocellular Antoni B areas with myxoid stroma, cyst formation, stromal hemorrhage, and calcification (*Figure 9-19*). Thick-walled vessels with hyalinized walls and fibrin deposition are scattered throughout the lesion, but more evident in Antoni B foci. Mitoses are absent or rare. Rare subtypes of schwannoma described in the lung include the cellular variant with fascicles of uniform spindled Schwann cells and absence of Verocay body formation,[103] and the melanotic psammomatous schwannoma, which is associated with Carney complex, has an uncertain malignant potential, and is histologically characterized by psammomatous calcifications and melanin deposition.[104]

Immunohistochemical profile

These lesions demonstrate an identical immunoprofile as extrapulmonary examples. Tumors show diffuse expression of S-100 protein. Collagen IV immunostaining is characteristically pericellular. Variable expression of glial fibrillary acidic protein and CD57 is evident. The fibrous capsule contains a variable number of thin spindled (perineural) fibroblasts that express epithelial membrane antigen.

Clinical outcome

Schwannomas are cured with complete surgical excision including bronchoscopic and laser resection.[102]

MENINGIOMA

Extracranial and extraspinal tumors with histological features identical to prototypic dural-based meningiomas are rare lesions that mostly occur in the head and neck region in association with peripheral nerves. Even more rare are meningiomas primary to the lung. Metastasis from a central nervous system meningioma requires exclusion as the lung is involved in about 60% of metastatic meningioma.[105] The cell of origin for primary pulmonary meningioma is presently undecided, but heterotopic arachnoid cell rests (minute meningothelial nodules) and pluripotential mesenchymal cells are the current two main contenders.[106] However, a recent molecular study showed that minute meningothelial nodules lack the high frequency loss of heterozygosity in chromosome 1p, 14q, and 22q that typify conventional meningioma[107] suggesting that these commonly encountered lesions are probably not the precursor of pulmonary meningioma.

Clinical Features

Primary pulmonary meningioma is a disease of the adult population (peak incidence in the sixth decade of life). The majority of patients are asymptomatic and the tumor is identified radiologically.[108] The lesion is almost always sporadic.

Imaging

Plain radiograph and computerized tomography demonstrate a nondescript, well-circumscribed nodule.[109] Increased metabolic activity by tumor on positron emission tomography has been reported in a case of a benign primary pulmonary meningioma.[110,111]

Gross Features

Grossly, pulmonary meningiomas are typically solitary lesions measuring less than 1 to 12 cm in diameter[108] and appear as well-circumscribed, unencapsulated nodules with a granular cut surface. The majority of meningiomas are located in the peripheral.[109]

Microscopic Features

Microscopically, most primary pulmonary meningiomas are of the transitional-type (*Figure 9-21*) and feature nests of cytologically bland spindled to ovoid cells arranged in a focally whorled pattern with variable number of psammomatous calcifications.[112] Cells have eosinophilic to amphophilic cytoplasm and a centrally placed oval nuclei with an occasional intranuclear inclusion. The fibrous meningioma is the second most common subtype reported and is composed of elongated spindle cells arranged in collagen-rich fascicles without a whorled configuration or presence of psammomatous calcifications.[112] The chordoid meningioma, characterized by cords and nests of spindled and epithelioid meningeal cells in a myxoid stroma associated with a lymphoplasmacytic inflammatory infiltrate, has been described in the literature[113]

Immunohistochemical Profile

Meningiomas diffusely express epithelial membrane antigen, vimentin, progesterone receptor, CD56 and variably express for S-100 protein.[112,114]

Clinical Outcome

Meningiomas with benign histological features and a peripheral location are cured with wedge resection. Lobectomy should be reserved for centrilobular lesions.[109]

PARAGANGLIOMA

Paragangliomas are tumors derived from paraganglion cells (*Figure 9-22*), which are modified neuroendocrine cells of neural crest origin that form aggregates, adjacent to the sympathetic chain (sympathetic chromaffin bodies) or along nerves and vessels in the head and neck region and thorax (parasympathetic nonchromaffin or glomus bodies). Unlike the sympathetic paragangliomas, the latter group including thoracic tumors usually does not cause systemic hypertension. Published epidemiologic data on primary pulmonary paraganglioma is difficult to verify because the term *chemodectoma* was used in the old literature for cases of paraganglioma, and histological overlap with the more common

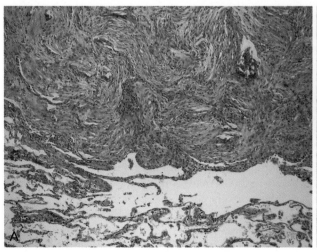
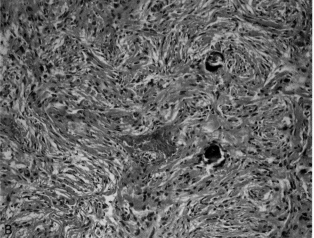

FIGURE 9-21 Meningioma: A. Well-delineated nodule from the adjacent lung parenchyma. B. Nests of cytologically bland spindled to ovoid cells with psammomatous calcifications.

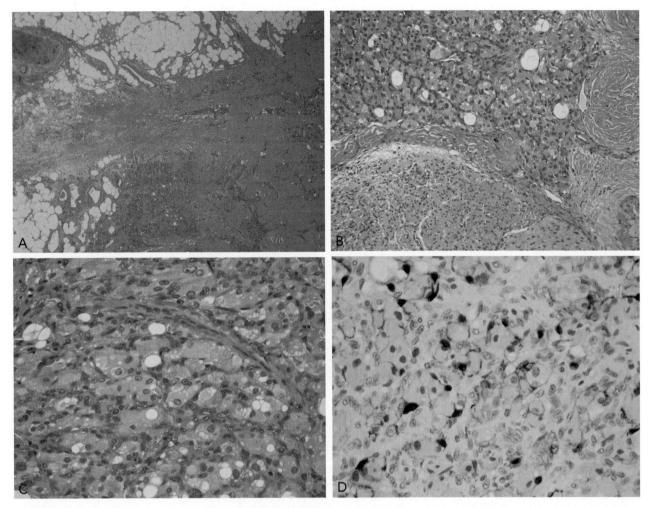

FIGURE 9-22 Paraganglioma: **A.** Low power of this mediastinal lesion with a densely sclerotic stroma. Bronchial cartilage seen in the upper left corner. **B, C.** Medium to high magnification of round to ovoid cells with lightly eosinophilic to clear cytoplasm arranged in solid, rounded aggregates which are surrounded by thin fibrovascular septa. Associated nerve bundles seen (B). **D.** S100 immunostain highlights the sustentacular cells.

neuroendocrine tumor, carcinoid, makes evaluation of many purported cases found in the literature difficult to accept as paraganglioma. Consequently, the diagnosis of paraganglioma should not be rendered unless keratin immunostaining excludes carcinoid (as well as gangliocytic paraganglioma), and no spindle cell component, or perivascular pseudorosette, trabecular, pseudoglandular, or linear (ribbon-like) cell arrangements are identified.

Clinical Features

Based on case reports in the English language literature, pulmonary paraganglioma mainly affects middle-aged adults with a strong predilection for females.[115] In nearly one-half of cases and particularly those with peripherally located lesions, the tumor was discovered incidentally. Chest pain, cough, dyspnea, or pneumonia are presenting symptoms in the remaining cases.[115]

Imaging

Imaging detects a nondescript, well-delineated solitary opaque mass located at the periphery of the lung. In one reported case, positron emission tomography showed increased uptake in the lesion.[115]

Gross Features

Tumors reported in the literature range in size from about 1 to 13 cm.[115] Oftentimes, the tumor is associated with a bronchus or pulmonary vessel.[115] Grossly, the mass is well circumscribed, unencapsulated with a pink-tan homogenous cut surface.

Microscopic Features

Paragangliomas are well-circumscribed nodules consisting of round to ovoid cells with lightly eosinophilic to clear cytoplasm arranged in solid, rounded aggregates ("zellballen" pattern) which are surrounded by thin fibrovascular septa. Cell nuclei are hyperchromatic with finely dispersed chromatin and occasionally have intranuclear inclusions. Degenerative nuclear atypia is sometimes observed. One histologic feature noted in paraganglioma is the presence of one cell partially enveloping another cell in a "ball-in-glove" configuration.

Immunohistochemical Profile

Tumor cells express chromogranin, synaptophysin, CD56, and neuron-specific enolase, but not keratin.[116] Spindled dendritic cells at the interface of the fibrovascular septa and tumor aggregates are usually imperceptible on light microscopic examination but are highlighted with S-100 protein.[116]

Clinical Outcome

The overwhelming majority of purported cases of paraganglioma are successfully treated with lobectomy, wedge resection, and even enucleation.

GLOMUS TUMOR

Glomus tumors are rare lesions that arise from the glomus body, a neuromuscular structure composed of modified smooth muscle cells that is normally found in the finger tips, palmar surface of the hand, and toes, and functions in heat regulation. Despite near absence of the glomus body in other regions of the body, glomus tumors have been found in viscera, central nervous system, bone, and mediastinum. This section concentrates on intrapulmonary and tracheal glomus tumors.

Clinical Features

Primary pulmonary glomus tumor occurs primarily in adults and has a peak incidence in the fifth and sixth decades of life. The process shows a strong male predominance. The tumor arises primarily in the lung parenchyma, less often in bronchial submucosa, and rarely in the trachea. Patients with peripheral lesions are usually asymptomatic, while individuals with bronchial-based tumors more often present with hemoptysis, cough, and infrequently, chest pain and dyspnea.[117]

Imaging

Imaging typically demonstrates a well-delineated, nondescript nodular lesion.

Gross Features

Glomus tumors range from less than 1 cm to almost 10 cm. with over one-half of reported cases measuring 3 cm or less in dimension.[117] Grossly, the intrapulmonary glomus tumor is a well-circumscribed, lobulated nodule with a gray-white to yellow-tan cut surface and foci of hemorrhage. Endotracheal lesions have a polypoid configuration.

Microscopic Features

The vast majority of cases reported in the literature are the conventional glomus tumor consisting of a sheet-like proliferation of cuboidal cells with eosinophilic to clear cytoplasm, distinct cell borders, and a rounded, centrally placed, cytologically bland nucleus (*Figure 9-23*). Reticulin and periodic acid-Schiff histochemical stains highlight basement membrane

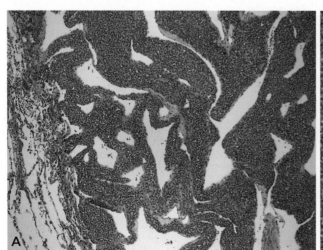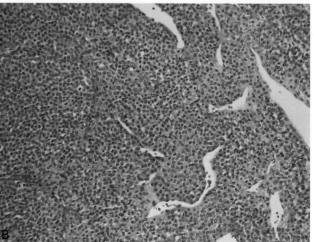

FIGURE 9-23 Glomus tumor: A, B. Low and medium magnification of a well-delineated nodule composed of sheet-like proliferation of cuboidal cells with eosinophilic to clear cytoplasm, distinct cell borders, and a rounded, centrally placed, cytologically bland nucleus.

material surrounding individual cells. The cellular nodules are intimately associated with rounded and irregularly contoured, hemangiopericytoma-like ("staghorn") vessels. Degenerative nuclear atypia and oncocytic change are uncommon histologic findings in glomus tumor. Glomangioma features ectatic vessels with a thin encircling cuff of glomus cells.[118-120] Glomus tumor with a component of spindled myoid cells is termed glomangiomyoma.[121]

Immunohistochemical Profile

Glomus cells express smooth muscle actin, vimentin, and collagen type IV (in a pericellular fashion). Variable expression of caldesmon and calponin is identified, but desmin is typically negative.[122]

Clinical Outcome

Glomus tumor, glomangioma, and glomangiomyoma are benign entities requiring complete surgical excision.

PERIVASCULAR EPITHELIAL CELL TUMORS (PEComas) OF THE LUNG

Perivascular epithelioid cell tumors, or PEComas, are uncommon spindled and epithelioid cell mesenchymal neoplasms found virtually in all body sites and characterized morphologically by a distinctive epithelioid cell (with no counterpart in normal tissue) having the potential for dual immunoexpression of myogenic (smooth muscle actin and calponin) and melanocytic (HMB-45 and Melan-A) proteins. The prototypic PEComa, the angiomyolipoma (AML) of the kidney, was first described and later associated with the tuberous sclerosis complex in the early 1900s.[123] In the 1970s, the clear cell "sugar" tumor (CCST) of the lung[124] and lymphangioleiomyomatosis (LAM)[125] were delineated as distinct but separate clinicopathologic entities. Pea et al in 1991[126] identified a peculiar HMB-45 immunoexpressing perivascular epithelioid cell that was found in both AML and CCST and, later, discovered in LAM.[126] This section focuses on the two main PEComas of the lung: lymphangiomyomatosis and clear cell "sugar" tumor.

Lymphangioleiomyomatosis

Lymphangioleiomyomatosis (LAM) is a rare condition that occurs almost exclusively in women of reproductive age[127] and typically affects the lungs and the axial thoracoabdominal lymphatic system. The process is sporadic in about 85% of cases, but in the remaining 15%, the condition is associated with the autosomal dominant tuberous sclerosis complex caused by *TSC-1* or *TSC-2* gene mutations. Approximately 2% to 3% of tuberous sclerosis patients develop this lesion[128,129] including males and children.[129] The mutations responsible for the syndrome result in loss of suppressor proteins, hamartin (encoded by the *TSC1* gene) and tuberin (encoded by *TSC2* gene), and tumor cell proliferation and growth through a downstream effector, mammalian target of rapamycin (*mTOR*).[130] One study found that sporadic LAM and coexisting renal AML both have a somatic *TSC2* gene mutations and suggested the possibility that pulmonary LAM may arise from migrating lesional cells from renal angiomyolipoma.[131]

Clinical features

Sporadic and tuberous sclerosis–associated LAM arises primarily in women between ages of 20 and 50 years.[13] LAM causes progressive destruction of the lung parenchyma by promoting the formation of cystically altered air spaces, resulting in dyspnea on exertion, hemothorax, chylous pleural effusions, and pneumothorax.[128] Extrapulmonary manifestations in both sporadic and syndromal LAM includes chylous ascites, resulting in abdominal distention and pain, lymphedema, and lymphadenopathy (due to thoracoabdominal lymph node involvement by LAM).

Imaging

The classic triad of radiographic findings for LAM includes a reticular interstitial pattern, chylous pleural effusion, and pneumothorax.[132] In advance disease, plain radiographs detect "honey-comb" change in the lung parenchyma with minimal fibrosis.[128] High-resolution computerized tomography scan shows multiple, bilateral, well-defined, thin-walled cysts (*Figure 9-24*) measuring between 0.2 and 6 cm.[128]

Gross features

Grossly, a variable number of thin-walled, well-defined cysts are present throughout all lung fields and may impart a "honey-comb" appearance to the lung in more advanced cases.

Histologic features

Microscopically, LAM demonstrates a nodular and plaque-like proliferation of plump spindled myoid cells with vaguely fibrillated and variably vacuolated eosinophilic cytoplasm and nuclei with focally irregular contours surrounding cystically dilated air spaces (*Figure 9-24*). A population of epithelioid appearing cells with clear to vacuolated cytoplasm is admixed with the spindled element. Hemosiderin and/or fresh blood is variably deposited in and around the lesional tissue.

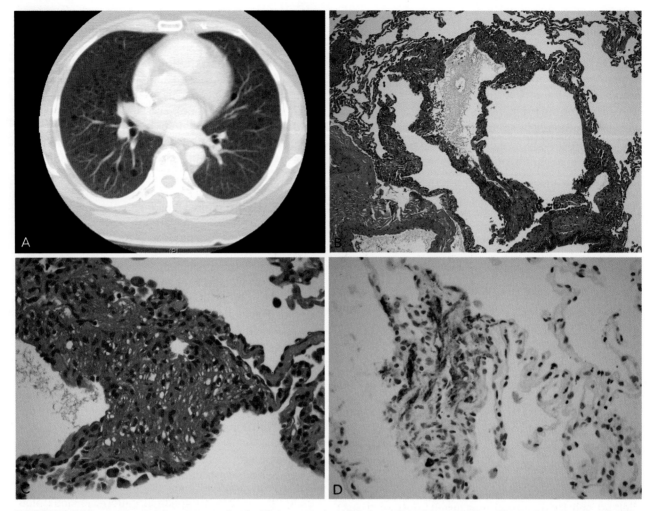

FIGURE 9-24 Lymphangioleiomyomatosis: A. High-resolution CT scan showing multiple, bilateral, well-defined, thin-walled cysts. B. Proliferation of plump spindled myoid cells surrounding cystically dilated air spaces. C. High magnification of spindle cells with a vaguely fibrillated and variably vacuolated eosinophilic cytoplasm and nuclei with focally irregular contours. D. HMB-45 immunoexpression of the spindle cells.

Immunohistochemical profile

Similar to other perivascular epithelioid cell tumors (PEComas), the key lesion cells coexpress smooth muscle markers, smooth muscle actin and calponin, and less often caldesmon and desmin, and melanocyte-related markers, Melan-A (MART-1), HMB-45, and microphthalmia transcription factor. Endocrine receptors such as ER and PR are frequently expressed in the lesion (*Figure 9-25*). Cathepsin-K is also typically expressed in cells of LAM.[133]

Clinical outcome

Prognosis of patients with LAM is variable with a 10-year survival between 70% and 80%.[134,135] Treatment for the condition is mainly supportive, but hormonal manipulation (eg, oophorectomy, progesterone or tamoxifen administration, or use of gonadotrophin-releasing hormone agonists) has been used with limited success.[136]

Promising results with mTOR inhibitors have been documented.[137] However, patients with advanced stage LAM and ensuing respiratory failure ultimately require lung transplant.[138]

Benign Clear Cell (Sugar) Tumor (Monotypic Angiomyolipoma)

Clinical features

This PEComa is an extremely rare lung tumor and is considered a monocellular or monotypic variant of AML.[139] The lesion has a wide age distribution, but commonly affects patients in the sixth decade of life, and shows a slight female bias. The tumors are usually small, solitary, peripheral nodules that are detected radiologically.[140] Rare cases of clear cell (sugar) tumor are associated with tuberous sclerosis complex and LAM of the lung.[141]

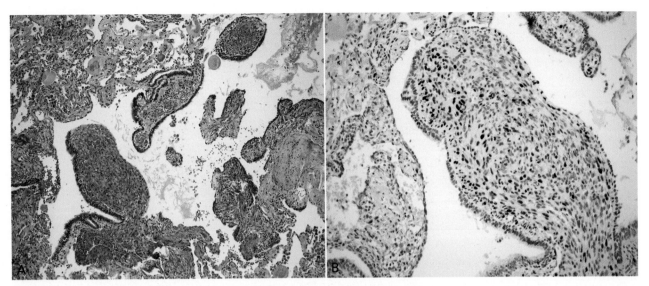

FIGURE 9-25 Lymphangioleiomyomatosis: **A.** H&E section of the patient with LAM showing proliferation of plump spindled myoid cells surrounding cystically dilated air spaces. **B.** Expression of ER within the lesional cells.

Imaging

On imaging, the tumor presents as a round, homogenous, well-circumscribed nodule. Due to the high vascularity of the lesion, the clear cell (sugar) tumor is frequently hyperintense on computerized tomography with contrast. Increased positron emission tomography uptake by a clear cell (sugar) tumor has been reported[142]

Gross features

Grossly, clear cell (sugar) tumor is generally small (median size of 2 cm), but the lesion ranges from millimeters to 6.5 cm.[140] The tumor is well circumscribed with a solid, pink to gray translucent, glistening cut surface.

Microscopic features

Microscopically, clear cell (sugar) tumor of the lung is composed of sheets of round to oval cells with lightly eosinophilic to clear (glycogen-rich) cytoplasm and well-defined cell borders. Nuclei are rounded with variably sized nucleoli and can demonstrate mild to moderate cytological atypia (*Figure 9-26*). Tumor cells occasionally demonstrate nuclear condensation of eosinophilic cytoplasm and arachnoidal extensions of cytoplasm to the cell membrane ("spider cells").[140] A prominent network of thin-walled, sinusoidal vessels characteristically surround nests of cells. One reported clear cell (sugar) tumor contained mature adipose tissue, thus showing histologic overlap with AML.[139] Periodic acid-Schiff histochemical staining typically demonstrates an abundance of intracytoplasmic glycogen.[140]

Immunohistochemical profile

Similar to other PEComas, tumor cells express smooth muscle markers, smooth muscle actin and calponin, and less often caldesmon and desmin, along with melanocyte-related markers, Melan-A (MART-1), HMB-45, and microphthalmia transcription factor .CD1a[143] and cathepsin-K[144] are both expressed in cells of clear cell (sugar) tumor of the lung.

Clinical outcome

Surgical resection is the mainstay of therapy for clear cell (sugar) tumor of the lung and is curative in all cases exhibiting benign histology.[1]

MULTIFOCAL MULTINODULAR PNEUMOCYTE HYPERPLASIA

Multifocal multinodular pneumocyte hyperplasia (MMPH) is a rare, but relatively unique respiratory epithelial cell proliferation associated with tuberous sclerosis complex[145] One study demonstrated loss of heterozygosity on genes TSC1 and TSC2 in cells of multifocal multinodular pneumocyte hyperplasia from patients with tuberous sclerosis complex.[146]

Clinical Features

Multifocal multinodular pneumocyte hyperplasia occurs primarily in women and has a peak incidence in the fourth decade of life.[147] Respiratory signs and symptoms in patients with multifocal multinodular pneumocyte hyperplasia are mostly related to the coexisting manifestations of tuberous sclerosis and/or LAM.

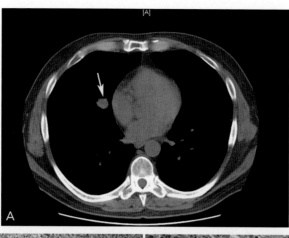

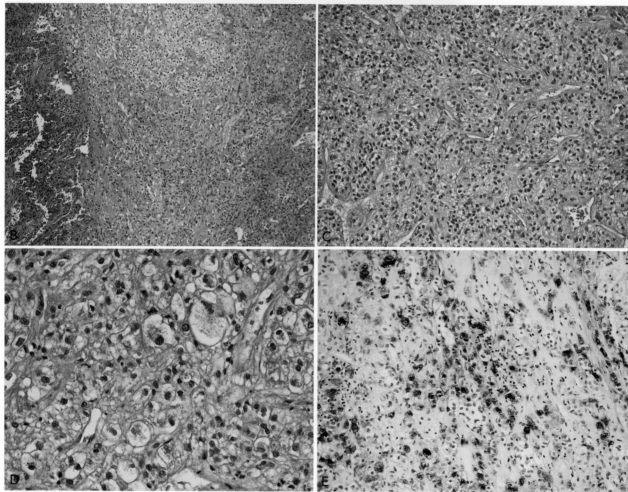

FIGURE 9-26 Clear cell tumor: A. CT scan of the chest with a solitary, peripherally located, well-delineated mass. B. Low power of lung with the unencapsulated sheets of neoplastic cells without necrosis. C. Sheets of round to oval cells with lightly eosinophilic to clear (glycogen-rich) cells, surrounded by a prominent network of thin-walled, sinusoidal vessels. D. High power demonstrates well-defined cell borders, eosinophilic to clear cytoplasm and linear extensions of cytoplasm from the nucleus to the cell membrane ("spider cells"). E. Melanocytic marker HMB-45 expression in some of the tumor cells.

Imaging

Plain radiograph and computerized tomography discloses a nondescript lower lobe or diffuse reticulonodular infiltrative pattern.[147]

Gross Features

Within the lung parenchyma are multiple sharply demarcated and randomly distributed nodules ranging in size from 1 to 3 mm in diameter.

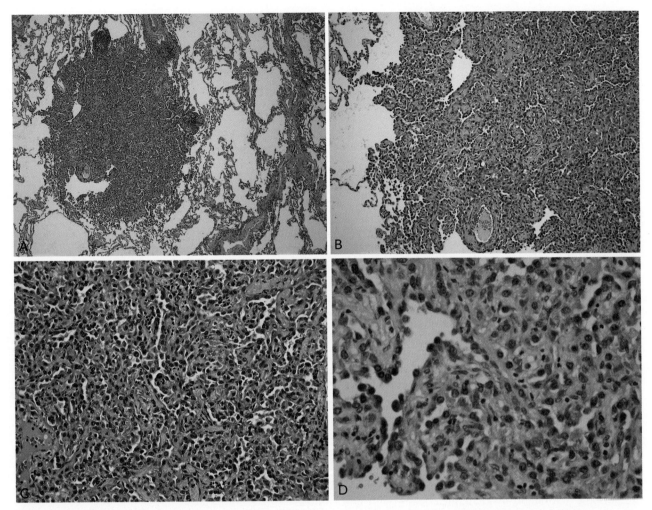

FIGURE 9-27 Micronodular pneumocyte hyperplasia: A. Low magnification of micronodule with 1-mm well-defined nodular aggregate of alveolar pneumocytes. B-D. Medium- to high-power magnification with cleft like space, prominent alveolar pneumocyte hyperplasia with occasional intranuclear inclusion.

Microscopic Features

The process begins as a modest proliferation of type II pneumocytes along alveolar septa and later forming cellular aggregates within the alveolar walls. Microscopically, the nodules are composed of plump type II pneumocytes with abundant eosinophilic cytoplasm and cytologically bland, vesicular nuclei harboring prominent nucleoli, and an occasional eosinophilic intranuclear cytoplasmic inclusion (*Figure 9-27*). Notably, the proliferation is well delineated from the surrounding lung tissue.

Immunohistochemical Profile

The cells exhibit an immunohistochemical profile of type II pneumocytes with broad-spectrum keratin, TTF-1, epithelial membrane antigen, and surfactant apoprotein B expression.

Clinical Outcome

Multifocal multinodular pneumocyte hyperplasia is considered a benign hamartomatous process. Prognosis of patients with the condition depends on the other manifestations of the tuberous sclerosis complex.

GRANULAR CELL TUMOR

Granular cell tumor is a benign and relatively rare mesenchymal neoplasm of purported Schwann cell derivation. The tumor affects superficial soft tissues, especially in the head and neck region, breast, tongue, and viscera. Approximately 6% to 10% of reported cases involve the lung.[148]

Clinical Features

Granular cell tumor primarily affects adults and has a peak incidence in the fourth and fifth decades of life.

The vast majority of intrapulmonary lesions are endobronchial, but the process also affects the trachea and rarely, peripheral lung.[148] Granular cell tumors are typically solitary lung lesions, but multiple tumors arise in approximately 25% of patients.[148]

Imaging

Plain radiographs typically disclose a well-delineated, nondescript nodular lesion. Larger tumors that cause bronchial obstruction are infiltrative processes that result in distal atelectasis and mimic lung carcinoma.

Gross Features

Granular cell tumors of the lung range in size from under 1 to 6.5 cm with a median size of about 1 cm.[148] Macroscopically, the process is usually well circumscribed, but occasionally ill defined, and has a tan-white to pink-yellow cut surface.[148] Endobronchial lesions oftentimes have a nodular or papillary configuration.

Microscopic Features

The tumor consists of epithelioid to spindled mesenchymal cells with abundant, coarsely granular, brightly eosinophilic cytoplasm and round to oval, cytologically bland nuclei possessing small nucleoli (*Figure 9-28*). Large cytoplasmic granules with surrounding haloes representing secondary lysosomes are characteristic. Periodic acid-Schiff histochemical stain (with and without diastase treatment) highlights innumerable granules within the cytoplasm. Mitotic activity is minimal. The cells infiltrate a fibrotic stroma in nests and as individual cells. Involvement of peripheral nerve twigs

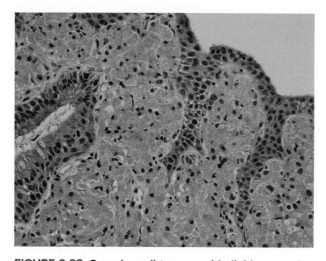

FIGURE 9-28 Granular cell tumor: epithelioid mesenchymal cells with abundant, coarsely granular, brightly eosinophilic cytoplasm and round to oval, cytologically bland nuclei. Overlying epithelium with squamous metaplasia.

is a common feature. Overlying bronchial mucosa occasionally undergoes squamous metaplasia, but pseudoepitheliomatous hyperplasia is typically not observed.[148]

Immunohistochemical Profile

Tumor cells show strong and diffuse expression of S-100 protein, α-inhibin, and calretinin.[148,149] As electron microscopy reveals an overabundance of cytoplasmic lysosomes, CD68 is also strongly expressed.[148,150]

Clinical Outcome

Granular cell tumor is typically benign and curable with surgical excision including bronchoscopic and "sleeve" resection, and laser therapy.[148]

REFERENCES

1. Travis WD, Brambilla E, Muller-Hermelink HK, et al. *Pathology and Genetics. Tumours of the Lung, Pleura, Thymus and Heart.* Lyon, France: IARC Press; 2004.
2. Moran CA, Suster S, Askin FB, Koss MN. Benign and malignant salivary gland-type mixed tumors of the lung. Clinicopathologic and immunohistochemical study of eight cases. *Cancer.* May 15, 1994;73(10):2481-2490.
3. Sakamoto H, Uda H, Tanaka T, Oda T, Morino H, Kikui M. Pleomorphic adenoma in the periphery of the lung. Report of a case and review of the literature. *Arch Pathol Lab Med.* April 1991;115(4):393-396.
4. Wenig BM, Hitchcock CL, Ellis GL, Gnepp DR. Metastasizing mixed tumor of salivary glands. A clinicopathologic and flow cytometric analysis. *Am J Surg Pathol.* September 1992;16(9):845-858.
5. Moran CA. Primary salivary gland-type tumors of the lung. *Semin Diagn Pathol.* May 1995;12(2):106-122.
6. Ang KL, Dhannapuneni VR, Morgan WE, Soomro IN. Primary pulmonary pleomorphic adenoma. An immunohistochemical study and review of the literature. *Arch Pathol Lab Med.* May 2003;127(5):621-622.
7. Fechner RE, Bentinck BR, Askew JB Jr. Acinic cell tumor of the lung. A histologic and ultrastructural study. *Cancer.* February 1972;29(2):501-508.
8. Moran CA, Suster S, Koss MN. Acinic cell carcinoma of the lung ("Fechner tumor"). A clinicopathologic, immunohistochemical, and ultrastructural study of five cases. *Am J Surg Pathol.* November 1992;16(11):1039-1050.
9. Sabaratnam RM, Anunathan R, Govender D. Acinic cell carcinoma: an unusual cause of bronchial obstruction in a child. *Pediatr Dev Pathol.* September-October 2004;7(5):521-526.
10. Ukoha OO, Quartararo P, Carter D, Kashgarian M, Ponn RB. Acinic cell carcinoma of the lung with metastasis to lymph nodes. *Chest.* February 1999;115(2):591-595.
11. Chuah KL, Yap WM, Tan HW, Koong HN. Recurrence of pulmonary acinic cell carcinoma. *Arch Pathol Lab Med.* July 2006;130(7):932-933.
12. Ritter JH, Nappi O. Oxyphilic proliferations of the respiratory tract and paranasal sinuses. *Semin Diagn Pathol.* May 1999;16(2):105-116.
13. Colby TV, Koss MN, Travis WD. *Tumors of the Lower Respiratory Tract.* Washington, DC: Armed Forces Institute of Pathology; 1995.

14. Laforga JB, Aranda FI. Multicentric oncocytoma of the lung diagnosed by fine-needle aspiration. *Diagn Cytopathol.* July 1999;21(1):51-54.

15. Antonescu CR, Zhang L, Chang NE, et al. EWSR1-POU5F1 fusion in soft tissue myoepithelial tumors. A molecular analysis of sixty-six cases, including soft tissue, bone, and visceral lesions, showing common involvement of the EWSR1 gene. *Genes Chromosomes Cancer.* December 2010;49(12):1114-1124.

16. Chand M, Mann JM, Sabayev V, et al. Endotracheal myoepithelioma. *Chest.* July 2011;140(1):242-244.

17. Cagirici U, Sayiner A, Inci I, Veral A. Myoepithelioma of the lung. *Eur J Cardiothorac Surg.* February 2000;17(2):187-189.

18. Veeramachaneni R, Gulick J, Halldorsson AO, Van TT, Zhang PL, Herrera GA. Benign myoepithelioma of the lung: a case report and review of the literature. *Arch Pathol Lab Med.* November 2001;125(11):1494-1496.

19. Kourda J, Ismail O, Smati BH, Ayadi A, Kilani T, El Mezni F. Benign myoepithelioma of the lung - a case report and review of the literature. *Cases Journal.* 2010;3(1):25.

20. Hornick JL, Fletcher CD. Myoepithelial tumors of soft tissue: a clinicopathologic and immunohistochemical study of 101 cases with evaluation of prognostic parameters. *Am J Surg Pathol.* September 2003;27(9):1183-1196.

21. Higashiyama M, Kodama K, Yokouchi H, et al. Myoepithelioma of the lung: report of two cases and review of the literature. *Lung Cancer.* April 1998;20(1):47-56.

22. Miura K, Harada H, Aiba S, Tsutsui Y. Myoepithelial carcinoma of the lung arising from bronchial submucosa. *Am J Surg Pathol.* September 2000;24(9):1300-1304.

23. Karpathiou G, Sivridis E, Mikroulis D, Froudarakis M, Giatromanolaki A. Pulmonary mucus gland adenomas: are they always of endobronchial localization? *Case Rep Pathol.* 2013;2013:239173.

24. Ferguson CJ, Cleeland JA. Mucous gland adenoma of the trachea: case report and literature review. *J Thorac Cardiovasc Surg.* February 1988;95(2):347-350.

25. England DM, Hochholzer L. Truly benign "bronchial adenoma". Report of 10 cases of mucous gland adenoma with immunohistochemical and ultrastructural findings. *Am J Surg Pathol.* August 1995;19(8):887-899.

26. Kwon JW, Goo JM, Seo JB, Seo JW, Im JG. Mucous gland adenoma of the bronchus: CT findings in two patients. *J Comput Assist Tomogr.* September-October 1999;23(5):758-760.

27. Couraud S, Isaac S, Guibert B, Souquet PJ. Bronchial mucous gland adenoma revealed following acute pneumonia. *Interact Cardiovasc Thorac Surg.* March 2012;14(3):347-349.

28. Chang T, Husain AN, Colby T, et al. Pneumocytic adenomyoepithelioma: a distinctive lung tumor with epithelial, myoepithelial, and pneumocytic differentiation. *Am J Surg Pathol.* April 2007;31(4):562-568.

29. Tsuji N, Tateishi R, Ishiguro S, Terao T, Higashiyama M. Adenomyoepithelioma of the lung. *Am J Surg Pathol.* August 1995;19(8):956-962.

30. Fletcher JA, Pinkus GS, Donovan K, et al. Clonal rearrangement of chromosome band 6p21 in the mesenchymal component of pulmonary chondroid hamartoma. *Cancer Res.* November 15 1992;52(22):6224-6228.

31. Arrigoni MG, Woolner LB, Bernatz PE, Miller WE, Fontana RS. Benign tumors of the lung. A ten-year surgical experience. *J Thorac Cardiovasc Surg.* October 1970;60(4):589-599.

32. Gjevre JA, Myers JL, Prakash UB. Pulmonary hamartomas. *Mayo Clin Proc.* January 1996;71(1):14-20.

33. Blair TC, McElvein RB. Hamartoma of the lung. A clinical study of 25 cases. *Dis Chest.* September 1963;44:296-302.

34. Siegelman SS, Khouri NF, Scott WW Jr, et al. Pulmonary hamartoma: CT findings. *Radiology.* August 1986;160(2):313-317.

35. Gaerte SC, Meyer CA, Winer-Muram HT, Tarver RD, Conces DJ Jr. Fat-containing lesions of the chest. *Radiographics.* October 2002;22 Spec No:S61-S78.

36. Liebow AA, Hubbell DS. Sclerosing hemangioma (histiocytoma, xanthoma) of the lung. *Cancer.* January-February 1956;9(1):53-75.

37. Yousem SA, Wick MR, Singh G, et al. So-called sclerosing hemangiomas of lung. An immunohistochemical study supporting a respiratory epithelial origin. *Am J Surg Pathol.* August 1988;12(8):582-590.

38. Satoh Y, Tsuchiya E, Weng SY, et al. Pulmonary sclerosing hemangioma of the lung. A type II pneumocytoma by immunohistochemical and immunoelectron microscopic studies. *Cancer.* September 15, 1989;64(6):1310-1317.

39. Devouassoux-Shisheboran M, Hayashi T, Linnoila RI, Koss MN, Travis WD. A clinicopathologic study of 100 cases of pulmonary sclerosing hemangioma with immunohistochemical studies: TTF-1 is expressed in both round and surface cells, suggesting an origin from primitive respiratory epithelium. *Am J Surg Pathol.* July 2000;24(7):906-916.

40. Katzenstein AL, Gmelich JT, Carrington CB. Sclerosing hemangioma of the lung: a clinicopathologic study of 51 cases. *Am J Surg Pathol.* August 1980;4(4):343-356.

41. Vaideeswar P. Sclerosing hemangioma with lymph nodal metastases. *Indian J Pathol Microbiol.* July-September 2009;52(3):392-394.

42. Muraoka M, Oka T, Akamine S, et al. Endobronchial lipoma: review of 64 cases reported in Japan. *Chest.* January 2003;123(1):293-296.

43. Moran CA, Suster S, Koss MN. Endobronchial lipomas: a clinicopathologic study of four cases. *Mod Pathol.* February 1994;7(2):212-214.

44. Boland JM, Fritchie KJ, Erickson-Johnson MR, Oliveira AM, Colby TV, Folpe AL. Endobronchial lipomatous tumors: clinicopathologic analysis of 12 cases with molecular cytogenetic evidence supporting classification as "lipoma". *Am J Surg Pathol.* November 2013;37(11):1715-1721.

45. Sakaguchi Y, Isowa N, Tokuyasu H, Miura H. A resected case of solitary pulmonary capillary hemangioma showing pure ground glass opacity. *Ann Thorac Cardiovasc Surg.* 2014;20 suppl:578-581.

46. Maeda R, Isowa N, Sumitomo S, Matsuoka K. Pulmonary cavernous hemangioma. *Gen Thorac Cardiovasc Surg.* April 2007;55(4):177-179.

47. Weissferdt A, Moran CA. Primary vascular tumors of the lungs: a review. *Ann Diagn Pathol.* August 2010;14(4):296-308.

48. Cottin V, Dupuis-Girod S, Lesca G, Cordier JF. Pulmonary vascular manifestations of hereditary hemorrhagic telangiectasia (rendu-osler disease). *Respiration.* 2007;74(4):361-378.

49. Abrahams NA, Colby TV, Pearl RH, Chipps BE, Juris AL, Leslie KO. Pulmonary hemangiomas of infancy and childhood: report of two cases and review of the literature. *Pediatr Dev.* May-June 2002;5(3):283-292.

50. Faul JL, Berry GJ, Colby TV, et al. Thoracic lymphangiomas, lymphangiectasis, lymphangiomatosis, and lymphatic dysplasia syndrome. *Am J Respir Crit Care.* March 2000;161(3 pt 1):1037-1046.

51. Limmer S, Krokowski M, Kujath P. Pulmonary lymphangioma. *Ann Thorac Surg.* January 2008;85(1):336-339.

52. Tazelaar HD, Kerr D, Yousem SA, Saldana MJ, Langston C, Colby TV. Diffuse pulmonary lymphangiomatosis. *Hum Pathol.* December 1993;24(12):1313-1322.

53. Miettinen M, Wang ZF. Prox1 transcription factor as a marker for vascular tumors-evaluation of 314 vascular endothelial and 1086 nonvascular tumors. *Am J Surg Pathol.* March 2012;36(3):351-359.

54. Sanlialp I, Karnak I, Tanyel FC, Senocak ME, Buyukpamukcu N. Sclerotherapy for lymphangioma in children. *Int J Pediatr Otorhinolaryngol.* July 2003;67(7):795-800.

55. Carney JA, Sheps SG, Go VL, Gordon H. The triad of gastric leiomyosarcoma, functioning extra-adrenal paraganglioma and pulmonary chondroma. *N Engl J Med.* June 30, 1977;296(26): 1517-1518.

56. Carney JA. The triad of gastric epithelioid leiomyosarcoma, pulmonary chondroma, and functioning extra-adrenal paraganglioma: a five-year review. *Medicine.* May 1983;62(3):159-169.

57. Rodriguez FJ, Aubry MC, Tazelaar HD, Slezak J, Carney JA. Pulmonary chondroma: a tumor associated with Carney triad and different from pulmonary hamartoma. *Am J Surg Pathol.* December 2007;31(12):1844-1853.

58. Terada T. Vascular leiomyoma of the lung arising from pulmonary artery. *Int J Clin Exp Pathol.* 2013;6(1):97-99.

59. White SH, Ibrahim NB, Forrester-Wood CP, Jeyasingham K. Leiomyomas of the lower respiratory tract. *Thorax.* April 1985;40(4):306-311.

60. Jautzke G, Muller-Ruchholtz E, Thalmann U. Immunohistological detection of estrogen and progesterone receptors in multiple and well differentiated leiomyomatous lung tumors in women with uterine leiomyomas (so-called benign metastasizing leiomyomas). A report on 5 cases. *Pathol Res Pract.* March 1996;192(3):215-223.

61. Kir G, Cetiner H, Gurbuz A, Eren S. Immunohistochemical profile of intravenous leiomyomatosis. *Eur J Gynaecol Oncol.* 2004;25(4):481-483.

62. Semeraro D, Gibbs AR. Pulmonary adenoma: a variant of sclerosing haemangioma of lung? *J Clin Pathol.* November 1989;42(11):1222-1223.

63. Burke LM, Rush WI, Khoor A, et al. Alveolar adenoma: a histochemical, immunohistochemical, and ultrastructural analysis of 17 cases. *Hum Pathol.* February 1999;30(2):158-167.

64. Yousem SA, Hochholzer L. Alveolar adenoma. *Hum Pathol.* October 1986;17(10):1066-1071.

65. Sak SD, Koseoglu RD, Demirag F, Akbulut H, Gungor A. Alveolar adenoma of the lung. Immunohistochemical and flow cytometric characteristics of two new cases and a review of the literature. *APMIS.* December 2007;115(12):1443-1449.

66. Kuwahara M, Nagafuchi M, Rikimaru T, Iwasaki A, Shirakusa T. Pulmonary papillary adenoma. *Gen Thorac Cardiovasc Surg.* October 2010;58(10):542-545.

67. Fukuda T, Ohnishi Y, Kanai I, et al. Papillary adenoma of the lung. Histological and ultrastructural findings in two cases. *Acta Pathol Jpn.* January 1992;42(1):56-61.

68. Fine G, Chang CH. Adenoma of type 2 pneumocytes with oncocytic features. *Arch Pathol Lab Med.* August 1991;115(8):797-801.

69. Allen TC, Amrikachi M, Cagle PT. Pulmonary sclerosing papillary adenoma. *Pathol Int.* July 2013;63(7):364-367.

70. Flieder DB, Koss MN, Nicholson A, Sesterhenn IA, Petras RE, Travis WD. Solitary pulmonary papillomas in adults: a clinicopathologic and in situ hybridization study of 14 cases combined with 27 cases in the literature. *Am J Surg Pathol.* November 1998;22(11):1328-1342.

71. Tryfon S, Dramba V, Zoglopitis F, et al. Solitary papillomas of the lower airways: epidemiological, clinical, and therapeutic data during a 22-year period and review of the literature. *J Thorac Oncol.* April 2012;7(4):643-648.

72. Popper HH, el-Shabrawi Y, Wockel W, et al. Prognostic importance of human papilloma virus typing in squamous cell papilloma of the bronchus: comparison of in situ hybridization and the polymerase chain reaction. *Hum Pathol.* November 1994;25(11):1191-1197.

73. Cerfolio RJ, Allen MS, Nascimento AG, et al. Inflammatory pseudotumors of the lung. *Ann Thorac Surg.* April 1999;67(4):933-936.

74. Snyder CS, Dell'Aquila M, Haghighi P, Baergen RN, Suh YK, Yi ES. Clonal changes in inflammatory pseudotumor of the lung: a case report. *Cancer.* November 1, 1995;76(9):1545-1549.

75. Yousem SA, Shaw H, Cieply K. Involvement of 2p23 in pulmonary inflammatory pseudotumors. *Hum Pathol.* April 2001;32(4): 428-433.

76. Borczuk AC. Benign tumors and tumorlike conditions of the lung. *Arch Pathol Lab Med.* July 2008;132(7):1133-1148.

77. Kobashi Y, Fukuda M, Nakata M, Irei T, Oka M. Inflammatory pseudotumor of the lung: clinicopathological analysis in seven adult patients. *Int J Clin Oncol.* December 2006;11(6):461-466.

78. Meis JM, Enzinger FM. Inflammatory fibrosarcoma of the mesentery and retroperitoneum. A tumor closely simulating inflammatory pseudotumor. *Am J Surg Pathol.* December 1991;15(12):1146-1156.

79. Coffin CM, Watterson J, Priest JR, Dehner LP. Extrapulmonary inflammatory myofibroblastic tumor (inflammatory pseudotumor). A clinicopathologic and immunohistochemical study of 84 cases. *Am J Surg Pathol.* August 1995;19(8):859-872.

80. Rohrlich P, Peuchmaur M, Cocci SN, et al. Interleukin-6 and interleukin-1 beta production in a pediatric plasma cell granuloma of the lung. *Am J Surg Pathol.* May 1995;19(5):590-595.

81. Pettinato G, Manivel JC, De Rosa N, Dehner LP. Inflammatory myofibroblastic tumor (plasma cell granuloma). Clinicopathologic study of 20 cases with immunohistochemical and ultrastructural observations. *Am J Clin Pathol.* November 1990;94(5):538-546.

82. Cook JR, Dehner LP, Collins MH, et al. Anaplastic lymphoma kinase (ALK) expression in the inflammatory myofibroblastic tumor: a comparative immunohistochemical study. *Am J Surg Pathol.* November 2001;25(11):1364-1371.

83. Hussong JW, Brown M, Perkins SL, Dehner LP, Coffin CM. Comparison of DNA ploidy, histologic, and immunohistochemical findings with clinical outcome in inflammatory myofibroblastic tumors. *Mod Pathol.* March 1999;12(3):279-286.

84. Coffin CM, Humphrey PA, Dehner LP. Extrapulmonary inflammatory myofibroblastic tumor: a clinical and pathological survey. *Semin Diagn Pathol.* May 1998;15(2):85-101.

85. Yousem SA, Flynn SD. Intrapulmonary localized fibrous tumor. Intraparenchymal so-called localized fibrous mesothelioma. *Am J Clin Pathol.* March 1988;89(3):365-369.

86. Aufiero TX, McGary SA, Campbell DB, Phillips PP. Intrapulmonary benign fibrous tumor of the pleura. *J Thorac Cardiovasc Surg.* August 1995;110(2):549-551.

87. Rao N, Colby TV, Falconieri G, Cohen H, Moran CA, Suster S. Intrapulmonary solitary fibrous tumors: clinicopathologic and immunohistochemical study of 24 cases. *Am J Surg Pathol.* February 2013;37(2):155-166.

88. Geramizadeh B, Banani A, Moradi A, Hosseini SM, Foroutan H. Intrapulmonary solitary fibrous tumor with bronchial involvement: a rare case report in a child. *J Pediatr Surg.* January 2010;45(1):249-251.

89. Briselli M, Mark EJ, Dickersin GR. Solitary fibrous tumors of the pleura: eight new cases and review of 360 cases in the literature. *Cancer.* June 1 1981;47(11):2678-2689.

90. Moran CA, Suster S, Koss MN. The spectrum of histologic growth patterns in benign and malignant fibrous tumors of the pleura. *Semin Diagn Pathol.* May 1992;9(2):169-180.

91. Schirosi L, Lantuejoul S, Cavazza A, et al. Pleuro-pulmonary solitary fibrous tumors: a clinicopathologic, immunohistochemical, and molecular study of 88 cases confirming the prognostic value of de Perrot staging system and p53 expression, and evaluating the role of c-kit, BRAF, PDGFRs (alpha/beta), c-met, and EGFR. *Am J Surg Pathol.* November 2008;32(11):1627-1642.

92. England DM, Hochholzer L, McCarthy MJ. Localized benign and malignant fibrous tumors of the pleura. A clinicopathologic review of 223 cases. *Am J Surg Pathol.* August 1989;13(8):640-658.

93. Meyerson SL, D'Amico TA. Intrathoracic desmoid tumor: brief report and review of literature. *J Thorac Oncol.* June 2008;3(6):656-659.

94. Wilson RW, Gallateau-Salle F, Moran CA. Desmoid tumors of the pleura: a clinicopathologic mimic of localized fibrous tumor. *Mod Pathol.* January 1999;12(1):9-14.

95. Andino L, Cagle PT, Murer B, et al. Pleuropulmonary desmoid tumors: immunohistochemical comparison with solitary fibrous tumors and assessment of beta-catenin and cyclin D1 expression. *Arch Pathol Lab Med.* October 2006;130(10):1503-1509.

96. Wilson RW, Moran CA. Epithelial-myoepithelial carcinoma of the lung: immunohistochemical and ultrastructural observations and review of the literature. *Hum Pathol.* May 1997;28(5):631-635.

97. Ng TL, Gown AM, Barry TS, et al. Nuclear beta-catenin in mesenchymal tumors. *Mod Pathol.* January 2005;18(1):68-74.

98. Perez-Montiel MD, Plaza JA, Dominguez-Malagon H, Suster S. Differential expression of smooth muscle myosin, smooth muscle actin, h-caldesmon, and calponin in the diagnosis of myofibroblastic and smooth muscle lesions of skin and soft tissue. *Am J Dermatopathol.* April 2006;28(2):105-111.

99. Brodsky JT, Gordon MS, Hajdu SI, Burt M. Desmoid tumors of the chest wall. A locally recurrent problem. *J Thorac Cardiovasc Surg.* October 1992;104(4):900-903.

100. Takeda S, Miyoshi S, Minami M, Matsuda H. Intrathoracic neurogenic tumors—50 years' experience in a Japanese institution. *Eur J Cardiothorac Surg.* October 2004;26(4):807-812.

101. Unger PD, Geller GA, Anderson PJ. Pulmonary lesions in a patient with neurofibromatosis. *Arch Pathol Lab Med.* August 1984;108(8):654-657.

102. Ohtsuka T, Nomori H, Naruke T, Orikasa H, Yamazaki K, Suemasu K. Intrapulmonary schwannoma. *Jpn J Thorac Cardiovasc Surg.* March 2005;53(3):154-156.

103. Domen H, Iwashiro N, Kimura N, et al. Intrapulmonary cellular schwannoma. *Ann Thorac Surg.* October 2010;90(4):1352-1355.

104. Lin YF, Hsi SC, Chang JL, Huang CH. Intrapulmonary psammomatous melanotic schwannoma. *J Thorac Cardiovasc Surg.* January 2009;137(1):e25-e27.

105. Karasick JL, Mullan SF. A survey of metastatic meningiomas. *J Neurosurg.* February 1974;40(2):206-212.

106. Marchevsky AM. Lung tumors derived from ectopic tissues. *Semin Diagn Pathol.* May 1995;12(2):172-184.

107. Ionescu DN, Sasatomi E, Aldeeb D, et al. Pulmonary meningothelial-like nodules: a genotypic comparison with meningiomas. *Am J Surg Pathol.* February 2004;28(2):207-214.

108. Cesario A, Galetta D, Margaritora S, Granone P. Unsuspected primary pulmonary meningioma. *Eur J Cardiothorac Surg.* March 2002;21(3):553-555.

109. Incarbone M, Ceresoli GL, Di Tommaso L, et al. Primary pulmonary meningioma: report of a case and review of the literature. *Lung Cancer.* December 2008;62(3):401-407.

110. Cura M, Smoak W, Dala R. Pulmonary meningioma: false-positive positron emission tomography for malignant pulmonary nodules. *Clin Nucl Med.* October 2002;27(10):701-704.

111. Meirelles GS, Ravizzini G, Moreira AL, Akhurst T. Primary pulmonary meningioma manifesting as a solitary pulmonary nodule with a false-positive PET scan. *J Thorac Imaging.* August 2006;21(3):225-227.

112. Moran CA, Hochholzer L, Rush W, Koss MN. Primary intrapulmonary meningiomas. A clinicopathologic and immunohistochemical study of ten cases. *Cancer.* December 1, 1996;78(11):2328-2333.

113. Rowsell C, Sirbovan J, Rosenblum MK, Perez-Ordonez B. Primary chordoid meningioma of lung. *Virchows Arch.* March 2005;446(3):333-337.

114. Masago K, Hosada W, Sasaki E, et al. Is primary pulmonary meningioma a giant form of a meningothelial-like nodule? A case report and review of the literature. *Case Rep Oncol.* May 2012;5(2):471-478.

115. Zhang JJ, Liu T, Peng F. Primary paraganglioma of the lung: a case report and literature review. *J Int Med Res.* 2012;40(4):1617-1626.

116. Shibahara J, Goto A, Niki T, Tanaka M, Nakajima J, Fukayama M. Primary pulmonary paraganglioma: report of a functioning case with immunohistochemical and ultrastructural study. *Am J Surg Pathol.* June 2004;28(6):825-829.

117. Ariizumi Y, Koizumi H, Hoshikawa M, et al. A primary pulmonary glomus tumor: a case report and review of the literature. *Case Rep Pathol.* 2012;2012:782304.

118. Tang CK, Toker C, Foris NP, Trump BF. Glomangioma of the lung. *Am J Surg Pathol.* March 1978;2(1):103-109.

119. Rossle M, Bayerle W, Lohrs U. Glomangioma of the lungs: a rare differential diagnosis of a pulmonary tumour. *J Clin Pathol.* September 2006;59(9):1000.

120. Santambrogio L, Nosotti M, Palleschi A, Gazzano G, De Simone M, Cioffi U. Primary pulmonary glomangioma: a coin lesion negative on PET study. Case report and literature review. *Thorac Cardiovasc Surg.* September 2011;59(6):380-382.

121. Katabami M, Okamoto K, Ito K, Kimura K, Kaji H. Bronchogenic glomangiomyoma with local intravenous infiltration. *Eur Respir J.* November 2006;28(5):1060-1064.

122. Folpe AL, Fanburg-Smith JC, Miettinen M, Weiss SW. Atypical and malignant glomus tumors: analysis of 52 cases, with a proposal for the reclassification of glomus tumors. *Am J Surg Pathol.* January 2001;25(1):1-12.

123. Folpe AL, Kwiatkowski DJ. Perivascular epithelioid cell neoplasms: pathology and pathogenesis. *Hum Pathol.* January 2010;41(1):1-15.

124. Liebow AA, Castleman B. Benign clear cell ("sugar") tumors of the lung. *Yale J Biol Med.* February-April 1971;43(4-5):213-222.

125. Frack MD, Simon L, Dawson BH. The lymphangiomyomatosis syndrome. *Cancer.* August 1968;22(2):428-437.

126. Pea M, Bonetti F, Zamboni G, et al. Melanocyte-marker-HMB-45 is regularly expressed in angiomyolipoma of the kidney. *Pathology.* July 1991;23(3):185-188.

127. Taylor JR, Ryu J, Colby TV, Raffin TA. Lymphangioleiomyomatosis. Clinical course in 32 patients. *N Engl J Med.* November 1 1990;323(18):1254-1260.

128. Chorianopoulos D, Stratakos G. Lymphangioleiomyomatosis and tuberous sclerosis complex. *Lung.* July-August 2008;186(4):197-207.

129. Johnson SR. Lymphangioleiomyomatosis. *Eur Respir J.* May 2006;27(5):1056-1065.

130. Goncharova EA, Goncharov DA, Eszterhas A, et al. Tuberin regulates p70 S6 kinase activation and ribosomal protein S6 phosphorylation. A role for the TSC2 tumor suppressor gene in pulmonary lymphangioleiomyomatosis (LAM). *J Biol Chem.* August 23, 2002;277(34):30958-30967.

131. Carsillo T, Astrinidis A, Henske EP. Mutations in the tuberous sclerosis complex gene TSC2 are a cause of sporadic pulmonary lymphangioleiomyomatosis. *Proc Natl Acad Sci U S A.* May 23, 2000;97(11):6085-6090.

132. Aberle DR, Hansell DM, Brown K, Tashkin DP. Lymphangiomyomatosis: CT, chest radiographic, and functional correlations. *Radiology.* August 1990;176(2):381-387.

133. Chilosi M, Pea M, Martignoni G, et al. Cathepsin-k expression in pulmonary lymphangioleiomyomatosis. *Mod Pathol.* February 2009;22(2):161-166.

134. Urban T, Lazor R, Lacronique J, et al. Pulmonary lymphangioleiomyomatosis. A study of 69 patients. Groupe d'Etudes et de Recherche sur les Maladies "Orphelines" Pulmonaires (GERM"O"P). *Medicine.* September 1999;78(5):321-337.

135. Matsui K, Beasley MB, Nelson WK, et al. Prognostic significance of pulmonary lymphangioleiomyomatosis histologic score. *Am J Surg Pathol.* April 2001;25(4):479-484.

136. Clarke BE. Cystic lung disease. *J Clin Pathol.* October 2013;66(10):904-908.

137. Taveira-DaSilva AM, Hathaway O, Stylianou M, Moss J. Changes in lung function and chylous effusions in patients with lymphangioleiomyomatosis treated with sirolimus. *Ann Intern.* June 21, 2011;154(12):797-805, W-292-793.

138. Ryu JH, Moss J, Beck GJ, et al. The NHLBI lymphangioleiomyomatosis registry: characteristics of 230 patients at enrollment. *Am J Respir Crit Care.* January 1, 2006;173(1):105-111.

139. Bonetti F, Pea M, Martignoni G, et al. Clear cell ("sugar") tumor of the lung is a lesion strictly related to angiomyolipoma--the concept of a family of lesions characterized by the presence of the perivascular epithelioid cells (PEC). *Pathology.* July 1994;26(3):230-236.

140. Gaffey MJ, Mills SE, Askin FB, et al. Clear cell tumor of the lung. A clinicopathologic, immunohistochemical, and ultrastructural study of eight cases. *Am J Surg Pathol.* March 1990;14(3):248-259.

141. Flieder DB, Travis WD. Clear cell "sugar" tumor of the lung: association with lymphangioleiomyomatosis and multifocal micronodular pneumocyte hyperplasia in a patient with tuberous sclerosis. *Am J Surg Pathol.* October 1997;21(10):1242-1247.

142. Zarbis N, Barth TF, Blumstein NM, Schelzig H. Pecoma of the lung: a benign tumor with extensive 18F-2-deoxy-D-glucose uptake. *Interact Cardiovasc Thorac Surg.* October 2007;6(5):676-678.

143. Adachi Y, Horie Y, Kitamura Y, et al. CD1a expression in PEComas. *Pathol Int.* March 2008;58(3):169-173.

144. Rao Q, Cheng L, Xia QY, et al. Cathepsin K expression in a wide spectrum of perivascular epithelioid cell neoplasms (PEComas): a clinicopathological study emphasizing extrarenal PEComas. *Histopathology.* March 2013;62(4):642-650.

145. Popper HH, Juettner-Smolle FM, Pongratz MG. Micronodular hyperplasia of type II pneumocytes--a new lung lesion associated with tuberous sclerosis. *Histopathology.* April 1991;18(4):347-354.

146. Hayashi T, Kumasaka T, Mitani K, Yao T, Suda K, Seyama K. Loss of heterozygosity on tuberous sclerosis complex genes in multifocal micronodular pneumocyte hyperplasia. *Mod Pathol.* September 2010;23(9):1251-1260.

147. Muir TE, Leslie KO, Popper H, et al. Micronodular pneumocyte hyperplasia. *Am J Surg Pathol.* April 1998;22(4):465-472.

148. Deavers M, Guinee D, Koss MN, Travis WD. Granular cell tumors of the lung. Clinicopathologic study of 20 cases. *Am J Surg Pathol.* June 1995;19(6):627-635.

149. Fine SW, Li M. Expression of calretinin and the alpha-subunit of inhibin in granular cell tumors. *Am J Clin Pathol.* February 2003;119(2):259-264.

150. Le BH, Boyer PJ, Lewis JE, Kapadia SB. Granular cell tumor: immunohistochemical assessment of inhibin-alpha, protein gene product 9.5, S100 protein, CD68, and Ki-67 proliferative index with clinical correlation. *Arch Pathol Lab Med.* July 2004;128(7):771-775.

10 Metastatic Neoplasms

Leslie A. Litzky

TAKE HOME PEARLS

- Routinely consider the possibility of metastatic disease in every case.
- Recognize the metastatic tumor histologic mimics for each type of primary lung tumor (and the primary lung tumor mimics of metastatic disease).
- Always obtain clinical and radiographic information prior to finalization of diagnosis.
- Do not use the latency period to discount metastatic disease.
- Be familiar with the recommended immunohistochemical panels and be aware of uncommon variants of primary lung tumors or extrapulmonary primaries.
- Make the effort to obtain prior slides and paraffin blocks for histologic comparison, taking into account the effects of prior treatment and latency interval on differentiation and immunophenotype.

INTRODUCTION

The recognition of metastatic disease in the lung is essential to patient care and is likely to assume even greater significance as patient survival continues to improve and the field of targeted therapeutics evolves. And yet, in many circumstances, distinguishing extrapulmonary metastasis from a primary lung tumor remains a challenging area for practicing pathologists. Access to the lung may be obtained by vascular/lymphatic invasion, airway spread, pleural seeding, or direct tumor extension. Metastases to the lung are

the most common malignancy involving the lung. It is easy to lose sight of this fact in the hectic daily routine of evaluating samples that are frequently presented to the pathologist as suspicious for a primary lung tumor. There are a few key steps in the approach to metastatic tumors that will help minimize diagnostic difficulties. It is useful to routinely consider the possibility of metastatic disease in each and every case as there are potential metastatic tumor histologic mimics for every type of primary lung tumor. Following initial histologic evaluation, it is always prudent to consider the final diagnosis is light of the clinical and radiographic findings and to make the extra effort to obtain that information if not provided. Patients and clinicians may not be aware of how long the time interval can be for the recurrence of malignant disease and may not include some piece of relevant history until prompted by an inquiry for clinical correlation. In some instances, the presence of an extrapulmonary primary may not be clinically apparent at the time of evaluation and the suggestion that the tumor may represent metastatic disease will result in additional radiographic or endoscopic workup. Pathologists should be familiar with the recommended immunohistochemical panels that support the diagnosis of a primary lung tumor or other common extrapulmonary primaries. Current literature should be regularly reviewed with the understanding that there are many exceptions and caveats in the interpretation of immunohistochemical stains. Uncommon variants of primary lung tumors and uncommon variants of extrapulmonary primaries may not show the expected immunophenotype and poorly differentiated tumors may not have as robust an immunophenotype as their better differentiated counterparts. As difficult as it is to keep up with the continuous stream of publications on tumor immunohistochemistry, pathologists should make every effort to familiarize themselves with this literature and to critically assess the supportive immunohistochemical data in each individual case. Extensive therapy over a prolonged period of time may also affect the immunophenotype. Finally, it is a time-honored and time-tested principle that obtaining the prior slides and paraffin blocks for histologic comparison and possible additional ancillary studies is one of the best ways to avoid making a false assumption that will result in an interpretative error.

EXCLUSION OF PRIMARY PULMONARY CARCINOMA

It is easier to approach the broad topic of excluding a primary pulmonary carcinoma by first summarizing what is often considered to be typical of primary pulmonary carcinomas and what clues might prompt the pathologist to consider metastasis from an extrapulmonary primary (*Table 10-1*). Clinical history—in particular smoking history—is an obvious piece of relevant information. Worldwide, it is estimated that 85% of lung cancer in men and slightly less than 50% of lung cancer in women are tobacco-smoking related.[1] A significant smoking history notwithstanding, it is important to consider the alternative possibility of metastasis from another smoking-related tumor such as a head and neck squamous cell carcinoma that may be clinically occult or the prior relevant history simply not disclosed. Neither should the absence of a smoking history dissuade one from the diagnosis of lung cancer, depending on the radiographic features and correlative data. The

characteristic "spiculated" radiographic appearance of primary lung cancers and the usual more "rounded" and "circumscribed" appearance of metastases is a similarly significant piece of information. However, it should be understood that these radiographic criteria are based on series in which the most frequent tumors are nonsmall cell carcinomas, and the less common lung tumors are not well represented. There are exceptions in both instances where a metastasis can appear more spiculated and a lung primary more rounded.[2] Multiple pulmonary nodules without a dominant lung mass favor metastatic disease whereas mediastinal and hilar adenopathy favor a pulmonary primary. These are not invariable radiographic findings, however, and occasional metastatic tumors may have significant hilar or mediastinal adenopathy. Cavitation does occur in metastatic disease but is far more commonly seen with a pulmonary primary. Calcification is similarly very rare in metastatic disease. A detailed radiographic assessment of the thorax may reveal pleural, mediastinal, lower neck/thyroid, or intravascular abnormalities that suggest an alternative primary and secondary involvement of the lung. Major metastatic patterns and their characteristic features will be reviewed in separate sections with the acknowledgment that overlap in these patterns exists.

On a histologic basis, it is often true that primary lung carcinomas that have grown slowly over some period of years will elicit a desmoplastic stromal response and some degree of inflammation as well as an area of central fibrosis. By contrast, many metastatic lesions will lack an area of central fibrosis and may be better demarcated from the surrounding lung tissue. An unambiguous and contiguous in situ component—either squamous cell carcinoma in situ (in the case of squamous cell carcinoma) or a peripheral nonmucinous lepidic growth pattern (in the case of adenocarcinoma)—establish the diagnosis of a lung primary. Because it is common for metastatic parenchymal nodules to begin as intravascular or intralymphatic tumor emboli, the presence of significant lymphovascular invasion adjacent to the tumor mass is a typical finding. Metastatic nodules are frequently subpleural and often show conspicuous visceral pleural invasion. Histologically, it may be fairly obvious that the tumor is metastatic but often enough the histologic appearance is or could be consistent with some subtype of a primary lung carcinoma. Whether or not potentially confirmatory ancillary studies (most often immunohistochemistry) are pursued at this juncture will depend on the availability of such ancillary studies, as well as cost considerations, therapeutic impact, and (in the current era of personalized diagnostics) whether the sample is to be preferentially reserved for molecular analysis.

Assuming that immunohistochemical studies are indicated, the selection of an appropriate immunohistochemical panel will depend on the histologic

Table 10-1 Exclusion of Primary Lung Carcinoma or Findings Favoring Metastatic Tumor

- Clinical history with particular attention to tobacco use and prior malignancies
- Radiologic appearance with specific reference to mass circumscription, location, distribution, lymphadenopathy, and other intrathoracic or extrathoracic abnormalities
- Lack of unambiguous and contiguous in situ component—either squamous cell carcinoma in situ (in the case of squamous cell carcinoma) or a peripheral nonmucinous lepidic growth pattern (in the case of adenocarcinoma)
- Conspicuous intravascular or intralymphatic tumor emboli and subpleural location
- Histologic appearance integrated with immunophenotype and other ancillary studies

appearance of the tumor and the differential diagnosis that is generated based on that histology and any additional patient history. Specific tumors of origin will be covered in the subsequent sections but as a fundamental differential diagnostic approach, it is possible to group tumors into general categories such as primary pulmonary adenocarcinoma and its variants versus metastasis, primary squamous cell carcinoma and its variants versus metastasis, primary pulmonary large cell carcinoma versus other undifferentiated/ pleomorphic large cell tumors, primary sarcomatoid carcinomas versus other spindle cell tumors, primary carcinoid tumors versus metastases with endocrine/ neuroendocrine features, and primary pulmonary high-grade neuroendocrine tumors versus other small round cell tumors. This conceptual framework provides a practical departure point for generating a differential diagnosis and for ordering ancillary studies but it is not meant to constrain the diagnostic evaluation as circumstances dictate.

SOLITARY METASTASIS

The solitary pulmonary nodule is a routine problem in medical centers where there is frequent radiographic surveillance for patients with prior malignancies or simply just a high frequency of radiographic studies done for some other indication. Although estimates vary, one study from a high volume medical center reported the incidence of solitary metastasis involving the lungs as 3.5%.[3] This possibility of solitary metastasis is high enough to maintain a reasonable index of suspicion for metastasis-particularly when there is relevant clinical history and suggestive radiographic or histologic findings (*Table 10-2*). Most patients with solitary metastasis are asymptomatic—as are most patients with solitary pulmonary nodules. As discussed previously, radiologists will typically favor a pulmonary primary when the lesion appears "spiculated" and favor metastasis when the lesion is well circumscribed with smooth borders. Nevertheless, smoothly contoured primary lung tumors do occur as do metastases with irregular borders—thereby necessitating thoughtful histological

Table 10-2   Solitary Metastasis

- Most patients asymptomatic
- Estimates of incidence vary but generally within the single digit range (2%-9%) of patients who present with solitary pulmonary nodules
- Usually well circumscribed with smooth contours
- Most common extrapulmonary primary sites are colon, kidney, breast, skin (melanoma), and soft tissue (sarcomas)

evaluation, comparison with any prior material, and immunohistochemical studies as well. In patients with a known prior extrapulmonary malignancy, there is often concern that a new, well-circumscribed solitary pulmonary nodule represents a metastasis. Although in any specific individual case this may be less likely on a statistical basis, the anxiety and uncertainty over the radiographic findings will nevertheless lead to a sampling or excision in many circumstances (*Figure 10-1A and B*). On occasion, the gross appearance suggests a specific metastatic tumor (*Figure 10-1C*). In other instances, the nodule is nondescript but suggests metastasis or is more consistent with a primary lung tumor (*Figure 10-1D and E*). The most common extrapulmonary primary sites to present as solitary metastases are colon, kidney, breast, skin (melanoma), and soft tissue (sarcomas).

MULTIPLE METASTASES

Multiple pulmonary parenchymal nodules is the most common pattern of metastatic tumor spread and exclusive involvement of the lungs is seen in a significant number of cases (*Table 10-3*). The vast majority of these patients will either have a known prior history of malignancy or are diagnosed with a synchronous primary. Most patients are asymptomatic. The typical presenting symptoms can be correlated with the size and location of the nodules. Airway involvement may result in wheezing, cough, or hemoptysis. Pleural or chest wall involvement may result in pleural effusion, chest wall pain, or a Pancoast syndrome. Spontaneous pneumothorax is an extremely rare presentation but does occur. The average size range for metastatic parenchymal nodules is 1 to 2 cm but there is variability with some metastatic tumor nodules below the detection limits for high-resolution CT (0.5 cm or less) and other metastatic tumors that are so large as to nearly occupy the entire lung. A miliary distribution pattern has also been described. These radiographic features are reflected in the gross findings typically seen at autopsy where numerous relatively well-circumscribed nodules are apparent. Following the normal regional perfusion patterns of the lung, there is a preference for lower lung zone involvement over the upper lung zones and the subpleural regions are often affected (*Figure 10-2*). Histologically, the parenchymal nodules destroy the underlying pulmonary architecture and adjacent lymphovascular invasion is often easily identified. Unusual patterns of parenchymal involvement include lepidic, interstitial, or intra-alveolar spread. The most common primary sites in order of frequency are breast, colon, stomach, pancreas, kidney, skin (melanoma), prostate, liver, thyroid, adrenal gland, male and female genital tracts.[1]

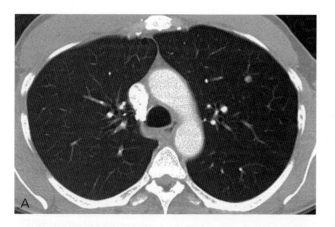

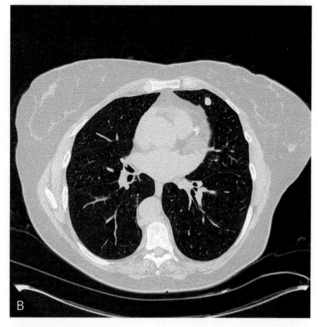

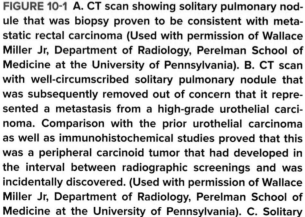

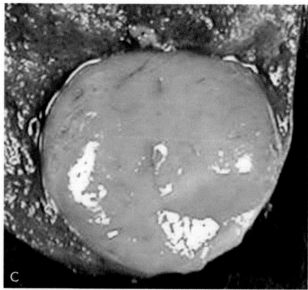

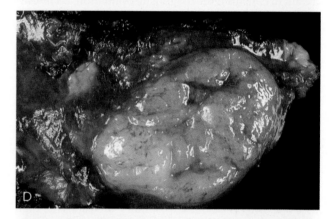

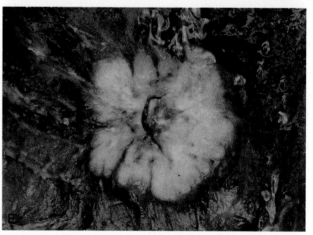

FIGURE 10-1 A. CT scan showing solitary pulmonary nodule that was biopsy proven to be consistent with metastatic rectal carcinoma (Used with permission of Wallace Miller Jr, Department of Radiology, Perelman School of Medicine at the University of Pennsylvania). B. CT scan with well-circumscribed solitary pulmonary nodule that was subsequently removed out of concern that it represented a metastasis from a high-grade urothelial carcinoma. Comparison with the prior urothelial carcinoma as well as immunohistochemical studies proved that this was a peripheral carcinoid tumor that had developed in the interval between radiographic screenings and was incidentally discovered. (Used with permission of Wallace Miller Jr, Department of Radiology, Perelman School of Medicine at the University of Pennsylvania). C. Solitary pulmonary nodule, metastatic Hürthle cell carcinoma. The nodule is well circumscribed and has a distinctive mahogany color typical of a tumor with oncocytic features. D. Solitary pulmonary nodule, metastatic urothelial carcinoma. This nodule is well circumscribed but has a nondescript gross appearance. Immunohistochemical stains were required to confirm the primary site. E. Solitary pulmonary nodule, primary pulmonary adenocarcinoma. This nodule has an irregular border that is typical of pulmonary primaries. Microscopic sections showed a solid predominant pattern. The tumor cells were positive for TTF-1 and Napsin A, supporting the diagnosis.

Table 10-3 Multiple Metastases

- Most common pattern of metastatic tumor spread
- Exclusive involvement of the lungs in a significant number of cases
- Vast majority of patients have a known prior history of malignancy or are diagnosed with a synchronous primary
- Most patients are asymptomatic
- Average size range 1-2 cm
- Preference for lower lung zone and subpleural regions
- Relatively well-circumscribed parenchymal nodules most characteristic
- Unusual patterns include lepidic, interstitial, or intra-alveolar spread
- Common primary sites include breast, colon, stomach, pancreas, kidney, skin (melanoma), prostate, liver , thyroid, ovary, and uterus

Table 10-4 Lymphangitic Spread of Metastatic Tumor

- Distinctive clinical presentation and radiographic findings with poor prognosis
- CT scans show nonuniform nodular thickening of the interlobular septa and bronchovascular bundles with preservation of the alveolated lung parenchyma
- Gross thickening of the interlobular septa, bronchovascular connective tissue, and subpleural connective tissue
- Tumor cells permeate lymphatic spaces with or without a desmoplastic reaction or the formation of larger tumor nodules
- Most common primary sites include breast, stomach, lung, pancreas, prostate, uterus, and colon

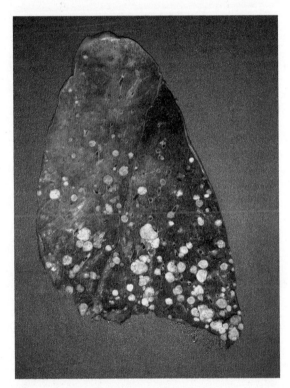

FIGURE 10-2 Autopsy lung showing widely metastatic follicular carcinoma of the thyroid. Note the lower lobe predominance of the tumor nodules.

LYMPHANGITIC SPREAD OF METASTATIC TUMOR

Although less common than parenchymal nodules, lymphangitic spread of metastatic tumor is an important and distinctive pattern in terms of clinical presentation, radiographic findings, and poor prognosis (*Table 10-4*). Most instances of lymphangitic spread begin as hematogenous tumor that extends into the interstitium and follows the normal lymphatic distribution of the lung. The lymphatic involvement results in thickening of the interlobular septa, bronchovascular connective tissue, and subpleural connective tissue. The radiographic appearance reflects this pattern of spread and the CT findings include nonuniform nodular thickening of the interlobular septa and bronchovascular bundles with preservation of the alveolated lung parenchyma (*Figure 10-3A*). The insidious onset of dyspnea, along with the fact that pleural effusions or hilar/mediastinal adenopathy are present in a minority of patients, may make lymphangitic carcinomatosis difficult to diagnose prior to the more obvious and pre-terminal phase of rapid progressive dyspnea. Although occasionally subtle, the thickening of the interlobular septa and bronchovascular bundles can be grossly appreciated (*Figure 10-3B*). Microscopically, the tumor cells permeate the lymphatic spaces with or without a desmoplastic reaction or the formation of larger tumor nodules (*Figure 10-3C-E*). Lymphangitic spread can be seen with any kind of metastatic tumor but the most common primary sites include breast, stomach, lung, pancreas, prostate, uterus, and colon.

VASCULAR METASTASES

Large tumor emboli occluding the main pulmonary arteries are rare but have been reported with tumors arising in the right side of the heart or pulmonary trunk as well as with tumors such as renal cell carcinomas or hepatocellular carcinomas that are known for their tendency to invade the large systemic veins. Microscopic

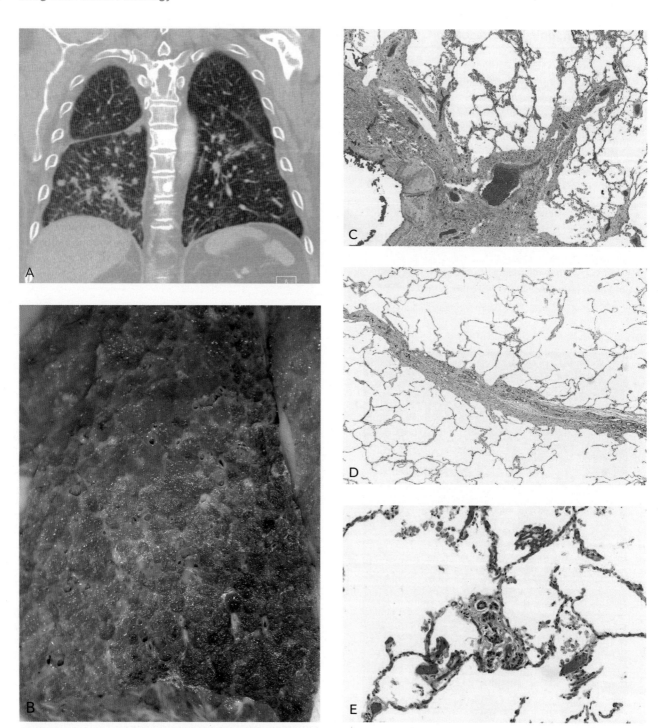

FIGURE 10-3 **A.** CT scan showing lymphangitic carcinoma with a septal and bronchovascular pattern. The patient presented with dyspnea and a history of prostate cancer. (Used with permission of Wallace Miller Jr, Department of Radiology, Perelman School of Medicine at the University of Pennsylvania). **B.** Autopsy lung with septal prominence as a result of lymphangitic spread of prostate cancer. **C.** Tumor spreading within the lymphatics in a bronchovascular distribution (H&E, 22×). **D.** Tumor spreading within septal lymphatics (H&E, 30×). **E** Small acinar glands typical of prostatic adenocarcinoma (H&E, 100×).

tumor emboli are common in autopsy studies but the entity of microscopic thrombotic tumor microangiopathy represents a distinct subset of patients who typically present with sudden onset of pulmonary hypertension and right-sided heart failure as well as sudden death (*Table 10-5*).[4] In some instances, the tumor emboli result in pulmonary infarcts with symptoms of pleuritic chest pain and hemoptysis. The initial clinical suspicion is usually pulmonary embolism and many cases are only diagnosed at postmortem examination. Radiographically, the diagnosis is suggested indirectly by the findings of pulmonary hypertension. The gross

Table 10-5 Vascular Metastases

- Large tumor emboli occluding the main pulmonary arteries are rare
- Microscopic tumor emboli are common in autopsy studies
- Tumor-related thrombotic pulmonary microangiopathy a distinct entity and presentation with acute onset of pulmonary hypertension and right-sided heart failure as well as sudden death
- Microscopic findings of tumor-related thrombotic pulmonary microangiopathy are prominent fibrointimal hyperplasia and organizing thrombi within the small pulmonary arteries and arterioles that may or may not be associated with a large number of tumor cells
- Gastric and breast carcinomas are most common tumors associated with this syndrome
- Prognosis dismal even if identified premortem

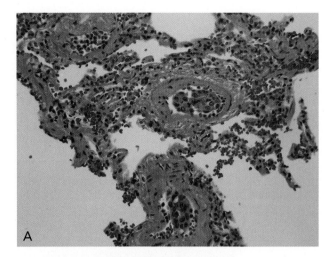

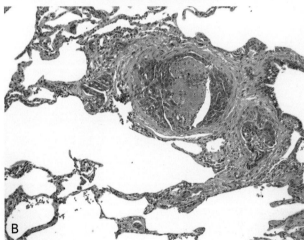

FIGURE 10-4 Vascular invasion: A. metastatic breast carcinoma. Small pulmonary arterial vessels are filled with clusters of tumor cells (H&E, 200×). B. Metastatic breast carcinoma. The tumor cells with fibrin and necrosis (H&E, 100×).

findings are equally inconspicuous unless there are thromboemboli in larger arteries or pulmonary infarcts. Microscopic sections show prominent vascular involvement with involvement of numerous small pulmonary arteries and arterioles (*Figure 10-4A*). The clusters of tumor cells often occlude the vascular lumens. Fibrin is intermixed with the tumor cells and there is often fibrointimal hyperplasia (*Figure 10-4B*). The most common tumors associated with this syndrome are gastric and breast carcinomas but a range of other tumor types have been reported. Even when this entity is identified premortem, the prognosis is dismal and many cases have been documented in association with sudden death.

ENDOBRONCHIAL METASTASES

Some tumors have a tendency for spread to the submucosal lymphatics or vasculature of the large airways and with subsequent expansile polypoid growth may mimic a primary tumor of the bronchus (*Table 10-6*). Alternatively, permeation of the submucosa with tumor can lead to concentric narrowing of the airway without a large mass. Direct extension from other mediastinal tumors, the esophagus, or pleura as well as aerogenous spread from an upper airway malignancy are also considerations. The clinical presentation of endobronchial metastasis does not differ from the clinical presentation of primary endobronchial tumors. Patients may present as an asymptomatic radiographic finding or with dyspnea, wheezing, infection, and hemoptysis (*Figure 10-5A*). A wide variety of tumors have been reported as endobronchial metastases with the most common primaries representing breast, bone, soft tissue, colon, kidney, and skin (melanoma) (*Figure 10-5B and C*).[5-7] The interval between the diagnosis of the original tumor and presentation of endobronchial metastasis can extend

Table 10-6 Endobronchial Metastases

- The clinical and radiographic presentation of endobronchial metastasis does not differ from the clinical presentation of primary endobronchial tumors
- Interval between the diagnosis of the original tumor and presentation of endobronchial metastasis can extend far beyond the a mean of 4-5 years
- Bronchoscopy may show expansile polypoid growth or concentric narrowing of the airway without a large mass
- Most common primary pulmonary endobronchial tumors are squamous cell carcinomas, neuroendocrine tumors, and salivary gland–type tumors
- Other types of endobronchial tumors such as sarcomas and non-salivary gland–type adenocarcinomas should prompt consideration of metastatic disease
- Most common metastases are breast, bone, soft tissue, colon, kidney, and skin (melanoma)
- Differential diagnosis may include direct extension from other mediastinal tumors, the esophagus, or pleura as well as airway spread from a head and neck tumor

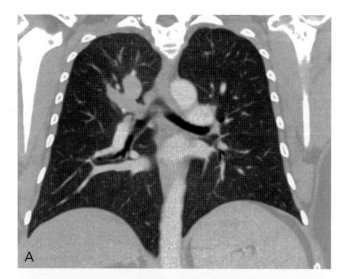
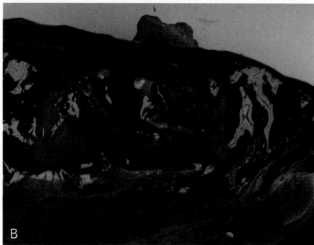
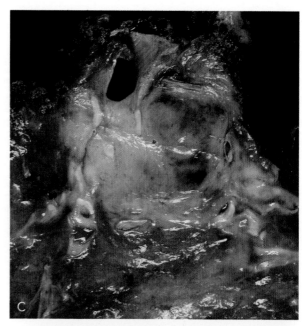
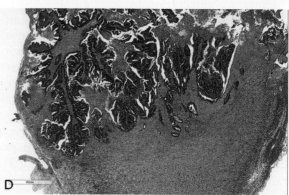

FIGURE 10-5 A. CT scan showing metastatic endobronchial tumor (malignant melanoma). (Used with permission of Wallace Miller Jr, Department of Radiology, Perelman School of Medicine at the University of Pennsylvania). B. Metastatic endobronchial tumor, renal cell carcinoma. C. Metastatic endobronchial tumor, malignant melanoma. D. Metastatic colonic adenocarcinoma to the trachea. A primary adenocarcinoma would be extremely unusual in this location and immunohistochemical stains can be useful in this instance to confirm the site of origin (H&E, 27×).

far beyond the reported mean of 4 to 5 years. It is useful to remember that the most common primary endobronchial tumors are squamous cell carcinomas, neuroendocrine tumors, and salivary gland–type tumors. Other types of endobronchial tumors (for example, sarcomas and non-salivary gland–type adenocarcinomas) should prompt a consideration of metastatic disease and additional clinical history, if not initially or incompletely provided (*Figure 10-5D*).

TUMORS OF ORIGIN

Lung

When a patient presents with a dominant lung mass and multiple satellite nodules, it is reasonable to conclude that the lung is the primary site on a clinical basis.

Table 10-7 Primary Lung Tumors

- Differential diagnosis and immunohistochemical workup should be centered on the histologic appearance within the framework below and any prior history of malignancy
- Primary pulmonary adenocarcinoma and its variants vs metastases
- Primary squamous cell carcinoma and its variants vs metastases
- Primary large cell carcinoma vs metastatic undifferentiated/pleomorphic large cell tumors
- Pulmonary sarcomatoid carcinoma vs metastatic spindle cell tumors
- Primary carcinoid tumors vs metastatic tumors with well-differentiated neuroendocrine/endocrine features
- Primary pulmonary high-grade neuroendocrine carcinomas vs other small round cell tumors

Pathologically confirming that the lung is the primary site may prove to be more difficult, however, depending on the microscopic features (*Table 10-7*). The topic of primary lung tumors is very broad and includes many unusual variants. A comprehensive discussion of primary lung tumors will not be attempted within the confines of this chapter. The focus here is to provide a practical approach and to highlight important diagnostic pitfalls in routine evaluation.

Pulmonary adenocarcinoma is the most common type of lung tumor in many countries (*Figure 10-6A*). Thyroid transcription factor 1 (TTF-1) is the usual first step in the immunohistochemical evaluation to determine site of origin.[8] TTF-1 has great utility but the limits of this stain's sensitivity and specificity are not always well appreciated, particularly by clinicians. Although infrequent, some ovarian tumors, endometrial tumors, breast carcinomas, colonic adenocarcinomas, and a subset of cholangiocarcinomas may be TTF-1 positive as well.[9-15] There are two main antibody clones commercially available and it has been documented that the type of clone may greatly influence the prevalence of TTF-1 expression in other tumors.[16] One should be aware of this when evaluating clinical material as well

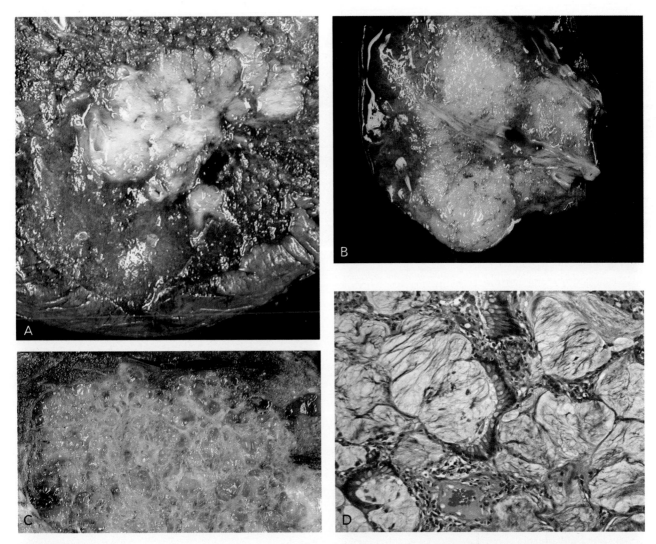

FIGURE 10-6 A. Primary pulmonary adenocarcinoma. Note the irregular margins. **B.** Invasive mucinous adenocarcinoma consistent with pulmonary primary. This large 5-cm lung mass was positive for TTF-1 and CK7 but negative for TTF-1. The patient underwent a right middle lobectomy with subsequent chemotherapy and XRT for tumor size and N1-positive nodes. A completion pneumonectomy was performed 22 months later. The patient was still alive with isolated brain metastases 3 years later following the pneumonectomy. **C.** Invasive mucinous (colloid) carcinoma. This tumor was TTF-1 negative. The patient was a nonsmoker and 7 years S/P a Whipple for a node negative well-differentiated mucinous (colloid) adenocarcinoma of the ampulla. An isolated metastasis from a pancreatic primary was favored on a clinical basis although no therapy was instituted due the patient's advanced age. **D.** Pulmonary adenocarcinoma with enteric differentiation (H&E, 200×).

CHAPTER 10

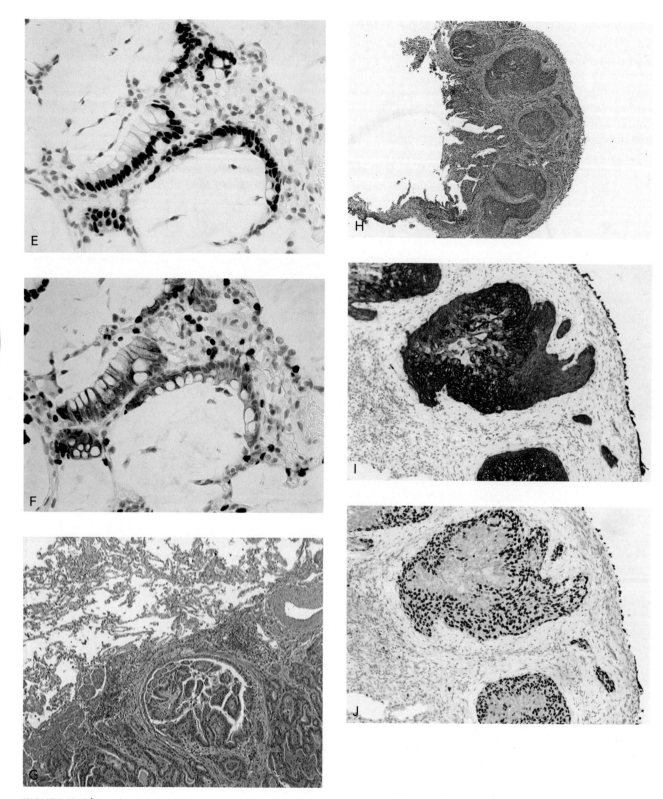

FIGURE 10-6 (*Continued*) **E. Pulmonary adenocarcinoma with enteric differentiation. The tumor cells are strongly positive for CDX2 (200×). F. Pulmonary adenocarcinoma with enteric differentiation. There is no nuclear positivity for TTF-1 (200×). G. Metastatic papillary carcinoma of the thyroid (H&E, 100×). H. Metastatic thyroid carcinoma. This biopsy is from a patient with a long-standing history of papillary carcinoma of the thyroid and multiple courses of treatment. The patient had known metastatic disease but there was one nodule in the lung that was more spiculated and considered to be suspicious for a primary lung cancer (H&E, 40×). I. Metastatic thyroid carcinoma. The tumor cells were strongly positive for CK5/6 (100×). J. Metastatic thyroid carcinoma. The tumor cells were strongly positive for p63 (pictured here) and TTF-1 (100×).**

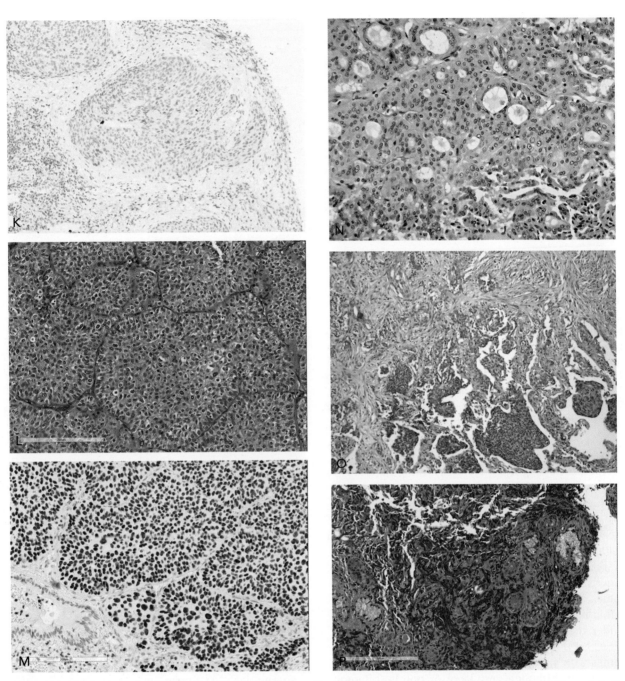

FIGURE 10-6 (Continued) K. Metastatic thyroid carcinoma. The tumor cells were negative for Napsin A, thyroglobulin, PAX8, and calcitonin. The decision was made to excise the nodule . The resection specimen showed classic papillary carcinoma of the thyroid admixed with a solid squamous component. Review of the original thyroid primary showed a very focal solid squamous component. **L.** Metastatic urothelial carcinoma (H&E, 200×). The nests of cell are squamoid in appearance with the nests separated by a delicate fibrovascular network. **M.** Metastatic urothelial carcinoma. The tumor cells are strongly positive for GATA3, supporting the diagnosis (200×). **N.** Metastatic thyroid carcinoma. This biopsy was submitted as an endobronchial mass and could easily be mistaken for an oncocytic carcinoid tumor. The patient was noted to have a history of a metastatic Hürthle cell carcinoma of the thyroid and a thyroglobulin was strongly positive, confirming the diagnosis (H&E, 400×). **O.** Metastatic medullary carcinoma. This neuroendocrine proliferation was initially interpreted as DIPNECH and multiple microcarcinoids on the basis of strong TTF-1 positive staining, along with positive synaptophysin and chromogranin staining. It was then discovered that the patient had a prior history of medullary carcinoma of the thyroid and calcitonin stains were performed. The tumor cells were strongly positive for calcitonin, supporting the diagnosis (H&E, 100×). **P.** Metastatic prostatic adenocarcinoma misdiagnosed as small cell carcinoma. This biopsy was from a patient with a referral diagnosis of small cell carcinoma. Note the misleading "crush" artifact that is present. It was unclear if immunohistochemical stains had been done on the prior outside material. Additional clinical information was provided at the time of rebiopsy that the patient also had a history of prostate cancer (H&E, 200×).

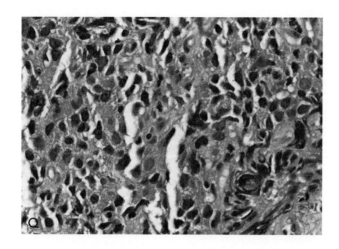

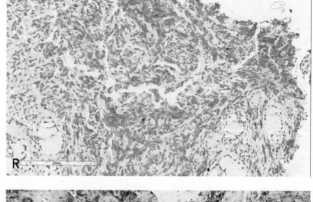

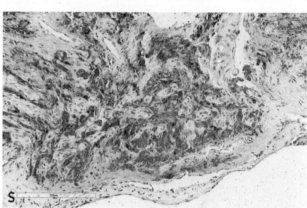

FIGURE 10-6 (*Continued*) **Q. Metastatic prostatic adeno-carcinoma. Although it is hard to assess the nuclear detail, there is a suggestion of more cytoplasm than is character-istic of a small cell carcinoma (H&E, 400×). R. Metastatic prostatic adenocarcinoma. Immunostaining was CD56 was negative as were synaptophysin, chromogranin, and TTF-1 (200×). S. Metastatic prostatic adenocarcinoma. The tumor cells are strongly positive for PSA, supporting the diagnosis (200×).**

as when reviewing the literature. Adding Napsin A to the immunohistochemical workup provides about an incremental increase in sensitivity for pulmonary adenocarcinomas but introduces a whole other set of specificity concerns that must be sorted out.[8] Both renal cell and thyroid carcinomas can be Napsin A positive, as well as an assorted minority of breast carcinomas, pancreaticobiliary primaries, and colonic adenocarci-nomas. Although it might seem logical that surfactant antibodies would be useful, these antibodies have only moderate sensitivity and specificity.[17,18]

Sorting out the differential diagnosis for adenocarci-nomas with variable glandular and solid patterns can be difficult. Although very large or poorly differenti-ated pulmonary adenocarcinomas may have necrosis, prominent necrosis is a frequent feature of metastatic disease. When faced with a tumor showing an acinar, cribriform, or solid pattern that cannot be demon-strated to be TTF-1 positive, cytokeratin 7 (CK7) and cytokeratin 20 (CK20) can be used in an attempt to further narrow the differential diagnosis. This type of algorithmic immunohistochemical analysis using CK7/CK20-positive/negative patterns with supplementation of additional markers as needed has been summarized in other reviews.[19,20] As a general (and fortunate) rule, most primary pulmonary adenocarcinomas will be TTF-1 positive and CK7 positive but there is clearly a sub-set of lung adenocarcinomas that are not (*Figure 10-6B*

and C). Lung primaries with enteric differentiation may have an immunophenotype (CK7 negative/CK20, MOC2, and CDX-2 positive) that is indistinguish-able from metastatic colorectal carcinomas and can only be sorted out on a clinicoradiologic basis alone (*Figure 10-6D-F*).[21] The differential diagnosis of TTF-1–negative/CK7-positive tumors can be equally as challenging. This category will still include a subset of often poorly differentiated pulmonary adenocarcino-mas as well as a wide array of extrapulmonary primaries. These extrapulmonary primaries include gastric or pancreaticobiliary carcinomas, urothelial carcinomas, breast carcinomas, endocervical/cervical carcinomas, endometrial carcinomas, ovarian carcinomas, malig-nant mesothelioma, salivary gland tumors, and thyroid carcinomas. Further details as to the subsequent workup for this category of tumors will be provided in other sections on tumor origin and there are some newer markers such as GATA3 that have helped narrow this dif-ferential diagnosis. However, sensitivity and specificity limits for newer markers are still evolving and caution is recommended in interpretation. It is generally true that it is difficult to extrapolate the data to poorly differentiated tumors of any primary site or to rely on the published sensitivity/specificity data in metastatic sites. In some instances, it is simply best to be cautious and convey to the clinician that the site of origin cannot be confirmed on a histologic/immunophenotypic basis alone.

Better differentiated adenocarcinomas with specific histologic features are often more straightforward. The most common diagnostic considerations for tumors with papillary/micropapillary features include lung, thyroid, breast, ovary, and kidney. Malignant mesothelioma might also be a consideration depending on the radiologic appearance. Nearly all papillary/micropapillary pulmonary primaries are TTF-1 positive as are well-differentiated thyroid papillary carcinomas (*Figure 10-6G*). While the addition of thyroglobulin often helps resolve this issue, it should be remembered that thyroid carcinomas may not be thyroglobulin positive or may lose thyroglobulin positivity over time. Paired box 8 (PAX8), a relatively new marker that is expressed in some tumors of the thyroid (as well as some GYN and renal tumors), may be useful in this instance.[22] As mentioned previously, some ovarian tumors, endometrial tumors, and breast carcinomas may be TTF-1 positive. TTF-1 positivity is extremely rare in renal cell carcinomas and has not been reported in malignant mesothelioma to date.[16] Signet ring cells are common in extrapulmonary primaries such as the stomach, other luminal gastrointestinal sites, breast, and pancreas, but primary pulmonary adenocarcinomas can have prominent signet ring cell features. EML4-ALK fusions are associated with some of these pulmonary primaries and therefore identification of the primary site may have particularly significant therapeutic implications. This may be difficult on an immunohistochemical basis alone because of the overlap in immunohistochemical profiles. About 85% of signet ring cell adenocarcinomas of the lung will be TTF-1 positive.[19] Clear cell change is seen in multiple types of primary pulmonary carcinomas including adenocarcinomas, squamous cell carcinomas, and neuroendocrine tumors. Nevertheless, metastasis from an extrapulmonary primary is a leading consideration in tumors with prominent clear cells. The most common clear cell tumor in the lung is metastatic renal cell carcinoma but clear cell change has been reported in tumors from nearly every primary site. Other major primary sites to consider for tumors with clear cell change include the adrenal cortex and salivary glands.

Confirming the diagnosis on a histologic basis alone of a primary pulmonary squamous cell carcinoma is nearly always impossible. The usual immunohistochemical panel used to support squamous differentiation in the lung consists of CK5/6 and p63 or p40 (or both p63 and p40 depending on the particular laboratory). It has been reported that a small percentage of pulmonary squamous cell carcinomas are TTF-1 positive but there is variability in the literature with questions raised as to whether some of the positivity represents entrapped background lung or antibody specificity.[23] The occasional biopsy/resection will show a clearcut in situ component but otherwise the diagnosis defaults to the clinical history, physical examination, and radiographic findings. The differential diagnosis will include intrathoracic and extrathoracic carcinomas with squamous differentiation as well as other malignancies with an epithelioid appearance. This latter category includes malignant mesothelioma, malignant melanoma, germ cell tumors, and urothelial carcinoma. Head and neck primaries, as well as malignant melanoma, will be covered in separate sections. In each instance, integrating the clinical and radiographic information is essential. All too often the pathologist is left with the false assumption that the lesional material represents a classic pulmonary primary when in fact there are clinical or radiographic findings that would suggest otherwise. Within the thorax, special attention should be paid to any esophageal, pleural, mediastinal, or lower neck abnormalities. An esophageal squamous cell primary must be determined on clinical grounds but the paired staining of p63 with CK5/6 is useful in excluding malignant mesothelioma.[24] CD5 is expressed in a significant percentage of thymic carcinomas of different subtypes; however, a small percentage of pulmonary squamous carcinomas are also positive for CD5.[25] In these circumstances, the diagnosis of thymic carcinoma most often defaults to the radiographic findings. There are a number of markers that may prove helpful in diagnosing a germ cell tumor with the biggest pitfall being a failure to consider the possibility in the appropriate clinical setting.[20] The same is true for the recently described entity of NUT midline carcinoma which should be included within the differential diagnosis of any poorly differentiated epithelioid mediastinal tumor, regardless of age.[26,27] Metastatic thyroid carcinoma is typically considered in a TTF-1–positive tumor but what might be less obvious is that thyroid tumors (or any tumor with squamous differentiation) can be CK5/6 and p63 positive as well (*Figure 10-6H-K*). GATA3 has good sensitivity and specificity for breast and urothelial carcinomas—two primary sites that, as an aside, can be radiographically occult by initial evaluation unless particular attention is directed toward them. Up until the introduction of GATA3, metastatic urothelial carcinoma was difficult to distinguish from a lung primary, given that both can be CK5/6 and p63 positive (*Figure 10-6L and M*).

By definition, primary pulmonary large cell carcinoma does not show specific evidence of glandular or squamous differentiation.[1] Leaving aside the issue recently raised as to whether this category which encompasses a number of variants (large cell neuroendocrine carcinoma, basaloid carcinoma, lymphoepithelioma-like carcinoma, clear cell carcinoma, and large cell carcinoma with rhabdoid phenotype) should be retained, the more fundamental issue is that these primary pulmonary tumors are highly pleomorphic and therefore the differential diagnosis must be expanded to include a wide variety of tumors.[28] The differential diagnosis will include other poorly differentiated carcinomas, germ cell tumors, malignant melanoma, malignant mesothelioma, malignant lymphoma, and epithelioid sarcomas. Recommended immunohistochemical panels have been summarized in other publications.[19,20] The most pertinent point is to avoid concluding that cytokeratin positivity supports a diagnosis of carcinoma when the clinical history, radiographic findings, or histologic appearance might suggest otherwise. In the particular instance of a sarcoma, specific translocation studies may be diagnostic. The same cautionary point is to be made in regard to hematopoietic malignancies, not all of which are LCA positive and some of which may be EMA or CK positive.

The immunohistochemical workup and differential diagnosis for a primary pulmonary sarcomatoid carcinoma and other spindle cell tumors has similar caveats in terms of immunohistochemical interpretation. The differential diagnosis will include primary pulmonary sarcomatoid carcinoma, metastatic sarcomatoid carcinoma, malignant mesothelioma, metastatic sarcoma, and primary pulmonary sarcomas. This topic has been reviewed in depth in other publications.[29-31] Although extensive sampling may be helpful in defining a tumor's lineage, this is not an option in smaller samplings and it simply may not be possible to come to a definitive diagnosis in this instance. In larger samples, immunohistochemical stains and molecular studies can reliably classify many sarcomatoid lesions. One study of pulmonary sarcomatoid carcinomas has demonstrated that TTF-1 is superior to Napsin A, with an overall sensitivity of about 60% for TTF-1.[32]

There is a spectrum of primary pulmonary neuroendocrine tumors that includes low-grade (typical carcinoid), intermediate-grade (atypical carcinoid), and high-grade neuroendocrine tumors (large cell neuroendocrine carcinoma and small cell carcinoma). The differential diagnosis and most common extrapulmonary primary sites will differ according to the histologic grade. Before considering this differential diagnosis, it is worth acknowledging that even when the differential diagnosis is restricted to the primary lung tumors, it can be difficult to recognize and grade a pulmonary neuroendocrine tumor, particularly in a small sampling. In this regard, the immunohistochemical panel commonly applied to subclassify nonsmall cell lung (NSCLC) tumors may aid in the separation of pulmonary neuroendocrine tumors from other NSCLCs. One recent study indicates that pulmonary neuroendocrine tumors have a distinct but nonspecific immunohistochemical profile (Napsin A–/p40–/p63–/CK5/6–/ TTF-1±).[33] Ki-67 immunostaining, especially in smaller samples, is helpful in further subclassifying neuroendocrine tumors into low- or high-grade neuroendocrine carcinomas.[34] The occasionally difficult classification of pulmonary neuroendocrine tumors has been reviewed and the focus here will be on differential diagnosis.[35]

In addition to typical and atypical pulmonary carcinoid tumors, the differential diagnosis of a low to intermediate-grade neuroendocrine tumor in the lung includes other metastatic well-differentiated neuroendocrine carcinomas, metastatic carcinomas such as breast or prostate, salivary gland tumors such as adenoid cystic carcinoma (either primary or metastatic), paraganglioma, sclerosing hemangioma, and smooth muscle tumors (*Figure 10-6N*). The latter differential of a smooth muscle tumor is most frequently encountered in the instance of peripheral carcinoid with a spindle cell appearance. The use of immunohistochemical stains to confirm neuroendocrine differentiation (chromogranin, synaptophysin, and CD56) is a potential pitfall. Other types of carcinomas can show evidence of neuroendocrine differentiation and there are other nonepithelial tumors that are positive for these markers. The differential diagnosis of carcinoid tumors (usually atypical carcinoid tumor) from metastatic breast carcinoma can be problematic, particularly in the absence of clinical history. Estrogen and progesterone staining can be seen in primary pulmonary neuroendocrine tumors, although strong and diffuse ER/PR positivity combined with TTF-1 negativity favors breast carcinoma on a probabilistic basis.[36,37] While TTF-1 appears to be relatively specific for pulmonary carcinoids when compared with other metastatic well-differentiated neuroendocrine tumors, it is not especially sensitive with a wide range of positivity reported in the literature for pulmonary primaries and rare reports of TTF-1–positive nonpulmonary tumors described.[38-40] Peripheral typical carcinoids are reported to be far more frequently TTF-1 positive than those in a central location.[41] A panel of immunostains that includes CDX-2, PDX-1, NESP-55, and TTF-1 has been reported to be useful in distinguishing well-differentiated neuroendocrine tumors of the gastrointestinal tract and pancreas from lung.[42] Even small neuroendocrine tumor proliferations (diffuse idiopathic neuroendocrine cell hyperplasia [DIPNECH] and microcarcinoids) may prove to be problematic. There are reports of DIPNECH radiographically diagnosed as diffuse metastatic disease and there are occasional metastatic well-differentiated neuroendocrine carcinomas that mimic DIPNECH and microcarcinoids (*Figure 10-6O*).[43]

As with all immunohistochemical stains, a single positive marker should not be interpreted independently from other markers and the clinical context. In the final analysis, clinical history and additional radiographic findings may provide the weightiest evidence in favor of a primary or metastatic disease.

At the high-grade neuroendocrine tumor end of the spectrum, the differential diagnosis includes metastatic carcinomas from extrapulmonary primaries and other malignant small round cell tumors. This latter category includes malignant lymphoma, malignant melanoma, malignant mesothelioma (small cell variant), rhabdomyosarcoma, Ewing sarcoma/PNET, neuroblastoma, hepatoblastoma, desmoplastic small round cell tumor (DSRCT), mesenchymal chondrosarcoma, small cell osteosarcoma, and Wilms tumor. The general workup for a malignant small round cell tumor has been reviewed but a few general points will be emphasized.[19,20] Depending on the clinical circumstances, radiographic features and histologic appearance, an important first step is to ascertain that the tumor is indeed cytokeratin positive using a broad cytokeratin cocktail and an initial small panel may also include S-100 and CD45. Subsequent to that determination, other cytokeratin pairings such as CK7 and CK20 or CK5/6 and p63 will help separate out the entities such as Merkel cell carcinoma and basaloid squamous cell carcinoma. TTF-1 positivity should not be relied upon to distinguish a primary pulmonary small cell carcinoma from an extrapulmonary site and "crush artifact" should never be considered diagnostic for small cell carcinoma (*Figure 10-6P-S*). Nevertheless, while the histologic appearance of small cell carcinoma is virtually identical regardless of the primary site, the clinical circumstances and radiologic appearance are rarely so confusing. The vast majority of pulmonary small cell lung carcinomas occur in patients with a significant smoking history and the usual patient presents with advanced stage disease. Most small cell carcinomas of the lung are centrally located and have significant associated mediastinal lymph node adenopathy. The typical radiographic appearance of metastatic small cell carcinoma from an extrapulmonary site is multiple pulmonary nodules without mediastinal lymph node enlargement. Conspicuous or dominant mediastinal/pleural masses, particularly in a patient without a classic history for a primary pulmonary small cell carcinoma, is often an indication for a more extensive immunohistochemical panel where stains such as desmin, WT-1, and CD99 might be added. As with better differentiated neuroendocrine tumors, the use of immunohistochemical stains to confirm neuroendocrine differentiation (chromogranin, synaptophysin, and CD56) is a potential pitfall if it is not correlated with other immunohistochemical stains that support tumor lineage. Many entities in the malignant small round cell tumor category show variable positivity with neuroendocrine markers and the occasional small cell carcinoma may be negative for these markers.

Colorectal Carcinomas

The lung is the most common extra-abdominal site of metastasis for colorectal carcinoma and it is important to recognize that pulmonary metastasis can and does occur in the absence of metastatic disease to the liver (*Table 10-8*). Compared to colonic adenocarcinoma,

Table 10-8 Colorectal Carcinomas

- Lung most common extra-abdominal site of metastasis for colorectal carcinoma
- Pulmonary metastasis can occur in the absence of metastatic disease to the liver
- Metastatic colorectal carcinoma most frequent as a solitary nodule or multiple nodules
- Usual confirmatory immunohistochemical panel includes TTF-1, CDX2, CK7, and CK20
- In some cases, distinguishing a pulmonary primary from a metastatic colorectal primary can be challenging
- Variants of primary pulmonary adenocarcinomas include enteric differentiation (PAED), numerous signet ring cells, or colloid adenocarcinoma
- In these mucinous variants of pulmonary adenocarcinoma, immunohistochemistry may be of no utility and the diagnosis must be integrated with the clinical and radiologic findings

rectal carcinomas have a higher risk of developing lung metastases.[44] One large epidemiologic study that focused on survival data following pulmonary metastasectomy reported about an 11% incidence of synchronous lung metastasis and about a 6% 5-year cumulative rate of metachronous lung metastasis.[44] Metastatic colorectal carcinoma is most frequently encountered as a solitary nodule or multiple nodules. Endobronchial disease is far less frequent but should be considered in the differential diagnosis of an adenocarcinoma involving the airway in the appropriate clinical setting (*Figure 10-7A*). Although intrathoracic lymph node metastasis is also far less frequent, there is a significant incidence of regional lymph node metastasis in the patient in pulmonary resections for metastatic disease.[45] In many instances, the confirmation of metastatic disease is straightforward—particularly when integrated with the clinical history and radiographic information (*Figure 10-7B and C*). Though by no means pathognomonic, necrosis is typical of metastatic colorectal primaries. The usual confirmatory immunohistochemical panel includes TTF-1, CDX2, CK7, and CK20 (*Figure 10-7D-H*). Nevertheless, distinguishing a pulmonary primary from a metastatic colorectal primary can be challenging, given the number of histologic variants in both sites and the overlap in immunohistochemical profiles. Primary pulmonary adenocarcinomas can show extensive enteric differentiation (PAED) or consist of numerous signet ring cells or appear as a colloid adenocarcinoma.[21,46] In these mucinous variants of pulmonary adenocarcinoma, immunohistochemistry may be of no utility in distinguishing between the two primary sites and the diagnosis typically will default to clinical and radiologic correlation.

CHAPTER 10

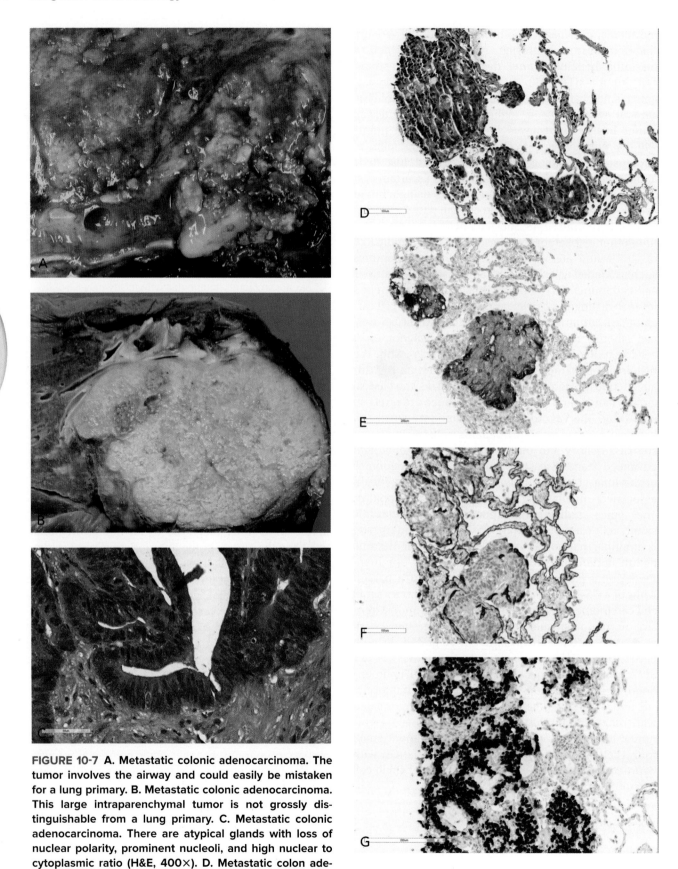

FIGURE 10-7 A. Metastatic colonic adenocarcinoma. The tumor involves the airway and could easily be mistaken for a lung primary. **B.** Metastatic colonic adenocarcinoma. This large intraparenchymal tumor is not grossly distinguishable from a lung primary. **C.** Metastatic colonic adenocarcinoma. There are atypical glands with loss of nuclear polarity, prominent nucleoli, and high nuclear to cytoplasmic ratio (H&E, 400×). **D.** Metastatic colon adenocarcinoma in lung (H&E, 200×). **E.** Metastatic colonic adenocarcinoma in lung. The tumor cells are CK20 positive, supporting the diagnosis (200×). **F.** Metastatic colonic adenocarcinoma in lung. The tumor cells are CK7 negative, supporting the diagnosis (200×).

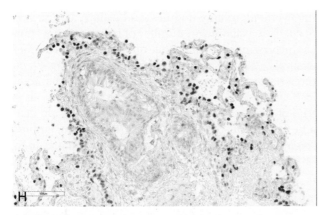

FIGURE 10-7 (*Continued*) **G. Metastatic colonic adeno-carcinoma in lung. The tumor cells are CDX2 positive, supporting the diagnosis (200×). H. Metastatic colonic adenocarcinoma in lung. The tumor cells are TTF-1 negative, supporting the diagnosis (200×).**

Head and Neck

A pulmonary nodule in a patient with a (usually) known head and neck primary is a common diagnostic dilemma (*Table 10-9*). This section focuses on the most common histology of head and neck squamous cell carcinoma (HNSCC); tumors with salivary gland features will be covered in a subsequent section. Aside from a clearcut transition from in situ to invasive squamous cell carcinoma, there is no other conclusive morphologic means of differentiating a primary pulmonary squamous cell carcinoma from a head and neck squamous cell carcinoma metastasis. Given that this feature is rarely present in small samplings or even larger resections, it is essential to integrate the clinical history and radiologic studies into the final diagnostic interpretation. The epidemiology of HNSCC has changed over the past 20 years with a rise in disease associated with human papillomavirus (HPV) and a decline in tobacco-related disease. Simultaneous, synchronous, or metachronous pulmonary tumors is an ongoing management issue, particularly given the increased survival rates in heads and neck patients.[47] The presence or absence of cervical lymph node metastases is relevant as is the appearance and location of the lung lesion and the hilar/mediastinal lymph node status. Most patients with HNSCC develop cervical lymph node metastasis prior to pulmonary disease. The disease-free interval is also considered. A new lung primary is conventionally favored after 2 to 5 years; however, late metastasis from an HNSCC does occur. For a solitary pulmonary nodule, the usual strategy in operable patients is resection with pathologic evaluation (*Figure 10-8*). Even after the pulmonary nodule is resected, histologic and immuno-histochemical evaluation are most often of no utility. There are studies that have proposed various molecular

Table 10-9 Head and Neck Squamous Cell Carcinoma

- A solitary pulmonary nodule in a patient with known head and neck primary a common diagnostic dilemma
- Aside from a clearcut transition from in situ to invasive squamous cell carcinoma, there is no other conclusive morphologic means of differentiating a primary pulmonary squamous cell carcinoma from a head and neck squamous cell carcinoma metastasis
- Essential to integrate the clinical history and radiologic studies into the final diagnostic interpretation
- Epidemiology of HNSCC has changed with a rise in disease associated with human papillomavirus (HPV) and a decline in tobacco-related disease
- Presence or absence of cervical lymph node metastases relevant as is appearance and location of the lung lesion and the hilar/mediastinal lymph node status
- Most patients with HNSqCC develop cervical lymph node metastasis prior to pulmonary disease
- Disease-free interval important with a new lung primary conventionally favored after 2-5 years
- Late metastasis from an HNSCC does occur
- For a solitary pulmonary nodule, the usual strategy in operable patients is resection with pathologic evaluation
- It is possible in equivocal clinicopathological circumstances and when the distinction is critical for treatment or prognosis to use clonality studies for distinguishing a pulmonary primary from HNSCC metastasis

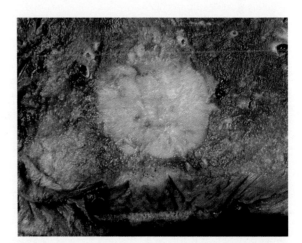

FIGURE 10-8 **Metastatic squamous cell carcinoma. The patient, a former 60 pack-year smoker, presented with a tonsillar primary 2 years prior, which was treated with resection and neck dissection as well as chemotherapy and XRT. The primary tumor was high-grade and nonke-ratinizing with focal spindle cell features. Angiolymphatic invasion was noted at the time within the primary and multiple nodes were positive. The resected left lower lobe lung nodule was histologically identical with prominent lymphovascular invasion and was diagnosed as metastatic squamous cell carcinoma.**

strategies to separate a primary squamous cell carcinoma of the lung from a metastasis from the head and neck but these techniques have not been incorporated into robust routine clinical assays. It is possible in equivocal clinicopathological circumstances and when the distinction is critical for treatment or prognosis to use clonality studies for differentiation.[48] High-risk HPV in situ hybridization has been proposed as a means of analyzing tumors in patients with oropharyngeal squamous cell carcinoma who develop a squamous cell carcinoma in their lungs.[49]

Malignant Melanoma

Primary pulmonary melanomas have been reported, but they are exceptionally rare and the majority of melanomas diagnosed in the lung are metastatic or presumed to be metastatic (*Table 10-10*). The usual presentation is multiple intrapulmonary nodules but other patterns such as lymphangitic spread, endobronchial

involvement, miliary nodules, and solitary nodules do occur.[50] In a significant number of instances, the clinical history may be somewhat remote and obscure, for example, "skin lesion of back removed years ago," and often only offered upon further inquiry by the pathologist. Other than a tendency for circumscription—as is true of many other metastatic tumors—there are usually no specific gross features to suggest melanoma (*Figure 10-9A and B*). On occasion, pigmentation may be grossly obvious and can be seen microscopically. In

Table 10-10 Malignant Melanoma

- The vast majority of melanomas diagnosed in the lung are metastatic
- Multiple intrapulmonary nodules are the usual presentation
- Other patterns such as lymphangitic spread, endobronchial involvement, miliary nodules, and solitary nodules do occur
- Metastatic melanoma is often amelanotic and misdiagnosis best avoided by a high degree of suspicion when encountering any poorly differentiated tumor of the lung—whether epithelioid, sarcomatoid, biphasic, or malignant small round cell in appearance
- In a patient with a known history of melanoma, even a solitary pulmonary nodule should be considered suspicious for metastasis until proven otherwise
- Any tumor that proves to be TTF-1, CK7, CK5/6, and p63 (or p40) negative should not be automatically assumed to be a poorly differentiated nonsmall cell carcinoma
- Immunohistochemical panel should include a robust cytokeratin cocktail and an expanded panel of markers such as S-100, HMB-45, and Melan-A/MART-1
- A small percentage of melanomas can be focally cytokeratin positive or S-100 negative and some lung carcinomas may be S-100 positive
- Some melanomas can be p63 positive
- Over time and often with multiple courses of treatment, late metastatic disease may lose some degree of immunoreactivity with the more frequently used melanoma markers
- Other melanoma markers such as MITF-2, tyrosinase, or Sox-10 may be necessary when there is a high index of suspicion for metastatic melanoma

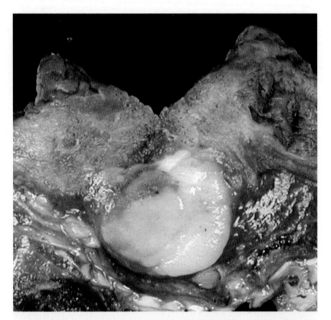

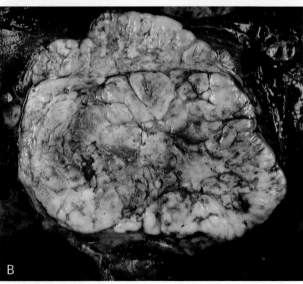

FIGURE 10-9 A. Metastatic malignant melanoma. Solitary pulmonary nodule without any remarkable gross features. The circumscription of the nodule would certainly raise the possibility of metastatic disease. B. Metastatic malignant melanoma. Large mass without any remarkable gross features that would help in the distinction from a lung primary.

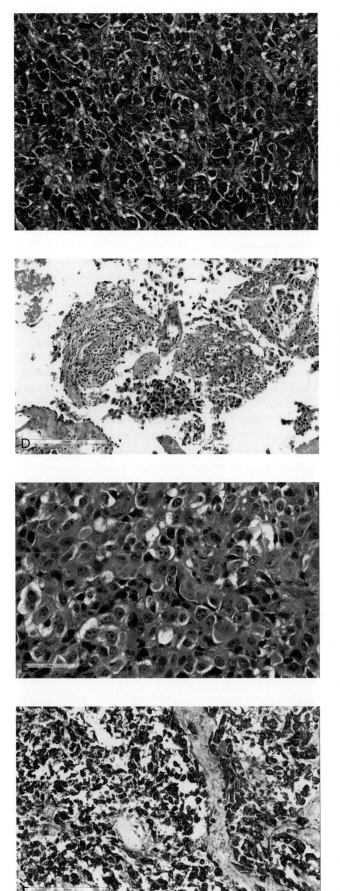

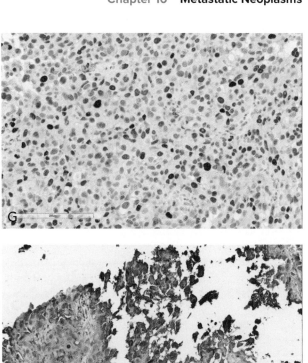

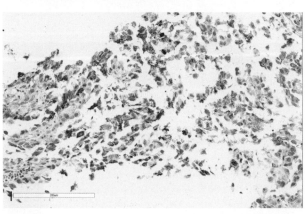

CHAPTER 10

FIGURE 10-9 (*Continued*) **C.** Metastatic melanoma. Large epithelioid tumor cells with obvious melanin pigment (H&E, 200×). **D.** Metastatic malignant melanoma. Endobronchial biopsy showing clusters of poorly differentiated epithelioid tumor cells (H&E, 200×). **E.** Metastatic malignant melanoma. Higher magnification of better preserved area showing pleomorphic epithelioid tumor cells with vesicular nuclei and prominent nucleoli. There is no evidence of melanin pigment (H&E, 400×). **F.** Metastatic malignant melanoma. Positive staining using a sensitive cytokeratin cocktail is a potential pitfall (pancytokeratin, 200×). **G.** Metastatic malignant melanoma. Positive p63 staining is a potential pitfall (p63, 200×). **H.** Metastatic malignant melanoma. An additional panel of three affirmative melanoma markers (see I and J) and less sensitive cytokeratin cocktail (K) confirm the diagnosis of metastatic malignant melanoma (S-100, 200×). **I.** Metastatic malignant melanoma. The tumor cells are positive for **HMB45** (200×).

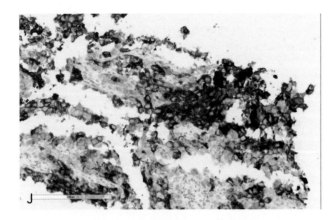

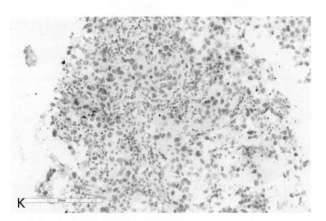

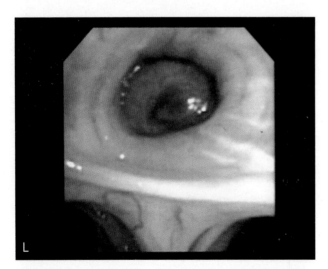

FIGURE 10-9 (*Continued*) J. Metastatic malignant mela-noma. The tumor cells are positive for Melan A (200×). K. Metastatic malignant melanoma. The tumor cells are negative for AE1/3 (200×). L. Endobronchial tumor diag-nosed as metastatic malignant melanoma. Following histopathologic confirmation of melanoma (D-K), the phy-sician requested further history from the patient (who had previously reported only a history of "skin cancer") and the physician re-reviewed the bronchoscopic findings that in retrospect suggested a more unusual endobronchial nodule.

this instance, metastatic melanoma is readily diagnosed by the identification of melanin within the tumor and confirmed by immunohistochemistry (*Figure 10-9C*). Unfortunately metastatic melanoma is often amelanotic and misdiagnosis is best avoided by a high degree of suspicion when encountering any poorly differentiated tumor of the lung—whether epithelioid, sarcomatoid, biphasic, or malignant small round cell in appearance. In a patient with a known history of melanoma, even a solitary pulmonary nodule should be considered suspi-cious for metastasis until proven otherwise. Although limited immunohistochemical panels on small samples are to be encouraged for tissue preservation and subse-quent molecular studies, it is easy to get into difficulties when the selection of immunohistochemical stains is too restricted. Any tumor that proves to be TTF-1, CK7, CK5/6, and p63 (or p40) negative should not be auto-matically assumed to be a poorly differentiated nons-mall cell carcinoma. Conversely, strong p63 staining alone should not be taken as confirmation of squamous differentiation. In these instances, the next step should be a robust cytokeratin cocktail and an expanded panel of markers such as S-100, HMB-45, and Melan-A/ MART-1. As with any immunohistochemical panel, exception to these general rules must be kept in mind. A small percentage of melanomas can be focally cyto-keratin positive or S-100 negative and some lung carci-nomas may be S-100 positive (*Figure 10-9D-L*).[19] Some melanomas can be p63 positive.[51] Finally, it should be noted that over time and often with multiple courses of treatment, late metastatic disease may lose some degree of immunoreactivity with the more frequently used markers (S-100, HMB-45, and Melan A). Other markers such as MITF-2, tyrosinase, or Sox-10 may be necessary when there is a high index of suspicion. Sox-10 has been shown to have slightly higher sensitivity for detection of invasive melanoma (97%), as compared with S100 (91%).[52]

Renal Cell Carcinoma

Renal cell carcinoma (RCC) is one of the most common tumors to metastasize to the lung—both at the time of initial diagnosis and many years after the initial primary presentation (*Table 10-11*). Metastases may present as a solitary pulmonary nodule or as multiple intra-parenchymal nodules. Renal cell carcinoma is one of the most common tumors to present as an endobron-chial lesion, often as a late manifestation of the disease (*Figure 10-10A*).[53] If available, comparison with the pri-mary renal cell tumor is helpful but in some instances many years will have passed and the primary may not be available for comparison. Immunohistochemistry is recommended for renal tumor histologic subtyping

Table 10-11 Renal Cell Carcinoma

- Renal cell carcinoma (RCC) is one of the most common tumors to metastasize to the lung—both at the time of initial diagnosis and many years after the initial primary diagnosis
- Metastases may present as a solitary pulmonary nodule or as multiple intraparenchymal nodules
- Renal cell carcinoma is one of the most common tumors to present as an endobronchial lesion, often as a late manifestation of the disease
- Immunohistochemistry is recommended for renal tumor histologic subtyping with the confirmatory immunohistochemical panel varying according to histologic subtype
- The diversity of renal tumor histologic subtypes must be considered when deciding on an appropriate immunohistochemical panel to confirm or exclude metastasis
- Common clear cell renal cell carcinomas are typically positive for RCC and PAX 2 or 8
- Both PAX2 and PAX8 are diagnostically useful markers for metastatic renal tumors
- PAX8 appears to be more sensitive but adding PAX2 occasionally increases the diagnostic yield in a small subset of metastatic RCCs
- Positivity for PAX2 and PAX8 will vary more among other subtypes such as chromophobe RCC or collecting duct RCC
- TTF-1 has good sensitivity and specificity if the differential diagnosis is a lung primary
- Napsin A has no discriminatory value if the differential diagnosis is a lung primary

with the confirmatory immunohistochemical panel varying according to histologic subtype.[54] This diversity of renal tumor histologic subtypes must be considered when deciding on an appropriate immunohistochemical panel to confirm or exclude metastasis. Common clear cell renal cell carcinomas are typically positive for RCC(m), and PAX 2 or 8 (*Figure 10-10B-F*). Positivity for PAX2 and PAX8 will vary more among other subtypes such as chromophobe RCC or collecting duct RCC.[55] Both PAX2 and PAX8 are diagnostically useful markers for metastatic renal tumors. PAX8 appears to be more sensitive but adding PAX2 occasionally increases the diagnostic yield in a small subset of metastatic RCCs.

Breast

Involvement of the lung by mammary carcinoma is common, either at the time of presentation or after any years from the time of initial diagnosis (*Table 10-12*). Although parenchymal nodules are most frequently seen, lymphangitic spread, tumor emboli, endobronchial

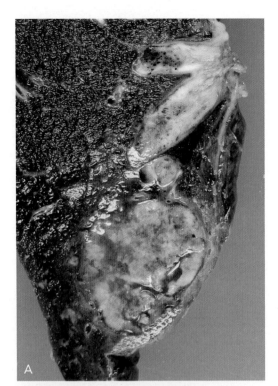

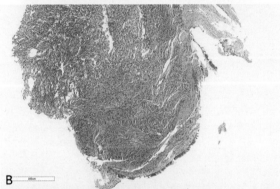

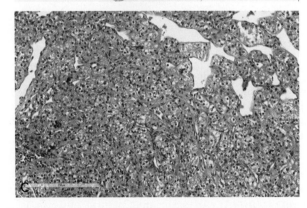

FIGURE 10-10 **A. Metastatic renal cell carcinoma. Note both the endobronchial component as well as the large intraparenchymal mass. B. Metastatic renal cell carcinoma. The tumor extensively involves the bronchial submucosa (H&E, 50×). C. Metastatic renal cell carcinoma. Conventional clear cell type (H&E, 200×).**

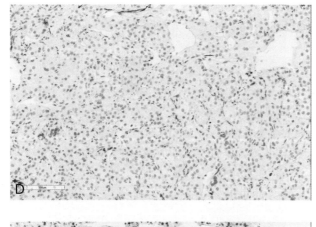

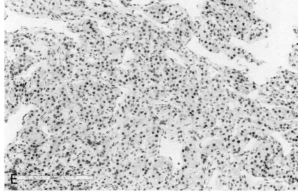

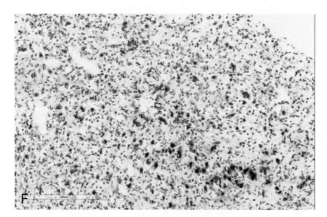

Table 10-12 Breast Carcinoma

- Involvement of the lung by mammary carcinoma is common, either at the time of presentation or after many years from the time of initial diagnosis
- Parenchymal nodules most frequently seen
- Breast carcinoma is one of the most common tumors to present as lymphangitic spread, tumor emboli, or endobronchial involvement
- Using latency is not a reliable criterion in determining the primary site
- Oligometastatic disease can be difficult to recognize and to confirm by immunohistochemistry
- Breast carcinomas can mimic any number of primary lung tumors including those with squamous or neuroendocrine differentiation as well as adenocarcinoma
- Direct histologic comparison with the breast primary is useful as well any information regarding the results of prior hormone receptor status with the caveat that the receptor status in the metastasis may not be concordant with the breast primary
- Breast carcinomas and pulmonary adenocarcinomas share the same cytokeratin (CK) 7 positive/ cytokeratin (CK) 20 negative profile and therefore other immunohistochemical markers must be used to support the site of origin
- Markers that are commonly used include TTF-1, Napsin A, gross cystic disease fluid protein-15, mammoglobin, estrogen receptor, and GATA3
- TTF-1 can be positive in a small percentage of breast carcinomas
- Estrogen and progesterone staining can be seen in both pulmonary adenocarcinomas as well as primary pulmonary neuroendocrine tumors
- GATA3 expression is a useful marker for metastatic breast carcinoma, particularly in triple-negative and metaplastic carcinomas

FIGURE 10-10 (*Continued*) **D. Metastatic renal cell carcinoma. The tumor cells are negative for CK7 (200×). E. Metastatic renal cell carcinoma. The tumor cells are positive for PAX8 (200×). F. Metastatic renal cell carcinoma. The tumor cells are positive for RCC (200×).**

involvement, and direct chest wall invasion do occur (*Figure 10-11A*). An associated pleural effusion is a prominent feature in about half of patients with metastatic breast carcinoma. In addition, there appears to be a true association of breast cancer and breast cancer treatment with lung cancer that is not confounded by misdiagnosis.[56] Using latency is not a reliable criterion for assignment of primary status and misdiagnosis has significant clinical implications. Oligometastatic

disease can be difficult to recognize and to confirm by immunohistochemistry. Breast carcinomas can mimic any number of primary lung tumors including those with squamous or neuroendocrine differentiation as well as adenocarcinoma. Direct histologic comparison with the breast primary is useful as well any information regarding the results of prior hormone receptor status with the caveat that the receptor status in the metastasis may not be concordant with the breast primary. Reported ER/PR receptor primary/metastatic tumor discordant estimates vary greatly with HER2 discordant status reported far less frequently.[57] Breast carcinomas and pulmonary adenocarcinomas share the same CK7-positive/CK20-negative profile and therefore other immunohistochemical markers must be used to support the site of origin. Markers that are commonly used include TTF-1, Napsin A, gross cystic disease fluid

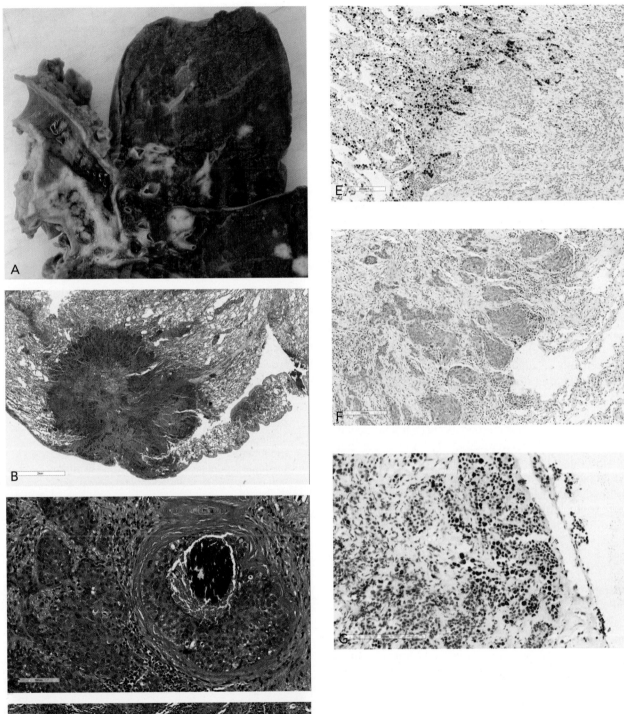

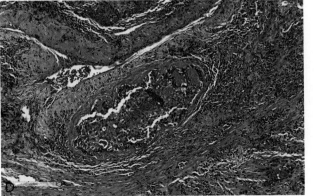

FIGURE 10-11 A. Metastatic breast carcinoma. Autopsy lung showing advanced disease with multiple parenchymal nodules as well as lymph node involvement. **B.** Metastatic breast carcinoma. Wedge resection showing relatively well-circumscribed subpleural nodule (H&E, 12×). **C.** Metastatic breast carcinoma. Nests of tumor cells with prominent comedo necrosis and calcifications (H&E, 200×). **D.** Metastatic breast carcinoma. Prominent lymphovascular invasion (H&E 100×). **E.** Metastatic breast carcinoma. Negative TTF-1 stain in tumor cells (100×). **F.** Metastatic breast carcinoma. BRST2 negative (100×). **G.** Metastatic breast carcinoma. Positive GATA3 (200×).

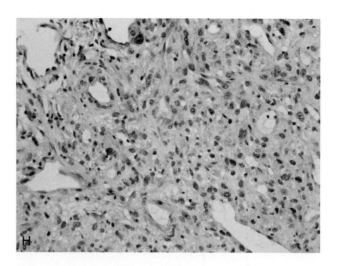

FIGURE 10-11 (*Continued*) H. This core needle biopsy of a very large pulmonary mass in a woman with a smoking history and a "history of breast cancer" was favored to be a primary sarcomatoid carcinoma on the basis of its large size and location. An extensive immunohistochemical panel was positive only for vimentin, CD68, D2-40, factor XIIIa (stromal), thrombomodulin (stromal), desmin (focal), and calretinin (focal). Multiple cytokeratins were negative. The prior slides were obtained and it was recognized that her "breast cancer" was a malignant phyllodes tumor that was identical to the lung mass (H&E, 200×).

protein-15, mammoglobin, estrogen receptor, and GATA3 (*Figure 10-11B-G*).[58,59] It should be noted that TTF-1 can be positive in a small percentage of breast carcinomas (2.4%), using one antibody clone that is commercially available and widely used.[14] Estrogen and progesterone staining can be seen in both pulmonary adenocarcinomas as well as primary pulmonary neuroendocrine tumors.[36,60] GATA3 expression can be useful as a marker for metastatic breast carcinoma, particularly in triple-negative and metaplastic carcinomas which tend to lack specific markers of breast origin.[61] Clarifying what type of "breast" cancer is essential. Although far less common, phyllodes tumors do metastasize to the lung and may mimic a sarcomatoid tumor (*Figure 10-11H*).

Prostate

Prostate specific markers are robust and should be liberally included in diagnostic panels, as it is certainly possible for a prostatic primary to be occult or clinically remote. The most common metastatic pattern for prostatic adenocarcinoma is lymphangitic spread with rare occasional instances of parenchymal nodules, endobronchial tumors, and lymph node metastases (*Table 10-13*). Characteristic histologic patterns of prostatic adenocarcinoma—microacinar, tubulopapillary (glandular), or carcinoid-like features—do overlap with primary pulmonary adenocarcinomas and neuroendocrine tumors (*Figure 10-12A and B*).[62] Careful attention to nuclear features (uniform round nuclei with prominent nucleoli) and cellular details (intraluminal blue mucin and prominent cell borders) may also prompt recognition in the instance of an occult or remote primary (*Figure 10-12C*). Metastatic prostatic duct adenocarcinoma shows histologic features similar to metastatic colonic adenocarcinoma. A high index of suspicion in any patient with a prior history

Table 10-13 Prostatic Adenocarcinoma

- Prostatic specific markers (prostate-specific antigen [PSA] and prostate-specific acid phosphatase [PSAP]) are robust and should be included in diagnostic panels when the clinical history or histology suggests the diagnosis
- The most common pattern for metastatic prostatic adenocarcinoma is lymphangitic spread
- Characteristic histologic patterns of prostatic adenocarcinoma—microacinar, tubulopapillary (glandular), or carcinoid-like features—overlap with primary pulmonary adenocarcinomas and neuroendocrine tumors
- Careful attention to nuclear features (uniform round nuclei with prominent nucleoli) and cellular details (intraluminal blue mucin and prominent cell borders) may also prompt recognition of prostatic adenocarcinoma in the instance of an occult or remote primary
- Metastatic prostatic duct adenocarcinoma shows histologic features similar to metastatic colonic adenocarcinoma
- Only a small percentage (<5%) of poorly differentiated prostatic adenocarcinomas are completely negative for all prostatic markers

of prostatic adenocarcinoma is important and, fortunately, positive staining for prostate-specific antigen (PSA) and prostate-specific acid phosphatase (PSAP) persists in the majority of metastatic prostatic adenocarcinomas. Given their high sensitivity and specificity, immunohistochemical stains are very reasonable to perform even when the histologic appearance does not obviously suggest a prostatic primary (*Figure 10-12D*). When properly titrated so that the positive PSA control appropriately shows strong staining of benign prostatic

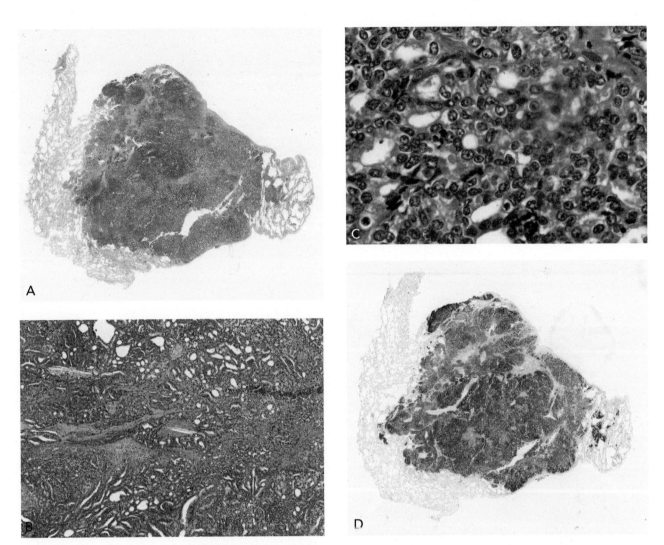

FIGURE 10-12 **A. Metastatic prostate cancer presenting as a solitary pulmonary nodule (H&E, 3×). B. Metastatic prostate cancer. There is prominent cribriform architecture and small glands, suggesting the diagnosis of prostatic adenocarcinoma (H&E, 40×). C. Metastatic prostate cancer. High power shows the round nuclei with prominent nucleoli (H&E, 400×). D. Metastatic prostate cancer. The tumor cells are strongly positive for PSA, confirming the diagnosis (3×).**

glands, strong focal cytoplasmic staining can be seen even in most poorly differentiated prostatic adenocarcinomas.[63] There is a small percentage (<5%) of poorly differentiated prostatic adenocarcinomas that are completely negative for all prostatic markers, and therefore, particularly in a small biopsy, the possibility of metastatic disease should not be excluded with a compelling clinical history.[64]

Sarcoma

In most instances of metastatic sarcoma to the lung, a previous history of a primary sarcoma is well known and there is no diagnostic difficulty (*Table 10-14*). Primary pulmonary sarcomas are rare and must be substantiated by obtaining the prior history and ascertaining that an extrapulmonary site has been clinically

and radiographically excluded. Radiographically and grossly, metastatic sarcomas are usually well circumscribed and solid. Solitary and multiple nodules are the most common patterns (*Figure 10-13A-E*). Cystic lesions, with or without pneumothorax, do occur and are a potential diagnostic pitfall. Another notable exception is angiosarcoma which can present as diffuse pulmonary hemorrhage or thromboembolic disease (*Figure 10-13F*). The histologic appearance of metastatic sarcomas may be less straightforward, particularly if the patient has had a protracted course with recurrences and additional therapy. Any number of high-grade sarcomas can show foci of osseous or cartilaginous differentiation, paucicellular fibrous areas, a hemangiocytoma-like pattern, and cystic hemorrhage. Extensive sampling of any sarcomatoid lesion in the lung is essential and, in these instances, it is best to

Table 10-14 Sarcomas

- In most instances of metastatic sarcoma to the lung, a previous history of a primary sarcoma is well known and there is no diagnostic difficulty
- Solitary and multiple nodules are the most common patterns
- Cystic sarcomas, with or without pneumothorax, are a potential diagnostic pitfall.
- Extensive sampling of any sarcomatoid lesion in the lung is essential and it is best to obtain the primary tumor for review and proper subclassification. The histologic appearance of metastatic sarcomas may change over time and with therapy
- Spindle cell lesions in women can be problematic, especially without an adequate gynecologic history
- Both high- and low-grade uterine smooth muscle tumors metastasize to the lung
- Smooth muscle or endometrial stromal sarcoma metastasis may present as cystic lung disease and represent potential mimics of pulmonary lymphangioleiomyomatosis. Knowledge of the clinical history, radiographic features, and a careful scrutiny of the histology along with a panel of immunohistochemical stains will be helpful in diagnostically difficult cases

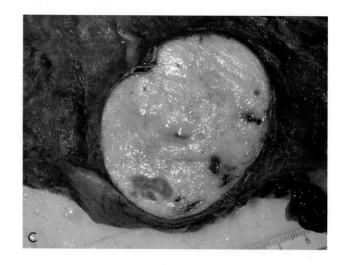

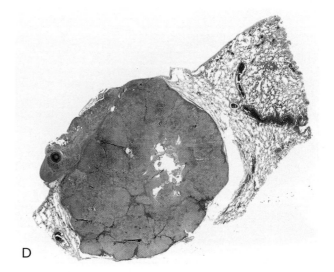

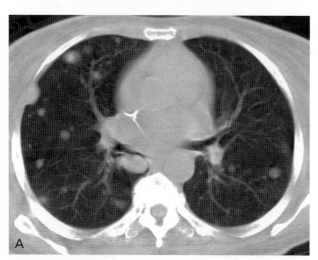

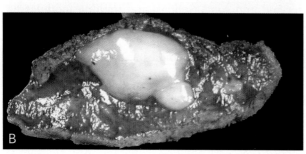

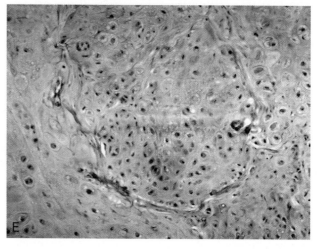

FIGURE 10-13 **A.** CT radiograph showing multiple nodules of metastatic sarcoma. (Used with permission of Wallace Miller Jr, Department of Radiology, Perelman School of Medicine at the University of Pennsylvania). **B.** Metastatic leiomyosarcoma. **C.** Metastatic sarcoma. The patient had a history of a primary gluteal sarcoma. The primary was not available for review and the patient had multiple treatment regimens. At autopsy, the tumor showed only focal smooth muscle differentiation. **D.** Metastatic chondrosarcoma (H &E, 10×). **E.** Metastatic chondrosarcoma. The lesion was composed entirely of malignant cartilage (H&E 100×).

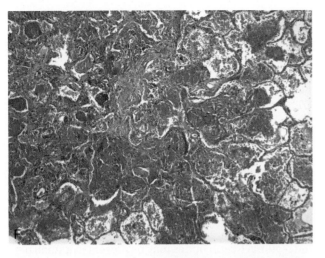

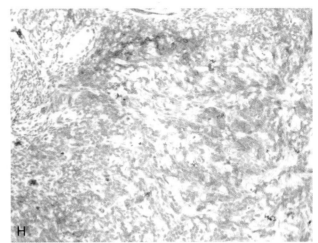

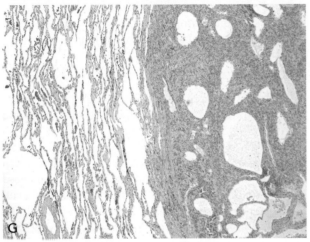

FIGURE 10-13 (*Continued*) F. Metastatic angiosarcoma. This pattern of organizing hemorrhage is typical of metastatic angiosarcoma and makes recognition of the malignant cells difficult (H&E, 50×). G. Metastatic endometrial stromal sarcoma (H&E, 50×). H. Metastatic endometrial sarcoma. The tumor cells are positive for CD10, supporting the diagnosis (200×).

obtain the primary tumor for review and proper sub-classification. Primary leiomyoma or leiomyosarcoma of the lung should be considered quite rare with the burden of proof focused on the rigorous exclusion of metastatic disease. Spindle cell lesions in women can be problematic, especially when a prior gynecologic history is either unknown or dismissed. Both high-grade and low-grade uterine smooth muscle tumors metastasize to the lung. These patients are generally asymptomatic and present with an incidental radiographic finding of solitary or multiple rounded opacities. The entity of "benign metastasizing leiomyoma" with its entirely bland histologic appearance has generated controversy over the years. Current evidence supports the concept that these low-grade smooth muscle neoplasms are metastatic rather than a primary benign tumor.[65-68] It is speculated that some cases represent metastases from very a well-differentiated uterine leiomyosarcoma and some may be the result of intravascular leiomyomatosis of the uterus or from embolization during myomectomy. Also in women, smooth muscle or endometrial stromal sarcoma metastasis may

present as cystic lung disease and represent potential mimics of the cystic interstitial lung disease, pulmonary lymphangioleiomyomatosis. Knowledge of the clinical history, radiographic features, and a careful scrutiny of the histology along with a panel of immunohistochemical stains will be helpful in diagnostically difficult cases. An immunohistochemical panel that includes smooth muscle actin, desmin, HMB-45, ER/PR receptors, and CD10 is useful in distinguishing these entities (*Figure 10-13G and H*).[69]

Other

The preceding sections have provided details on common metastatic tumors, particularly those that are likely to be resected for diagnostic and/or therapeutic purposes. The focus has also been on tumors that are most likely to present with late metastatic disease in which the prior history of malignancy and the latency period tend to be discounted. Other organ sites were not covered in more detail because of low incidence or the likelihood of presenting with more obvious clinical history and pulmonary involvement in the setting of widespread disease. Ovarian, endometrial, hepatocellular, and nonseminomatous testicular germ cell tumors fall into this latter category. Although there is no substitute for an astute histologic evaluation that incorporates a rational panel of immunohistochemical stains, diagnostic errors will be further reduced by attention to the clinical history and the review of prior material.

MALIGNANT SALIVARY GLAND–TYPE TRACHEOBRONCHIAL TUMORS

The mixed seromucinous glands that are found in the submucosa of the trachea and large bronchi are believed to give rise to a variety of salivary gland–like tumors, histologically indistinguishable from their major salivary gland counterparts. Salivary gland carcinomas represent less than 1% of all lung carcinomas, with mucoepidermoid carcinoma and adenoid cystic carcinoma being the most common subtypes.[70] The clinical presentation and growth pattern make these primary salivary gland–type tumors of the lung a distinctive subgroup of epithelial tumors of the lung. The characteristic pattern of central airway involvement is of major significance in distinguishing these tumors from metastasis from a salivary gland primary. Most metastases from primary salivary gland carcinomas are located in the peripheral lung and usually represent late disease. A specific awareness of these primary pulmonary tumors will avoid a misdiagnosis of metastatic disease, despite the complete overlap in morphology. As important, the recognition of these tumors and their separation from other nonsmall lung carcinomas has significant therapeutic and prognostic implications.

Adenoid Cystic Carcinoma

Clinical features of adenoid cystic carcinoma

Adenoid cystic carcinoma is quite rare, representing less than 0.2% of all primary lung tumors[70] The tumor typically presents in the fourth and fifth decades of life but there is a wide age range from young adults to older patients. There is an equal gender distribution. A majority of cases originate intraluminally with only a few peripheral cases reported. The typical presenting symptoms such as wheezing, progressive dyspnea, stridor, cough, and hemoptysis reflect the intraluminal tumor growth. Long-term survival can be achieved with adequate resection but local late (greater than 10 years) recurrences do occur following resection.[71-74] The most common site of disseminated disease is the lung parenchyma itself.

Imaging features of adenoid cystic carcinoma

The most frequent locations of primary pulmonary adenoid cystic carcinomas are in the lower trachea, mainstem bronchi, and the lobar bronchi (*Figure 10-14A*).[75] Routine radiographs are usually interpreted as normal. CT scans demonstrate an intraluminal mass of soft-tissue attenuation with submucosal involvement and extension through the tracheal wall, a diffuse or circumferential airway wall thickening, a soft-tissue mass filling the airway, or a homogeneous mass encircling the airway with wall thickening in the transverse and longitudinal planes. The intraluminal mass is variable in shape and can be either polypoid or broad based with smooth, lobulated, or irregular margins. Metastasis to the regional lymph nodes may be present in a small percentage of cases at the time of diagnosis. Tumor in the lobar or segmental bronchi may show distal atelectasis, postobstructive pneumonia, or air trapping.

Gross features of adenoid cystic carcinoma

Adenoid cystic carcinoma has a variable growth pattern. Some tumors are grossly nodular and exophytic with minimal invasion of the bronchus, whereas others have a mixed nodular/infiltrative or predominantly infiltrative growth pattern (*Figure 10-14B*). The intraluminal mass can have smooth, irregular, or lobulated borders and the mass often infiltrates the airway wall. Some tumors cause localized circumferential thickening of the airway wall or multifocal narrowing with generalized airway constriction. There may be lymph node involvement, usually by direct extension, and some tumors have a tendency to radially spread into the adjacent parenchyma rather than along the airways. The microscopic extent of invasion nearly always exceeds that which is grossly apparent. By contrast, metastatic lesions are usually peripheral.

Histologic features of adenoid cystic carcinoma

The tumor cells are small with a relatively high nuclear/cytoplasmic ratio but nuclear pleomorphism and mitoses are rare. Characteristic mucinous cysts of varying size are present within the tubular and cribriform patterns. Poorly differentiated tumors have a significant component of solid tumor nests (*Figure 10-14B-E*). Like their salivary gland counterparts, adenoid cystic carcinomas show conspicuous perineural invasion. Until recently there were no reports of TTF-1 positivity in adenoid cystic carcinomas from any primary site or in subsequent metastasis. One study of 12 cases has now reported TTF-1 positivity in adenoid cystic carcinomas metastatic to the lung but no TTF-1 positivity in any of the primary sites (including three lung primaries).[76] The study used two different TTF-1 antibody clones and

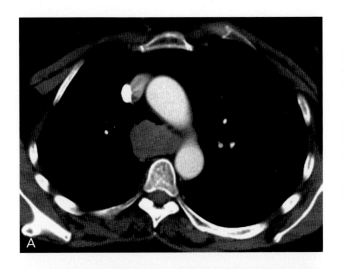

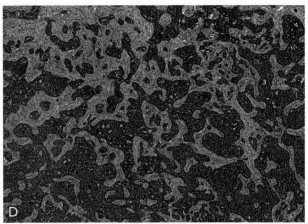

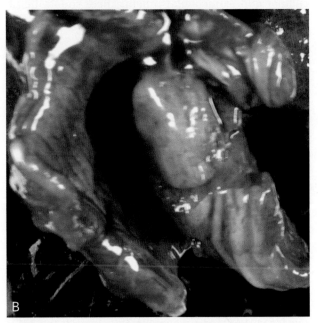

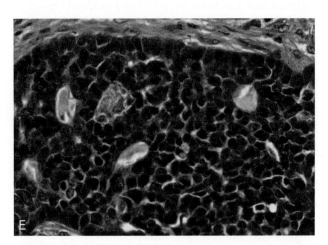

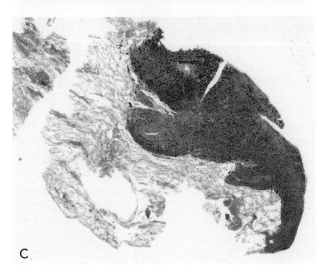

FIGURE 10-14 **A. CT** scan showing adenoid cystic carcinoma of trachea. (Used with permission of Wallace Miller Jr, Department of Radiology, Perelman School of Medicine at the University of Pennsylvania). **B.** Primary pulmonary adenoid cystic carcinoma. Left upper lobe sleeve lobectomy showing the polypoid endobronchial component. Microscopically, the tumor extended beyond the bronchial wall cartilage and into the underlying peribronchial soft tissue with perineural invasion. **C.** Metastatic adenoid cystic carcinoma from a salivary gland carcinoma of the tongue. The solitary 2.6 cm parenchymal nodule is peripherally located with significant visceral pleural invasion (H&E, 3×). **D.** Metastatic adenoid cystic carcinoma from a salivary gland carcinoma of the tongue. Although a focal cribriform and tubular pattern can be appreciated, most of the tumor c ells are arranged in solid nests, as is typical in higher grade lesions (H&E, 40×). **E.** Metastatic adenoid cystic carcinoma from a salivary gland carcinoma of the tongue. High power showing the relative uniformity of the tumor cells and a relatively high nuclear/cytoplasmic ratio. Nuclear pleomorphism and mitoses are rare. The histologic features are otherwise indistinguishable from a primary pulmonary tumor (H&E, 400×).

the micrographs show staining within the center of the metastatic tumors in the lung that does not appear to be from entrapped pneumocytes. The significance of this finding is unclear.

Mucoepidermoid Carcinoma

Clinical features of mucoepidermoid carcinoma

Mucoepidermoid carcinomas account for approximately 0.1% to 0.2% of lung cancers.[70,77] The age at presentation is variable but almost half of patients with mucoepidermoid carcinoma occur in patients under 30 years of age and it is a common tumor in the pediatric population. There is no gender predilection. Some patients with this tumor may be asymptomatic but classically patients present with symptoms of bronchial obstruction due to the tumor's characteristic endobronchial location. Symptoms include wheezing, cough, hemoptysis, and episodes of postobstructive pneumonia. There are two grading systems that have been used to categorize these tumors.[78,79] Both classifications clearly demonstrate that lower grade tumors, which are usually confined to the bronchus and only rarely have regional lymph node metastasis, have an excellent prognosis following complete excision. Higher grade tumors can have a more aggressive course and the data suggest that closer long-term clinical follow-up is indicated for these patients.[72-74,80] t(11;19)(q21;p13) is characteristic of mucoepidermoid carcinoma both within the salivary gland and in other organ sites including the lung.[81] FISH to detect MAML2 rearrangement using a MAML2-11q21 break-apart probe can be used to support a diagnosis of mucoepidermoid carcinoma in the lung.[80]

Imaging features of mucoepidermoid carcinoma

Although the CT manifestations are variable and nonspecific, the common finding is a central solitary well-defined ovoid or rounded intraluminal mass.[82] Distal pneumonia or atelectasis is typical, although the radiographic findings may be subtle and identified only in retrospect.

Gross features of mucoepidermoid carcinoma

Mucoepidermoid carcinomas usually arise from the segmental and subsegmental bronchi, but can involve the trachea as well (*Figure 10-15A*). They range in size from a few millimeters to up to 6 cm and grow as polypoid masses with a tan or gray surface. On cross-section, the tumor may appear more mucoid or cystic than the more common nonsmall cell carcinomas of the lung.

Histologic features of mucoepidermoid carcinoma

Initial pathology-based evaluations of pulmonary mucoepidermoid carcinoma divided the tumors into low- and high-grade tumors and this was incorporated into the current 2004 WHO classification.[1] Other studies have used the Brandwein classification for salivary gland tumors that sets forth criteria for low-, intermediate-, and high-grade tumors. By definition, the tumor is composed of a variable number of mucin-secreting, squamous and intermediate cells (*Figure 10-15B-D*). The intermediate cells have a polygonal shape and eosinophilic cytoplasm, but lack obvious squamous or glandular differentiation. The mucinous component consists of well-differentiated glands, with both intracellular and extracellular mucin. There should be no keratinization, squamous pearl formation, or an overlying in situ squamous cell carcinoma component. Some tumors are associated with a prominent lymphocytic infiltrate.[83] The Brandwein classification assigns a point value for specific histologic features such as <25% cystic component.[79] In a large and well-characterized pathology series, an intermediate grade was assigned largely because of tumor invasion in small nests and islands but occasionally due to a limited intracystic component.[80] This series also looked at immunohistochemical staining patterns and incorporate FISH analysis for MALM2 rearrangement. As in other series, the pulmonary mucoepidermoid tumors were TTF-1 negative. P63 and p40 staining was present but variable. It may be difficult to distinguish mucoepidermoid carcinoma from other tumors, particularly in a small sampling. It is useful to note that all of the tumors in this series that were reconfirmed to be mucoepidermoid carcinoma upon careful histologic review were positive for MALM2 rearrangement. This suggests that FISH to detect MAML2 rearrangement may have diagnostic utility in difficult cases.

PLEUROPULMONARY THYMOMA

Thymomas are tumors that are derived from the epithelial elements of the thymus and represent the most common tumor of the anterior mediastinum. Although metastatic thymoma to the lung or pleura is more common and should certainly be considered in a patient with a large anterior mediastinal mass or a prior history of mediastinal thymoma, primary pleural or primary intrapulmonary thymomas have been documented.[84-96] These tumors are rare and generally believed to arise from ectopic thymic tissue in the pleura or pulmonary parenchyma.[97] In some of the initial reports, it is difficult to exclude the possibility of a primary mediastinal mass but subsequent studies have made it clear

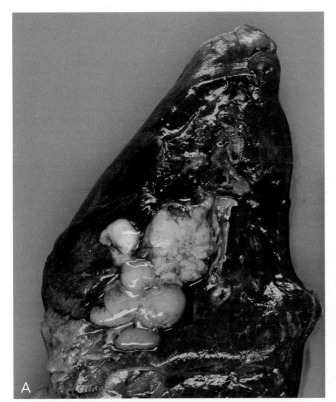

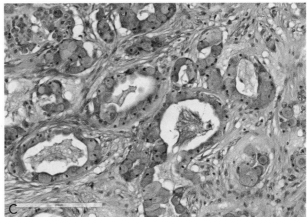

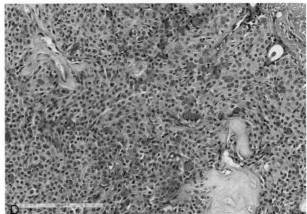

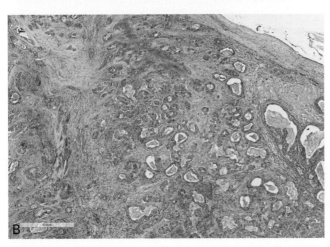

FIGURE 10-15 A. Primary pulmonary mucoepidermoid carcinoma. Right lower lobectomy showing a large endobronchial tumor with significant distal mucus plugging. B. Primary pulmonary mucoepidermoid carcinoma. There is an admixture of well-differentiated mucinous glands and an intermediate cell component involving the bronchial submucosa (H&E 40×). C. Primary pulmonary mucoepidermoid carcinoma. Well-differentiated mucinous glands with both intracellular and extracellular mucin (H&E, 200×). D. Primary pulmonary mucoepidermoid carcinoma. Intermediate cell component with polygonal cells containing eosinophilic cytoplasm and without cytologic atypia. There is no keratinization or squamous pearl formation (H&E, 200×).

that primary pulmonary and pleural thymomas, histologically indistinguishable from classic mediastinal thymomas, do exist. As always, the diagnosis rests on thorough correlation with the clinicoradiologic findings as well as careful gross examination of any resected specimen.

Clinical Features of Pleuropulmonary Thymoma

Primary pulmonary thymomas most commonly present as an incidentally discovered radiographic mass, with a minority presenting with hemoptysis, recurrent pneumonia, chest pain or in association with

paraneoplastic syndromes such as myasthenia gravis or Good syndrome. The median age of presentation was 50, with a range from 14 to 77 years and a roughly equal gender distribution. The absence of a primary mediastinal mass was documented either radiographically or by surgical exploration.

Primary pleural thymomas have presented in patients as increasing dyspnea, chest pain, or nonspecific symptoms such as fever and weight loss. An occasional patient was asymptomatic. In the limited number of cases that have been reported, the median decade of presentation was the sixth with an age range from 19 to 75 years and an equal gender distribution.

CHAPTER 10

Imaging Features of Pleuropulmonary Thymoma

The majority of primary pulmonary thymomas have been reported as peripheral lesions with a few localized to the hilum. Two were reported as unilateral but multifocal. The tumors ranged in size from 1.5 to almost 13 cm, with a median of 3 cm. Primary pleural thymomas can present as diffuse pleural thickening, a solitary ill-defined pleural mass or a large pleural effusion. Encasement of the lung can be partial or extensive, mimicking malignant mesothelioma.

Gross Features of Pleuropulmonary Thymoma

Gross descriptions are limited and consist of a non-specific description of firm tissue with a white to tan/yellow-gray appearance. The gross growth patterns reflect the previously described imaging features.

Histologic Features of Pleuropulmonary Thymoma

It is typically the low power appearance of prominent lobular architecture or organoid pattern as well as the characteristic fibrous bands that prompt initial consideration of the diagnosis of thymoma. On higher power, a dense and prominent lymphoid component along with the neoplastic epithelial component can be appreciated. Immunohistochemical stains can be used to characterize the background lymphoid population and cytokeratin stains can be used to highlight the epithelial component. Pleuropulmonary thymomas of all thymoma histologic subtypes (WHO A, AB, B1, B2, and B3) have been reported and the differential diagnosis will therefore vary depending on the thymic epithelial tumor subtype and the tumor location.[1] Focal membranous staining of thymic epithelial cells with CD20 as well as a lack of calretinin nuclear positivity are the main findings which favor a diagnosis of a thymic epithelial tumor over malignant mesothelioma.[95] Unlike their mediastinal counterparts, these tumors are frequently not encapsulated and therefore the usual staging criteria for thymomas cannot be applied. The limited number of cases with a variable degree of follow-up makes it difficult to draw statistically valid conclusions about long-term prognosis.

SUMMARY

The usual types of metastatic tumor spread in the lung and the typical presentation of metastases from the most common primary sites have been reviewed. Diagnostic errors can be avoided by careful consideration of the histopathologic features in conjunction with adequate clinical history and radiologic interpretation. An awareness of unusual subtypes of common tumors as well as unusual clinical circumstances will further enhance diagnostic accuracy.

REFERENCES

1. Travis WD, Brambilla E, Muller-Hermelink HK, et al. Tumours of the lung. In: Travis WD, Brambilla E, Muller-Hermelink HK, et al, eds. *Pathology and Genetics of Tumours of the Lung, Pleura, Thymus and Heart*. Lyon, France: IARC Press; 2004. *WHO Health Organization Classification of Tumours*.
2. Hirakata K, Nakata H, Haratake J. Appearance of pulmonary metastases on high-resolution CT scans: comparison with histopathologic findings from autopsy specimens. *Am J Roentgenol*. 1993;161:37-43.
3. Viggiano RW, Swenson SJ, Rostenow EC. Evaluation and management of solitary and multiple pulmonary nodules. *Clin Chest Med*. 1992;13:83-95.
4. Pinckard JK, Wick M. Tumor-related thrombotic pulmonary microangiopathy: review of pathologic findings and pathophysiologic mechanisms. *Ann Diagn Pathol*. 2000;4:154-157.
5. Heitmiller R, Marasco W, Hruban R, Marsh B. Endobronchial metastasis. *J Thorac Cardiovasc Surg*. 1993;106:537-542.
6. Katsimbri PP, Bamias AT, Froudarakis ME, Peponis IA, Constantopoulos SH, Pavlidis NA. Endobronchial metastases secondary to solid tumors: report of eight cases and review of the literature. *Lung Cancer*. 2000;28:163-170.
7. Sørensen JB. Endobronchial metastases from extrapulmonary solid tumors. *Acta Oncol*. 2004;43:73-79.
8. Bishop JA, Sharma R, Illei PB. Napsin A and thyroid transcription factor-1 expression in carcinomas of the lung, breast, pancreas, colon, kidney, thyroid, and malignant mesothelioma. *Hum Pathol*. 2010;41:20-25.
9. Comperat E, Zhang F, Perrotin C, et al. Variable sensitivity and specificity of TTF-1 antibodies in lung metastatic adenocarcinoma of colorectal origin. *Mod Pathol*. 2005;18:1371-1376.
10. Siami K, McCluggage WG, Ordonez NG, et al. Thyroid transcription factor-1 expression in endometrial and endocervical adenocarcinomas. *Am J Surg Pathol*. 2007;31:1759-1763.
11. Kubba LA, McCluggage WG, Liu J, et al. Thyroid transcription factor-1 expression in ovarian epithelial neoplasms. *Mod Pathol*. 2008;21:485-490.
12. Zhang PJ, Gao HG, Pasha TL, Litzky L, Livolsi VA. TTF-1 expression in ovarian and uterine epithelial neoplasia and its potential significance, an immunohistochemical assessment with multiple monoclonal antibodies and different secondary detection systems. *Int J Gynecol Pathol*. 2009;28:10-18.
13. Klingen TA, Chen Y, Gundersen MD, Aas H, Westre B, Sauer T. Thyroid transcription factor-1 positive primary breast cancer: a case report with review of the literature. *Diagn Pathol*. 2010;5:37.
14. Robens J, Goldstein L, Gown AM, Schnitt SJ. Thyroid transcription factor-1 expression in breast carcinomas. *Am J Surg Pathol*. 2010;34:1881-1885.
15. Surrey LF, Frank R, Zhang PJ, Furth EE. TTF-1 and Napsin-A are expressed in a subset of cholangiocarcinomas arising from the gallbladder and hepatic ducts: continued caveats for utilization of immunohistochemistry panels. *Am J Surg Pathol*. 2014;38:224-227.
16. Ordóñez NG. Value of thyroid transcription factor-1 immunostaining in tumor diagnosis: a review and update. *Appl Immunohistochem Mol Morphol*. 2012;20:429-444.

17. Nicholson AG, McCormick CJ, Shimosato Y, Butcher DN, Sheppard MN. The value of PE-10, a monoclonal antibody against pulmonary surfactant, in distinguishing primary and metastatic tumours. *Histopathology.* 1995;27:57-60.

18. Bejarano PA, Baughman RP, Biddinger PW, et al. Surfactant proteins and thyroid transcription factor-1 in pulmonary and breast carcinomas. *Mod Pathol.* 1996; 9:445-452.

19. Jagirdar J. Application of immunohistochemistry to the diagnosis of primary and metastatic carcinoma to the lung. *Arch Pathol Lab Med.* 2008;132:384-396.

20. Bahrami A, Truong LD, Ro JY. Undifferentiated tumor. True identity by immunohistochemistry. *Arch Pathol Lab Med.* 2008; 132:326-348.

21. Rossi G, Murer B, Cavazza A, et al. Primary mucinous (so-called colloid) carcinomas of the lung: a clinicopathologic and immunohistochemical study with special reference to CDX-2 homeobox gene and MUC2 expression. *Am J Surg Pathol.* April 2004;28(4):442-452.

22. Laury AR, Perets R, Piao H, et al. A comprehensive analysis of PAX8 expression in human epithelial tumors. *Am J Surg Pathol.* 2011;35:816-826.

23. Ordóñez NG. Thyroid transcription factor-1 is not expressed in squamous cell carcinomas of the lung: an immunohistochemical study with review of the literature. *Appl Immunohistochem Mol Morphol.* 2012;20:525-530.

24. Husain AN, Colby T, Ordóñez NG, et al. Guidelines for pathologic diagnosis of malignant mesothelioma: 2012 update of the consensus statement from the International Mesothelioma Interest Group. *Arch Pathol Lab Med.* 2013;137(5):647-667.

25. Saad RS, Landreneau RJ, Liu Y, Silverman JF. Utility of immunohistochemistry in separating thymic neoplasms from germ cell tumors and metastatic lung cancer involving the anterior mediastinum. *Appl Immunohistochem Mol Morphol.* 2003;11:107-112.

26. Evans AG, French CA, Cameron MJ, et al. Pathologic characteristics of NUT midline carcinoma arising in the mediastinum. *Am J Surg Pathol.* 2012;36:1222-1227.

27. Gökmen-Polar Y, Cano OD, Kesler KA, Loehrer PJ, Badve S. NUT midline carcinomas in the thymic region. *Mod Pathol.* May 23, 2014. doi:10.1038/modpathol.2014.63. [Epub ahead of print].

28. Weissferdt A. Large cell carcinoma of lung: on the verge of extinction? *Semin Diagn Pathol.* June 12, 2014 [Epub ahead of print].

29. Litzky LA. Pulmonary sarcomatous tumors. *Arch Pathol Lab Med.* 2008;132:1104-1117.

30. Franks TJ, Galvin JR. Sarcomatoid carcinoma of the lung: histologic criteria and common lesions in the differential diagnosis. *Arch Pathol Lab Med.* 2010;134:49-54.

31. Travis WD. Sarcomatoid neoplasms of the lung and pleura. *Arch Pathol Lab Med.* 2010;134:1645-1658.

32. Terra SB, Aubry MC, Yi ES, Boland JM. Immunohistochemical study of 36 cases of pulmonary sarcomatoid carcinoma—sensitivity of TTF-1 is superior to napsin. *Hum Pathol.* 2014;45:294-302.

33. Zhang C, Schmidt LA, Hatanaka K, Thomas D, Lagstein A, Myers JL. Evaluation of Napsin A, TTF-1, p63, p40, and CK5/6 immunohistochemical stains in pulmonary neuroendocrine tumors. *Am J Clin Pathol.* 2014; 142:320-324.

34. Pelosi G, Rodriguez J, Viale G, Rosai J. Typical and atypical pulmonary carcinoid tumor overdiagnosed as small-cell carcinoma on biopsy specimens: a major pitfall in the management of lung cancer patients. *Am J Surg Pathol.* 2005;2:179-187.

35. Rekhtman N. Neuroendocrine tumors of the lung: an update. *Arch Pathol Lab Med.* 2010;134:1628-1638.

36. Sica G, Wagner PL, Altorki N, Port J, et al. Immunohistochemical expression of estrogen and progesterone receptors in primary pulmonary neuroendocrine tumors. *Arch Pathol Lab Med.* 2008;132:1889-1895.

37. Vollmer RT. Primary lung cancer vs. metastatic breast cancer: a probabilistic approach. *Am J Clin Pathol.* 2009;132:391-395.

38. Oliveira AM, Tazelaar HD, Myers JL, Erickson LA, Lloyd RV. Thyroid transcription factor-1 distinguishes metastatic pulmonary from well-differentiated neuroendocrine tumors of other sites. *Am J Surg Pathol.* 2001;25:815-819.

39. Cai YC, Banner B, Glickman J, Odze RD. Cytokeratin 7 and 20 and thyroid transcription factor 1 can help distinguish pulmonary from gastrointestinal carcinoid and pancreatic endocrine tumors. *Hum Pathol.* 2001;32:1087-1093.

40. Matoso A, Singh K, Jacob R, et al. Comparison of thyroid transcription factor-1 expression by 2 monoclonal antibodies in pulmonary and nonpulmonary primary tumors. *Appl Immunohistochem Mol Morphol.* 2010;18:142-149.

41. Du EZ, Goldstraw P, Zacharias J, et al. TTF-1 expression is specific for lung primary in typical and atypical carcinoids: TTF-1 positive carcinoids are predominantly in peripheral location. *Hum Pathol.* 2004;35:825-831.

42. Srivastava A, Hornick JL. Immunohistochemical staining for CDX-2, PDX-1, NESP-55, and TTF-1 can help distinguish gastrointestinal carcinoid tumors from pancreatic endocrine and pulmonary carcinoid tumors. *Am J Surg Pathol.* 2009; 33:626-632.

43. Darvishian F, Ginsberg MS, Klimstra DS, Brogi E. Carcinoid tumorlets simulate pulmonary metastases in women with breast cancer. *Hum Pathol.* 2006;37:839-844.

44. Mitry E, Guiu B, Cosconea S, Jooste V, Faivre J, Bouvier A. Epidemiology, management and prognosis of colorectal cancer with lung metastases: a 30-year population-based study. *Gut.* 2010; 59:1383-1388.

45. Bölükbas S, Sponholz S, Kudelin N, Eberlein M, Schirren J. Risk factors for lymph node metastases and prognosticators of survival in patients undergoing pulmonary metastasectomy for colorectal cancer. *Ann Thorac Surg.* 2014;97:1926-1932.

46. Inamura K, Satoh Y, Okumura S, et al. Pulmonary adenocarcinomas with enteric differentiation: histologic and immunohistochemical characteristics compared with metastatic colorectal cancers and usual pulmonary adenocarcinomas. *Am J Surg Pathol.* 2005;29:660-665.

47. Douglas WG, Rigual NR, Loree TR, Wiseman SM, Al-Rawi S, Hicks WL Jr. Current concepts in the management of a second malignancy of the lung in patients with head and neck cancer. *Curr Opin Otolaryngol Head Neck Surg.* 2003;11:85-88.

48. Geurts TW, van Velthuysen ML, Broekman F, et al. Differential diagnosis of pulmonary carcinoma following head and neck cancer by genetic analysis. *Clin Cancer Res.* 2009;15:980-985.

49. Bishop JA, Ogawa T, Chang X, et al. HPV analysis in distinguishing second primary tumors from lung metastases in patients with head and neck squamous cell carcinoma. *Am J Surg Pathol.* 2012; 36:142-148.

50. Patnana M, Bronstein Y, Szklaruk J, et al. Multimethod imaging, staging, and spectrum of manifestations of metastatic melanoma. *Clin Radiol.* 2011;66:224-236.

51. Matin RN, Chikh A, Chong SLP, et al. P63 is an alternative p53 repressor in melanoma that confers chemoresistance and a poor prognosis. *J Exp Med.* 2013;210:581-603.

52. Nonaka D, Chiriboga L, Rubin BP. Sox10: a pan-schwannian and melanocytic marker. *Am J Surg Pathol.* 2008;32:1291-1298.

53. Khattak MA, Fisher RA, Pickering LM, Gore ME, Larkin JM. Endobronchial metastases from renal cell carcinoma: a late manifestation of the disease with an increasing incidence. *BJU Int.* 2012;110:1407-1408.

54. Tan PH, Cheng L, Rioux-Leclercq N, et al. Renal tumors: diagnostic and prognostic biomarkers. *Am J Surg Pathol.* 2013; 37:1518-1531.

55. Ozcan A, de la Roza G, Ro JY, Shen SS, Truong LD. PAX2 and PAX8 expression in primary and metastatic renal tumors: a comprehensive comparison. *Arch Pathol Lab Med.* 2012;13:1541-1551.

56. Tennis M, Singh B, Hjerpe A, et al. Pathological confirmation of primary lung cancer following breast cancer. *Lung Cancer.* 2010;69:40-45.

57. Curtit E, Nerich V, Mansi L, et al. Discordances in estrogen receptor status, progesterone receptor status, and HER2 status between primary breast cancer and metastasis. *Oncologist.* 2013;18:667-674.

58. Yang M, Nonaka D. A study of immunohistochemical differential expression in pulmonary and mammary carcinomas. *Mod Pathol.* 2010; 23:64-661.

59. Kawaguchi KR, Lu FI, Kaplan R, et al. In search of the ideal immunopanel to distinguish metastatic mammary carcinoma from primary lung carcinoma: a tissue microarray study of 207 cases. *Appl Immunohistochem Mol Morphol.* August 2013 (epub ahead of print).

60. Dabbs DJ, Landreneau RJ, Liu Y, et al. Detection of estrogen receptor by immunohistochemistry in pulmonary adenocarcinoma. *Ann Thorac Surg.* 2002;73:403-405.

61. Cimino-Mathews A, Subhawong AP, Ilei PB, et al. GATA3 expression in breast carcinoma: utility in triple-negative, sarcomatoid, and metastatic carcinomas. *Hum Pathol.* 2013;44:1341-1349.

62. Copeland JN, Amin MB, Humphrey PA, Tamboli P, Ro JY, Gal AA. The morphologic spectrum of metastatic prostatic adenocarcinoma to the lung: special emphasis on histologic features overlapping with other pulmonary neoplasms. *Am J Clin Pathol.* 2002;117:552-557.

63. Brimo F, Epstein JI. Immunohistochemical pitfalls in prostate pathology. *Hum Pathol.* 2012;43:313-324.

64. Chuang AY, DeMarzo AM, Veltri RW, Sharma RB, Bieberich CJ, Epstein JI. Immunohistochemical differentiation of high-grade prostate carcinoma from urothelial carcinoma. *Am J Surg Pathol.* 2007;31:1246-1255.

65. Tietze L, Gunther K, Horbe A, et al. Benign metastasizing leiomyoma. A cytogenetically balanced but clonal disease. *Hum Pathol.* 2000;31:126-128.

66. Patton KT, Cheng L, Papavero V, et al. Benign metastasizing leiomyoma: clonality, telomere length and clinicopathologic analysis. *Mod Pathol.* 2006;19:130-140.

67. Nucci MR, Drapkin R, Dal Cin P, Fletcher CD, Fletcher JA. Distinctive cytogenetic profile in benign metastasizing leiomyoma: pathogenetic implications. *Am J Surg Pathol.* 2007;31:737-743.

68. Nuovo GJ, Schmittgen TD. Benign metastasizing leiomyoma of the lung: clinicopathologic, immunohistochemical, and microRNA analyses. *Diagn Mol Pathol.* 2008;17:145-150.

69. Aubry MC, Myers JL, Colby TV, Leslie KO, Tazelaar HD. Endometrial stromal sarcoma metastatic to the lung—a detailed analysis of 16 patients. *Am J Surg Pathol.* 2002;26:440-449.

70. Colby TV, Koss MN, Travis WD. *Tumors of the Lower Respiratory Tract, Atlas of Tumor Pathology.* Third series, fascicle 13. Washington, DC: Armed Forces Institute of Pathology; 1994.

71. Moran CA, Suster S, Koss MN. Primary adenoid cystic carcinoma of the lung. A clinicopathologic and immunohistochemical study of 16 cases. *Cancer.* 1994; 73:1390-1397.

72. Molina JR, Aubry MC, Lewis JE, et al. Primary salivary gland-type lung cancer: spectrum of clinical presentation, histopathologic and prognostic factors. *Cancer.* 2007;110:2253-2259.

73. Kang D-Y, Yoon YS, Kim HK, et al. Primary salivary gland-type lung cancer: surgical outcomes. *Lung Cancer.* 2011;72:250-254.

74. Zhu F, Liu Z, Hou Y, et al. Primary salivary gland-type lung cancer: clinicopathological analysis of 88 cases from China. *J Thorac Oncol.* 2013;8:1578-1584.

75. Kwak SH, Lee KS, Chung MJ, Jeong YJ, Kim GY, Kwon OJ. Adenoid cystic carcinoma of the airways: helical CT and histopathologic correlation. *AJR.* 2004;183:277-281.

76. An J, Park S, Sung SH, Cho MS, Kim SC. Unusual expression of thyroid transcription factor 1 and napsin A in metastatic adenoid cystic carcinoma of extrapulmonary origin in the lung. *Am J Clin Pathol.* 2014;141:712-717.

77. Heitmiller RF, Mathisen DJ, Ferry JA, Mark EJ, Grillo HC. Mucoepidermoid lung tumors. *Ann Thorac Surg.* 1989;47:394-399.

78. Yousem SA, Hochholzer L. Mucoepidermoid carcinoma of the lung. *Cancer.* 1987;60:1346-1352.

79. Brandwein MS, Ivanov K, Wallace DI, et al. Mucoepidermoid carcinoma: a clinicopathologic study of 80 patients with special reference to histological grading. *Am J Surg Pathol.* 2001; 25:835-845.

80. Roden AC, García JJ, Wehrs RN, et al. Histopathologic, immunophenotypic and cytogenetic features of pulmonary mucoepidermoid carcinoma. *Mod Pathol.* April 18, 2014. [Epub ahead of print].

81. Achcar Rde O, Nikiforova MN, Dacic S, Nicholson AG, Yousem SA. Mammalian mastermind like 2 11q21 gene rearrangement in bronchopulmonary mucoepidermoid carcinoma. *Hum Pathol.* 2009;40:854-860.

82. Lia X, Zhang W, Wua X, Suna C, Chena M, Zenga Q. Mucoepidermoid carcinoma of the lung: common findings and unusual appearances on CT. *Clin Imag.* 2012;36:8-13.

83. Shilo K, Foss RD, Franks TJ, DePeralta-Venturina M, Travis WD. Pulmonary mucoepidermoid carcinoma with prominent tumor-associated lymphoid proliferation. *Am J Surg Pathol.* 2005;29:407-411.

84. Payne CB, Morningstar WA, Chester EH. Thymoma of the pleura masquerading as diffuse mesothelioma. *Am J Res Dis.* 1960;94:441-446.

85. Yeoh CB, Ford JM, Lattes R, Wylie RH. Intrapulmonary thymoma. *J Thorac Cardiovasc Surg.* 1966;51:131-136.

86. Kung IT, Loke SL, So SY, Lam WK, Mok CK, Khin MA. Intrapulmonary thymoma: report of two cases. *Thorax.* 1985; 40:471-474.

87. Honma K, Shimada K. Metastasizing ectopic thymoma arising in the right thoracic cavity and mimicking diffuse pleural mesothelioma. An autopsy study of a case with review of the literature. *Wien Klin Wochenschr.* 1986;98:14-20.

88. Green WR, Pressoir R, Gumbs RV, Warner O, Naab T, Qayumi M. Intrapulmonary thymoma. *Arch Pathol Lab Med.* 1987;111:1074-1076.

89. Fukayama M, Maeda Y, Funata N, et al. Pulmonary and pleural thymoma. Diagnostic application of lymphocyte markers to the thymoma of unusual site. *Am J Clin Pathol.* 1988;89:617-621.

90. Moran CA, Travis WD, Rosado-de-Christenson M, Koss MN, Rosai J. Thymomas presenting as pleural tumors. Report of eight cases. *Am J Surg Pathol.* 1992;16:138-144.

91. James CL, Iyer PV, Leong AS. Intrapulmonary thymoma. *Histopathology.* 1992;21:175-177.

92. Moran CA, Suster S, Fishback NF, Koss MN. Primary intrapulmonary thymoma: a clinicopathologic and immunohistochemical study of eight cases. *Am J Surg Pathol.* 1995;19: 304-312.

93. Veynovich B, Masetti P, Kaplan PD, Jasnosz KM, Yousem SA, Landreneau RJ. Primary pulmonary thymoma. *Ann Thor Surg.* 1997;64:1471-1473.

94. Fushimi H, Tanio Y, Kotoh K. Ectopic thymoma mimicking diffuse pleural mesothelioma: a case report. *Hum Pathol.* 1998;29:409-410.

95. Attanoos RL, Galateau-Salle F, Gibbs AR, Muller S, Ghandour F, Dojcinov SD. Primary thymic epithelial tumors of the pleura mimicking malignant mesothelioma. *Histopathology.* 2002;41:42-49.

96. Myers PO, Kritikos N, Bongiovanni M, et al. Primary intrapulmonary thymoma: a systematic review. *Eur J Surg Oncol.* 2007;33:1137-1141.

97. Marchevsky AM. Lung tumors derived from ectopic issues. *Semin Diagn Pathol.* 1995;172-184.

11 Pleura

Alain C. Borczuk

TAKE HOME PEARLS

- Diffuse malignant mesothelioma is an uncommon, aggressive malignant neoplasm that arises from mesothelial cells which line the pleural, pericardial, and abdominal cavity, with an incidence rate of less than 1 in 100,000.
- After an increase in malignant mesothelioma in men during the 1970s into the early 1990s, there has been a steady decrease. The incidence in women has been level over the same time period, and at a significantly lower rate.
- Mortality from malignant mesothelioma is high, with 5-year survival rates under 10%.
- The classic description of malignant pleural mesothelioma is a thickening in the pleural space with encasement of the lung by a rind-like visceral pleura.
- The majority of mesotheliomas have epithelioid histology (about 70%-75%), with biphasic histology (10%-15%) and sarcomatoid histology (10%) making up the remainder.
- The range of epithelioid histologic patterns of malignant mesothelioma is quite large and therefore overlap with patterns of carcinoma is quite frequent. Therefore, immunohistochemistry is typically employed to diagnose malignant mesothelioma.
- Immunohistochemical markers of mesothelial differentiation include calretinin and WT1 (nuclear) as well as cytokeratin 5/6 and D2-40 (podoplanin). None of these markers are sufficiently sensitive or specific to be used alone and a minimum of two mesothelial markers is recommended, although more may be needed in some cases.

- As a result of the significant morphologic overlap between atypical mesothelial cells and malignant mesothelial cells, cytologic and cytomorphologic features are unreliable in the differential diagnosis of mesothelial hyperplasia and malignant mesothelioma.
- Other pleural neoplasms that may enter into the differential of malignant mesothelioma include *pseudomesotheliomatous carcinoma, localized malignant mesothelioma, well-differentiated papillary mesothelioma, solitary fibrous tumor, malignant solitary fibrous tumor, synovial sarcoma, and vascular sarcomas.*

DIFFUSE MALIGNANT MESOTHELIOMA (DMM)

Epidemiology and Demographics

Diffuse malignant mesothelioma (DMM) is an aggressive malignant neoplasm arising from mesothelial cells which line the pleural, pericardial, and abdominal cavity. It is an uncommon malignancy, with an incidence rate of less than 1 in 100,000, with estimates ranging from 2 to 3 per million to as high as 17 per million in selected populations. Pleural malignant mesothelioma is more common in men than women, and in North America this ratio is in the range of 4:1 and 5:1. The disease occurs across a wide age range, with case reports in children, but a measurable incidence in the population begins at age 35 and peaks in the late 1970s and early 1980s.[1,2]

An increase in cases was seen in men during the 1970s into the early 1990s, with a steady decrease since then. The incidence in women has been level over the same time period, and at a significantly lower rate. Mortality from malignant mesothelioma is high, with 5-year survival rates under 10%. This mortality rate is largely unchanged in this treatment resistant disease.[2]

Etiologies of Diffuse Malignant Mesothelioma

Mesothelioma is associated with exposure to asbestos. Studies from the Northwest Cape province of South Africa in adults who lived near asbestos mines as children[3] and among insulation workers in NY exposed during the 1940s[4] showed an increased relative risk of development of malignant mesothelioma. Asbestos is divided broadly into serpentine types (eg, chrysotile) and amphibole types (eg, amosite, crocidolite, anthophyllite, tremolite, and actinolite); it appears that the highest risk of MM is associated with amphibole types.[5-9] In autopsy series, cases of MM show increased amphibole fibers when compared to nondisease controls, and chrysotile loads are similar in cases and controls. Differences in fiber properties and fiber clearance from the lung are cited to account for this difference in exposure risk.[10] Contamination of chrysotile and non-asbestos minerals with amphibole asbestos has been put forth as the explanation for mesothelioma risk among workers in chrysotile asbestos (or nonasbestos) mines.

A significant interval or latency between exposure and development of disease has been noted, with an interval of over 20 years associated with the highest relative risk.[11] The attributable risk of asbestos in mesothelioma development varies by gender and location of the mesothelioma, with asbestos exposure having the highest relationship to male gender and pleural disease. For example, the attributable risk of asbestos exposure in men with pleural mesothelioma is nearly 90%, while just under 25% in women. There is also risk of pleural mesothelioma from cohabitant exposure in households with an asbestos worker.[12]

When examining the lower mesothelioma attribution to asbestos in women and in nonpleural mesothelioma, it is likely that other etiologies exist other than asbestos exposure.[13] Another mineral fiber, erionite, has been found to cause mesothelioma in Turkey, with similar latency but higher rate of disease association. Erionite is also found in the United States, in North Dakota and some Western states.[14] Radiation exposure, either occupational or associated with radiation therapy for other malignancies, has been shown to increase risk of malignant mesothelioma. Studies of radiation-treated lymphoma, breast carcinoma, and testicular carcinoma show a subsequent increased risk of malignant mesothelioma.[15-22] While chronic serosal inflammation, certain chemical exposures and viral infection with SV40

have all been raised as possible etiologies, the evidence for these causes remains limited and controversial.

There is a recent report of a genetic predisposition for malignant mesothelioma as part of a new cancer syndrome associated with BRCA1-associated protein 1 (BAP1) germline mutations. These patients are at increased risk for uveal melanoma and malignant mesothelioma and there appears to be possible increased risk as well for renal cell carcinoma, lung adenocarcinoma, meningioma, and pigmented skin lesions.[23-25]

Clinical Features and Imaging

Patients with pleural mesothelioma often present with respiratory complaints (dyspnea), which can be related to pleural effusion in many cases. Chest pain can also be a presenting symptom. Some patients are asymptomatic with an incidentally discovered effusion. Some patients experience weight loss. Physical examination findings, when present, also relate to pleural effusion.

Various methodologies can be used to image the chest in malignant mesothelioma. Chest x-ray may be useful in identifying pleural effusion and masses/pleural thickening can be suggested by this method. Computed tomography can better delineate and more accurately define the changes seen by chest x-ray, including pleural thickening, pleural effusion, and reduced lung volumes. Magnetic resonance imaging may also be useful. PET scanning has been used to assess extent of disease.[26]

Gross Findings

The classic description of malignant pleural mesothelioma is a thickening in the pleural space with encasement of the lung by a rind-like visceral pleura (*Figure 11-1A*). The tumor can be seen growing into interlobar fissures. Disease is asymmetric and often unilateral. Advanced disease can spread through the intercostal spaces and into the chest wall (*Figure 11-1B*). The tumor can also grow in a nodular pattern or can form additional small nodules over other less involved areas in otherwise rind-like cases (*Figure 11-1C*). Hyalinized pleural plaques, which are white plate-like thickenings over the parietal pleura and diaphragmatic surface, can become invaded by mesothelioma.

Rare cases of malignant mesothelioma are characterized by a single mass lesion without the diffuse thickening or satellite nodules. This is called localized malignant mesothelioma (see later section).

Histologic Features of Diffuse Malignant Mesothelioma

The major subtypes of malignant mesothelioma are epithelioid and spindled/sarcomatoid, with combinations

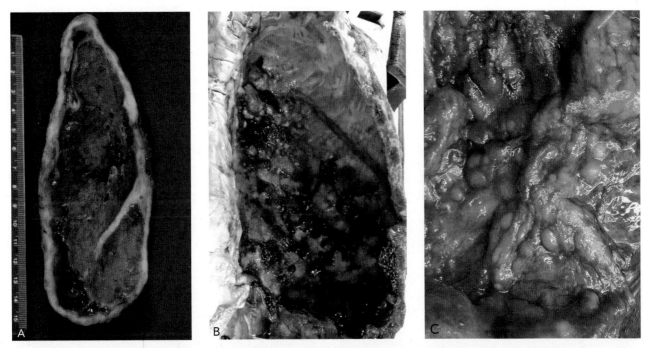

FIGURE 11-1 Gross appearance of diffuse malignant mesothelioma. **(A)** Lung with marked circumferential pleural thickening, gray-white, and extending down the interlobar fissure. **(B)** The left parietal pleura and posterior chest wall exposed during autopsy examination reveals hemorrhagic, nodular, and white plaque-like thickenings of malignant mesothelioma invading into the chest wall. **(C)** The visceral pleura of the lung has a nodular, not rind-like growth pattern.

termed biphasic. The majority of mesotheliomas are epithelioid (roughly 70%-75%), with biphasic tumors (10%-15%) and sarcomatoid tumors (10%) representing the minority.

However, patterns of growth within each major subtype have been described (*Figure 11-2*). Tumors of pure epithelioid histology can have patterns described as papillary (*Figure 11-2A*—cells growing along exophytic fronds with vascular cores), tubulopapillary

(a mixture of gland-like formations and papillary structures) and solid (*Figure 11-2B*—sheets or nests of polygonal epithelioid cells). However, the range of epithelioid patterns is quite large and therefore overlap with patterns of carcinoma is quite frequent. Such patterns include micropapillary (*Figure 11-2C*—small tufts without fibrovascular cores), trabecular (cord like), acinar (*Figure 11-2D*—gland forming), and adenomatoid (*Figure 11-2E*—flat cells lining small

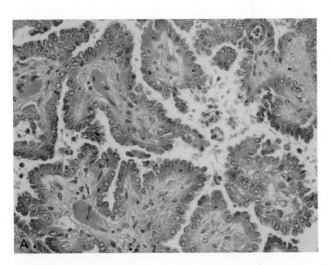
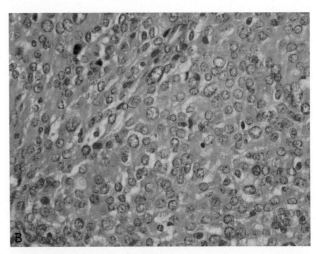

FIGURE 11-2 Architectural patterns of malignant mesothelioma, epithelioid type. **(A)** The papillary pattern is characterized by a single or stratified layer of atypical mesothelial cells with irregular outpouchings on a fibrovascular core. **(B)** The solid subtype shows sheet-like cellular growth.

spaces). Some cases can have abundant extracellular hyaluronic acid matrix (*Figure 11-2F*) and rare cases can produce intracellular mucin; others have abundant psammoma bodies (*Figure 11-2G*). Some cellular features of epithelioid subtype include clear cell (*Figure 11-3A*—mimicking renal cell carcinoma), deciduoid/hepatoid (*Figure 11-3B*—abundant eosinophilic cytoplasm), signet ring (*Figure 11-3C*—intracytoplasmic vacuole), small cell (*Figure 11-3D*—higher nuclear to cytoplasmic ratio, no molding or karyorrhexis) , rhabdoid (*Figure 11-3E*—large cells with ball like deeply eosinophilic cytoplasm), and pleomorphic

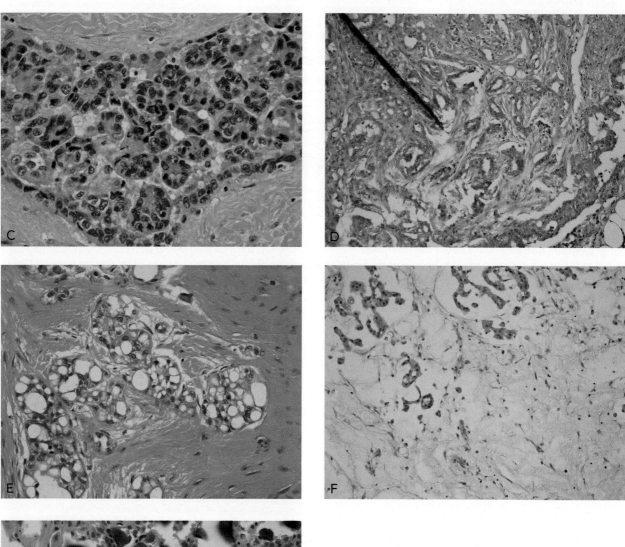

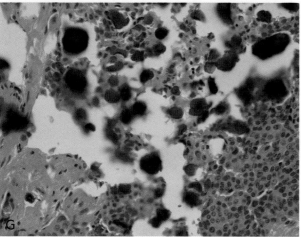

FIGURE 11-2 (*Continued*) **(C)** The micropapillary pattern shows small clusters of cells in radial or petal-like arrangements without a fibrovascular core. **(D)** The tubular pattern shows gland-shaped structures, some of which are fused. **(E)** The adenomatoid pattern grows as flat cells surrounding a microcystic space. **(F)** Some cases have abundant extracellular material, with tumor cells in clusters, appearing to "float" within it. **(G)** Abundant psammoma bodies are seen in this tumor.

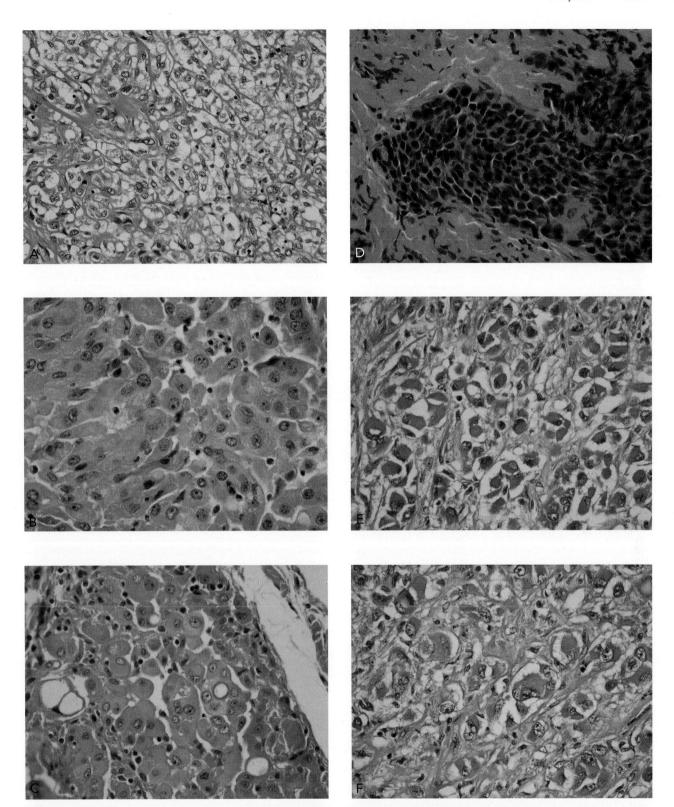

FIGURE 11-3 Cellular patterns of malignant mesothelioma, epithelioid type. (A) Clear cell change can be seen, mimicking renal cell carcinoma. (B) Abundant eosinophilic cytoplasm characterizes the deciduoid pattern (C) Signet ring-like vacuoles, some expansile in the cytoplasm, are seen in this tumor. These are typically not mucicarmine positive. (D) The small cell histology is cellular with high nuclear to cytoplasmic ratio, but without karyorrhexis or nuclear molding. (E) Rhabdoid appearing cells also contain eosinophilic cytoplasm, but this is a ball-like structure rather than diffuse eosinophilia. (F) Pleomorphic tumors have little architecture, and show enlarged irregular nuclei.

Table 11-1 Epithelioid Malignant Mesothelioma—Architectural and Cellular Patterns

Architectural	Cellular
Papillary/tubulopapillary	Clear cell
Solid	Deciduoid
Trabecular	Signet ring
Acinar	Small cell
Micropapillary	Rhabdoid
Adenomatoid	Pleomorphic
Adenoid cystic	
Abundant extra cellular matrix	
Psammomatous	

(*Figure 11-3F*—irregular, bizarre nuclei). The importance of these subtypes is largely the awareness of their existence to avoid misclassification as a carcinoma (see section on immunohistochemistry).

A complexity of this classification is that some patterns refer to architectural features, while others to cellular features (*Table 11-1*). As a result combinations are frequent, and can be even in the same part of the tumor. For example, deciduoid histology can be solid, papillary, and acinar (not limited to these). It is unclear whether further subtyping results in better prognostic stratification.

The cells of mesothelioma often have deceptively uniform nuclei with moderate amounts of cytoplasm; mitotic rate is often low. These are factors that can make cytologic detection of disease especially difficult, and the morphologic overlap with reactive mesothelium can be challenging in tissue samples of reactive pleural conditions.

Tumors with spindle cell histology are called sarcomatoid. Sarcomatoid mesothelioma (SM) can be composed of atypical spindle cells without further characterization or differentiation, which is the most common spindled pattern (*Figure 11-4A*). These tumors are generally sufficiently cellular that they are recognized as neoplastic. More difficult are cases that have very bland spindle cells with minimal atypia amidst abundant acellular collagen, termed desmoplastic pattern. These desmoplastic mesotheliomas grow in a storiform pattern (*Figure 11-4B*) and can be intermixed with hyalinized pleural plaque obscuring their malignant nature even further. This disorganized growth, presence of bland necrosis (*Figure 11-4C*), and invasion into adipose tissue (*Figure 11-4D*) or lung are all features that confirm malignancy in these tumors. While desmoplastic areas can be seen focally, the desmoplastic mesothelioma

category is applied when this pattern represents 50% or more of the tumor.[27]

Some tumors have a combination of epithelioid and spindled patterns, and these are called malignant mesothelioma, biphasic type. It is required that either component (epithelioid or spindled) comprise at least 10% of the tumor to qualify for a biphasic designation.

Rare mesotheliomas can have heterologous elements like bone or cartilage and are usually part of biphasic or sarcomatoid mesothelioma (*Figure 11-4E*).[28]

One uncommon and challenging subtype is the lymphohistiocytoid subtype which has been historically placed in the sarcomatoid group (*Figure 11-4F*). These tumors have abundant lymphocytic infiltration, and the tumor cells themselves have resemblance to Reed-Sternberg cells or cells of large cell lymphoma. It is proposed that these tumors are better placed in the epithelioid category as they appear to have more favorable prognosis than the other sarcomatoid mesotheliomas.[29-31]

Another complicated subtype includes tumors with large, anaplastic, giant, or pleomorphic cells, mentioned in the epithelioid section. These tumors can have either epithelioid or spindle cell components. These pleomorphic mesotheliomas are currently classified in the epithelioid subtype, but their poorer prognosis suggests that they behave in a similar fashion to tumors with a biphasic histology.[32,33]

Immunohistochemical Features of Diffuse Malignant Mesothelioma

The diagnosis of malignant mesothelioma is confirmed using immunohistochemistry tests (*Table 11-2*). As the differential diagnosis is often with adenocarcinoma, a combination of markers indicating either mesothelial origin or epithelial origin is used. Markers of mesothelial differentiation include calretinin and WT1 (nuclear) as well as cytokeratin 5/6 and D2-40 (podoplanin). None of these markers are sufficiently sensitive or specific to be used alone; a minimum of two mesothelial markers is recommended, although more may be needed in some cases. Markers of carcinoma differentiation include MOC31, BG8, CEA, CD15, B72.3, and BEREP4. It is of note that MOC31 and BerEP4 recognize the same protein, and produce fairly similar results, so one but not both of these two should be performed in the same panel. None of these markers are sufficiently specific for adenocarcinoma to be used alone; a minimum of two carcinoma markers is recommended and many cases require a larger panel.[34]

Increasingly, markers associated with organ-specific cellular differentiation are used in conjunction with general carcinoma markers as they can provide organ

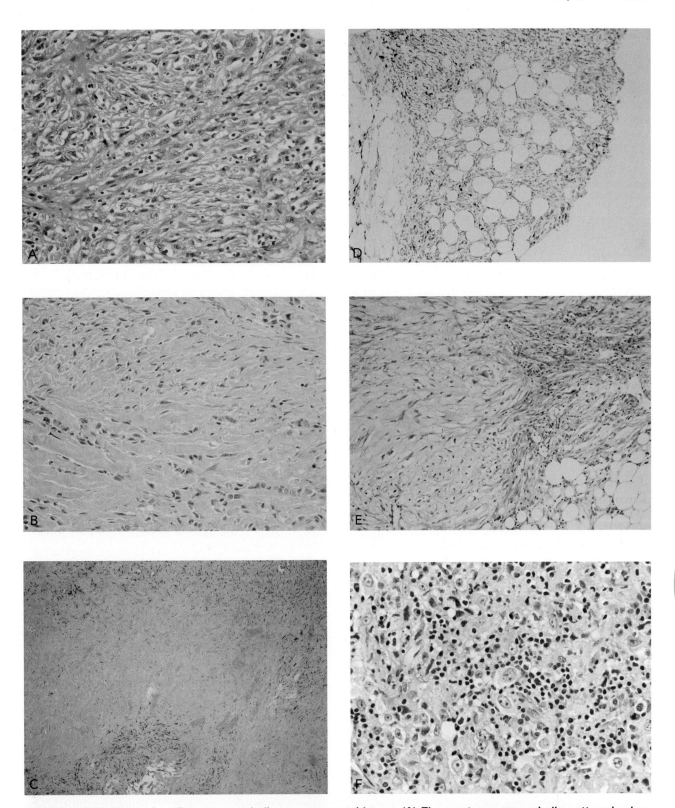

FIGURE 11-4 Patterns of malignant mesothelioma, sarcomatoid type. **(A)** The most common spindle pattern is characterized by atypical spindle cells, vaguely in fascicular bundles. **(B)** Desmoplastic mesothelioma is characterized by dense collagen and relatively bland spindle cells. **(C)** Bland infarct-like necrosis is seen in desmoplastic mesothelioma. **(D)** Cytokeratin stain highlights bland spindle cells invading adipose tissue. **(E)** Heterologous elements such as immature cartilage can rarely be seen in sarcomatoid mesothelioma. **(F)** Hodgkin-like cells amidst lymphocytic stroma is characteristic of lymphohistiocytoid malignant mesothelioma.

Table 11-2 Markers Useful in Panels in the Diagnosis of Malignant Pleural Mesothelioma and Its Mimics

Mesothelioma	Adenocarcinoma	Organ-Specific/ Adenocarcinoma	Squamous CA	Vascular Sarcoma	Synovial Sarcoma	Solitary Fibrous Tumor
Calretinin	BG8	TTF1	P40/p63	CD34	CD99	CD34
WT1	MOC31/BerEP4	Napsin A	MOC31	CD31	CD56	STAT6
D240	CEA	Pax8	BG8			
CK 5/6	CD15	Estrogen receptor				
	B72.3	Progesterone receptor				

of origin specificity. For example, since lung adenocarcinoma is frequently in the differential diagnosis of mesothelioma, thyroid transcription factor 1, a marker of type 2 pneumocytes and small airway cells, is used since it is positive in lung adenocarcinoma and negative in mesothelioma. Napsin A is chosen for similar reasons in this setting. Other markers of potential use include PAX8 to distinguish mesothelioma from renal cell carcinoma and female genital tract adenocarcinoma or hormone receptors to distinguish from breast and gynecological cancer.

Because of the reactivity for CK5/6 in mesothelioma and the overlap with squamous cell carcinoma, IHC for p63 or p40 may help distinguish squamous carcinoma from mesothelioma; MOC31 and BG8 may also be helpful in this setting.

The immunohistochemistry panels described above to characterize mesothelial differentiation have reduced sensitivity in sarcomatoid mesothelioma. Calretinin reacts with some but not all sarcomatoid mesotheliomas, and nonspecific cytoplasmic (not the specific nuclear) staining for WT1 occurs in a higher number of cases.[35] D240 may be the most sensitive of the mesothelial markers in this setting,[35] but is less specific as D240 can stain a wide variety of tumors including tumors of endothelial origin. In many cases, the most useful marker in the diagnosis of SM is cytokeratin, with a panel of negative carcinoma markers. This emphasizes that this diagnosis is in partly one of exclusion, as sarcomatoid carcinomas and some sarcomas will be cytokeratin positive, and some SM will be keratin negative. One cannot overemphasize the added value of extensive sampling to reveal a better differentiated or epithelioid area than a quixotic pursuit of a wider IHC panel in an exclusively sarcomatoid area.

With those observations in mind, however, several spindle cell tumors/sarcomas enter the differential diagnosis of sarcomatoid mesothelioma. Solitary fibrous tumors are typically cytokeratin negative. They are positive for CD34 while SMs are negative; in challenging cases STAT6 IHC has been found to be useful as solitary fibrous tumors harbor a fusion protein which

is the result of an NAB-STAT6 translocation (see later section). Synovial sarcoma (SS) can also be found in the chest wall and can mimic mesothelioma; the frequent cytokeratin reactivity of synovial sarcoma also creates a diagnostic difficulty, as can occasional calretinin staining in SS. Bcl2 is not useful in the differential with SS as mesotheliomas can be positive, but CD99 and CD56 may be useful as they are not frequently reported as positive in MM. TLE1 IHC which is frequently positive in SS has also been described in MM.[36] However, there are usually morphologic differences in the epithelioid and spindle areas of synovial sarcoma from mesothelioma and the characteristic X:18 translocation with SYT-SSX fusion can be detected to confirm the diagnosis. Primitive neuroectodermal tumors can occur in the pleura and chest wall and can enter the differential diagnosis of MM variants (eg, small cell variant).[37,38] While usually cytokeratin negative, a significant proportion can be immunoreactive for cytokeratin. While the IHC panel approach can be helpful (eg, positive synaptophysin, FLI1 and CD99, usually negative in MM), difficult cases can be resolved through FISH study, looking for EWS1 translocations.

Epithelioid Diffuse Malignant Mesothelioma Versus Reactive Mesothelial Hyperplasia

As a result of the significant morphologic overlap between atypical mesothelial cells and malignant mesothelial cells, cytologic and cytomorphologic features are unreliable in the differential diagnosis of mesothelial hyperplasia and malignant mesothelioma. Several parameters have been proposed, and require an integrated diagnostic approach.[39,40] Reactive proliferations are often quite cellular, and in biopsy samples relatively large but uniform collections of atypical cells can occur, but do not invade underlying tissue (*Figure 11-5A*). An important observation is that reactive processes are zonal; the reactive mesothelial cells grow in layers relative to the surface. In reactive processes there can be fibrin and reactive granulation tissue; this granulation tissue is characterized by regularly spaced vascularity, parallel to each other but perpendicular to the surface. With chronic processes this layering occurs beneath the surface and this can mimic invasion (*Figure 11-5B*); however, careful examination, a good-sized sample and sometimes immunohistochemistry can highlight the layered appearance (*Figure 11-5C*). Parameters that

deviate away from such orderly growth include dense or haphazard involvement of pleural tissue, expansile cellular growth (*Figure 11-5D*), and complex architectures (*Figure 11-5E*). Mesothelial proliferations in an absence of inflammation and reactive pleuritis raise suspicion for malignancy, as does necrosis. In fact, large expansile nodules are considered sufficient for the diagnosis

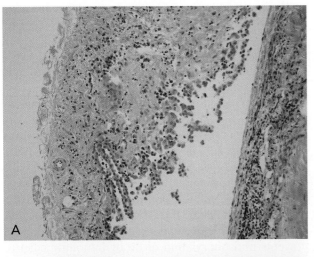
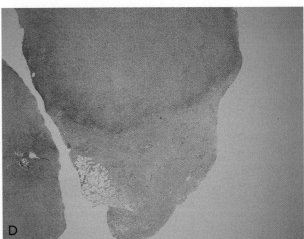
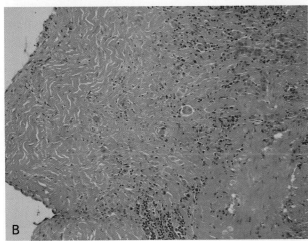
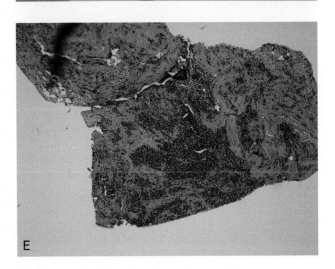
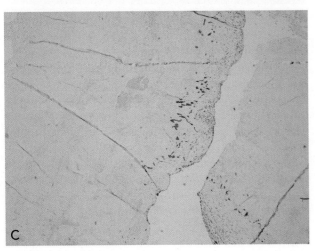

FIGURE 11-5 Reactive mesothelial hyperplasia and malignant mesothelioma. (A) Mesothelial cells proliferate along pleural surfaces. Morphologically, these cells can be as atypical as malignant mesothelioma, but without invasion. **(B)** Reactive proliferations can become embedded in stroma and therefore mimic invasion patterns such as trabecular and micropapillary. **(C)** Cytokeratin immunohistochemistry can help in demonstrating a layered linear appearance in these proliferations. **(D)** While invasion is a critical parameters, expansile nodular growth is an important criterion of malignancy. **(E)** Expansile and irregular complex growth, away from the surface, is also a feature of malignancy.

of malignant mesothelioma, once the cells are determined to be of mesothelial lineage.

However, invasion remains a critical parameter, and to some extent the description of disordered and expansile growth in pleural connective tissue speaks to the suggestion of invasion. However, unequivocal invasion of adipose tissue, skeletal muscle, stromal tissue or lung is in support of malignancy; in the case of stromal tissue invasion, care must be taken to observe disordered, not layered growth. Recent descriptions of tissue vacuolization mimicking adipose tissue ("fake fat") must also be taken into account.

Some markers may prove helpful in this determination, and IHC for p53, desmin, GLUT-1, IMP3, and CD146 have all been proposed in this context. In addition, a high rate of homozygous p16 deletion is considered strong support for malignant mesothelioma. All of these adjunctive approaches are best performed on tissue samples with a high morphologic suspicion for mesothelioma, and perform as supportive or confirmatory tests rather than stand-alone evidence.[41-44]

Molecular Features of Diffuse Malignant Mesothelioma

The cytotoxic effect of asbestos on cells and the subsequent effects on cellular survival have been implicated in the pathogenesis of malignant mesothelioma. Specifically, generation of reactive oxygen molecules have been shown to cause DNA damage, with activation of NFKB and AP-1 pathways found to enhance cellular survival. Chronic activation of macrophages and other inflammatory cells may provide an environment conducive to mesothelial cellular survival.[45] Interestingly, activating oncogenic mutations (eg, EGFR,KRAS) have not been described in mesothelioma, and mutations otherwise commonly seen in solid tumors, such as p53 mutation, are not frequently described in MM. While receptor tyrosine kinase pathways are activated in MM, such as EGFR, VEGFR, PDGFR, HGF and IGF, targeting these pathways, while under continued investigation, have had limited success in therapeutic response.

The molecular pathogenesis of mesothelioma does surround loss of tumor suppressor gene function, often by deletion.[46] NF2 losses (22q12.1 deletion) are a frequent alteration in MM,[47,48] and resultant loss and truncation of merlin (NF2 protein) is seen.[49] More recent data indicate nonsense and missense mutations also occur in this gene, resulting in loss of function, and when all gene deleterious alterations are combined, this is reported in up to 60% of MM. NF2 regulates cell growth signaling via the Hippo pathway, and inhibits a transcriptional program mediated by YAP1. Loss of NF2 supports cellular survival, invasion, and growth, and its frequent loss in MM suggests that this is a critical

pathway in mesothelioma development. Mutations in LATS2, also in this pathway, have been described in a smaller number of cases.

Somatic mutations in BAP1 occur in about 20% of MM in Caucasian patients, and this rate may be higher in Asian populations.[50] Heterozygous deletions in BAP1 are also described and when combined, roughly 40% of pleural MMs have BAP1 alteration.[49] Individual studies have shown increased sporadic BAP1-positive MM in smokers and in epithelioid subtype, but these findings remain preliminary.[51] As mentioned previously, germline mutations in BAP1 have been identified as a new familial cancer syndrome, which includes MM, uveal melanomas, cutaneous pigmented lesion, meningioma, and some carcinomas (lung, renal).[23-25]

Frequent deletion in chromosome 9p21 leads to loss of p16 (*CDKN2a*) and p14 as well as the nearby gene p15. Deletion of this locus (homozygous deletion) occurs in over 70% of cases, and may approach 100% in sarcomatoid MM.[52-54] In addition, p16 mutation and gene silencing promoter hypermethylation also occur.[55]

The losses in 9p21 impact two critical tumor suppressor pathways of Rb and p53. The tumor suppressor gene *CDKN2a* is a cyclin-dependent kinase inhibitor that prevents phosphorylation of Rb by inhibiting cdk4/6. This keeps cells from entering the cell cycle, and loss of p16 results in cdk4/6 activation, Rb phosphorylation, and ultimately cell cycle progression. Loss of p14 results in loss of the tumor suppressor effects of p53, as p14 normally plays a role in p53 stabilization.

Loss of *CDKN2a* locus through homozygous deletion may predict poor prognosis in malignant pleural mesothelioma, and a high number of cells showing homozygous deletion may be useful in distinction of reactive from malignant mesothelial proliferations.[54,56-59]

SARCOMATOUS MALIGNANT MESOTHELIOMA VERSUS FIBROUS PLEURITIS

This can be an extremely challenging distinction, and this is especially true in desmoplastic MM; useful criteria in this differential are summarized in *Table 11-3*. The gross appearance can include diffuse thickening and opacity of the pleura space (*Figure 11-6A*). Since once again cellular features are less important than architectural features and tumor stromal interaction, sample size needs to be sufficient to assess architecture and relations to adjacent structures.

The key feature to the diagnosis of fibrous pleurisy is zonation (*Figure 11-6B*). Fibrin can be present, as can granulation tissue and stromal cellularity, but these features are most prominent along the pleural surface and become less prominent in deeper layers. The granulation tissue has uniform vascularity perpendicular to

Table 11-3 **Histologic Features Useful in the Distinction of Sarcomatoid MM and Fibrous Pleurisy**

Cellular zonation
Uniformly spaced capillaries, perpendicular to the surface
Sharp, noninvasive interface with adipose tissue
Uniform thickening
No nodular/haphazard proliferation
No necrosis away from the surface
Zonal cytokeratin immunohistochemistry[a]
No cytokeratin-positive cells in adipose tissue

[a]Cytokeratin zonality not always present. When helpful, gradient of cytokeratin reactivity, decreasing into deeper layers.

the surface, and this too resolves in the deeper tissue (*Figure 11-6C*). The process is often uniformly thickened, and the mesothelial proliferation is therefore not nodular/expansile. The spindle cells can be layered but are not storiform, the cellularity decreases in deeper areas and shows a sharp (*Figure 11-6D*). Necrosis can be present at the surface of fibrous pleurisy, but in MM necrosis can be anywhere in the layers with infarct-like features (bland necrosis). As in reactive mesothelial hyperplasia, definitive evidence of invasion can be a critical feature in favor of malignancy. Invasion of adipose tissue is a key finding, and cytokeratin immunohistochemistry can highlight this feature (see *Figure 11-4D*). Cytokeratin immunohistochemistry can also be zonal in some cases of fibrous pleurisy, but this can be inconsistent. When helpful,

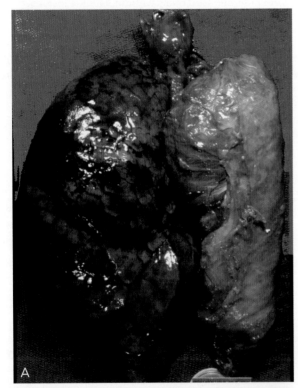

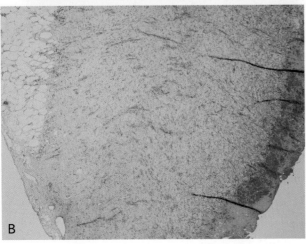

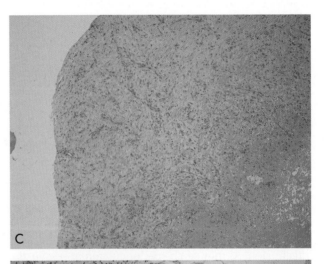

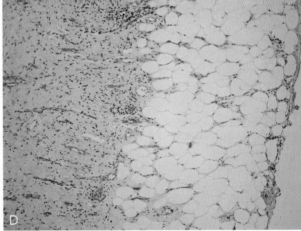

FIGURE 11-6 Gross and histologic features of fibrous pleurisy. **(A)** Fibrous pleuritis/pleurisy can involve the pleural space, causing diffuse unilateral adhesion, thickening, and opacity, like malignant mesothelioma. **(B)** Fibrous pleuritis shows uniform thickening as well as zonation. **(C)** Surface regions show evenly spaced parallel capillaries, perpendicular to the surface. **(D)** In contrast to mesothelioma, fibrous pleurisy becomes less cellular at the interface with adipose tissue, and a sharp demarcation.

cytokeratin is most intense toward the surface, decreasing into deeper layers. However, the finding of cytokeratin-positive cells in the deeper layers is not supportive of MM, but extension of cytokeratin-positive spindle cells into adipose tissue is very supportive of the diagnosis.

PSEUDOMESOTHELIOMATOUS CARCINOMA

Some cases of pulmonary and nonpulmonary carcinomas involve the pleural space in a diffuse rind-like pattern.[60] While the majority of these cases are adenocarcinomas, this can occur with other histologic patterns as well. In lung cases, the lung primary may be a small peripheral tumor which becomes difficult to resolve from the adjacent rind-like thickening. In such cases, it is critical to recognize this possibility and perform the immunohistochemistry panels that distinguish carcinoma from mesothelioma.

LOCALIZED MALIGNANT MESOTHELIOMA

Clinical Features of Localized Malignant Mesothelioma (LMM)

This is a histologic malignant mesothelioma that presents as a mass lesion rather than a diffuse rind-like or multinodular thickening. As a result, these tumors are often asymptomatic, and are not associated with pleural effusion. As they can be pedunculated or sessile, the clinical impression may include a pleural-based tumor, a pulmonary tumor, a chest wall tumor, or a mediastinal tumor, depending on where they arise. Such tumors have also been described in the pericardium and abdomen.[61]

LMM patients have an average age of 62, which is comparable to DMM, but the male to female ratio is only slight male predominant. Perhaps related to this gender observation is that LMM is not associated with asbestos exposure; the male predominance in DMM is largely attributed to occupational asbestos exposure.

The identification of this category is the result of the better prognosis associated with this growth pattern. Prognosis in this group is not determined by histologic subtype. There is potential for surgical cure in this disease if completely resected.

Gross Features of Localized Malignant Mesothelioma

This diagnosis is hinged on a single mass lesion, on or in the pleura without diffuse spread or satellite nodules

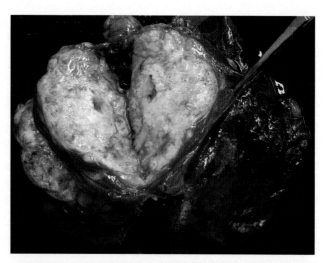

FIGURE 11-7 Localized malignant mesothelioma is a discrete pleural-based mass without satellite lesions.

(*Figure 11-7*). They can invade into adjacent structures, however. This category should not be used for mesothelioma with small satellite lesions but with one dominant nodule.

Histologic and Immunohistochemistry Features of Localized Malignant Mesothelioma

The histology and immunohistochemistry profile of LMM is the same as for DMM. Interestingly, these tumors can be epithelioid, biphasic, or sarcomatoid, despite their localized presentation.

WELL-DIFFERENTIATED PAPILLARY MESOTHELIOMA (WDPM)

Clinical Features of Well-Differentiated Papillary Mesothelioma

This is a bland papillary mesothelial proliferation and is often an incidental finding. However, the propensity of this tumor for superficial spread without invasion can lead to presentation with pleural effusion. Patients can present with symptoms related to pleural effusion such as shortness of breath. This tumor is rare in the pleura and more commonly encountered in the abdomen, where it is often an incidental finding during abdominal surgery.[62]

While abdominal disease does not appear to be related to asbestos exposure, asbestos relationship has been suggested in pleural disease. This tumor has a favorable prognosis but can recur, requiring repeated resections.[63-65]

Gross Features of Well-Differentiated Papillary Mesothelioma

The typical appearance of this tumor is either single growths of millimeter size (subcentimeter), multiple growths of millimeter/subcentimeter size, or less discrete small thickenings imparting a velvety quality to the otherwise smooth pleural surface. Controversial is whether there is an upper limit to the tumor size in WDPM, but this has not been established. However, all cases certainly warrant extensive sampling to rule out malignant mesothelioma and this applies to tumors over 2.0 cm.

Histologic Features of Well-Differentiated Papillary Mesothelioma

These tumors are composed of papillary structures lined by a single layer of bland mesothelial cells that are flat to cuboidal. They have a pattern of exophytic growth (*Figure 11-8A*). The papillary structures have cores, and these fibrovascular cores can be myxoid and filled with foamy macrophages. The critical feature of this tumor is the bland nature of the nuclei. The nuclei are small and round, and the chromatin relatively uniform (*Figure 11-8B*). The nuclear contours are relatively smooth, and nucleoli are absent or indistinct. In contrast, papillary MM shows greater nuclear atypia with some stratification (*Figure 11-8C*). Mitotic activity is absent to very low. Invasion into underlying stroma can be seen and such cases should be designated as WDPM with invasion. While invasion does not upgrade a tumor to malignant mesothelioma, it may be that WDPM with invasion has a higher rate of recurrence.[63]

Immunohistochemical Features of Well-Differentiated Papillary Mesothelioma

These tumors show immunohistochemistry profiles as expected for mesothelial cells including calretinin, WT1, D240, and cytokeratin 5/6 and negative carcinoma markers.

SOLITARY FIBROUS TUMOR

Clinical Features of Solitary Fibrous Tumor

Solitary fibrous tumors (SFTs) are spindle cell neoplasms that generally arise from the visceral pleura (80%), but can occur elsewhere including lung, mediastinum, and parietal pleura/chest wall. They can occur at any age, but

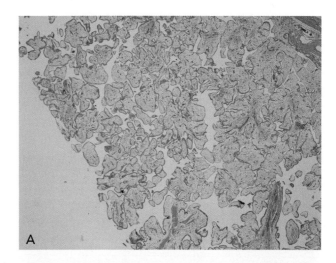

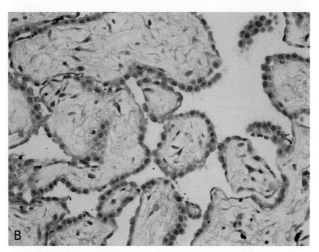

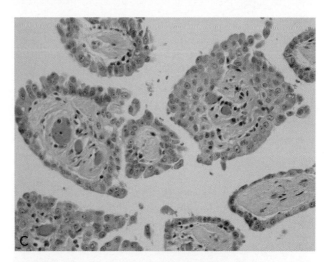

FIGURE 11-8 The histology of well-differentiated papillary mesothelioma. (A) Arborizing exophytic papillary proliferations are typical of WDPM. (B) Papillary structures of WDPM are lined by single layers of flat relatively bland cells. (C) In contrast, papillary malignant mesothelioma shows asymmetric stratification of epithelium, and in addition, nuclear atypia is more marked, with nuclei showing nucleoli.

are usually seen in adults , independent of gender, with an average age of 55.[66,67] They are generally low-grade, slow-growing tumors; they are usually discovered incidentally. In some cases, patients develop chest pain, cough, dyspnea, or fever[67,68]; in rarer instances patients develop hypoglycemia (about 4% of cases), related to tumoral product of insulin-like growth factor.[69]

Gross Features of Solitary Fibrous Tumor

These are solitary tumors and generally well circumscribed. They can be pedunculated and in some cases such a pedicle can be identified as a surgical margin (*Figure 11-9A*). Their cut surface is gray and whorled (*Figure 11-9B*). Cystic degeneration, hemorrhage, and

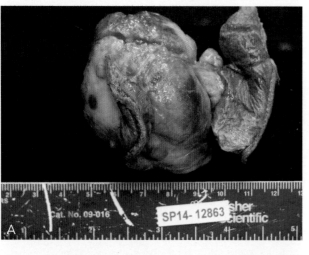
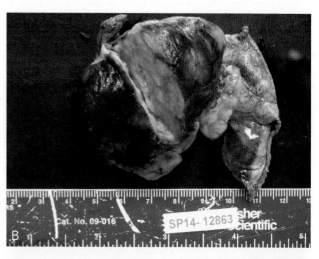
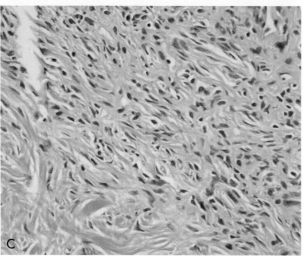
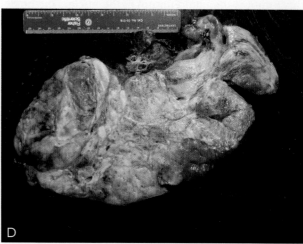
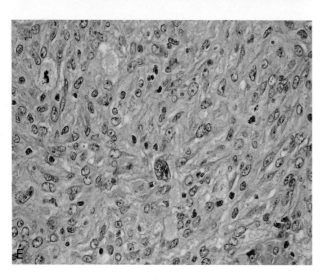

FIGURE 11-9 Features of benign and malignant solitary fibrous tumor. (A) Benign solitary fibrous tumors are circumscribed and often pedunculated pleural-based masses. (B) On cut surface, tumors are whorled and gray-white (C) Histologically, bland spindle cells are seen amidst fibrous stroma, showing variable cellularity. (D) Malignant solitary fibrous tumors are generally larger, not pedunculated and can be seen invading lung tissue. Necrosis and variegated cut surface are more often present. (E) The histology image shows greater cellularity, marked pleomorphism, and mitotic activity.

calcification can be present. Tumors can have a wide range of size at presentation and large series report an average of 6.0 cm. Lack of pedicle and large size (>10 cm) are two proposed criteria predictive of recurrence.[70]

Histologic Features of Solitary Fibrous Tumor

The classic histology is a variably cellular spindle cell neoplasm composed of fibroblastic cells. While typical cases have cellular and paucicellular areas (*Figure 11-9C*), dense cellularity which is fibrosarcoma like should raise concern for malignancy. The cells do not organize into discrete fascicles or bundles, and the variable cellularity is characterized by paucicellular areas with hyalinized stroma. The tumor also has prominent branching vessels, sometimes with perivascular fibrosis. In benign tumors, mitotic rate is usually low (<4 in 10 HPF); while no single criterion predicts malignancy, a higher mitotic rate should raise a suspicion of malignancy.

Immunohistochemical Features of Solitary Fibrous Tumor

Solitary fibrous tumors are typically cytokeratin negative, while positive for CD34 and bcl2.[71] More recently, a characteristic[72] NAB2-STAT6 fusion was identified in solitary fibrous tumor, and the resultant aberrant expression of STAT6 can be detected by immunohistochemistry in 98% of cases.[73] STAT6 IHC is generally negative in other spindle cell tumors including sarcomatoid mesothelioma; it was found rarely in dedifferentiated liposarcoma and in one case of a fibrous histiocytoma.

MALIGNANT SOLITARY FIBROUS TUMOR

Clinical Features of Malignant Solitary Fibrous Tumor

These tumors are generally larger than their benign counterparts, and more likely to exhibit chest wall invasion. In one series, age over 55 was more often associated with malignancy.[74] Presenting symptoms overall do not predict recurrence; it is noted that in one series pleural effusion was associated with recurrence.[70] In a multicenter series of 50 malignant SFTs, mean age was 65 with no gender predilection, with 25% having pleural effusion.[75] Incomplete resection including chest wall invasion and malignant pleural effusion were associated with recurrence.

Gross Features of Malignant Solitary Fibrous Tumor

Malignant SFTs were larger (mean size 12.8 cm) and less likely to be pedunculated (22%) than benign SFTs

Table 11-4 Proposed Criteria for Malignant Solitary Fibrous Tumor

Criterion	England[67]	de Perrot[71]	Tapias (≥ 3 points)[70]
>4 mitoses in 10 HPF	X	X	1
Necrosis	X	X	1
Hypercellularity	X	X	1
Nuclear atypia	X	X	
No pedicle/sessile		X	1
Nonvisceral pleural origin			1
Size >10 cm			1

(*Figure 11-9D*). Malignant SFTs were more likely to arise from parietal pleura than benign SFTs, although visceral pleura remains the most common site. Malignant SFTs were more likely to have hemorrhage or necrosis.[74,75]

Histologic Features of Malignant Solitary Fibrous Tumor

Malignant solitary fibrous tumors frequently have areas of high cellularity (*Figure 11-9e*), and in some cases this hypercellularity mimics areas of other types of sarcoma such as dedifferentiated liposarcoma or fibrosarcoma.[74] Hemorrhage and necrosis are more commonly seen, and increased mitotic rate of >4 in 10 HPF. In one series, the average mitotic rate was 10 in 10 HPF in malignant SFTs.[75] While nuclear atypia was cited in earlier studies as part of malignant SFTs, it may be that this is not independent of other criteria; also, hypercellularity with overlapping nuclei may be more important than atypia in this prediction. Criteria used in the distinction of benign from malignant SFT are summarized in *Table 11-4*.

Immunohistochemical Features of Malignant Solitary Fibrous Tumor

The IHC of malignant SFT is the same as that of solitary fibrous tumor.

SYNOVIAL SARCOMA

Clinical Features of Synovial Sarcoma

Primary pleuropulmonary synovial sarcoma is an uncommon tumor, and represents an unusual but well-described location for this sarcoma, which is typically in the extremities. The average age is 42, with equal rates in men and women. These tumors are not found incidentally, and typical presenting symptoms include dyspnea, chest pain, cough, or hemoptysis. Synovial sarcoma presents as a mass lesion, without radiologic calcification or cavitation; pleural effusion is common. Pulmonary involvement, abdominal spread, and notably lymph node metastasis can be seen at presentation or with recurrence. These tumors are difficult to treat neoplasms, with a significant recurrence rate and with a high mortality rate (40%-50%).[76-81]

Gross Features of Synovial Sarcoma

These tumors are generally large, with an average size of 7.5 cm. They can have a fleshy tan cut surface with areas of softening and hemorrhage, but have also been described as rubbery.

Histologic Features of Synovial Sarcoma

Synovial sarcoma can be monophasic or biphasic. Pleuropulmonary synovial sarcomas are usually monophasic (92%). In this regard, they enter the differential diagnosis of sarcomatoid mesothelioma and sarcomatoid carcinoma. Monophasic tumors are spindle cell tumors with dense cellularity composed of interlacing fascicles. These packed fascicles tend to be more cellular than most spindle cell neoplasms in the differential of SS (*Figure 11-10A*). Myxoid areas can be present. Collagen can be fine and interlacing between individual cells or more moderate but still diffusely interspersed. Entrapped epithelial structures such as pneumocytes are often present (*Figure 11-10B* and *C*), and should not be mistaken for biphasic histology. Hemangiopericytoma-like vasculature is frequently present as dilated staghorn vessels (*Figure 11-10D*). Microscopic calcification and cyst formation can be seen. Patterns that can cause diagnostic confusion include Verocay-like areas, rosettes, microcysts, and rhabdoid histology. Biphasic tumors have gland-forming spaces and papillary structures can be seen.

Mitotic activity is usually present, but can be highly variable, from 2 in 10 HPF to over 40 in 10 HPF. About one-quarter of thoracic synovial sarcomas are characterized as Grade 3/poorly differentiated tumors using FNCLCC grading classification. In such tumors, densely cellular areas appear as small round cells with scant collagen. Such cellular areas can have the more rhabdoid appearing cells.

Immunohistochemical Features of Synovial Sarcoma

By immunohistochemistry, at least one epithelial marker is frequently positive (up to 90%) including pancytokeratin, cytokeratin 7, cytokeratin 5/6, BerEP4, or epithelial membrane antigen[78,82] (*Figure 11-10E*). Also, positive are bcl2, CD99, and CD56 and these markers can lead to confusion with other small blue cell tumors in small samples; usually larger samples will reveal spindle cell areas not typical of PNET or small cell carcinoma. CD99 is usually negative in mesothelioma, and has been reported as negative in small cell type mesothelioma which is in the differential of SS.[83] CD56 is reported as negative in mesothelioma in two series.[84,85] S100 and calretinin can also be positive, so that differentiation from MPNST, melanoma, and mesothelioma also requires a panel approach. TLE1 has emerged as a useful and specific marker for synovial sarcoma; however, some mesothelioma cases can be positive so in this site this is an important pitfall.[36] WT1, SMA, desmin, and CD34 are usually negative.

The chromosomal translocation t(X:18)(p11;q11) is seen in the majority of cases, and this results in SYT/SSX1 and SYT/SSX2 fusions. Overall while there are trends in fusion type and clinicopathologic features, there is sufficient overlap in these features so as to limit their utility in prognostication.[78]

VASCULAR SARCOMA (INCLUDING EPITHELIOID HEMANGIOENDOTHELIOMA AND ANGIOSARCOMA)

Clinical Features of Vascular Sarcoma

This is a rare entity in the pleura, but described cases are mostly in men aged 55 to 71. All were symptomatic, some with chest pain, pleural effusion, and hemothorax. There was a history of asbestos exposure in several cases and some postradiation cases. In contrast to the favorable prognosis and female predominance of pulmonary epithelioid hemangioendothelioma (EHE), pleural EHE-like and epithelioid angiosarcomas have a male predominance and a poor prognosis. Lung, liver, and nodal metastasis have been described.[86-88]

Gross Features of Vascular Sarcoma

This tumor type can involve the pleura in a diffuse pattern (*Figure 11-11A*) and with both smooth and nodular appearance. This may resemble malignant mesothelioma. Vascular tumors can be grossly red and hemorrhagic, but this is not always the case.

Histologic Features of Vascular Sarcoma

Two patterns of vascular pleural tumors have been described. One pattern resembles EHE in other organs, in that there are relatively bland nests of cells in small clusters with a prominent vacuolar space. These spaces

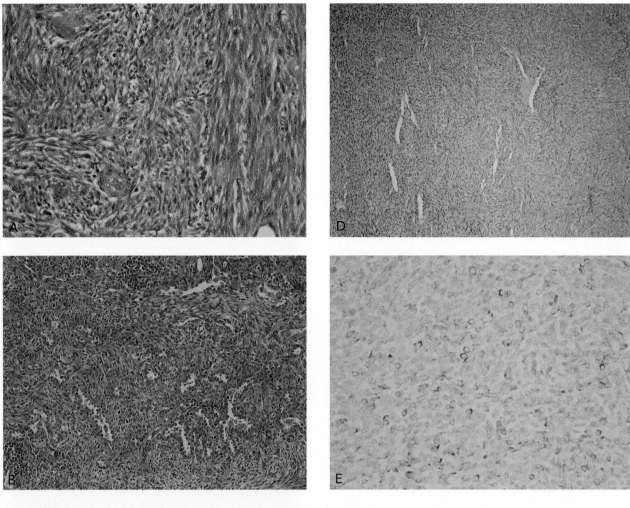

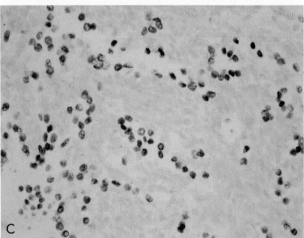

FIGURE 11-10 Histologic features of synovial sarcoma. **(A)** Densely cellular spindle cell neoplasm with interlacing bundles of cells with moderate atypia. **(B)** Invasion of monophasic synovial sarcoma into lung tissue entraps pneumocytes but is not evidence of biphasic growth pattern. **(C)** Thyroid transcription factor 1 immunohistochemistry confirms the epithelioid cells as pneumocytes and not tumor cells. **(D)** "Hemangiopericytoma"-like vessels are the characteristic seen in monophasic synovial sarcoma **(E)** Cytokeratin immunohistochemistry is frequently positive, even in poorly differentiated areas.

are variably filled with the debris of red blood cells (*Figure 11-11B*). In some cases, nests with clear cell histology can be seen. However, many of the cells lack these specific features and are epithelioid, mimicking carcinoma or mesothelioma (*Figure 11-11C,D*). In the epithelioid angiosarcoma pattern, papillary projections are seen as well as dilated spaces lined by high cuboidal

and hobnail-shaped cells. These cells can have prominent nucleoli with significant atypia (*Figure 11-11E,F*). Desmoplastic stroma can outstrip the neoplastic cellularity, sometimes obscuring it. Red blood cells can be prominent and can also be seen within cytoplasmic vacuoles. The vacuoles should not be mucicarmine positive. Some cases have pseudoglandular structures

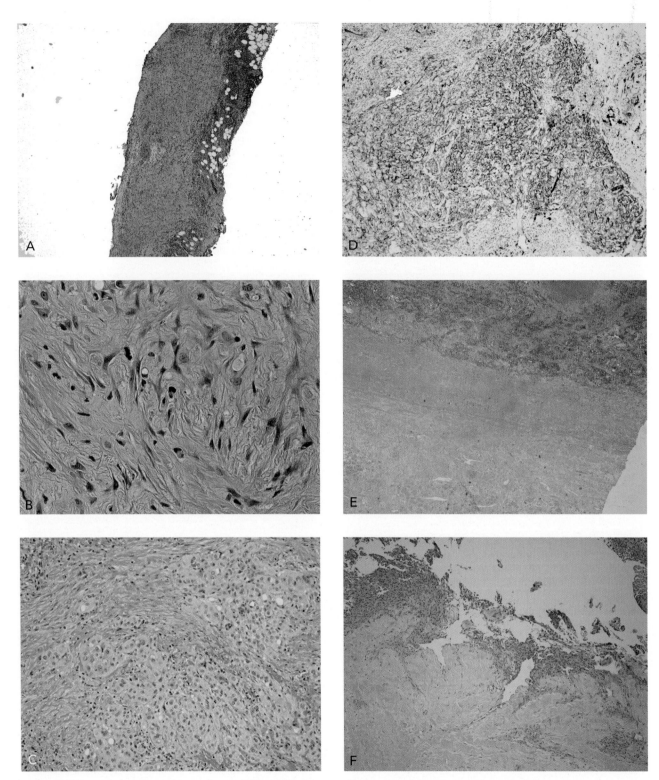

FIGURE 11-11 Histologic features of vascular sarcoma in the pleura. (A) A low power view of a pleural stripping shows a diffuse thickening. (Used with permission of Fabrizio Remotti). **(B)** A mixture of spindled and plumper vaguely nested cells are seen, some with intracytoplasmic vacuoles. These vacuoles are abortive blood vessels and can occasionally contain a degenerated red blood cell in this EHE-like vascular sarcoma. **(C)** Some areas can consist of purely epithelioid cells, and this can mimic mesothelioma. Vacuoles are present, but this can also occur in mesothelioma **(D)** CD31 immunohistochemistry (shown) is strongly positive in these cells and along with **CD34** confirmed the endothelial differentiation in this tumor. **(E)** A higher grade angiosarcoma invades along the pleural surface showing pseudomesotheliomatous growth. **(F)** In areas, growth of tumor along surfaces mimics mesothelioma.

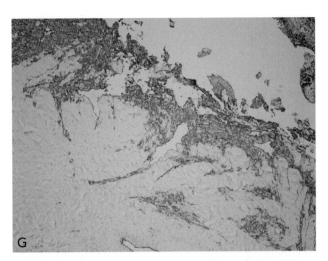
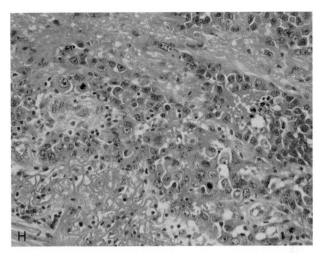

FIGURE 11-11 (*Continued*) **(G) Immunohistochemistry for CD34 (shown) and CD31 confirms the endothelial differentiation. (H) High-grade angiosarcoma shows highly atypical cuboidal cells with formation of irregular spaces consistent with abortive vascular channels.**

and can mimic mesothelioma and adenocarcinoma. These pseudoglandular structures are lined by cuboidal cells, sometimes with hobnail morphology and high-grade nuclei.

Immunohistochemical Features of Vascular Sarcoma

Endothelial markers such as CD31 and CD34 should be positive (*Figure 11-11G,H*). Cytokeratin can be positive at a weak to intermediate intensity. Translocations in WWTR1-CAMTA1[89,90] were described in two pleural EHE examined and YAP1-TFE3 translocations[91] have been described in EHE including pulmonary EHE, but not specifically in the more aggressive pleural EHE.

OTHER PRIMARY NEOPLASMS OF THE PLEURA

Adenomatoid Tumor

These benign gland forming mesothelial proliferations are rare in the pleural space and more commonly seen in the genitourinary system. They are not associated with asbestos exposure. They are small visceral pleural-based nodules, under 3.0 cm, most often representing incidental findings (*Figure 11-12A*). Histologically, adenomatoid tumors are tubule-forming mesothelial proliferations (*Figure 11-12B*) composed of bland cells that by immunohistochemistry are mesothelial. The cells are bland and can contain vacuoles or eosinophilic cytoplasm.[92]

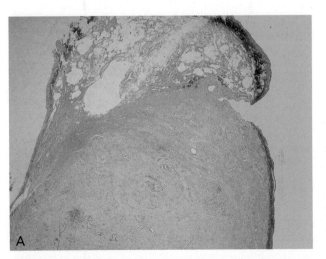
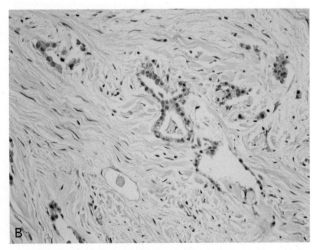

FIGURE 11-12 Histologic features of adenomatoid tumor. (A) Low-power view shows lung tissue with attached well-circumscribed pleural-based mass. (B) High magnification shows well-formed tubular structures lined by bland mesothelial cells.

Calcifying Fibrous Pseudotumor of Pleura

This is an uncommon but well-described cause of a pleural-based mass lesion.[93] These tumors are seen in young adults and once identified usually are persistent but do not show significant interval growth. Imaging can detect calcification in some lesions. Grossly, these are well-circumscribed masses composed of gray-white band-like areas (*Figure 11-13A*). Histologically, these tumors are characterized by a mass of paucicellular dense collagen with bland spindle cells and small calcifications which are lamellated. Surrounding the mass, at the peripheral rim is a reactive lymphocytic population. Invasion of spindle cell into adipose tissue is not seen, and significant cellularity or fascicular growth of spindle cells is not seen (*Figure 11-13B-D*). These are benign tumors, but are resected because of

persistent nonregression of a mass lesion. They can be multiple.[94] They do not recur if completely excised and do not metastasize.

Pleuropulmonary Blastoma

This is a pediatric tumor, with most cases presenting prior to age 10, and with equal gender distribution.[95] These tumors range from grossly cystic neoplasms, mimicking pediatric congenital pulmonary adenomatoid malformations, to solid and higher grade malignant tumors. Prognosis is overall poor, although possibly better for cystic lesions. The tumors are therefore divided into Type 1 (cystic), Type 2 (solid and cystic), and Type 3 (solid). Histologically, these tumors can be cystic, with entrapped epithelial lining with underlying blastemal cells with higher cellularity (*Figure 11-14A*) near epithelial surface ("cambium

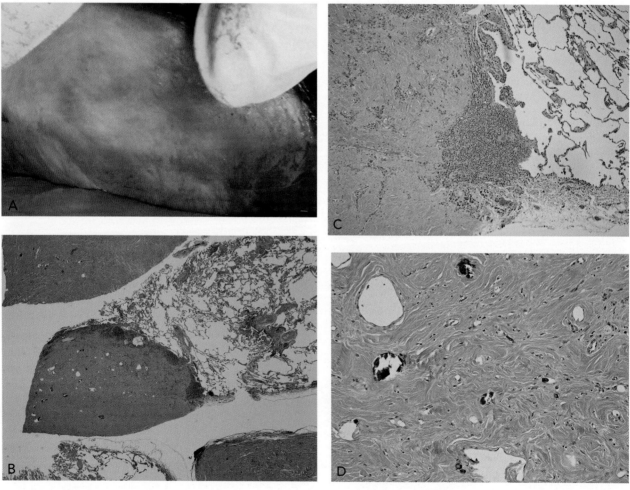

FIGURE 11-13 Gross and histologic features of calcifying fibrous pseudotumor of pleura. **(A)** The cut surface of this well-circumscribed mass lesion shows a gray-white fibrous appearance. **(B)** These fibrous lesions are circumscribed and attached to the pleural surface. **(C)** The periphery of the fibrous lesion characteristically shows a rim of lymphocytic/plasmacytic inflammation. **(D)** The center of the lesion shows dense collagenized tissue with scant spindle cell proliferation and distinctive lamellated calcifications.

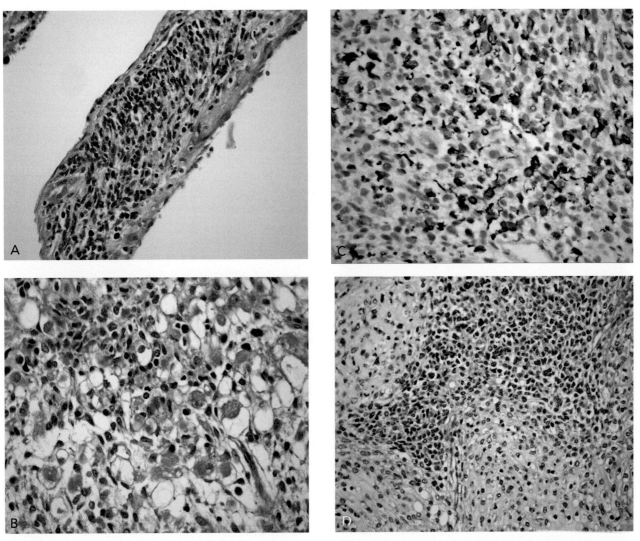

FIGURE 11-14 Histologic features of pleuropulmonary blastoma (PPB). **(A)** The walls of a cystic PPB are filled with cellular areas that have immature cells in a band-like layer resembling developmental structures and sometimes referred to as a "cambium" layer. **(B)** Frequent skeletal muscle differentiation can be seen. **(C)** Muscle differentiation can be confirmed by immunohistochemistry, with desmin (shown), myogenin, or MyoD1. **(D)** Solid PPB have extensive sheet-like areas of primitive blastemal-like cells and can also contain heterologous elements, like the malignant cartilage shown in this panel.

layer"). Foci of rhabdomyoblastic differentiation can be seen (*Figure 11-14B* and *C*). In higher grade lesions, cyst formation is less apparent and replaced by solid growing areas of highly cellular primitive appearing blastemal cells, with overt areas of rhabdomyosarcomatous and malignant cartilaginous foci (*Figure 11-14D*). Immunohistochemistry can confirm myoid differentiation using desmin, MyoD1, and myogenin. Molecular testing has identified evidence of mutations in Dicer1, a gene whose function is ribonuclease activity critical to the processing of microRNA during development, including lung development. Mutations in Dicer1 have been identified as germline mutations in patients with pleuropulmonary blastoma, as well as both sporadic and germline mutations in patients with Sertoli cell tumors of the ovary.[96,97] Other rare tumors have

also been described in this syndrome including cystic nephroma, Wilms tumor, and medulloepithelioma.[98]

Lymphoma

The pleura can be the primary site for lymphoma. Pyothorax-associated lymphoma is associated with long-term chronic pleuritis, usually over 10 years after initial injury.[99] It is described in older patients, is male predominant and most cases reported are from Japan. These present as nodular masses with associated chest pain and constitutional symptoms. This is an EBV-associated B-cell lymphoma and histologically resembles other large B-cell lymphomas. Like other large B-cell lymphomas, therapeutic responses can be achieved and with such responses, 5-year survival can be as high as 50%. Primary effusion lymphomas (PELs) are also described in this site.[100] PELs are generally diagnosed in persistent pleural effusions that harbor malignant lymphoid cells characterized on smears, flow cytometry, and molecular study. Solid nodules are not seen at presentation but can occur later. PELs are associated with immunosuppression, most commonly due to HIV/AIDS, and evidence for HHV8 infection can be demonstrated using immunohistochemistry for latency-associated nuclear antigen, a virally encoded protein expressed in transformed tumor cells. The cells typically have an immunoblastic appearance, are CD45 positive, but often difficult to further assign lineage as B or T cell. It is an aggressive tumor with a poor prognosis despite initial therapeutic responses.

NONNEOPLASTIC PATHOLOGY OF THE PLEURA

Reactive Mesothelial Hyperplasia

Various injuries to the pleura can result in proliferation of mesothelial cells. These injuries can be traumatic (pneumothorax, postsurgical), related to lung infarct, inflammatory, immunological, infectious, and neoplastic from nonmesothelial malignancies. The mesothelial proliferations can be cytologically atypical, and due to the chronic nature of the insult can entrap mesothelial cells in multiple layers, mimicking invasion. Mitotic activity does not help distinguish benign from malignant proliferations. While not usually forming expansile nodules, these proliferations can be papillary, tubule forming, or solid, with overlap of patterns with malignant mesothelioma.

These proliferations require assessment of architecture as well as surrounding tissue and therefore a significant sample must be processed. Individual high power fields of reactive mesothelial proliferations will show patterns of growth and nuclear atypia convincing for malignancy. However, the distribution of these nests amidst otherwise reactive appearing granulation tissue–like stroma, and association of uniformly spaced vessels perpendicular to the pleural surface are critical observations. In addition, despite significant entrapment by organization, morphologic assessment enhanced by immunohistochemistry can convincingly demonstrate an organized layered appearance to these atypical nests. In addition, there is often a zonal distribution of cellularity, with the greatest proliferation near the pleural surface, decreasing into deeper tissue.

Fibrous Pleuritis

Fibrous pleuritis is the organization that occurs after hemorrhagic or fibrinous pleuritis, often with recurrent pleural effusions. It is a chronic process, and can result in significant proliferation followed by progressively dense fibrosis. This fibrosis can be rind like and can encase the lung, similar to the pattern of malignant mesothelioma.

Causes of fibrous pleuritis include collagen vascular disease, chronic empyema, medications, and asbestos exposure.

The gross appearance of fibrous pleuritis is a thickening and complete opacification of the pleura. The pleural surface is white/off-white and shaggy. Nodules are not usually present. Dense collagenized pleural plaques are white, raised, and thickened; these have a shiny surface and can be seen on the visceral and parietal pleural surfaces, including the surface of the diaphragm. The histology of fibrous pleuritis varies with the activity of the process and its chronicity.

REFERENCES

1. International Agency for Research and Cancer. Cancer incidence in 5 continents. Volume X (electronic version). http://ci5.iarc.fr. Accessed July 2014.
2. Surveillance, Epidemiology, and End Results (SEER) Program. SEER*Stat Database: Populations - Total U.S. (1969-2012) <Single Ages to 85+, Katrina/Rita Adjustment> - Linked To County Attributes - Total U.S., 1969-2012 Counties, National Cancer Institute, DCCPS, Surveillance Research Program, Surveillance Systems Branch, released April 2014. www.seer.cancer.gov.
3. Wagner JC, Sleggs CA, Marchand P. Diffuse pleural mesothelioma and asbestos exposure in the North Western Cape Province. *Br J Ind Med.* October 1960;17:260-271.
4. Selikoff IJ, Churg J, Hammond EC. Asbestos exposure and neoplasia. *JAMA.* April 6 1964;188:22-26.
5. McDonald AD. Mineral fibre content of lung in mesothelial tumours: preliminary report. *IARC Sci Publ.* 1980(30):681-685.
6. McDonald AD. Malignant mesothelioma in Quebec. *IARC Sci Publ.* 1980(30):673-680.
7. McDonald AD, McDonald JC. Malignant mesothelioma in North America. *Cancer.* October 1, 1980;46(7):1650-1656.
8. McDonald JC. Asbestos-related disease: an epidemiological review. *IARC Sci Publ.* 1980(30):587-601.
9. McDonald JC, McDonald AD. Epidemiology of mesothelioma from estimated incidence. *Prev Med.* September 1977;6(3):426-442.
10. McDonald JC, Liddell FD, Gibbs GW, Eyssen GE, McDonald AD. Dust exposure and mortality in chrysotile mining, 1910-75. *Br J Ind Med.* February 1980;37(1):11-24.
11. Rake C, Gilham C, Hatch J, Darnton A, Hodgson J, Peto J. Occupational, domestic and environmental mesothelioma risks in the British population: a case-control study. *Br J Cancer.* April 7 2009;100(7):1175-1183.
12. Spirtas R, Heineman EF, Bernstein L, et al. Malignant mesothelioma: attributable risk of asbestos exposure. *Occup Environ Med.* December 1994;51(12):804-811.
13. Jasani B, Gibbs A. Mesothelioma not associated with asbestos exposure. *Arch Pathol Lab Med.* March 2012;136(3):262-267.
14. Carbone M, Baris YI, Bertino P, et al. Erionite exposure in North Dakota and Turkish villages with mesothelioma. *Proc Natl Acad Sci U S A.* August 16 2011;108(33):13618-13623.
15. Cavazza A, Travis LB, Travis WD, et al. Post-irradiation malignant mesothelioma. *Cancer.* April 1 1996;77(7):1379-1385.

16. De Bruin ML, Burgers JA, Baas P, et al. Malignant mesothelioma after radiation treatment for Hodgkin lymphoma. *Blood*. April 16 2009;113(16):3679-3681.

17. Fung C, Fossa SD, Beard CJ, Travis LB. Second malignant neoplasms in testicular cancer survivors. *J Natl Compr Canc Netw*. April 2012;10(4):545-556.

18. Ng AK, Travis LB. Subsequent malignant neoplasms in cancer survivors. *Cancer J*. November-December 2008;14(6):429-434.

19. Schairer C, Hisada M, Chen BE, et al. Comparative mortality for 621 second cancers in 29356 testicular cancer survivors and 12420 matched first cancers. *J Natl Cancer Inst*. August 15 2007;99(16):1248-1256.

20. Teta MJ, Lau E, Sceurman BK, Wagner ME. Therapeutic radiation for lymphoma: risk of malignant mesothelioma. *Cancer*. April 1 2007;109(7):1432-1438.

21. Travis LB, Andersson M, Gospodarowicz M, et al. Treatment-associated leukemia following testicular cancer. *J Natl Cancer Inst*. July 19 2000;92(14):1165-1171.

22. Tward JD, Wendland MM, Shrieve DC, Szabo A, Gaffney DK. The risk of secondary malignancies over 30 years after the treatment of non-Hodgkin lymphoma. *Cancer*. July 1 2006;107(1):108-115.

23. Testa JR, Cheung M, Pei J, et al. Germline BAP1 mutations predispose to malignant mesothelioma. *Nat Genet*. October 2011;43(10):1022-1025.

24. Cheung M, Talarchek J, Schindeler K, et al. Further evidence for germline BAP1 mutations predisposing to melanoma and malignant mesothelioma. *Cancer Genet*. May 2013;206(5):206-210.

25. Abdel-Rahman MH, Pilarski R, Cebulla CM, et al. Germline BAP1 mutation predisposes to uveal melanoma, lung adenocarcinoma, meningioma, and other cancers. *J Med Genet*. December 2011;48(12):856-859.

26. Armato SG 3rd, Labby ZE, Coolen J, et al. Imaging in pleural mesothelioma: a review of the 11th International Conference of the International Mesothelioma Interest Group. *Lung Cancer (Amsterdam, Netherlands)*. November 2013;82(2):190-196.

27. Wilson GE, Hasleton PS, Chatterjee AK. Desmoplastic malignant mesothelioma: a review of 17 cases. *J Clin Pathol*. April 1992;45(4):295-298.

28. Klebe S, Brownlee NA, Mahar A, et al. Sarcomatoid mesothelioma: a clinical-pathologic correlation of 326 cases. *Mod Pathol*. March 2010;23(3):470-479.

29. Henderson DW, Attwood HD, Constance TJ, Shilkin KB, Steele RH. Lymphohistiocytoid mesothelioma: a rare lymphomatoid variant of predominantly sarcomatoid mesothelioma. *Ultrastruct Pathol*. 1988;12(4):367-384.

30. Yao DX, Shia J, Erlandson RA, Klimstra DS. Lymphohistiocytoid mesothelioma: a clinical, immunohistochemical and ultrastructural study of four cases and literature review. *Ultrastruct Pathol*. July-August 2004;28(4):213-228.

31. Galateau-Salle F, Attanoos R, Gibbs AR, et al. Lymphohistiocytoid variant of malignant mesothelioma of the pleura: a series of 22 cases. *Am J Surg Pathol*. May 2007;31(5):711-716.

32. Kadota K, Suzuki K, Sima CS, Rusch VW, Adusumilli PS, Travis WD. Pleomorphic epithelioid diffuse malignant pleural mesothelioma: a clinicopathological review and conceptual proposal to reclassify as biphasic or sarcomatoid mesothelioma. *J Thorac Oncol*. May 2011;6(5):896-904.

33. Ordonez NG. Pleomorphic mesothelioma: report of 10 cases. *Mod Pathol*. July 2012;25(7):1011-1022.

34. Husain AN, Colby T, Ordonez N, et al. Guidelines for pathologic diagnosis of malignant mesothelioma: 2012 update of the consensus statement from the International Mesothelioma Interest Group. *Arch Pathol Lab Med*. May 2013;137(5):647-667.

35. Chirieac LR, Pinkus GS, Pinkus JL, Godleski J, Sugarbaker DJ, Corson JM. The immunohistochemical characterization of sarcomatoid malignant mesothelioma of the pleura. *Am J Cancer*. 2011;1(1):14-24.

36. Matsuyama A, Hisaoka M, Iwasaki M, Iwashita M, Hisanaga S, Hashimoto H. TLE1 expression in malignant mesothelioma. *Virchows Arch*. November 2010;457(5):577-583.

37. Jurgens H, Bier V, Harms D, et al. Malignant peripheral neuroectodermal tumors. A retrospective analysis of 42 patients. *Cancer*. January 15 1988;61(2):349-357.

38. Gu M, Antonescu CR, Guiter G, Huvos AG, Ladanyi M, Zakowski MF. Cytokeratin immunoreactivity in Ewing's sarcoma: prevalence in 50 cases confirmed by molecular diagnostic studies. *Am J Surg Pathol*. March 2000;24(3):410-416.

39. Cagle PT, Churg A. Differential diagnosis of benign and malignant mesothelial proliferations on pleural biopsies. *Arch Pathol Lab Med*. November 2005;129(11):1421-1427.

40. Churg A, Colby TV, Cagle P, et al. The separation of benign and malignant mesothelial proliferations. *Am J Surg Pathol*. September 2000;24(9):1183-1200.

41. Minato H, Kurose N, Fukushima M, et al. Comparative immunohistochemical analysis of IMP3, GLUT1, EMA, CD146, and desmin for distinguishing malignant mesothelioma from reactive mesothelial cells. *Am J Clin Pathol*. January 2014;141(1):85-93.

42. Lagana SM, Taub RN, Borczuk AC. Utility of glucose transporter 1 in the distinction of benign and malignant thoracic and abdominal mesothelial lesions. *Arch Pathol Lab Med*. July 2012;136(7):804-809.

43. Monaco SE, Shuai Y, Bansal M, Krasinskas AM, Dacic S. The diagnostic utility of p16 FISH and GLUT-1 immunohistochemical analysis in mesothelial proliferations. *Am J Clin Pathol*. April 2011;135(4):619-627.

44. Kato Y, Tsuta K, Seki K, et al. Immunohistochemical detection of GLUT-1 can discriminate between reactive mesothelium and malignant mesothelioma. *Mod Pathol*. February 2007;20(2):215-220.

45. Mossman BT, Shukla A, Heintz NH, Verschraegen CF, Thomas A, Hassan R. New insights into understanding the mechanisms, pathogenesis, and management of malignant mesotheliomas. *Am J Pathol*. April 2013;182(4):1065-1077.

46. Sekido Y. Molecular pathogenesis of malignant mesothelioma. *Carcinogenesis*. July 2013;34(7):1413-1419.

47. Bianchi AB, Mitsunaga SI, Cheng JQ, et al. High frequency of inactivating mutations in the neurofibromatosis type 2 gene (NF2) in primary malignant mesotheliomas. *Proc Natl Acad Sci U S A*. November 21 1995;92(24):10854-10858.

48. Cheng JQ, Lee WC, Klein MA, Cheng GZ, Jhanwar SC, Testa JR. Frequent mutations of NF2 and allelic loss from chromosome band 22q12 in malignant mesothelioma: evidence for a two-hit mechanism of NF2 inactivation. *Genes Chromosomes Cancer*. March 1999;24(3):238-242.

49. Bott M, Brevet M, Taylor BS, et al. The nuclear deubiquitinase BAP1 is commonly inactivated by somatic mutations and 3p21.1 losses in malignant pleural mesothelioma. *Nat Genet*. July 2011;43(7):668-672.

50. Yoshikawa Y, Sato A, Tsujimura T, et al. Frequent inactivation of the BAP1 gene in epithelioid-type malignant mesothelioma. *Cancer Sci*. May 2012;103(5):868-874.

51. Zauderer MG, Bott M, McMillan R, et al. Clinical characteristics of patients with malignant pleural mesothelioma harboring somatic BAP1 mutations. *J Thorac Oncol*. November 2013;8(11):1430-1433.

52. Xio S, Li D, Vijg J, Sugarbaker DJ, Corson JM, Fletcher JA. Codeletion of p15 and p16 in primary malignant mesothelioma. *Oncogene*. August 3, 1995;11(3):511-515.

53. Illei PB, Rusch VW, Zakowski MF, Ladanyi M. Homozygous deletion of *CDKN2A* and codeletion of the methylthioadenosine phosphorylase gene in the majority of pleural mesotheliomas. *Clin Cancer Res*. June 2003;9(6):2108-2113.

54. Lopez-Rios F, Chuai S, Flores R, et al. Global gene expression profiling of pleural mesotheliomas: overexpression of aurora

kinases and P16/*CDKN2A* deletion as prognostic factors and critical evaluation of microarray-based prognostic prediction. *Cancer Res.* March 15, 2006;66(6):2970-2979.

55. Wu D, Hiroshima K, Matsumoto S, et al. Diagnostic usefulness of p16/*CDKN2A* FISH in distinguishing between sarcomatoid mesothelioma and fibrous pleuritis. *Am J Clin Pathol.* January 2013;139(1):39-46.

56. Dacic S, Kothmaier H, Land S, et al. Prognostic significance of p16/*cdkn2a* loss in pleural malignant mesotheliomas. *Virchows Arch.* December 2008;453(6):627-635.

57. Illei PB, Ladanyi M, Rusch VW, Zakowski MF. The use of *CDKN2A* deletion as a diagnostic marker for malignant mesothelioma in body cavity effusions. *Cancer.* February 25 2003;99(1):51-56.

58. Musti M, Kettunen E, Dragonieri S, et al. Cytogenetic and molecular genetic changes in malignant mesothelioma. *Cancer Genet Cytogenet.* October 1, 2006;170(1):9-15.

59. Chiosea S, Krasinskas A, Cagle PT, Mitchell KA, Zander DS, Dacic S. Diagnostic importance of 9p21 homozygous deletion in malignant mesotheliomas. *Mod Pathol.* June 2008;21(6):742-747.

60. Attanoos RL, Gibbs AR. 'Pseudomesotheliomatous' carcinomas of the pleura: a 10-year analysis of cases from the Environmental Lung Disease Research Group, Cardiff. *Histopathology.* November 2003;43(5):444-452.

61. Allen TC, Cagle PT, Churg AM, et al. Localized malignant mesothelioma. *Am J Surg Pathol.* July 2005;29(7):866-873.

62. Malpica A, Sant'Ambrogio S, Deavers MT, Silva EG. Well-differentiated papillary mesothelioma of the female peritoneum: a clinicopathologic study of 26 cases. *Am J Surg Pathol.* January 2012;36(1):117-127.

63. Churg A, Allen T, Borczuk AC, et al. Well-differentiated papillary mesothelioma with invasive foci. *Am J Surg Pathol.* July 2014;38(7):990-998.

64. Chen X, Sheng W, Wang J. Well-differentiated papillary mesothelioma: a clinicopathological and immunohistochemical study of 18 cases with additional observation. *Histopathology.* April 2013;62(5):805-813.

65. Galateau-Salle F, Vignaud JM, Burke L, et al. Well-differentiated papillary mesothelioma of the pleura: a series of 24 cases. *Am J Surg Pathol.* April 2004;28(4):534-540.

66. Magdeleinat P, Alifano M, Petino A, et al. Solitary fibrous tumors of the pleura: clinical characteristics, surgical treatment and outcome. *Eur J Cardiothorac Surg.* June 2002;21(6):1087-1093.

67. England DM, Hochholzer L, McCarthy MJ. Localized benign and malignant fibrous tumors of the pleura. A clinicopathologic review of 223 cases. *Am J Surg Pathol.* August 1989;13(8):640-658.

68. Briselli M, Mark EJ, Dickersin GR. Solitary fibrous tumors of the pleura: eight new cases and review of 360 cases in the literature. *Cancer.* June 1 1981;47(11):2678-2689.

69. Hajdu M, Singer S, Maki RG, Schwartz GK, Keohan ML, Antonescu CR. IGF2 over-expression in solitary fibrous tumours is independent of anatomical location and is related to loss of imprinting. *J Pathol.* July 2010;221(3):300-307.

70. Tapias LF, Mino-Kenudson M, Lee H, et al. Risk factor analysis for the recurrence of resected solitary fibrous tumours of the pleura: a 33-year experience and proposal for a scoring system. *Eur J Cardiothorac Surg.* July 2013;44(1):111-117.

71. de Perrot M, Fischer S, Brundler MA, Sekine Y, Keshavjee S. Solitary fibrous tumors of the pleura. *Ann Thorac Surg.* July 2002;74(1):285-293.

72. Chmielecki J, Crago AM, Rosenberg M, et al. Whole-exome sequencing identifies a recurrent NAB2-STAT6 fusion in solitary fibrous tumors. *Nat Genet.* February 2013;45(2):131-132.

73. Doyle LA, Vivero M, Fletcher CD, Mertens F, Hornick JL. Nuclear expression of STAT6 distinguishes solitary fibrous tumor from histologic mimics. *Mod Pathol.* March 2014;27(3):390-395.

74. Demicco EG, Park MS, Araujo DM, et al. Solitary fibrous tumor: a clinicopathological study of 110 cases and proposed risk assessment model. *Mod Pathol.* September 2012;25(9):1298-1306.

75. Lococo F, Cesario A, Cardillo G, et al. Malignant solitary fibrous tumors of the pleura: retrospective review of a multicenter series. *J Thorac Oncol.* November 2012;7(11):1698-1706.

76. Hartel PH, Fanburg-Smith JC, Frazier AA, et al. Primary pulmonary and mediastinal synovial sarcoma: a clinicopathologic study of 60 cases and comparison with five prior series. *Mod Pathol.* July 2007;20(7):760-769.

77. Suster S, Moran CA. Primary synovial sarcomas of the mediastinum: a clinicopathologic, immunohistochemical, and ultrastructural study of 15 cases. *Am J Surg Pathol.* May 2005;29(5):569-578.

78. Begueret H, Galateau-Salle F, Guillou L, et al. Primary intrathoracic synovial sarcoma: a clinicopathologic study of 40 t(X;18)-positive cases from the French Sarcoma Group and the Mesopath Group. *Am J Surg Pathol.* March 2005;29(3):339-346.

79. Okamoto S, Hisaoka M, Daa T, Hatakeyama K, Iwamasa T, Hashimoto H. Primary pulmonary synovial sarcoma: a clinicopathologic, immunohistochemical, and molecular study of 11 cases. *Hum Pathol.* July 2004;35(7):850-856.

80. Essary LR, Vargas SO, Fletcher CD. Primary pleuropulmonary synovial sarcoma: reappraisal of a recently described anatomic subset. *Cancer.* January 15 2002;94(2):459-469.

81. Zeren H, Moran CA, Suster S, Fishback NF, Koss MN. Primary pulmonary sarcomas with features of monophasic synovial sarcoma: a clinicopathological, immunohistochemical, and ultrastructural study of 25 cases. *Hum Pathol.* May 1995;26(5):474-480.

82. Miettinen M, Limon J, Niezabitowski A, Lasota J. Calretinin and other mesothelioma markers in synovial sarcoma: analysis of antigenic similarities and differences with malignant mesothelioma. *Am J Surg Pathol.* May 2001;25(5):610-617.

83. Ordonez NG. Mesotheliomas with small cell features: report of eight cases. *Mod Pathol.* May 2012;25(5):689-698.

84. Chu PG, Arber DA, Weiss LM. Expression of T/NK-cell and plasma cell antigens in nonhematopoietic epithelioid neoplasms. An immunohistochemical study of 447 cases. *Am J Clin Pathol.* July 2003;120(1):64-70.

85. Ioachim HL, Pambuccian SE, Hekimgil M, Giancotti FR, Dorsett BH. Lymphoid monoclonal antibodies reactive with lung tumors. Diagnostic applications. *Am J Surg Pathol.* January 1996;20(1):64-71.

86. Crotty EJ, McAdams HP, Erasmus JJ, Sporn TA, Roggli VL. Epithelioid hemangioendothelioma of the pleura: clinical and radiologic features. *AJR Am J Roentgenol.* December 2000;175(6):1545-1549.

87. Zhang PJ, Livolsi VA, Brooks JJ. Malignant epithelioid vascular tumors of the pleura: report of a series and literature review. *Hum Pathol.* January 2000;31(1):29-34.

88. Lin BT, Colby T, Gown AM, et al. Malignant vascular tumors of the serous membranes mimicking mesothelioma. A report of 14 cases. *Am J Surg Pathol.* December 1996;20(12):1431-1439.

89. Tanas MR, Sboner A, Oliveira AM, et al. Identification of a disease-defining gene fusion in epithelioid hemangioendothelioma. *Sci Transl Med.* August 31 2011;3(98):98ra82.

90. Errani C, Zhang L, Sung YS, et al. A novel WWTR1-CAMTA1 gene fusion is a consistent abnormality in epithelioid hemangioendothelioma of different anatomic sites. *Genes Chromosomes Cancer.* August 2011;50(8):644-653.

91. Antonescu CR, Le Loarer F, Mosquera JM, et al. Novel YAP1-TFE3 fusion defines a distinct subset of epithelioid hemangioendothelioma. *Genes Chromosomes Cancer.* August 2013;52(8):775-784.

92. Minato H, Nojima T, Kurose N, Kinoshita E. Adenomatoid tumor of the pleura. *Pathol Int.* August 2009;59(8):567-571.

93. Pinkard NB, Wilson RW, Lawless N, et al. Calcifying fibrous pseudotumor of pleura. A report of three cases of a newly described entity involving the pleura. *Am J Clin Pathol.* February 1996;105(2):189-194.

94. Shibata K, Yuki D, Sakata K. Multiple calcifying fibrous pseudotumors disseminated in the pleura. *Ann Thorac Surg.* February 2008;85(2):e3-e5.

95. Priest JR, McDermott MB, Bhatia S, Watterson J, Manivel JC, Dehner LP. Pleuropulmonary blastoma: a clinicopathologic study of 50 cases. *Cancer.* July 1 1997;80(1):147-161.

96. Heravi-Moussavi A, Anglesio MS, Cheng SW, et al. Recurrent somatic DICER1 mutations in nonepithelial ovarian cancers. *N Engl J Med.* January 19 2012;366(3):234-242.

97. Hill DA, Ivanovich J, Priest JR, et al. DICER1 mutations in familial pleuropulmonary blastoma. *Science.* August 21 2009;325(5943):965.

98. Slade I, Bacchelli C, Davies H, et al. DICER1 syndrome: clarifying the diagnosis, clinical features and management implications of a pleiotropic tumour predisposition syndrome. *J Med Genet.* April 2011;48(4):273-278.

99. Aozasa K, Takakuwa T, Nakatsuka S. Pyothorax-associated lymphoma: a lymphoma developing in chronic inflammation. *Adv Anat Pathol.* November 2005;12(6):324-331.

100. Nador RG, Cesarman E, Chadburn A, et al. Primary effusion lymphoma: a distinct clinicopathologic entity associated with the Kaposi's sarcoma-associated herpes virus. *Blood.* July 15 1996;88(2):645-656.

Bacterial and Mycobacterial Diseases

Andrew Paul Norgan and Timothy Craig Allen

TAKE HOME PEARLS

- GMS and silver impregnation stains are useful for the identification of gram-positive organisms in tissue.
- Bacteria enter the lungs through the bronchi (aerogenous spread or aspiration), bloodstream (hematogenous seeding or septic emboli) or by direct extension from neighboring structures (neck, chest wall, diaphragm, and mediastinum)
- Risks for bacterial pneumonia include young age (infants and children less than 2 years of age), age >65, being immunocompromised (HIV/AIDS, organ transplant, chemotherapy, long-term steroid use), being malnourished, having an underlying cardiopulmonary conditions (asthma, chronic obstructive pulmonary disease, congestive heart failure, cystic fibrosis), and being a smoker.
- Community-acquired pneumonia from all causes is the leading cause of infection-related death in the United States, and remains a leading cause of death worldwide.
- Pneumonia from all causes is the single largest contributor to mortality of children <5 worldwide; approximately 1 to 2 million children who die annually from pneumonia, with 50% of deaths attributed to *Streptococcus pneumoniae* and *Haemophilus influenzae* type B.
- Sputum Gram stain, with its low cost and rapid turnaround time, is the mainstay of morphologic diagnosis of bacterial pneumonia.
- With the exception of the *Corynebacterium* spp and *Bacillus anthracis*, the gram-positive bacilli are primarily opportunistic or incidental pathogens of low virulence.
- Currently, over 2 billion people (or roughly a third of the world population) are latently infected with *Mycobacterium tuberculosis* and there are approximately 9 million new infections each year.
- Active tuberculosis is associated with significant acute and chronic impairments in lung function, including cavity formation, fibrosis, emphysema, and bronchiectasis.
- Elderly Caucasian women with slender body habitus are at increased risk for developing a nodular bronchiectatic *Mycobacterium avium-intracellulare* complex infection, also termed Lady Windermere syndrome.

SPECIMEN HANDLING ISSUES

All specimens must be handled utilizing universal precautions in order to prevent skin and mucous membrane exposure to organisms. Whenever possible, all specimens designated for infectious workup should be handled for processing within a biological safety hood, and specifically specimens designated for mycobacterial workup should be.

Because there is both patient risk and expense in obtaining cytologic, biopsy, or excisional material for infectious workup, care must be taken to maximize its utility. A pathologist's assistance in deciding the division of excised tissue for infectious workup versus histologic examination often helps maximize tissue utility.

BACTERIAL DISEASE

Many of the bacteria that cause human disease primarily or secondarily involve the lungs. Pneumonia, in its varied manifestations, is the most common consequence of pulmonary involvement by nonmycobacterial pathogens. Mycobacteria, by contrast, typically cause granulomatous disease. Integration of the pattern of inflammation with the microscopic appearance of the pathogenic organisms can often provide clues helpful in rendering a final diagnosis.

Classification of Bacterial Pneumonia

Numerous systems for the classification of bacterial pneumonia exist, including anatomic, clinical, etiological, epidemiological, and pathological. Diagnostic accuracy is enhanced by a comprehensive understanding of both pathological and clinical classifications of pneumonia, which together often lead to the causative agent. When a microorganism is present, morphology alone sometimes leads to an accurate final diagnosis. More commonly, morphology, the pattern of inflammation, and the clinical situation are combined with epidemiologic risk factors to suggest a specific pathogen or group of pathogens.

Anatomical classification of pneumonia includes lobar, multilobar, bronchial, or interstitial. Histologically, pneumonia can broadly be grouped into categories of nonnecrotizing or necrotizing, with acute or chronic inflammatory infiltrates that are granulomatous, neutrophilic, lymphoplasmacytic, or histiocytic.

Clinical classification combines elements of epidemiology and temporality, leading to groupings that include community-acquired pneumonia (CAP), health care-associated pneumonia (HCAP), hospital-acquired pneumonia (HAP), ventilator-associated pneumonia (VAP), and aspiration pneumonia. Such classifications are useful in defining the most likely organisms involved in a given infection, which drives the choice of an empiric treatment.

Pathogenesis of Bacterial Pneumonia

Bacteria enter the lungs through the bronchi (aerogenous spread or aspiration), bloodstream (hematogenous seeding or septic emboli) or by direct extension from neighboring structures (neck, chest wall, diaphragm and mediastinum). The route of arrival often influences the resulting pathology. Bronchopneumonia is most commonly associated with a centrilobular origin of infection, which then extends outward from the secondary lobule of the lung. Intra-alveolar connections (so-called "pores of Kohn") allow fluid, infecting organisms, and immune cells to spread throughout a lobe, resulting in a typical lobar pneumonia. If multiple lobules are seeded, multilobar pneumonia may occur.

In contrast, hematogenous dissemination, by contrast, often results in a diffuse multifocal or miliary pattern of disease. The miliary pattern (termed such due to its gross resemblance to small millet seeds) is created by multiple or innumerable small foci of disease that involve the lungs bilaterally. The pattern results from the deposition of blood-borne microorganisms in small arterioles of the lungs. Septic emboli usually cause fewer total nodules, and larger pulmonary vessels may be involved; occasionally, radiography shows a "feeding vessel sign" with either a pulmonary artery or vein appearing to enter or exit a nodule.[1] Direct extension usually results in abscess formation, with the abscess extending from the primary site of infection. When the pleural space is involved, effusion or empyema frequently occurs.

The most common method of pneumonia spread is aerogenous. The respiratory tract has several mechanical and immunological barriers that must be overcome in order for a pathogen to establish an infection. Primary barriers to infection include the hairs the nasal tract, mucociliary escalator of the respiratory tract, secreted proteins (lysozyme, transferrin, immunoglobulin A, defensins), toll-like receptors, and alveolar macrophages.[2-5] These mechanical and chemical barriers will often clear microorganisms that enter the respiratory tract before they reach the alveoli of secondary lobules. Within the secondary lobule, many organisms are cleared by alveolar macrophages before an infection can be established.

Organisms that fail to be cleared by alveolar macrophages result in toll-like receptor signaling, macrophage activation, neutrophil chemotaxis and the influx of dendritic cells, and T and B lymphocytes, resulting in the development of acute pneumonia. The majority of acute infections will be cleared, often with little residual damage to the lung parenchyma. However, not all infections are cleared, and organisms capable of achieving a balance with the host immune response may establish a permanent presence within lung, a process known as colonization. Colonization frequently occurs in the setting of chronic lung diseases such as COPD and cystic fibrosis, and it is a risk factor for future acute exacerbations.[6,7] In contrast, some organisms such as *Mycobacterium tuberculosis* or *Mycobacterium avium-intracellulare* typically establish a persistent infection in the absence of homeostasis with the host immune system, leading to a chronic inflammatory response with progressive damage, including bronchiectasis and fibrosis.

Risk Factors for Developing Bacterial Pneumonia

Risk for bacterial pneumonia include young age (infants and children less than 2 years of age), age >65,

Table 12-1 Risk Factors for Developing Bacterial Pneumonia

Age less than 2 or greater than 65 years
Immunocompromised (HIV/AIDS patient, organ transplant recipient, undergoing chemotherapy)
Malnourished
Underlying cardiopulmonary condition (asthma, chronic obstructive pulmonary disease, congestive heart failure, cystic fibrosis)
Smoker
Impaired cough reflex (intrinsic, medication induced, or alcohol induced)
Placed on a ventilator
Viral upper respiratory tract infection (predisposes to secondary bacterial pneumonia)

being immunocompromised (HIV/AIDS, organ transplant, chemotherapy, long-term steroid use, and being malnourished), and those with underlying cardiopulmonary conditions (asthma, chronic obstructive pulmonary disease, congestive heart failure, cystic fibrosis) and smokers.[8-11] In addition, mechanical factors such as impaired cough reflex (intrinsic or due to sedating medications or alcohol), chronic aspiration, limited mobility, and being placed on ventilator are risk factors for developing pneumonia.[12,13] Viral upper respiratory tract infections impair the mucociliary elevator system and predispose to development of secondary bacterial pneumonias[14] (*Table 12-1*).

Exogenous Bacterial Pneumonia

Bacterial infections within the lower respiratory tract may arise from exogenous or endogenous sources; however, exogenous sources are less common. Organisms typically associated with exogenous bacterial pneumonia include infections with *Mycobacterium* sp, Legionnaire disease, *Yersinia pestis* infection, and anthrax.

Endogenous Bacterial Pneumonia

Endogenous bacterial pneumonias are more common, and some endogenous bacterial pneumonias, for example, *Streptococcus pneumoniae* pneumonia, may be limited by the use of vaccinations. Other common endogenous bacterial pneumonia–causing organisms include enteric gram-negative bacilli, *Staphylococcus aureus*, and *Haemophilus influenzae*. These pneumonias occur due to spread of bacterial organisms from the upper airway or gastrointestinal tract to the lower respiratory tract.

Inflammatory Responses to Bacterial Pneumonia

The primary immune cell of the lung is the alveolar macrophage (AM). Failure of alveolar macrophages to control microorganisms in the alveoli leads to macrophage activation via toll-like receptors and secretion of inflammatory cytokines such as tumor necrosis factor α, interleukin-1β, interleukin-6, and interlukin-8.[15-17] These factors, in turn, recruit circulating polymorphonuclear neutrophils (PMNs) to the alveoli. PMNs phagocytize microorganisms and release further cytokines to promote further immune activation.[18,19] The elaboration of cytokines by responding immune cells leads to both systemic symptoms (fever and chills) and local inflammatory response. Inflammation-associated increases in vascular permeability result in the entry of fibrin-rich plasma into the alveolar spaces. As with bacteria, the pores of Kohn allow fluid to move between alveolar airspaces throughout an affected lobe, resulting in lobar consolidation.

Secondary Bacterial Pneumonia

Damage to the normal defense barriers of the lung predisposes to the development of bacterial pneumonia. The term *secondary bacterial pneumonia* is applied to bacterial infections occurring immediately after or concomitantly with an initial viral infection, most commonly the influenza virus.[14] Influenza virus is estimated to cause approximately 25,000 deaths and 200,000 hospitalizations per year in the United States.[20-22] A primary complication of influenza virus infection, and source of significant mortality, is secondary bacterial infection.[23] The most common organisms involved are *Streptococcus pneumonia*, *Staphylococcus aureus*, and *Haemophilus influenzae*.[24] Secondary pneumonia by *S aureus* was first described after the 1918 influenza pandemic, during which it was associated with near total mortality.[14,25] Methicillin-resistant *Staphylococcus aureus* (MRSA) coinfections during recent influenza seasons have shown mortality of as high as 50% during recent influenza epidemics.[26]

Etiologies of Community-Acquired Bacterial Pneumonia

The causative agents of community-acquired bacterial pneumonia have traditionally been divided into "typical" and "atypical" groups.[27,28] Typical pathogens include *S pneumoniae*, *H influenzae*, *S aureus*, group A streptococci, *Moraxella catarrhalis*, and aerobic gram-negative bacteria.[27,29,30] Atypical pathogens include *M pneumoniae*, *Legionella* spp, *Chlamydophila pneumoniae*, and *C psittaci*.[28,31] Historically, a microbiological diagnosis has been obtained in only 50% of CAP cases; molecular diagnostics have improved the detection rate to around 60% to 80% in some cases, but an etiology is often not identified in a large minority.[30] Where the etiological agent is known, typical pathogens have been identified in approximately 80% of CAP worldwide, with atypical pathogens responsible for the remained.[32] This distribution may be slowly evolving as molecular diagnostics make the laboratory detection of atypical pathogens more reliable.[30]

Worldwide, *S pneumoniae* is the most common cause of CAP and is responsible alone for approximately one-third to one-half of cases.[33,34] *H influenzae* is the second most common typical pathogen. Mycoplasma pneumonia and *Chlamydophila pneumoniae* are the predominant atypical organisms causing CAP; the incidence of CAP caused by atypical pathogens appears to be increasing as detection has improved.[30,34] Anaerobic bacteria are involved for 10% to 20% of CAP.[34,35]

Demographics of Community-Acquired Bacterial Pneumonia

The incidence of CAP in the United States is not definitively known (CAP is not a reportable disease), but is estimated to be approximately 4 to 5 million cases per year.[36,37] In the United States, around 80% of community-acquired pneumonia is treated in the outpatient setting; mortality for outpatients is around <2%.[34,38] The 20% of community-acquired pneumonia patients who are hospitalized have a significantly higher mortality rate, 10% to 50%.[34,38] CAP from all causes is the leading cause of infection-related death in the United States, and remains a leading cause of death worldwide. The worldwide incidence of lower respiratory infections (including bacterial pneumonia) is around 450 million cases.[39] Patients with an age >65 or <5 are at particular risk for morbidity and mortality. Pneumonia from all causes is the single largest contributor to mortality of children <5 worldwide; approximately 1 to 2 million children who die annually from pneumonia, with 50% of deaths attributed to *Streptococcus pneumoniae* and *Haemophilus influenzae* type B.[40,41]

Etiologies of Nosocomial Bacterial Pneumonia

Six organisms are responsible for the approximately 80% of HABP and VABP.[42] In the United States, these organisms listed by declining incidence are Staphylococcus aureus (generally methicillin-resistant or MRSA), and gram-negative bacilli (*Pseudomonas aeruginosa, Klebsiella* species, *Escherichia coli, Acinetobacter* species, and *Enterobacter* species).[42] In Asia, gram-negative organisms predominate, with *Pseudomonas* spp and *Acinetobacter baumannii* more prevalent than MRSA.[43] Other causative organisms include *Serratia* species,

Stenotrophomonas maltophilia, S pneumoniae, and *Haemophilus influenzae.*[42]

Demographics of Nosocomial Bacterial Pneumonia

Hospital-acquired pneumonia is the second most common nosocomial infection in the United States.[44] The worldwide incidence of hospital-acquired bacterial pneumonia is estimated to be 5 to 20 per 1000 hospitalizations, with significant regional variability.[43,44] Mechanical ventilation increases the risk of developing hospital-acquired pneumonia by 6- to 20-fold.[44] The estimated mortality attributable to hospital-acquired pneumonias is approximately 30% to 50%.[44]

Clinical Features of Bacterial Pneumonia

Bacterial pneumonia is defined by a number of clinical features and specific radiographic findings.

Signs and symptoms of bacterial pneumonia

Signs and symptoms of bacterial pneumonia vary with the etiology of infection. Nonspecific symptoms present in most cases of typical pneumonia are fever, cough, shortness of breath, and sputum production.[34] Physical examination signs can include crackles, dullness to percussion, decreased breath sounds, bronchial breath sounds, and pleural rub. Atypical pneumonia may present with dry cough, muscle aches, arthralgias, pharyngitis, and rash (Mycoplasma pneumonia).[28] Signs of lobar consolidation are usually absent on physical examination. *Legionella* spp cause a severe pneumonia that usually presents with extrapulmonary signs and symptoms that help distinguish it from typical or other atypical infections, including mental confusion, bradycardia, abdominal pain and diarrhea, hyponatremia, hematuria, elevated creatinine, and elevated liver enzymes.[28]

Laboratory tests in the diagnosis of bacterial pneumonia

In community-acquired pneumonia not requiring hospitalization, laboratory testing is often not required. Laboratory testing routinely performed in hospitalized patients includes blood culture, sputum culture and Gram stain, and pneumococcal and *Legionella* urine antigen detection.[45] In addition, pathogen nucleic acid amplification (single pathogen or multiplex) from nasopharyngeal swabs, expectorated or induced sputum samples is increasingly available.[46,47] In general, approximately 50 to 60% of bacterial infections will be diagnosed by laboratory testing. Sputum culture and blood cultures are particularly insensitive, rendering a diagnosis in less than 20% of cases.[48]

Imaging features of bacterial pneumonia

Chest radiograph is the preferred imaging modality for the initial diagnosis of bacterial pneumonia.[48] Typical findings include segmental or lobar consolidation (lobar pneumonia), interstitial infiltrates (atypical pneumonia), bronchopneumonia (hospital-acquired pneumonia), and occasionally cavitation (hospital-acquired and aspiration pneumonia) and/or pleural effusion.[49,50] A negative chest x-ray does not rule out pneumonia; patients with initially negative chest x-rays will often have subsequently positive films after rehydration or the passage of time.[51]

Computed tomography (CT) scanning of the lungs is more sensitive than plain radiographs for the diagnosis of pneumonia, but due to issues such as cost, radiation exposure, and availability, it is not recommended as a first-line modality.[48,52]

Pulmonary Function Tests in the Diagnosis of Bacterial Pneumonia

Pulmonary function testing is rarely used in the diagnosis of bacterial pneumonia, but may play a role in assisting with the diagnosis of pneumonia in select situations (eg, HIV/AIDS). Bacterial pneumonia impacts many aspects of lung function. The filling of the lungs with fluid (consolidation) directly decreases total lung capacity (TLC), vital capacity (VC), and lung compliance, roughly in proportion to the volume of lung affected.[53] The primary defect in lung function that results in hypoxemia is intrapulmonary arterial shunt, with a lesser contribution from ventilation and perfusion mismatch.[54,55] In some pneumonias (eg, *Pneumocystis* spp pneumonia), hypoxia appears to be related primarily to a defect in diffusing capacity (measured as diffusing capacity of carbon monoxide [DL_{CO}]).[56] Reductions in forced vital capacity and forced expiratory volume have been noted as a consequence of airway inflammation or diffuse involvement of pneumonia.

Diagnostic Difficulties With Bacterial Pneumonia

Several factors complicate the diagnosis of bacterial pneumonia. First, many of the clinical signs and symptoms of pneumonia (fevers, chills, and cough) are nonspecific, and observed in viral upper respiratory tract or other infections. Secondly, radiologic findings may lag behind the development of pneumonia, or be obscured by comorbidities.

Even in the setting of clinically apparent pneumonia, laboratory confirmation is often challenging. Sputum Gram stain is insensitive, but does offer specificity of around 90% for pneumococcal pneumonia.[34] Blood cultures have similarly poor diagnostic sensitivity,

estimated to be less than 20%.[34] Sputum cultures have poor sensitivity as well, and are often contaminated by oropharyngeal flora that can make it difficult to distinguish pathogens from commensal organisms. Some pathogens (eg, *Legionella*) require special media or culture conditions to be reliably recovered from respiratory specimens—these can be missed if not specifically ordered by the clinical provider or if alternative testing methods (antigen testing or PCR) are not employed.

The development of nucleic acid amplification and probe-based nucleic acid technologies has markedly improved the ability of the laboratory to diagnose pneumonia.[57] The continued development and deployment of rapid multiplex PCR assays is likely to lead to continued improvements the diagnostic rate of pneumonia in the future.[46,47,57]

Prognostic Factors for Bacterial Pneumonia

Bacterial pneumonia has a widely varied outcome. The variation in outcome is due in part to host factors and in part to the causative organism. Among patients who are not hospitalized, mortality is <2%.[38] Mortality in patients hospitalized in general care units is approximately 14%, while patients requiring ICU level care experience a mortality rate as high as 50%.[45,58]

Two predictive indexes to determine the prognosis of a given case of bacterial pneumonia have been extensively studied. The CURB-65 system utilizes five factors to predict a risk for increased mortality: blood urea nitrogen greater than 20 mg/dL, diastolic blood pressure less than 60 mm Hg, respiratory rate >30/min, new confusion, and age >65; presence of three or more factors indicates severe disease, and should prompt assessment for ICU admission.[58] Mortality at 30 days associated with three or more characteristics is 17% to 57%.[59]

An alternative system, the Pneumonia Severity Index (PSI), uses a large number of factors including sex, age, nursing home residence, comorbid conditions, physical examination findings, and laboratory and radiographic findings to generate a composite score. The composite score is then used to group patients into five classes, with predicted 30-day mortality increasing from 0.1% in the least severe cases to 27% in the most severe cases.[60] As with the CURB-65 system, age is an important factor (eg, for a patient with an age >65, age will be the single largest contributor to a PSI score).

Laboratory Diagnosis of Bacterial Pneumonia

The laboratory diagnosis of bacterial pneumonia incorporates elements of direct observation, culture, and—increasingly—molecular testing.

Morphologic identification of bacterial pneumonia

Sputum Gram stain is the mainstay of morphologic diagnosis of bacterial pneumonia.[61-63] While there have been variable reports of the clinical utility of sputum Gram stains, the low cost and rapid turnaround time of Gram stains have ensured that they continue to be analyzed within most clinical microbiology laboratories. A major problem with Gram stains of tracheal secretions or sputum is contaminated by nonpathogenic respiratory tract flora. Most laboratories employ acceptance criteria to disregard specimens with too many squamous cells or bacterial morphologies.[64] Gram stain morphology is sometimes also used in the identification of cultured organisms, although molecular methods such as mass spectrometry are displacing morphologic and biochemical identification methods.[57]

Special stains for the diagnosis of bacterial pneumonia

Aside from the traditional Gram stain, there are few special stains employed in the microbiology laboratory for the diagnosis of bacterial pneumonia from sputum samples or blood bottles. In contrast, a pathologist examining tissue specimens may benefit greatly from the use of special stains in assisting with a diagnosis.

Gram-positive bacteria are often readily identified on a hematoxylin- and eosin-stained section when they are examined at higher magnifications. There are two tissue Gram stains in routine use: Brown-Brenn and Brown-Hopps.[65] The primary difference is sensitivity for certain gram-negative organisms, which is improved in the Brown-Hopps version (at the cost of some gram-positive sensitivity).[65] Giemsa staining is useful primarily for the identification of intracellular bacteria or bacterial inclusions (eg, *Rickettsiae*).[66]

A Gomori methenamine silver (GMS) stain, routinely used in the diagnosis of fungal microorganisms, may be of particular utility in identifying small gram-positive organisms or the filamentous gram-positive organisms *Actinomyces* and *Nocardia*.[66] GMS stains the gram-positive cell wall, and stain deposits artifactually increase the apparent size of the organism, rendering detection easier in some circumstances.

Other silver stains, such as the Warthin-Starry, Dieterle, and Steiner and Steiner are useful in the detection gram-negative organisms such as *Helicobacter pylori*, pathogenic spirochetes, *Rickettsiae* , *Bartonella*, and Donovan bodies (bacterial inclusions of granuloma inguinale) that either stain poorly or not at all with traditional Gram stains.[66,67]

Finally, acid-fast stains are essential in the identification of mycobacteria, and may be useful in the identifications of several nonmycobacterial organisms.

The three primary acid-fast stains employed are the hot Ziehl-Neelsen, cold Kinyoun, and the "gentler" modified acid-fast Fite stain. Tuberculous and most nontuberculous mycobacteria are identified by the standard ZN stain.[66] *Mycobacterium leprae*, however, will decolorize in the more stringent ZN and requires the Fite method.[66] Other bacteria identifiable with modified acid-fast stains include *Nocardia*, *Rhodococcus*, and *Legionella micadei*.[66]

Occasionally, a combination of morphological and staining characteristics may allow for a firm microbial identification to be rendered from direct observation of tissue. More commonly, histopathological examination of tissue will allow for the formation of a differential diagnosis of infection, with confirmation through correlation of culture information, molecular testing from fresh or formalin fixed specimens, and use of immunohistochemical stains.

Molecular testing for the diagnosis of bacterial pneumonia

Physician ordered molecular testing for bacterial pneumonia has been somewhat limited in its utility due to the diversity of pathogens that cause bacterial pneumonia and fact that most molecular tests (nucleic acid amplification/detection or antigen detection assays) currently available are targeted at a single microorganism.[57,68] As multiplex nucleic acid amplification/detection assays become more commonplace, the utility of molecular testing is likely to increase.[46,47] For example, the FilmArray system can detect three pathogenic bacteria (*Mycoplasma*, *Chlamydophila,* and *Bordetella*) and 21 viruses from a nasal pharyngeal swab in approximately 1 hour.[46]

Rapid antigen detection is another method commonly used in the diagnosis of bacterial pneumonia. Pneumococcal antigen and *Legionella* antigen are commercially available.[57]

For the pathologist, molecular testing for bacterial pneumonia involves either immunohistochemical stains or in situ hybridization.[69] Neither is commonly employed and nor widely available, and these techniques are routinely employed only in specialized referral centers such as the CDC Infectious Disease Pathology Branch.

Focal Bacterial Pneumonia

Focal (or lobar) pneumonia suggests the radiological pattern of lobar consolidation within one lobe (multilobar or bilateral pneumonia involves more than one lobe).[50] A characteristic of lobar pneumonia is bronchial sparing; the bronchus is surrounded by consolidated lung parenchyma, appearing as air filled outlines of bronchial spaces or an "air bronchogram."[50] This

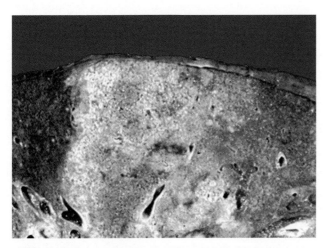

FIGURE 12-1 Gross image of lobar pneumonia showing consolidation within one lobe.

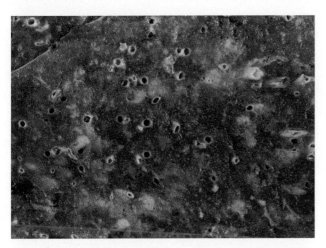

FIGURE 12-2 Gross image of bronchopneumonia showing bronchi at the center of the inflammatory response.

pattern contrasts with bronchopneumonia, in which the bronchi are the center of the inflammatory response (*Figures 12-1* and *12-2*).

Round Pneumonia

Round pneumonia describes a form of lobar pneumonia commonly seen predominantly in children in the posterior lung fields; however, the entity has also been described in adults.[49,70,71] The description "round" refers to a well-defined opacity within a lobe that does not involve the entire lobe. In contrast to the situation in adults, where infection and inflammation (and consolidation) spreads throughout a lobe via the pores of Kohn and canals of Lambert, the inflammation of round pneumonia is thought to be confined by incomplete development of those channels. As in lobar pneumonia, air bronchograms are often seen.

Lobar Pneumonia

As with its radiographic appearance, the pathophysiology of lobar pneumonia is well defined. Lobar pneumonia results from acute inflammation within the air spaces that cause them to fill with a protein and cell-rich inflammatory fluid. This fluid can track through the lobe via the pores of Kohn and canals of Lambert that normally allow for collateral airflow.

Lobar pneumonias evolve through four stages: consolidation, red hepatization, gray hepatization, and resolution.[72] A wide-variety of organisms can produce a lobar pattern of pneumonia.

Organisms

The most common cause of a lobar pattern of infection is *Streptococcus pneumoniae*. Other pathogens that can cause a lobar pattern include staphylococci, other streptococci, and gram-negative organisms such as *Klebsiella pneumonia*, *Legionella pneumophila*, *Haemophilus influenzae*, and *Pseudomonas aeruginosa*.[50] *Mycobacterium tuberculosis* infection can also manifest with a lobar pattern.[50]

Red hepatization

Red hepatization refers to the gross appearance of a lung early in the process of consolidation. The reddish color likely stems from capillary congestion and red cells filling the airspaces as they extravasate along with neutrophils and plasma into the airspaces. As consolidation progresses and the infection begins to resolve, fibrinopurulent exudates form within the alveoli and begin to organize, leading to gray hepatization.

Gray hepatization

Gray hepatization refers to the gross appearance of the lung as organization continues, red cells degenerate, and macrophages replaces neutrophils within the airspaces. In typical cases of lobar pneumonia, macrophages accomplish the progressive digestion and removal of the organizing alveolar exudates, leading to final resolution of the infection.

Resolution

A typical lobar pneumonia can completely resolve, as the inflammatory process does not disrupt the underlying alveolar architecture. This is consistent with studies of pulmonary function after uncomplicated pneumonia, which have showed that the usual course is a complete restoration of function. Necrosis is infrequently seen, and an elastin stain can verify preservation of the alveolar architecture.

CHAPTER 12

Bronchopneumonia

In contrast to lobar pneumonia, which begins as an infection within the airspaces, usually within a single lobe of the lung, bronchopneumonia refers to a pattern of pneumonia in which the infection extends from airways into the lung parenchyma.[52] Also known as lobular pneumonia, bronchopneumonia is generally characterized by the involvement of numerous lobules within a lobe. The extension of many small opacities from the airways has given rise to the description "tree-in-bud" pattern when observed by computed tomography images of the lungs.[52] With time, a bronchopneumonia may spread to involve an entire lobe—and thus be radiographically indistinguishable from a lobar pneumonia. As with lobar pneumonia, this pattern of infection can be seen with a variety of infecting organisms; however, it is generally more associated with hospital-acquired infections caused by *Staphylococcus aureus*, *Klebsiella*, *E coli*, and *Pseudomonas*, and anaerobic bacteria, it is less commonly seen with *Streptococcus pneumoniae*.[52]

Necrotizing Bacterial Pneumonia and Lung Abscess

In contrast to the typical pattern of lobar pneumonia previously discussed, necrotizing bacterial pneumonias and bacterial lung abscesses cause permanent destruction of lung parenchyma. Histologically, there is diffuse inflammation and necrosis, along with focal vasculitis. When severe, necrotizing pneumonia may lead to cavitation and abscess formation.[73,74] Acutely, necrotic abscess appears as a thin-walled cavity filled with neutrophils, fibrin, hemorrhage, and cellular debris can be seen. Chronic abscesses show replacement of neutrophils with macrophages, and organization in the surrounding lung parenchyma with fibroblast proliferation and deposition of collagen. With resolution of infection, abscess cavities are often replaced by fibrous tissue over a period of months or years. A cavity that fails to undergo fibrosis may develop an epithelial lining.

The most common cause of a necrotizing pneumonia or lung abscess is aspiration, and anaerobic or mixed infections involving anaerobes are usually at fault.[73-75] Other etiologies of necrotizing infections include lung infarction or hemorrhage with superimposed infection, infectious thromboemboli, and direct extension from adjacent infected tissue. Host factors that contribute to the development of lung abscess include (diabetes, alcoholism, impaired cough or swallowing, and immunosuppression).

Acute Bacterial Pneumonia

Acute pneumonia refers to pneumonia of less than 3 weeks' duration. Acute bacterial pneumonias are divided into typical and atypical categories on the basis of presentation.

Chronic Bacterial Pneumonia

Chronic bacterial pneumonia (lasting longer than 3 weeks in duration) is indicative either of a slowly resolving typical pneumonia,[76] or of the involvement of organisms such as *Mycobacterium tuberculosis*, atypical mycobacteria, or the filamentous bacteria *Nocardia* spp and *Actinomyces* spp

Organizing Pneumonia

Organizing pneumonia refers to the presence of organized plugs of granulation tissue within the distal airspaces (also termed Masson bodies) or bronchiolar lumen[77,78] (*Figures 12-3* and *12-4*). This is a nonspecific

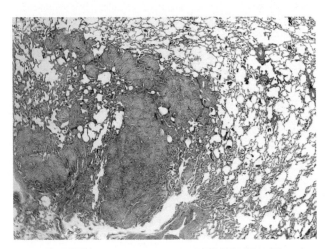

FIGURE 12-3 Medium power of organizing pneumonia showing organized plugs of granulation tissue within the distal airspaces.

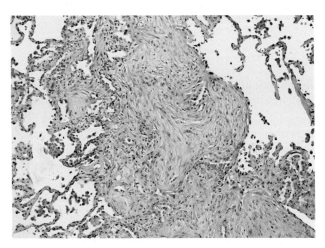

FIGURE 12-4 Higher power image of organizing pneumonia showing granulation tissue within distal airspaces.

pathological pattern that can be caused by many different processes that cause injury to the lung—among them bacterial infection.[79] Organizing pneumonia usually results from infections that damage the underlying alveolar architecture and fail to resolve, leading to prolonged inflammation and fibrosis.

Aspiration Pneumonia

Aspiration of oral and/or gastric contents can cause direct chemical injury to the lung (pneumonitis), primarily from gastric acid.[80] Pneumonitis quickly leads to an acute exudative response, with edema, congestion, and alveolar necrosis within 4 hours, neutrophil infiltration within 24 to 48 hours and hyaline membranes within 72 hours. Aspiration pneumonitis can resolve without further sequelae, or lead to fibrosis, depending on the severity of the injury.

Aspiration pneumonia can develop secondary to pneumonitis or independently of pneumonitis by direct seeding of the lungs with oral flora. In hospitalized patients (usually on multiple medications including gastric acid inhibitors), there can be significant colonization of the stomach by gram-negative organisms that can subsequently seed the lungs after an aspiration event. Pathologic hallmarks of aspiration pneumonia are necrosis, cavitation, and abscess formation.[74,80]

It has been generally thought that aspiration pneumonias were primarily caused by anaerobic organisms. More recent studies have shown that gram-negative organisms likely play a significant role in aspiration pneumonias.

Bacterial Pneumonia From Gram-Positive Cocci

Gram-positive cocci are significant contributors to community- and hospital-acquired pneumonias worldwide. *Streptococcus pneumoniae* is the leading cause of community-acquired pneumonia in the world, while *Staphylococcus aureus* (usually methicillin-resistant or MRSA) is a major contributor to hospital-acquired pneumonias. As a general rule, most gram-positive organisms are visible by staining with tissue Gram stain (B-H and/or B-B) or GMS (*Table 12-2*).

Streptococcus pneumoniae

S pneumoniae is an encapsulated diplococcus in short pairs or chains that appears gram-positive or gram variable on staining. Pneumococci are lancet shaped, and the capsule may be visible as a faint clearing around the cells on Gram stain. In immunocompetent adults, *S pneumoniae* usually causes a lobar pneumonia that heals by resolution. Infections in children, the elderly, and immunocompromised hosts are associated with increased

Table 12-2 Bacterial Pneumonia From Gram-Positive Cocci

Streptococcus pneumonia *Staphylococcus aureus*

β-Hemolytic streptococci
  Streptococcus pyogenes
  Streptococcus agalactiae

Anaerobic cocci
  Finegoldia magna
  Parvimonas micra
  Peptostreptococcus anaerobius

mortality. Strains of *S pneumoniae* with increased virulence (eg, type 3) have been described, and are associated with necrotizing infections and sepsis.[81-83]

Staphylococcus aureus

S aureus is a highly virulent organism that grows in grape-like gram-positive clusters of cocci. The organism stains gram-positive, although in tissue Gram staining may be variable; GMS staining is often useful to highlight the organisms when they are not abundant or well visualized by Gram stain.[66] *S aureus* is the most common cause of hospital-acquired pneumonia in Western countries, and typically causes a necrotizing bronchopneumonia.[42] Isolates from cases of hospital-acquired pneumonia are usually methicillin resistant (MRSA). In contrast to *S aureus*, the coagulase-negative staphylococci (eg, *Staphylococcus epidermidis* and *Staphylococcus lugdunensis*) are not typically respiratory tract pathogens.

In addition to necrotizing pulmonary infections, *Staphylococcus aureus* is the most common organism identified in botryomycosis, a rare bacterial infection that resembles *Actinomyces* infections.[84-86] Botryomycosis is characterized by the formation of eosinophilic granules (similar to the sulfur granules formed by *Actinomyces*) filled with *S aureus* or other organisms (eg, *E coli*, *Pseudomonas aeruginosa*).[84,85] The granules are located within a neutrophilic abscess and are often surrounded by eosinophilic Splendor-Hoeppli material.[85] Organism identification often requires culture, as the morphology of the organism can be distorted in granules. Botryomycosis occurs in immunocompromised hosts, and requires surgical excision for treatment.[86,87] The radiographic appearance of botryomycosis is not specific, and may resemble carcinoma, fungal or tubercular infections.[88]

β-Hemolytic streptococci

Streptococcus pyogenes and *Streptococcus agalactiae* are the most common β-hemolytic streptococci involved in pulmonary infections; however, other species of β-hemolytic streptococci also cause pulmonary disease.[89-92] The key morphological characteristic of the streptococci in blood or broth cultures, the formation of long chains of cocci, is rarely apparent in tissue sections.

S pyogenes (Group A) is a highly virulent pathogen associated with pneumonia in hospitalized or immunocompromised hosts, children, and after viral infections.[89,90,93] Pneumonia caused by *S pyogenes* is usually rapidly progressive, with edema, hemorrhage, and abscess formation; empyema and septicemia are frequently present.[93,94] *S agalactiae* (Group B) is a significant cause of neonatal sepsis and pneumonia, with a high associated mortality.[95] Increasingly, Group B streptococci are also being identified as a cause of invasive infections, including pneumonia, in elderly adults.[96] Other streptococci, including members of Group C, D, and F, have been reported in primary or polymicrobial pneumonias.[91,92,97] The viridans group Streptococci (usually α-hemolytic rather than β) are normal flora and infrequently primary pulmonary pathogens. Viridans streptococci have been reported to cause pneumonia in children and immunocompromised hosts, and are frequently isolated from polymicrobial pneumonias.[98,99]

Anaerobic cocci

Finegoldia magna (previously *Peptostreptococcus magnus*), *Parvimonas micra*, and *Peptostreptococcus anaerobius* are the most common anaerobic gram-positive cocci isolated from aspiration-related abscesses.[100,101] The organisms are normal flora, and usually cause infections only in immunocompromised hosts and those with altered mental status and/or swallowing disorders leading to chronic aspiration. Anaerobic bacteria are usually found as part of a polymicrobial infection that includes gram-negative anaerobes (eg, *Bacteroides*, *Prevotella*, and *Fusobacterium*) and aerobic bacteria (commonly *Staphylococcus* spp, *Streptococcus* spp, and Enterobacteriaceae).[100-102]

Histopathologically, aspiration pneumonias are characterized by acute inflammation and necrosis with abscess formation; chronic inflammation results in fibrosis and scar formation. Granulomatous inflammation may be seen if food particles have been aspirated.[103]

Bacterial Pneumonia From Gram-Positive Bacilli

With the exception of the *Corynebacterium* spp and *Bacillus anthracis*, the gram-positive bacilli are primarily opportunistic or incidental pathogens of low virulence (*Table 12-3*).

Corynebacteria

The corynebacteria are a genus of small, nonmotile gram-positive rods. Non-diphtheriae species are normal flora

Table 12-3 Bacterial Pneumonia From Gram-Positive Bacilli

Corynebacteria
Nocardiosis
Actinomyces
Rhodococcus
Bacillus species
Bacillus anthracis
Bacillus cereus

within the respiratory tract. *C diphtheriae*, when infected with a diphtheria toxin encoding phage, is the causative agent of diphtheria.[104,105] Diphtheria is primarily a disease upper respiratory tract, with marked inflammation, necrosis, and fibrinopurulent pseudomembrane formation.[106] Involvement of the lower respiratory tract is by direct extension, with airway-centered disease that extends into the lung parenchyma (a bronchopneumonia pattern). Diphtheria is rare since the widespread use of vaccination with diphtheria toxoid, although recent epidemics have occured.[104] Non-diphtheriae *Corynebacterium*, including *C pseudodiphtheriticum*, *C jeikeium*, and others are causative agents of pneumonia, usually in the elderly, immunocompromised hosts, or those with preexisting lung disease.[107-110]

Nocardiosis

The *Nocardia* spp are gram-positive filamentous bacteria that are respiratory pathogens of immunocompromised hosts (eg, organ transplant recipients, chronic steroid or immunosuppressant use) or those with preexisting lung disease.[111-113] *Nocardia* infections can present with either an acute or chronic course and are characterized by extensive necrosis and occasional granuloma formation.[114] *Nocardia* are poorly stained on hematoxylin- and eosin-stained sections, but are easily visualized with Gram or GMS stains. The organisms are partially acid fast, and stain with a beaded pattern by modified acid-fast staining (Fite); they may occasionally be visualized on tissue AFB stains that use weaker acid decolorizers.[66] In contrast to *Actinomyces* infections, *Nocardia* rarely form sulfur granules.[114]

Actinomyces

The *Actinomyces* are facultatively anaerobic branching filamentous gram-positive bacilli, morphologically similar to the *Nocardia*.[114] *Actinomyces* are normal flora in the oropharyngeal tract, and usually cause infection only after penetrating trauma, in immunocompromised hosts, or within preexisting lung pathology.[115] Actinomycosis is a chronic necrotizing infection with microabscess formation, fibrosis, and cavitation.[114,115]

The organisms can be locally invasive. *Actinomyces* infections are often characterized by the formation of tight amorphous aggregations of organisms with identifiable peripheral filaments (grossly yellow, these carry the misnomer "sulfur granules").[115,116] The bacilli are visualized with Gram and GMS stains, but are usually not acid fast (in contrast to *Nocardia*).[66]

Rhodococcus

Rhodococcus (formerly *Corynebacterium*) equi is a small, pleomorphic gram-positive coccobacillus that is an important veterinary pathogen; in humans *Rhodococcus* causes chronic opportunistic infections primarily in immunocompromised hosts.[117-119] The organisms can be visualized by Gram, GMS, and modified acid fast (eg, Fite) stains.[117] *Rhodococcus* can be found in almost any organ system, but pulmonary involvement is present in approximately 80% of cases involving immunocompromised hosts.[117,120] Infections are characterized by neutrophilic infiltration, microabscesses, necrosis, and sheets of histiocytes with foamy eosinophilic cytoplasm and abundant phagocytized coccobacilli.[121] The phagocytosed bacteria are thought to persist intracellularly due to impaired phagolysosome maturation.[121] Michaelis-Guttman bodies can sometimes be seen; these are calcified phagolysosomes that stain with PAS and Von Kossa calcium stains.[122,123] The presence of persistent phagocytized organisms and MG bodies is termed malakoplakia; this finding is not specific to *Rhodococcus* and is also seen in mycobacterial or some gram-negative infections.[119] Rarely, *Rhodococcus* infections lead to infectious pseudotumors (dense spindle cell proliferations that mimic sarcomas).[124]

Bacillus species

The *Bacillus* species are large, aerobic, gram-positive spore-forming rods. *Bacillus anthracis* (causative agent of anthrax), and *B cereus*, are the primary respiratory pathogens of the *Bacillus* genera.[125,126] In the case of anthrax, infection can occur by three routes: direct inoculation of the skin (cutaneous anthrax), ingestion (gastrointestinal anthrax), and inhalation (pulmonary anthrax).[125] Pulmonary infection is caused by inhalation of spores, which then germinate in the lungs to produce a rapidly growing infection or by hematogenous dissemination from another site (eg, gastrointestinal anthrax).[125,127] Pulmonary anthrax causes an initial localized hemorrhagic pneumonia as inhaled spores geminate and the bacilli elaborate the toxins, edema factor, lethal factor, and protective antigen.[128] The organism spreads via the lymphatics to the mediastinal lymph nodes, with associated hemorrhagic pulmonary and mediastinal lymphadenitis and mediastinitis (leading to the characteristic mediastinal thickening on chest radiograph or CT).[128,129] Further hematogenous dissemination of the bacilli results in septicemia and death.

Non-anthracis *Bacillus* species, such as *Bacillus cereus* (well known as a cause of toxin-mediated food poisoning), *B subtilis*, and *B sphaericus*, are opportunistic, and infrequent, respiratory pathogens.[126,130]

Bacterial Pneumonia From Other Gram-Positive Bacilli

Clostridium species

The *Clostridium* are gram-positive anaerobic spore-forming bacilli (the spores of *Clostridium* spp are rarely visible in tissue). The *Clostridium* spp are rarely associated with pulmonary infections. *Clostridium perfringens* pleuropulmonary disease is characterized by necrotizing pneumonia with pleural involvement, usually in the setting of penetrating trauma, invasive procedures in the chest cavity, or septicemia.[131,132]

Listeria monocytogenes

Listeria monocytogenes is a small gram-positive *Bacillus* that is a rare cause of pneumonia. *Listeria* pneumonia has been reported in immunocompromised hosts, transplant recipients, and in the setting of multisystem disease.[133-136] Histologically, *Listeria* pneumonia is characterized by necrosis, microabscess formation, and granulomas.[136]

Lactobacillus

Lactobacillus species are long, slender gram-positive rods that are normal flora of the gastrointestinal and urogenital tracts. *Lactobacillus* spp are rarely pathogens, but have been reported to cause pneumonia in immunocompromised hosts and ventilated patients.[137-139] Interestingly, *Lactobacillus* species probiotics have also been administered to ventilated patients in an effort to reduce colonization by more pathogenic organisms, with some success.[140] There is a single report of probiotic-associated *Lactobacillus* pneumonia.[141]

Bacterial Pneumonia Gram-Negative Organisms

In contrast to the gram-positive bacteria, where *Streptococcus* pneumonia and *Staphylococcus aureus* are by far the most common causes of gram-positive bacterial pneumonia, many gram-negative bacteria cause serious lower respiratory tract infections (*Table 12-4*).

Escherichia coli

E coli is a gram-negative *Bacillus* associated commonly with ventilator-associated pneumonia and pneumonias

Table 12-4 Bacterial Pneumonia From Gram-Negative Organisms

Escherichia coli
Klebsiella pneumonia
Neisseria species
Serratia
Enterobacter
Proteus
Yersinia pestis
Haemophilus influenzae
Legionella
Pseudomonas aeruginosa
Burkholderia species
  Burkholderia cepacia
  Burkholderia pseudomallei
Bordetella pertussis
Brucella
Chlamydophila pneumoniae

in immunocompromised hosts, those with preexisting lung disease.[43,142] *Escherichia coli* pneumonias are associated with severe disease, rapid progression, bacteremia, and high mortality.[143] Histologically, there is acute inflammation with abundant monocytes and hemorrhage.[144]

Klebsiella pneumoniae

Klebsiella pneumoniae are encapsulated short gram-negative rods. Like *E coli, Klebsiella* is a common cause of nosocomial pneumonia and pneumonia in immunocompromised hosts.[145,146] The organisms can be visualized with Gram or GMS stains, and occasionally display bipolar Gram staining. Histologically, *Klebsiella pneumonia* shows hemorrhage and necrosis, with abundant acute inflammation and disruption of the alveolar septa.[147] Abscess formation can occur, but is more common in mixed infections with anaerobes. Reminiscent of tuberculosis, sputum from infected patients can be mucoid and red.[145]

Neisseria species

Neisseria are gram-negative encapsulated diplococci. The organisms are visible in tissue sections by Gram staining. *N meningitides* is most commonly associated with meningococcal meningitis, but infrequently causes a primary pneumonia.[148,149] Meningococcal pneumonia is associated with older age patients and *Neisseria* bacteremia.[149] Serogroup Y is the most common serogroup recovered from pneumonia patients, and is associated with severe disease.[149,150]

Serratia

Serratia are gram-negative bacilli that cause ventilator-associated pneumonias.[151] *Serratia* spp cause

hemorrhagic bronchopneumonia, with acute inflammation, variable pulmonary large vessel vasculitis, microabscess formation, and cavitation.[152,153]

Enterobacter

The *Enterobacter* species are short encapsulated gram-negative rods that cause hospital-acquired and ventilator-associated pneumonias.[154,155] Risk factors for infection include old age, preexisting lung disease (eg, COPD), and endotracheal intubation (VAP).[155] Community-acquired *Enterobacter* infections have been reported, but are rare.[156] *Enterobacter* spp cause necrotizing pneumonia with abscess formation and cavitation.

Proteus

Proteus spp are gram-negative bacilli that cause hospital-acquired and ventilator-associated pneumonias.[42,157] *Proteus* pneumonia is characterized by a mixed mononuclear and polymorphonuclear cell infiltrate, hemorrhage, and areas of necrosis. Abscess formation can occur.[158]

Yersinia pestis

The *Yersinia*, including *Y pestis, Y pseudotuberculosis,* and *Y enterocolitica,* are gram-negative bacilli that diverse diseases.[159] *Y pestis* is the causative agent of plague, which has three forms: bubonic, septicemic, and pneumonic. Pneumonic plague occurs secondarily by hematogenous dissemination to the lungs, or primarily (less common) by inhalation of infected aerosols or secretions, without treatment mortality is 100%.[159,160] Plague bacilli in the respiratory tract persist in alveolar macrophages and rapidly replicate. Clinically, there is copious production of bloody sputum.[159] On histological sections, abundant bacilli and necrotizing hemorrhage are seen.

Haemophilus influenzae

Haemophilus influenzae is a small gram-negative rod that causes community- and hospital-acquired pneumonias in children and those with immunosuppression or preexisting lung disease.[30,43,161] Vaccination has reduced the incidence of *H influenzae* serotype B infections, but has had no impact on the incidence of infections with nonencapsulated (nontypable) strains.[162,163] In tissue sections, the diminutive organism can be visualized by tissue Gram stain, but may be better seen with silver impregnation stains such as Warthin-Starry.

Legionella

The *Legionella* are slender waterborne gram-negative rods that cause severe community- or institutionally acquired pneumonia.[164] *Legionella pneumophila* is the etiologic agent of the self-limiting upper respiratory infection "Pontiac fever," and of the pneumonia "Legionnaires disease."[165,166] *Legionella pneumophila* pneumonia is usually severe, requiring hospitalization and intensive care.[167] *Legionella micdadei* is the etiologic agent of "Pittsburgh pneumonia," a severe pneumonia in immunocompromised hosts.[168] *Legionella* bacteria Gram stain poorly, and are better visualized in tissue with silver impregnation stains. In contrast to L. pneumophila, L. micdadei stains with modified acid-fast staining (Fite) in addition to silver impregnation.[61,169]

Legionella cause a lobular or multilobular pneumonia that can quickly progress to confluence.[170] Necrosis and abscess formation are common features.[171] Histologically, *Legionella* pneumonia is characterized by an infiltrate of neutrophils and macrophages, small vessel vasculitis, and necrotic destruction of the septal architecture.[170]

Pseudomonas aeruginosa

Pseudomonas aeruginosa is a gram-negative *Bacillus* that is a major cause of acute hospital- and ventilator-associated pneumonia, and chronic pneumonia in populations with preexisting lung disease (eg, cystic fibrosis, COPD).[42,172] *Pseudomonas* pulmonary infections are particularly problematic for patients with cystic fibrosis, as once the organism colonizes the lung it can mutate into mucoid strains that are resistant to treatment and lead to lifelong chronic infections.[173] *Pseudomonas* pneumonia is characterized by radiologically by multiple nodular opacities and bronchopneumonia pattern; pulmonary effusions are frequently present.[174] Histologically displays an abundant infiltrate of neutrophils and macrophages, hemorrhage, necrosis, and destruction of alveolar septal architecture.[175]

Burkholderia species

B cepacia is a slender gram-negative rod that colonizes the lungs of individuals with cystic fibrosis or other immunosuppressive conditions such as chronic granulomatous disease.[176] It causes a spectrum of disease, ranging from acute suppurative infection to chronic necrotizing granulomatous pneumonia. Histologically, features of necrotizing bronchopneumonia and necrotizing granulomatous pneumonia can both be seen.[177]

B pseudomallei is the causative agent of "melioidosis," a systemic infection characterized by abscess formation in multiple organs; pneumonia is the most common presenting sign and is seen in approximately 50% of patients.[178] The disease is most prevalent in South East Asia, but is also found in Central and South America.[178-180] Melioidosis infectious most often resolve after an acute phase, but persist in approximately 10% of cases. Radiologically, acute pulmonary disease is characterized by a bronchopneumonia pattern with abscess formation and honeycombing.[181] Chronic infections form lung nodules similar in clinical appearance to tuberculosis or malignancy. Acute melioidosis pathology shows an acute mixed inflammatory infiltrate with giant cells containing phagocytized bacilli in a background of necrosis with abscess formation.[182] Chronic pulmonary disease shows abundant giant cells with necrosis and granuloma formation.[182]

Bordetella pertussis

Bordetella pertussis, causative agent of whooping cough (pertussis), is a small gram-negative coccobacillus. Pertussis primarily affects the upper respiratory tract, but infections (particularly in infants) can progress to a necrotizing bronchopneumonia.[183] Histology shows abundant leukocytosis in the alveolar spaces and surrounding lymphovasculature, hemorrhage, and fibrinous edema.[183] The airways are the primary site of infection, and bacteria may be visible in the cilia of the respiratory tract, within the alveolar spaces, or within alveolar macrophages.[183] A characteristic finding is a dense luminal aggregates of leukocytes within the small lymphovacsulature.[183]

Brucella

Brucella are tiny, slender gram-negative coccobacilli that are intracellular pathogens of the reticuloendothelial system. *Brucella* species reside within zoonotic reservoirs, and generally infect by direct contact with host species (cattle, pigs, goats) or through ingestion or inhalation of contaminated host products.[184] *Brucella* pulmonary involvement is rare, involving from 1% to 15% of cases.[185-187] The manifestations of *Brucella* involvement in the respiratory tract are myriad, and include bronchopneumonia, interstitial pneumonia, and granulomatous nodularity with hilar and paratracheal adenopathy reported.[185] Miliary disease has been reported. Histopathologically, *Brucella* pulmonary infections are characterized by a mainly mononuclear infiltrate, with granuloma formation reported in some cases.[185]

Chlamydophila and Chlamydia

Chlamydophila pneumoniae (formerly *Chlamydia*) is a major cause of atypical community-acquired pneumonia.[32] The Chlamydiaceae (*Chlamydophila* and *Chlamydia*) are obligate intracellular pathogens with a unique biphasic life cycle consisting of elementary and reticulate forms.[188-190] The infectious elementary body is hearty and persists in the environment, essentially fulfilling the role of bacterial spore. Once inhaled and phagocytosed by the respiratory epithelium or alveolar macrophages, the elementary body converts into a reticulate body that replicates within the phagosomes of infected cells. After replication, reticulate bodies transform again into infectious elementary bodies, and are released from the cell by exocytosis or lysis to infect new hosts.[190]

Chlamydophila pneumoniae is responsible for approximately 10% of community-acquired pneumonias.[188] Clinical presentation is variable, and can range from mild cough and malaise that can last for weeks to more severe pneumonia.[188] *Chlamydophila psittaci* is associated with pneumonia in individuals exposed to psittacine (parrots) or other birds.[189]

Both organisms cause a pneumonia histopathologically characterized by an acute airway-centered neutrophilic infiltrate that is replaced after a week by a macrophage response.[191,192] In Psittacosis, pathognomonic intracytoplasmic inclusions (Levinthal-Cole-Lillie bodies) can sometimes be seen in Giemsa-stained alveolar macrophages recovered by BAL.[192]

Chlamydia trachomatis is primarily an ocular and genital pathogen, but can cause pneumonia in neonates, usually 4 to 16 weeks of age.[193,194] The Chlamydaciae may be visualized in tissue with Giemsa, Papanicolaou, HE, and WS stains, but are rarely seen by light microscopy due to their small size.[66]

Pneumonia From Obligately Anaerobic Bacteria

Obligate anaerobes usually infect the lung within the context of an aspiration event that causes an initial chemical injury and subsequent edema, which in turn creates a nonaerated environment for growth. Gram-positive cocci anaerobes implicated in aspiration pneumonias include *Finegoldia magna*, *Parvimonas micra*, and *Peptostreptococcus anaerobius*.[100,101] The gram-positive anaerobic bacilli are rarely a cause of primary pneumonia in the lungs, although the *Clostridium* may cause pneumonia after hematogenous dissemination or by direct extension from the abdomen.[131,132] Anaerobic gram-negative bacilli, including *Fusobacterium nucleatum*, and *Prevotella melaninogenica*, *Bacteroides* species, are frequently isolated from pulmonary abscesses.[73,100-102]

The *Actinomyces*, gram-positive nonspore-forming filamentous rods that are predominantly anaerobic, cause a necrotizing pneumonia, often within the context of a polymicrobial infection.[114,115]

Lung Involvement With Other Bacterial Infections

Bartonella henselae (cat scratch disease)

Bartonella henselae is a small gram-negative rod and causative agent of "cat scratch disease," a systemic illness involving fever and lymphadenopathy.[195] Classically,

infected lymph nodes often show suppurative granulomas and stellate microabscesses. Respiratory involvement is by hematogenous seeding, and presents with a multinodular pattern.[196] Histopathologically, the pulmonary nodules are characterized by a mixed inflammatory infiltrate of neutrophils, lymphocytes, and foamy macrophages in a background of patchy necrosis.[196] The organisms are generally not visible by H&E or Gram or Giemsa staining, but can be visualized silver impregnation stains such as Warthin-Starry.[196,197]

Tropheryma whipplei (Whipple disease)

Tropheryma whipplei is a gram-positive bacterium in the Actinomycete family.[198] *Tropheryma* is generally considered to be of low virulence, but does cause the "Whipple disease," a multiorgan disease characterized by polyarthritis, diarrhea, and lymphadenopathy and weight loss.[198] In addition, *T whipplei* is an important cause of culture negative endocarditis.[199] A chronic cough, interstitial pneumonia, and sarcoid-like nodular pulmonary presentation have also been described for the disease.[200-202] In the lungs, *Tropheryma* infections are characterized by interstitial infiltrates and granulomas (sarcoid is an important differential diagnosis).[202] Pulmonary involvement for *T whipplei* is diagnosed using molecular methods such as PCR, as microscopic diagnosis of extraintestinal Whipple disease has been difficult.[200,201,203] Gastrointestinal biopsy demonstrating characteristic PAS-positive inclusions in foamy macrophages can also be helpful in establishing presence of the disease.[202]

MYCOBACTERIAL DISEASE

The *Mycobacterium tuberculosis* complex includes the human pathogens *M tuberculosis*, *M africanum*, *M canetti*, *M caprae*, and *M pneumoniae*, human and animal pathogen *M bovis*, and the primarily rodent pathogen *M microti*.[204] *Mycobacterium tuberculosis* (MTB) infections have plagued humans since the advent of civilization, and emerged perhaps as long as 500,000 years ago.[205] Currently, over 2 billion people (or roughly a third of the world population) are latently infected with MTB and there are approximately 9 million new infections each year.[206,207] Primary infection with tuberculosis leads to overt clinical disease in only 10% of cases; the majority of primary MTB infections resolve in latency. Latent infections have an estimated 10% lifetime risk of reactivation (5% in the first year and 5% thereafter), with higher risk of progression to active disease (approximately 10% per year) in the setting of HIV/AIDS or chronic immunosuppression.[208,209]

Tuberculosis was historically a chronic and incurable disease. The discovery streptomycin, the first effective antitubercular chemotherapeutic, in the 1940s gave rise to hope that tuberculosis might not only be cured, but eliminated.[210] Unfortunately, in only a few short years streptomycin-resistant MTB strains were reported. Resistant strains of MTB have emerged in lockstep with the development of new therapies, and within the greater tuberculosis epidemic, there is a second epidemic of multidrug (MDR) and extensively drug-resistant (XDR) strains of the disease.[211,212]

Tuberculosis

Pathogenesis of tuberculosis

The pathogenicity of tuberculosis stems less from its virulence than from its intrinsic resistance to the host immune defense. Tuberculosis bacilli, once inhaled, are engulfed by type II alveolar macrophages and other host phagocytic cells.[213] Ingestion of the mycobacteria leads to recruitment of innate immune cells, including neutrophils and monocytes.[214] Through a number of mechanisms, MTB prevents phagosome maturation and fusion with host lysosomes, thereby avoiding destruction.[215] Indeed, MTB actively replicates with host phagocytic cells, eventually leading to cell death and release of the organisms. The failure of the innate immune response to clear the organism leads to the activation of adaptive immunity.

The adaptive immune response to tuberculosis is complex, but centers on the activation of macrophages by CD4+ T cells through the secretion of interferon gamma and TNF-α.[216,217] The complex of T cells and activated macrophages usually checks disease progression in immunocompetent hosts, although MTB infections are rarely cleared completely. Instead, local cytokines lead to the further influx of monocytes, which fuse when activated to form syncytial giant cells at the periphery of the lesion. The constellation of focal central necrosis, peripheral giant cells, and lymphohistiocytic inflammation is termed the tuberculoid granuloma.

Tuberculoid granulomas are not static structures, but rather represent a homeostatic equilibrium between the bacilli and the adaptive immune system. Recent data have suggested that granulomas may be directly induced by mycobacteria, perhaps as a mechanism to isolate the bacilli from additional immune response.[218,219]

Risk factors for developing tuberculosis

The risk for developing tuberculosis can be divided into the risk of infection with MTB, and the risk of progression to active disease once infected. Similarly, risk factors can be divided into host factors and environmental factors. Host and environmental risk factors for infection with MTB are primarily related to exposure, risk

Table 12-5 Risk Factors for Developing Tuberculosis

Host Factors
  Young age
  Malnutrition
  Immunosuppressed condition
  Diabetes mellitus
  Renal failure requiring hemodialysis
  Gastrointestinal resection
  Carcinoma of the head and neck
  Alcohol use
  Active smoking
  Intravenous drug use
  Mining
  Silicosis

Environmental Factors
  Low socioeconomic status
  Exposure to air pollution
  Living in crowded and poorly ventilated conditions
    (eg, incarceration)

factors living in a highly endemic area, close and sustained contact with an infected individual, working in health care, and living in crowded and poorly ventilated conditions[209,220,221] (*Table 12-5*).

Host factors that contribute to the development of active MTB infection include young age, malnutrition, immunosuppressive conditions (HIV/AIDS or other), diabetes mellitus, renal failure requiring hemodialysis, gastrointestinal resection, and carcinoma of the head and neck.[209,220] Additional risks include alcohol use, active smoking, intravenous drug use, mining, and silicosis.[209,220,222,223] Certain ethnic populations, such as indigenous North Americans and indigenous Australians are at higher baseline risk of developing active TB.[209] Environmental risk factors associated with an increased risk of active MTB include low socioeconomic status (likely a composite factor for other risks), exposure to air pollution, and living in crowded and poorly ventilated conditions (eg, incarceration).[209]

Etiologies of tuberculosis

Although the majority of tuberculosis is caused by MTB, organisms of the tuberculosis complex other than MTB can cause tuberculosis-like infections. *M bovis* was previously a significant source of zoonotic *Mycobacterium* infection, primarily through consumption of contaminated raw milk. The advent of pasteurization has significantly reduced the incidence of *M bovis* infections, which make up less than 1.8% of tuberculosis outside of Africa and 2.8% within Africa.[224,225] *Mycobacterium africanum* is responsible for up to 50% of tuberculosis in West Africa.[226] *M microti* and *M caprae* cause rare cases of tuberculosis in humans.[225,227]

Demographics of tuberculosis

It is estimated that 2 billion people are infected with MTB, and the vast majority of those infections are latent. Data from 2013 showed an incidence of 9 million new MTB infections worldwide (approximately 13% were also HIV positive), with 1.5 million MTB-related deaths (approximately 360,000 with HIV).[228] Among individuals coinfected with HIV (approximately 300 million people), tuberculosis remains the leading cause of death. In the United States, the rate of tuberculosis cases in 2013 was 3 per 100,000.[229]

Clinical features of tuberculosis

Tuberculosis is known as one of the "great mimickers" in medicine; it can infect any organ system with varied presentations.

Signs and symptoms of tuberculosis

Primary tuberculosis infection may be asymptomatic, or present with symptoms of an atypical community-acquired pneumonia, with nonproductive cough and limited radiological findings.[230] The classical signs of active pulmonary tuberculosis infection include fever, weight loss, night sweats, malaise, and persistent cough.[231] Mucoid bloodstained sputum is characteristic, but not always present. Erosion of a tubercle through pulmonary vessels can lead to frank hemoptysis.[232] Although local destruction and cavitation can occur, dyspnea is usually a late feature of the disease. When the pleura is involved, pleuritic chest pain and reduced chest expansion can be noted. Extrapulmonary disease has innumerable presentations, depending on the system involved.

Laboratory tests in the diagnosis of tuberculosis

Clinical testing for MTB exposure is centered on the tuberculin skin test (TST). The Mantoux method of the TST utilizes an intradermal injection of a purified tuberculin to elicit a wheal and flare indicative of delayed-type hypersensitivity in previously exposed individuals.[233] The TST is common, but somewhat limited by a tendency toward false-positive (prevalent in BCG vaccinated populations) and false-negative (more common in children, the elderly, and immunocompromised individuals) results, and a lack of specificity for MTB.[233] Newer interferon-gamma release assays (IGRA) also depend on the elicitation of a delayed-type hypersensitivity response, but utilize antigens that are more specific for MTB and specifically do not cross-react with the BCG vaccine strain of *M bovis*.[234,235] IGRAs are generally superior to TSTs in terms of sensitivity and specificity for the diagnosis of latent tuberculosis infections, but can have indeterminate results in the immunosuppressed.[234] As with TSTs, IGRA assays cannot distinguish between latent and active TB.[234]

Diagnosis of active infection requires either isolation of the MTB complex organism or detection of its nucleic acid, from clinical samples.[236] The classical method of tuberculosis diagnosis is the morphological identification of MTB in acid-fast (Ziehl-Neelsen or Kinyoun) stained sputum samples.[237] Fluorescence microscopy, utilizing auramine O or auramine and rhodamine stained specimens, has recently supplanted acid-fast staining as the preferred method of microscopic diagnosis due to increased sensitivity with comparable specificity.[238] In addition to microscopy, nucleic acid amplification testing (NAAT) from direct clinical specimens can be performed to aid in detection; NAAT tests tend to be highly sensitive (>90%) and specific (>90%) in smear positive disease, but have variable sensitivity (60%-70%) in smear negative disease.[239] Recently, utilization of sensitive and specific NAAT (real-time PCR or line probe assays) that incorporate combined diagnosis and resistance gene testing directly from clinical specimens has become more commonplace.[240-242]

Mycobacterial culture can be performed using solid or liquid media (or often, both). Liquid media has advantages over solid media in both in terms of increased sensitivity (near 90%) and in reduced time to detection, but can have higher rates of contamination in some settings.[243] The chief limitation of mycobacterial culture is the slow-growing nature of the organism; mean detection time for culture is around 10 to 13 days.[243,244] Growth from a positive culture may undergo species level identification via molecular probes, nucleotide sequencing, or protein mass spectrometry.[245]

Many rapid antigen and antibody detection systems have been developed for MTB diagnosis, but in general these have not performed with sufficient sensitivity or specificity as compared to sputum smear microscopy to supplant direct diagnosis.[246]

Imaging features of tuberculosis

Chest x-ray has been used as an adjunct to tuberculin skin testing for tuberculosis screening, and in conjunction with sputum smear microscopy for diagnosis of active tuberculosis.[247,248] Reports of the sensitivity and specificity of chest x-ray are variable, but agreement with sputum smear microscopy is generally high.[248] The imaging features of tuberculosis vary with the temporality and course of infection. Primary tuberculosis infections may be undetectable, or manifest as patchy or lobar consolation in any lobe (right middle lobe is most common), mediastinal adenopathy (more common in children), and pleural effusion (ipsilateral to site of disease and more common in adults); the findings of primary tuberculosis are more common in the setting of AIDS.[249,250] The majority of primary infections (>95%) resolve, usually with granuloma formation, fibrosis, and calcification. A radiographically visible primary parenchymal lesion is referred to as a Ghon focus or lesion and when combined with ipsilateral mediastinal adenopathy is termed a primary or Ghon complex.[251] A calcified and fibrosed Ghon complex is known as a Ranke complex.[251,252] Parenchymal lesions are more common in adults, while children are more likely to manifest mediastinal adenopathy. Primary infection is less commonly associated with cavitation, pleural effusions, or a military pattern, although all of these may be seen.

Reactivation tuberculosis (postprimary) or reinfection is classically characterized by parenchymal nodules in the apical and posterior segments of upper lobes, or less commonly, the superior segments of the lower lobes.[251] As in primary infection, the lesions can appear as ill defined or patchy opacities. Cavitation is seen in one-quarter to one-half of cases.[251] Bronchial spread is common in post-primary tuberculosis, giving rise to a "tree-in-bud" imaging pattern of well-defined nodules associated with bronchi (and also explaining the high infectivity associated with this stage of infection).[251] Mediastinal adenopathy and pleural effusions are uncommon in post-primary TB. Miliary tuberculosis is an uncommon presentation of primary or post-primary tuberculosis; it is characterized by the presence of numerous small 1 to 3 mm noncalcified nodules throughout the lungs (and occasionally other organs).[251,252] The miliary pattern confers a poor prognosis as it represents hematogenous dissemination of the organism.[253]

Pulmonary function tests in the diagnosis of tuberculosis

Active tuberculosis is associated with significant acute and chronic impairments in lung function. Sequelae of infection, in particular in the setting of cavitating disease, can include fibrosis, emphysema, and bronchiectasis.[254,255] Pulmonary function deficits after severe tuberculosis pulmonary disease are global, and include reduction in forced vital capacity, forced expiratory volume, and diffusing capacity.[255-257]

Routes of tuberculosis spread

Pulmonary tuberculosis occurs when *Mycobacterium tuberculosis* enters the body through inhalation, or ingestion followed by aspiration. Initial dissemination is usually lymphatic to local and mediastinal lymph nodes, although hematogenous dissemination also occurs. Once a pulmonary infection is established, bronchial spread of the organism to other areas within the lungs is common. Bronchial spreading seeds the airways with bacteria, allowing for respiratory transmission of the organism.

Diagnostic difficulties with tuberculosis

The diagnosis of tuberculosis has been historically challenging, and remains so today. Clinically, the disease has few pathognomic characteristics, and signs and symptoms overlap with those seen in other infections or malignancy. Screening tests for tuberculosis, such as the tuberculin skin test, are of limited utility in settings of high endemicity, areas with routine use of BCG vaccination, and in the setting of AIDS. Although interferon-gamma release assays are improved in their ability to distinguish disease caused by tuberculosis complex mycobacterium from vaccination or infection with non-tuberculous mycobacteria, they share the limitation of TSTs in not being able to distinguish latent from active disease. Sputum smears are useful in defining active disease, but have limited sensitivity. Due to the nature of mycobacteria, culture, when diagnostic, is slow (average time to diagnosis of 2 weeks). Molecular testing from direct clinical specimens is rapid and specific, but like sputum smear microscopy, it has limited sensitivity there is a low burden of organisms in the sputum.

Prognostic factors for tuberculosis

Prognostic factors indicative of increased risk of tuberculosis morbidity and mortality include host, disease, and social factors. Host factors include increased duration of illness prior to therapy, older age at diagnosis, male sex, HIV coinfection, active smoking, and low body weight.[258-261] Disease factors include late presentation or increased duration of illness prior to therapy, initial sputum smear positive for AFB or smear status unknown, disseminated tuberculosis, tuberculosis meningitis, and interruption of antibiotic therapy.[258-261] Social factors lack of a treatment supporter.[258-261] In the United States, US birth and use of directly observed therapy were also negative prognostic factors.[258]

Primary tuberculosis

Primary tuberculosis infection is initiated by inhalation of mycobacterial bacilli within respiratory droplet nuclei. Tuberculosis bacilli that enter the alveoli are engulfed by resident macrophages, but are often able to survive and replicate intracellular until development of cell-mediated immunity. Cell-mediated immunity leads to activation of macrophages, destruction of most of the infecting organisms, and granuloma formation with peripheral giant cells.[207] The tubercular granuloma (or tuberculoma or tubercle) walls off the infection and generally prevents further spread in most cases.[262] Radiographically, the resolved primary lesion is known as a Ghon focus.[251] Histologically, the periphery of the tubercular granuloma is comprised of primarily of Langhans type multinucleated giant cells with peripherally arranged nuclei (a consequence of fusion of activated macrophages) and epithelioid macrophages, with admixed T cells and scant plasma cells.[207] The center of the granuloma is necrotic, with amorphous eosinophilic (caseous) material.[207]

More often in children and then in adults, the organism traffics to the ipsilateral mediastinal lymph nodes before the cell-mediated response is able to arrest the infection, leading to ipsilateral mediastinal adenopathy.[251] The combination of a Ghon focus and calcified mediastinal nodes is known as a Ranke complex.[251]

Cavitation and pleural effusions are uncommon in primary infections, but are reported in approximately 20% of cases.[251] Miliary spread is rare, but more common in immunocompromised hosts.[253]

Approximately 90% of primary infections will resolve with the establishment of a latent infection.[207] The latent infection is kept in check by constant activity of the host immune system; disruption of the host immune system predisposes to reactivation.

Reactivation/reinfection (post-primary or secondary) tuberculosis

Post-primary tuberculosis occurs in one of three ways, through either an uncontrolled primary infection, reactivation of a latent primary infection, or exogenous reinfection.[263-265] Most reactivation disease occurs within 2 years of primary infection.[206] Compromise of the immune system at a later date can also prompt the reemergence of a dormant infection.[266] It is unclear how long tuberculosis bacilli may remain viable in tubercular granulomas, but reactivation disease has occurred decades after primary exposure.[267,268] The degree to which reactivation versus reinfection contributes to post-primary tuberculosis has not been well characterized, but is clearly dependent on the prevalence of active tuberculosis in the region of interest.[264,265]

Secondary tuberculosis is associated with an initial foamy macrophage predominant pneumonia that progresses to caseating necrosis and fibrosis.[269] The process is usually centered within the apical and posterior segments of the upper lobe of the lung, but airway involvement can lead to tuberculous bronchopneumonia (with a tree-in-bud pattern) that can progress to involve entire segments and lobes.[269] As the lesion progresses, cavitation can occur, with thin- or thick-walled cavities surrounded granulation tissue and fibrosis. If the pleura is involved, diffuse thickening and pleural adhesions result.

Miliary tuberculosis

Miliary disease is a rare manifestation of tuberculosis, accounting for only 1% to 2% of cases, which is associated with high mortality.[253] The radiographic and pathologic appearance of miliary tuberculosis arises from the identification of innumerable small (1-3 mm) well-defined foci of infection (tubercles) in the lungs or other visceral organs. Miliary disease occurs as the result of uncontrolled hematogenous spread of mycobacterium throughout the body. Miliary tuberculosis implies a defect in cell-mediated immunity, and risk factors include malnutrition, HIV/AIDS, immunosuppressive use, rheumatologic diseases, underlying malignancy, and others.[253]

Progressive fibrocavitary tuberculosis

If unchecked, post-primary tuberculosis frequently leads to progressive fibrocavitary tuberculosis, a state of chronic inflammation leading to the destruction of lung parenchyma by chronic granuloma formation, caseous necrosis and cavitation.[269] Repeated rounds of inflammation and healing lead to scarring, volume loss, calcification, bronchiectasis, and bronchostenosis.[270,271] Histologically, there are large areas of caseous necrosis surrounded by fibrotic bands. The areas of necrosis frequently cavitate, leading to a thick-walled lesion with granulomas interspersed within the wall. Cavitary lesions either persist, or are less frequently replaced with fibrous tissue.[269] Tuberculous bacilli multiply in cavitary lesions, which serve as a source of bacteria for bronchial seeding when cavities communicate with the airways.[272] Seeding of the airways leads to chronic airway inflammation, local spread of the disease, and also increased sputum bacterial counts and overall infectivity.[272] Fibrocavitary lesions can also communicate with the pulmonary arterial vasculature, leading to a Rasmussen aneurysm and the risk of severe uncontrolled hemoptysis.[273]

Pleural involvement with tuberculosis

Pleural tuberculosis is a manifestation of extrapulmonary disease that occurs in approximately 20% to 30% of tuberculosis infections.[274,275] It can be seen in both primary and post-primary infections, and frequently occurs in the absence of detectable pulmonary parenchymal lesions on chest x-ray.[276] Tuberculous pleuritis is frequently associated with low organism burden, and diagnosis can be difficult. Culture of pleural fluid is positive in only 12% to 40% of cases of pleural tuberculosis, while nucleic acid amplification testing and smear microscopy are usually negative.[277,278] Sputum microscopy or nucleic acid testing, similarly, is usually negative in cases of pleural tuberculosis, although induced sputum microscopy and culture may be more sensitive.[279]

Tuberculous pleuritis is characterized by an exudative lymphocyte-predominant effusion. Biochemical analyses of pleural fluid demonstrating elevations in adenosine deaminase and/or interferon-gamma levels are sensitive and specific markers of tuberculosis infection.[280]

Histologically, the presence of caseating granulomas within pleural specimens raises suspicion for the disease, while demonstration of AFB is diagnostic. Biopsy histopathology has a reported sensitivity for detection of MTB of approximately 50%; this is significantly improved by incorporation of data from biopsy culture and nucleic acid testing of biopsy specimens.[281]

Tuberculosis in cancer patients

The interplay between tuberculosis and cancer has been historically complex, with observations suggesting both a causative role in terms of lung cancer and an increase in tuberculosis rates among those with certain malignancies.

There is a significant body of literature showing an association between tuberculosis and the development of lung cancer.[282-285] It is generally assumed this increased risk stems from repeated rounds of tuberculosis-associated inflammation. A systemic review of studies from the past 50 years calculated a 1.8-fold increase in the risk of developing adenocarcinoma of the lung (interestingly, there was no significant association with other variants of lung cancer).[286]

In addition to lung cancer, hematologic malignancy, head and neck cancers, and digestive tract lesions have been shown to confer an increased risk for the development of active tuberculosis.[287] Hematologic malignancies have been associated as much as a 50- to 100-fold increased rate of active tuberculosis in populations at high risk for latent tuberculosis.[288] The increased risk conferred by aerodigestive tract malignancies is less, but still significant.[287,289] The mechanism of this increased risk is unclear, although in the case of hematologic tumors is most likely immune system dysfunction.

Tuberculosis in patients with HIV

HIV coinfection increases both the risk of progression of primary MTB infection, and the risk of reactivation disease; overall the risk of developing active tuberculosis in the setting of coinfection is approximately 20- to 37-fold.[290] The mechanism by which HIV coinfection exacerbates MTB infection has not been fully elucidated, but likely involves the destruction of CD4+ T cells by the HIV virus; both incidence of tuberculosis and tuberculosis-associated mortality vary directly with CD4+ T-cell count.[291] The elimination of helper T cells diminishes the ability of the immune system to generate a delayed-type hypersensitivity response that is necessary for formation and maintenance of granulomas, and in function of tuberculosis screening assays.[292,293]

In addition to increasing the risk of the development of active disease, HIV coinfection is associated with an increased duration of infectivity, absent or nonspecific pulmonary symptoms, increased pulmonary tuberculosis severity, increased risk of disseminated disease, increased treatment failure, and increased MTB-associated mortality.[294] Indeed, TB is leading killer of HIV-infected individuals worldwide. WHO estimates

that of 9 million new tuberculosis infections in 2013, 1.17 million were in individuals with HIV.[228]

Tuberculosis treatment

Latent tuberculosis is treated with either isoniazid or rifampin, or a combination of isoniazid and rifapentine over a period of 3 to 9 months depending on the regimen.[295,296] Active tuberculosis treatment generally is more complicated, with first-line therapy consisting of a 6-month regimen four oral drugs: isoniazid and rifampin (for 6 months), plus pyrazinamide and ethambutol (for 2 initial months).[297] Daily therapy is optimal for all patients and should be used in the initial phase for patients with HIV or living in HIV endemic areas.

Approximately 3% to 4% of new patients and 20% of previously treated patients worldwide will carry multidrug-resistant (MDR) tuberculosis (MDR is resistant to at least isoniazid and rifampin).[298] In some regions, the rate of MDR-TB in previously treated cases was as high as 50%.[298,299] Second-line agents for tuberculosis treatment include injectables (kanamycin, amikacin, capreomycin, streptomycin), fluoroquinolones (levofloxacin, moxifloxacin, ofloxacin), oral bacteriostatic agents (para-aminosalicylic acid, cycloserine, terizidone, ethionamide, prothionamide), and agents with potential activity (eg, clofazimine, clarithromycin).[297] Drug susceptibility testing should be conducted if there is concern for MDR-TB or treatment failure. A drug regimen for MDR-TB generally consists of four drugs, with any active first-line agent and the sequential addition of an injectable agent, fluoroquinolone, and oral bacteriostatic agent as necessary to reach four drugs.[297]

Drug-resistant tuberculosis

Mycobacterium tuberculosis is notorious for the development of resistance to antimicrobial agents. Multidrug-resistant TB (MDR-TB) is defined by clinical resistance to at least the first-line agent's isoniazid and rifampin; 3% to 4% of new TB cases are MDR.[299] Resistance to isoniazid and rifampin, plus resistance to a fluoroquinolone and one of three injectable drugs (amikacin, kanamycin, or capreomycin) is termed extensively drug-resistant (XDR).[299] XDR-TB, a subset of MDR-TB, accounts for only 5% of overall drug-resistant cases, but greater than 10% of cases in some areas such as Eastern Europe and Central Asia.[299] Mortality rates for XDR TB are comparable to those of TB before the advent of antibiotics, and reach 90% in the setting of HIV coinfection.[297,299]

Laboratory diagnosis of tuberculosis

Morphologic identification of tuberculosis

Mycobacterium tuberculosis is a gram-positive non-spore-forming slender *Bacillus* (approximately 1 to 4 μm in length and 0.5 μm in diameter). Mycobacteria do not Gram stain well due to waxy substances (mycolic acids) in the cell wall, but retain the dye fuchsin in the presence of an acid-alcohol decolorizer (hence, "acid fast").[300,301] The tuberculosis bacillus can be identified by direct examination of sputum or other tissue sources by acid-fast or fluorescence staining.

Special stains for the diagnosis of tuberculosis

Auramine O and auramine-rhodamine are fluorescent stains used for the diagnosis of MTB from smears or tissue.[302,303] MTB can also be visualized by acid-fast methods, including Ziehl-Neelsen, cold Kinyoun method, or various modified Ziehl-Neelsen stains such as Fite (which either contain reduced acid or additional oils) (*Figure 12-5*). The modified acid-fast stains also detect *Mycobacterium leprae* or *Nocardia* spp.

Molecular testing for the diagnosis of tuberculosis

Nucleic acid amplification tests (NAAT), including transcription-mediated amplification and PCR, are sensitive and specific assays that have long been used to aid in the diagnosis of MTB directly from clinical specimens or from culture.[237] PCR combined with Sanger sequencing has provided the mainstay of sequence-based resistance gene testing to date, but is likely to be supplanted in time by targeted and whole genome sequencing as costs continue to decrease.[304,305] Several of the newer rapid NAATs also incorporate resistance gene testing, either for first- or second-line drugs. The Xpert system, a cartridge-based PCR assay that simultaneously detects MTB and genetic rifampin resistance, has been recommended by WHO since 2010 and is now widely deployed worldwide.[306] Additional rapid assays for resistance testing include line probe assays (which utilize PCR and probe hybridization for visualization) that test for mutations that confer resistance to rifampin, rifampin and isoniazid, or second-line TB drugs.[242,307,308]

Distinct from nucleic acid–based methods, proteomic identification of Mycobacteria is now being incorporated into the clinical microbiology laboratory.[245] Although currently limited to cultured specimens, mass spectrometry is a rapid method for providing species level organism identification.

Issues regarding culture for tuberculosis

Mycobacterial culture is more sensitive than direct examination, and remains in many cases gold standard for TB diagnosis. However, several characteristics of mycobacteria complicate the culture process. Because of the nature of the organism, growth of *Mycobacterium tuberculosis* on solid media can take from 4 to 8 weeks. Liquid culture is both more sensitive and significantly faster, often turning positive within 10 days, but is more susceptible than solid media to contamination.[243] Culture of the organism creates a serious risk for laboratory-based infections, and is preferably conducted in biosafety level 3 facilities.

Gross features of tuberculosis granulomas

Tuberculous granulomas are round, variably sized, firm, and tan-colored nodules. Some nodules, usually those larger in size, may be soft and tan-white (caseous necrosis).

Histologic features of tuberculosis granulomas

Tuberculous granulomas are characterized by a central area of caseous necrosis surrounded by a periphery of multinucleated giant cells (Langhans type) and chronic inflammation characterized by epithelioid macrophages, T cells, and few plasma cells.

Special stains

Carbol fuchsin–based acid-fast stains form the mainstay of MTB detection in tubercular granulomas.[301] The Ziehl-Neelsen stain is most commonly used, with the cold Kinyoun modification preferable in some areas. Modified acid-fast methods, such as Fite-Faraco will also stain *Mycobacterium tuberculosis*, in addition to organisms such as *Mycobacterium leprae* and nonmycobacterial acid-fast organisms (eg, *Nocardia, Rhodococcus, Legionella micdadei*).[301,309] Auramine-based fluorescent stains can also be used on FFPE tissue specimens, and is generally more sensitive than acid-fast stains.[310]

Immunohistochemical stains for tuberculosis proteins (eg, MPT64) have been described, and are more sensitive and specific than acid-fast staining.[311] Sensitive and specific in situ hybridization methods have also been described. Of note, routine evaluation of a granuloma should include GMS and PAS stains to rule out fungal organisms.

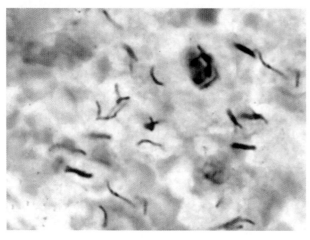

FIGURE 12-5 High power image of Ziehl-Neelsen stain showing *Mycobacterium tuberculosis* organisms.

Mycobacterial Pseudotumor

Inflammatory pseudotumors can arise in all organisms of the body by various mechanisms. Infection, often in the setting of profound immunosuppression, may contribute to pseudotumor development, although the overall incidence remains low.

Epidemiology of mycobacterial pseudotumor

Mycobacterial pseudotumor is a rare entity, with fewer than 50 cases in the literature.[312,313] There are few estimates of incidence, although various reports have suggested that bronchopulmonary pseudotumor may occur in up to 2% to 4% of cases active pulmonary tuberculosis.[313] Mycobacterial pseudotumors have been reported throughout the body, although there are little data on organ-specific incidence.

Demographics of mycobacterial pseudotumor

Mycobacterial pseudotumor is usually seen in immunosuppressed hosts (ie, HIV/AIDS, posttransplant or malignancy).[314-317] It has also been observed in babies that have received the BCG vaccination.[318]

Mycobacterial organisms causing of mycobacterial pseudotumor

Mycobacterium tuberculosis, *Mycobacterium avium-intracellulare* complex, *Mycobacterium chelonae*, *M kansasii*, *M haemophilum*, and *M simiae* have been reported as causative agents of pseudotumor.[312,318-322] Given the large number of organisms that can cause inflammatory pseudotumors, including fungi and viruses, it is likely that infection with other mycobacterial species has the potential to lead to pseudotumor formation.

Diagnostic criteria of mycobacterial pseudotumor

Mycobacterial pseudotumor can mimic a variety of entities radiologically, and is ultimately a histologic diagnosis.[323] The combination of pseudotumor histology and evidence of mycobacterial infection, either microbiologic or by direct examination of the tissue, is sufficient to render the diagnosis.

Clinical features of mycobacterial pseudotumor

The clinical features of mycobacterial pseudotumor depend largely on the location of the mass. Spindle cell pseudotumors of infectious origin have been described throughout the body, including lymph nodes, skin, lung, bone, brain, spleen, and retroperitoneum.[314-316,324-326] The lesions are benign, but may be symptomatic by local mass effect.[317,321] As the lesions are clinically difficult to distinguish from malignancy, they will often prompt a full workup that includes imaging, biopsy, and potential resection.

Imaging features of mycobacterial pseudotumor

The imaging features of mycobacterial pseudotumor are nonspecific. Plain x-ray or CT shows solid nodules or nonspecific masses.[323]

Gross features of mycobacterial pseudotumor

Mycobacterial pseudotumors are grossly round to oval, white, gray, or tan nodules or masses.[312] They can be firm to rubbery in consistency, or are softer if areas of coagulative necrosis are present.

Histologic features of mycobacterial pseudotumor

Mycobacterial pseudotumor is characterized by a nodular lesion comprised of vague fascicles of benign appearing spindle cell in a storiform pattern.[316] Langhans giant cells and areas of caseous necrosis may be identified, and are helpful in directing the diagnosis.[312] A chronic inflammatory cell infiltrate of plasma cells and lymphocytes is often present; however, the foamy histiocytes that often characterize a mycobacterial infection are not found.[312,327] The lesions often contain abundant acid-fast bacilli within the spindle cell, although this is not universal and molecular detection of *Mycobacterium* may be required. The differential diagnosis includes inflammatory pseudotumors of other origins, inflammatory myofibroblastic tumor, and intranodal Kaposi sarcoma, and others.[314,328,329] MPT is distinguished from intranodal Kaposi sarcoma by an absence of mitosis in MPT.[314]

Cytologic features of mycobacterial pseudotumor

Fine needle aspiration of a mycobacterial pseudotumor shows spindle cell and granulomatous inflammation with a background of mixed inflammatory cells consisting primarily of epithelioid histiocytes and lymphocytes.[322] The cells display relatively bland cytology, although mild reactive atypia can be present.[322] The foamy histiocytes of tuberculoid granulomas are usually absent.[327] There should be no multinucleated tumor cells or mitoses.[322]

Immunohistochemical features of mycobacterial pseudotumor

The spindle cells of mycobacterial pseudotumor are positive for CD68 and CD163, variably positive for S100, and negative for factor XIIIa, CD34, smooth muscle actin, vimentin, and desmin.[322,325,330] They are immunochemically distinct from Kaposi sarcoma, which is CD31 and CD34 positive, negative for CD68 and S100.[314]

Molecular features of mycobacterial pseudotumor

Mycobacterial pseudotumors are reactive, and not characterized by distinct molecular features.

Nontuberculous Mycobacteria

Although *Mycobacterium tuberculosis* is by far the most prolific and deadly of the mycobacterial pathogens, nontuberculosis mycobacteria (NTM) are significant causes of disease worldwide. NTM are soil and water microorganisms that are ubiquitous in the environment and capable of causing disease in both immunocompetent and immunocompromised hosts. Pulmonary infection is the most common manifestation of NTM disease, but skin and soft tissue infections, lymphadenitis, and disseminated infections also occur.[331] *Mycobacterium avium-intracellulare* complex (MAC) organisms are responsible for between 40% and 80% of NTM-caused pulmonary disease worldwide.[332,333] The other causative agents vary significantly geographically; *M chelonae/abscesses*, *M fortuitum*, and *M kansasii* are the most commonly isolated organisms in the United States, Australia, and Asia, while *M malmoense*, *M gordonae*, *M kansasii*, and *M xenopi* are common in Europe.[332,333]

Pathogenesis of nontuberculous mycobacterial lung disease

NTM, and in particular MAC, most often cause an extended course of chronic lung disease. The pathogenesis of NTM lung disease is imperfectly understood, but appears to include pathogen-mediated immune dysfunction leading to intracellular survival and replication, and ultimately chronic infection.[334]

MAC classically causes an upper lobe cavitary infection (reminiscent of tuberculosis), but can also cause a nodular bronchiectatic infection without lobar preference.[335,336] In elderly Caucasian women, a bronchiectatic nodular disease that predominantly affects that middle lobe and lingula has been described; this presentation has sometimes been called "Lady Windermere syndrome" after the Oscar Wilde character.[337,338] In addition, MAC has been implicated as the cause of a noninfectious allergic lung disease, "Hot Tub lung."[339,340]

Risk factors for developing nontuberculous mycobacterial lung disease

The vast majority of NTM pulmonary infections develop in immunocompromised hosts and those with chronic lung disease. Risk factors include HIV/AIDS, history of smoking or alcoholism, cystic fibrosis, COPD or bronchiectasis, and use of TNF-α antagonists.[341-344] In addition, elderly Caucasian women with slender body habitus are at increased risk for developing a nodular bronchiectatic MAC infection (Lady Windermere syndrome).[331,341]

Etiologies of nontuberculous mycobacterial lung disease

MAC, *M kansasii*, *M chelonae/abscessus*, and *M fortuitum* are common causes of NTM pulmonary disease in North America.[332,333] *M malmoense* and *M xenopi* are more common strains in Europe.[332,333] Other strains that have been isolated include *M asiaticum*, *M celatum*, *M chelonae*, *M haemophilum*, *M scrofulaceum*, *M shimoidei*, *M simiae*, *M smegmatis*, and *M szulgai*.[333]

Common nontuberculous mycobacteria causing lung disease

MAC, *M kansasii*, *M chelonae/abscessus*, and *M fortuitum* are the most common etiological agents of NTM pulmonary disease in North America.[332,333] *M malmoense* and *M xenopi* are more commonly in Europe.[332,333]

Demographics of nontuberculous mycobacterial lung disease

Unlike MTB, NTM pulmonary infections have been increasing in prevalence over the past few decades. Estimates of the incidence of NTM pulmonary disease in the United States overall vary widely, and range from 1.4 to 6.7 per 100,000.[332] Age is a considerable risk factor for NTM, and prevalence among those aged greater than 59 is 26.7 per 100,000.[345] For age 65 and older, prevalence has been reported as high as 47 per 100,000.[342] Geographically, South East and Western Coastal United States have the highest prevalence of NTM pulmonary disease.[342] For patients greater than 65, women are 1.4 times more likely to be NTM pulmonary disease cases than men, but men are 1.8 times more likely to die from NTM pulmonary infections.[342]

Clinical features of nontuberculous mycobacterial lung disease

NTM pulmonary disease is defined by slow onset and nonspecific symptoms.

Signs and symptoms of nontuberculous mycobacterial lung disease

Pulmonary infection with NTM has variable presentations. Limited disease (Lady Windermere syndrome) can present similar to a recurrent bronchitis.[346] More severe infections present with a tuberculosis-like disease characterized by chronic productive cough, fevers, night sweats, weight loss, lethargy, and malaise.[346,347] Hemoptysis is less common than with MTB.

Laboratory tests in the diagnosis of nontuberculous mycobacterial lung disease

Laboratory diagnosis of NTM mycobacteria is similar to that of MTB, and involves either direct visualization of the organism from a clinical or culture specimens by microscopy, or detection by nucleic acid amplification from clinical or culture specimens, or paraffin embedded tissues.[348,349] Similar to MTB, culture is usually conducted using both liquid and solid culture media. Identification of NTM at the species level can be achieved by nucleic acid hybridization (with or without prior amplification), line probe assays, sequencing, or mass spectrometry.[350,351]

Imaging features of nontuberculous mycobacterial lung disease

Active NTM pulmonary disease may be without diagnostic abnormality, particularly in immunocompromised patients, or display patchy airspace opacities, ill-defined nodules, and bronchiectasis with diffuse bronchial wall thickening.[352,353] Limitation of bronchiectatic disease to the right middle lobe and lingua is characteristic of infection in elderly Caucasian women.[352,353] Cavitary disease (usually MAC) is less common, and presents with upper lung zone cavitation with volume loss and fibrosis (similar in appearance to MTB).[352,353] CT has an important role in the diagnosis of NTM infections, as important findings are often not visible on plain chest x-ray.[354]

Solitary pulmonary nodules

NTM pulmonary disease may manifest as solitary pulmonary nodule (SPN) on imaging.[355] There are no distinct radiographic features that definitively distinguish an SPN caused by nontuberculous mycobacterium from a tuberculoma or malignancy, and nodules displaying increased 18F-fluorodeoxyglucose uptake have been reported.[356,357] Histologically, SPN caused by NTM often show chronic granulomatous inflammation (impossible to distinguish from granulomas caused by MTB), with or without detectable acid-fast bacilli.[355]

Chronic progressive disease

Progressive MAC usually occurs in middle-age to elderly men with additional risk factors such as alcoholism, smoking, and chronic lung disease.[346] Much like MTB, progressive MAC is characterized by an upper lobe predominance with cavitation and fibrosis. Bronchiectasis and nodular infiltrates are often also present.[346,347]

Chronic bronchiolitis with bronchiectasis

In immunocompetent hosts, elderly women, those with thoracic skeletal deformities, MAC can present as an initial bronchiolitis that develops over time into a multinodular bronchiectasis.[346,347] Progression of this disease is usually slow; cavitation may present late in the disease.[347] There is some data to suggest CFTR gene mutations may also contribute to bronchiectatic MAC.

Disseminated disease

Rarely seen in immunocompetent hosts, disseminated *Mycobacterium avium* complex infection is an important complication of advanced HIV in patients with fewer than 50 CD4+ T cells per microliter of blood.[358-360] Macrolide prophylaxis for patients with T-lymphocyte counts below 50 per microliter was previously the mainstay of prevention for disseminated MAC, but since the advent of highly active antiretroviral therapy the incidence of disseminated MAC has greatly diminished, and is now approximately 0.5 per 100 person-years.[359] Disseminated MAC is associated with nonspecific B symptoms and increased mortality (independent of CD4+ T-cell count).[359]

As with other form of NTM disease, MAC is contracted from the environment by inhalation or ingestion.[361] Dissemination occurs by lymphohematogenous spread from the initial site of infection and can involve any organ system, although infection of the spleen, liver, and reticuloendothelial system is most common.[362] Histologically, abundant acid-fast bacilli within monocytes or macrophages can be seen.[363] Within lymph nodes or other tissues, the bacilli can grow in large sheets that displace the normal cellular architecture.[363]

Hypersensitivity pneumonitis—"hot tub lung"

The pathophysiology of MAC-related hypersensitivity pneumonitis is not well understood, and displays features of both a hypersensitivity reaction and infection.[364-366] The disease involves exposure to water sources of MAC (eg, hot tub, pool) combined with subacute hypersensitivity-like pneumonitis. For diagnosis, MAC should be isolated from the patient and radiographic and/or pathological evidence of hypersensitivity pneumonitis should be present. Histologically, there is granulomatous inflammation reminiscent of hypersensitivity pneumonitis.[367]

Pulmonary function tests in the diagnosis of nontuberculous mycobacterial lung disease

A small study of 15 women with bronchiectatic MAC infection, but not preexisting lung disease, showed MAC infection was associated with an increased residual volume and decreased expiratory flow.[368] There was no observed decrease in total lung capacity, FEV_1, or DL_{CO}.[368] A larger study of 68 patients, with approximately one-third fibrocavitary disease and two-thirds bronchiectatic disease reported a yearly decline in FEV_1 and FVC associated with MAC infection.[369]

CHAPTER 12

Prognostic factors for nontuberculous mycobacterial lung disease

Negative prognostic factors for all-cause mortality of NTM infections include male sex, age ≥65, the presence of a significant comorbidities, BMI ≤18.5, and radiographic features consistent with fibrocavitary disease or fibrocavitary disease combined with nodular-bronchiectatic disease.[343,370] *M xenopi* infection was a negative prognostic factor in one study.[343]

Gross features of nontuberculous mycobacterial lung disease

The gross appearance of an NTM pulmonary infection varies, both with the severity of the disease, immune function of the host, and type of disease presentation. Less severe NTM infections, or disseminated infections in immunocompromised hosts, may have no overt or limited gross pulmonary pathologic findings.[371] Occasionally, NTM infections may manifest grossly as a solitary pulmonary nodule or in a multinodular military pattern.[371]

Gross findings in fibrocavitary are similar to those of tuberculosis; characteristic features include upper lobe predominant cavitation and gray-tan fibrosis. In contrast, nodular and bronchiectatic disease is characterized by airway-centered pathology including dilated and ectatic bronchi, thickened bronchial walls, and peribronchiolar granulomas and fibrosis[371] (*Figure 12-6*).

Histologic features of nontuberculous mycobacterial lung disease

Fibrocavitary NTM disease has a histologic appearance indistinguishable from that of post-primary tuberculosis. It is characterized microscopically by noncaseating or caseating granulomas, necrosis, cavitation, and fibrosis.

Nodular-bronchiectatic NTM lung disease is characterized by progressive destruction of the bronchial cartilage and smooth muscle, respiratory mucosal ulceration, and narrowing of the airways.[372] Microscopically, there is robust chronic lympho- and monocytic infiltrate with noncaseating epithelioid or caseating granulomas and bronchial wall thickening, necrosis, and obliteration. As the disease progresses, cavity formation and fibrosis are seen.[371,372] As with tuberculosis, necrotic materials in cavities serve as a chronic source of organisms for bronchial dissemination of disease. Submucosal granulomas can exert a mass effect leading to airway stenosis. Emphysema and organizing pneumonia are sometimes present.[372]

Special stains

NTM can be visualized by fluorescent (eg, auramine) or acid-fast stains (eg, Ziehl-Neelsen or Fite-Faraco).[373] Immunohistochemical and in situ hybridization detection methods are available for nontuberculous mycobacteria, but are not currently in common usage.[374-376]

REFERENCES

1. Dodd JD, Souza CA, Müller NL. High-resolution MDCT of pulmonary septic embolism: evaluation of the feeding vessel sign. *Am J Roentgenol.* 2006;187:623-629.
2. Boyton RJR, Openshaw PJP. Pulmonary defences to acute respiratory infection. *Br Med Bull.* 2002;61:1-12. http://bmb.oxford journals.org/content/61/1/1.short. Accessed October 10, 2014.
3. Diamond G, Legarda D, Ryan LK. The innate immune response of the respiratory epithelium. *Immunol Rev.* 2000;173:27-38.
4. Schwartz DA, Quinn TJ, Thorne PS, Sayeed S, Yi AK, Krieg AM. CpG motifs in bacterial DNA cause inflammation in the lower respiratory tract. *J Clin Invest.* 1997;100:68-73.
5. Singh PK, Jia HP, Wiles K, et al. Production of beta-defensins by human airway epithelia. *Proc Natl Acad Sci U S A.* 1998;95:14961-14966.
6. Smith JJ, Travis SM, Greenberg EP, Welsh MJ. Cystic fibrosis airway epithelia fail to kill bacteria because of abnormal airway surface fluid. *Cell.* 1996;85:229-236.
7. Pier GB. Role of the cystic fibrosis transmembrane conductance regulator in innate immunity to Pseudomonas aeruginosa infections. *Proc Natl Acad Sci U S A.* 2000;97:8822-8828.
8. Grant CC, Emery D, Milne T, et al. Risk factors for community-acquired pneumonia in pre-school-aged children. *J Paediatr Child Health.* 2012;48(5):402-412.
9. Farr BM, Woodhead MA, MacFarlane JT, et al. Risk factors for community-acquired pneumonia diagnosed by general practitioners in the community. *Respir Med.* 2000;94(5):422-427.

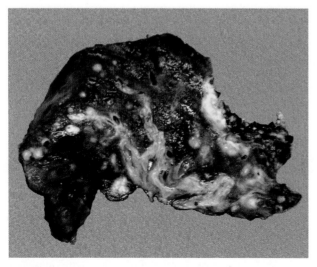

FIGURE 12-6 Gross image of lobectomy involved with *Mycobacterium avium-intracellulare* complex disease, showing diffuse bronchiectasis.

10. Torres A, Peetermans WE, Viegi G, Blasi F. Risk factors for community-acquired pneumonia in adults in Europe: a literature review. *Thorax.* 2013;68(11):1057-1065.

11. Almirall J, Bolíbar I, Serra-Prat M, et al. New evidence of risk factors for community-acquired pneumonia: a population-based study. *Eur Respir J.* 2008;31(6):1274-1284.

12. Hunter JD. Ventilator associated pneumonia. *Postgrad Med J.* 2006;82(965):172-178.

13. Samokhvalov A V, Irving HM, Rehm J. Alcohol consumption as a risk factor for pneumonia: a systematic review and meta-analysis. *Epidemiol Infect.* 2010;138(12):1789-1795.

14. Rothberg MB, Haessler SD, Brown RB. Complications of viral influenza. *Am J Med.* 2008;121(4):258-264.

15. Bowden DH. The alveolar macrophage. *Environ Health Perspect.* 1984;55:327-341.

16. Goldstein E, Lippert W, Warshauer D. Pulmonary alveolar macrophage. Defender against bacterial infection of the lung. *J Clin Invest.* 1974;54(3):519-528.

17. Ryan LK, Golenbock DT, Wu J, Vermeulen MW. Characterization of proinflammatory cytokine production and CD14 expression by murine alveolar macrophage cell lines. In *Vitro Cell Dev Biol Anim.* 1997;33(8):647-653.

18. Reutershan J, Basit A, Galkina E V, Ley K. Sequential recruitment of neutrophils into lung and bronchoalveolar lavage fluid in LPS-induced acute lung injury. *Am J Physiol Lung Cell Mol Physiol.* 2005;289(5):L807-L815.

19. Sibille Y, Reynolds HY. Macrophages and polymorphonuclear neutrophils in lung defense and injury. *Am Rev Respir Dis.* 1990;141(2):471-501.

20. Thompson M, Shay D, Zhou H, et al. Estimates of deaths associated with seasonal influenza—United States, 1976–2007. *MMWR Morb Mortal Wkly Rep.* 2010;59:1057-1062. http://www.ncbi.nlm.nih.gov/pubmed/20798667.

21. Thompson WW, Weintraub E, Dhankhar P, et al. Estimates of US influenza-associated deaths made using four different methods. *Influenza Other Respir Viruses.* 2009;3(1):37-49.

22. Thompson WW, Shay DK, Weintraub E, et al. Influenza-associated hospitalizations in the United States. *JAMA.* 2004;292(11):1333-1340.

23. McCullers J a. The co-pathogenesis of influenza viruses with bacteria in the lung. *Nat Rev Microbiol.* 2014;12(4):252-262.

24. Metersky ML, Masterton RG, Lode H, File TM, Babinchak T. Epidemiology, microbiology, and treatment considerations for bacterial pneumonia complicating influenza. *Int J Infect Dis.* 2012;16(5):e321-e331.

25. Morens DM, Taubenberger JK, Fauci AS. Predominant role of bacterial pneumonia as a cause of death in pandemic influenza: implications for pandemic influenza preparedness. *J Infect Dis.* 2008;198(7):962-970.

26. Kallen AJ, Brunkard J, Moore Z, et al. Staphylococcus aureus community-acquired pneumonia during the 2006 to 2007 influenza season. *Ann Emerg Med.* 2009;53(3):358-365.

27. Mandell LA. Epidemiology and etiology of community-acquired pneumonia. *Infect Dis Clin North Am.* 2004;18(4):761-776.

28. Cunha BA. The atypical pneumonias: clinical diagnosis and importance. *Clin Microbiol Infect.* 2006;12(suppl 3):12-24.

29. Apisarnthanarak A, Mundy LM. Etiology of community-acquired pneumonia. *Clin Chest Med.* 2005;26(1):47-55.

30. Johansson N, Kalin M, Tiveljung-Lindell A, Giske CG, Hedlund J. Etiology of community-acquired pneumonia: increased microbiological yield with new diagnostic methods. *Clin Infect Dis.* 2010;50(2):202-209.

31. Thibodeau KP, Viera AJ. Atypical pathogens and challenges in community-acquired pneumonia. *Am Fam Physician.* 2004;69(7):1699-1706.

32. Marrie TJ, Costain N, La Scola B, et al. The role of atypical pathogens in community-acquired pneumonia. *Semin Respir Crit Care Med.* 2012;33(3):244-256.

33. Wiemken TL, Peyrani P, Ramirez JA. Global changes in the epidemiology of community-acquired pneumonia. *Semin Respir Crit Care Med.* 2012;33(3):213-219.

34. File TM. Community-acquired pneumonia. *Lancet.* 2003;362(9400):1991-2001.

35. Yamasaki K, Kawanami T, Yatera K, et al. Significance of anaerobes and oral bacteria in community-acquired pneumonia. *PLoS One.* 2013;8(5).

36. Mandell LA. Spectrum of microbial etiology of community-acquired pneumonia in hospitalized patients: implications for selection of the population for enrollment in clinical trials. *Clin Infect Dis.* 2008;47(suppl 3):S189-S192.

37. Niederman MS, McCombs JS, Unger AN, Kumar A, Popovian R. The cost of treating community-acquired pneumonia. *Clin Ther.* 1998;20:820-837.

38. Welte T, Köhnlein T. Global and local epidemiology of community-acquired pneumonia: the experience of the CAPNETZ Network. *Semin Respir Crit Care Med.* 2009;30(2):127-135.

39. WHO. Revised global burden of disease 2002 estimates. 2004. http://www.who.int/healthinfo/global_burden_disease/estimates_regional_2002_revised/en/ .

40. Rudan I, O'Brien KL, Nair H, et al. Epidemiology and etiology of childhood pneumonia in 2010: estimates of incidence, severe morbidity, mortality, underlying risk factors and causative pathogens for 192 countries. *J Glob Health.* 2013;3:010401.

41. Rudan I, Boschi-Pinto C, Biloglav Z, Mulholland K, Campbell H. Epidemiology and etiology of childhood pneumonia. *Bull World Health Organ.* 2008;86:408-416.

42. Jones RN. Microbial etiologies of hospital-acquired bacterial pneumonia and ventilator-associated bacterial pneumonia. *Clin Infect Dis.* 2010;51(suppl 1):S81-S87.

43. Chawla R. Epidemiology, etiology, and diagnosis of hospital-acquired pneumonia and ventilator-associated pneumonia in Asian countries. *Am J Infect Control.* 2008;36(4, suppl 2):S93-S100.

44. American Thoracic Society; Infectious Diseases Society of America. Guidelines for the management of adults with hospital-acquired, ventilator-associated, and healthcare-associated pneumonia. *Am J Respir Crit Care Med.* 2005;171:388.

45. Remington LT, Sligl WI. Community-acquired pneumonia. *Curr Opin Pulm Med.* 2014;20(3):215-224.

46. Babady NE. The FilmArray respiratory panel: an automated, broadly multiplexed molecular test for the rapid and accurate detection of respiratory pathogens. *Expert Rev Mol Diagn.* 2013;13(8):779-788.

47. Abdeldaim GMK, Strålin K, Korsgaard J, Blomberg J, Welinder-Olsson C, Herrmann B. Multiplex quantitative PCR for detection of lower respiratory tract infection and meningitis caused by Streptococcus pneumoniae, Haemophilus influenzae and Neisseria meningitidis. *BMC Microbiol.* 2010;10:310.

48. Mandell L a, Wunderink RG, Anzueto A, et al. Infectious Diseases Society of America/American Thoracic Society consensus guidelines on the management of community-acquired pneumonia in adults. *Clin Infect Dis.* 2007;44(suppl 2):S27-S72.

49. Franquet T. Imaging of pneumonia: trends and algorithms. *Eur Respir J.* 2001;18(1):196-208.

50. Vilar J, Domingo ML, Soto C, Cogollos J. Radiology of bacterial pneumonia. *Eur J Radiol.* 2004;51:102-113.

51. Maughan BC, Asselin N, Carey JL, Sucov A, Valente JH. False-negative chest radiographs in emergency department diagnosis of pneumonia. *R I Med J.* 2014;97(8):20-23.

52. Washington L, Palacio D. Imaging of bacterial pulmonary infection in the immunocompetent patient. *Semin Roentgenol.* 2007;42(2):122-145.

53. Light RB. Pulmonary pathophysiology of pneumococcal pneumonia. *Semin Respir Infect.* 1999;14(3):218-226.

54. Gea J, Roca J, Torres A, Agustí AG, Wagner PD, Rodriguez-Roisin R. Mechanisms of abnormal gas exchange in patients with pneumonia. *Anesthesiology.* 1991;75(5):782-789.

55. Rodriguez-Roisin R, Roca J. Update '96 on pulmonary gas exchange pathophysiology in pneumonia. *Semin Respir Infect.* 1996;11(1):3-12.

56. Mitchell DM, Fleming J, Harris JR, Shaw RJ. Serial pulmonary function tests in the diagnosis of P. carinii pneumonia. *Eur Respir J Off J Eur Soc Clin Respir Physiol.* 1993;6(6):823-827. http://erj.ersjournals.com/content/6/6/823.short. Accessed October 9, 2014.

57. Gaydos CA. What is the role of newer molecular tests in the management of CAP? *Infect Dis Clin North Am.* 2013;27(1):49-69.

58. Sligl WI, Marrie TJ. Severe community-acquired pneumonia. *Crit Care Clin.* 2013;29(3):563-601.

59. Lim WS, van der Eerden MM, Laing R, et al. Defining community acquired pneumonia severity on presentation to hospital: an international derivation and validation study. *Thorax.* 2003;58:377-382.

60. Fine MJ, Auble TE, Yealy DM, et al. A prediction rule to identify low-risk patients with community-acquired pneumonia. *N Engl J Med.* 1997;336(4):243-250.

61. Rosón B, Gudiol F. Utility of Gram stain and sputum culture in the management of community-acquired pneumonia. *Clin Pulm Med.* 2003;10(1):1-5.

62. Rosón B, Carratalà J, Verdaguer R, et al. Prospective study of the usefulness of sputum Gram stain in the initial approach to community-acquired pneumonia requiring hospitalization. *Clin Infect Dis.* 2000;31(4):869-874.

63. Mayer J. Laboratory diagnosis of nosocomial pneumonia. *Semin Respir Infect.* 2000;15:119-131.

64. Anevlavis S, Petroglou N, Tzavaras A, et al. A prospective study of the diagnostic utility of sputum Gram stain in pneumonia. *J Infect.* 2009;59(2):83-89.

65. Engbaek K, Johansen K, Jensen M. A new technique for Gram staining paraffin-embedded tissue. *J Clin Pathol.* 1979;32(2):187-190.

66. Woods GLG, Walker DDH. Detection of infection or infectious agents by use of cytologic and histologic stains. *Clin Microbiol Rev.* 1996;9(3):382-404.

67. Gupta E, Bhalla P, Khurana N, Singh T. Histopathology for the diagnosis of infectious diseases. *Indian J Med Microbiol.* 2009;27(2):100-106.

68. Werno AM, Murdoch DR. Medical microbiology: laboratory diagnosis of invasive pneumococcal disease. *Clin Infect Dis.* 2008;46:926-932.

69. Guarner J, Packard MM, Nolte KB, et al. Usefulness of immunohistochemical diagnosis of Streptococcus pneumoniae in formalin-fixed, paraffin-embedded specimens compared with culture and gram stain techniques. *Am J Clin Pathol.* 2007;127:612-618.

70. Wagner AL, Szabunio M, Hazlett KS, Wagner SG. Radiologic manifestations of round pneumonia in adults. *Am J Roentgenol.* 1998;170:723-726.

71. Kim YW, Donnelly LF. Round pneumonia: imaging findings in a large series of children. *Pediatr Radiol.* 2007;37:1235-1240.

72. Tuomanen EEI, Austrian R, Masure HR, Epstein F. Pathogenesis of pneumococcal infection. *N Engl J Med.* 1995;332(19): 1280-1284.

73. Bartlett JG. The role of anaerobic bacteria in lung abscess. *Clin Infect Dis.* 2005;40(7):923-925.

74. Johanson WG Jr, Harris GD, Johanson WG. Aspiration pneumonia, anaerobic infections, and lung abscess. *Med Clin North Am.* 1980;64:385-394.

75. Puligandla PS, Laberge JM. Respiratory infections: pneumonia, lung abscess, and empyema. *Semin Pediatr Surg.* 2008;17:42-52.

76. Kirtland SSH. A clinical profile of chronic bacterial pneumonia: report of 115 cases. *Chest.* 1994;106(1):15.

77. Drakopanagiotakis F, Polychronopoulos V, Judson MA. Organizing pneumonia. *Am J Med Sci.* 2008;335:34-39.

78. Epler GR. Bronchiolitis obliterans organizing pneumonia. *Arch Intern Med.* 2001;161:158-164.

79. Cordier JF. Cryptogenic organizing pneumonia. *Clin Chest Med.* 2004;25:727-738.

80. Marik PE. Pulmonary aspiration syndromes. *Curr Opin Pulm Med.* 2011;17:148-154.

81. Kadioglu A, Weiser JN, Paton JC, Andrew PW. The role of Streptococcus pneumoniae virulence factors in host respiratory colonization and disease. *Nat Rev Microbiol.* 2008;6:288-301.

82. Weinberger DM, Harboe ZB, Sanders EAM, et al. Association of serotype with risk of death due to pneumococcal pneumonia: a meta-analysis. *Clin Infect Dis.* 2010;51:692-699.

83. Ahl J, Littorin N, Forsgren A, Odenholt I, Resman F, Riesbeck K. High incidence of septic shock caused by Streptococcus pneumoniae serotype 3 - a retrospective epidemiological study. *BMC Infect Dis.* 2013;13:492.

84. Winslow DJ. Botryomycosis. *Am J Pathol.* 1959;35(1):153-167.

85. Bersoff-Matcha SJ, Roper CC, Liapis H, Little JR. Primary pulmonary botryomycosis: case report and review. *Clin Infect Dis.* 1998;26:620-624.

86. Katapadi K, Pujol F, Vuletin JC, Katapadi M, Pachter BR. Pulmonary botryomycosis in a patient with AIDS. *Chest.* 1996;109:276-278.

87. Paz HL, Little BJ, Ball WC, Winkelstein JA. Primary pulmonary botryomycosis; A manifestation of chronic granulomatous disease. *Chest.* 1992;101(4):1160-1162.

88. Ariza-Prota MA, Pando-Sandoval A, García-Clemente M, Jiménez H, Álvarez-Álvarez C, Casan-Clara P. Primary pulmonary botryomycosis: a bacterial lung infection mimicking lung cancer. *Int J Tuberc Lung Dis.* 2013;17:992-994.

89. Muller MP, Low DE, Green KA, et al. Clinical and epidemiologic features of group a streptococcal pneumonia in Ontario, Canada. *Arch Intern Med.* 2003;163:467-472.

90. Deutscher M, Lewis M, Zell ER, Taylor TH, Van Beneden C, Schrag S. Incidence and severity of invasive streptococcus pneumoniae, group a streptococcus, and group b streptococcus infections among pregnant and postpartum women. *Clin Infect Dis.* 2011;53:114-123.

91. Pathak V, Hurtado Rendon IS, Smina M. Necrotizing pneumonia caused by Group C streptococci in a young adult. *Respir Care.* 2012;57:454-456.

92. Shinzato T, Saito A. The Streptococcus milleri group as a cause of pulmonary infections. *Clin Infect Dis.* 1995;21 (suppl 3):S238-S243.

93. Al-Kaabi N, Solh Z, Pacheco S, Murray L, Gaboury I, Le Saux N. A comparison of group A Streptococcus versus Streptococcus pneumoniae pneumonia. *Pediatr Infect Dis J.* 2006;25:1008-1012.

94. Cengiz AB, Kanra G, Caḡlar M, Kara A, Güçer Ş, Ince T. Fatal necrotizing pneumonia caused by group A streptococcus. *J Paediatr Child Health.* 2004;40:69-71.

95. Rudiger M, Some M, Jarstrand C, et al. Group B streptococcal pneumonia in the newborn. *Semin Respir Med.* 1979;1: 99-105.

96. Edwards MS, Baker CJ. Group B streptococcal infections in elderly adults. *Clin Infect Dis.* 2005;41:839-847.

97. Rose HD, Allen JR, Witte G. Streptococcus zooepidemicus (group C) pneumonia in a human. *J Clin Microbiol.* 1980;11:76-78.

98. Marrie TJ. Bacteremic community-acquired pneumonia due to viridans group streptococci. *Clin Investig Med.* 1993;16:38-44.

99. Freitas M, Castelo A, Petty G, Gomes CE, Carvalho E. Viridans streptococci causing community acquired pneumonia. *Arch Dis Child.* 2006;91:779-780.

CHAPTER 12

100. DiBardino DM, Wunderink RG. Aspiration pneumonia: a review of modern trends. *J Crit Care.* 2014.

101. Boyanova L, Djambazov V, Gergova G, et al. Anaerobic microbiology in 198 cases of pleural empyema: a Bulgarian study. *Anaerobe.* 2004;10:261-267.

102. Wang J-L, Chen K-Y, Fang C-T, Hsueh P-R, Yang P-C, Chang S-C. Changing bacteriology of adult community-acquired lung abscess in Taiwan: Klebsiella pneumoniae versus anaerobes. *Clin Infect Dis.* 2005;40:915-922.

103. Yousem SA, Faber C. Histopathology of aspiration pneumonia not associated with food or other particulate matter: a clinicopathologic study of 10 cases diagnosed on biopsy. *Am J Surg Pathol.* 2011;35:426-431.

104. Mokrousov I. Corynebacterium diphtheriae: genome diversity, population structure and genotyping perspectives. *Infect Genet Evol.* 2009;9:1-15.

105. Wagner PL, Waldor MK. Bacteriophage control of bacterial virulence. *Infect Immun.* 2002;70:3985-3993.

106. Hadfield T, McEvoy P. The pathology of diphtheria. *J Infect Dis.* 2000;20306(suppl 1):3-7. http://jid.oxfordjournals.org/content/181/Supplement_1/S116.short. Accessed October 9, 2014.

107. Díez-Aguilar M, Ruiz-Garbajosa P, Fernández-Olmos A, et al. Non-diphtheriae Corynebacterium species: an emerging respiratory pathogen. *Eur J Clin Microbiol Infect Dis.* 2013;32:769-772.

108. Chiner E, Arriero JM, Signes-Costa J, et al. Corynebacterium pseudodiphtheriticum pneumonia in an immunocompetent patient. *Monaldi Arch Chest Dis.* 1999;54:325-327.

109. Djossou F, Bézian M-C, Moynet D, Le Flèche-Matéos A, Malvy D. Corynebacterium mucifaciens in an immunocompetent patient with cavitary pneumonia. *BMC Infect Dis.* 2010;10:355.

110. McNaughton RD, Villanueva RR, Donnelly R, Freedman J, Nawrot R. Cavitating pneumonia caused by Corynebacterium group JK. *J Clin Microbiol.* 1988;26:2216-2217.

111. Marrie TJ. Pneumonia caused by Nocardia species. *Semin Respir Infect.* 1994;9:207-213.

112. Brugnano R, Cozzari M, Bruna Pasticci M, et al. Nocardia asteroides pneumonia in a renal transplant recipient: diagnostic and therapeutic considerations. *J Nephrol.* 1995;0:273-276.

113. Jonsson S, Wallace RJ, Hull SI, Musher DM. Recurrent Nocardia pneumonia in an adult with chronic granulomatous disease. *Am Rev Respir Dis.* 1986;133:932-934.

114. Yildiz O, Doganay M. Actinomycoses and Nocardia pulmonary infections. *Curr Opin Pulm Med.* 2006;12:228-234.

115. Wong VK, Turmezei TD. Actinomycosis. *BMJ.* 2011;343 (d6099):1-7.

116. Susaki K, Bandoh S, Fujita J, et al. A case of pulmonary actinomycosis, who expectorated sulfur granules, caused by Actinomyces odontolyticus and Actinomyces meyeri. *Nihon Kokyuki Gakkai Zasshi.* 2005;43:231-235.

117. Weinstock DM, Brown AE. Rhodococcus equi: an emerging pathogen. *Clin Infect Dis.* 2002;34:1379-1385.

118. Johnson DH, Cunha BA. Rhodococcus equi pneumonia. *Semin Respir Infect.* 1997;12:57-60.

119. Mosser DM, Hondalus MK. Rhodococcus equi: an emerging opportunistic pathogen. *Trends Microbiol.* 1996;4:29-33.

120. Kedlaya I, Ing MB, Wong SS. Rhodococcus equi infections in immunocompetent hosts: case report and review. *Clin Infect Dis.* 2001;32:E39-E46.

121. Yamshchikov AV, Schuetz A, Lyon GM. Rhodococcus equi infection. *Lancet Infect Dis.* 2010;10:350-359.

122. Kwon KY, Colby TV. Rhodococcus equi pneumonia and pulmonary malakoplakia in acquired immunodeficiency syndrome: pathologic features. *Arch Pathol Lab Med.* 1994;118:744-748.

123. Van Hoeven KH, Dookhan DB, Petersen RO. Cytologic features of pulmonary malakoplakia related to Rhodococcus equi in an immunocompromised host. *Diagn Cytopathol.* 1996;15:325-328.

124. Akilesh S, Cross S, Kimmelshue K, Kirmani N, Dehner LP, El-Mofty SK. Pseudotumor of the Tracheal-Laryngeal Junction with Unusual Morphologic Features Caused by Rhodococcus equi Infection. *Head Neck Pathol.* 2011;5:395-400.

125. Penn CC, Klotz SA. Anthrax pneumonia. *Semin Respir Infect.* 1997;12:28-30.

126. Hoffmaster AR, Hill KK, Gee JE, et al. Characterization of Bacillus cereus isolates associated with fatal pneumonias: strains are closely related to Bacillus anthracis and Harbor B. anthracis virulence genes. *J Clin Microbiol.* 2006;44:3352-3360.

127. Meric M, Willke A, Muezzinoglu B, Karadenizli A, Hosten T. A case of pneumonia caused by Bacillus anthracis secondary to gastrointestinal anthrax. *Int J Infect Dis.* 2009;13.

128. Abramova FA, Grinberg LM, Yampolskaya OV, Walker DH. Pathology of inhalational anthrax in 42 cases from the Sverdlovsk outbreak of 1979. *Proc Natl Acad Sci U. S. A.* 1993;90:2291-2294.

129. Kyriacou DN, Yarnold PR, Stein AC, et al. Discriminating inhalational anthrax from community-acquired pneumonia using chest radiograph findings and a clinical algorithm. *Chest.* 2007;131:489-496.

130. Avashia SB, Riggins WS, Lindley C, et al. Fatal pneumonia among metalworkers due to inhalation exposure to Bacillus cereus Containing Bacillus anthracis toxin genes. *Clin Infect Dis.* 2007;44:414-416.

131. Palmacci C, Antocicco M, Bonomo L, Maggi F, Cocchi A, Onder G. Necrotizing pneumonia and sepsis due to Clostridium perfringens: a case report. *Cases J.* 2009;2:50.

132. Chen CH, Ho SY, Lin KH. Necrotizing pneumonia associated with septicemia caused by Clostridium perfringens: a case report. *J Intern Med Taiwan.* 2011;22:287-291.

133. Garcia-Montero M, Rodriguez-Garcia JL, Calvo P, et al. Pneumonia caused by Listeria monocytogenes. *Respiration.* 1995;62:107-109.

134. Whitelock-Jones L, Carswell J, Rasmussen KC. Listeria pneumonia. A case report. *S Afr Med J.* 1989;75:188-189.

135. De Sá FRN, Sztajnbok J, De Almeida JFL, Troster EJ, Vaz FAC. Listeria monocytogenes pneumonia in a cirrhotic child. *Int J Clin Pract.* 2004;58:536-538.

136. Stamm AM, Dismukes WE, Simmons BP, et al. Listeriosis in renal transplant recipients: report of an outbreak and review of 102 cases. *Rev Infect Dis.* 1982;4(3):665-682.

137. Jones SD, Fullerton DA, Zamora MR, Badesch DB, Campbell DN, Grover FL. Transmission of Lactobacillus pneumonia by a transplanted lung. *Ann Thorac Surg.* 1994;58:887-889.

138. Wood GC, Boucher BA, Croce MA, Fabian TC. Lactobacillus species as a cause of ventilator-associated pneumonia in a critically ill trauma patient. *Pharmacotherapy.* 2002;22:1180-1182.

139. Fruchart C, Salah A, Gray C, et al. Lactobacillus species as emerging pathogens in neutropenic patients. *Eur J Clin Microbiol Infect Dis.* 1997;16:681-684.

140. Morrow LE, Kollef MH, Casale TB. Probiotic prophylaxis of ventilator-associated pneumonia: a blinded, randomized, controlled trial. *Am J Respir Crit Care Med.* 2010;182:1058-1064.

141. Doern CD, Nguyen ST, Afolabi F, Burnham CAD. Probiotic-associated aspiration pneumonia due to Lactobacillus rhamnosus. *J Clin Microbiol.* 2014;52:3124-3126.

142. Messika J, Magdoud F, Clermont O, et al. Pathophysiology of Escherichia coli ventilator-associated pneumonia: implication of highly virulent extraintestinal pathogenic strains. *Intensive Care Med.* 2012;38:2007-2016.

143. Okimoto N, Hayashi T, Ishiga M, et al. Clinical features of Escherichia coli pneumonia. *J Infect Chemother.* 2010;16:216-218.

144. Tillotson J, Lerner A. Pneumonias caused by gram negative bacilli. *Medicine (Baltimore)*. 1966;45(1):65-76. http://journals.lww.com/md-journal/Abstract/1966/01000/Pneumonias_Caused_By_Gram_Negative_Bacilli.3.aspx. Accessed October 22, 2014.

145. Prince SE, Dominger KA, Cunha BA, Klein NC. Klebsiella pneumoniae pneumonia. *Hear Lung J Acute Crit Care*. 1997;26:413-417.

146. Podschun R, Ullmann U. Klebsiella spp. as nosocomial pathogens: epidemiology, taxonomy, typing methods, and pathogenicity factors. *Clin Microbiol Rev*. 1998;11:589-603.

147. Tsai Y-F, Ku Y-H. Necrotizing pneumonia: a rare complication of pneumonia requiring special consideration. *Curr Opin Pulm Med*. 2012;18:246-252.

148. Lewis JF, Arnold C, Alexander J. Meningococcal pneumonia. *Am J Clin Pathol*. 1973;59:388-390.

149. Winstead JM, McKinsey DS, Tasker S, De Groote MA, Baddour LM. Meningococcal pneumonia: characterization and review of cases seen over the past 25 years. *Clin Infect Dis*. 2000;30:87-94.

150. Romero-Gomez MP, Rentero Z, Paño JR, Mingorance J. Bacteraemic pneumonia caused by Neisseria meningitidis serogroup Y. *Respir Med Case Reports*. 2012;5:23-24.

151. Jabeen Z, Asif R, Kadri SM, Alam Shah B, Tabasum S. Serratia marcescens pneumonia. *JK Pract*. 2004;11:200.

152. Goldstein JD, Godleski JJ, Balikian JP, Herman PG. Pathologic patterns of Serratia marcescens pneumonia. *Hum Pathol*. 1982;13:479-484.

153. Balikian JP, Herman PG, Godleski JJ. Serratia pneumonia. *Radiology*. 1980;137:309-311.

154. Karnad A, Alvarez S, Berk SL. Enterobacter pneumonia. *South Med J*. 1987;80:601-604.

155. Hennigs JK, Baumann HJ, Schmiedel S, et al. Characterization of enterobacter cloacae pneumonia: a single-center retrospective analysis. *Lung*. 2011;189:475-483.

156. Boyer A, Amadeo B, Vargas F, et al. Severe community-acquired Enterobacter pneumonia: a plea for greater awareness of the concept of health-care-associated pneumonia. *BMC Infect Dis*. 2011;11:120.

157. Okimoto N, Hayashi T, Ishiga M, et al. Clinical features of Proteus mirabilis pneumonia. *J Infect Chemother*. 2010;16:364-366.

158. Tillotson JR, Lerner AM. Characteristics of pneumonias caused by Bacillus proteus. *Ann Intern Med*. 1968;68(2):287-294. http://annals.org/article.aspx?articleid=682037. Accessed October 23, 2014.

159. Rollins SE, Rollins SM, Ryan ET. Yersinia pestis and the plague. *Am J Clin Pathol*. 2003;119(suppl 1):S78-S85.

160. Krishna G, Chitkara RK. Pneumonic plague. *Semin Respir Infect*. 2003;18:159-167.

161. Cordero E, Pachón J, Rivero A, et al. Haemophilus influenzae pneumonia in human immunodeficiency virus-infected patients. The Grupo Andaluz para el Estudio de las Enfermedades Infecciosas. *Clin Infect Dis*. 2000;30:461-465.

162. Hershckowitz S, Elisha MB, Fleisher-Sheffer V, Barak M, Kudinsky R, Weintraub Z. A cluster of early neonatal sepsis and pneumonia caused by nontypable Haemophilus influenzae. *Pediatr Infect Dis J*. 2004;23:1061-1062.

163. Murphy TF, Faden H, Bakaletz LO, et al. Nontypeable Haemophilus influenzae as a pathogen in children. *Pediatr Infect Dis J*. 2009;28:43-48.

164. Carratalà J, Garcia-Vidal C. An update on Legionella. *Curr Opin Infect Dis*. 2010;23:152-157.

165. Pancer K, Stypułkowska-Misiurewicz H. Pontiac fever—nonpneumonic legionellosis. *Przegl Epidemiol*. 2003;57:607-612.

166. Diederen BMW. Legionella spp. and Legionnaires' disease. *J Infect*. 2008;56:1-12.

167. Vergis EN, Akbas E, Yu VL. Legionella as a cause of severe pneumonia. *Semin Respir Crit Care Med*. 2000;21:295-304.

168. Fang GD, Yu VL, Vickers RM. Infections caused by the Pittsburgh pneumonia agent. *Semin Respir Infect*. 1987;2:262-266.

169. Hilton E, Freedman RA, Cintron F, Isenberg HD, Singer C. Acid-fast bacilli in sputum: a case of Legionella micdadei pneumonia. *J Clin Microbiol*. 1986;24:1102-1103.

170. Winn WC, Myerowitz RL. The pathology of the Legionella pneumonias. A review of 74 cases and the literature. *Hum Pathol*. 1981;12:401-422.

171. Johnson KM, Huseby JS. Lung abscess caused by Legionella micdadei. *Chest*. 1997;111:252-253.

172. Fujitani S, Sun HY, Yu VL, Weingarten JA. Pneumonia due to pseudomonas aeruginosa: Part I: epidemiology, clinical diagnosis, and source. *Chest*. 2011;139:909-919.

173. Pritt B, O'Brien L, Winn W. Mucoid Pseudomonas in cystic fibrosis. *Am J Clin Pathol*. 2007;128:32-34.

174. Shah RM, Wechsler R, Salazar AM, Spirn PW. Spectrum of CT findings in nosocomial Pseudomonas aeruginosa pneumonia. *J Thorac Imaging*. 2002;17:53-57.

175. Takajo D, Iwaya K, Katsurada Y, et al. Community-acquired lobar pneumonia caused by Pseudomonas aeruginosa infection in Japan: a case report with histological and immunohistochemical examination. *Pathol Int*. 2014;64(5):224-230.

176. Lipuma JJ. Update on the Burkholderia cepacia complex. *Curr Opin Pulm Med*. 2005;11:528-533.

177. Belchis DA, Simpson E, Colby T. Histopathologic features of Burkholderia cepacia pneumonia in patients without cystic fibrosis. *Mod Pathol*. 2000;13:369-372.

178. Wiersinga WJ, Currie BJ, Peacock SJ. Melioidosis. *N Engl J Med*. 2012;367:1035-1044.

179. Currie BJ. Melioidosis: an important cause of pneumonia in residents of and travellers returned from endemic regions. *Eur Respir J*. 2003;22:542-550.

180. Inglis TJJ, Rolim DB, Sousa ADQ. Melioidosis in the Americas. *Am J Trop Med Hyg*. 2006;75:947-954.

181. Lim KS, Chong VH. Radiological manifestations of melioidosis. *Clin Radiol*. 2010;65:66-72.

182. Wong KT, Puthucheary SD, Vadivelu J. The histopathology of human melioidosis. *Histopathology*. 1995;26:51-55.

183. Paddock CD, Sanden GN, Cherry JD, et al. Pathology and pathogenesis of fatal Bordetella pertussis infection in infants. *Clin Infect Dis*. 2008;47(3):328-338.

184. Franco MP, Mulder M, Gilman RH, Smits HL. Human brucellosis. *Lancet Infect Dis*. 2007;7:775-786.

185. Pappas G, Bosilkovski M. Brucellosis and the respiratory system. *Clin Infect Dis*. 2003;37(7):e95-e99. http://cid.oxfordjournals.org/content/37/7/e95.short. Accessed October 9, 2014.

186. Sanford JP. Brucella pneumonia. *Semin Respir Infect*. 1997;12:24-27.

187. Hatipoglu CA, Bilgin G, Tulek N, Kosar U. Pulmonary involvement in brucellosis. *J Infect*. 2005;51:116-119.

188. Burillo A, Bouza E. Chlamydophila pneumoniae. *Infect Dis Clin North Am*. 2010;24:61-71.

189. Stewardson AJ, Grayson ML. Psittacosis. *Infect Dis Clin North Am*. 2010;24:7-25.

190. Hammerschlag MR. The intracellular life of chlamydiae. *Semin Pediatr Infect Dis*. 2002;13:239-248.

191. Blasi F, Aliberti S, Allegra L, et al. Chlamydophila pneumoniae induces a sustained airway hyperresponsiveness and inflammation in mice. *Respir Res*. 2007;8:83.

192. McGavran MH, Beard CW, Berendt RF, Nakamura RM. The pathogenesis of psittacosis. *Am J Pathol*. 1962;40(6):653-670.

193. Hess DL. Chlamydia in the neonate. *Neonatal Netw*. 1993;12:9-12.

194. Takase Y, Khono T, Kinoshita T, Niki T. Investigation of Chlamydia trachomatis pneumonia in children. *Kansenshogaku Zasshi.* 1990;64:1177-1183.

195. Chomel BB, Boulouis HJ, Breitschwerdt EB. Cat scratch disease and other zoonotic Bartonella infections. *J Am Vet Med Assoc.* 2004;224:1270-1279.

196. Caniza MA, Granger DL, Wilson KH, et al. Bartonella henselae: etiology of pulmonary nodules in a patient with depressed cell-mediated immunity. *Clin Infect Dis.* 1995;20:1505-1511.

197. Caponetti GC, Pantanowitz L, Marconi S, Havens JM, Lamps LW, Otis CN. Evaluation of immunohistochemistry in identifying bartonella henselae in cat-scratch disease. *Am J Clin Pathol.* 2009;131:250-256.

198. Fenollar F, Lagier JC, Raoult D. Tropheryma whipplei and Whipple's disease. *J Infect.* 2014;69:103-112.

199. Geißdörfer W, Moos V, Moter A, et al. High frequency of Tropheryma whipplei in culture-negative endocarditis. *J Clin Microbiol.* 2012;50:216-222.

200. Bousbia S, Papazian L, Auffray JP, et al. Tropheryma whipplei in patients with pneumonia. *Emerg Infect Dis.* 2010;16:258-263.

201. Kelly CA, Egan M, Rawlinson J. Whipple's disease presenting with lung involvement. *Thorax.* 1996;51:343-344.

202. Dutly F, Altwegg M. Whipple's disease and "Tropheryma whippelii." *Clin Microbiol Rev.* 2001;14:561-583.

203. Fenollar F, Ponge T, La Scola B, Lagier JC, Lefebvre M, Raoult D. First isolation of Tropheryma whipplei from bronchoalveolar fluid and clinical implications. *J Infect.* 2012;65:275-278.

204. Brosch R, Gordon S V, Marmiesse M, et al. A new evolutionary scenario for the Mycobacterium tuberculosis complex. *Proc Natl Acad Sci U. S. A.* 2002;99:3684-3689.

205. Donoghue HD. Human tuberculosis—an ancient disease, as elucidated by ancient microbial biomolecules. *Microbes Infect.* 2009;11:1156-1162.

206. Zumla A, Raviglione M, Hafner R, von Reyn CF. Tuberculosis. *N Engl J Med.* 2013;368:745-755.

207. Lawn SD, Zumla AI. Tuberculosis. *Lancet.* 2011;378:57-72.

208. Horsburgh CR. Priorities for the treatment of latent tuberculosis infection in the United States. *N Engl J Med.* 2004;350:2060-2067.

209. Narasimhan P, Wood J, Macintyre CR, Mathai D. Risk factors for tuberculosis. *Pulm Med.* 2013;2013:1-11.

210. Streptomycin in Tuberculosis Trials Committee, Committee S in TT. Streptomycin treatment of pulmonary tuberculosis: a Medical Research Council Investigation. *BMJ.* 1948;2:769-782.

211. Johnson R, Streicher EM, Louw GE, Warren RM, van Helden PD, Victor TC. Drug resistance in Mycobacterium tuberculosis. *Curr Issues Mol Biol.* 2006;8:97-112.

212. Gandhi NR, Nunn P, Dheda K, et al. Multidrug-resistant and extensively drug-resistant tuberculosis: a threat to global control of tuberculosis. *Lancet.* 2010;375:1830-1843.

213. Bermudez LE, Goodman J. Mycobacterium tuberculosis invades and replicates within type II alveolar cells. *Infect Immun.* 1996;64:1400-1406.

214. Bhatt K, Salgame P. Host innate immune response to Mycobacterium tuberculosis. *J Clin Immunol.* 2007;27:347-362.

215. Rohde K, Yates RM, Purdy GE, Russell DG. Mycobacterium tuberculosis and the environment within the phagosome. *Immunol Rev.* 2007;219:37-54.

216. Allie N, Grivennikov SI, Keeton R, et al. Prominent role for T cell-derived tumour necrosis factor for sustained control of Mycobacterium tuberculosis infection. *Sci Rep.* 2013;3:1809.

217. Flynn JL, Chan J, Triebold KJ, Dalton DK, Stewart TA, Bloom BR. An essential role for interferon gamma in resistance to Mycobacterium tuberculosis infection. *J Exp Med.* 1993;178:2249-2254.

218. Ulrichs T, Kaufmann SHE. New insights into the function of granulomas in human tuberculosis. *J Pathol.* 2006;208:261-269.

219. Russell DG, Cardona P-J, Kim M-J, Allain S, Altare F. Foamy macrophages and the progression of the human tuberculosis granuloma. *Nat Immunol.* 2009;10:943-948.

220. Davies PDO. Risk factors for tuberculosis. *Monaldi Arch Chest Dis.* 2005;63:37-46.

221. Gessner BD, Weiss NS, Nolan CM. Risk factors for pediatric tuberculosis infection and disease after household exposure to adult index cases in Alaska. *J Pediatr.* 1998;132:509-513.

222. Tekkel M, Rahu M, Loit HM, Baburin A. Risk factors for pulmonary tuberculosis in Estonia. *Int J Tuberc Lung Dis.* 2002;6:887-894.

223. Coker R, McKee M, Atun R, et al. Risk factors for pulmonary tuberculosis in Russia: case-control study. *BMJ.* 2006;332:85-87.

224. Cosivi O, Grange JM, Daborn CJ, et al. Zoonotic tuberculosis due to Mycobacterium bovis in developing countries. *Emerg Infect Dis.* 1999;4:59-70.

225. Müller B, Dürr S, Alonso S, et al. Zoonotic Mycobacterium bovis—induced tuberculosis in humans. *Emerg Infect Dis.* 2013;19:899-908.

226. De Jong BC, Antonio M, Gagneux S. Mycobacterium africanum—review of an important cause of human tuberculosis in West Africa. *PLoS Negl Trop Dis.* 2010;4(9):e744.

227. Panteix G, Gutierrez MC, Boschiroli ML, et al. Pulmonary tuberculosis due to Mycobacterium microti: a study of six recent cases in France. *J Med Microbiol.* 2010;59(pt 8):984-989.

228. WHO. Global Tuberculosis Report. 2014. 2014:1-171. http://www.who.int/tb/publications/global_report/en/. Accessed October 27, 2014.

229. Maher D, Uplekar M, Blanc L, Raviglione M. Treatment of tuberculosis. *BMJ.* 2003; Oct 11;327(7419):822-823. http://www.bmj.com/content/327/7419/822.short. Accessed October 9, 2014.

230. Schlossberg D. Acute tuberculosis. *Infect Dis Clin North Am.* 2010;24:139-146.

231. Barker RD. Clinical tuberculosis. *Medicine.* 2012;40:340-345.

232. Middleton JR, Sen P, Lange M, Salaki J, Kapila R, Louria DB. Death-producing hemoptysis in tuberculosis. *Chest.* 1977;72:601-604.

233. Nayak S, Acharjya B. Mantoux test and its interpretation. *Indian Dermatol. Online J.* 2012;3:2.

234. Madariaga MG, Jalali Z, Swindells S. Clinical utility of interferon gamma assay in the diagnosis of tuberculosis. *J Am Board Fam Med.* 2007;20:540-547.

235. Pottumarthy S, Morris AJ, Harrison AC, Wells VC. Evaluation of the tuberculin gamma interferon assay: potential to replace the mantoux skin test. *J Clin Microbiol.* 1999;37:3229-3232.

236. Lange C, Mori T. Advances in the diagnosis of tuberculosis. *Respirology.* 2010;15:220-240.

237. Rodrigues C, Vadwai V. Tuberculosis: laboratory diagnosis. *Clin Lab Med.* 2012;32:111-127.

238. Steingart KR, Henry M, Ng V, et al. Fluorescence versus conventional sputum smear microscopy for tuberculosis: a systematic review. *Lancet Infect Dis.* 2006;6:570-581.

239. Shingadia D. The diagnosis of tuberculosis. *Pediatr Infect Dis J.* 2012;31:302-305.

240. Niemz A, Boyle DS. Nucleic acid testing for tuberculosis at the point-of-care in high-burden countries. *Expert Rev Mol Diagn.* 2012;12(7):687-701.

241. Steingart KR, Schiller I, Horne DJ, Pai M, Boehme CC, Dendukuri N. Xpert® MTB/RIF assay for pulmonary tuberculosis and rifampicin resistance in adults. *Cochrane Database Syst Rev.* 2014;1:CD009593.

242. Şkenders GK, Holtz TH, Riekstina V, Leimane V. Implementation of the INNO-LiPA Rif. TB® line-probe assay in rapid detection of multidrug-resistant tuberculosis in Latvia. *Int J Tuberc Lung Dis.* 2011;15:1546-1553.

CHAPTER 12

243. Chihota VN, Grant AD, Fielding K, et al. Liquid vs. solid culture for tuberculosis: performance and cost in a resource-constrained setting. *Int J Tuberc Lung Dis*. 2010;14:1024-1031.

244. Pfyffer GE, Welscher HM, Kissling P, et al. Comparison of the mycobacteria growth indicator tube (MGIT) with radiometric and solid culture for recovery of acid-fast bacilli. *J Clin Microbiol*. 1997;35:364-368.

245. Balada-Llasat JM, Kamboj K, Pancholi P. Identification of mycobacteria from solid and liquid media by matrix-assisted laser desorption ionization-time of flight mass spectrometry in the clinical laboratory. *J Clin Microbiol*. 2013;51:2875-2879.

246. World Health Organization. *Laboratory-Based Evaluation of 19 Commercially Available Rapid Diagnostic Tests for Tuberculosis*. Geneva : World Health Organization. 2008;1-80. http://apps.who.int/iris/handle/10665/43967. Accessed October 28, 2014.

247. Hoa NB, Cobelens FG, Sy DN, Nhung NV., Borgdorff MW, Tiemersma EW. Yield of interview screening and chest X-ray abnormalities in a tuberculosis prevalence survey. *Int J Tuberc Lung Dis*. 2012;16:762-767.

248. Van Cleeff MRA, Kivihya-Ndugga LE, Meme H, Odhiambo JA, Klatser PR. The role and performance of chest X-ray for the diagnosis of tuberculosis: a cost-effectiveness analysis in Nairobi, Kenya. *BMC Infect Dis*. 2005;5:111.

249. Lee KS, Song KS, Lim TH, Kim PN, Kim IY, Lee BH. Adult-onset pulmonary tuberculosis: findings on chest radiographs and CT scans. *Am J Roentgenol*. 1993;160:753-758.

250. Jones BE, Ryu R, Yang Z, et al. Chest radiographic findings in patients with tuberculosis with recent or remote infection. *Am J Respir Crit Care Med*. 1997;156:1270-1273.

251. Leung A. Pulmonary tuberculosis: the essentials. *Radiology*. 1999;210(2):307-322. http://pubs.rsna.org/doi/full/10.1148/radiology.210.2.r99ja34307. Accessed October 29, 2014.

252. Yeon JJ, Lee KS. Pulmonary tuberculosis: up-to-date imaging and management. *Am J Roentgenol*. 2008;191:834-844.

253. Sharma SK, Mohan A, Sharma A, Mitra DK. Miliary tuberculosis: new insights into an old disease. *Lancet Infect Dis*. 2005;5:415-430.

254. Pasipanodya JG, Miller TL, Vecino M, et al. Pulmonary impairment after tuberculosis. *Chest*. 2007;131(6):1817-1824.

255. Hnizdo E, Singh T, Churchyard G. Chronic pulmonary function impairment caused by initial and recurrent pulmonary tuberculosis following treatment. *Thorax*. 2000;55:32-38.

256. De Rosa M, Ciappi G. Respiratory function impairment in pulmonary tuberculosis. *Rays*. 1998;23:87-92. http://www.ncbi.nlm.nih.gov/pubmed/9673138.

257. Lee EJ, Lee SY, In KH, et al. Routine pulmonary function test can estimate the extent of tuberculous destroyed lung. *Sci World J*. 2012;2012:1-5.

258. Horne DJ, Hubbard R, Narita M, Exarchos A, Park DR, Goss CH. Factors associated with mortality in patients with tuberculosis. *BMC Infect Dis*. 2010;10:258.

259. Burton NT, Forson A, Lurie MN, Kudzawu S, Kwarteng E, Kwara A. Factors associated with mortality and default among patients with tuberculosis attending a teaching hospital clinic in Accra, Ghana. *Trans R Soc Trop Med Hyg*. 2011;105:675-682.

260. Nahid P, Jarlsberg LG, Rudoy I, et al. Factors associated with mortality in patients with drug-susceptible pulmonary tuberculosis. *BMC Infect Dis*. 2011;11:1.

261. Yen Y-F, Yen M-Y, Shih H-C, et al. Prognostic factors associated with mortality before and during anti-tuberculosis treatment. *Int J Tuberc Lung Dis*. 2013;17:1310-1316.

262. Russell DG. Who puts the tubercle in tuberculosis? *Nat Rev Microbiol*. 2007;5:39-47.

263. Lambert ML, Hasker E, Van Deun A, Roberfroid D, Boelaert M, Van der Stuyft P. Recurrence in tuberculosis: relapse or reinfection? *Lancet Infect Dis*. 2003;3:282-287.

264. Jasmer RM, Bozeman L, Schwartzman K, et al. Recurrent tuberculosis in the United States and Canada: relapse or reinfection? *Am J Respir Crit Care Med*. 2004;170:1360-1366.

265. Andrews JR, Noubary F, Walensky RP, Cerda R, Losina E, Horsburgh CR. Risk of progression to active tuberculosis following reinfection with Mycobacterium tuberculosis. *Clin Infect Dis*. 2012;54:784-791.

266. Scanga CA, Mohan VP, Joseph H, Yu K, Chan J, Flynn JL. Reactivation of latent tuberculosis: variations on the cornell murine model. *Infect Immun*. 1999;67:4531-4538.

267. Walter ND, Painter J, Parker M, et al. Persistent latent tuberculosis reactivation risk in united states immigrants. *Am J Respir Crit Care Med*. 2014;189:88-95.

268. Gengenbacher M, Kaufmann SHE. Mycobacterium tuberculosis: success through dormancy. *FEMS Microbiol Rev*. 2012;36:514-532.

269. Hunter RL. Pathology of post primary tuberculosis of the lung: an illustrated critical review. *Tuberculosis*. 2011;91:497-509.

270. Jordan TS, Spencer EM, Davies P. Tuberculosis, bronchiectasis and chronic airflow obstruction. *Respirology*. 2010;15:623-628.

271. Hunter RL. On the pathogenesis of post primary tuberculosis: the role of bronchial obstruction in the pathogenesis of cavities. *Tuberculosis*. 2011;91(suppl 1):S6-S10.

272. Palaci M, Dietze R, Hadad DJ, et al. Cavitary disease and quantitative sputum bacillary load in cases of pulmonary tuberculosis. *J Clin Microbiol*. 2007;45:4064-4066.

273. Picard C, Parrot A, Boussaud V, et al. Massive hemoptysis due to Rasmussen aneurysm: detection with helicoidal CT angiography and successful steel coil embolization. *Intensive Care Med*. 2003;29:1837-1839.

274. Light RW. Update on tuberculous pleural effusion. *Respirology*. 2010;15:451-458.

275. Ferrer J. Pleural tuberculosis. *Eur Respir J*. 1997;10:942-947.

276. Seiscento M, Vargas FS, Bombarda S, et al. Pulmonary involvement in pleural tuberculosis: how often does it mean disease activity? *Respir Med*. 2011;105(7):1079-1083.

277. Moon JW, Chang YS, Kim SK, et al. The clinical utility of polymerase chain reaction for the diagnosis of pleural tuberculosis. *Clin Infect Dis*. 2005;41:660-666.

278. Porcel JM, Palma R, Valdés L, Bielsa S, San-José E, Esquerda A. Xpert° MTB/RIF in pleural fluid for the diagnosis of tuberculosis. *Int J Tuberc Lung Dis*. 2013;17:1217-1219.

279. Conde MB, Loivos AC, Rezende VM, et al. Yield of sputum induction in the diagnosis of pleural tuberculosis. *Am J Respir Crit Care Med*. 2003;167:723-725.

280. Krenke R, Korczyński P. Use of pleural fluid levels of adenosine deaminase and interferon gamma in the diagnosis of tuberculous pleuritis. *Curr Opin Pulm Med*. 2010;16:367-375.

281. Hasaneen NA, Zaki ME, Shalaby HM, El-Morsi AS. Polymerase chain reaction of pleural biopsy is a rapid and sensitive method for the diagnosis of tuberculous pleural effusion. *Chest*. 2003;124:2105-2111.

282. Harikrishna J, Sukaveni V, Kumar DP, Mohan A. Cancer and tuberculosis. *JIACM*. 2012;13(2):142-144.

283. Cicenas S, Vencevicius V. Lung cancer in patients with tuberculosis. *World J Surg Oncol*. 2007;5:22.

284. Zheng W, Blot WJ, Liao ML, et al. Lung cancer and prior tuberculosis infection in Shanghai. *Br J Cancer*. 1987;56:501-504.

285. Emgels EA, Min S, Chapman RS, et al. Tuberculosis and subsequent risk of lung cancer in Xuanwei, China. *Int J Cancer*. 2009;124:1183-1187.

286. Liang H-Y, Li X-L, Yu X-S, et al. Facts and fiction of the relationship between preexisting tuberculosis and lung cancer risk: a systematic review. *Int J Cancer*. 2009;125(12):2936-2944.

287. Wu CY, Hu HY, Pu CY, et al. Aerodigestive tract, lung and haematological cancers are risk factors for tuberculosis: an 8-year population-based study. *Int J Tuberc Lung Dis*. 2011;15:125-130.

288. Kamboj M, Sepkowitz KA. The risk of tuberculosis in patients with cancer. *Clin Infect Dis.* 2006;42(11):1592-1595.

289. Kuo SC, Hu YW, Liu CJ, et al. Association between tuberculosis infections and non-pulmonary malignancies: a nationwide population-based study. *Br J Cancer.* 2013;109(1):229-234.

290. Getahun H, Gunneberg C, Granich R, Nunn P. HIV infection-associated tuberculosis: the epidemiology and the response. *Clin Infect Dis.* 2010;50(suppl 3):S201-S207.

291. Pawlowski A, Jansson M, Sköld M, Rottenberg ME, Källenius G. Tuberculosis and HIV Co-Infection. *PLoS Pathog.* 2012;8:e1002464.

292. Cobelens FG, Egwaga SM, van Ginkel T, Muwinge H, Matee MI, Borgdorff MW. Tuberculin skin testing in patients with HIV infection: limited benefit of reduced cutoff values. *Clin Infect Dis.* 2006;43:634-639.

293. Jones S, De Gijsel D, Wallach FR, Gurtman AC, Shi Q, Sacks H. Utility of QuantiFERON-TB Gold in-tube testing for latent TB infection in HIV-infected individuals. *Int J Tuberc Lung Dis.* 2007;11:1190-1195.

294. Kwan C, Ernst JD. HIV and tuberculosis: a deadly human syndemic. *Clin Microbiol Rev.* 2011;24:351-376.

295. Cohn D, O'Brien R, Geiter L. Targeted tuberculin testing and treatment of latent tuberculosis infection. *MMWR Morb Mortal.* 2000;49:1-51.

296. Report MW. Recommendations for use of an isoniazid-rifapentine regimen with direct observation to treat latent Mycobacterium tuberculosis infection. *MMWR Morb Mortal Wkly.* Rep. 2011;60:1650-1653. http://www.ncbi.nlm.nih.gov/pubmed/22157884.

297. The World Health Organization. *Treatment of Tuberculosis: Guidelines.* Geneva; 2010:1-160.

298. Zignol M, van Gemert W, Falzon D, et al. Surveillance of anti-tuberculosis drug resistance in the world: an updated analysis, 2007-2010. *Bull World Health Organ.* 2012;90:111-119.

299. World Health Organization. *Multidrug and Extensively Drug-Resistant TB (M/XDR-TB): 2010 Global Report on Surveillance and Response.* 2010:57. http://whqlibdoc.who.int/publications/2010/9789241599191_eng.pdf.

300. Brennan PJ, Nikaido H. The envelope of mycobacteria. *Annu Rev Biochem.* 1995;64:29-63.

301. Reynolds J, Moyes RB, Breakwell DP. Differential staining of bacteria: acid fast stain. *Curr Protoc Microbiol.* 2009;Appendix 3:Appendix 3H.

302. Anthony RM, Kolk AHJ, Kuijper S, Klatser PR. Light emitting diodes for auramine O fluorescence microscopic screening of Mycobacterium tuberculosis. *Int J Tuberc Lung Dis.* 2006;10:1060-1062.

303. McCarter YS, Robinson A. Detection of acid-fast bacilli in concentrated primary specimen smears stained with rhodamine-auramine at room temperature and at 37 degrees C. *J Clin Microbiol.* 1994;32:2487-2489.

304. Patnaik M, Liegmann K, Peter JB. Rapid detection of smear-negative Mycobacterium tuberculosis by PCR and sequencing for rifampin resistance with DNA extracted directly from slides. *J Clin Microbiol.* 2001;39:51-52.

305. Köser CU, Bryant JM, Becq J, et al. Whole-genome sequencing for rapid susceptibility testing of M. tuberculosis. *N Engl J Med.* 2013;369:290-292.

306. Van Rie A, Page-Shipp L, Scott L, Sanne I, Stevens W. Xpert(®) MTB/RIF for point-of-care diagnosis of TB in high-HIV burden, resource-limited countries: hype or hope? *Expert Rev Mol Diagn.* 2010;10:937-946.

307. Huang WL, Chen HY, Kuo YM, Jou R. Performance assessment of the GenoType MTBDRplus test and DNA sequencing in detection of multidrug-resistant Mycobacterium tuberculosis. *J Clin Microbiol.* 2009;47:2520-2524.

308. Brossier F, Veziris N, Aubry A, Jarlier V, Sougakoff W. Detection by GenoType MTBDRsl test of complex mechanisms of resistance to second-line drugs and ethambutol in multidrug-resistant Mycobacterium tuberculosis complex isolates. *J Clin Microbiol.* 2010;48:1683-1689.

309. Lee HN, Embi CS, Vigeland KM, White CR. Concomitant pulmonary tuberculosis and leprosy. *J Am Acad Dermatol.* 2003;49:755-757.

310. Bhatia VN, Rao S, Saraswathi G. Auramine staining in histopathology sections. *Indian J Lepr.* 1987;59:386-389.

311. Hunter RL, Jagannath C, Actor JK. Pathology of postprimary tuberculosis in humans and mice: contradiction of long-held beliefs. *Tuberculosis.* 2007;87:267-278.

312. Androulaki A, Papathomas TG, Liapis G, et al. Inflammatory pseudotumor associated with Mycobacterium tuberculosis infection. *Int J Infect Dis.* 2008;12(6):607-610.

313. Agarwal R, Srinivas R, Aggarwal AN. Parenchymal pseudotumoral tuberculosis: case series and systematic review of literature. *Respir Med.* 2008;102(3):382-389.

314. Logani S, Lucas DR, Cheng JD, Ioachim HL, Adsay NV. Spindle cell tumors associated with mycobacteria in lymph nodes of HIV-positive patients: "Kaposi sarcoma with mycobacteria" and "mycobacterial pseudotumor." *Am J Surg Pathol.* 1999;23:656-661.

315. Basilio-de-Oliveira C, Eyer-Silva WA, Valle HA, Rodrigues AL, Pinheiro Pimentel AL, Morais-De-Sá CA. Mycobacterial spindle cell pseudotumor of the appendix vermiformis in a patient with aids. *Braz J Infect Dis.* 2001;5:98-100.

316. Philip J, Beasley MB, Dua S. Mycobacterial spindle cell pseudotumor of the lung. *Chest.* 2012;142:783-784.

317. Patel S, Pfeffer M. A small bowel obstruction caused by mycobacterial spindle cell pseudotumor. *J Hosp Med.* 2012;7:S291-S292. http://ovidsp.ovid.com/ovidweb.cgi?T=JS&PAGE=reference&D=emed10&NEWS=N&AN=70698462.

318. Suchitha S, Sheeladevi CS, Manjunath GV, Sunila R. BCG induced Mycobacterial Spindle cell Pseudotumor in an infant. *Indian J Tuberc.* 2009;56:104-107.

319. Youssef D, Ilyas S, Chaudhary H, Al-Abbadi MA. Myocbacterium-avium intracellulare associated inflammatory pseudotumor of the anterior nasal cavity. *Head Neck Pathol.* 2011;5:296-301.

320. Wood C, Nickoloff BJ, Todes-Taylor NR. Pseudotumor resulting from atypical mycobacterial infection: a "histoid" variety of Mycobacterium avium-intracellulare complex infection. *Am J Clin Pathol.* 1985;83:524-527.

321. Phowthongkum P, Puengchitprapai A, Udomsantisook N, Tumwasorn S, Suankratay C. Spindle cell pseudotumor of the brain associated with Mycobacterium haemophilum and Mycobacterium simiae mixed infection in a patient with AIDS: the first case report. *Int J Infect Dis.* 2008;12:421-424.

322. Holmes BJ, Subhawong AP, Maleki Z. Mycobacterial spindle cell pseudotumor: atypical mycobacterial infection mimicking malignancy on fine needle aspiration. *Diagn Cytopathol.* 2013;42(9):772-774.

323. Patnana M, Sevrukov AB, Elsayes KM, Viswanathan C, Lubner M, Menias CO. Inflammatory pseudotumor: the great mimicker. *Am J Roentgenol.* 2012;198.

324. Rahmani M, Alroy J, Zoukhri D, Wein RO, Tischler AS. Mycobacterial pseudotumor of the skin. *Virchows Arch.* 2013;463:843-846.

325. Suster S, Moran CA, Blanco M. Mycobacterial spindle-cell pseudotumor of the spleen. *Am J Clin Pathol.* 1994;101:539-542.

326. Morrison A, Gyure KA, Stone J, et al. Mycobacterial spindle cell pseudotumor of the brain: a case report and review of the literature. *Am J Surg Pathol.* 1999;23:1294-1299.

327. Corkill M, Stephens J, Bitter M. Fine needle aspiration cytology of mycobacterial spindle cell pseudotumor. A case report. *Acta Cytol.* 1995;39:125-128. http://www.ncbi.nlm.nih.gov/entrez/query.fcgi?cmd=Retrieve&db=PubMed&dopt=Citation&list_uids=7847000.

CHAPTER 12

328. Kovach SJ, Fischer AC, Katzman PJ, et al. Inflammatory myofi-broblastic tumors. *J Surg Oncol.* 2006;94:385-391.

329. Chen KTK. Mycobacterial spindle cell pseudotumor of lymph nodes. *Am J Surg Pathol.* 1992;16(3):276-281.

330. Ohara K, Kimura T, Sakamoto K, Okada Y. Nontuberculous mycobacteria-associated spindle cell pseudotumor of the nasal cavity: a case report. *Pathol Int.* 2013;63:266-271.

331. Cassidy PM, Hedberg K, Saulson A, McNelly E, Winthrop KL. Nontuberculous mycobacterial disease prevalence and risk factors: a changing epidemiology. *Clin Infect Dis.* 2009;49: e124-e129.

332. Kendall BA, Winthrop KL. Update on the epidemiology of pulmonary nontuberculous mycobacterial infections. *Semin Respir Crit Care Med.* 2013;34:87-94.

333. Hoefsloot W, Van Ingen J, Andrejak C, et al. The geographic diversity of nontuberculous mycobacteria isolated from pulmonary samples: an NTM-NET collaborative study. *Eur Respir J.* 2013;42:1604-1613.

334. Rocco JM, Irani VR. Mycobacterium avium and modulation of the host macrophage immune mechanisms. *Int J Tuberc Lung Dis.* 2011;15:447-452.

335. Glassroth J. Pulmonary disease due to nontuberculous mycobacteria. *Chest.* 2008;133:243-251.

336. Inderlied CB, Kemper CA, Bermudez LE. The Mycobacterium avium complex. *Clin Microbiol Rev.* 1993;6:266.

337. Reich JM, Johnson RE. Mycobacterium avium complex pulmonary disease presenting as an isolated lingular or middle lobe pattern; The Lady Windermere syndrome. *Chest.* 1992;101: 1605-1609.

338. Bhatt SP, Nanda S, Kintzer JS. The Lady Windermere syndrome. *Prim Care Respir J.* 2009;18:334-336.

339. Waller EA, Roy A, Brumble L, Khoor A, Johnson MM, Garland JL. The expanding spectrum of Mycobacterium avium complex-associated pulmonary disease. *Chest.* 2006;130:1234-1241.

340. Embil J, Warren P, Yakrus M, et al. Pulmonary illness associated with exposure to Mycobacterium-avium complex in hot tub water: hypersensitivity pneumonitis or infection? *Chest.* 1997;111:813-816.

341. Chan ED, Iseman MD. Underlying host risk factors for nontuberculous mycobacterial lung disease. *Semin Respir Crit Care Med.* 2013;34:110-123.

342. Adjemian J, Olivier KN, Seitz AE, Holland SM, Prevots DR. Prevalence of nontuberculous mycobacterial lung disease in U.S. Medicare beneficiaries. *Am J Respir Crit Care Med.* 2012;185(8):881-886.

343. Andréjak C, Thomsen V, Johansen IS, et al. Nontuberculous pulmonary mycobacteriosis in Denmark: incidence and prognostic factors. *Am J Respir Crit Care Med.* 2010;181:514-521.

344. Field SK, Fisher D, Cowie RL. Mycobacterium avium complex pulmonary disease in patients without HIV infection. *Chest.* 2004;126(2):566-581.

345. Prevots DR, Shaw PA, Strickland D, et al. Nontuberculous mycobacterial lung disease prevalence at four integrated health care delivery systems. *Am J Respir Crit Care Med.* 2010;182: 970-976.

346. Chitty SA, Ali J. Mycobacterium avium complex pulmonary disease in immunocompetent patients. *South Med J.* 2005;98: 646-652.

347. Weiss CH, Glassroth J. Pulmonary disease caused by nontuberculous mycobacteria. *Expert Rev Respir Med.* 2012;6:597-612; quiz 613.

348. Somoskovi A, Salfinger M. Nontuberculous mycobacteria in respiratory infections: advances in diagnosis and identification. *Clin Lab Med.* 2014;34:271-295.

349. Van Ingen J. Diagnosis of nontuberculous mycobacterial infections. *Semin Respir Crit Care Med.* 2013;34:103-109.

350. Somoskovi A, Mester J, Hale YM, Parsons LM, Salfinger M. Laboratory diagnosis of nontuberculous mycobacteria. *Clin Chest Med.* 2002;23:585-597.

351. Shitikov E, Ilina E, Chernousova L, et al. Mass spectrometry based methods for the discrimination and typing of mycobacteria. *Infect Genet Evol.* 2012;12:838-845.

352. Levin DL. Radiology of pulmonary Mycobacterium avium-intracellulare complex. *Clin Chest Med.* 2002;23:603-612.

353. Wittram C, Weisbrod GL. Mycobacterium avium complex lung disease in immunocompetent patients: radiography-CT correlation. *Br J Radiol.* 2002;75:340-344.

354. Ellis SM, Hansell DM. Imaging of non-tuberculous (atypical) mycobacterial pulmonary infection. *Clin Radiol.* 2002;57:661-669.

355. Gribetz AR, Damsker B, Bottone EJ, Kirschner PA, Teirstein AS. Solitary pulmonary nodules due to nontuberculous mycobacterial infection. *Am J Med.* 1981;70:39-43.

356. Hahm CR, Park HY, Jeon K, et al. Solitary Pulmonary Nodules Caused by Mycobacterium tuberculosis and Mycobacterium avium Complex. *Lung.* 2010;188:25-31.

357. Nakagawa N, Tanino Y, Inokoshi Y, et al. Solitary pulmonary nodule due to Mycobacterium intracellulare showing intense uptake on 18F-fluorodeoxyglucose-positron emission tomography. *Nihon Kokyuki Gakkai Zasshi.* 2009;47:122-127.

358. Corti M, Palmero D. Mycobacterium avium complex infection in HIV/AIDS patients. *Expert Rev Anti Infect Ther.* 2008;6:351-363.

359. Karakousis PC, Moore RD, Chaisson RE. Mycobacterium avium complex in patients with HIV infection in the era of highly active antiretroviral therapy. *Lancet Infect Dis.* 2004;4:557-565.

360. Nightingale SD, Byrd LT, Southern PM, Jockusch JD, Cal SX, Wynne BA. Incidence of Mycobacterium avium-intracellulare complex bacteremia in human immunodeficiency virus-positive patients. *J Infect Dis.* 1992;165:1082-1085.

361. Horsburgh RC. Mycobacterium avium complex infection in the acquired immunodeficiency syndrome. *N Engl J Med.* 1991;324:1332-1338.

362. Torriani FJ, McCutchan JA, Bozzette SA, Grafe MR, Havlir DV. Autopsy findings in AIDS patients with Mycobacterium avium complex bacteremia. *J Infect Dis.* 1994;170:1601-1605.

363. Horsburgh CR. The pathophysiology of disseminated Mycobacterium avium complex disease in AIDS. *J Infect Dis.* 1999;179(suppl):S461-S465.

364. Cappelluti E, Fraire AE, Schaefer OP. A case of "hot tub lung" due to Mycobacterium avium complex in an immunocompetent host. *Arch Intern Med.* 2003;163:845-848.

365. Aksamit TR. Hot tub lung: infection, inflammation, or both? *Semin Respir Infect.* 2003;18:33-39.

366. Hanak V, Kalra S, Aksamit TR, Hartman TE, Tazelaar HD, Ryu JH. Hot tub lung: presenting features and clinical course of 21 patients. *Respir Med.* 2006;100:610-615.

367. Cheung OY, Muhm JR, Helmers RA, et al. Surgical pathology of granulomatous interstitial pneumonia. *Ann Diagn Pathol.* 2003;7:127-138.

368. Yamazaki Y, Kubo K, Fujimoto K, Matsuzawa Y, Sekiguchi M, Honda T. Pulmonary function tests of Mycobacterium avium-intracellulare infection: correlation with bronchoalveolar lavage fluid findings. *Respiration.* 2000;67(1):46-51.

369. Lee M-R, Yang C-Y, Chang K-P, et al. Factors associated with lung function decline in patients with non-tuberculous mycobacterial pulmonary disease. *PLoS One.* 2013;8(3):e58214.

370. Hayashi M, Takayanagi N, Kanauchi T, Miyahara Y, Yanagisawa T, Sugita Y. Prognostic factors of 634 HIV-negative patients with Mycobacterium avium complex lung disease. *Am J Respir Crit Care Med.* 2012;185(5):575-583.

371. O'Connell ML, Birkenkamp KE, Kleiner DE, Folio LR, Holland SM, Olivier KN. Lung manifestations in an autopsy-based series

of pulmonary or disseminated nontuberculous mycobacterial disease. *Chest.* 2012;141:1203-1209.

372. Fujita J, Ohtsuki Y, Shigeto E, et al. Pathological findings of bronchiectases caused by Mycobacterium avium intracellulare complex. *Respir Med.* 2003;97(8):933-938.

373. Den Hertog AL, Daher S, Straetemans M, Scholing M, Anthony RM. No added value of performing Ziehl-Neelsen on auramine-positive samples for tuberculosis diagnostics. *Int J Tuberc Lung Dis.* 2013;17:1094-1099.

374. Ulrichs T, Lefmann M, Reich M, et al. Modified immunohistological staining allows detection of Ziehl-Neelsen-negative Mycobacterium tuberculosis organisms and their precise localization in human tissue. *J Pathol.* 2005;205:633-640.

375. Goel MM, Budhwar P. Immunohistochemical localization of mycobacterium tuberculosis complex antigen with antibody to 38 kDa antigen versus Ziehl Neelsen staining in tissue granulomas of extrapulmonary tuberculosis. *Indian J Tuberc.* 2007;54:24-29.

376. Jeyanathan M, Alexander DC, Turenne CY, Girard C, Behr MA. Evaluation of in situ methods used to detect Mycobacterium avium subsp. paratuberculosis in samples from patients with Crohn's disease. *J Clin Microbiol.* 2006;44:2942-2950.

13 Fungal Diseases

Rodolfo Laucirica and Charles E. Stager

TAKE HOME PEARLS

- Invasive fungal infections of the lower respiratory tract are termed mycoses.
- Mycoses can be divided into two broad categories: endemic fungal infections are usually localized to specific geographic regions where the soil and climate conditions are optimal for fungal growth. Opportunistic fungal infections involve ubiquitous fungi and occur primarily in immunocompromised hosts.
- A number of reagents, stains, and media are utilized when isolating and identifying pathogenic molds and yeasts from tissue samples or secretions. Nonselective, selective, and differential media are used for isolation and presumptive identification of some pulmonary pathogens. Serologic assays have proven useful for some invasive fungal infections.
- The development of nucleic acid probes has advanced the identification of dimorphic fungi once they are recovered in culture. There are a number of PCR-based assays reported in the literature that have been highly sensitive and specific for fungal detection and identification when testing various specimen types.
- *Pneumocystis* pneumonia or pneumocystosis is a form of pneumonia caused by *Pneumocystis jiroveci* (formerly known as *Pneumocystis carinii*) that occurs in the immunocompromised.
- Species of *Aspergillus* are ubiquitous molds and are the most common invasive molds worldwide.
- Forms of pulmonary aspergillosis include fungus balls, hypersensitivity reactions such as allergic bronchopulmonary aspergillosis, eosinophilic pneumonia, and bronchocentric granulomatosis and several invasive diseases including acute invasive aspergillosis, necrotizing pseudomembranous tracheobronchitis, and chronic necrotizing aspergillosis.
- With acute invasive aspergillosis, the characteristic gross finding is the presence of target lesions in the lung consisting of a nodular pulmonary infarct associated with thrombosis secondary to vascular invasion by fungal hyphae.
- *Histoplasma* is the most common pulmonary infection worldwide, most common endemic mycosis in AIDS patients, and most prevalent endemic mycosis in the United States.
- The primary clinical forms of pulmonary histoplasmosis include acute self-limited disease, chronic cavitary, progressive disseminated, and mediastinal histoplasmosis.
- Coccidioidomycosis is endemic throughout the southwestern United States, northern and central Mexico, and parts of Central and South America. Coccidioidomycosis can manifest itself in one of three clinical forms: primary pulmonary disease (most common), progressive pulmonary disease, or disseminated coccidioidomycosis.
- Hematogenous dissemination of *Candida* results in a bilateral miliary pattern with numerous discrete nodules (abscesses with organisms) involving the lung parenchyma. Angioinvasion leads to hemorrhagic infarction of the involved lung. Airway-associated spread of *Candida* may result in acute bronchopneumonia that is primarily localized to the lower lobes.

- The incidence of cryptococcosis has steadily increased primarily due to the use of corticosteroids, improved patient survival with certain malignancies, and the onset of AIDS/HIV.
- Cryptococcal infection has two primary clinical forms: pulmonary infection and cerebromeningeal infection due to hematogenous spread from the lung.
- Pulmonary sporotrichosis usually results from inhalation of spores of *S schenckii* causing caseous, necrotizing, or suppurative-type granulomas.
- Zygomycosis is a potentially fatal infection caused by fungi of the class Zygomycetes, comprised of the orders Mucorales and Entomophthorales. Pulmonary zygomycosis occurs most often in neutropenic patients receiving chemotherapy and those undergoing hematopoietic stem cell transplants.
- Pulmonary zygomycosis is characterized by angioinvasion associated with thrombosis and hemorrhagic infarction of the lung tissue distal to the involved blood vessel. Granulomatous vasculitis may also be present.
- The histologic reaction to pulmonary blastomycosis is typically suppurative, with a marked neutrophil response associated with abscess formation. Necrotizing granulomatous inflammation has also been described with this fungal pathogen.
- Dematiaceous fungi are septate fungi that have brown-black cell walls due to the presence of a melanin-like pigment.

INTRODUCTION

Pulmonary fungal infections are less common than bacterial and viral infections but may pose significant problems in diagnosis and treatment. With respect to the respiratory tract, pathogenic fungi usually cause infections when airborne spores reach the lung or paranasal sinuses. Invasive fungal infections of the lower respiratory tract (termed mycoses) can be divided into two broad categories: endemic or opportunistic. Endemic fungal infections are usually localized to specific geographic regions where the soil and climate conditions are optimal for fungal growth. For example, coccidioidomycosis is commonly found in the southwestern and western regions of the United States whereas histoplasmosis is frequently seen in states along the Ohio River valley and lower Mississippi River. In contrast, opportunistic fungal infections involve ubiquitous fungi and occur primarily in immunocompromised hosts. Chemotherapy, immunosuppressive treatments, prolonged corticosteroid therapy, stem cell transplantation, congenital immune deficiency syndromes, and AIDS represent risk factors that predispose patients to acquire opportunistic fungal infections. In these patients, fungal infections need to be treated aggressively due to the

Table 13-1 Examples of Endemic and Opportunistic Fungi

Endemic	Opportunistic
Histoplasma	*Aspergillus*
Coccidioides	*Cryptococcus*
Blastomyces	*Candida*
Paracoccidioides	*Pneumocystis*
	Zygomycosis (Mucormycosis)

high rate of morbidity and mortality associated with this form of fungal disease. Examples of opportunistic fungal infections include invasive aspergillosis and systemic candidiasis. *Table 13-1* lists common endemic and opportunistic fungal pathogens.

CLINICAL FEATURES

The clinical features associated with fungal infections will depend in large part on known risk factors, age, and immune status of the patient. These parameters will dictate the severity of the disease and potential etiologic agents.[1-3] For example, in patients who are immunocompetent, it may be difficult to establish the diagnosis morphologically since the number of organisms may be quite small. In such cases, cultures and serologic data coupled with the clinical information may be needed to confirm the diagnosis. However, with immunocompromised patients where there may be large numbers of organisms, morphologic assessment of tissue samples may be all that is needed to establish the diagnosis (see the Laboratory Diagnosis section). Clinical findings associated with fungal infections will vary depending on the immunologic status of the host. They include nonspecific features such as fever, chills, myalgias, pleuritic chest pain, and cough (can be nonproductive or productive). However, some patients may be entirely asymptomatic. The radiologic picture can also be quite variable depending on the offending organism and stage of the disease. Radiologic changes include confluent areas of consolidation, nodular interstitial opacities, and solid or cavity masses. The distribution of these changes may also be organism dependent. For example, *Aspergillus*, *Cryptococcus*, and *Blastomyces* usually affect the upper lobes while *Coccidioides* affects the hilar and lower lobes. Finally, acute histoplasmosis has been associated with a bilateral military pattern that can mimic mycobacterial infections.[4] Patients who develop pneumonia as a complication of fungal infections may show a restrictive pattern with pulmonary function tests (PFTs). The latter is characterized by reduced total lung capacity (TLC). However, PFTs are usually not required when evaluating patients for fungal infections of the lung.

LABORATORY DIAGNOSIS

There are a variety of methods by which one can establish the diagnosis of fungal infections. The most common and frequently used method involves morphologic evaluation of tissue samples obtained by pulmonologists, radiologists, or surgeons. If the lesion is involving a bronchus or alveolar tissue adjacent to a major airway, an endobronchial or transbronchial biopsy may often yield diagnostic information. Pulmonologist can also use bronchioalveolar lavages (BALs) to sample lesions in the distal airways including the respiratory bronchiole, alveolar ducts, and alveoli. Subpleural lesions can be evaluated by CT-guided fine needle aspiration (FNA) or video-assisted thoracoscopic (VATS) biopsies. Depending on the type of material obtained, the specimen can be processed in the cytology (BAL or FNA) or histology laboratory (tissue biopsy). In addition to routine stains performed on tissue samples, special stains such as Grocott-Gomori methenamine silver (GMS), periodic acid-Schiff (PAS), and mucicarmine stains are frequently employed to identify fungal pathogen (see below). These sampling methods are also useful to obtain sterile tissue for culture and other ancillary studies such as immunofluorescence and molecular testing.

All types of pulmonary specimens should be submitted to the microbiology laboratory in sterile containers. BALs, bronchial washings, and pleural fluids should be centrifuged prior to microscopic examination and culture. A wet prep of these specimens, as well as tissue impression smears, can be stained with calcofluor white (with or without KOH). Lung tissue should be inoculated in the appropriate media within 15 minutes of arrival to the laboratory. Other pulmonary specimens such as BALs, washings, aspirates, and sputum should be inoculated within 2 hours. For samples obtained after hours or on weekends, they can be stored at 4°C for up to 24 hours. Fresh tissue should be ground for recovery of *Histoplasma capsulatum* and minced for other fungal pathogens.[5]

A number of reagents, stains, and media are utilized when isolating and identifying pathogenic molds and yeasts from tissue samples or secretions. Properly processed and stained clinical specimens can be examined by direct microscopy and may provide presumptive identification of some fungal pathogens and aid in the selection of the appropriate growth media.[5,6]

Reagents

A. *N*-acetyl-L-cysteine and dithiothreitol. These are mucolytic agents used to prepare sputum specimens for detection of fungi, including *Pneumocystis jiroveci*, for microscopic examination.
B. Potassium hydroxide (10%) with lactophenol cotton blue. This agent is used to prepare wet mounts of fungal growth. Aniline (cotton blue) stains the cell wall of the fungi blue.
C. India ink or nigrosin. These agents are used on wet mounts for detection of the polysaccharide capsule of *Cryptococcus neoformans* and *Cryptococcus gattii*.

Stains

A. Mucicarmine stain. This stain is used to differentiate *C neoformans* from other nonencapsulated yeast of similar size and shape. The polysaccharide capsule stains deep rose to red.
B. Periodic acid-Schiff (PAS) stain. This stain is used to detect yeast and fungal hyphae. Periodic acid hydrolyses the cell wall, permitting the modified Schiff reagent to impart a pink to magenta color to the yeast and hyphal structures.
C. Grocott-Gomori methenamine silver (GMS) stain. This stain is commonly employed to identify yeast or hyphae from a variety of fungal pathogens. The fungal elements stain black against a pale green background.
D. Calcofluor white stain. Calcofluor white stains cellulose and chitin in the fungal cell wall. A fluorescent microscope with ultraviolet (UV) or blue-purple excitation and special filters are required to visualize fungi using this stain. Fungal elements, including *P jiroveci* cysts, stain blue-white against a dark background. The cyst walls of *P jiroveci* demonstrate a "double-parenthesis"-like form with this stain. Other yeast will frequently demonstrate budding with intense internal staining.
E. Giemsa stain. The Giemsa stain is used to stain bone marrow, buffy coat, and tissue specimens. Giemsa will stain the intracellular yeast forms of *H capsulatum* blue, surrounded by a clear halo representing the cell wall. Giemsa will also stain trophozoites of *P jiroveci*.

Media for Primary Isolation

Specimens from nonsterile pulmonary sites are inoculated onto media containing agents to suppress growth of bacteria and some saprophytic fungi. Nonselective, selective, and differential media are used for isolation and presumptive identification of some pulmonary pathogens (*Table 13-2*). Specimens should be incubated at 30°C or at room temperature for 3 to 4 weeks.

A. Brain heart infusion agar (BHI) medium, with or without 10% sheep blood. The medium is used for all fungi, including the fastidious dimorphic fungi. This

Table 13-2 Routine and Specialized Media for Culture of Pulmonary Specimens

	Routine Media			Specialized Media							
	SABHI	**IMA**	**BHIA**	**Inhibited by Cycloheximide**	**Kelly**	**BGCA**	**CM**	**YEPA**	**CGBB**	**BN**	**CA**
H capsulatum	✓	✓	✓	No	✓	✓		✓			
B dermatitidis	✓	✓	✓	No	✓	✓		✓			
C immitis/ posadasii	✓	✓	✓	No	✓		✓				
P brasiliensis	✓	✓	✓	No	✓		✓				
S schenckii	✓	✓	✓	No	✓	✓					
Aspergillus sp	✓	✓		Yes							
C neoformans/ gattii	✓	✓		Yes					✓	✓	
Candida sp	✓	✓		Yes[a]							✓
Zygomycetes	✓	✓		Yes							
P boydii	✓	✓		No							
Fusarium sp	✓	✓		Yes[a]							

SABHI, Sabouraud brain heart infusion agar; IMA, inhibitory mold agar; BHI, brain heart infusion agar; Kelly, Kelly medium; BGCA, blood-glucose-cysteine agar; CM, converse medium; YEPA, yeast extract phosphate agar, CGBB, canavanine glycine bromthymol blue agar; BN, birdseed agar-Niger seed agar; CA, chromogenic agar.
[a]Variably sensitive to cycloheximide.

medium can be made selective by adding chloramphenicol and gentamicin to inhibit gram-positive and gram-negative bacteria.

B. Sabouraud brain heart infusion agar (SABHI) medium. SABHI, with or without antibacterial agents or cycloheximide, is used for cultivation of all fungi, including dimorphic fungi. Sheep blood can be added to better recover fastidious fungi and enhance the growth of *H capsulatum*. This medium can be made selective by adding chloramphenicol, penicillin, streptomycin, or cycloheximide. Aerobic actinomycetes can be inhibited by the antibiotics. Cycloheximide can inhibit some pulmonary pathogens including *Aspergillus*, some dematiaceous fungi, *Pseudallescheria, Scopulariopsis, Zygomycetes,* and yeasts such as some *Candida* spp and *C neoformans*.

C. Inhibitory mold agar (IMA) medium. IMA is an enriched medium and can be made selective by adding chloramphenicol and gentamicin to inhibit gram-positive and gram-negative bacteria. IMA is composed of casein and animal tissue.

Specialized Media

A. Kelly medium. This medium is composed of beef extract, peptone, sodium chloride, and starches, and is used to culture dimorphic fungi.

B. Blood-glucose-cysteine agar medium. This medium is composed of a tryptose blood agar base mixed with L-cysteine and sheep blood. Penicillin is added to inhibit some bacteria. The medium is used in the conversion of mold to yeast for *Blastomyces dermatitidis, H capsulatum, Paracoccidioides brasiliensis,* and *Sporothrix schenckii*.

C. Converse medium. This is a liquid medium composed of glucose, ammonium acetate, magnesium sulfate, potassium phosphate, zinc sulfate, and tamol. The medium is used to convert the mold phase of *Coccidioides immitis* to spherule formation.

D. Yeast extract phosphate agar medium with ammonium. The medium is used to recover *H capsulatum* and *B dermatitidis* from contaminated specimens.

E. Canavanine glycine bromthymol blue agar medium. This medium is used to differentiate *C neoformans* from *C gattii*. *C neoformans* imparts a greenish-yellow color to the medium while *C gattii* turns the medium a cobalt blue.

F. Birdseed agar-Niger seed agar medium. This is a selective medium used to differentiate *Cryptococcus* spp. Of the *Cryptococcus* spp, only *C neoformans* produces the enzyme phenol oxidase which breaks down the seed substrate, leading to the production of melanin pigment. The pigment is taken up by the yeast cell wall, imparting a tan to brown color to the colonies.

G. Chromogenic agar medium. Proprietary chromogenic agents provide a medium for isolation and differentiation of relevant *Candida* sp found in pulmonary specimens. The medium contains chloramphenicol to inhibit bacteria. Various yeasts produce a characteristic color that, together with morphology, provides a reliable presumptive identification of clinically important *Candida* sp.

Nonculture Based Methods

Serologic assays have proven useful for some invasive fungal infections. The detection of a specific antibody response can be performed rapidly and is noninvasive. However, the presence of antibodies does not always correlate with invasive disease and when patients are immunocompromised, antibodies may not be formed.[7] Serologic tests for the detection of *C immitis* and *H capsulatum* are highly useful but are of less utility if the pulmonary infection is due to other fungi. Serology testing for *B dermatitidis* has little clinical utility because of lack of sensitivity and cross-reactivity that occurs with other fungal agents.[8]

Direct fluorescence antibody kits are commercially available for *P jiroveci* but not for other fungi causing pulmonary infections.

Immunohistochemistry (IHC) is a valuable ancillary tool that, in conjunction with routine and special stains, can aid in the diagnosis of fungal infections.[9-11] Immunohistochemistry involves antibodies binding to specific antigens in tissues or cytologic samples. The antibody can be conjugated to an enzyme such as peroxidase, which can catalyze a color-producing reaction. Alternatively, the antibody can be tagged to a fluorophore such as fluorescein. The antibodies are then detected with a fluorescent microscope or by chromogenic signal amplification. These IHC assays are technically simple and can be performed on smears or on paraffin-embedded tissue sections. The antigenicity does not appear to be affected when tissues are stored in formalin or paraffin-embedded specimens.[12] Consequently, these fixed specimens can be sent to reference labs for IHC testing. The Centers for Disease Control (CDC), Division of Mycotic Diseases, offers a broad range of IHC assays for pathogenic fungi.

Antigen detection assays for early detection of invasive fungal infections include the galactomannan assay for *Aspergillus*, and the β-D-glucan assay for fungi, urinary, serum, BAL, and CSF antigen tests for *H capsulatum*, *B dermatitidis*, *C immitis,* and *C neoformans*. The detection of fungal antigens in body fluids requires a relatively large amount of antigen, which may limit assay sensitivity.[8]

Molecular methods may be useful when fungi are not detected by histochemical or immunohistochemical stains or are present in small numbers, stain poorly, have an atypical morphology similar to other fungi, or cannot be cultured.[13]

In situ hybridization (ISH) uses complementary sequences of nucleotides on chromosomes to impart

specificity.[14] A fluorescent or chromogenic agent binds to a portion of a chromosome which has a complementary sequence. ISH has been used to detect fungi in tissue and has been shown to detect *B dermatitidis*, *C immitis*, *C neoformans,* and several *Candida* spp.[15,16]

The development of nucleic acid probes has advanced the identification of dimorphic fungi once they are recovered in culture. The GenProbe AccuProbe assay (Hologic Diagnostics, San Diego, CA) can be performed in about 2 hours. A chemiluminescent-labeled DNA probe, specific for target fungal rRNA, is incubated with a lysate of the organism. The probe has sensitivity similar to that of the historic and more labor-intensive exoantigen test but demonstrates slightly less specificity, depending on the fungus tested. The probe has demonstrated 100% specificity for *H capsulatum* and *C immitis*. However, specificity for *B dermatitidis* is 99.7% because there is cross-reactivity with *Paracoccidioides brasiliensis*.[17-19]

There are a number of PCR-based assays reported in the literature that have been highly sensitive and specific for fungal detection and identification when testing various specimen types (eg, serum, plasma, BAL, tissue).[20] Because there has been a lack of standardization and clinical validation, they are not part of the consensus criteria for defining an invasive fungal infection.[21] However, PCR-based methods can improve both the sensitivity and specificity of histopathologic evaluations.[22,23] Detection of fungal DNA in tissue, whether fresh, formalin fixed or paraffin embedded, has been described.[24] Finally, the combination of universal primers for fungi, which target 18S rRNA, and sequencing the amplified product, has broadened the diagnosis of fungal infections.[20,25,26]

FUNGAL DISEASES

Pneumocystis jiroveci *Pneumonia*

Pneumocystis pneumonia or pneumocystosis is a form of pneumonia caused by *Pneumocystis jiroveci* (formerly known as *Pneumocystis carinii*). Once considered to be a protozoan, *P jiroveci* has now been reclassified as a fungus.[27] *Pneumocystis* is a relatively rare infection in people with a normal immune system. However, it is common among people with weakened immune systems, such as premature or severely malnourished children, the elderly, patients treated with immunosuppressive therapies, and those with collagen-vascular diseases. It is also a frequent cause of pneumonia in HIV/AIDS patients.[28]

There are at least two different life forms of *Pneumocystis*: trophozoites and cysts. The cysts are thick walled and have up to eight intracystic bodies (sporozoites) while the trophic form measures about

2 µm, possesses a single nucleus, and is surrounded by a plasma membrane.[28,29] The exact route of *Pneumocystis* infection is not completely understood. Some researchers believe that aerosolized particles are transmitted from host to host with initial infections occurring in infancy or early childhood, with reactivation later in life during periods of immune suppression. Others believe that early childhood infections are not the source of infections later in life; rather the disease is reacquired if the host lacks T-cell-based immune responses necessary for effective defense.[29-31] Once inhaled, *Pneumocystis* has considerable tropism for the lung. However, extrapulmonary dissemination has been reported in patients with advanced HIV infection.[32,33] Once inside the lung, the trophozoites bind tightly to the alveolar epithelial cells. This attachment promotes the transition of the organism from the trophic to the cyst form and also leads to suppression of epithelial cell growth and production of inflammatory mediators, culminating in lung injury and impaired gas exchange.[29,34]

The clinical manifestations of *Pneumocystis jiroveci* pneumonia (PJP) are variable depending on the immune status of the hosts. At one extreme, the symptoms and signs are minimal, whereas at the other, there is rapidly progressive respiratory failure. Typical findings include nonproductive cough, dyspnea, and fever. Tachypnea is present and crackles may be heard on auscultation.

Early in the course of the disease, chest radiographs may show bilateral hazy or ground glass opacities involving the perihilar regions. Over time, these changes can progress to diffuse areas of consolidation involving the lower or upper lobes. High-resolution CT (HRCT) scans demonstrate bilateral ground glass attenuation that has a geographic distribution with sharply demarcated borders.[35,36]

The classic pattern of injury associated with PJP consists of intra-alveolar foamy exudates that can be seen in either tissue biopsies or BAL-derived samples (*Figure 13-1A* and *B*). With tissue biopsies, the exudate is usually accompanied by mild chronic interstitial inflammation and type 2 pneumocyte hyperplasia. The foamy spaces represent negative images of *Pneumocystis* cysts. These cysts are round to oval, measure 5 to 7 µm and may have prominent grooves or condensed areas representing collapse of the cyst wall[37] (*Figure 13-2*). The intra-alveolar exudates of PJP need to be differentiated from other intra-alveolar-associated patterns of lung injury including pulmonary edema and pulmonary alveolar proteinosis (PAP). The exudates with pulmonary edema do not have a granular appearance while the exudates of PAP although granular does not have a foamy appearance.

Atypical forms of lung injury associated with PJP include diffuse alveolar damage, interstitial fibrosis, organizing pneumonia, lymphocytic interstitial

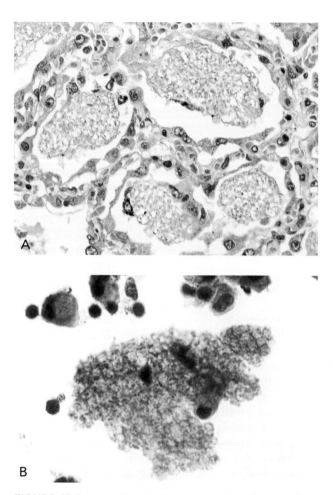

FIGURE 13-1 **Intra-alveolar foamy exudate characteristic of PJP in tissue (A) and BAL (B) samples. The empty spaces represent negative images of the *Pneumocystis* cysts.**

pneumonia, granulomatous inflammation, military disease, microcalcifications, vasculitis associated with cavitary lesions, and minimal change histology (*Table 13-3*). The granulomas may be either necrotizing or non-necrotizing, so other infectious agents such as mycobacteria and *Histoplasma* need to be considered in the differential diagnosis. These unusual patterns of *Pneumocystis* infection are more frequently seen in HIV-infected patients.[38] Of these histologic findings, the most frequent patterns associated with AIDS patients are interstitial fibrosis and organizing pneumonia. They represent 63% and 36%, respectively, of lung biopsy findings from AIDS patients infected with *Pneumocystis*.[38] In both cases, there are plugs of loose connective tissue (organizing fibrosis) in either the pulmonary interstitium or within alveolar spaces. This most likely represents two end points of the same disease process that initially begins within alveolar spaces and is ultimately incorporated into the adjacent interstitium.

Trophozoites of *P jiroveci* are 1 to 5 µm, pleomorphic and contain a single nucleus. *P jiroveci* cysts are

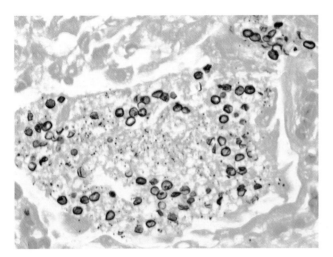

FIGURE 13-2 The GMS stain highlights the round and cup-shaped cysts. Grooves and dot-like condensed areas of the cyst wall are seen along lower half of this photograph.

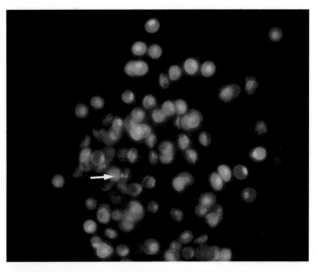

FIGURE 13-3 Arrow points to the "double comma" morphology of the cyst wall in a BAL sample from an HIV patient (calcofluor white stain).

thick walled, rounded, and approximately 5 to 8 μm in size, although thin-walled cysts also exist. Cysts and trophozoites are found in the lungs and many other extrapulmonary specimens, especially in immunocompromised patients.[39]

A variety of stains have been used to detect *Pneumocystis* in clinical specimens. These stains include GMS, Giemsa, or Giemsa-like stains and calcofluor white. GMS stains the cyst wall black but trophozoites are not visible with this stain. The GMS stain

highlights the grooves in the cyst wall that impart a wrinkled appearance to the cyst[40] (*Figure 13-2*). As illustrated in *Figure 13-3* with the calcofluor white stain, the cyst wall thickenings may have a "double comma" morphology. Calcofluor white is a fluorescent stain, whose active ingredient is Cellufluor. Cellufluor binds to β-linked polysaccharides such as chitin and cellulose in the cyst wall of *Pneumocystis*.[41] Giemsa and rapid Giemsa-like stains do not stain the cyst wall but rather stain the nuclei of *Pneumocystis* trophozoites a reddish-purple and stain the cytoplasm a light blue. There are approximately 10-fold more trophic forms than cysts in infected specimens.[42] Immunofluorescent stains, both direct and indirect, employing monoclonal antibodies, are available commercially for the direct detection of *Pneumocystis* in clinical specimens[43] (*Figure 13-4*).

Table 13-3 Patterns of Injury With *Pneumocystis* Infection

Intra-alveolar foamy exudate (classic pattern of lung injury)
Diffuse alveolar damage
Interstitial fibrosis
Organizing pneumonia
Granulomatous inflammation
Lymphocytic interstitial pneumonia
Subpleural emphysematous blebs
Miliary disease
Microcalcifications
Vasculitis and necrotizing cavitary lesions
Minimal change histology

Used with permission from Lung infections. In: Travis WD, Colby TV, Koss MN, Rosado-de-Christenson ML, Müller NL, King TE, eds. Non-neoplastic Disorders of the Lower Respiratory Tract. Bethesda, MD: American Registry of Pathology/Armed Forces Institute of Pathology; 2002:592-638.

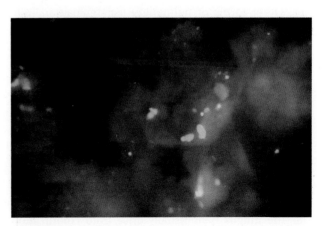

FIGURE 13-4 Several cysts are visible with a direct immunofluorescent stain.

Procop et al[44] compared four different stains for detection of *P jiroveci* in 313 respiratory specimens. A direct fluorescent monoclonal antibody had the highest sensitivity (90.8%) but the lowest specificity (81.9%). The sensitivity and specificity for the calcofluor white stain, GMS stain, and a Giemsa-like stain were 73.8% and 99.6%; 79.4% and 99.2%; and 49.2% and 99.6%, respectively.

β-D-glucan is a cell wall component of many fungi, including *Pneumocystis*. A meta-analysis of 12 studies found that the β-D-glucan assay was sensitive in detecting *P jiroveci* in clinical specimens.[45]

The detection of *P jiroveci* using direct or nested PCR has been reported.[46,47] The use of quantitative PCR to differentiate colonization from infection may become useful,[48] but the presence of an amplified product has not been strictly correlated with infection.[49,50] A few reference laboratories do offer quantitative and/or qualitative PCR for *P jiroveci*.

Aspergillosis

Species of *Aspergillus* are ubiquitous molds and are the most common invasive molds worldwide. Although they are the second most common fungal pathogens after *Candida* sp, *Aspergillus* spp are more commonly isolated from the lung. There are several species of *Aspergillus*, but *A fumigatus* is the one most often seen in the clinical laboratory and is the most frequent species isolated from lungs of immunocompromised patients. Other species of *Aspergillus* encountered in the clinical laboratory include *flavus* and *niger*.[51]

Humans usually acquire the disease through inhalation of spores. Therefore, the lungs are typically the site of primary infection. Once inside the host, pulmonary aspergillosis can evolve into one of several forms, depending to some extent on the immunologic status of the host. The most frequent form of infection is the formation of fungus balls within the lung parenchyma after colonization of major airways or preexisting cavities. Other forms of pulmonary aspergillosis include hypersensitivity reactions such as allergic bronchopulmonary aspergillosis, eosinophilic pneumonia, and bronchocentric granulomatosis and several invasive diseases including acute invasive aspergillosis, necrotizing pseudomembranous tracheobronchitis, and chronic necrotizing aspergillosis (*Table 13-4*).[52]

The clinical and radiologic findings of pulmonary aspergillosis will vary depending on which form of the disease is present. Patients with aspergillomas (fungus balls) may be asymptomatic or may present with extensive and potentially life-threatening hemoptysis if the Aspergilloma erodes into a major blood vessel. The fungus balls usually arise from colonization of preexisting cavities that have formed due to a variety of causes such as tuberculosis, sarcoidosis, chronic

Table 13-4 Patterns of Injury With Pulmonary Aspergillosis

Fungus ball
Allergic bronchopulmonary aspergillosis
Eosinophilic pneumonia
Mucoid impaction
Bronchocentric granulomatosis
Hypersensitivity pneumonitis
Acute invasive aspergillosis
Necrotizing pseudomembranous tracheobronchitis
Chronic necrotizing aspergillosis
Bronchopleural fistula
Empyema

Used with permission from Lung infections. In: Travis WD, Colby TV, Koss MN, Rosado-de-Christenson ML, Müller NL, King TE, eds. Non-neoplastic Disorders of the Lower Respiratory Tract. Bethesda, MD: American Registry of Pathology/Armed Forces Institute of Pathology; 2002:592-638.

lung abscess, histoplasmosis, and neoplasms.[53,54] Radiologically, the fungus ball arises within preexisting intraparenchymal cavities or bronchiectatic airways. The Aspergilloma is usually located in the upper lobes and presents as a rounded nodule outlined by a rim of air ("air-crescent" sign).[55]

The hypersensitivity reactions associated with *Aspergillus* sp usually manifest themselves in one of two ways: allergic bronchopulmonary aspergillosis or hypersensitivity pneumonitis. Allergic bronchopulmonary aspergillosis is typically found in chronic asthmatics and those with cystic fibrosis that develop hypersensitivity to a variety of fungal pathogens, especially *Aspergillus fumigatus*.[56,57] Patients with allergic bronchopulmonary aspergillosis characteristically display elevation of IgE and IgG antibodies to *Aspergillus* and central bronchiectasis.[58,59] The radiologic findings include bronchiectasis (bilateral/upper lobe predominant), centrilobular nodules, and mucoid impaction.[58] Hypersensitivity pneumonitis (HP), also known as extrinsic allergic alveolitis, represents a diffuse interstitial granulomatous disease resulting from an immunologic reaction to an inhaled organic antigen or simple chemicals. There are a variety of examples of HP including "farmer's lung," "bird fancier's lung, and "maple bark stripper's disease."[60,61] Although the antigens in all these cases are different, the resulting pattern of lung injury is similar. In the case of *Aspergillus*, the precipitating event is the inhalation of spores leading to HP in the appropriately sensitized individual. The radiologic changes of acute or subacute HP on HRCT consist of diffuse and bilateral centrilobular nodular opacities which reflect the presence of alveolitis.[62] In the chronic stage of the disease, fibrosis usually develops that has a reticular pattern and is located in the mid and lower lung zones.[63]

The invasive forms of pulmonary aspergillosis tend to occur in immunocompromised patients such as those receiving chemotherapy or immunosuppressive drugs or HIV-infected individuals. The three most important forms of invasive disease include acute invasive aspergillosis, necrotizing pseudomembranous tracheobronchitis, and chronic necrotizing aspergillosis. Patients can present with nonspecific findings that include productive or nonproductive cough and dyspnea. In addition, high fever, pleuritic pain, and pleural friction rubs have also been described in patients with acute invasive aspergillosis.[64] Radiologic findings include multifocal, bilateral opacities that can progress to confluent nodules over time. Surrounding these areas of consolidation are ground glass attenuations, referred to on HRCT as "halo signs."[65,66]

Regardless of the clinical presentation, pathologic confirmation of aspergillosis usually requires morphologic assessment of cytologic or tissue biopsy samples. The hyphae of *Aspergillus* spp are septate and branching and 3 to 6 μm in width. Branching is usually dichotomous at 45° angles (*Figure 13-5*). The hyphal form of *Aspergillus* needs to be differentiated from other fungi such as *Fusarium* sp and *Pseudallescheria boydii*. While the width and hyphal contours of these three fungi overlap, the branching pattern with *Fusarium* is at right angle while the hyphae of *Pseudallescheria boydii* are arranged haphazardly.[67]

Although *Aspergillus* hyphae are visible with routine H&E stains, they are more easily seen with GMS or PAS stains (*Figures 13-6*). The hyphae of most species of *Aspergillus* are indistinguishable. Therefore, speciation is based on the morphology of the fruiting bodies or conidial heads (*Figure 13-7*). These structures are only

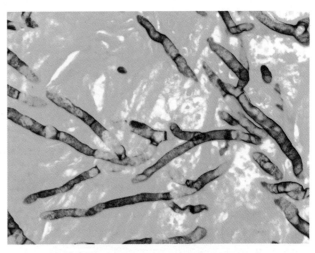

FIGURE 13-6 The dichotomous branching and septation of *Aspergillus* hyphae are easily seen in this GMS preparation.

seen when the organism is exposed to air, such as cavities associated with fungus balls or necrotizing pseudomembranous tracheobronchitis where a layer of fungal organisms grows along the tracheal or bronchial mucosal surface (*Figure 13-9*). With acute invasive aspergillosis, the characteristic gross finding is the presence of target lesions in the lung. The target lesion consists of a nodular pulmonary infarct associated with thrombosis secondary to vascular invasion by fungal hyphae. These target lesions have a pale center surrounded by a hemorrhagic rim (*Figure 13-8*). They are usually multiple and peripherally located. Histologic assessment of these lesions confirms the presence of large

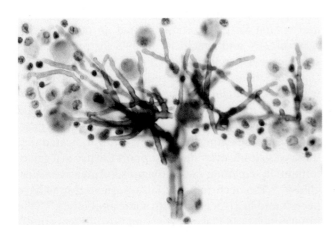

FIGURE 13-5 Numerous hyphal structures with rigid walls and 45° branching are seen in this BAL sample from an HIV patient (Papanicolaou stain).

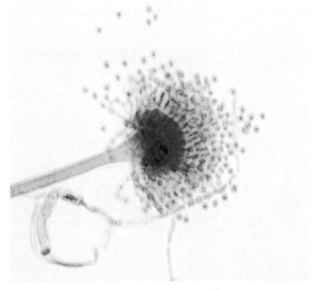

FIGURE 13-7 Culture of *Aspergillus* illustrating a fruiting body. The conidial head consists of a vesicle with stigmata and chains of conidia along the surface of the fruiting body (lactophenol cotton blue stain).

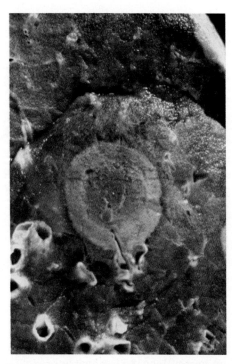

FIGURE 13-8 This gross photograph illustrates the "targetoid" lesion that is the characteristic of aspergillosis in the lung. Note the thrombus in the lower half of the hyperemic center of this lesion.

number of *Aspergillus* organisms in the occluded blood vessel and infarcted lung (*Figure 13-9*). Chronic necrotizing aspergillosis is characterized by the presence of necrotizing granulomatous inflammation within the lung parenchyma or distal airways. The organisms are usually found in areas of tissue necrosis.[68,69] Patients with HP-associated aspergillosis have a bronchiolocentric chronic interstitial pneumonia associated with

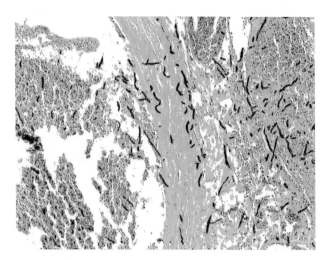

FIGURE 13-9 The corresponding histology shows numerous fungal organisms migrating from the thrombus (left side) across the blood vessel and into the adjacent infarcted lung (GMS stain).

ill-defined granulomas and organizing pneumonia. This pattern of lung injury can be seen in other forms of HP-associated diffuse parenchymal lung diseases. Therefore, appropriate serologic testing and/or morphologic identification of the organism is imperative to arrive at the correct diagnosis.[70,71]

Aspergillus sp usually grows rapidly on a variety of media, but are inhibited by cycloheximide. Laboratory tests for allergic bronchopulmonary aspergillosis include immediate skin test reactivity to *Aspergillus* antigens, precipitating serum antibodies to *A fumigatus*, serum total IgE >417 IU/mL (>1000 ng/mL), peripheral blood eosinophilia >5/mm^3, and elevated serum IgE and IgG to *A fumigatus*.[67,72,73] Serologic tests for *Aspergillus* using immunodiffusion, complement fixation, and ELISA are commercially available.

Galactomannan is a component of fungal cell walls that can be detected by a sandwich-like EIA in serum or plasma,[74] BAL fluid,[75,76] and CSF.[77] An *Aspergillus* quantitative galactomannan EIA should be used in conjunction with other diagnostic tests. Using an EIA for galactomannan, it has been reported that two consecutive serum specimens with a test optical reading of 0.5 or greater provided the highest test accuracy.[78] Consequently, it is recommended that two consecutive positive results are required for classification as a true positive result. The galactomannan EIA performed with serum may be positive before an invasive infection with *Aspergillus* sp and may be used in monitoring and preemptive treatment.[79,80] Galactomannan EIA testing in BAL fluid has also been shown to have clinical value in the management of patients with invasive aspergillosis,[81] and Penack et al reported that testing of BAL fluid increased the sensitivity of the EIA compared with serum alone from 71% to 100%.[82] Treatment with antifungal agents reduces the sensitivity of the galactomannan EIA. The sensitivity of the test was 52% in patients receiving antifungal therapy versus 89% in those who were not.[83]

A published meta-analysis of 27 studies showed that testing for galactomannan had an overall sensitivity of 71% and specificity of 89% for proven cases of invasive aspergillosis when used for surveillance.[84] Galactomannan has been reported to correlate well with clinical outcome.[85] The European Conference on Infections in Leukemia established evidence-based recommendations for the use of biomarkers in the diagnosis of invasive fungal infections. They indicated that there was strong evidence to support the use of a galactomannan screening test for diagnosis of invasive aspergillosis.[86] The occurrence of false-positive results have been found in association with some antibiotics,[87-89] the intravenous fluid PlasmaLyte[90] and the different cutoffs of positivity among studies.[91] The monoclonal antibody in the Platelia *Aspergillus* EIA (Biorad Laboratories, Hercules, CA) assay cross-reacts with galactomannan in

Penicillium sp, *Paecilomyces, Alternaria, Trichosporon, Botrytis, Wallemia, Cladosporium,* and *Histoplasma*.[92-94]

Polymerase chain reaction (PCR) testing has been performed with mixed results in patients with invasive aspergillosis. Using BAL-derived samples, Luong et al[95] tested lung transplant recipients and found that pan-*Aspergillus* PCR had a sensitivity of 100% for invasive pulmonary aspergillosis, while the sensitivity was 85% for an *Aspergillus*-specific PCR. On the other hand, Buess et al[96] found that with immunocompromised patients, that nested PCR for *Aspergillus* was negative for three of three patients with proven invasive pulmonary aspergillosis and the sensitivity for 53 patients with a high suspicion of invasive disease by chest x-ray or CT scan was only 28% by PCR. However, another publication found that a combination of PCR and galactomannan antigen EIA detected 100% of invasive aspergillosis cases, with a positive predictive value of 75.1%.[97] In addition, based on a meta-analysis, it has been proposed that a single negative PCR test is adequate to exclude a diagnosis of invasive aspergillosis, whereas two PCR-positive results are required to confirm diagnosis.[98]

There are no commercial kits available for *Aspergillus* PCR. Some reference labs offer qualitative PCR for *Aspergillus* as well as universal primers for fungi with sequencing of any amplified product for a definitive identification, frequently to species.

Histoplasmosis

Histoplasmosis is caused by the dimorphic fungus *Histoplasma capsulatum*. *Histoplasma* lives naturally in the soil, and is the most common pulmonary infection worldwide, most common endemic mycosis in AIDS patients, and most prevalent endemic mycosis in the United States.[99,100] In the United States, *Histoplasma* is endemic in certain regions of the country, especially the Mississippi and Ohio River valleys. Infections develop when *Histoplasma* microconidia present in contaminated bird droppings or bat guano are inhaled into the lungs. Once inside the lungs, they transform into the yeast form of this organism. The yeasts are then ingested by macrophages and spread to adjacent lymph nodes and throughout the reticuloendothelial system. In order to survive within the host, *H capsulatum* has evolved several defense strategies including mechanisms for modulating its microenvironmental pH level and resistance to host degradative enzymes and nutrient starved conditions.[101]

The primary clinical forms of pulmonary histoplasmosis include acute self-limited disease, chronic cavitary, progressive disseminated, and mediastinal histoplasmosis.[4,102,103] The spectrum of disease is directly tied to the immunologic status of the patient. Most patients with acute self-limited disease are asymptomatic. However, if exposed to large numbers of

organisms, patients may complain of fever, chills, myalgia, and a nonproductive cough. Over the course of the disease, chest radiographs display pulmonary nodules which may or may not calcify areas of cavitation and ipsilateral hilar adenopathy.[66]

Chronic cavitary histoplasmosis may arise from an acute infection or develop after a long period of latency. It usually occurs in adults and may mimic tuberculosis from a clinical and radiologic standpoint. The histoplasmin skin test and the histoplasmin complement fixation test are positive in more than 80% of cases and sputum cultures are usually positive for *Histoplasma capsulatum*. The disease usually affects the upper lobes and patients may develop fibrocavity lesions.[104,105]

Progressive disseminated histoplasmosis is characteristically seen in immunocompromised patients. The clinical picture reflects the aggressive course of the disease with patients developing hemoptysis, weight loss, diarrhea, anemia, purpura, lymphadenopathy, and oropharyngeal ulcers. The mortality rate may reach 80% in untreated patients primarily due to respiratory complications.[4] The radiologic findings with disseminated histoplasmosis include bilateral military or diffuse reticular and nodular opacities which may progress to areas of airspace consolidation.[105,106]

The clinical findings in mediastinal histoplasmosis may be quite variable depending on the stage of the disease. Early in the course of the infection patients may be asymptomatic, but as the disease progresses patients complain of cough, dyspnea, chest pain, and hemoptysis.[107,108] The radiologic findings can also vary. Patients with granulomatous mediastinal disease usually have soft tissue masses that are located in the mid portion of the mediastinum. Over time, these soft tissue masses may undergo calcification. The mediastinal granulomas may also be associated with hilar adenopathy.[109,110] Chest radiographs of patients with fibrosing (sclerosing) mediastinal histoplasmosis may be normal or demonstrate mediastinal or hilar nodal enlargement. There may also be atelectasis due to airway obstruction and interstitial edema/infiltrates due to vascular occlusion by the fibrous tissue[105,109,111]. The fibrous proliferation is thought to represent an abnormal immunologic response to *Histoplasma* antigens.[112]

The pathologic response to histoplasmosis depends to a large extent on the immunologic status of the host. Immunocompetent patients usually develop necrotizing and nonnecrotizing granulomas. The latter may mimic sarcoidosis. These granulomas may appear as solitary lesions, military nodules, or cavitary lesions. With chronic infections, the granulomas may undergo fibrosis, often in a laminar pattern. In addition, these fibrotic granulomas are also prone to calcify. In patients with impaired immunity, there is a pronounce macrophage response without granulomatous inflammation. Dissemination leads to lesions in the bone marrow,

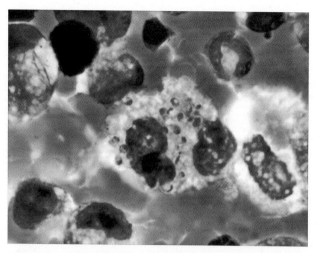

FIGURE 13-10 Numerous intracellular round to oval yeasts are present in macrophages from a BAL sample of a patient with histoplasmosis (modified Giemsa stain).

skin, adrenal glands, lymph nodes, liver, spleen, GI tract, and other sites.[110,113] Confirmation of the diagnosis requires identification of the organism in tissue or cytologic samples. *Histoplasma capsulatum* are yeasts measuring 2 to 5 μm, with narrow-based unequal budding. They may be seen in routine stains and when numerous, appear as small round to ovoid structures within macrophages (*Figure 13-10*). A clear space or artifactual "halo" may be seen on H&E-stained sections due to retraction of the basophilic cytoplasm from the poorly stained cell wall[4] (*Figure 13-11*). Scant number of single yeast forms may be present in old granulomas, making it difficult to establish the diagnosis. Hyphal forms have been rarely seen in cases of intravascular infections.[114] GMS, PAS, and calcofluor stains are useful to highlight the yeasts

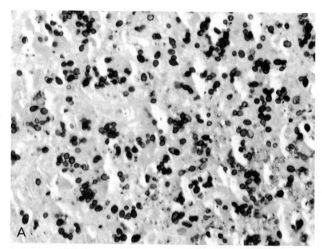

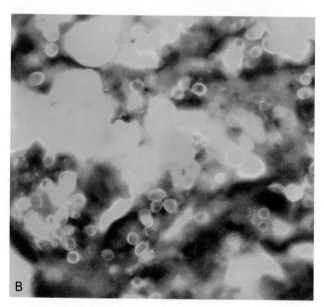

FIGURE 13-12 The corresponding GMS (A) and calcofluor white (B) stain of *Figure 13-11* illustrates numerous budding yeasts. The morphology and size of the yeasts are compatible with *Histoplasma*.

in tissue sections or BAL samples (*Figure 13-12A and B*). It is rare to find yeasts forms in sputum or pleural fluid specimens.

Although occasional intracellular forms of *B dermatitidis* are similar in size (2-5 μm) to *H capsulatum*, most measure 8 to 15 μm and divide by broad-based budding (*Table 13-5*). They also have thick double-contoured cell walls. Capsule-deficient *Cryptococcus neoformans/gattii* is usually weakly positive with mucicarmine and the yeast forms are more variable in size, ranging from 2 to 20 μm. Although the yeast forms of *Candida* sp (2-6 overlap μm) with *H capsulatum*, the presence of pseudohyphae should confirm the diagnosis of *Candida* sp. Yeasts of *P marneffei* are similar in size to *H capsulatum* and are often intracellular.

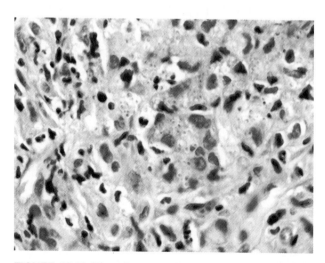

FIGURE 13-11 *Histoplasma* granuloma in a lung biopsy from an HIV patient. Note the "clear halos" around the yeast forms due to cytoplasmic retraction (hematoxylin-eosin stain).

Table 13-5 Morphology of Fungal Yeasts

Fungus	Size (µm)	Budding	Pseudohyphae/Hyphae
H capsulatum	2–5	Single, narrow	Rare
B dermatitidis	8–15	Single, broad	Rare
C neoformans	2–20	Single, narrow	Rare
Candida sp	2–6	Single, narrow	Yes (pseudohyphae)
P marneffei	2–6	No	Yes (short hyphae)

Used with permission from Lung infections. In: Travis WD, Colby TV, Koss MN, Rosado-de-Christenson ML, Müller NL, King TE, eds. Non-neoplastic Disorders of the Lower Respiratory Tract. Bethesda, MD: American Registry of Pathology/Armed Forces Institute of Pathology; 2002:592-638.

However, no budding is seen and short hyphal forms of this organism also exist (*Table 13-5*). Endospores of *Coccidioides* can also be confused with *Histoplasma* yeast.[4,115]

H capsulatum can be more readily cultured from patients with chronic infection. In general, colonies can develop in 3 to 7 days, but some strains may require 4 to 6 weeks to grow. *H capsulatum* can form sterile hyphae, in which case identification can be made with the GenProbe AccuProbe assay, which has largely replaced exoantigen testing.[116]

Serologic tests for histoplasmosis most often use H and M antigens, which are obtained from an extract of *H capsulatum* mycelia. The immunodiffusion test (IM) can be performed with serum or CSF, is qualitative, and is highly specific for detection of antibodies to the H and M antigens.[117] However, in acute infections, the ID test is not very sensitive[118,119] as only 7% of serum specimens from patients with acute infection have any immunodiffusion bands.[120] Upon infection, the M band appears before the H band and can indicate an acute infection, a chronic progressive infection or a past infection. After disease resolution, the antibody to the M antigen can persist up to 3 years, while H antibody can persist for 1 to 2 years. Upon infection, an H band indicates active disease and generally will appear in 2 to 3 weeks. The presence of both H and M bands is considered to be conclusive for the diagnosis of histoplasmosis if the clinician determines that it is consistent with the patient's clinical course of disease.[121-123]

The complement fixation (CF) test employs an extract of *H capsulatum* mycelia and a second antigen obtained from a suspension of *Histoplasma* yeast cells.[124,125] For patients with pulmonary infection with *H capsulatum*, serum is used in testing. The CF test is quantitative, which allows the clinician to follow the titers over different stages of infection and treatment. If the CF test is negative during the acute phase of infection, additional specimens should be tested 3 or 4 weeks later in that CF antibodies turn positive, generally 3 to 6 weeks after onset of infection. After that time, repeated tests will remain positive for months.[126] If the patient

has a 1:32 or greater titer or a fourfold increase in titer, it would indicate an active infection.[121] The CF test detects cross-reactions from other fungal infections, such as blastomycosis, candidiasis, coccidioidomycosis, and paracoccidioidomycosis.[127] The CF test is more sensitive than the immunodiffusion test but less specific.[128]

A third-generation quantitative EIA for detection of *H capsulatum* galactomannan antigen in urine, serum, or BAL fluid was introduced in 2007.[129] A multicenter evaluation of patients with various forms of pulmonary histoplasmosis and who were tested with a third-generation *Histoplasma* galactomannan EIA with urine or serum was reported.[130] For patients with acute pulmonary histoplasmosis, 80% were positive for antigen if both urine and serum were tested.[130,131] In patients with proven or probable cases of progressive disseminated histoplasmosis, antigenuria was detected in 92%, including 95% of those with AIDS, 93% who were immunocompromised, and 73% of those who were not immunocompromised.[130] In combining patients with all forms of pulmonary histoplasmosis, antigenuria was detected in 50% of immunocompromised patients and 41% on nonimmunocompromised patients, whereas the results of tests for antibodies were positive in 90% of immunocompromised and 91% of nonimmunocompromised patients. However, a few cases were positive only with antigenuria.[130] Consequently, it is recommended to test for antigenuria and serum antibodies. BAL specimens were reported positive for *Histoplasma* antigen in 90% of patients with pulmonary histoplasmosis.[132] When using the *Histoplasma* EIA, cross-reactive antigens were detected in 90% of patients with blastomycosis,[129,133] 80% of patients with paracoccidioidomycosis and *P marneffei* infection, 60% with coccidioidomycosis,[129,133] and about 10% of those with aspergillosis.[133]

The GenProbe AccuProbe assay has been used by clinical labs for a number of years for identification of *H capsulatum* from culture. One study correctly identified 41 of 41 *H capsulatum* culture isolates.[133]

There are no FDA-approved PCR-based molecular methods for identification of *H capsulatum* in tissue or body fluids and reports of laboratory-based tests have shown inconsistent results. There are a few reference laboratories that offer PCR-based tests for *H capsulatum*. They will amplify DNA with universal primers for fungi from fungal colonies, fresh tissue, body fluids, or formalin-fixed tissue. There are a limited number of reference laboratories that will also test paraffin-embedded tissue sections. If an amplified product is obtained, it is sequenced for definitive identification.

Coccidioidomycosis

Coccidioidomycosis is a systemic mycosis caused by the dimorphic fungus, *Coccidioides immitis* or *Coccidioides posadasii*.[134] The filamentous (mycelial) form of this fungus thrives in dry, hot desert soil and is endemic throughout the southwestern United States, northern and central Mexico, and parts of Central and South America.[135-139] In the United States, it is estimated that 100,000 new cases of infection occur annually, 35,000 of which are from the state of California.[139] Humans acquire the disease by inhaling infective arthroconidia (spores). Once in the lung, each arthroconidia transforms into multinucleated spherical structures termed spherules. Over time, these spherules grow and divide internally producing large numbers of endospores (800–1000 endospores/mature spherule). Once the endospores are released, they can reinfect locally or spread to other sites via the blood and lymphatic circulation.

Coccidioidomycosis can manifest itself in one of three clinical forms: primary pulmonary disease, progressive pulmonary disease, or disseminated coccidioidomycosis. Primary pulmonary coccidioidomycosis is the most common form of this disease. It is characterized by pulmonary findings that appear 1 to 3 weeks after exposure to the fungus. About 60% patients infected with *Coccidioides* are asymptomatic and spontaneously cured without no clinical or radiologic manifestations. The remaining 40% generally present with symptoms of acute respiratory disease accompanied by fever, night sweats, and cough or pleuritic chest pain. The signs and symptoms usually appear 10 to 15 days after exposure and the severity of the disease parallels the infective fungal load and immunologic status of the patient. In addition to these nonspecific findings, about 20% of patients develop allergic manifestations in the form of erythema multiforme or erythema nodosum. These findings are mostly frequently reported in young Caucasian females.[4,139] Most patients with primary pulmonary disease recover spontaneously without evidence of persistent disease. Primary pulmonary infection with *Coccidioides* results in radiologic findings similar to those encountered in patients with acute histoplasmosis. Chest radiographs show patchy, unilateral, perihilar, or lower lobe consolidation. Approximately 5% of patients develop solitary nodules

that are asymptomatic in most patients. Another 5% of patients develop thin-walled cysts which may resolve spontaneously or persists for years.[139,140]

Progressive pulmonary coccidioidomycosis is generally chronic and develops after the first infection, the symptoms of which do not resolve after the first 2 months. This form of coccidioidomycosis may present as nodular or cavitary lesions or as cavitary lung disease with fibrosis. Due to its chronic progression, progressive pulmonary coccidioidomycosis constitutes an important differential diagnosis with pulmonary tuberculosis.[141,142] Depending on which form of the disease is present, radiologic studies show well-defined, solitary peripheral nodules or unilateral or bilateral apical consolidation, which may cavitate. Complications of these cavity lesions include pleural effusions, pneumothorax, or bronchopleural fistulas if the cavities rupture into the pleural space. In addition, mycetomas may also occur within the cavitary lesions.[4,139,140]

Disseminated infection is the rarest form of primary pulmonary coccidioidomycosis. It occurs in less than 1% of infected patients. Risk factors include race (more common in African Americans versus Caucasians), Group B blood type, diabetes mellitus, hematologic neoplasms, HIV infection, and transplantation. Also, women in their second and third trimesters of pregnancy are at increased risk for disseminated coccidioidomycosis.[141,142] Lesions are found in a variety of sites including the skin, central nervous system, genitourinary system, and bone.[139,141,142] In HIV patients with low CD4 counts (less than 250/mm^3), this disease may be rapidly progressive and fatal.[4] Radiologically, the lungs from patients with disseminated disease have bilateral, diffuse miliary reticular and nodular interstitial opacities.[66]

Acute coccidioidomycosis is characterized by an acute suppurative pneumonitis where the distal airspaces are filled with a neutrophilic infiltrate. As the disease progresses from an acute to chronic stage, necrotizing granulomas are formed which correspond to the nodular lesions seen radiologically. Over time, these granulomas may cavitate and become fibrotic. Subpleural fibrocaseous nodules have also been described in patients with chronic progressive coccidioidomycosis. These nodules consist of a central zone of necrosis surrounded by a dense collagenous fibrous capsule. Although the histologic picture can vary depending on the stage of the disease, identification of the fungus is required to confirm the diagnosis. The organisms are usually found within the neutrophilic infiltrate or in the necrotizing component of the granulomas. In tissue sections and cytologic samples, *Coccidioides* consists of immature spherules, mature spherules, and endospores. The spherules are round to oval and range from 30 to 200 μm in size. Mature spherules have a 1- to 2-μm-thick refractile wall and are filled

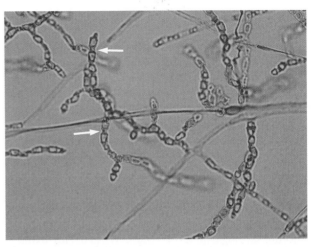

FIGURE 13-14 Mycelial form of *Coccidioides* illustrating chains of barrel-shaped arthroconidia. Arrows denote clear spaces between arthrospores within the hyphae (lactophenol cotton blue stain).

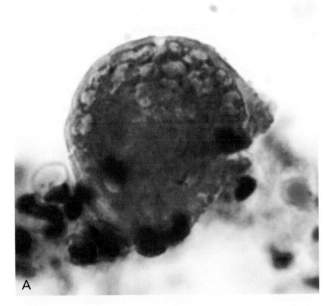

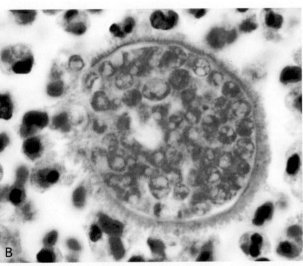

FIGURE 13-13 An FNA-derived sample (A) and corresponding cell block (B) illustrating a spherule of *Coccidioides* containing numerous endospores from an immunocompromised patient with miliary coccidioidomycosis (hematoxylin-eosin stain).

with endospores (*Figure 13-13A* and *B*). In contrast, immature spherules are devoid of endospores and are smaller than their mature counterparts. The uninucleate endospores measure 2 to 5 µm in diameter. All three yeast forms of this fungus are visible with routine stains. In addition, GMS and PAS stains endospores but the spherule wall stains only with GMS. The mycelial form of *Coccidioides* consists of septate hyphae that measure 2 to 4 µm in thickness and chains of barrel-shaped arthroconidia (*Figure 13-14*). Hyphae and arthroconidia are found in 10% to 30% of cavitary lesions,

particularly if they open into major airways.[142] Given the multiple yeast forms seen in *Coccidioides*, it may be confused with other pathogenic fungi (*Table 13-4*). The endospores of *Coccidioides* may be distinguished from *Histoplasma* and *Cryptococcus* by the presence of budding in the latter two. Immature spherules may be confused with *Blastomyces* due to their similar sizes. However, the presence of broad-based budding aids in distinguishing *Blastomyces* from the immature spherules of *Coccidioides*.[4]

Coccidioides spp grow rapidly on almost all routine culture media. On microscopic examination, the hyphae are thin and septate. Thick-walled arthroconidia, alternating with thin-walled empty cells are formed within the hyphae within 10 to 14 days. The arthroconidia are barrel shaped, 2.5 to 4 µm by 3 to 6 µm in size.[143] The production of arthroconidia within hyphae appears similar in *Coccidioides* sp and *Malbranchia*. However, *Malbranchia* does not produce spherules with endospores and the fungus does yield a negative result with exoantigen or DNA probe assays.[144] Spherules can be formed in culture when incubated at 37°C to 40°C on special synthetic media.[143]

Serology tests commonly used to aid in the diagnosis of coccidioidomycosis include latex agglutination (LA) immunodiffusion (ID), complement fixation (CF), and enzyme immunoassay (EIA). The LA assay is highly sensitive but has demonstrated high false-positive rates. A positive LA test must be confirmed by an alternate test for coccidioidal IgM and IgG antibodies[145] and consequently is not commonly used. The ID assay is qualitative and detects IgM in most patients in 1 to 2 weeks after onset of symptoms, may persist for several months and sometimes even longer with pulmonary or disseminated disease.[146] The CF assay is quantitative and reactions are scored as 0 (no fixation of complement), 1+, 2+, 3+, or 4+ at a given serial dilution of serum. A 4+ reaction is significant, whereas 3+ is significant only if the ID assay is also positive. 2+ or 1+ are not significant. A titer of greater than 1:16 in serum often indicates a disseminated infection. However, a lower titer can also indicate a disseminated infection.[147] Serology assays have demonstrated good sensitivity when both CF and ID are used in combination.[146] However, a negative serology test does not exclude infection with *Coccidioides*. A *Coccidioides* EIA to detect IgG and IgM is commercially available. The EIA IgG appears comparable in sensitivity to ID and CF, but the EIA IgM may give false-positive results and should be confirmed with another serologic method. The EIA is not useful in determining antibody titer.[148] Immunocompetent patients were more likely to be seropositive than immunosuppressed patients. When ID, CF, and EIA were considered as a whole, with immunocompromised patients, the sensitivity of the serologic evaluation increased, but was not statistically significant.[149] Among HIV patients with coccidioidomycosis, 60 of 88 (68%) had IgM or IgG serum antibodies, whereas 21 patients (23%) had negative serologic tests, including 17 patients with pulmonary disease.[150]

Fluorescent antibody assays for detection of *C immitis* in infected tissue and antibody in serum have been reported,[146] but are not available commercially or at reference laboratories.

A *Coccidioides* Antigen EIA is available at a reference laboratory (MiraVista Diagnostics, Indianapolis, IN). The antigen detects 0.03 ng/mL of *Coccidioides* galactomannan in urine. Among 24 patients with coccidioidomycosis, 17 (71%) had a positive test. Most of these patients were immunosuppressed and had severe disease. A *Histoplasma* antigenuria assay was positive in 14 of 17 of these patients that were tested, indicating extensive cross-reactivity. The *Coccidioides* antigenuria EIA reacted with 3 of 28 (11%) of specimens from patients with other mycoses, including two with histoplasmosis.[151] The performance of the *Coccidioides* antigenuria EIA in immunocompetent patients has not been established.

For identification of *Coccidioides* from culture with mycelia, the GenProbe AccuProbe Assay provides rapid results with high sensitivity and specificity.[152] Other molecular methods for diagnosis of *Coccidioides* infection hold great promise. Real-time PCR, with primers amplifying a 170 base pair region of the internal transcribed spacer 2 region of *Coccidioides* was reported.[153] PCR correctly identified 40 *Coccidioides* sp from culture with 100% sensitivity and specificity. In addition, a total of 226 respiratory specimens were cultured and the specimens were directly tested by PCR for *Coccidioides*. PCR demonstrated 100% sensitivity and 98.4% specificity compared to culture. PCR and culture were performed on 66 fresh tissue specimens. PCR demonstrated a sensitivity of 92.9% and a specificity of 98.1% versus culture. Conventional nested and real-time PCR has been reported to correctly identify from culture 120 isolates of *C posadasii* and found no false positives.[154] Using primers that targeted the 18S ribosomal RNA genome, Japanese workers detected *Coccidioides* sp in four paraffin-embedded pulmonary tissue specimens.[155] Commercial PCR kits for detection of *C immitis*/*C posadasii* are not available. However, reference laboratories offer universal primers for fungi on BAL fluid, fresh tissue, or paraffin-embedded tissue. If an amplified product is obtained, sequencing is performed which can provide a definitive identification.

Candidiasis

Candidiasis is a fungal infection caused by yeasts that belong to the genus *Candida*. *Candida* spp are common commensal organisms found in the respiratory, gastrointestinal, and urinary tracts. Of the more than 80 recognized species of *Candida*, over 20 are known pathogens in humans. The two most common that are isolated from clinical specimens are *Candida albicans* and *Candida glabrata* (formerly *Torulopsis glabrata*).[156-158] Others include *C tropicalis*, *C pseudotropicalis*, *C krusei*, *C lusitaniae*, *C stellatoidea*, and *C guilliermondii*.[4]

Candida sp normally lives on the skin and mucous membranes without causing infection. They usually are not pathogenic unless the patient becomes immunodeficient and then the organism invades into the tissues. The trigger that converts *Candida* into an invasive pathogen may reside in the chemical composition of the cell wall. Podzorski et al postulate that catabolites of fungal mannan present in the cell wall may contribute significantly to suppression of cell-mediated immunity in candidiasis.[159]

The signs and symptoms of *Candida* infection depend on the area affected by the disease. Most candidal infections result in complications such as redness, itching, and discomfort. An example of localized infections includes oropharyngeal candidiasis, or thrush. This is commonly seen in young infants, patients treated with antibiotics or steroids, and those with immune deficiency states such as AIDS/HIV. Other localized examples are candidal esophagitis and vaginitis and onychomycosis. Primary pulmonary candidiasis is rare. However, 50% to 80% of patients with disseminated candidiasis can have pulmonary involvement.[157] The lung may be involved hematogenously or by aspiration from the upper airways. Patients with pulmonary disease usually present with fever and tachypnea.[160] The radiologic manifestation of pulmonary candidiasis includes bilateral or unilateral airspace consolidation. Pulmonary involvement may be lobar, segmental, or patchy. HRCT findings include bilateral nodular opacities, multifocal ground glass attenuation, and masses of variable size.[161]

The pathologic findings of candidiasis depend on the route of infection (hematogenous or airway inhalation) and the immune status of the patient. Hematogenous dissemination results in a bilateral miliary pattern of disease with numerous discrete nodules involving the lung parenchyma. Histologic examination of the nodules reveal abscesses associated with variable numbers of organisms. Angioinvasion may also be seen leading to hemorrhagic infarction of the involved lung. Airway-associated disease may result in acute bronchopneumonia that is primarily localized to the lower lobes. Morphologically, *Candida* spp are oval yeast-like cells that measure 2 to 6 μm and are usually accompanied by pseudohyphae (*Figure 13-15*). The latter represent elongated yeasts with areas of constriction at points of budding (*Figure 13-16*). All *Candida* spp can produce pseudohyphae, with the exception of *C glabrata*. *C albicans* and *C dubliniensis* are the only *Candida* sp that produces germ tubes.[162] Germ tubes are cylindrical filamentous forms that demonstrate no indentation at the site of attachment to the mother yeast cell (*Figure 13-17*). *Candida* sp stain with PAS, GMS, and Gram stains. *Candida* spp are separated from other yeast forms by the presence of pseudohyphae (*Table 13-5*). These pseudohyphae branch at acute angles, and this finding helps distinguish *Candida* sp from hyphal structures of *Aspergillus* that are septate and display dichotomous branching. Rarely, blastoconidia ("chlamydospore like") are seen in tissue sections. These may be confused with *Cryptococcus*, *Blastomyces*, and *Paracoccidioides* sp.[163] Other potential look-alikes include *H capsulatum*, *Trichosporon heigelii*, and *Malassezia furfur*. *Candida* sp can be distinguished

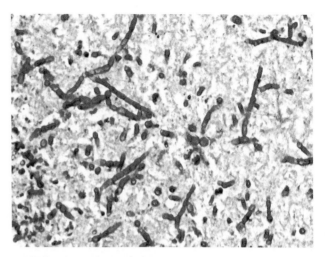

FIGURE 13-16 Photograph of a fungus ball from a patient with bronchocentric candidiasis. The pseudohyphae represent elongated yeasts with areas of constriction and points of budding (PAS stain).

from *Histoplasma* by their extracellular location and Gram stain positivity. The yeast form of *T beigelii* tends to be somewhat larger and more pleomorphic. *M furfur* forms distinctive unipolar broad-base buds but no pseudohyphae.[157,164]

Candida sp grows as moist, creamy colonies within 1 to 3 days at 25°C, 30°C, or 37°C. The addition of chromogens to the agar medium allows the direct detection of specific enzymatic activities characteristic of selected species of *Candida*. These media can be used for simultaneous isolation and presumptive identification of *C albicans*, *C krusei*, and *C tropicalis*. Use of these media shortens the

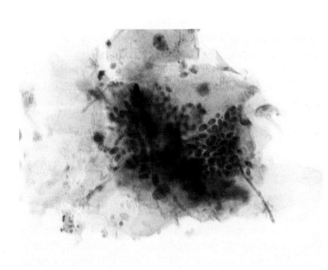

FIGURE 13-15 Positive sputum sample of *Candida* illustrating yeasts and pseudohyphae intermixed with squamous epithelial cells (Papanicolaou stain).

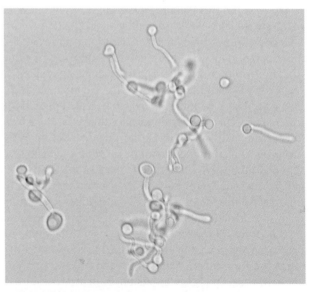

FIGURE 13-17 Wet mount of *Candida albicans* demonstrating numerous germ tube. The germ tube extends from the yeast cell with no constrictions.

time to presumptive identification and allows for easier detection of multiple *Candida* sp in a specimen.

Systemic candidiasis is often characterized by markedly elevated levels of antibodies recognizing *Candida* sp. However, interpretation of *Candida* antibodies is complicated by detection of *Candida* antibodies in 20% to 30% of healthy individuals and by the blunted responses in immunosuppressed patients at risk for systemic candidiasis.[165-167] Consequently, standard immunological tests usually have a low specificity and/ or sensitivity. *Candida* antibody results should be considered in the context of clinical findings and results from relevant laboratory tests, such as *Candida* antigen detection and/or culture. Antibody tests are available by ID, LA, and EIA from reference laboratories. Commercial kits are available to detect a cell-wall component, mannan, or a nonspecific fungal component, β-D-glucan. Studies have evaluated the detection of mannan in serum for diagnosis of invasive candidiasis in hematological and ICU patients and have demonstrated an overall sensitivity of 58% and specificity of 93%.[168-171] Of the various species of *Candida* that have been detected by the mannan assay, *C albicans* demonstrated the highest sensitivity and it was recommended to perform testing two to three times a week in high-risk patients.[170] In another study, a total of 83 serum specimens from seven neutropenic patients with invasive *C tropicalis* were tested with two Platelia *Candida* Mannan EIA's (Biorad Laboratories, Hercules, CA), one for detection of antigen in serum and the other for detection of antibodies in serum. In six patients, at least one positive test was obtained with sera collected, on average, 5 days (range, 2 to 10 days) prior to the first positive blood culture. As controls, 48 serum specimens from 12 febrile neutropenic patients with aspergillosis were tested with the two Platelia *Candida* assays. A low level of the antigen was detected in only one serum specimen and none showed significant *Candida* antibody titers. They concluded that the regular monitoring of both markers could contribute to the earlier diagnosis of *C tropicalis* systemic infections.[172] The Platelia *Candida* EIA now has a combined test that will detect both mannan antigen and antimannan antibody in serum. This assay has resulted in earlier diagnosis of invasive *Candida* infections compared to blood cultures.[173] When compared to imaging, the Platelia mannan antigen/antimannan antibody assay shorten significantly the median time to diagnosis of candidiasis for immunocompromised patients with hepatosplenic lesions.[170]

The Third European Conference on Infections in Leukemia reviewed and analyzed the literature concerning the performance of mannan antigen and antimannan antibody assays and concluded that both tests combined were useful for diagnosis of invasive candidiasis.[174]

There are several companies that manufacture a quantitative β-D-glucan EIA assay for testing in serum.

The Fungitell assay (Associates of Cape Cod, Inc, East Falmouth, MA) has been the most commonly used assay. For patients with a proven or probable invasive fungal infection, the assay has demonstrated an overall sensitivity of 77% and a specificity of 85%.[171,175,176] In patients treated with antifungal agents, the β-D-glucan titers show falling values and eventually become negative in favorable response to therapy.[171,175,176] False-positive results have been noted with treatment with β-lactam antibiotics, gram-negative bacteremia, abdominal surgery and with hemodialysis.[171,175,176] The β-D-glucan assay has not demonstrated false-positive results in patients colonized with *Candida* sp.[169,171,177,178]

An indirect immunofluorescence assay for *C albicans* IgG (Virvell Laboratories, Santa Fe Granada, Spain) can detect antibodies in serum against *C albicans* germ tubes. The sensitivity and specificity of the test has varied from 77% to 89% and 91% to 100%, respectively.[179] One study evaluated the combination of the IFA IgG assay and the β-D-glucan assay in 176 nonneutropenic patients with severe abdominal conditions on the third day after admission to the ICU and twice a week for the next 4 weeks. They found a sensitivity of 90.3%, a specificity of 54.8%, a positive predictive value of 42.4%, and a negative predictive value of 93.9% for invasive *Candida* infections.[180]

In a series of 55 patients with candidiasis, PCR was more sensitive compared to the β-D-glucan assay for diagnosis of invasive candidiasis (80% vs 56%) and deep-seated candidiasis (89% vs 53%). They found that the greatest sensitivity was obtained by combining blood culture with PCR or β-D-glucan, 98% and 79%, respectively.[181]

Cryptococcosis

Pulmonary cryptococcosis is caused by inhalation of spores of *Cryptococcus* sp. There are over 30 species of *Cryptococcus* and the two that are most frequently associated with human and animal infections are *C neoformans* and *C gattii*. Of these two species, *C neoformans* is the more common pathogen associated with human disease.[182]

Cryptococcus is distributed worldwide and the yeast is usually found in soil contaminated with bird droppings. Although cases of *Cryptococcus* were infrequently reported in the medical literature in the United States in the 1940s and 1950s, the incidence of cryptococcosis has steadily increased primarily due to the use of corticosteroids, improved patient survival with certain malignancies, and the onset of AIDS/HIV. The incidence of potentially life-threatening cryptococcal disease among AIDS patients is estimated to be 6% to 10% in the United States, Western Europe, and Australia. It is two to three times higher in sub-Saharan Africa where the incidence varies between

15% to 30%. Despite aggressive therapy, 30% to 60% of these patients succumb to their disease within 12 months of diagnosis.[183,184]

The pathogenesis of cryptococcosis is determined by three broad factors: the status of the host defense mechanism, the virulence of the strain of *C neoformans*, and the size of the inoculum.[185,186] Of these three factors, the integrity of the host defense mechanism is of paramount importance for disease progression. Crucial to the host defense mechanism is an intact cell-mediated immune (CMI) system in order to provide the host the ability to resist infection. The high susceptibility of adults with AIDS to cryptococcosis provides compelling clinical evidence for the importance of an intact CMI system. *C neoformans* is unique among the pathogenic fungi because the yeast is surrounded by an antiphagocytic polysaccharide capsule. Host resistance to cryptococcal infections is dependent on natural defense mechanisms that cope with this essential fungal virulence factor. This can be accomplished in one of three ways: (1) activation of the alternative complement pathway leading to deposition of the opsonic ligand iC3b at the capsular surface, (2) presence of essential cytokines which upregulate the efficiency of complement-dependent phagocytosis, and (3) availability of phagocytic cells whose complement receptors are capable of appropriate upregulation.[187]

Cryptococcal infection has two primary clinical forms: pulmonary infection and cerebromeningeal infection due to hematogenous spread from the lung.[188] Other sites of infection that have been reported in immunocompromised patients include the adrenals, heart liver, lymph nodes, joints, and kidneys.[185,186,188] Patients with primary pulmonary cryptococcosis are usually asymptomatic. When symptoms are present they include cough, chest pain, sputum production, weight loss, fever, and hemoptysis. Other less common symptoms include dyspnea and night sweats.[185,186,188] Most patients (70%–90%) with cerebromeningeal involvement present with signs and symptoms of subacute meningitis or meningoencephalitis, such as headache, fever, lethargy, coma, personality changes, and memory loss.[189] Examination of the cerebrospinal fluid will show increase protein, mononuclear pleocytosis, and a reduced glucose level.

The radiologic manifestations of pulmonary cryptococcosis are usually localized to the upper lung lobes. They include nodules or masses that may or may not have well-defined borders. In addition, there may also be unilateral or bilateral parenchymal consolidation which may contain air bronchograms. Cavitation, calcification, and pleural effusions are rarely seen pulmonary cryptococcal infections.[190,191] Immunocompromised patients with disseminated disease may exhibit diffuse, bilateral reticular, and nodular interstitial densities or diffuse military nodules. Bilateral parenchymal

consolation may also occur within disseminated form of pulmonary cryptococcosis.[190]

The histologic findings of cryptococcal infection depend on the immune status of the patient. Patients with intact immune systems usually have fibrocaseous granulomas or granulomatous pneumonia, whereas immunocompromised patients have extensive tissue infiltration by organisms in a pneumonic fashion or mucoid infiltrates with minimal tissue response. Regardless of the histologic pattern of response, confirmation of cryptococcal infection requires identification of the yeast in tissue or cytologic samples. The organisms are round, budding yeast forms which usually measure 4 to 7 μm in diameter, but range from 2 to 20 μm (*Table 13-5*). The yeast is eosinophilic to basophilic, oval to elliptical in shape, and occasionally appears refractile. Budding is usually single and narrow based. The cells appear to have a halo that represents the thick mucinous capsule characteristic of this organism (*Figure 13-18A* and *B*). The capsule can be visualized

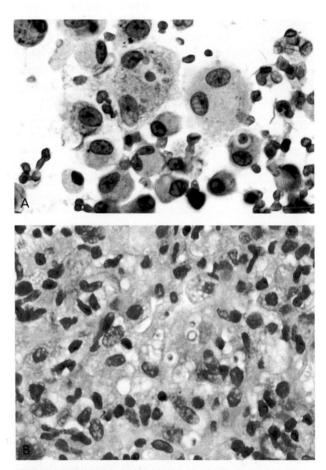

FIGURE 13-18 **BAL sample from a transplant patient illustrating several cryptococcal organisms within alveolar macrophages (A) (Papanicolaou stain). The corresponding tissue biopsy depicts a granuloma containing numerous *Cryptococcus* (B) (hematoxylin-eosin stain). Note the clear halo representing the thick mucinous capsule characteristic of this organism.**

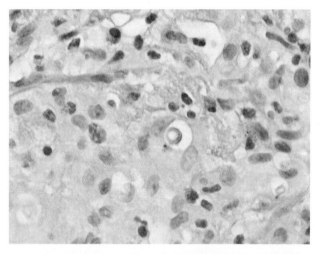

FIGURE 13-19 The mucin stain highlights the mucinous capsule of *Cryptococcus* (mucicarmine stain).

with a variety of stains including mucicarmine, PAS, and Alcian blue (*Figure 13-19*). It is important to remember that a capsule-deficient form of *Cryptococcus* is found in immunocompromised patients. Given the lack of a mucinous capsule, mucicarmine stains will no longer be useful in recognizing the organisms. In these cases, Fontana-Masson stains, immunohistochemistry, or cultures may be necessary to establish the diagnosis.

Given the variable morphology of *Cryptococcus*, it may be confused with a variety of yeast-forming fungi.[192] The presence of the thick mucinous capsule is a valuable clue in differentiating *Cryptococcus* from other fungi. However, problems arise when trying to differentiate the capsule-deficient form from other fungal yeasts. Capsule-deficient *C neoformans* may be confused with *H capsulatum*, *B dermatitidis*, *S schenckii*, *Candida* sp, and *C immitis*. The Fontana-Masson stain may be helpful in separating the cell-deficient form of *Cryptococcus* from these other fungi since it stains the yeast cell wall and not the capsule.[193] However, sporotrichosis and immature spherules of *C immitis* also stain with the Fontana-Masson stain. From a morphologic standpoint, the distinctive cigar-shaped budding of *S schenckii* and broad-based budding of *B dermatitidis* help differentiate these two fungi from *C neoformans*.

C neoformans/gattii grows well on standard mycology media within 2 to 10 days. A primary medium, Birdseed-Niger seed agar, will enhance detection of these species. The yeast grow equally well at 25°C and 37°C.

Serum antibodies to *Cryptococcus* are not very helpful in diagnosing and deciding treatment for cryptococcosis but are offered by reference labs. Currently, the most commonly used diagnostic tests for *C neoformans/gattii* involve detection of their polysaccharide antigen and include latex agglutination (LA), EIA, and a lateral flow assay (LFA). *Cryptococcus* serum antigen assays are not very sensitive in detecting cryptococcal pneumonia in immunocompetent patients. If these patients are asymptomatic and have a negative serum antigen test, they do not necessarily need a screening lumbar puncture to rule out CNS disease. However, if the immunocompetent patient is antigen positive, dissemination from the lungs is more likely.[194,195] In patients that have HIV, antigen tests are very sensitive in detecting cryptococcal pneumonia and are moderately sensitive in those with other underlying immunocompromising conditions.[196-200] When these patients have cryptococcal pneumonia, it is recommended to obtain CSF, whether the antigen test on serum is positive or negative, to rule out CNS disease, even if they have no symptoms, since cryptococcal meningitis would have a different treatment program.[201] The LFA has been demonstrated to be more sensitive than LA or EIA and can provide both a qualitative and quantitative result in 10 minutes. Quantitative titers are ascertained by serial dilution of the serum and determining the highest dilution that produces a positive result.[202-205] However, the cryptococcal antigen titer is not very precise for use in following therapy.[206] Infections with *Trichosporon asahii* or the bacteria *Stomatococcus* or *Capnocytophaga* has resulted in false-positive cryptococcal antigen tests.[207-209]

There are no commercial PCR kits for *C neoformans/gattii*. But reference laboratories do offer PCR for these fungi.

Sporotrichosis

Sporotrichosis is a disease caused by the dimorphic fungus, *Sporothrix schenckii*. This fungus is found in decaying vegetation, sphagnum moss, and soil.[210,211] Infection usually occurs as a result of cutaneous injury due to thorns, splinters, barbs, etc, that are contaminated from exposure to soil or plant material. Animal to human transmission has also been documented via scratches or bites from infected animals.[212] Although it is distributed worldwide, the majority of cases have been reported from endemic areas in the United States (Oklahoma, Missouri, Mississippi River valley), South America (Brazil, Peru, and Columbia), India, Japan.[213-215] Although the incidence of sporotrichosis is difficult to access, in a remote area of Peru, it is estimated to be approximately 50 to 60 cases/100,000 population.[215]

Sporotrichosis most commonly involves the skin, subcutaneous tissue, and lymphatics. Pulmonary involvement usually results from inhalation of spores of *S schenckii*. Rarely, this organism can disseminate to other sites such as the bones, meninges, and gastrointestinal tract. The disseminated form of this disease has been described in immunocompromised individuals such as alcoholics, diabetics, patients with hematologic malignancies, those receiving corticosteroid therapy, and AIDS/HIV.[213,216] Patients with pulmonary disease usually have symptoms that mimic tuberculosis and include dyspnea, cough, purulent sputum, hemoptysis, fever, night sweats, and weight loss.[217]

The radiologic manifestations of pulmonary sporotrichosis include parenchymal nodules or masses that may undergo cavitation. Diffuse reticular and nodular opacities can also be present. In addition, hilar and mediastinal adenopathy may occur as a component of the parenchymal disease or as an isolated finding.[218]

Histologically, caseous, necrotizing, or suppurative-type granulomas are usually seen in pulmonary sporotrichosis. The yeasts are round, oval, or cigar-shaped and measure 2 to 6 μm in diameter, but can be up to 10 μm. The buds appear elongated or "teardrop" in shape, or they have narrow-based attachments with a "pipe-stem" appearance.[216,219] The yeast forms of *S schenckii* may be difficult to find in tissue sections since they are usually few in number. One important clue for the diagnosis of sporotrichosis is the presence of asteroid bodies in the tissue sections. However, these asteroid bodies are not specific for *S schenckii*, as they can be seen in a variety of granulomatous-related lung diseases such as sarcoidosis. In cytologic samples, the organism stain with calcofluor white (with or without KOH). The yeasts can be seen in H&E stained sections, but are best visualized with GMS or PAS stains.[220]

Given the small size of the yeasts of *S schenckii*, they may be confused with other fungi such as *H capsulatum* and acapsular *Cryptococcus*. However, the elongated, cigar-shaped morphology of *S schenckii* yeasts is not seen with *H capsulatum*. Differentiation from capsule-deficient *Cryptococcus* may be more difficult, as both stain with the Fontana-Masson stain (see cryptococcosis). *S schenckii* may also be confused with Hamazaki-Wesenberg bodies, which also have an elongated cigar-shaped appearance. However, these structures have a yellow-brown color, lack budding, and are smaller than the yeasts of *S schenckii*.[216,219]

Culture is considered the gold standard for the diagnosis of sporotrichosis. The mold phase of *Sporothrix* grows within 5 days of inoculation on standard mycology media at 25°C to 30°C. A wet mount of the mold phase demonstrates hyaline septate hyphae that produce at right angles thin conidiophores. The tip of the conidiophores bare many small tear-shaped or almost round conidia forming a rosette-like cluster (*Figure 13-20*). The mold phase can be converted to the yeast phase on brain heart infusion agar or on blood agar at 37°C. It may require several transfers to obtain a good yeast phase. The yeasts are round, oval, or fusiform with buds and can vary in size (1-3×3-10 μm).[221]

Serology is not useful in the diagnosis of sporotrichosis and is not available at reference labs. Reference labs do offer universal primers for fungi for cultures, BAL fluid, fresh tissue, and paraffin-embedded tissue.

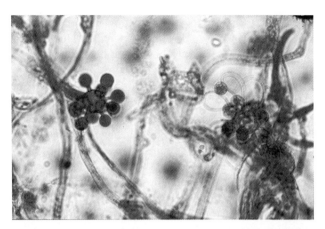

FIGURE 13-20 **Mold phase of *Sporothrix* demonstrating hyphae and a cluster of conidia protruding from a central conidiophore (lactophenol cotton blue stain).**

If an amplified product is obtained, it is sequenced for definitive identification.

Paracoccidioidomycosis

Pulmonary paracoccidioidomycosis (South American blastomycosis) is an infection caused by the thermally dimorphic fungus, *Paracoccidioides brasiliensis*. *P brasiliensis* is endemic in the tropical and subtropical regions of Latin America, extending from Mexico to Argentina. However, it does not occur in every country within this geographic distribution. Brazil accounts for 80% of reported cases; Columbia and Venezuela arc the next most frequent sites of infection.[222,223] Although the true incidence of the disease is not known, within in endemic areas the incidence is believed to be three cases per 100,000 inhabitants.[224]

P brasiliensis occurs as a mycelium in nature, the saprobiotic form of this fungus. The infectious cycle begins with inhalation of conidia (4 μm) or mycelial fragments which are deposited in the distal portions of the lung parenchyma. There, the conidia transform into yeast cells which can disseminate other sites such as lymph nodes, bone, and skin through the lymphatic and venous circulation. Animal-to-human or human-to-human transmission of this fungus has not been reported.[222,225,226]

Two primary clinical forms of paracoccidioidomycosis infections occur in humans. There is an acute/subacute or juvenile and a chronic or adult form. In addition, a subclinical or asymptomatic infection also exists that can be documented by a positive skin test in 10% of the population of Brazil and Colombia.[185,227] The juvenile form represents only 3% to 5% of all cases.[222] This form progresses rapidly (weeks to months) and is marked by involvement of the reticuloendothelial system (spleen, liver, lymph nodes, and bone marrow).

The adult form occurs in more than 90% of patients, most of whom are males and progresses slowly, taking up to several years to become fully established.[222] In contrast to the juvenile form, the lungs represent a primary focus of disease in the adult stage, and in approximately 25% of cases, is the only organ system involved.[222] Respiratory symptoms are nonspecific and include weight loss, chronic cough, fever, and shortness of breath. The radiologic findings of paracoccidioidomycosis are indistinguishable from other fungal infections and can mimic tuberculosis and sarcoidosis. They include nodular, infiltrative, fibrotic, or cavitary lesions. Bilateral linear and reticular opacities and airspace consolidation have also been reported. The lesions are preferentially located in the central and lower portions of the lungs, with sparing of the apices.[228,229]

The histologic changes range from an acute suppurative bronchopneumonia to a granulomatous and fibrosing process. The granulomas may be ill defined or well formed. The yeast cells of *P brasiliensis* are spherical, vary markedly in size (4-60 μm) and have multiple buds attached by narrow necks ("ship's or pilot's wheel" morphology). The presence of multiple buds can provide presumptive identification of paracoccidioidomycosis when found in tissue.[230,231] The yeast wall is thick and doubly contoured. Germ tubes and short hyphal fragments may be seen in lung specimens from immunocompromised patients.[227,232] The number of organisms varies, depending on the stage of the disease. If the infection is active, the organisms can be seen with routine H&E stains. However, in the chronic stage few organisms are present necessitating the use of special stains such as calcofluor white (with or without KOH), GMS, or PAS. The differential includes cryptococcosis, blastomycosis, and sporotrichosis.[227] The characteristic budding and lack of staining with mucicarmine helps separate *P brasiliensis* from *C neoformans*.

The diagnosis of paracoccidioidomycosis is determined by the isolation of the fungus in clinical specimens. *P brasiliensis* grows slowly in culture, generally requiring 20 to 30 days. Mold to yeast conversion requires incubation at 37°C on an enriched medium such as brain heart infusion agar and generally requires 10 to 20 days. At 37°C, the mother yeast cell appears spherical or oval and is 3 to 30 μm in diameter. The mother yeast cell produces multiple buds with a narrow base of attachment.[116]

Double immunodiffusion (DID) serology has been reported for diagnosis, treatment, and monitoring patients with paracoccidioidomycosis.[233] However, studies have demonstrated false-negative results.[234] Counterimmunoelectrophoresis is about as sensitive as DID but shows no enhancement of specificity.[234] EIA assays have shown cross-reactivity with sera from a variety of different fungal infections.[235] Serology assays are not available at reference labs. There are several reports that have described the detection of *P brasiliensis* antigen in urine, CSF, and BAL specimens[236,237] and the decline of antigen levels in serum during effective therapy.[238,239] However, antigen testing for *P brasiliensis* infection is not a routine diagnostic test and is not available at reference labs.

In patients infected with *P brasiliensis*, PCR assays have been reported on sputa, CSF, and paraffin-embedded tissue.[240,241] However, routine use of molecular diagnosis is not performed in clinical labs. Reference labs offer universal primers for fungi on cultures, BAL fluid, fresh tissue, or paraffin-embedded tissue. If an amplified product is obtained, sequencing is performed and can provide a definitive identification.

Zygomycosis (Mucormycosis)

Zygomycosis is a potentially fatal infection caused by fungi of the class *Zygomycetes*, comprised of the orders *Mucorales* and *Entomophthorales*. Of these two orders, the majority of human infections are caused by *Mucorales* (mucormycosis). Among this order, *Rhizopus oryzae* (*Rhizopus arrhizus*) is by far the most common cause of infection. Other less frequently isolated organisms include *Absidia corymbifera*, *Apophysomyces elegans*, *Cokeromyces*, *Syncephalastrum*, and *Cunninghamella* sp.[242-245] The *Zygomycetes* are ubiquitous in nature and are found in decaying organic matter. Cases have been reported worldwide, in both developed and developing countries. In developed countries, mucormycosis is primarily seen in patients with diabetes mellitus or those with hematologic malignancies receiving chemotherapy or transplant recipients receiving immunosuppressive drugs. Mucormycosis has also been rarely described in patients with AIDS/HIV. In developing countries, the disease is mostly frequently seen in patients with uncontrolled diabetes or trauma[242,243,246,247]. In the United States, the estimated incidence of mucormycosis is 1.7 cases per million people per year, which translates to about 500 cases per year.[248]

In order to cause disease, agents of mucormycosis must extract from the host sufficient iron for growth, evade the host's phagocytic system (mononuclear cells and neutrophils), and gain access to the vascular system for dissemination.[243] Given that iron is required for growth of this organism, presence of elevated available serum iron has been linked to increase susceptibility to mucormycosis. The iron chelating drug, deferoxamine, and diabetic ketoacidosis are two examples that lead to increase iron either by providing this nutrient directly to the fungus (deferoxamine) or possibly through releasing iron from binding proteins in the presence of acidosis.[249,250] The host's phagocytic system is the major defense mechanism against mucormycosis. Neutropenic or immunosuppressed patients cannot mount an effective defense against this organism. In addition, impaired phagocytic activity has also been seen in patients with hyperglycemia and acidosis.[251] Finally, the *Zygomycetes*, like *Aspergillus* sp, are angio-invasive fungal organisms. Studies of *R oryzae* have documented their ability to adhere to endothelial cells and subendothelial matrix proteins in order to facilitate their hematogenous dissemination from the site of origin to other target organs.[252,253]

Most human infections result from inhalation of sporangiospores that have been released in the air, through inoculation of organisms into disrupted skin or mucosa, or ingestion is possible. Once inside the host, the most frequent reported sites of infection include the sinuses (39%), lungs (24%), and skin (19%). Based on these sites of infection and clinical presentation, invasive mucormycosis is classified into one of the following six categories: (1) rhinocerebral (most common form in diabetics), (2) pulmonary, (3) cutaneous, (4) gastrointestinal, (5) disseminated, and (6) rare forms (endocarditis, osteomyelitis, peritonitis, renal infections).[243,246,254]

Pulmonary zygomycosis occurs most often in neutropenic patients receiving chemotherapy and those undergoing hematopoietic stem cell transplants.[243] Symptoms include fever, dyspnea, cough, and pleuritic chest pain. Endobronchial zygomycosis can cause airway obstruction leading to lung collapse. Invasion of hilar blood vessels may result in massive hemoptysis.[246,255] The radiologic findings include, in descending order of frequency: lobar consolidation, isolated masses, nodular disease, and cavitation. Wedge-shaped infarcts and hilar or mediastinal lymphadenopathy have also been reported.[256] On CT scans, the presence of a reversed halo sign characterized by a focal area of ground glass attenuation surrounded by a ring of consolidation is more frequently seen in patients infected with zygomycosis compared to other invasive pulmonary fungal pathogens.[257]

Pulmonary zygomycosis is characterized by angio-invasion associated with thrombosis and hemorrhagic infarction of the lung tissue distal to the involved blood vessel. Granulomatous vasculitis may also be present. The hyphae are broad ranging from 5 to 25 μm. Due to their thin walls, the hyphae frequently appear twisted or folded. The branching pattern is irregular, but 90° branching does occur.[258] When cut on cross section, the hyphae often appear round or oval with clear centers (*Figure 13-21A* and *B*). If the fungus is exposed to ambient air, fruiting bodies or chlamydoconidium may be seen. These structures range in size from 15 to 30 μm. The fungus is visible with routine H&E stains as wells as PAS and GMS stains. The primary differential diagnosis involves *Aspergillus* sp. The presence of septation, rigid walls, and 45° branching would favor a diagnosis of aspergillosis over zygomycosis. Spherical to ovoid, 15 to 30 μm in diameter, thick-walled, hyaline

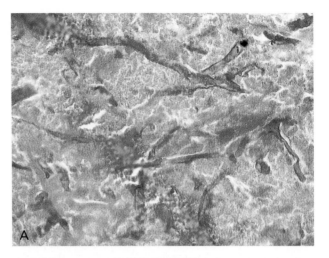

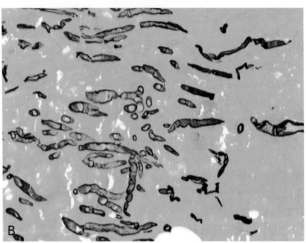

FIGURE 13-21 (A) Cell block from an **FNA** biopsy from a transplant patient with pulmonary zygomycosis (hematoxylin-eosin stain). There are numerous broad, twisted, and branched hyphae that are highlighted in the corresponding GMS stain preparation **(B)**.

chlamydospores can be found in tissue. They are PAS and H&E positive but stain poorly with GMS. Sometimes, the chlamydospores do not stain and appear as empty rings. The chlamydospores can resemble immature spherules and arthroconidia of *C immitis* or yeast forms of *B dermatitidis*. In pulmonary infections, chlamydospores can be located in alveoli and bronchial lumens.

Zygomycetes do not survive more than a few hours at 4°C. If culture is delayed, storage at room temperature is recommended.[259] Zygomycetes have thin-walled hyphae which become easily damaged when biopsies are taken or during tissue preparation in the lab. Tissue should be gently minced and thin slices placed onto the culture medium.[259,260] Only 15% to 25% of cases yield a positive culture.[261] Definitive identification of zygomycetes requires isolation of colonies on standard fungal media. Fungal media with antibiotics can be used with sputum or BAL specimens. However, fungal media should not contain cycloheximide, which will inhibit Zygomycetes growth. Zygomycetes grow within 3 to 5 days at 25°C or 30°C. In addition, they can also grow at 54°C to 58°C, a useful distinguishing characteristic to separate this organism from other pathogenic fungi. Zygomycetes are common in the environment, so a positive culture from nonsterile site does not always indicate infection.[262]

Antibodies to zygomycetes have been reported by ELISAs, DID, and immunoblot analysis.[263,264] However, these serological tests have not been clinically validated and are not available commercially or at reference labs. Antigen and immunohistochemistry for Zygomycetes are under investigation but are not available commercially or at reference labs. There are a number of publications using in situ hybridization or PCR for detection and identification of zygomycetes in tissue or body fluids.[265-269] However, no commercial kits are available. Reference labs do offer PCR for zygomycetes. Universal primers for fungi with sequencing of amplified products are also available at reference labs.

Blastomycosis

Pulmonary blastomycosis is an infection caused by inhalation of the dimorphic fungus, *B dermatitidis*. *B dermatitidis* is endemic to north central United States and southern central Canada, with somewhat lower-level endemicity in the southeastern United States.[270,271] Endemic disease has also been reported in other countries such as Africa, India, South America, and Israel.[272] In the United States, the incidence of blastomycosis has been rising in some regions of the country, particularly in the Midwest. For example, in Illinois the number of cases reported to the Department of Public Health in 2004 was 94 while during the previous 10 years, 500 cases were reported to public health authorities.[273]

B dermatitidis resides in soil or organic matter. The mycelial form releases infective conidia which are subsequently inhaled by a susceptible host. Once inside the lungs, the conidia transform themselves into the pathogenic yeast phase within the distal airways. The phagocytic action of alveolar macrophages, neutrophils, and monocytes provides natural resistance to infection with conidia of *B dermatitidis*, and alveolar macrophages have also been shown to inhibit the transformation of conidia to the pathogenic yeasts.[274,275] If the host fails to contain the infection, lymphohematogenous dissemination to other sites such as the skin, bones, and genitourinary system can occur.

The consequences of infection with *B dermatitidis* are variable and range from subclinical infection to fatal disseminated disease. Symptoms of acute infection are similar to that of an acute bacterial pneumonia and include fever, cough, myalgia, and pleurisy.[276] Chronic infection is more common and patients complain of

productive cough, low-grade fever, hemoptysis, weight loss, and pleuritic chest pain. Blastomycosis has also been reported in patients with AIDS/HIV and those receiving prolonged corticosteroid therapy or cytotoxic drugs for hematologic or solid malignancies. In these cases, the disease is usually much more aggressive compared to infections involving immunocompetent hosts.[185]

The radiologic changes associated with pulmonary blastomycosis may present as focal or diffuse areas of parenchymal consolidation, which typically affects the upper lobes. Solitary or multiple nodules or masses occur in about 30% of cases and if associated with hilar and/or mediastinal lymphadenopathy, can mimic a neoplastic process. A miliary pattern similar to that of miliary tuberculosis is seen in up to 11% of cases, and cavitation has reported in about 6% to 37% of cases.[277-279] CT features of blastomycosis include air bronchograms, localized nodules or masses, and areas of consolidation.[280]

The histologic reaction to pulmonary blastomycosis is typically suppurative, with a marked neutrophil response associated with abscess formation. Necrotizing granulomatous inflammation has also been described with this fungal pathogen. Over time, these granulomas may become fibrotic and cavitary. The number of yeast forms can vary depending on the stage of the disease. Usually, they are more numerous in the acute versus chronic stage of the disease. The yeasts are oval and refractile with double-contoured walls and display broad-based budding (*Figure 13-22A* and *B*). They can be found inside or outside of macrophages and typically measure 8 to 15 μm, but can range up to 30 μm in size.[273,281] Rarely, germ tubes, multiple buds, pseudohyphae, and septate hyphae are seen in tissue. If numerous, the yeasts can be seen with routine H&E stains. Special stains that are useful in identifying this organism include GMS and PAS stains.[282] The larger yeast forms of *B dermatitidis* need to be differentiated from capsule-deficient *C neoformans*. The presence of broad-based budding is a useful clue in differentiating these two organisms. In addition, the Fontana-Masson stain is positive with *C neoformans*, but negative with *B dermatitidis*. Given the variable size of the yeasts, other fungal pathogens that may be mistaken for *B dermatitidis* are *C immitis* and *H capsulatum*.[282]

A single sputum specimen has yielded a positive culture in up to 75% of patients, while the positivity rate for multiple specimens was as high as 86%. BAL specimens can yield a positive culture in up to 92% of patients.[282] Since sputum, BAL, or bronchial wash specimens can be contaminated with bacteria or colonizing yeast, growth media should contain antibacterial agents and cycloheximide.[283] Sterile lung tissue should be cultured on nonselective media. *B dermatitidis* is not known to colonize patients or contaminate clinical specimens, so

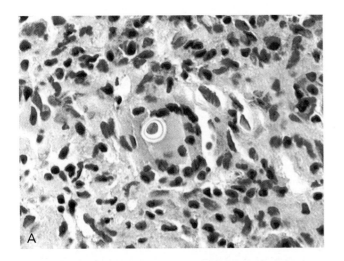

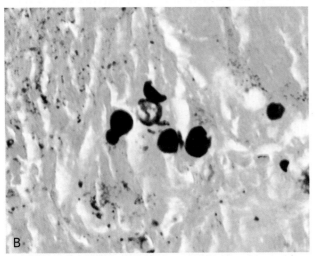

FIGURE 13-22 Multinucleated giant cell with an engulfed yeast of *Blastomyces*. Note the thick refractile wall surrounding the yeast cell (A) (hematoxylin-eosin stain). The GMS stain illustrates the characteristic broad-based budding of *Blastomyces* yeasts (B).

growth of the organism in culture confirms the diagnosis. Growth can occur in several days but can require up to 4 weeks when incubated at room temperature or 30°C. For definitive identification, the hyphal growth can be converted to the characteristic yeast form if grown at 37°C on media such as brain heart infusion agar with sheep blood. The yeast form generally grows in 2 to 3 days, although some isolates require several weeks. They appear as a buttery-like soft colony with a tan color. *B dermatitidis* hyphal growth can also be identified in a matter of hours with the GenProbe AccuProbe assay.[20] False-positive *B dermatitidis* results have been reported with *P braziliense*[284] and *Gymnascella hyalmospora*.[285] There is only a single reported case of *G hyalmospora* causing a pulmonary infection.[286]

Serologic testing by ID, CF, and EIA assays are generally not useful in the diagnosis of blastomycosis.[286]

While purified surface antigens for *B dermatitidis* have somewhat improved these assays, there is still extensive cross-reactivity with other fungi, including *H capsulatum*.[287] ID assays have good specificity for *B dermatitidis* but sensitivity is in the range of 2%8 to 64%.[26,27] CF tests have both poor specificity and low sensitivity, while EIAs have a fair specificity but a very poor sensitivity.[287-291] The MiraVista Blastomyces dermatitidis Quantitative Antigen EIA is used to assist in blastomycosis diagnosis, in monitoring therapy to determine when treatment can be stopped and to diagnose relapse of infection. The assay requires a minimum of 0.5 mL for urine and BAL specimens an 1.0 mL for serum, CSF, and other body fluids. It is recommended that both serum and urine specimens be tested in parallel. Detection of *B dermatitidis* antigenuria in 27 patients recently diagnosed with blastomycosis was 85%, while 50 control patients were negative for antigenuria.[292] To monitor therapy with antifungal agents, it is recommended to collect specimens at least 14 days after starting therapy and testing this specimen, as well as the last positive specimen in parallel. For those receiving antifungal therapy, antigen levels declined for those on effective therapy and increased with treatment failure.[293,294] PCR-based molecular diagnostic tests have been performed on various body fluids (eg, sputum, pleural fluid, BAL fluid, bronchial washes) and paraffin-embedded tissue.[295-298] There are a few reference labs that offer molecular diagnostic tests that can identify *B dermatitidis*. The reference labs will perform universal primers for fungi on cultures, BAL fluid, pleural fluid, tissue, or paraffin-embedded tissue. The amplified product is then sequenced for definitive identification of almost all fungi, including *B dermatitidis*. These tests have not been FDA approved but have been validated by the labs.

Pseudallescheriasis

Pseudallescheriasis is an infection caused by the dematiaceous fungus *Pseudallescheria boydii*, which represents the sexual state of the fungus *Scedosporium apiospermum*. Dematiaceous fungi are septate fungi that have brown-black cell walls due to the presence of a melanin-like pigment. Other dematiaceous fungal pathogens include *Bipolaris*, *Exophiala*, *Alternaria*, *Xylohypha*, and *Curvularia*. These dematiaceous fungi are associated with a variety of diseases including chromoblastomycosis, mycetomas, and phaeohyphomycosis. The latter is characterized by deep infections involving the eyes, skin, respiratory system, brain, and bone.[299-303]

P boydii is a ubiquitous filamentous fungus that is commonly found in temperate climates. It is usually present in soil, sewage, polluted waters, and the manure of farm animals.[304] In the United States, this organism is prevalent in the southern United States and California, but human infections have been described in the northern United States as well.[304] Within these geographic regions, *P boydii* infections are most frequently seen in immunocompromised patients or those with hematologic malignancies.[305-307] Given the significant risk factor of immunosuppression and development of invasive disease, the virulence of this fungus may be related to interactions between the cell wall and human monocytes. Bittencourt et al isolated and characterized an α-glucan from the cell wall of *P boydii* to determine its role in the induction of innate immune response.[308] They discovered that soluble α-glucan leads to a dose-dependent inhibition of phagocytosis fungal fruiting bodies (conidial phagocytosis). In addition, there was a decrease in the rate of phagocytosis when α-glucan was removed from the conidial surface by enzymatic digestion. This interaction may play a role in internalization of *P boydii* by macrophages. Other substances which may also be involved in the pathogenesis of pseudallescheriasis include interleukins 6, 8, and 15.[304]

Infections caused by *P boydii* can be localized with extension into deep soft tissues or disseminate hematogenously to other sites such as the bone/joints, abdomen, central nervous system, eye, and lymph nodes. The disseminated form of this disease is mostly seen among immunocompromised patients.

Pulmonary *Pseudallescheria* occurs when conidia enter the respiratory tract via inhalation. Germination of conidia results in hyphal invasion of the lower respiratory tract. Predisposing factors that lead to colonization of the respiratory tract include tuberculosis, sarcoidosis, and previous bacterial infections that result in cysts and cavities.[309] Patients may have no or minimal symptoms. Some may develop an allergic reaction to the fungus (allergic bronchopulmonary pseudallescheriasis). In these cases, patients may display expiratory wheezing, dyspnea, persistent cough with adherent sputum, and eosinophilia.[310,311] The radiologic findings are similar to those of aspergillosis. They include fungus balls within preexisting cavities, bronchiectasis, and abscesses with central cavitation.[312]

P boydii hyphae are septate and branching. However, in contrast to *Aspergillus*, the branching pattern has a haphazard arrangement.[313] The hyphae are narrow, measuring 2 to 5 μm in diameter. Conidia may also be present, usually within fungus balls. They are ovoid and measure 5 to 10 μm, and are located terminally or laterally on short conidiophores. *P boydii* can be visualized with routine H&E stains or special stains such as GMS and PAS in either histologic or cytologic samples. Although the branching pattern between *Aspergillus* and *Pseudallescheria* is different, there is some overlap in the branching pattern, especially with *A fumigatus*.[314] In these cases, examination of the conidia may be helpful in separating these fungi. Otherwise, culture will be needed for definitive diagnosis.

Colonies of *P boydii* grow rapidly at 25°C or 30°C and mature in 2 to 3 weeks. At 37°C, colonies are yeast-like, white, heaped, wrinkled, or folded. Mold to yeast conversion occurs on enriched media such as brain heart infusion agar following 10 to 20 days of incubation. The mother yeast cell produces multiple buds which surround the whole surface. The daughter cells are attached to the mother cell by a narrow neck portion. Before the bud is detached from the mother cell, secondary buds may form, producing short chains of yeast cells. Immunohistochemistry and direct immunofluorescence tests have been used for fungal identification,[315,316] but are not commercially available. Serologic or antigen tests are not used in clinical diagnosis and molecular tests are not available commercially. Reference labs do offer universal primers for fungi from culture, BAL fluid, fresh tissue, or paraffin-embedded tissue.

Fusariosis

Fusariosis is a mycosis caused by *Fusarium* sp, which are ubiquitous soil saprophytes. Within this genus, there are three species that are frequently implicated in human infections: *Fusarium solani*, *Fusarium oxysporum*, and *Fusarium moniliforme*.[317] *Fusarium* spp are widely distributed in soil, plants, and air. They are common in tropical and temperate regions but are also found in the desert, alpine, and artic regions.[318] Wind and rain effectively disperse *Fusarium* sp. This is one reason why a survey of airborne fungi conducted in the United States documented that *Fusarium* spp were more commonly recovered from air samples than were *Aspergillus* sp.[319] The pathogenesis of human infections may be related to substances produced by this fungus. Studies have shown that *Fusarium* sp produces cyclosporine A, trichothecene, and fumonisin, which enhance the pathogenic potential of this fungus. Trichothecene and fumonisin are mycotoxins which act to suppress cellular immunity and cause tissue breakdown.[317,320]

Risk factors for infection vary depending on the immunologic state of the host. Tissue breakdown from direct trauma, the presence of a foreign body in a colonized patient, severe burns in previously healthy individuals are the usual risk factors in nonimmunosuppressed patients. Disseminated disease is frequently seen in immunocompromised patients. The latter include neutropenic states, hematologic malignancies, and transplant recipients.[317,321,322] Disseminated infection usually presents with persistent fever refractory to antibacterial and antifungal agents, myalgias, and signs and symptoms related to multiorgan involvement. Although this fungus infects multiple sites, the most frequent sites of disseminated disease are the skin, sinuses, and lungs. Pleuritic chest pain, fever, cough, and hemoptysis occur in patients with pulmonary involvement. The clinical picture can mimic pulmonary aspergillosis.[322] However, in contrast to aspergillosis, infection with *Fusarium* sp is associated skin and subcutaneous lesions and positive blood cultures.[322-324] Radiologic manifestations of pulmonary fusarial infection mimic aspergillosis and include nonspecific infiltrates (most commonly) to nodular and/or cavitary lesions.[317]

In tissue, the hyphae of *Fusarium* sp are septate, measure 3 to 8 μm in diameter, and branch at acute or right angles. The branches may show prominent constrictions at their site of origin. In addition, the production of both macroconidia (multicellular, banana-like clusters) and microconidia (unicellular, ovoid to cylindrical spores) are characteristic of this fungus. Although both *Aspergillus* sp and *Fusarium* sp have septate branched hyphae, the presence of both 45°C and 90°C branching with *Fusarium* sp is a helpful clue to distinguish this fungus from *Aspergillus* sp. In cases where this is difficult, cultures or immunohistochemistry may be needed to confirm the diagnosis.[325]

Fusarium sp grows rapidly at 25°C or 30°C C. The hyphae are hyaline, septate and may produce intercalated or terminal chlamydoconidium. They are two or more celled, thick-walled, smooth, and cylindrical or sickle-shaped and tend to accumulate in balls or rafts. Most species produce chains of microconidia which are 2-4 × 4-8 μm in size and are formed on long or short conidiophores.[326]

Serologic tests for *Fusarium* sp are not used for clinical diagnosis and serology or immunohistochemistry kits are not commercially available. β-D-Glucan is a cell-wall constituent of many pathogenic fungi and is detectable in patients serum during invasive disease, including *Fusarium* sp.[327] Two-hundred eighty-three patients who had acute myeloid leukemia or myelodysplasia syndrome and who were receiving antifungal prophylaxis had serum specimens tested for β-D-glucan with the Fungitell assay. The assay was positive a median of 10 days before the clinical diagnosis in 100% of patients of proven or probable invasive fungal infection. This included cases of candidiasis, fusariosis, trichosporonosis, and aspergillosis.[328]

There are no FDA approved molecular tests for *Fusarium* sp. Reference labs offer universal primers for fungi on cultures, tissue, and paraffin-embedded tissue with sequencing of amplified amplicons.

REFERENCES

1. Dunn DL. Diagnosis and treatment of opportunistic infections in immunocompromised patients. *Am Surg.* 2000;66(2):117.
2. Dichter JR, Levine SJ, Shelhamer JH. Approach to the immunocompromised host with pulmonary symptoms. *Hematol Oncol Clin North Am.* 1993;7(4):887.
3. Wilson WR, Cockerill FR, Rosenow AC. Pulmonary disease in the immunocompromised host. *Mayo Clin Proc.* 1985;60(9):610.
4. Lung infections. In: Travis WD, Colby TV, Koss MN, Rosado-de-Christenson ML, Müller NL, King TE, eds. *Non-neoplastic Disorders of the Lower Respiratory Tract.* Bethesda, MD: American Registry of Pathology/Armed Forces Institute of Pathology; 2002:592-638.
5. Sutton DA. Specimen collection, transport and processing: mycology. In: Murray PR, ed-in-chief. *Manual of Clinical Microbiology.* 9th ed. Washington, DC: American Society for Microbiology; 2007:1728-1732.
6. LaRocco MT. Reagents, stains and media: mycology. In: Murray PR, ed-in-chief. *Manual of Clinical Microbiology.* 9th ed. Washington, DC: American Society for Microbiology; 2007:1737-1744.
7. Joos L, Tamm M. Breakdown of pulmonary host defense in the immunocompromised host: cancer chemotherapy. *Proc Am Thorac Soc.* 2005;2(5):445.
8. Shea YR. Algorithms for detection and identification of fungi. In: Murray PR, ed-in-chief. *Manual of Clinical Microbiology.* 9th ed. Washington, DC: American Society for Microbiology; 2007:1745-1761.
9. Eyzaguirre E, Hague AK. Application of immunohistochemistry to infections. *Arch Pathol Lab Med.* 2008;132(3):424.
10. Reiss E, de Repentigny L, Kuykendall RJ, et al. Monoclonal antibodies against Candida tropicalis mannan: antigen detection by enzyme immunoassay and immunofluorescence. *J Clin Microbiol.* 1986;24(5):796.
11. Blumenfeld W, Kovacs JA. Use of monoclonal antibody to detect Pneumocystis carinii in induced sputum and bronchoalveolar lavage fluid by immunoperoxidase staining. *Arch Pathol Lab Med.* 1988;112(12):1233.
12. Taylor CR, Shan-Rong S, Barr NJ. Techniques for immunohistochemistry: principles, pitfalls and standardization. In: Dabbs DJ, ed. *Diagnostic Immunohistochemistry. Theranostic and Genomic Applications.* 3rd ed. Philadelphia, PA: Saunders Elsevier; 2010:1-41.
13. Relman DA, Falkow S. Identification of uncultured microorganisms: expanding the spectrum of characterized microbial pathogens. *Infect Agents Dis.* 1992;1(5):245.
14. McNicol AM, Farquharson MA. In situ hybridization and its diagnostic applications in pathology. *J Pathol.* 1997;182(3):250.
15. Hayden RT, Qian X, Procop GW, Roberts GD, Lloyd RV. In situ hybridization for the identification of filamentous fungi in tissue section. *Diagn Mol Pathol.* 11(2):119.
16. Hayden RT, Qian X, Roberts GD, Lloyd RV. In situ hybridization for the identification of yeast-like organisms in tissue sections. *Diagn Mol Pathol.* 10(1):15.
17. Walsh TJ, Chanock SJ. Diagnosis of invasive fungal infections: advances in nonculture systems. *Curr Clin Top Infect Dis.* 1998;18:101.
18. Padhye AA, Smith G, McLaughlin D, Standard PG, Kaufman L. Comparative evaluation of a chemiluminescent DNA probe and an exoantigen test for rapid identification of Histoplasma capsulatum. *J Clin Microbiol.* 1992;30(12):3108.
19. Padhye AA, Smith G, Standard PG, McLaughlin D, Kaufman L. Comparative evaluation of chemiluminescent DNA probe assay and exoantigen tests for rapid identification of Blastomyces dermatitidis and Coccidioides immitis. *J Clin Microbiol.* 1994;32(4):867.
20. White PL, Perry MD, Barnes RA. An update on the molecular diagnosis of invasive fungal disease. *FEMS Microbiol Lett.* 2009;296(1):1.
21. De Pauw B, Walsh TJ, Donnelly JP, et al. Revised definitions of invasive fungal disease from the European Organization of Research and Treatment of Cancer/Invasive Fungal Infections Cooperative Group and the National Institute of Allergy and Infectious Diseases Mycoses Study Group (EORTC/MSG) Consensus Group. *Clin Infect Dis.* 2008;46(12):1813.

22. Ehrlich GD, Alexa-Sirko D. PCR and its role in clinical diagnostics. In: Ehrlich GD, Greenberg SJ, eds. *PCR-based Diagnosis in Infectious Disease*. Boston, MA: Blackwell Scientific Publications; 1994:3-18.

23. Arends MJ, Bird CC. Recombinant DNA technology and its diagnostic applications. *Histopathology*. 1992;21(4):303.

24. Guedes HL, Guimarães AJ, Muniz Mde M, et al. PCR assay for identification of Histoplasma capsulatum based on the nucleotide sequence of the M antigen. *J Clin Microbiol*. 2003;41(2):535.

25. Hsiao CR, Huang L, Bouchara JP, et al. Identification of medically important molds by an oligonucleotide assay. *J Clin Microbiol*. 2005;43(8):3760.

26. Yeo SF, Wong B. Current status of nonculture methods for diagnosis of invasive fungal infections. *Clin Microbiol Rev*. 2002;15(3):465.

27. Stringer J, Beard CB, Miller RF. A new name (*Pneumocystis jiroveci*) for pneumocystis from humans. *Emerg Infect Dis*. 2002;8(9):891.

28. Watts JC, Chandler FW. Pneumocystosis. In: Connor DH, Chandler FW, Manz HJ, et al, eds. *Pathology of Infectious Diseases*. Stamford, CT: Appleton & Lange; 1997:11-19.

29. Carmona EM, Limper AH. Update on the diagnosis and treatment of *Pneumocystis* pneumonia. *Ther Adv Resp Dis*. 2011;5(1):41.

30. Demanche C, Wanert F, Barthélemy M, et al. Molecular and serologic evidence of Pneumocystis circulation in a social organization of health macaques (*Macaca fascicularis*). *Microbiology*. 2005;151(pt 9):3117.

31. Icenhour CR, Rebholz SL, Collins MS, Cushion MT. Early acquisition of *Pneumocystis carinii* in neonatal rats as evidenced by PCR and oral swabs. *Eukaryot Cell*. 2002;1(3):414.

32. Hagmann S, Merali S, Sitnitskya Y, et al. *Pneumocystis carinii* infection presenting as an intra-abdominal cystic mass in a child with acquired immunodeficiency syndrome. *Clin Infect Dis*. 2001;33(8):1424.

33. Panos GZ, Karydis I, Velakoulis SE, Falagas ME. Multi-skeletal *Pneumocystis jiroveci* (*carinii*) in an HIV-seropositive patient. *Int J STD AIDS*. 2007;18(2):134.

34. Thomas CF, Limper AH. Current insights into the biology and pathogenesis of *Pneumocystis* pneumonia. *Nature Rev Microbiol*. 2007;5(4):298.

35. Boiselle PM, Crans CA Jr, Kaplan MA. The changing face of Pneumocystis carinii pneumonia in AIDS patients. *AJR AM J Roentgenol*. 1999;172(5):1301.

36. Bergin CJ, Wirth RL, Berry GJ, Castellino RA. Pneumocystis carinii pneumonia: CT and HRCT observations. *J Comput Assist Tomogr*. 1990;14(5):756.

37. Bedrossian CW. Ultrastructure of Pneumocystis carinii: a review of internal and surface characteristics. *Semin Diagn Pathol*. 1989;6(3):212.

38. Travis WD, Pittaluga S, Lipschik GY, et al. Atypical pathologic manifestations of Pneumocystis carinii pneumonia in the acquired immunodeficiency syndrome. Review of 123 lung biopsies from 76 patients with emphasis on cysts, vascular invasion, vasculitis, and granulomas. *Am J Surg Pathol*. 1990;14(7):615.

39. Cushion MT. Pneumocystis. In: Murray PR, ed-in-chief. *Manual of Clinical Microbiology*. 9th ed. Washington, DC: American Society for Microbiology; 2007:11789-1801.

40. Raab SS, Cheville JC, Bottles K, Cohen MB. Utility of Gomori methenamine silver stain in bronchoalveolar lavage. *Mod Pathol*. 1994;7(5):599.

41. Fraire AE, Kemp B, Greenberg SD, et al. Calcofluor white stain for the detection of Pneumocystis carinii in transbronchial lung biopsy specimens: a study of 68 cases. *Mod Pathol*. 1997;10(4):395.

42. Ng VL, Yajko DM, Hadley WK. Update on laboratory tests for the diagnosis pulmonary disease in HIV-1 infected individuals. *Semin Respir Infect*. 1993;8(2):86.

43. Khan MA, Farrag N, Butcher P. Detection of Pneumocystis carinii pneumonia: immunofluorescence staining, simple PCR or nPCR. *J Infect*. 1999;39(1):77.

44. Procop GW, Haddad S, Quinn J, et al. Detection of Pneumocystis jiroveci in respiratory specimens by four staining methods. *J Clin Microbiol*. 2004;42(7):3333.

45. Onishi A, Sugiyama D, Kogata Y, et al. Diagnostic accuracy of serum 1,3-beta-D-glucan for Pneumocystis jiroveci pneumonia, invasive candidiasis, and invasive aspergillosis: systematic review and meta-analysis. *J Clin Microbiol*. 2012;50(1):7.

46. Durand-Joly I, Chabé M, Soula F, et al. Molecular diagnosis of Pneumocystis pneumonia. *FEMS Immunol Med Microbiol*. 2005;45(3):405.

47. Wakefield AE, Pixley FJ, Banerji S, et al. Amplification of mitochondrial ribosome RNA sequences from Pneumocystis carinii DNA of rat and human origin. *Mol Biochem Parasitol*. 1990;43(1):69.

48. Alanio A, Desoubeaux G, Sarfati C, et al. Real-time PCR assay-based strategy for differentiation between active Pneumocystis jiroveci pneumonia and colonization in immunocompromised patients. *Clin Microbiol Infect*. 2011;17(10):1531.

49. Kovacs JA, Gill VJ, Meshnick S, Masur H. New insights into transmission, diagnosis and drug treatment of Pneumocystis carinii pneumonia. *JAMA*. 2001;286(19):2450.

50. Olsson M, Strålin K, Holmberg H. Clinical significance of nested polymerase chain reaction and immunofluorescence for detection of Pneumocystis carinii pneumonia. *Clin Microbiol Infect*. 2001;7(9):492.

51. Latge J. Aspergillus fumigatus and aspergillosis. *Clin Micro Rev*. 1999;12(2):310.

52. Al-Alawi A, Ryan CF, Flint JD, Müller NL. Aspergillus-related lung disease. *Can Respir J*. 2005;12(7):377.

53. Tomlinson JR, Sahn SA. Aspergilloma in sarcoid and tuberculosis. *Chest*. 1987;92(3):505.

54. Raz R, Ephros M, Or R, Polacheck I. Primary pulmonary aspergilloma: case report and review of the literature. *Isr J Med Sci*. 1986;22(5):400.

55. Gefter WB. The spectrum of pulmonary aspergillosis. *J Thorac Imaging*. 1992;7(4):56.

56. Bosken CH, Myers JL, Greenberger PA, Katzenstein AL. Pathologic features of allergic bronchopulmonary aspergillosis. *Am J Surg Pathol*. 1988;12(3):216.

57. Fink JN. Allergic bronchopulmonary aspergillosis. *Chest*. 1985;87(1 suppl):81s.

58. Glimp RA, Bayer AS. Fungal pneumonias. Part 3. Allergic bronchopulmonary aspergillosis. *Chest*. 1981;80(1):85.

59. Ward S, Heyneman LE, Lee MJ, et al. Accuracy of CT in the diagnosis of allergic bronchopulmonary aspergillosis in asthmatic patients. *AJR Am J Roentgenol*. 1999;173(4):937.

60. Ando M, Suga M, Kohrogi A. A new look at hypersensitivity pneumonitis. *Curr Opin Pulm Med*. 1999;5(5):299.

61. Reynolds HY. Hypersensitivity pneumonitis: correlation of cellular and immunologic changes with clinical phases of disease. *Lung*. 1998;166(4):189.

62. Hansell DM, Wells AU, Padley SP, Müller NL. Hypersensitivity pneumonitis: correlation of individual CT patterns with functional abnormalities. *Radiology*. 1996;199(1):123.

63. Lynch DA, Newell JD, Logan PM, et al. Can CT distinguish hypersensitivity pneumonitis from idiopathic pulmonary fibrosis? *AJR Am J Roentgenol*. 1995;165(4):807.

64. Chandler FW, Watts JC. Fungal infections. In: Dail DH, Hammer SP, eds. *Pulmonary Pathology*. 2nd ed. New York, NY: Springer-Verlag; 1994:351-427.

65. Goyal R, White CS, Templeton PA, et al. High attenuation mucous plugs in allergic bronchopulmonary aspergillosis: CT appearance. *J Comput Assist Tomogr.* 1992;16(4):649.
66. McAdams HP, Rosado-de-Christenson ML, Lesar M, et al. Thoracic mycoses from opportunistic fungi: radiologic-pathologic correlation. *Radiographics.* 1995;15(2):255.
67. Stevens DA, Moss RB, Kurup VP, et al. Allergic bronchopulmonary aspergillosis in cystic fibrosis—state of the art. Cystic Fibrosis Foundation Consensus Conference. *Clin Infect Dis.* 2003;37(suppl 3):S225.
68. Sugino K, Hasegawa C, Sano G, Homma S. Pathophysiological study of chronic necrotizing pulmonary aspergillosis. *Jpn J Infect Dis.* 2008;61(6):450.
69. Lovrenski A, Panjković M, Eri Z, et al. Chronic necrotizing pulmonary aspergillosis. *Vojnosanit Pregl.* 2011;68(11):988.
70. Bains SN, Judson MA. Allergic bronchopulmonary aspergillosis. *Clin Chest Med.* 2012;33(2):265.
71. Matsuse H, Tsuchida T, Fukahori S, et al. Dissociation between sensitizing and colonizing fungi in patients with allergic bronchopulmonary aspergillosis. *Ann Allergy Asthma Immunol.* 2013;111(3):190.
72. Greenberger PA, Patterson R. Diagnosis and management of allergic bronchopulmonary aspergillosis. *Ann Allergy.* 1986;56(6):444.
73. Riscili BP, Wood KL. Noninvasive pulmonary Aspergillus infection. *Clin Chest Med.* 2009;30(2):315.
74. Maertens J, Verhaegen J, Lagrou K, Van Eldere J, Boogaerts M. Screening for circulating galactomannan as a noninvasive diagnostic tool for invasive aspergillosis in prolonged neutropenic patients and stem cell transplantation recipients: a prospective validation. *Blood.* 2001;97(6):1604.
75. Sanguinetti M, Posteraro B, Pagano L, et al. Comparison of real-time PCR, conventional PCR, and galactomannan antigen detection by enzyme-linked immunosorbent assay using bronchoalveolar lavage fluid samples from hematology patients for diagnosis of invasive pulmonary aspergillosis. *J Clin Microbiol.* 2003;41(8):3922.
76. Clancy CJ, Jaber RA, Leather HL, et al. Bronchoalveolar lavage galactomannan in diagnosis of invasive pulmonary aspergillosis among solid-organ transplant patients. *J Clin Microbiol.* 2007;45(6):1759.
77. Viscoli C, Machetti M, Gazzola P, et al. Aspergillus galactomannan antigen in the cerebrospinal fluid of bone marrow transplant recipients with probable cerebral aspergillosis. *J Clin Microbiol.* 2002;40(4):1496.
78. Maertens JA, Klont R, Masson C, et al. Optimization of the cutoff value for the Aspergillus double-sandwich enzyme immunoassay. *Clin Infect Dis.* 2007;44(10):1329.
79. Herbrecht R, Letscher-Bru V, Oprea C, et al. Aspergillus galactomannan detection in the diagnosis of invasive aspergillosis in cancer patients. *J Clin Oncol.* 2002;20(7):1898.
80. Mennink-Kersten MA, Donnelly JP, Verweij PE. Detection of circulating galactomannan for the diagnosis and management of invasive aspergillosis. *Lancet Infect Dis.* 2004;4(6):349.
81. Musher B, Fredricks D, Leisenring W, et al. Aspergillus galactomannan enzyme immunoassay and quantitative PCR for the diagnosis of invasive aspergillosis with bronchoalveolar lavage fluid. *J Clin Microbiol.* 2004;42(12):5517.
82. Penack O, Rempf P, Graf B, Blau IW, Thiel E. Aspergillus galactomannan testing in patients with long-term neutropenia: implications for clinical management. *Ann Oncol.* 2008;19(5):984.
83. Marr KA, Laverdiere M, Gugel A, Leisenring W. Antifungal therapy decreases sensitivity of the Aspergillus galactomannan enzyme immunoassay. *Clin Infect Dis.* 2005;40(12):1762.
84. Pfeiffer CD, Fine JP, Safdar N. Diagnosis of invasive aspergillosis using a galactomannan assay: a meta-analysis. *Clin Infect Dis.* 2006;42(10):1417.
85. Miceli MH, Grazziutti ML, Woods G, et al. Strong correlation between serum aspergillus galactomannan index and outcome of aspergillosis in patients with hematological cancer: clinical and research implications. *Clin Infect Dis.* 2008;46(9):1412.
86. Marchetti O, Lamoth F, Mikulska M, et al. ECIL recommendations for the use of biological markers for the diagnosis of invasive fungal diseases in leukemic patients and hematopoietic SCT recipients. *One Marrow Transplant.* 2012;47(2):846.
87. Viscoli C, Machetti M, Cappellano P, et al. False-positive galactomannan platelia Aspergillus test results for patients receiving piperacillin-tazobactam. *Clin Infect Dis.* 2004;38(6):913.
88. Adam O, Aupérin A, Wilquin F, et al. Treatment with pipperacillin-tazobactam and false-positive Aspergillus galactomannan antigen test results for patients with hematological malignancies. *Clin Infect Dis.* 2004;38(6):917.
89. Mattei D, Rapezzi D, Mordini N, et al. False-positive Aspergillus galactomannan enzyme-linked immunosorbent assay results in vivo during amoxicillin-clavulanic acid treatment. *J Clin Microbiol.* 2004;42(11):5362.
90. DelBono V, Mikulska M, Viscoli C. Invasive aspergillosis: diagnosis, prophylaxis and treatment. *Curr Opin Hematol.* 2008;15(6):586.
91. Almyroudis NG, Segal BH. Prevention and treatment of invasive fungal diseases in neutropenic patients. *Curr Opin Infect Dis.* 2009;22(4):385.
92. Stynen D, Sarfati J, Goris A, et al. Rat monoclonal antibodies against Aspergillus galactomannan. *Infect Immunol.* 1992;60(6):2237.
93. Swanink CM, Meis JF, Rijs AJ, Donnelly JP, Verweij PE. Specificity of a sandwich enzyme-linked immunosorbent assay for detecting Aspergillus galactomannan. *J Clin Microbiol.* 1997;35(1):257.
94. Wheat LJ, Hackett E, Darkin M, et al. Histoplasmosis-associated cross-reactivity in the BioRad Platelia Aspergillus enzyme immunoassay. *Clin Vaccine Immunol.* 2007;14(5):638.
95. Luong ML, Clancy CJ, Vadnerkar A, et al. Comparison of an Aspergillus real-time polymerase chain reaction assay with galactomannan testing of bronchoalveolar lavage for detection of invasive pulmonary aspergillosis in lung transplant recipients. *Clin Infect Dis.* 2011;52(10):1218.
96. Buess M, Cathomas G, Halter J, et al. Aspergillus PCR in bronchoalveolar lavage for detection of invasive pulmonary aspergillosis in immunocompromised patients. *BMC Infect Dis.* 2012;12:237.
97. Cuenca-Estrella M, Meije Y, Diaz-Pedroche C, et al. Value of serial quantification of fungal DNA by a real-time PCR-based technique for early diagnosis of invasive aspergillosis in patients with febrile neutropenia. *J Clin Microbiol.* 2009;47(2):379.
98. Mengoli C, Cruciani M, Barnes RA, Loeffler J, Donnelly JP. Use of PCR for diagnosis of invasive aspergillosis: systemic review and meta-analysis. *Lancet Infect Dis.* 2009;9(2):89.
99. Wheat J. Endemic mycosis in AIDS: a clinical review. *Clin Micro Rev.* 1995;8(1):146.
100. Chu JH, Feudtner C, Hedon K, et al. Hospitalizations for endemic mycoses: a population-based national study. *Clin Infect Dis.* 2006; 42(6):822.
101. Woods JP, Heinecke EL, Luecke JVV, et al. Pathogenesis of *Histoplasma capsulatum. Semin Respir Infect.* 2001;16(2):91.
102. Goldman M, Johnson PC, Sarosi GA. Fungal pneumonias. The endemic mycoses. *Clin Chest Med.* 1999;20():507.
103. Goodwin RA, Shapiro JL, Thurman GH. Disseminated histoplasmosis. *Medicine.* 1980;59(1):1.
104. Corti ME, Cendoya Ca, Soto I, et al. Disseminated histoplasmosis and AIDS: clinical aspects and diagnostic methods for early detection. *AIDS Patient Care STDS.* 2000;14(3):149.
105. Conces DJ Jr. Histoplasmosis. *Semin Roentgenol.* 1996; 31(1):14.
106. Pugsley HE, Brown AS, Cheung OT. Chronic cavity histoplasmosis of the lung. *Can Med Assoc J.* 1963; 88(13):646.

107. Loyd JE, Tillman BF, Atkinson JB, et al. Mediastinal fibrosis complicating histoplasmosis. *Medicine.* 1988;67(5):295.

108. Mathisen DJ, Grillo HC. Clinical manifestation of mediastinal fibrosis and histoplasmosis. *Ann Thorac Surg.* 1992;54(6):1053.

109. Gurney JW, Conces DJ. Pulmonary histoplasmosis. *Radiology.* 1996;199(2):297.

110. Subramanian S, Abraham OC, Rupali P, et al. Disseminated histoplasmosis. *J Assoc Physicians India.* 2005;45:185.

111. McNeeley MF, Chung JH, Bhalla S, et al. Imaging of granulomatous fibrosing mediastinitis. *AJR Am J Roentgenol.* 2012;199(2):319.

112. Bonifaz A, Chang P, Moreno K, et al. Disseminated cutaneous histoplasmosis in acquired immunodeficiency syndrome: report of 23 cases. *Clin Exp Dermatol.* 2009;34(4):481.

113. McLeod DS, Mortimer RH, Perry-Keene DA, et al. Histoplasmosis in Australia: report of 16 cases and literature review. *Medicine (Baltimore).* 2011;90(1):61.

114. Hutton JP, Durham JB, Miller DP, Everett ED. Hyphal forms of Histoplasma capsulatum. A common manifestation of intravascular infections. *Arch Pathol Lab Med.* 1985;109(4):330.

115. Gupta N, Arora S, Rajwanshi A, Nijhawan R, Srinivasan R. Histoplasmosis cytodiagnosis and review of the literature with special emphasis on differential diagnosis on cytomorphology. *Cytopathology.* 2010;21(4):240.

116. Larone DH, Mitchell TB, Walsh TJ. Histoplasma, blastomyces, coccidioides, and other dimorphic fungi causing systemic mycoses. In: Murray, ed-in-chief. *Manual of Clinical Microbiology.* 7th ed. Washington, DC: American Society for Microbiology; 1999:1259-1274.

117. Jacobson ES, Straus SE. Serologic tests for histoplasmosis. *Ann Intern Med.* 1983;98(4):560.

118. Wheat J, French ML, Kohler RB, et al. The diagnostic laboratory tests for histoplasmosis: analysis of experience in a large urban outbreak. *Ann Inter Med.* 1982;97(5):680.

119. Schubert JH, Wiggins GI. Preliminary studies of H and M components of histoplasmin for skin tests and serology. *Am Rev Respir Dis.* 1965;92(4):640.

120. Wheat LJ. Laboratory diagnosis of histoplasmosis: update 2000. *Semin Respir Infect.* 2001;16(2):131.

121. Kaufman L. Laboratory methods for the diagnosis and confirmation of systemic mycosis. *Clin Infect Dis.* 1992;14(suppl 1):S23.

122. Klite PD. The interpretation of agar-gel precipitin reactions in histoplasmosis. *J Lab Clin Med.* 1965;66(5):780.

123. Davies SF. Serodiagnosis of histoplasmosis. *Semin Respir Infect.* 1986;1(1):9.

124. Pine L, Malcolm GB, Gross H, Gray SB. Evaluation of purified H and M antigens of histoplasmin as reagents in the complement fixation test. *Sabouraudia.* 1978;16(4):257.

125. Campbell CC. Use of yeast phase antigens in a complement fixation test for histoplasmosis. IV. Results with ground yeast phase antigens in serial specimens of serum from thirty-seven patients. *Public Health Monogr.* 1956;70(39):140.

126. Wheat J. Histoplasmosis. Experience during outbreaks in Indianapolis and review of the literature. *Medicine (Baltimore).* 1997;76(5):339.

127. Wheat J, French ML, Kamel S, Tewari RP. Evaluation of cross-reactions in Histoplasma capsulatum serologic tests. *J Clin Microbiol.* 1986;23(3):493.

128. Bauman DS, Smith CD. Comparison of immunodiffusion and complement fixation tests in the diagnosis of histoplasmosis. *J Clin Microbiol.* 1976;2(2):77.

129. Connolly PA, Durkin MM, Lemonte AM, Hockett EJ, Wheat LJ. Detection of histoplasma antigen by a quantitative enzyme immunoassay. *Clin Vaccine Immunol.* 2007;14(12):1587.

130. Hage CA, Ribes JA, Wengenack NL, et al. Multicenter evaluation of tests for diagnosis of histoplasmosis. *Clin Infect Dis.* 2011;53(5):448.

131. Swartzentruber S, Rhodes L, Kurkjian K, et al. Diagnosis of acute pulmonary histoplasmosis by antigen detection. *Clin Infect Dis.* 2009;49(12):1878.

132. Hage CA, Davis TE, Fuller D, et al. Diagnosis of histoplasmosis by antigen detection in BAL fluid. *Chest.* 2010;137(3):623.

133. Huffnagle KE, Gander RM. Evaluation of Gen-Probe Histoplasma capsulatum and Cryptococcus neoformans AccuProbes. *J Clin Microbiol.* 1993;31(2):419.

134. Fisher M, Koenig TJ, White JW. Molecular and phenotypic description of *Coccidioides posadasii* sp nov., previously recognized as the non-California population of *Coccidioides immitis.* *Mycologia.* 20002;94():73.

135. Fisher FS, Bultman MW, Johnson SM, et al. Coccidioides niches and habitat parameters in the southwestern United Sates: a matter of scale. *Ann N Y Acad Sci.* 2007;1111:47.

136. Brown J, Benedict K, Park BJ, Thompson GR 3rd. Coccidioidomycosis: epidemiology. *Clin Epidermiol.* 2013; 25(5):185.

137. Deus Fiho Ad. Chapter 2: Coccidioidomycosis. *J Bras Pneumol.* 2009;35(9):920.

138. Batra P. Pulmonary coccidioidomycosis. *J Thorac Imaging.* 1992;7(4):29.

139. Stevens DA. Coccidioidomycosis. *N Engl J Med.* 1995;332 (16):1077.

140. Galgiani JN, Ampel NM, Catanzaro A, et al. Practice guideline for the treatment of coccidioidomycosis. Infectious Diseases Society of America. *Clin Infect Dis.* 2000;30(4):658.

141. Ampel NM. Coccidioidomycosis. In: Sarosi GA, Davies SF, eds. *Fungal Disease of the Lung.* 3rd ed. Philadelphia, PA: Lippincott William & Wilkins; 2000:59-78.

142. Pappagianis D, Chandler FW. Coccidioidomycosis. In: Connor DH, Chandler F.W, Manz HJ, et al eds. *Pathology of Infectious Disease.* Stamford, CT: Appleton & Lange; 1997:977-987.

143. Rippon JW. Coccidioidomycosis. In: *Wonsierioicz M: Medical Mycology, the Pathogenic Fungi and the Pathogenic Actinomycetes.* Philadelphia, PA: WB Saunders Company-Harcourt Brace Jaovanovich; 1988:433-473.

144. Pan S, Sigler L, Cole GT. Evidence for a phylogenetic connection between Coccidioides immitis and Uncinocarpus reesii (Onygenaceae). *Microbiology.* 1994;140(pt 6):1481.

145. Davies SF, Sarosi GA. Role of serodiagnostic tests and skin tests in the diagnosis of fungal disease. *Clin Chest Med.* 1987;8(1):135.

146. Pappagianis D, Zimmer BL. Serology of coccidioidomycosis. *Clin Microbiol Rev.* 1990;3(3):247.

147. Stevens DA. Coccidioides immitis. In: Mandell GL, Bennett JE, Dolin R, eds. *Principles and Practice of Infectious Diseases.* New York, NY: Churchill-Livingstone; 1995:2365-2373.

148. Kaufman L, Sekhon AS, Moledina N, Jalbert M, Pappaginas D. Comparative evaluation of commercial Premier EIA and microimmunodiffusion and complement fixation tests for Coccidioides immitis antibodies. *J Clin Microbiol.* 1995; 33(3):618.

149. Blair JE, Coakley B, Santelli AC, Hentz JG, Wengenack NL. Serologic testing for symptomatic coccidioidomycosis in immunocompetent and immunosuppressed hosts. *Mycopathologia.* 2006;162(5):317.

150. Singh VR, Smith DK, Lawrence J, et al. Coccidioidomycosis in patients infected with human immunodeficiency virus: review of 91 cases at a single institution. *Clin Infect Dis.* 1996;23(3):563.

151. Durkin M, Connolly P, Kuberski T, et al. Diagnosis of coccidioidomycosis with use of the Coccidioides antigen enzyme immunoassay. *Clin Infect Dis.* 2008;47(8):e69.

152. Stockman L, Clark KA, Hunt JM, Roberts GD. Evaluation of commercially available acridinium ester-labeled chemiluminescent DNA probes for culture identification of Blastomyces dermatitidis, Coccidioides immitis, Cryptococcus neoformans and Histoplasma capsulatum. *J Clin Microbiol.* 1993;31(4):845.

CHAPTER 13

153. Binnicker MJ, Buckwalter SP, Eisberner JJ, et al. Detection of Coccidioides species in clinical specimens by real-time PCR. *J Clin Microbiol.* 2007;45(1):173.

154. Bialek R, Kern J, Herrmann T, et al. PCR assays for identification of Coccidioides posadasii based on the nucleotide sequence of the antigen 2/proline-rich antigen. *J Clin Microbiol.* 2004;42(2):778.

155. Kishi K, Fujii T, Miyamoto A, Kohna T, Yoshimura K. Pulmonary coccidioidomycosis found in healthy Japanese individuals. *Respiratory.* 2008;13(2):252.

156. Chandler FW, Ajello L. Torulopsis. In: Connor DH, Chandler F.W, Manz HJ, et al, eds. *Pathology of Infectious Disease.* Stamford, CT: Appleton & Lange; 1997:1105-1108.

157. Luna MA. Candidiasis. In: Connor DH, Chandler FW, Manz HJ, et al, eds. *Pathology of Infectious Diseases.* Stamford, CT: Appleton & Lange; 1997:953-964.

158. Rosati LA, Leslie KO. Lung infections. In: Leslie KO, Wick MR, eds. *Practical Pulmonary Pathology. A Diagnostic Approach.* Philadelphia, PA: Churchill Livingstone; 2005:97-180.

159. Podzorski RP, Herron J, Fast DJ, Nelson RD. Pathogenesis of candidiasis. Immunosuppression by cell wall mannan catabolites. *Arch Surg.* 1989;124(11):1290.

160. Masur H, Rosen PP, Armstrong D. Pulmonary disease caused by Candida species. *Am J Med.* 1977;63(6):914.

161. McAdams HP, Rosado-de-Christenson ML, Lesar M, et al. Thoracic mycoses from opportunistic fungi: radiologic-pathologic correlation. *Radiographics.* 1995; 15(2):271.

162. Sullivan D, Coleman D. Candida dubliniensis: characteristics and identification. *J Clin Microbiol.* 1998;36(2): 329.

163. Alasio TM, Lento PA, Bottone EJ. Giant blastoconidia of *Candida albicans. Arch Pathol Lab Med.* 2003;127(7):868.

164. Warren NG, Hazen KC. Candida, Cryptococcus, and other yeasts of clinical importance. In: Murray, ed-in-chief. *Manual of Clinical Microbiology.* 7th ed. Washington, DC: American Society for Microbiology;1999:1184-1199.

165. Jones JM. Laboratory diagnosis of invasive candidiasis. *Clin Microbiol Rev.* 1900;3(1):32.

166. van Deventer AJ, van Vliet HJ, Voogd L, Hop WC, Goessens WH. Increased specificity of antibody detection in surgical patients with invasive candidiasis with cytoplasmic antigens depleted of mannan residues. *J Clin Microbiol.* 1993;31(4):994.

167. Zöller L, Krämer I, Kappe R, Sonntag HG. Enzyme immunoassay for invasive Candida infections: reactivity of somatic antigens of Candida albicans. *J Clin Microbiol.* 1991;29(9):1860.

168. Sendid B, Tabouret M, Poirot JL, et al. New enzyme immunoassay for sensitive detection of circulating Candida albicans mannan and antimannan antibodies: Useful combined test for diagnosis of systemic candidiasis. *J Clin Microbiol.* 1999;37(5):1510.

169. Alam FF, Mustafa AS, Khan ZU. Comparative evaluation of (1,3);B-D-glucan, mannan and anti-mannan antibodies, and Candida species-specific snPCR in patients with candidaemia. *BCM Infect Dis.* 2007;7:103.

170. Prella M, Bille J, Pugnale M, et al. Early diagnosis of invasive candidiasis with mannan antigenemia and antimannan antibodies. *Diagn Microbiol Infect Dis.* 2005;51(2):95.

171. Mokaddas E, Khan ZU, Ahmad S, Nampoory MR, Burhamah M. Value of (1,3)-b-D-glucan Candida mannan and Candida DNA detection in the diagnosis of candidaemia. *Clin Microbiol Infect.* 2011;17(10):1549.

172. Sendid B, Caillot D, Baccouch-Humbert B, et al. Contribution of the Platelia Candida-specific antibody and antigen tests to early diagnosis of systemic Candida tropicalis infection in neutropenic patients. *J Clin Microbiol.* 2003;41(19):4551.

173. Sendid B, Poirot JL, Tabouret M, et al. Combined detection of mannanaemia and antimannan antibodies as a strategy for the diagnosis of systemic infection caused by pathogenic Candida species. *J Med Microbiol.* 2002;51(5):433.

174. Mikulska M, Calandra T, Sanquinetti M, Poulain D, Viscoli C. Third European Conference on Infections in Leukemia Group. The use of mannan antigen and anti-mannan antibodies in the diagnosis of invasive candidiasis: recommendations from the Third European Conference on Infection in Leukemia. *Crit Care.* 2010;14(6):R222.

175. Ostrosky-Zeichner L, Alexander BD, Kett DH, et al. Multicenter clinical evaluation of the (1—3) beta-D-glucan assay as an aid to diagnosis of fungal infections in humans. *Clin Infect Dis.* 2005;41(5):654.

176. Koo S, Bryar JM, Page JH, Baden LR, Marty FM. Diagnostic performance of the (1—3)-b-D-glucan assay for invasive fungal disease. *Clin Infect Dis.* 2009;49(11):1650.

177. Odabasi Z, Mattiuzzi G, Estey E, et al. b-D-glucan as a diagnostic adjunct for invasive fungal infections: Validation, cutoff development, and performance in patients with acute myelogenous leukemia and myelodysplastic syndrome. *Clin Infect Dis.* 2004;39(2):199.

178. Mokaddas E, Burhamah MH, Khan ZU, Ahmad S. Levels of (1→3)-b-D-glucan, Candida mannan and Candida DNA in serum samples of pediatric cancer patients colonized with Candida species. *BMC Infect Dis.* 2010;10:292.

179. Zaragoza R, Pemán J, Quindós G, et al. Clinical significance of the detection of Candida albicans germ tube-specific antibodies in critically ill patients. *Clin Microbiol Infect.* 2009; 15(6):592.

180. León C, Ruiz-Santana S, Saavedra P, et al. Value of b-D-glucan and Candida albicans germ tube antibody for discriminating between Candida colonization and invasive candidiasis in patients with severe abdominal conditions. *Intensive Care Med.* 2012;38(8):1315.

181. Nguyen MH, Wissel MC, Shields RK, et al. Performance of real-time polymerase chain reaction, b-D-glucan assay, and blood cultures in the diagnosis of invasive candidiasis. *Clin Infect Dis.* 2012;54(9):1240.

182. Chayakulkeereen M, Perfect JR. Cryptococcosis. In: Hospenthal DR, Rinaldi MG, eds. *Diagnosis and Treatment of Human Mycosis.* Totowa, NJ: Human Press Inc; 2008:255-276.

183. Powderly WG. Crytoccoccal meningitis and AIDS. *Clin Infect Dis.* 1993;17(5):837.

184. Mitchell TG, Perfect JR. Cryptococcosis in the era of AIDS-100 years after the discovery of *Cryptococcus neoformans. Clin Microbiol Rev.* 1995;8(4):515.

185. Davies SF, Sarosi GA. Fungal infections. In: Murray JF, Nadel JA, Mason RJ, Boushey HA Jr, eds. *Textbook of Respiratory Medicine.* 3rd ed. Philadelphia, PA: WB Saunders; 2000:1107-1141.

186. Perfect JR. Cryptococcosis. *Infect Dis Clin North Am.* 1989;3(1):77.

187. Kozel TR. Opsonization and phagocytosis of *Cryptococcus neoformans. Arch Med Res.* 1993;24(3):211.

188. Campbell GD. Primary pulmonary cryptococcosis. *Am Rev Respir Dis.* 1966;94(2):236.

189. Lehmann PF, Morgan RJ, Freimer EH. Infection with *Cryptococcus neoformans* vs *gattii* leading to a pulmonary cryptococcoma and meningitis. *J Infect.* 1984;9(3):301.

190. Woodring JH, Ciporkin G, Lee C, et al. Pulmonary cryptococcosis. *Semin Roentgenol.* 1996;31(1):67.

191. Patz EF Jr, Goodman PC: Pulmonary cryptococcosis. *J Thorac Imaging.* 1992;7(4):51.

192. Chandler FW, Watts JC. Cryptococcus. In: Connor DH, Chandler FW, Manz HJ, et al eds. *Pathology of Infectious Diseases.* Stamford, CT: Appleton & Lange; 1997:989-997.

193. Ro JY, Lee SS, Ayala AG. Advantage of Fontana-Masson stain in capsule-deficient cryptococcal infection. *Arch Pathol Lab Med.* 1987;111(1):53.

194. Aberg JA, Mundy LM, Powderly WG. Pulmonary cryptococcosis in patients without HIV infection. *Chest.* 1999;115(3):734.

195. Baddley JW, Perfect JR, Oster RA, et al. Pulmonary cryptococcosis in patients without HIV infection: factors associated with disseminated disease. *Eur J Clin Microbiol Infect Dis.* 2008;27(10):937.

196. Pappas PG, Perfect JR, Cloud GA, et al. Cryptococcosis in human immunodeficiency virus-negative patients in the era of effective azole therapy. *Clin Infect Dis.* 2001;33(5):690.

197. Meyohas MC, Roux P, Bollens D, et al. Pulmonary cryptococcosis localized and disseminated infections in 27 patients with AIDS. *Clin Infect Dis.* 1995;21(3):628.

198. Finke R, Strobel ES, Kroepelin T, et al. Disseminated cryptococcosis in a patient with malignant lymphoma. *Mycoses.* 1988;(suppl 1):201.

199. Christoph I. Pulmonary Cryptococcus neoformans and disseminated Nocardia brasiliensis in an immunocompromised host. Case report. *NC Med J.* 1990; 51(5):219.

200. Jensen WA, Rose RM, Hammer SM, Karchmer AW. Serologic diagnosis of focal pneumonia caused by Cryptococcus neoformans. *Am Rev Respir Dis.* 1985; 132(1):189.

201. Singh N, Alexander BD, Lortholary O, et al. Pulmonary cryptococcosis in solid organ transplant recipients: clinical relevance of serum cryptococcal antigen. *Clin Infect Dis.* 2008; 46(2):12.

202. Kozei I, Bauman S. CrAg lateral flow assay for cryptococcus. *Expert Opin Med Diagn.* 2012; 6(3):245.

203. Jarvis JN, Percival A, Bauman S., et al. Evaluation of a novel point-of-care cryptococcal antigen test on serum, plasma, and urine from patients with HIV-associated cryptococcal meningitis. *Clin Infect Dis.* 2011; 53(10):1019.

204. Lindsley MD, Mekha N, Baggett HC, et al. Evaluation of a newly developed lateral flow immunoassay for the diagnosis of cryptococcosis. *Clin Infect Dis.* 2011;53(4):321.

205. Hansen J, Slechta ES, Marcellene A, et al. Large-scale evaluation of the immuno-mycologics lateral flow and enzyme-linked immunoassays for detection of cryptococcal antigen in serum and cerebrospinal fluid. *Clin Vaccine Immunol.* 2013; 20(1):52.

206. Jarvis JN, Lawn SD, Vogt M, et al. Screening for cryptococcal antigenemia in patients in South Africa. *Clin Infect Dis.* 2009;48(7):856.

207. Chanock SJ, Toltzis P, Wilson C. Cross-reactivity between Stomatococcus mucilaginosus and latex agglutination for cryptococcal antigen. *Lancet.* 1993;342(8879):1119.

208. McManus EJ, Jones JM. Detection of a Trichosporon beigelii antigen cross-reactive with Cryptococcus neoformans capsular polysaccharide in serum from a patient with disseminated Trichosporon infection. *J Clin Microbiol.* 1985; 21(5):681.

209. Westerink MA, Amsterdam D, Petell RJ, et al. Septicemia due to DF-2: cause of a false-positive cryptococcal latex agglutination result. *Am J Med.* 1987;83(1):155.

210. Kauffman CA, Hajjeh R, Chapman SW. Practice guidelines for the management of patients with sporotrichosis. *Clin Infect Dis.* 2000;30(4):684.

211. Al-Tawfiq JA, Wools KK. Disseminated sporotrichosis and *Sporothrix schenckii* fungemia as the initial presentation of human immunodeficiency virus infection. *Clin Infect Dis.* 1998;26(6):1403.

212. Reed KD, Moore FM, Geiger GE, Stemper M. Zoonotic transmission of sporoatrichosis: case report and review. *Clin Infect Dis.* 1993;16(3):384.

213. Kauffman CA. Sporotrichosis. *Clin Infect Dis.* 1999;29(2):231.

214. da Rosa AC, Scroferneker ML, Vettorato R, et al. Epidemiology of sporotrichosis: a study of 304 cases in Brazil. *J Am Acad Dermatol.* 2005:52(3 pt 1):451.

215. Pappas PG, Tellez I, Deep AE, et al. Sporotrichosis in Peru: description of an area of hypersensitivity. *Clin Infect Dis.* 2000;30(1):65.

216. Chandler FW, Watts JC. Sporotrichosis. In: Connor DH, Chandler F.W, Manz HJ, et al, eds. *Pathology of Infectious Disease.* Stamford, CT: Appleton & Lange; 1997:1089-1096.

217. England DM, Hochholtzer L. Sporothrix infection of the lung without cutaneous disease. Primary pulmonary sporotrichosis. *Arch Pathol Lab Med.* 1987;111(3):298.

218. Fraser RS, Müller NL, Colman N, Pare PD. Fungi and actinomyces. In: Fraser RS, Müller NL, Colman N, Pare ND, eds. *Fraser and Pare's Diagnosis of Diseases of the Chest.* 4th ed. Philadelphia, PA: WB Saunders; 1999;875-978.

219. England DM, Hichholzer L. Sporothrix infection of the lung without cutaneous disease. Primary pulmonary sporotrichosis. *Arch Pathol Lab Med.* 1987;111(3):298.

220. England DM, Hochholtzer L. Primary pulmonary sporotrichosis. A report of eight cases with clinicopathologic review. *Am J Surg Pathol.* 1985;9(3):193.

221. Larone DH. Thermally dimorphic fungi. In: *Larone DH: Medically Important Fungi. A Guide to Identification.* 2nd ed. Washington DC: American Society for Microbiology; 1993;77-169.

222. Brummer E, Castaneda E, Restrepo A. Paracoccidioidomycosis: an update. *Clin Microbiol Rev.* 1993;6(2):89.

223. Restrepo A. The ecology of Paracoccidioides brasiliensis: a puzzle still unsolved. *J Med Vet Mycol.* 1985;23(5):323.

224. Barrozo LV, Mendes RP, Marques SA, et al. Climate and acute/subacute paracoccidioidomycosis in a hyper-endemic area in Brazil. *Int J Epidemiol.* 2009;38(6):1642.

225. Bellissimo-Rodrigues F, Bollela VR, Da Fonseca BA, Martinez R. Endemic paracoccidioidomycosis: relationship between clinical presentation and patients' demographic features. *Med Mycol.* 2013;51(3):313.

226. Fortes MR, Miot HA, Kurokawa CS. Immunology of paracoccidioidomycosis. *An Bras Dermatol.* 2011;86(3):516.

227. Londero AT, Chandler FW. Paracoccidioidomycosis. In: Connor DH, Chandler FW, Manz HJ, et al, eds. *Pathology of Infectious Disease.* Stamford, CT: Appleton & Lange; 1997:1045-1053.

228. Restrepo A, Robledo R, Giraldo H, et al. The gamut of paracoccidioidomycosis. *Am J Med.* 1976;61(1):33.

229. Funari M, Kavakama J, Shikanai-Yasu MA, et al. Chronic pulmonary paracoccidioidomycosis (South American blastomycosis): high-resolution CT findings in 41 patients. *AJR Am J Roentgenol.* 1999;173(1):59.

230. deCamargo ZP. Serology of paracoccidioidomycosis. *Mycopathologia.* 2008;165(4-5):289.

231. del Negro GM, Garcia NM, Rodrigues EG, et al. The sensitivity, specificity and efficiency values of some serological tests used in the diagnosis of paracoccidioidomycosis. *Rev Inst Med Trop Sao Paulo.* 1991;33(4): 277.

232. Taborda AB, Arechavala AL. Paracoccidioidomycosis. In: Sarosi GA, Davis SF, eds. *Fungal Diseases of the Lung.* 2nd ed. New York, NY: Raven Press;1993:85-94.

233. Mendes-Giannini MJ, Camargo ME, Lacaz CS, Ferreira AW. Immunoenzymatic absorption test for serodiagnosis of paracoccidioidomycosis. *J Clin Microbiol.* 1984;20(8): 103.

234. Marques da Silva SH, Queiroz-Telles. Detection of circulating gp43 antigen in serum, cerebrospinal fluid and bronchoalveolar lavage fluid of patients with paracoccidioidomycosis. *J Clin Microbiol.* 2003;41(8): 3675.

235. Salina MA, Shikanai-Yasuda MA, Mendes RP, Barraviera B, Mendes-Giannini MJ. Detection of circulating Paracoccidioides brasiliensis antigen in urine of paracoccidioidomycosis patients before and during treatment. *J Clin Microbiol.* 1998;36 (6): 1723.

236. Gomez BL, Figueroa JI, Hamilton AJ, et al. Antigenemia in patients with paracoccidioidomycosis: detection of the 87-kilodalton determinant during and after antifungal therapy. *J Clin Microbiol.* 1998; 36(11):3309.

237. Marques da Silva SH, Queiroz-Telles F, Colombo AL, Blotta MH, Lopes JD, Camargo ZP. Monitoring of gp43 antigenemia in paracoccidioidomycosis patients during therapy. *J Clin Microbiol.* 2004; 42(6): 2419.

238. Gomes GM, Cisalpino PS, Taborda CP, et al. Polymerase chain reaction for diagnosis of paracoccidioidomycosis. *J Clin Microbiol.* 2000;38(12): 3478.

239. San-Blas G, Niño-Vega G, Baretto L, et al. Primers for the clinical detection of Paracoccidioides brasiliensis. *J Clin Microbiol.* 2005;43(8): 4255.

240. Calcagno AM, Niño-Vega G, San-Blas F, San-Blas G. Geographic discrimination of Paracoccidioides brasiliensis strains by randomly amplified polymorphic DNA analysis. *J Clin Microbiol.* 1998; 36(6): 1733.

241. Ricci G, Da Silva ID, Sano A, Borra RC, Franco M. Detection of Paracoccidioides brasiliensis by PCR in biopsies from patients with paracoccidioidomycosis: correlation with the histopathologic pattern. *Pathologica.* 2007; 99(2):41.

242. Ribes JA, Vanover-Sams CL, Baker DJ. Zygomycetes in human disease. *Clin Microbiol Rev.* 2000;13(2):236.

243. Spellberg B, Edwards J Jr, Ibrahim Ashraf. Novel perspectives on Mucormycosis: pathophysiology, presentation, and management. *Clin Microbiol Rev.* 2005;18(3):556.

244. Kwon-Chung KJ, Young RC, Orlando M. Pulmonary mucormycosis caused by Cunninghamella elegans in a patient with chronic myelogenous leukemia. *Am J Clin Pathol.* 1975;64(4):544.

245. Ventura GJ, Kantarjian HM, Anaissie E, et al. Pneumonia with Cunningham species in patients with hematologic malignancies. A case report and review of the literature. *Cancer.* 1986;58(7):1534.

246. Petrikkos G, Skiada A, Lortholary O, et al. Epidemiology and clinical manifestations of mucormycosis. *Clin Infect Dis.* 2012;54(S1):S23.

247. Antinori S, Nebuloni M, Magni C, et al. Trends in the postmortem diagnosis of opportunistic invasive fungal infections in patients with AIDS: a retrospective study of 1630 autopsies performed between 1984 and 2002. *Am J Clin Pathol.* 2009;132(2):221.

248. Rees JR, Pinner RW, Hajjeh RA, et al. The epidemiological features of invasive mycotic infections in the San Francisco Bay area. *Clin Infect Dis.* 1998,27(5).1130.

249. Boelaert JR, de Locht M, Van Cutsem J, et al. Mucormycosis during deferoxamine therapy is a siderophore-mediated infection. In vitro and in vivo animal studies. *J Clin Investig.* 1993;91(5):1979.

250. Artis WM, Fountain JA, Delcher HK, Jones HE. A mechanism of susceptibility to mucormycosis in diabetic ketoacidosis: transferrin and iron availability. *Diabetes.* 1982;31(12):1109.

251. Chinn RY, Diamond RD. Generation of chemotactic factors by *Rhizopus oryzae* in the presence and absence of serum: relationship to hyphal damage by human neutrophils and effects of hyperglycemia and ketoacidosis. *Infect Immun.* 1982;38(3):1123.

252. Bouchara JP, Oumeziane NA, Lissitzky JC, et al. Attachment of spores of the human pathogenic fungus *Rhizopus oryzae* to extracellular matrix components. *Eur J Cell Biol.* 1996;70(1):76.

253. Ibrahim AS, Spellberg B, Avanessian Y, et al. Rhizopus oryzae adheres to, is phagocytosed by, and damages endothelial cells in vitro. *Infect Immun.* 2005;73(2):778.

254. Torres-Narbona M, Guinea J, Martinez-Alarcon J, et al. Impact of mucormycosis on microbiology overload: a survey study in Spain. *J Clin Microbiol.* 2007;45(6):2051.

255. Passamonte PM, Dix JD. Nosocomial pulmonary mucormycosis with fatal hemoptysis. *Am J Med Sci.* 1985;289(2):65.

256. McAdams HP, Rosado de Christenson M, Strollo DC, Patz EF Jr. Pulmonary mucormycosis: radiologic findings in 32 cases. *AJR Am J Roentgenol.* 1997;168(6):1541.

257. Wahba H, Truong MT, Lei X. Reversed halo sign in invasive pulmonary fungal infections. *Clin Infect Dis.* 2008;46(11):1733.

258. Frater JL, Hall GS, Procop GW. Histologic features of zygomycosis. Emphasis on perineural invasion and fungal morphology. *Arch Pathol Lab Med.* 2001;125(3):375.

259. Richardson MD, Shankland GS. Rhizopus, Rhizomucor, Absidia, and other agents of systemic and subcutaneous zygomycosis. In: Murray, ed-in-chief. *Manual of Clinical Microbiology.* 7th ed. Washington, DC: American Society for Microbiology; 1999:1242-1258.

260. Chayakulkeeree M, Ghannoum M, Perfect JR. Zygomycosis: the re-emerging fungal infection. *Eur J Clin Microbiol Infect Dis.* 2006;25(4):215.

261. Chakrabarti A, Das A, Sharma A, et al. Ten years' experience in zygomycosis at a tertiary care centre in India. *J Infect.* 2001;42(4):261.

262. Torres-Narbona M, Guinea J, Martinez-Alarcón, et al. Workload and clinical significance of the isolation of zygomycosis in a tertiary general hospital. *Med Mycol.* 2008;46(3):225.

263. Ribes J, Vanover-Sams CL, Baker DJ. Zygomycetes in human disease. *Clin Microbiol Rev.* 2000;13(2):236.

264. Wysong DR, Waldorf AR. Electrophoresis and immunoblot analyses of Rhizopus arrhizus antigens. *J Clin Microbiol.* 1987;25(2):358.

265. Kasai M, Harrington SM, Francesconi A, et al. Detection of a molecular biomarker for Zygomycetes by quantitative PCR assays of plasma, bronchoalveolar lavage, and lung tissue in a rabbit model of experimental pulmonary zygomycosis. *J Clin Microbiol.* 2008;46(11):3690.

266. Machouart M, Larché J, Burton K, et al. Genetic identification of the main opportunistic Mucorales by PCR-restriction fragment length polymorphism. *J Clin Microbiol.* 2006;44(3):805.

267. Bialek R, Konrad F, Kern J, et al. PCR based identification and discrimination of agents of mucormycosis and aspergillosis in paraffin wax embedded tissue. *J Clin Pathol.* 2005;58(11):1180.

268. Dannaoui E, Schwarz P, Slany M, et al. Molecular detection and identification of Zygomycetes species from paraffin-embedded tissues in a murine model of disseminated zygomycosis: a collaborative European Society of Clinical Microbiology and Infectious Diseases (ESCMID) Fungal Infection Study Group (EFISG) evaluation. *J Clin Microbiol.* 2010;48(6):2043.

269. Hofman V, Dhouibi A, Butori C, et al. Usefulness of molecular biology performed with formaldehyde-fixed tissue in the diagnosis of combined pulmonary invasive mucormycosis and aspergillosis in an immunocompromised patient. *Diagn Pathol.* 2010;5:1.

270. Chu JH, Feudtner C, Heydon K, et al. Hospitalizations for endemic mycoses: a population-based national study. *Clin Infect Dis.* 2006;42(6):822.

271. Kaplan W, Clifford MK. Blastomycosis. I. A review of 198 collected cases in veterans administration hospitals. *Am Rev Respir Dis.* 1964;89:659.

272. Carman WF, Frean JA, Crewe-Brown HH. Blastomycosis in Africa. A review of known cases diagnosed between 1951 and 1987. *Mycopathologia.* 1989;107(1):25.

273. Saccente M, Woods GL. Clinical and laboratory update on blastomycosis. *Clin Microbiol Rev.* 2010;23(2):367.

274. Drutz DJ, Frey CL. Intracellular and extracellular defenses against *Blastomyces dermatitidis* conidia and yeasts. *J Lab Clin Med.* 1985;105(6):737.

275. Sugar AM, Picard M. Macrophage-and oxidant-mediated inhibition of the ability of live *Blastomyces dermatitidis* conidia to transform to the pathogenic yeasts phase: implications for the pathogenesis of dimorphic fungal infections. *J Infect Dis.* 1991;163(2):371.

276. Sarosi GA, Hammerman KJ, Tosh FE, Kronenberg RS. Clinical features of acute pulmonary blastomycosis. *N Engl J Med.* 1974;290(10):540.

277. Gadkowski LB, Stout JE. Cavitary pulmonary disease. *Clin Microbiol Rev.* 2008;21(2):305.

278. Patel RG, Patel B, Petrini MF, et al. Clinical presentation, radiographic findings, and diagnostic methods of pulmonary blastomycosis: a review of 100 consecutive cases. *South Med J.* 1999;92(3):289.

279. Kuzo RS, Goodman LR. Blastomycosis. *Semin Roentgenol.* 1996;31(1):45.

280. Winer-Muram HT, Rubin SA. Pulmonary blastomycosis. *J Thorac Imaging.* 1992;7(4):23.

281. Brandt ME, Warnock DW. Histoplasma, blastomyces, coccidioides, and other dimorphic fungi causing systemic mycoses. In: Murray PR, ed-in-chief. *Manual of Clinical Microbiology*, 9th ed. Washington, DC: American Society for Microbiology; 1857-1873.

282. Chandler FW. Blastomycosis. In: Connor DH, Chandler FW, Manz HJ, et al., eds. *Pathology of Infectious Diseases.* Stamford, CT: Appleton & Lange; 1997:943-951.

283. Martymowicz MA, Prakash UB. Pulmonary blastomycosis: an appraisal of diagnostic techniques. *Chest.* 2002;121(3):768.

284. Padhye AA, Smith G, Standard PG, McLaughlin D, Kaufman L. Comparative evaluation of chemiluminescent DNA probe assays and exoantigen tests for rapid identification of Blastomyces dermatitidis and Coccidioides immitis. *J Clin Microbiol.* 1994; 32(4): 867.

285. Iwen PC, Sigler L, Tatantolo S, et al. Pulmonary infections caused by Gymnasclla hyalinospora in patients with acute myelogenous leukemia. *J Clin Microbiol.* 2000;38(1):375.

286. Wheat LJ. Antigen detection, serology and molecular diagnosis of invasive mycoses in the immunocompromised host. *Transpl Infect Dis.* 2006;8(3):128.

287. Klein BS, Kuritsky JN, Chappell WA, et al. Comparison of the enzyme immunoassay, immunodiffusion and complement fixation tests in detecting antibody in human serum to the A antigen of Blastomyces dermatitidis. *Am Rev Respir Dis.* 1986;133(1):144.

288. Klein BS, Vergeront JM, Kaufman L, et al. Serological tests for blastomycosis: assessment during a large point-source outbreak in Wisconsin. *J Infect Dis.* 1987;155(2):262.

289. Bradsher RW, Pappas PG. Detection of specific antibodies in human blastomycosis by enzyme immunoassay. *South Med J.* 1995;88(12):1256.

290. Sekhon AS, Kaufman L, Kobayashi GS, Moledina NH, Jalbert M. The value of the Premier enzyme immunoassay for diagnosing Blastomyces dermatitidis infections. *J Med Vet Mycol.* 1995;33(2):123.

291. Durkin M, Witt J, LeMonte A, Wheat B, Connolly P. Antigen assay with the potential to aid in diagnosis of blastomycosis. *J Clin Microbiol.* 2004;42(10): 4873.

292. Bariola JR, Hage CA, Durkin M. Detection of Blastomyces dermatitidis antigen in patients with newly diagnosed blastomycosis. *Diagn Microbiol Infect Dis.* 2011;69(2):187.

293. Tarr M, Marcinak J, Mongkolrattanothaik K, et al. Blastomyces antigen detection for monitoring progression of blastomycosis in a pregnant adolescent. *Infect Dis Obstet Gynecol.* 2007;2007:89059.

294. Mongkolrattanothai K, Peev M, Wheat LJ, Marcinak J. Urine antigen detection of blastomycosis in pediatric patients. *Pediatr Infect Dis.* 2006;25(11): 1076.

295. Sandhu GS, Kline BC, Stockman L, Roberts GD. Molecular probes for diagnosis of fungal infections. *J Clin Microbiol.* 1995;33(11):2913.

296. Bialek R, Cirera AC, Herrmann T, et al. Nested PCR assays for detection of Blastomyces dermatitidis DNA in paraffin-embedded canine tissue. *J Clin Microbiol.* 2003;41(1):205.

297. Hayden RT, Qian X, Roberts GD, Lloyd RV. In situ hybridization for the identification of yeastlike organisms in tissue section. *Diagn Mol Pathol.* 2001;10(1):15.

298. Abbott JJ, Hamacher KL, Ahmed I. In situ hybridization in cutaneous deep fungal infections: a valuable diagnostic adjunct to fungal morphology and tissue cultures. *J Cutan Pathol.* 2006; 33(6):426.

299. Rossman SN, Cernoch PL, Davis JR. Dematiaceous fungi are an increasing cause of human disease. *Clin Infect Dis.* 1996;22(1):73.

300. Varkey JB, Perfect JR. Rare and emerging fungal pulmonary infections. *Semin Respir Crit Care Med.* 2008;29(2):121.

301. Walsh TJ, Groll AH. Emerging fungal pathogens: evolving challenges to immunocompromised patients for the twenty-first century. *Transpl Infect Dis.* 1999;1(4):247.

302. Fader RC, McGinnis MR. Infections caused by dematiaceous fungi: chromoblastomycosis and phaeohyphomycosis. *Infect Dis Clin North Am.* 1988;2(4):925.

303. Brandt ME, Warnock DW. Epidemiology, clinical manifestations, and therapy of infections caused by dematiaceous fungi. *J Chemother.* 2003;(suppl 2):36.

304. Cortez KJ, Roilides E, Quiroz-Telles F, et al. Infections caused by Scedosporium spp. *Clin Microbiol Rev.* 2008;21(1):157.

305. Sawada M, Isogai S, Miyake S, et al. Pulmonary pseudo-allescherioma associated with systemic lupus erythematosus. *Intern Med.* 1998;37(12):1046.

306. Walsh M, White L, Atkinson K, Enno A. Fungal Pseudoallescheria boydii lung infiltrates unresponsive to amphotericin B in leukemic patients. *Aust N Z J Med.* 1992;22(3):265.

307. Guerrero A, Torres P, Duran MT. Airborne outbreak of nosocomial Scedosporium prolificans infection. *Lancet.* 2001; 357(9264):1267.

308. Bittencourt VC, Figueiredo RT, da Silva RB, et al. An alpha-glucan of Pseudallescheria boydii is involved in fungal phagocytosis and Toll-like receptor activation. *J Biol Chem.* 2006;281226 (32):22614.

309. Bashir G, Shakeel S, Wani T, Kakru DK. Pulmonary pseudallescheriasis in a patient with healed tuberculosis. *Mycopathologia.* 2004;158(3):289.

310. Lake FR, Tribe AE, McAleer R, Froudist J, et al. Mixed allergic bronchopulmonary fungal disease due to Pseudallescheri boydii and Aspergillus. *Thorax.* 1990;45(6):489.

311. Miller MA, Greenberger PA, Amerian R, et al. Allergic bronchopulmonary mycosis caused by Pseudallescheri boydii. *Am Rev Respir Dis.* 1993;148(3):810.

312. Khurshid A, Barnett VT, Sekosan M, et al. Disseminated Pseudallescheri boydii infection in a nonimmunocompromised host. *Chest.* 1999;116(2):572.

313. Walts AE. Pseudallescheriasis. an underdiagnosed fungus? *Diagn Cytopathol.* 2001;25():153.

314. Hachimi-Idrissi S, Willemsen M, Desprechins B, et al. Pseudallescheri boydii and brain abscesses. *Pediatr Infect Dis.* 1990;9(10):737.

315. Kaufman L. Immunohistologic diagnosis of systemic mycosis. *Eur J Epidemiol.* 1992;8(3):377.

316. Kaufman L, Standard PG, Jalbert M, Kraft DE. Immunohistologic identification of Aspergillus spp. and other hyaline fungi by using polyclonal fluorescent antibodies. *J Clin Microbiol.* 1997;35(9):2206.

317. Diagnani MC, Anaissie EJ. Human fusariosis. *Clin Infect Microbiol.* 2004;10(S1):67.

318. Nelson PE, Diagnani MC, Anaissie EJ. Taxonomy, biology, and clinical aspects of Fusarium species. *Clin Microbiol Rev.* 1994;7(4):479.

319. Caplin I, Unger DL. Molds on the southern California deserts. *Ann Allergy.* 1983;50(4):260.

320. Sugiura Y, Barr JR, Barr DB, et al. Physiological characteristics and mycotoxins of human clinical isolates of *Fusarium* species. *Mycological Res.* 1999;103(11):1462.

321. Arney KL, Tiernan R, Judson MA. Primary pulmonary involvement of Fusarium solani in a lung transplant recipient. *Chest.* 1997;112(4):1128.

322. Boutati EI, Anaissie EJ. Fusarium, a significant emerging pathogen in patients with hematologic malignancy: ten years' experience at a cancer center and implications for management. *Blood.* 1997;90(3):999.

323. Nucci M, Anaissie E. Cutaneous infection by Fusarium species in healthy and immunocompromised hosts: implications for diagnosis and management. *Clin Infect Dis.* 2002; 35(8):909.

324. Caux F, Aractingi S, Baurmann H, et al. Fusarium solani cutaneous infection in a neutropenic patient. *Dermatology.* 1993;186(3):232.

325. Philips P, Weiner MH. Invasive aspergillosis diagnosed by immunohistochemistry with monoclonal and polyclonal reagents. *Hum Pathol.* 1987;18(10):1015.

326. Watts JC, Chandler FW, eds. *Pathology of Infectious Disease, Vol II.* Stamford, CT: Appleton & Lange; 1997:999-1001.

327. Yoshida M, Obayashi T, Iwama A, et al. Detection of plasma (1-3)-b-D-glucan in patients with Fusarium, Trichosporon, Saccharomyces and Acremonium fungaemias. *J Med Vet Mycol.* 1997;35(5):371.

328. Pazos C, Pontón J, Del Palacio A. Contribution of (1-3)-b-D-glucan chromogenic assay to diagnosis and therapeutic monitoring of invasive aspergillosis in neutropenic adult patients: a comparison with serial screening for circulating galactomannan. *J Clin Microbiol.* 2005;43(1):299.

CHAPTER 13

Viral, Parasitic, and Other Infectious Diseases

Sergio Piña-Oviedo and Blythe K. Gorman

TAKE HOME PEARLS

Viral Pneumonias

- Viral respiratory infections are the second most common respiratory infection following bacterial pneumonias. They may be found isolated or accompanied by bacterial pneumonia.
- Viral pneumonias are more frequent in young children, the elderly, patients with underlying lung disease (ie, COPD), and immunosuppressed individuals.
- Certain viruses (influenza, hantaviruses) may produce large-scale infectious outbreaks of pneumonia (epidemics) that may spread worldwide (pandemics).
- Viral pneumonia produces specific and nonspecific histopathologic changes in the lung.
- Nonspecific histopathologic changes include partial or complete necrosis of the bronchial or bronchiolar epithelium and diffuse alveolar damage, secondary to destruction of type II pneumocytes (surfactant-producing cells).
- Specific histopathologic changes include viral cytopathic effect reflected as nuclear and/or cytoplasmic inclusions in different cell types. However, not all viruses produce viral cytopathic effect.
- Diagnosis may be established by morphology if specific changes are found, but most of the time diagnosis relies on the clinical picture and serologic tests.
- Additional tests include immunohistochemistry for specific viral proteins, viral culture, or polymerase chain reaction to detect viral nucleic acids in respiratory secretions or lung tissue.

Mycoplasma, Chlamydial, and Rickettsial Pneumonias

- These organisms are small gram-negative intracellular bacteria that can infect the bronchial and alveolar epithelium, endothelial cells, and/or macrophages.
- *Mycoplasma* and *Chlamydophila pneumoniae* are the most common cause of atypical community-acquired pneumonia; *Chlamydia trachomatis* is a common cause of pneumonia in infants.
- Clinically, atypical pneumonias are characterized by mild nonspecific symptoms (mild fever, dry cough) with extrapulmonary symptoms, or may be asymptomatic, unless superinfection with other bacterial organisms occurs (*S pneumoniae*, *S aureus*).
- The radiologic findings may be far more concerning than the clinical symptoms and usually manifest as interstitial pneumonitis.
- Outbreaks of atypical pneumonia are less common than outbreaks of viral pneumonia.
- Some of these organisms are transmitted by zoonosis (*C psittaci*, the *Rickettsiae*, *Ehrlichia*, *Anaplasma*, and *Coxiella*).
- The histopathologic findings are not well characterized since atypical pneumonias are rarely fatal. Reported cases are characterized by nonspecific findings, that is peribronchiolar inflammation with different degrees of lymphohistiocytic inflammatory infiltrates with absence of neutrophils. Rickettsial pneumonias are characterized by lymphocytic vasculitis.

- Serologic tests and culture are cumbersome and nonspecific. Polymerase chain reaction is the fastest and preferred method for detection.
- Treatment includes the use of tetracyclines and macrolides, but not penicillins.

Parasitic Pneumonias

- Lung involvement by parasitic organisms is rare; the majority of cases occur as a secondary event after primary infection to other organs.
- Parasites that can produce pneumonia include *Plasmodium* spp, *Dirofilaria immitis*, *Trypanosoma cruzi*, *Ascaris lumbricoides*, *Entamoeba histolytica*, *Strongyloides stercoralis*, *Cryptosporidium*, *Capillaria aerophila,* and the microfilaria *Wuchereria bancrofti* and *Brugia malayi.*
- The clinical symptoms are nonspecific and vary from fever and cough to pulmonary edema to respiratory distress syndrome with or without peripheral eosinophilia.
- The radiologic findings are nonspecific but in certain circumstances may mimic a lung malignancy.
- Diagnosis can be obtained by recognition of the parasite in respiratory secretions or lung tissue accompanied by a granulomatous reaction and/or eosinophils (Loeffler syndrome).

VIRUSES

Approach to Pulmonary Viral Diseases

Viral pneumonias are among the most common respiratory infections affecting humans (range 5%-15%), after bacterial pneumonias. Common respiratory viruses (adenovirus, influenza, parainfluenza, respiratory syncytial virus) infect the immunocompetent host and usually produce a self-limiting disease with rare progression to pneumonia. In contrast, certain types of viruses (hantaviruses, henipaviruses, hemorrhagic fever viruses) may produce severe disease with acute respiratory failure, transmit rapidly, and produce large-scale infectious outbreaks. This situation is also true for common respiratory viruses, that is, influenza viruses, which may mutate and become aggressive with rapid transmission, leading to severe pulmonary infection and reaching pandemic levels with high mortality rates. A third group of viruses (herpes simplex virus, cytomegalovirus, varicella-zoster virus) will manifest as opportunistic pneumonia in immunocompromised individuals (transplant recipients, patients with acquired immunodeficiency syndrome, patients treated with steroids or immunomodulatory medications, patients with hematologic malignancies, etc) which is usually fatal if untreated. Young children (newborns and infants), the

elderly, and patients with underlying cardiopulmonary disease are also at risk for developing viral pneumonia. In fact, viruses are responsible for the majority of acute exacerbations occurring in patients with chronic bronchitis. Viruses alone can cause pneumonia but most of the times an accompanying bacterial infection is also present.

The diagnosis of viral pulmonary infection should be primarily suspected on clinical basis (age at presentation, associated concomitant disease, immunologic status, concomitant viral outbreaks in the community, etc) and confirmed by laboratory methods. The diagnosis may be established histologically if specific viral changes are obvious (viral cytopathic effect, see below). However, most of the time, confirmation of viral lung infection will rely on additional tests performed in respiratory secretions, serum or tissue, such as immunohistochemistry (IHC), serologic tests, antigen detection methods, viral culture, and molecular analyses.

Molecular Diagnosis of Viral Diseases

Molecular methods have replaced serologic tests, antigen detection methods, and viral cultures as the preferred methods for diagnosis of viral lung infections. These tests not only have higher sensitivity and specificity, but also yield results in a short period of time (usually few hours), which is crucial to initiate early antiviral treatment. Amplification of viral nucleic acids from respiratory secretions (bronchial brush, bronchoalveolar lavage) or fresh or formalin-fixed paraffin-embedded lung tissues can be obtained by the standard polymerase chain reaction (PCR) or reverse transcription-PCR (RT-PCR) with excellent and timely results. In addition, newly developed methods, such as multiplex RT-PCR, have the capability to detect more than one viral pathogen in clinical samples in a short period of time.[1] In situ hybridization has better sensitivity and specificity than IHC, but it is not as consistent and timely as PCR methodologies.

VIRAL PNEUMONIA

Viruses

Viruses are considered among the smallest infectious agents known to cause disease. Generally speaking, they are composed of RNA or DNA (single stranded, double stranded, circular) and viral proteins (capsid proteins, viral enzymes, etc) and may or may not be surrounded by a double-layered phospholipid membrane. Viruses contain surface proteins that are able to bind to proteins in the host cell membrane (receptor-ligand interaction) that will help the virus internalize, travel to the nucleus, and take advantage of the host cell machinery to replicate and expand forming new virions that will eventually destroy the cell and infect neighboring cells, perpetuating the cycle of infection. Viruses have the capability of infecting one or different cell types, including bronchial and alveolar epithelia. Certain viruses produce direct damage to the respiratory epithelial barrier with impairment of T cells and alveolar macrophages by different mechanisms.[2] These events facilitate colonization and superinfection of the lung parenchyma by bacterial organisms.

Viral Inclusions

Viral inclusions, also known as the viral cytopathic effect (VCE), represent the accumulation of millions of viral capsid proteins within a cell, and can be recognized histologically as round eosinophilic, basophilic, or amphophilic structures found in the cytoplasm, the nucleus, or both. They represent some of the specific changes seen in certain viral infections, some of which may be pathognomonic. For example, viral cytopathic changes seen in cytomegalovirus, herpes simplex, or adenovirus infection (nuclear and/or cytoplasmic inclusions) are characteristic for these diseases to suggest the diagnosis. Similarly, respiratory syncytial virus, measles, and other paramyxoviruses are usually associated with multinucleated giant cells with cytoplasmic or nuclear inclusions (so-called Warthin-Finkeldey cells). A list of the different types of inclusions seen in viral lung infection is shown in *Table 14-1*.

Table 14-1 Viral Pneumonias Showing Viral Cytopathic Effect

Virus	Cell Type/Cellular Location	Other Features
Cytomegalovirus	Alveolar epithelium and endothelial cells/nuclear and cytoplasmic	Single nuclear basophilic inclusion (~20 μm) with surrounding clear halo
		Multiple smaller cytoplasmic inclusions that are GMS and PAS positive; also highlighted with Giemsa or Wright stains in cytology preparations
Herpes simplex 1-2 and varicella-zoster virus	Bronchial and alveolar epithelium/nuclear	Three "Ms": multinucleation, molding, and margination at borders of necrotic lesions. Occasional single eosinophilic inclusion with clear halo (Cowdry A)
		VZV: accompanied by calcified necrotic nodules
Adenovirus	Alveolar epithelium/nuclear	Early infection: small, eosinophilic round inclusion with clear halo (Cowdry A)
		Late infection: smudgy basophilic chromatin (smudge cells)
		Ciliocytophthoria in BAL samples
Respiratory syncytial virus	Bronchial and alveolar epithelium/cytoplasmic	Syncytial cells: multinucleated with round to oval molded nuclei with clear chromatin; cytoplasm few or multiple small, round eosinophilic inclusions with paranuclear distribution, sometimes surrounded by cytoplasmic halo
Measles	Bronchial and alveolar epithelium/nuclear	Multinucleation (up to 50 nuclei) with nuclear eosinophilic inclusions; usually not molding (Warthin-Finkeldey cells)
Parainfluenza virus	Bronchial and alveolar epithelium/cytoplasmic	Early infection: mild increase in cytoplasm and nuclear enlargement
		Late infection: multinucleation (usually less than 10 nuclei), abundant cytoplasm with multiple small cytoplasmic eosinophilic inclusions and cytoplasmic vacuoles
Human metapneumovirus	Alveolar epithelium/nuclear	Smudge cells, similar to adenovirus (see text)
Hendra and Nipah viruses	Bronchial, alveolar, and endothelial cells/cytoplasmic	Multinucleated cells with round eosinophilic cytoplasmic inclusions
		Accompanied by thrombosis and microinfarcts (see text)
Influenza virus (H1N1)	Alveolar epithelial cells/nuclear	Glassy eosinophilic "pseudo-inclusions" with granular mitoses and hemophagocytosis (see text)

BAL, bronchoalveolar lavage.
Viruses that do not produce viral cytopathic changes include hantaviruses, hemorrhagic fever viruses, human bocaviruses, and influenza viruses (the latter show pseudoinclusions).

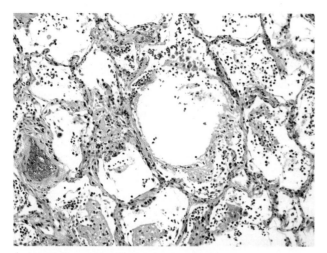

FIGURE 14-1 Histopathologic features of viral pneumonias, acute phase. Viruses can damage type II pneumocytes, the cells producing surfactant, and induce diffuse alveolar damage and the formation of hyaline membranes, also known as acute respiratory distress syndrome or **ARDS (H&E).**

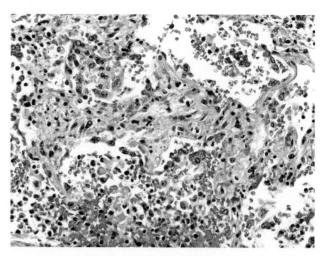

FIGURE 14-2 Histopathologic features of viral pneumonias, resolving phase. Once a viral infection has resolved, the lung parenchyma will develop features of interstitial fibroblastic proliferation and not uncommonly progress to interstitial pneumonia (H&E).

Histologic Features of Viral Pneumonia

Histopathologic features of viral pneumonia may be found throughout the lower respiratory tract, from the bronchial mucosa to the alveolar epithelium. They can be divided into general nonspecific changes present in most viral infections or in specific cytologic changes known as VCE in the form of nuclear and/or cytoplasmic inclusions (see above). General nonspecific features of viral pneumonia include partial or complete necrosis of the bronchial and bronchiolar epithelium and development of diffuse alveolar damage (DAD) during the acute phases or as proliferative changes in the resolving or chronic phases (*Figures 14-1 and 14-2*). Diffuse alveolar damage develops as a consequence of type II pneumocyte destruction by viruses, with decrease production of surfactant, eventual type I pneumocyte destruction, and hyaline membrane formation. In addition, there is usually abundant interstitial lymphocytic infiltrate, which may resolve or progress to pulmonary interstitial fibrosis. Several histologic changes suggestive or specific of particular viral infections are important clues to diagnosis.

Cytomegalovirus

Risk factors of cytomegalovirus lung infection

Human herpes virus type 5 or cytomegalovirus (CMV) is a DNA virus that commonly infects humans. In the past, CMV was known as salivary gland virus due to the frequent congenital salivary gland infection that occurred in newborns (so-called "congenital cytomegalic inclusion disease"). The Centers for Disease

Control and Prevention (CDC) reports that 50% to 80% adults at age 40 are infected with CMV in the United States.[3] The virus can be transmitted through secretions, mainly saliva, blood transfusions, and transplacentally. CMV infection is usually asymptomatic or may manifest as a mononucleosis-like picture with negative heterophile antibodies in immunocompetent individuals. The virus remains latent in the host indefinitely. However, newborns and immunosuppressed individuals, that is, HIV-infected patients with low CD4 counts (<50 cells/μL), patients with lymphoproliferative disorders or transplant recipients, are at increased risk for primary CMV infection and reactivation of prior infection. Immunosuppressants that diminish T-cell-mediated immunity, such as antithymocyte globulin, are associated with a higher rate of CMV reactivation, which may be latent in the host or the transplanted organ. CMV may also play a role in decreasing the T-cell response and favor superinfection with other opportunistic microorganisms, that is, *Pneumocystis jiroveci*, and produce severe interstitial pneumonia. CMV remains the most important pathogen following lung transplantation, either by direct damage to the lung after reactivation of the virus, or indirectly by enhanced allorecognition, facilitating the development of acute or chronic rejection.[4]

Clinical features of cytomegalovirus lung infection

Neonates or immunosuppressed patients with CMV infection may develop multisystem disease affecting any organ (retina, lung, liver, kidneys, adrenals, salivary gland, pancreas, and brain). CMV disease may occur in 40% of lung transplant recipients and in 15% to

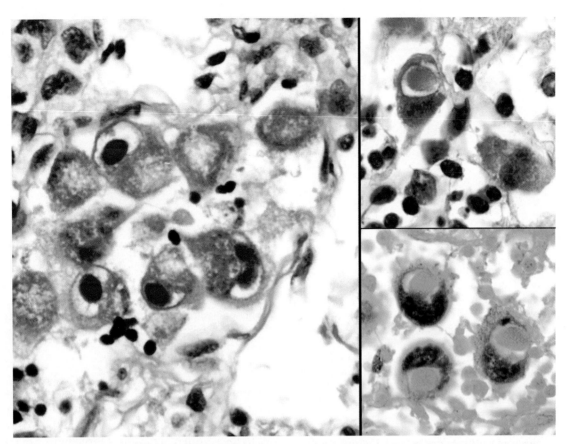

FIGURE 14-3 **Cytomegalovirus viral inclusions. Epithelial and endothelial cells show cellular enlargement (cytomegaly) with the presence of characteristic nuclear and cytoplasmic inclusions. The nuclear inclusion typically retracts from the nuclear membrane and gives the appearance of an "owl's eye" (H&E, left). The cytoplasmic inclusions are less commonly appreciated on H&E stain but can be highlighted with the periodic acid-Schiff (PAS, top right) or the Grocott methenamine silver (GMS) stains (bottom right). Because of these tinctorial properties, cytomegaloviral cellular changes were originally thought to represent a parasitic infection.**

20% of bone marrow transplant patients with a mortality rate of 85% without appropriate antiviral treatment. The highest risk of infection or reactivation occurs 1 to 3 months after transplantation.[5,6] Risk factors in these patients include the type of immunosuppressant used, presence of acute graft-versus-host disease (GVHD), older age, viremia, and pretransplant CMV antigenemia. Patients with CMV pneumonia primarily manifest systemic symptoms (fever, night sweats, malaise, anorexia, fatigue, arthralgias, myalgias) that precede pulmonary symptoms (tachypnea, hypoxia, and unproductive cough).

Imaging features of cytomegalovirus lung infection

Typical radiologic findings include bilateral interstitial or reticulonodular infiltrates that first appear in the lower lobes and later spread to the center of the lungs and then to the superior lobes.[7,8] A localized or nodular presentation is rare.

Cytologic and histologic features of cytomegalovirus lung infection

Microscopically, CMV infection has a pathognomonic VCE. CMV-infected cells show nuclear and cytoplasmic enlargement, with a single large, round basophilic or eosinophilic inclusion that fills the entire nucleus (~20 μm). The inclusion is separated from the nuclear membrane by an artifactual clear halo produced by formalin fixation, which creates the characteristic "owl's eye" appearance (*Figure 14-3*). Cytoplasmic inclusions, either small and granular or large, round, and eosinophilic, are not uncommonly seen in tissues, but are easily identified in cytologic specimens stained with metachromatic stains (Diff-Quick, Giemsa). These inclusions can be positive for periodic acid-Schiff (PAS) and Grocott methenamine silver (GMS) stains, which explains why CMV inclusions were mistaken for intracellular parasites in the past (*Figure 14-3*). Four patterns of CMV infection in the lung have been described: one with minimal inflammation and scattered cells showing

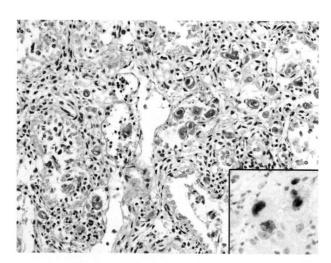

FIGURE 14-4 **Cytomegalovirus infection. Lung tissue from a case of disseminated cytomegaloviral infection in a death fetus. The lungs showed miliary-type spread of infection with foci of 10 to 20 cells with hallmark features of cytomegalovirus infection. Although the viral cytopathic effect is characteristic, immunohistochemistry is helpful to highlight infected cells that are not obviously recognized in areas of necrosis or with a prominent inflammatory background (inset).**

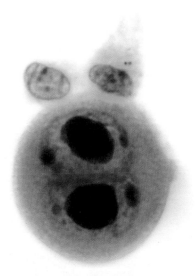

FIGURE 14-5 **Cytomegaloviral cytopathic effect in the bronchoalveolar lavage from a lung transplant recipient. Compare the size of the infected cell with normal adjacent cells (Papanicolaou stain).**

VCE; a pattern with diffuse interstitial pneumonia; an infection with miliary-type spread; and a hemorrhagic/necrotizing pneumonia[9] (*Figure 14-4*). The background of CMV pneumonia may range from minimal nonspecific changes to interstitial inflammation to DAD with hyaline membranes, intra-alveolar fibrin deposition, and diffuse hemorrhage and necrosis. In areas with abundant necrosis, CMV inclusions may not be obvious and the only feature suggestive of infection is the presence of enlarged cells with "smudgy" chromatin. Likewise, inclusions may be rare or not easily seen after antiviral therapy. CMV infection may be corroborated by IHC or immunofluorescence (IF) using monoclonal antibodies specific for CMV late proteins (ie, pp64, pp65) in lung tissue (*Figure 14-4*). In situ hybridization (ISH) is another technique for detection of CMV that is equally as effective as IHC; however, IHC is easier and faster to perform and interpret.[10] The specificity of IHC in tissue without CMV VCE is not known. Thus, it is not recommended to perform CMV IHC without clinical suspicion or histologic changes suggestive of CMV. CMV pneumonia may be diagnosed on bronchoalveolar lavage (BAL) (*Figure 14-5*), but the preferred method for diagnosis on these types of specimens is molecular analysis (see below).

Laboratory diagnosis of cytomegalovirus

Serologic tests for CMV detection include quantification of serum IgM and IgG specific antibodies and the CMV antigenemia assay. Enzyme-linked immunosorbent assay (ELISA) detects IgM anti-CMV antibodies in greater than 90% of adults with primary CMV infection. The presence of IgM anti-CMV antibodies in the serum of a newborn is diagnostic of congenital CMV infection. On the other hand, IgM titers may be low or absent in immunocompromised patients with active infection. A significant (fourfold) increase in IgG titers suggests recent infection with CMV, but IgG levels in immunocompromised patients are not reliable to detect reactivation of latent virus. Preferred methods for diagnosis are shell-vial viral culture or the CMV antigenemia assay. Viral culture is the gold standard diagnostic test but results are available only after 7 to 10 days. As treatment of patients with respiratory failure or severe pneumonia cannot be delayed, many patients are treated prophylactically if rapid assays are not available. The CMV antigenemia assay detects the viral protein pp65 in peripheral blood leukocytes using indirect IF. It is a rapid and sensitive test that allows detection of viral antigens during replication of the virus. It is one of the reference tests for monitoring CMV infection in immunosuppressed patients, particularly transplant recipients. The test correlates with worsening of clinical symptoms and with progression of disease, so it is useful to determine the need for antiviral therapy and to monitor the patient's response to antiviral treatment. Molecular tests for CMV detection include qualitative and quantitative (real-time) PCR. Real-time PCR uses specific primers for CMV early protein genes.

PCR can be used to quantitate the amount of CMV DNA, which increases immediately preceding symptoms of CMV disease and decreases after antiviral therapy.[11] Assessment of CMV DNA by PCR is more sensitive than the antigenemia test for detecting recurrent CMV disease in lung transplant patients.[11] PCR can be also performed on bronchoalveolar lavage specimens with excellent sensitivity, specificity, and positive predictive values.[12,13]

Treatment of cytomegalovirus lung infection

Treatment of CMV includes intravenous (IV) ganciclovir or oral valganciclovir (a ganciclovir prodrug). If resistance develops, alternative drugs include intravenous foscarnet or cidofovir for at least 3 to 6 weeks. Long-term maintenance therapy is usually indicated. Intravenous CMV immunoglobulin in combination with ganciclovir may decrease the incidence of CMV pneumonia in one-third of lung transplant patients.[4,5]

Prognosis of cytomegalovirus lung infection

Transplanted patients have a high mortality after developing CMV pneumonia even with antiviral treatment, and practically all patients will succumb to the disease if untreated. Thus, it is important for pathologists to recognize the features of CMV in surveillance lung transplant biopsies. Drug resistance to ganciclovir may develop, although it is rare. To further complicate the picture, CMV may produce immunosuppression leading to increased susceptibility to bacterial or fungal infections and GVHD in certain patients.[5]

Herpes Simplex Virus Type 1 and 2

Risk factors of herpes simplex virus lung infection

Herpes viruses are double-stranded DNA viruses that commonly infect humans. There are two serotypes of herpes simplex virus (HSV) that infect humans, HSV-1 and 2. These viruses are transmitted from person to person by direct contact with infected secretions or lesions. HSV-1 is more frequently isolated from oral lesions, whereas HSV-2 is more commonly detected in genital lesions. Nevertheless, HSV-1 may produce genital infection and vice versa. Healthy individuals infected with HSV-1 or 2 show either no symptoms or may develop mild skin lesions that may go unnoticed. Symptomatic disease includes the formation of blisters on or around the mouth and genitals and rarely malaise, fever, and lymphadenopathy. The virus remains latent in spinal ganglia after the initial infection and may reactivate sporadically or after immunosuppression. Concerning infections in immunocompetent hosts include herpetic keratitis, necrotizing tonsillitis, encephalitis, and aseptic meningitis. Neonates are at risk for encephalitis and disseminated infection after vaginal delivery from mothers with HSV-related genital lesions. Immunosuppressed individuals are at risk for herpes esophagitis, tracheobronchitis, HSV pneumonia, hepatitis, and disseminated infection.[6] Well-established risk factors for lower respiratory tract infection—usually caused by HSV-1—in patients with impaired immune systems or critically ill patients include intubation with aspiration of or contamination with oropharyngeal secretions.

Clinical features of herpes simplex virus lung infection

Mucocutaneous infection usually precedes HSV pneumonia[14] which occurs by hematogenous spread from oral or genital lesions. Outbreaks of HSV pneumonia in intensive care units have been related to nosocomial transmission of HSV through ventilators.[15] Individuals with extensive burns are also at risk for skin and lower respiratory tract infection. Pulmonary coinfection with *Pneumocystis jiroveci* is usually fatal. Clinical findings include development of fever, cough, dyspnea, and wheezing, with progression to hypoxia and the need for mechanical ventilation.[16]

Imaging features of herpes simplex virus lung infection

Three patterns of HSV pneumonia have been described by high-resolution computed tomography (HRCT) scan including predominant areas of diffuse or multifocal ground glass attenuation; predominant areas of multifocal peribronchial consolidations; and a mixed pattern.[17,18] Pleural effusions are not uncommon.[8]

Cytologic and histologic features of herpes simplex virus lung infection

The typical VCE in HSV infection is characterized by enlarged epithelial cells with nuclear amphophilic to eosinophilic "glassy" inclusions (Cowdry A inclusions) that displace the chromatin toward the periphery (margination) and sometimes leave a nuclear halo. HSV-infected cells are often multinucleated with compacted nuclei, each one containing a glassy inclusion (multinucleation and molding) (*Figure 14-6*). In immunocompromised patients, a pattern of extensive lung necrosis is suggestive of HSV infection. VCE is characteristically found at the periphery of the necrotic lesions, which may occur in part due to HSV-induced vasculitis. Histologically, HSV pneumonia may manifest in three different patterns, including a necrotizing tracheobronchitis, necrotizing pneumonia, and an interstitial pneumonia, all with variable proportion of cells showing VCE.[9] Necrotizing tracheobronchitis is characterized by extensive ulceration and necrosis of the lower respiratory tract mucosa and formation of fibrinopurulent

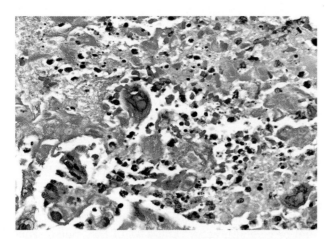

FIGURE 14-6 Herpes simplex virus, viral cytopathic effect, and necrotic changes. Infected respiratory bronchial epithelial cells demonstrates cellular enlargement with abundant eosinophilic cytoplasm, multinucleation, molding, and margination (the "three Ms"). Note the extensive necrosis and hemorrhage in the background (H&E).

exudate (*Figures 14-7 and 14-8*). Necrotizing pneumonia is mainly distributed around bronchi and is composed of extensive necroinflammatory infiltrates in the surrounding lung tissue. Interstitial pneumonia is usually diffuse and shows features of DAD with interstitial inflammation, interstitial edema, intra-alveolar fibrinous exudates with hemorrhage, and hyaline membrane formation. This pattern corresponds to the areas of ground glass attenuation observed on HRCT.[17] BAL may detect epithelial cells with VCE, which are more likely to be observed in immunosuppressed patients

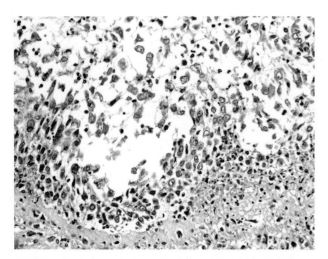

FIGURE 14-7 Herpes simplex virus, necrotizing tracheobronchitis. In this case of fatal pneumonia, the mucosa shows necrosis and sloughing of the bronchiolar epithelium with presence of several eosinophilic nuclear inclusions. The differential diagnosis includes herpes simplex, varicella-zoster virus or adenoviral infection (H&E). Immunohistochemical stains were positive for HSV1-2.

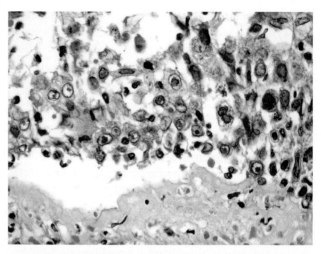

FIGURE 14-8 Herpes simplex virus, necrotizing tracheobronchitis. Higher magnification on the same case depicted in Figure 14-7 shows several eosinophilic inclusions in the bronchiolar respiratory cells (left) and occasional cells with typical herpes simplex inclusion (right). If only these features are seen, the differential diagnosis includes herpes simplex, varicella-zoster virus or adenoviral infections (H&E). Immunohistochemistry was positive for HSV1-2.

(*Figure 14-9*). In certain circumstances, the presence of extensive necrosis and few cells with VCE may suggest the possibility of adenoviral or varicella-zoster virus infection, which may be practically impossible to differentiate from HSV infection by morphology. In these circumstances, IHC and/or ISH for HSV-1/HSV-2 are extremely helpful.

Laboratory diagnosis of herpes simplex viruses

The gold standard test for diagnosis of acute HSV lesions in mucous membranes is the shell-vial culture. This technique requires centrifugation of the sample and inoculation of mink lung cells followed by detection of HSV-specific antigens by IHC. Ninety-nine percent (99%) of positive cultures are detected in less than 24 hours. Other methods include detection of HSV antigens on cells scraped from the base of mucocutaneous lesions by IF or ELISA. Test results by antigen detection are obtained within hours and have high specificity, but a sensitivity of 80%. On the other hand, determination of HSV antibody titers is less helpful to detect lung infection. Its major clinical utility is to identify seropositive organ transplant recipients who may need prophylactic antiviral therapy prior to transplantation.

For detection of HSV in cases of pneumonia or necrotizing tracheobronchitis, cells should be collected by bronchial washing or a BAL. Collection by this method

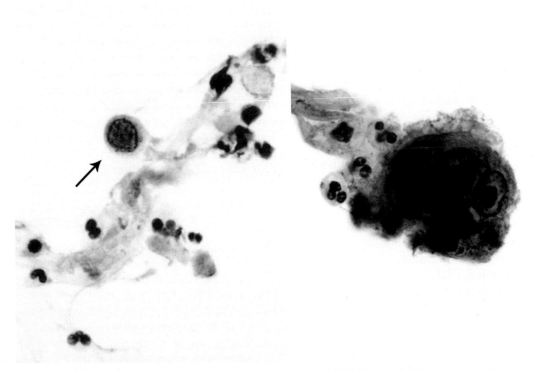

FIGURE 14-9 Herpes Simplex viral cytopathic effect in the BAL cytology specimen from an immunocompromised patient. A cell with no multinucleation shows a nuclear inclusion (left, arrow). Other areas of the specimen showed enlarged cells with multinucleation, molding, and margination (right) (Papanicolaou stain).

may be insufficient to allow diagnosis by culture or antigen detection. In this context, PCR is the preferred method for diagnosis and may improve the diagnostic yield of HSV testing by 50% in BAL specimens.[19] PCR for HSV uses flanking primers spanning the glycoprotein D region of HSV-1 and 2 viruses. HSV detection is confirmed by melting-curve analysis. Amplification of HSV DNA has high sensitivity and specificity and is excellent for providing a timely diagnosis. PCR is the recommended method for detection of HSV in AIDS patients and may identify the causative agent in the setting of pneumonia of unknown etiology when culture, antigen detection, and histology have failed and antiviral treatment is needed promptly. The only caveat of PCR is that sensitivity will depend on the amount HSV DNA present in a sample. An HSV-positive BAL is more likely to be found in immunosuppressed patients with acute respiratory disease or patients who develop unexplained ground glass attenuations on imaging.[19]

Treatment of herpes simplex virus lung infection

Antiviral treatment for HSV pneumonia includes the use of IV acyclovir, an inhibitor of the viral DNA polymerase. When administered early in HSV pneumonitis, acyclovir has been shown to modify the course of infection and to improve survival. Addition of respiratory ventilation and reduction of immunosuppression have also been recommended for management. However, acyclovir-resistant strains have been reported and represent a growing problem, particularly in solid-organ transplant recipients.[20] In this instance, treatment with vidarabine or foscarnet has been used.

Prognosis of herpes simplex virus lung infection

Early diagnosis and antiviral treatment of HSV pneumonia substantially modifies the course of infection. If untreated, HSV pneumonia usually progresses into refractory acute respiratory distress syndrome (ARDS) with limited treatment options and high (80%) mortality. Controversy exists regarding the relationship between viral load and poor outcome in critically ill patients in the intensive care unit (ICU) setting.[21-23] A recent study has pointed to the detection of HSV-1 DNA in few samples of idiopathic pulmonary fibrosis, suggesting a potential association between HSV-1 and fibrotic idiopathic interstitial pneumonia.[24] Further studies will be necessary to confirm these findings.

Adenovirus

Risk factors of adenovirus lung infection

Adenoviruses are enveloped double-stranded DNA viruses (60-80 nm) that were originally recognized to produce "adenoid degeneration" in adenoid tissue cultures, hence the name. These viruses are normally found in the respiratory and gastrointestinal tract and may produce sporadic or epidemic infections due to reactivation after a period of latency. Outbreaks of infection occur more commonly among people in close groups, such as those in day care, among military recruits, and students. Neonates, malnourished children, and immunocompromised patients are at risk of developing severe disease including pneumonia, encephalitis, or systemic infection. Recent data indicate that adenoviruses produce about 6% of acute respiratory disease in children younger than 5 years.[25] The prevalence of adenoviral pneumonia in children varies from region to region, causing approximately 2% of the pediatric pneumonias in Argentina[26] and up to 13% of those in South Africa.[27] More than 50 serotypes of adenovirus are known and only a third of them produce human disease. Serotypes 1, 2, 3, and 7 are associated with pneumonia in children and serotypes 3 and 7 are associated with development of acute respiratory failure.[28,29] On the other hand, serotypes 4 and 7 are more commonly detected in military personnel in the United States.[30] In adults, serotypes 3, 4, and 7 are the most commonly associated with pneumonia. In the United States, adenovirus serotype 14 has been recognized as a more virulent serotype that produces severe respiratory disease and pneumonia in immunocompetent adults including civilians and military trainees.[31-33] This serotype was originally identified in the United States in 2005 and outbreaks of febrile respiratory illness have been reported since then in Washington, Oregon, and Texas.[31] In a study from MD Anderson, adenoviral pneumonia was the second most common manifestation of infection in allogeneic hematopoietic stem cell transplant (HSCT) recipients, accounting for 24% of all infections, just after gastrointestinal infection.[34]

Clinical features of adenovirus lung infection

The clinical manifestations of adenoviral pneumonia in children are similar to those seen in bacterial pneumonia with fever, cough, rhinorrhea, and dyspnea usually accompanied by gastrointestinal symptoms and moderate leukocytosis.[28] In some instances, acute adenoviral pneumonia is difficult to distinguish from bacterial infections, and appropriate detection of the causal agent becomes crucial to initiate adequate therapy. Presence of dyspnea is a risk factor associated with ICU admission.[28]

Imaging features of adenovirus lung infection

Imaging studies in patients with adenoviral pneumonia may show different patterns of lung involvement, including bilateral patchy areas of consolidation, interstitial infiltration, and rarely lobar consolidation or diffuse areas of air space consolidation.[35] Children usually show severe hyperinflation and bilateral bronchopneumonia.[8] Adults and immunocompetent individuals who develop adenoviral pneumonia usually present with fever, cough, and dyspnea, and lymphopenia rather than leukocytosis. Patients often have bilateral interstitial infiltrates on chest radiographs.[16]

Cytologic and histologic features of adenovirus lung infection

The VCE in adenoviral infection includes the presence of nuclear inclusions similar to those seen in HSV infection. Two types of nuclear inclusions related to the time of infection have been described: in early infection, the cells have a single small, eosinophilic, round to oval inclusion surrounded by a clear halo (Cowdry A). At later stages, the inclusion becomes basophilic and larger, with disappearance of the halo and blurring of the borders between the inclusion and the nuclear membrane, giving the chromatin a "smudgy" appearance (smudge cells) (*Figure 14-10*). The infected cells may be only slightly larger than noninfected cells but never enlarge to the degree of HSV or CMV-infected cells. In BAL, adenoviral cytopathic effect may also be accompanied by ciliocytophthoria.

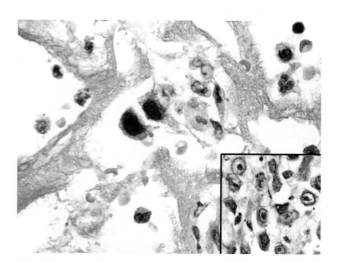

FIGURE 14-10 **Adenovirus. Cells with enlarged nucleus and smudgy chromatin are characteristic of adenoviral infection in late stages (so-called "smudge cells") (center). In early stages of infection, the smudge cells may not be present and only Cowdry type A inclusions, similar to those seen in Herpes simplex and varicella-zoster virus infection, are observed (inset, H&E).**

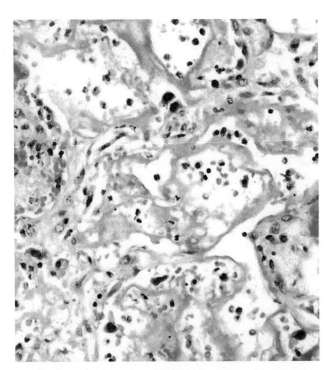

FIGURE 14-11 Adenovirus. Case of adenovirus pneumonia with diffuse alveolar damage and extensive necrosis (H&E). The necrosis seen in adenoviral infection has been referred to as "dirty" necrosis.

Adenovirus may affect the lung in two different or combined patterns, including an acute severe necrotizing pneumonia with or without necrotizing bronchitis and bronchiolitis, or an interstitial pattern with DAD, intra alveolar hemorrhage, and necrosis (*Figure 14-11*). Necrosis of bronchi is usually referred to as "dirty" necrosis due to the presence of karyorrhectic nuclei and cellular debris. The destruction of the respiratory mucosa is followed by deposition of acellular PAS-positive basement membrane-like material. Adenoviral VCE may only be obvious at the border of necrotic areas and distinction from HSV is impossible if no smudge cells are seen. Immunohistochemical stain for specific proteins of adenovirus (ie, E1A) will confirm infection by this pathogen.

Laboratory diagnosis of adenovirus

Several methods for detection of adenovirus infection are available, including viral antigen detection, serologic tests (IgM and IgG titers), viral culture, and PCR. For viral subtyping, hemagglutination-inhibition assays or neutralization with type-specific antisera are used. For viral culture, respiratory secretions are inoculated into specific cell lines and VCE is evaluated in 2 to 20 days. Rapid antigen detection, direct IF, and PCR methodologies will determine viral infection more rapidly. PCR is a more rapid and preferred method

for adenovirus detection. In a recent study involving immunocompromised children with viral pneumonia, PCR had high sensitivity and specificity (both above 80%) when viral culture and rapid antigen test were used as the gold standard.[13] Quantitative real-time PCR performed on HSCT recipients appears to be a good predictor of disease with plasma viral loads above 1000 copies/mL.[36] Multiplex RT-PCR with enzyme hybridization is a newly developed test that allows rapid detection of the most common viruses causing respiratory infections (influenza virus A and B, RSV, parainfluenza virus, human metapneumovirus, and rhinovirus), including adenovirus.[1]

Treatment of adenovirus lung infection

The antiviral drug of choice for adenoviral pneumonia is cidofovir. This drug inhibits viral replication and transcription and does not depend on the presence of viral enzymes. Early treatment with cidofovir and donor lymphocyte infusions show promising efficacy in HSCT recipients.[37,38] On the other hand, ribavirin and vidarabine are not effective for adenoviral pneumonia.[38]

Prognosis of adenovirus lung infection

Physicians should keep in mind adenovirus as the cause of lower respiratory infection in children that develop pneumonia with patchy infiltrates and have poor response to antibiotic therapy. Although rare, bronchiolitis obliterans is a well-known long-term respiratory complication from adenoviral pneumonia and close follow-up of these patients is needed. It is important to mention that if infection with adenovirus serotype 14 is suspected, immediate contact to the state health department should be established.[31]

Respiratory Syncytial Virus

Risk factors of respiratory syncytial virus lung infection

Respiratory syncytial virus (RSV) is a single-stranded RNA virus of the family *Paramyxoviridae* with a genome of approximately 15,000 nucleotides. The name of the virus derives from the identification of syncitia formation observed in cell cultures infected with the virus. Worldwide, RSV is the most common cause of lower respiratory infection in childhood (29%) just followed by influenza (17%),[39] and is the second most common viral pneumonia in older adults.[16] Viral outbreaks are more frequent during the winter season and decrease in the summer. There are two serologic groups of RSV, A and B, with no correlation with severity of symptoms. RSV is a major cause of nosocomial infection. Children younger than 6 months, those with low birth weight or congenital cardiac or pulmonary disease, are at risk for developing severe respiratory symptoms. By age 5, more than 80% of children have been exposed to and have developed incomplete immunity to RSV, and some children may manifest disease with milder symptoms. A risk of severe infection increases again at older ages (>65 years old) and in patients with underlying cardiac or lung disease (ie, chronic obstructive pulmonary disease) with a mortality rate ranging between 10% and 78%.[16] In immunocompromised adults (bone marrow transplant recipients, leukemia, AIDS patients) mortality ranges between 30% and 50%. Mortality is mostly related to severe lymphopenia, history of recent transplant (within the first month after transplantation), and older age.[16,40] Epidemics of RSV pneumonia affecting the elderly have been reported in nursing homes.

Clinical features of respiratory syncytial virus lung infection

In infants and young children, the clinical presentation of RSV infection typically includes a prodrome of upper respiratory symptoms with rhinorrhea, low-grade fever, and cough, and a later onset of lower respiratory symptoms including tachypnea, wheezing, and rales. Less than half of these patients will develop croup, bronchitis, bronchiolitis, pneumonia, or apnea requiring hospitalization. Older children without underlying problems may develop mild upper respiratory symptoms. Similar to children, adults may develop upper respiratory symptoms such as coryza and pharyngitis that precede lower respiratory symptoms including tracheobronchitis, bronchiolitis, and pneumonia. RSV infection of the lower respiratory tract can cause severe respiratory complications and high mortality, similar to seasonal influenza. Patients with RSV pneumonia typically present with fever, dyspnea, nonproductive cough, and wheezing, rales, and rhonchi on physical examination. Importantly, in adults with underlying cardiopulmonary disease, the symptoms of RSV infection may be poorly defined and difficult to identify. Occasionally, if clinical suspicion for viral pneumonia is low, such symptoms may be attributed to decompensation of the underlying cardiopulmonary problem rather than an acute viral infection. These patients usually present with long-standing respiratory tract infection with productive cough and wheezing. As mentioned above, immunocompromised adults will present with more severe symptoms and possibly with acute respiratory failure necessitating mechanical ventilation.

Imaging features of respiratory syncytial virus lung infection

Radiologically, RSV pneumonia typically presents with patchy bilateral alveolar infiltrates and an interstitial ground glass pattern of spread. Less often, the disease may manifest with small and ill-defined infiltrates.[35]

Cytologic and histologic features of respiratory syncytial virus lung infection

As mentioned previously, the name RSV denotes the typical VCE seen on viral cultures and on respiratory epithelial cells (ciliated cells, type I and type II pneumocytes) in vivo which consists in the formation of multinucleated giant cells (syncytial cells). The syncytial cells are not observed in all cases of RSV pneumonia but when present they are scattered throughout the bronchiolar and alveolar walls. Syncytial cells show multiple round-to-oval molded nuclei with intermediate-sized nucleoli and clear chromatin. The cytoplasm is abundant and may contain few or multiple characteristic small, round cytoplasmic eosinophilic inclusions, although they may be difficult to appreciate. These cytoplasmic inclusions are paranuclear and may be surrounded by a clear halo (*Figure 14-12*).

RSV usually manifests as necrotizing bronchiolitis or giant cell interstitial pneumonia.[9] In necrotizing bronchiolitis, there is circumferential inflammation in medium-sized airways with necrosis and abundant intraluminal debris composed of sloughed necrotic epithelium and inflammatory cells admixed with fibrin and mucus (*Figure 14-13*). The peribronchiolar inflammation is composed of macrophages and lymphocytes underneath the smooth muscle layer and neutrophils in the lamina propria and epithelium.[41] In vitro

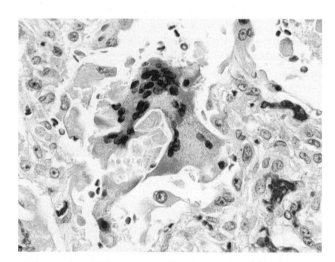

FIGURE 14-12 Respiratory syncytial virus. The viral cytopathic effect induced by this *Paramyxovirus* consists of markedly enlarged multinucleated cells (syncytial cells) with abundant eosinophilic—sometimes vacuolated—cytoplasm that may contain small eosinophilic inclusions. The nuclei show nuclear clearing but no nuclear inclusions are seen. Syncytial cells are not rigid and usually acquire the shape of the surrounding tissue (H&E).

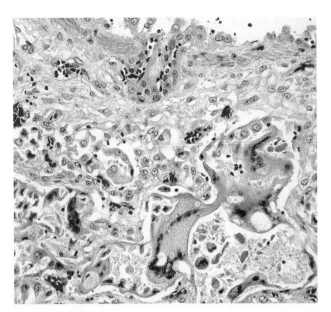

FIGURE 14-13 Respiratory syncytial virus. This terminal bronchiole shows surrounding inflammation, focal hemorrhage, and the presence of syncytial cells. The mucosa (top) shows marked reactive epithelium (H&E).

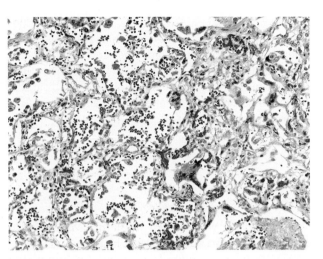

FIGURE 14-14 Giant cell pneumonia. There is diffuse alveolar damage with hyaline membrane formation, intra-alveolar hemorrhage, and scattered syncytial cells present in the alveolar walls. Case of respiratory syncytial virus pneumonia (H&E). Measles pneumonia and infections by other paramyxoviruses may be very similar.

experiments have shown that RSV is capable of sensitizing respiratory cells to apoptosis, supporting the concept of bronchiolar necrosis due to viral infection.[42] Enlargement of the bronchial-associated mucosal lymphoid tissue may worsen bronchiolar obstruction.[41] In giant cell interstitial pneumonia, there are increased numbers of syncytial cells and prominent DAD with associated inflammation and edema (*Figure 14-14*). This pattern is more commonly seen in immunocompromised patients. During the resolution phase, peribronchiolar fibrosis may occur and produce severe obstructive changes. When syncytial cells are found, the differential diagnosis should include other viral diseases that have multinucleated giant cells, including parainfluenza, measles, and herpes-zoster infection. Nonviral giant cell interstitial pneumonia should also be considered. However, syncytial cells may not be present in all cases and only the clinical picture, a high index of suspicion, and additional tests may aid in the diagnosis of the pathogen. IHC and/or IF for specific RSV antigens may be needed to establish diagnosis. In a series of pediatric autopsy cases with RSV pneumonia, IHC demonstrated RSV antigen in all ciliated cells but not in the basal cells of bronchioles. IHC also showed linear immunostaining in alveolar walls as well as in the intraluminal debris.

Laboratory diagnosis of respiratory syncytial virus

RSV can be isolated by viral culture from nasopharyngeal washes, tracheal secretions, or BAL with higher detection rate in the latter (89% of cases). However, due to the virus thermolability, this data may vary among laboratories. Inoculated cell lines will show the characteristic VCE and viral antigens may be detected by IF in 72 hours. Rapid detection is accomplished by ELISA with a sensitivity ranging from 80% to 90%. Antigen detection and viral culture are more reliable in young children and less useful in older children and adults. For the latter patients, multiplex RT-PCR should be considered.[1] Serologic tests are usually not used for diagnosis.

Treatment of respiratory syncytial virus lung infection

The only antiviral drug available for RSV pneumonia is ribavirin, a nucleoside analog of guanosine. An intravenous immunoglobulin that binds the membrane protein F from RSV (palivizumab) has also been used in the prevention of RSV infection. Treatment for RSV pneumonia in children includes the use of bronchodilators with the addition of ribavirin and palivizumab for infants and premature infants with acute severe disease or underlying risk factors. There is controversy regarding the treatment of RSV pneumonia in HSCT recipients. Use of aerosolized ribavirin and palivizumab may improve outcome in these patients, but recent guidelines recommend using these drugs with caution.[40]

Prognosis of respiratory syncytial virus lung infection

Factors associated with poor survival in RSV pneumonia include older age (>65 years old), radiologically confirmed pneumonia, requirement of mechanical ventilation, bacterial superinfection, and increased leukocytosis.[43] In HSCT recipients, lymphopenia, allogeneic transplant performed less than 1 month before infection, severe immunodeficiency and age >65 years have been associated with increased mortality.[40] RSV pneumonia may leave patients with residual disability from interstitial fibrosis. Patients may also be at risk of developing asthma later on.

Varicella-Zoster Virus

Risk factors of varicella-zoster virus lung infection

Varicella-zoster virus (VZV) or herpes virus type 5 causes chickenpox and shingles. Chickenpox occurs as a primary infection more commonly in children. The virus remains latent in the spinal cord ganglia and sporadically reactivates producing shingles, a limited form of VZV infection that presents with postherpetic neuralgia in a dermatomal distribution. The virus spreads by respiratory droplets and direct contact with skin lesions. Allegedly, primary infection never results in reinfection but this may not hold true. In the past, it was thought that chickenpox and shingles were different diseases, hence the names varicella (from the old term "variola") and zoster (a Greek term meaning "belt or girdle"). Chickenpox is a common infection in children with rare progression to VZV pneumonia. On the other hand, pneumonia is a major complication for adults infected with VZV, with VZV-related pneumonia reported in 10% to up to 50% of infected adult patients.[16,44,45] Smoking is a well-known risk factor for severe VZV pneumonia in immunocompetent adults. Third-trimester pregnant women, neonates infected before maternal antibodies against VZV have formed (usually within 4 days of delivery or 2 days postdelivery),[46] and immunosuppressed individuals are at higher risk of developing disseminated infection and pneumonia. These patients also have higher mortality rates (30%-40%) compared to the general population (10%). Adults with impaired-cell-mediated immunity and bone marrow transplant recipients have a higher risk of disseminated VZV infection and pneumonia (50%) compared to children with leukemia and solid tumors (30%).[45]

Clinical features of varicella-zoster virus lung infection

Clinically, patients with VZV develop low-grade fever, malaise, and a vesicular rash on the trunk and face that spreads centrifugally to the rest of the body with skin lesions at different stages of evolution.[45,47] VZV pneumonia develops 1 to 6 days later, after the previous symptoms are established, and is characterized by the eruption of new skin lesions, persistent fever, and dry cough. Patients later develop dyspnea, tachypnea, chest pain, and hemoptysis. Severe abdominal and/or back pain due to neuralgia is frequently seen 1 or 2 days prior to the onset of pneumonia.[45] Detection of several deep ulcers by bronchoscopy has been correlated with fatal outcomes in VZV pneumonia.[48]

Imaging features of varicella-zoster virus lung infection

Radiographic findings show ill-defined bilateral, nodular, or reticular infiltrates of different sizes. These lesions usually present with a peribronchial distribution and eventually extend throughout the lungs. Patients with previous history of VZV pneumonia may exhibit diffuse pulmonary punctate calcifications in chest radiographs that could erroneously be interpreted as a parasitic or granulomatous disease.[45,49] Similarly, HRCT scans from patients with VZV pneumonia will show multiple small (5-10 mm) lung nodules with or without surrounding ground glass attenuation, patchy ground glass attenuation, or coalescent nodules.[47,50]

Cytologic and histologic features of varicella-zoster virus lung infection

The histopathologic changes and VCE seen in VZV pneumonia are similar to those seen in HSV pneumonitis. The lung parenchyma will show diffuse hemorrhagic and necrotic foci that involve alveolar walls, blood vessels, and small bronchioles, correlating with the nodules seen on imaging. VZV nuclear inclusions and multinucleated giant cells identical to those seen in HSV infection may be found at the borders of necrotic areas, but are usually difficult to find. IHC for VZV may help identify infected cells and differentiate the VCE from HSV. In addition, there are interstitial mononuclear infiltrates with edema, intra-alveolar fibrin deposition and hemorrhage, type II pneumocyte hyperplasia, DAD, and hyaline membrane formation. Necrotizing bronchitis or bronchiolitis may occasionally be encountered. Resolved VZV lesions are composed of a fibrous capsule with a necrotic center that may calcify.

Laboratory diagnosis of varicella-zoster virus

The diagnosis of VZV is generally established on clinical basis. VZV can be isolated from bronchial wash and/or BAL by viral culture and rapid antigen detection by IF. As with HSV, PCR to detect viral nucleic acids is more sensitive and specific than antigen detection methods or viral culture.[51]

Treatment of varicella-zoster virus lung infection

Untreated adult VZV pneumonia is fatal in 10% of the cases. Treatment of VZV pneumonia includes the use of ventilatory support and IV acyclovir. Early treatment with acyclovir reduces mortality and visceral herpes zoster.[44,52] Use of VZV immunoglobulin produces transient passive immunity with a protective effect against VZV pneumonia.

Prognosis of varicella-zoster virus lung infection

Complications of VZV pneumonia include bacterial superinfection and sepsis.[45] In bone marrow transplant recipients, severe thrombocytopenia may complicate pulmonary hemorrhage and be followed by disseminated intravascular coagulopathy (DIC). Other complications such as syndrome of inappropriate antidiuretic hormone secretion (SIADH) and pulmonary embolus may develop.[45]

Hantavirus

Risk factors of hantavirus lung infection

Hantaviruses belong to the group of zoonotic viral infections. They are part of the family *Bunyaviridae*, which are enveloped viruses composed of three segments of negative sense RNA. The prefix "hanta" derives from the name "Hantaan," the Korean river where one of the first human epidemics occurred in 1982.[53] Hantaviruses produce an asymptomatic and persistent infection in rodents, with each virus species linked to a major rodent host species in a particular geographic location. The main risk factor for infection is traveling or living in areas where rodent exposure may occur.[54] Transmission occurs by inhalation of aerosolized excreta or rodent bites. The incubation period varies from 1 to 6 weeks. Hantaviruses can affect two different organs: (1) the kidney, producing hemorrhagic fever with renal syndrome (prevalent in Asia and Europe and produced by the Hataan, Seoul, Puumala, Dobrava virus, etc) and (2) the lung, causing hantavirus pulmonary syndrome (HPS, found in North and South America).[53]

The first outbreak of HPS in the United States occurred in May 1993, when several individuals presented with severe acute respiratory failure in the southwestern states of New Mexico, Arizona, Colorado, and Utah (also known as the Four Corners region). The causative agent of this acute respiratory disease was recognized as a new member of the *Hantavirus* genus. The virus was originally called Four Corners virus but was later renamed "Sin Nombre" virus (from the Spanish translation virus "without a name"). The reservoir for Sin Nombre virus was identified as the deer mouse, *Peromyscus maniculatus*. Although HPS had been sporadically reported in these areas before 1993, it is hypothesized that heavy rains increased food sources and rodents expanded their population, making contact with humans more frequently, which eventually progressed to an epidemic.

Thorough study of the clinical and laboratory features and pathologic findings of HPS was accomplished in the University of New Mexico.[55] Other related hantaviruses have been identified in the United States including the Bayou virus in Louisiana, the Black Creek Canal virus in Florida, and the New York virus in Northeast United States. In South America, several other hantaviruses producing HPS have also been recognized (Andes, Laguna Negra, Rio Mamore virus, etc).[56] Sin Nombre virus cannot be transmitted from human to human, but this type of transmission has been reported with Andes virus.[54] In October 2012, another outbreak of 10 confirmed cases of HPS caused by Sin Nombre virus occurred at Yosemite National Park, CA.[57,58]

Clinical features of hantavirus lung infection

Early manifestations of HPS include a vague prodrome of fever, chills, headaches, myalgias, nausea, and vomiting with severe back and hip pain for 1 to 7 days. Headache and abdominal pain may be prominent, followed by dry cough and shortness of breath that progress rapidly to acute respiratory failure and shock.[58] The majority of patients (80%-90%) will require hospitalization, mechanical ventilation, vasopressors, and extracorporeal membrane oxygenation in severe cases.[58-60] The mean age of presentation of HPS is 37 years with a 2:1 male to female ratio. Caucasians are the most commonly affected group followed by Native Americans and Hispanics. Characteristic laboratory findings include the tetrad of neutrophilia with a left shift, thrombocytopenia, hemoconcentration, and immunoblasts in the peripheral blood, accounting for >10% of all lymphoid cells.[55] The constellation of thrombocytopenia and fever in a patient with acute respiratory failure is highly sensitive for the diagnosis of HPS.[59]

Imaging features of hantavirus lung infection

Radiological findings of HPS include the presence of pronounced bilateral pulmonary interstitial infiltrates often with perihilar disease and progression to pulmonary edema with centrally located alveolar infiltrates.[8] Large pleural effusions are common but no cardiomegaly is seen. Rarely, consolidations may be observed.

Cytologic and histologic features of hantavirus lung infection

Sin Nombre virus does not cause any recognizable VCE on light microscopy. The virus can only be recognized by IHC or electron microscopy as inclusion bodies within pulmonary capillary endothelial cells. Pathologic findings seen in HPS include diffuse alveolar edema with alveolar fibrinous exudates. An intravascular and interstitial infiltrate composed of large immunoblast-type cells (CD8+ T cells)[61] may be seen and may even resemble a lymphoma. There is focal formation of hyaline membranes with minimal or no necrosis or acute inflammation. HPS has some histological differences with ARDS from other causes but may also represent an early phase in the ARDS spectrum (*Figure 14-1*). The presence of fibroblastic proliferation, type II pneumocyte hyperplasia, and alveolar wall atelectasis is characteristic of ARDS and rarely found in HPS, while the presence of immunoblast-type cells and positive IHC for hantaviral antigens in endothelial cells and alveolar macrophages is diagnostic of HPS.[61,62]

Laboratory diagnosis of hantaviruses

Laboratory diagnosis of HPS includes serologic tests and RT-PCR methods. In the acute phase, hantavirus-specific IgM titers can be detected in patients' sera by ELISA. Elevated IgG-specific antibodies can be detected during the resolving phases. RT-PCR can be used to confirm the presence of viral RNA in fresh frozen lung tissue or in peripheral blood mononuclear cells.

Treatment of hantavirus lung infection

Treatment of HPS is merely supportive with cardiovascular, respiratory, and renal support. Early supportive care may reduce mortality. Administration of fluids should be done with caution to avoid the risk of pulmonary edema. Patients usually require mechanical ventilation, vasopressors, and possibly extracorporeal mechanical ventilation.[58,60] No antiviral treatment has proven efficacious in HPS. Avoidance of rodents and preventive measures are the best methods to decrease transmission. HPS is a reportable disease to state health department in the United States.

Prognosis of hantavirus lung infection

The mortality rate of HPS is approximately 35%.[57] Patients who survive the acute phase will progress to a diuretic phase followed by rapid improvement and later to a convalescent phase, characterized by weakness and fatigue with slow recovery of the lung capacity.[58]

Influenza Viruses

Risk factors of influenza virus lung infection

Influenza viruses (from the Latin word *influentia*) are the most common cause of viral pneumonia in the general population. They belong to the family *Orthomyxoviridae* and contain eight segments of single-stranded negative-sense RNA. There are three serotypes: A, B, and C, with influenza A being the most virulent and clinically significant. They are enveloped viruses that contain the membranous glycoproteins hemagglutinin (H) and neuraminidase (N), which are major antigenic determinants. The different strains of influenza viruses are designated by the combination of H and N present on their surface. Currently, the two more common subtypes to produce seasonal influenza in humans are A H1N1 and A H3N2. Several other strains infect different species, such as birds, pigs, and other mammals. Influenza viruses can mutate easily by altering their surface antigens by two mechanisms: "antigenic drift" (spontaneous small mutations on the H protein resulting in resistant strains that produce seasonal epidemics) and "antigenic shift" (large mutations and recombination among influenza viruses from different species resulting in a new "hybrid" virus). Antigenic shift occurs occasionally and produces pandemics since the hosts will not have previous immunity to the new virus. Mortality rates range from 10% to 20% during outbreaks and as high as 50% during epidemics. The worst pandemic of influenza known to date occurred in 1918 when the flu caused >50 million deaths around the globe (the so-called Spanish flu).

Two influenza viruses are of bigger concern in humans: avian influenza H5N1, and the strain A H1N1 or swine flu. Avian influenza, a strain only supposed to infect birds, produced hundreds of cases of acute respiratory failure and severe pneumonia in Hong Kong in 1997. By 2010, avian influenza had caused disease in >500 people in several countries with mortality rates approaching 60%. Influenza H1N1 resulted from genetic recombination of a virus causing swine flu with strains that cause infection in birds and humans. In late March 2009, an outbreak of influenza was initially reported in Mexico and later in the United States. In a few weeks, the virus was identified as a novel swine-origin influenza A H1N1 virus.[63] The infection spread rapidly to other continents and was raised to the level of pandemic in June 2009 by the World Health Organization (WHO) with >200 countries affected.[64] Influenza virus H1N1 caused severe pneumonia in the young to middle age group (5-59 years), with the majority of deaths occurring in patients younger than 60 years (mortality rate of 87%).[65] By January 2010, WHO estimated that approximately 18,000 deaths were directly attributed to H1N1 infection. Mexico was among the countries with the greatest number of cases with severe clinical presentation and death.[63] H1N1 infection was declared in the post-pandemic period in August 2010.[64]. For further statistics review, the reader is referred to other sources.[16,64,66]

Recently, on April 1, 2013, an outbreak of a new avian influenza (strain H7N9) was reported in China. The majority of the 132 confirmed cases of infection reported contact with poultry. Most infected patients showed severe respiratory distress with 39 reported deaths.[67] The outbreak remitted after 1 month. No evidence of sustained of human-to-human spread was found and no cases were identified out of China.[68]

Individuals at risk for developing influenza pneumonia include young children (<5 years), patients with underlying cardiopulmonary disease, diabetes mellitus, immunosuppression, hemoglobinopathies, and those >65 years.[69] After RSV, influenza is the second most common cause of lower respiratory infection in childhood (17% of cases, worldwide).[39] Pregnant women, obese individuals, and indigenous populations had the poorest outcomes if infected with H1N1.[66] Epidemics and pandemics usually present in late winter and early spring.

Clinical features of influenza virus lung infection

Clinically, the only clue to suspect infection with influenza is a patient who presents with flu symptoms during the winter months, or when outbreak has been reported in the community. The incubation period of the disease is 1 to 3 days. Initially, influenza manifests by high-grade fever, chills, myalgias, arthralgias, cough, sore throat, and rhinorrhea that last 3 to 5 days. Pneumonia is characterized by persistent cough, sore throat, headache, myalgia, and malaise that develop after this period.[69,70] Symptoms may worsen with appearance of dyspnea and cyanosis sometimes with progression to respiratory failure. The most common complication of influenza pneumonia is bacterial superinfection caused by *S aureus*, *S pneumoniae* or *H influenzae*. Patients with avian influenza and H1N1 initially show similar symptomatology to seasonal influenza in addition to abdominal pain, vomiting, and diarrhea. Pneumonia develops in almost all patients and is characterized by cough, dyspnea, tachypnea, and chest pain that rapidly progresses to ARDS. Within 1 week of the onset of illness, patients with avian influenza will develop lymphopenia, thrombocytopenia, disseminated intravascular coagulation, multiorgan failure, and death. Patients with H1N1 may also develop lymphopenia and increased levels of lactate dehydrogenase and creatine kinase.[63] The severe presentation in H1N1 pneumonia does not appear to be secondary to viral genetic variation.[71]

Imaging features of influenza virus lung infection

Radiographic findings of influenza pneumonia include early perihilar infiltrates that eventually progress to diffuse bilateral interstitial infiltrates. Small centrilobular nodules corresponding to alveolar hemorrhage may be observed.[8] Avian influenza and H1N1 infection will demonstrate bilateral patchy interstitial infiltrates predominantly in the lower lobes that progress to diffuse interstitial infiltrates with linear, reticular, or nodular shadows.[63,66] Multifocal consolidation, pleural effusion,

and cavitations are not uncommonly seen in avian influenza pneumonia.[72]

Cytologic and histologic features of influenza virus lung infection

The histopathologic changes seen influenza pneumonia can be divided into those caused by the virus and those occurring after superimposed bacterial infection. Both coexist in the same patient in >50% of cases. Common but nonspecific changes caused by influenza include interstitial edema with a moderate mononuclear infiltrate, DAD, intra-alveolar hemorrhage, and hyaline membrane formation (*Figure 14-15*). These changes can be seen from day 2 of infection and up to day 13 of disease. The tracheobronchial tree may show squamous metaplasia, epithelial desquamation with submucosal edema, and chronic inflammation (tracheitis) as well as necrotizing bronchitis and bronchiolitis. No VCE or viral inclusions are seen. Bacterial superinfection occurs for two reasons: necrosis of the respiratory epithelial barrier and impairment of immunity caused by the virus.[2,73,74] Bacterial pneumonia will often obscure the viral changes. In addition to the findings described above, avian influenza may show patchy interstitial paucicellular fibrosis. Several histopathologic patterns of H1N1 pneumonia (DAD with hyaline membranes, organizing DAD, acute massive intra-alveolar edema with hemorrhage, neutrophilic bronchopneumonia and tracheobronchitis with minimal histologic changes in alveoli) have been reported in autopsy cases from Japan.[75] Cases from the initial outbreak in Mexico show alveolar macrophages with hemophagocytosis, cells

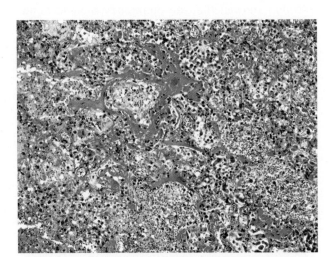

FIGURE 14-15 Influenza pneumonia from the outbreak in Mexico City in 2009. There is severe diffuse alveolar damage with prominent thick hyaline membranes, alveolar edema, and intra-alveolar hemorrhage (H&E). (Used with permission of Dr Javier Baquera Heredia, Hospital ABC, Mexico City, Mexico.)

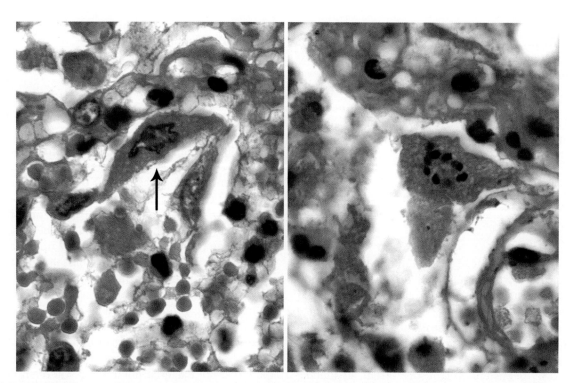

FIGURE 14-16 Influenza pneumonia. Cases from the outbreak in Mexico City in 2009 showed severe diffuse alveolar damage. Several cells showed irregular "raisinoid" nuclei with glassy "inclusion-like" eosinophilic material (left, arrow). In addition, several cells (possibly alveolar macrophages) showed granular mitoses reminiscent of those seen in astrocytes in demyelinating diseases. Abundant hemophagocytosis was also seen. (Used with permission of Dr Javier Baquera Heredia, Hospital ABC, Mexico City, Mexico.)

with eosinophilic "inclusion-like" glassy nuclei, and granular mitosis reminiscent of the ones seen in astrocytes in demyelinating diseases (personal communication) (*Figure 14-16*). However, an autopsy study from New Mexico including individuals who died after H1N1 infection showed that the pulmonary manifestations may be subtle (interstitial inflammation, edema, tracheobronchitis, and focal acute bronchopneumonia) if the time between onset of disease and death is very short.[76] Thus, pathologists should not always expect to see DAD when considering H1N1 influenza in the differential diagnosis of pneumonia.

Confirmatory diagnosis of influenza pneumonia requires detection of viral antigens by IHC due to lack of specific findings and VCE. Influenza viral antigens may show a different pattern of distribution based on the severity of the disease. Cases with a predominant DAD pattern show positive IHC in the tracheobronchial tree, type I and type II pneumocytes, alveolar macrophages, endothelial capillaries and even in hyaline membranes.[75,77,78] In contrast, cases with more predominant tracheitis and necrotizing bronchitis and bronchiolitis, the viral antigens are predominantly detected in the ciliated epithelium, submucosal glands, and gland ducts.[78,79] In the case of avian influenza H5N1, IHC is positive in alveolar epithelium and alveolar macrophages.[80]

Laboratory diagnosis of influenza viruses

Other methods of influenza detection include ISH and viral culture from nasal or throat swabs, nasal washes, and sputum. Viral culture shows positive results within 72 hours of inoculation in 90% of cases with the remaining cases showing positive results within 7 days. Serology methods are not recommended for diagnosis. The rapid test for influenza shows poor sensitivity (40%-80%) and high specificity (85%-100%) for seasonal and for H1N1 influenza, and is not used for detection of avian influenza. RT-PCR is the fastest and preferred method of detection for avian influenza and H1N1 infection. Multiplex RT-PCR with enzyme hybridization allows rapid detection of influenza A and B as well as for other common respiratory viruses.[1] Rapid isothermal amplification for detection of influenza A and B without RNA extraction is a promising technique that may render fast results (30 minutes) with sensitivities and specificities similar to PCR.[81]

Treatment of influenza virus lung infection

Treatment of influenza A flu symptoms includes supportive measures and use of the adamantane drugs, amantadine or rimantadine, within 48 hours of the onset of symptoms. Adamantanes block the ion-channel viral protein M2, interfering with the uncoating of the virus after its internalization within the cell. Viral resistance to adamantanes is not uncommon. Other antiviral medications effective for influenza A and B are the blockers of the N surface protein oseltamivir, zanamivir, and permivir.[82,83] These drugs prevent viral spread to neighboring cells. These medications have a lower rate of resistance but have a higher cost. Different combinations of these antiviral treatments should be given in influenza pneumonia even after the 48-hour window.[69] Administration of oseltamivir in avian influenza pneumonia even after the 48-hour window reduces the mortality in hospitalized patients. Combinations of oseltamivir and ribavirin may be required for resistant strains. H1N1 influenza pneumonia is treated with oseltamivir or zanamivir in all hospitalized patients, health care workers, or outpatients at risk for complications.[63] Corticosteroids are not beneficial in patients with H1N1 pneumonia.

Prognosis of influenza virus lung infection

Prognosis depends on many factors, such as the strain of influenza virus causing the infection, patient demographics, and patient comorbidities. Patients who present with respiratory failure or ARDS have a far worse prognosis.

Measles

Risk factors of measles lung infection

Measles is an enveloped, single-stranded RNA pleomorphic virus from the genus *Morbillivirus*, a member of the *Paramyxoviridae* family. It is the causative agent of rubeola or English measles. The virus is extremely infectious and humans are the only known natural reservoir. The incubation period is 10 to 14 days. Measles vaccination is highly protective against infection and viral complications. Pneumonia is the most common fatal complication.[84] Individuals at higher risk for pneumonia include children younger than 5 years, the elderly, pregnant women, immunosuppressed patients with hematologic malignancies, AIDS patients, and those who have not been vaccinated.[84-86] Severe disease is common in malnutrition, vitamin A deficiency, or vaccination failure.[84] Due to these reasons, a higher rate of complications and mortality is more commonly seen in developing countries, where measles is a public health problem.[84,87] The mortality rate of measles pneumonia is 40% in AIDS patients, 60% in infants, and 70% in patients with malignancy. Although the incidence of measles is low in developed countries, outbreaks of the disease may occur sporadically from importation of the virus from travelers to countries where measles is more prevalent. The CDC reported that during 2001 to 2008,

a median of 56 cases of measles occurred in the United States and 118 cases were reported during the first half of 2011, the highest since 1996.[88] From these cases, 89% were imported from abroad and the same percentage of patients were unvaccinated; 40% required hospitalization but pneumonia was rarely seen (<1%).[88] Outbreaks of measles have been reported during this decade in China,[89] Germany,[90] and Spain,[91] just to mention a few countries.

Clinical features of measles lung infection

Clinically, measles begins with a prodrome of fever, anorexia, coryza, cough, and conjunctivitis. Koplik spots may be seen 1 to 3 days before the appearance of a centrifugal maculopapular rash that lasts approximately 5 days. The virus is infective 3 to 5 days prior and 4 days postappearance of the rash. Approximately 3%—and up to 9%, based on the series[86]—of patients with measles will develop pneumonia with the majority of patients requiring hospitalization. Thirty percent to 50% of patients with measles pneumonia will develop bacterial superinfection due to *S pneumoniae, S aureus, H influenzae,* and *N. meningitides,*[85] which usually occurs 5 to 10 days after the onset of the rash. There are four clinical presentations of measles pneumonia: (1) measles-virus interstitial pneumonia, usually seen in immunocompromised patients (high levels of the type-2 pneumocyte secreted glycoprotein KL6 and associated with poor prognosis); (2) associated with bacterial superinfection, with clinical symptoms of bacterial pneumonia; (3) giant cell pneumonia (so-called Hecht pneumonia) that may develop before, during, after, or even without the maculopapular rash. Hecht pneumonia may be seen even 5 months after the initial symptoms; and (4) pneumonia of atypical measles (high fever, minimal or no exanthema, headache, arthralgias, and hepatitis, sometimes fatal).[8,84,92-94] Interestingly, progression to measles pneumonia in adults has been related to particular genotypes of the virus in China.[89] Complications of measles pneumonia include pneumomediastinum and mediastinal emphysema.

Imaging features of measles lung infection

Chest radiographs of patients with measles pneumonia show reticular and interstitial infiltrates and air space consolidation; children will also present with prominent hilar lymphadenopathy. CT scan shows ground glass attenuation, air space consolidation, and small centrilobular nodules scattered throughout the lung parenchyma. Pneumonia of atypical measles usually manifests as nodular consolidations that disappear quickly, hilar lymphadenopathy, and pleural effusion.[8]

Cytologic and histologic features of measles lung infection

The histopathologic findings seen in measles pneumonia may vary based on the duration of the disease and immunologic status of the patient.[93] The characteristic VCE consists of prominent multinucleation and enlargement of bronchial and alveolar epithelial cells. Measles giant cells may show up to 50 oval to round nuclei containing a homogeneous eosinophilic inclusion that may or may not be surrounded by a halo (so-called Warthin-Finkeldey cells). The nuclei may vary slightly in size but do not show molding as in HSV and VZV. In addition, measles giant cells have abundant eosinophilic cytoplasm that may show small eosinophilic inclusions, which are sometimes difficult to identify. Measles inclusions occasionally may be seen in alveolar macrophages and endothelial cells.[95] Measles pneumonia shows a pattern of acute necrotizing bronchitis and bronchiolitis with marked epithelial regeneration, reactive hyperplastic changes, multifocal squamous metaplasia, and peribronchial inflammatory infiltrates. There is characteristic cystic dilatation of mucous glands of the tracheobronchial tree.[92] Findings in the lung parenchyma include the presence of DAD accompanied by the previously described multinucleated giant cells (giant cell pneumonia). Areas of DAD that are rich in giant cells correspond to the centrilobular nodules seen on CT scan (see above). The amount of giant cells varies accordingly to the immune status of the patient, with abundant giant cells in more severe states of immunodeficiency and lesser amount—also with minimal or no nuclear inclusions—in immunocompetent individuals.[93] The latter patients may also exhibit a pattern of organizing DAD and interstitial pneumonia.[93] The differential diagnosis of measles pneumonia includes other giant cell viral pneumonias, such as VZV, RSV, and parainfluenza pneumonia, or noninfectious giant cell pneumonia (a type of pneumoconiosis). The latter has a different clinical presentation, history of exposure to hard metals and diffuse interstitial fibrosis, not typical of giant cell viral pneumonia (*Figure 14-17*). To rule out other viral pneumonias, clinical presentation and detection of viral antigens by IHC is extremely useful. Identification of measles VCE has been reported in a BAL sample from an immunocompromised patient.[96]

Measles virus can be confirmed by IHC or ISH. The viral proteins are seen in pneumocytes, alveolar macrophages, and pulmonary endothelial cells.[97] In vitro and in vivo studies in nonhuman primates have shown that alveolar macrophages and lung dendritic cells are the first cells to harbor the virus that later migrate to the bronchial-associated lymphoid tissue (BALT) and hilar lymph nodes.[98] Immunostaining for the nucleocapsid protein, hemagglutinin, and fusion proteins of measles localize to the nucleus and cytoplasm of infected cells,

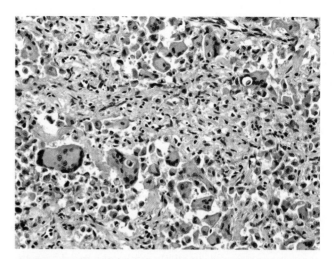

FIGURE 14-17 Giant cell interstitial pneumonia. This rare type of pneumoconiosis is secondary to long-term inhalation of heavy metals and should not be confused with giant cell pneumonia secondary to viral infection. No nuclear or cytoplasmic inclusions are seen. The clinical presentation is completely different to that seen in viral pneumonia. The differential diagnosis includes respiratory syncytial virus infection, measles pneumonia, and infection caused by other *Paramyxoviruses*.

respectively. Hemagglutinin is also detected at the luminal membrane in infected cells.[99]

Laboratory diagnosis of measles

Generally, measles infection is detected clinically but laboratory diagnosis is needed to detect measles pneumonia. The virus can be isolated from respiratory secretions by culture in approximately 6 to 10 days. Serology for measles-specific IgM antibodies may be used to confirm acute infection, whereas IgG titers confirm seroconversion after vaccination. PCR is the most rapid and preferred method of detection.

Treatment of measles lung infection

The treatment of measles pneumonia is based primarily on supportive measures but children and immunosuppressed patients may require intensive care unit management and ventilatory support. Vitamin A supplementation and antibiotic therapy for bacterial superinfection reduces mortality from measles pneumonia.[84] Aerosolized or IV ribavirin is the recommended therapy in children and immunocompromised patients. As mentioned previously, vaccination dramatically decreases the development of complications, including pneumonia.

Prognosis of measles lung infection

Pediatric patients that overcome measles pneumonia are at higher risk to develop constrictive bronchiolitis (bronchiolitis obliterans), mediated by cytokines and acute inflammatory cells.[100]

Human Parainfluenza Viruses

Risk factors of human parainfluenza virus lung infection

Parainfluenza viruses (PIV) are enveloped, nonsegmented, negative-stranded RNA virus of the family *Paramyxoviridae*, subfamily *Paramyxovirinae*. PIV were discovered in the late 1950s as ubiquitous viruses able to produce a clinical picture similar to influenza, but that differed from influenza in their biological properties,[101] hence the prefix "para-." There are four subtypes of PIV (types 1 to 4). PIV-1 and 3 belong to the genus *Respirovirus,* whereas PIV-2 and 4A and B are part of the genus *Rubulavirus.*[101] PIV-1 and 2 are the primary cause of laryngotracheobronchitis (croup) in children 6 months to 3 years of age. PIV-4 causes mild upper respiratory tract infection in children and adults. PIV-1 and 3 cause bronchiolitis in children aged 6 weeks to 2 years. PIV-3 is more likely to cause pneumonia in infants, adults, the elderly, and in 2% to 7% of immunocompromised individuals.[40] Major factors associated with PIV pneumonia in children are a young age at presentation, lack of previous exposure to PIV-3, and an underlying cardiopulmonary disease.[102] Immunosuppressed patients —including BMT, HSCRT, and solid-organ recipients—are at higher risk of developing severe pneumonia and respiratory failure (20%-50%) with high mortality rates compared to the general population. A study from MD Anderson Cancer Center showed that of 61 bone marrow transplant recipients with confirmed PIV in respiratory secretions, 44% developed pneumonia and 37% died.[103]

Clinical features of human parainfluenza virus lung infection

PIV infection is the second cause of bronchiolitis in children after RSV. The incubation period is 1 to 3 days. The clinical symptoms of bronchiolitis develop particularly in infants due to the small size of their terminal airways.[101] Common symptoms include fever, coryza, cough, and expiratory wheezing with later progression to tachypnea, muscle retractions, and trapping of air. Some patients may progress to respiratory failure and require hospitalization. Early PIV-3 infection in preterm infants may manifest with nonspecific symptoms, including apnea, bradycardia, and flu-like illness that may progress to respiratory distress in patients with underlying pulmonary disease.[104] The peak incidence of PIV pneumonia in children occurs at age 2 to 3 years. Clinically, pneumonia follows the previously described upper respiratory tract symptoms and is characterized by the fever, cough, shortness of breath, and detection of rales on physical examination. About a third of children with PIV pneumonia develop bacterial superinfection and 5% to 20% will demonstrate coinfection with another virus.[101] In immunocompetent adults, PIV pneumonia manifests with dry cough, hoarseness, and shortness of breath, all nonspecific symptoms seen in atypical pneumonias. PIV-3 pneumonia can manifest as a pertussis-like infection with paroxysmal and persistent cough with no lymphocytosis.[105] Bacterial superinfection also develops in adults, particularly the elderly. A case of hemorrhagic pneumonia has been described in a patient coinfected with PIV-4A and *Chlamydia pneumoniae*.[106] PIV is an opportunistic pathogen that causes severe and often fatal pneumonia in immunocompromised patients, that is, children with severe combined immunodeficiency, adults after solid organ or bone marrow transplant and hematologic malignancies). PIV pneumonia may be difficult to differentiate from other lung infections and coinfection with other viruses is not uncommon. However, the presence of upper respiratory tract symptoms, sinusitis, and wheezing prior to the development of pneumonia is highly suspicious for PIV infection. In a study of adult bone marrow transplant recipients, the most common symptoms associated with PIV pneumonia were fever, cough, shortness of breath, production of sputum, sinonasal congestion, rhinorrhea, and sore throat.[103] A study from 2001 showed that 24 of 32 (75%) lung transplant recipients presented with PIV infection with similar upper respiratory tract symptoms, as described above.[107]

Imaging features of human parainfluenza virus lung infection

On chest radiographs, PIV pneumonia initially manifests with hyperexpansion of the lungs—more common seen in children—and a spectrum of findings ranging from patchy to diffuse bilateral interstitial infiltrates, atelectasis, and pulmonary consolidation.[101,103] CT scan findings include diffuse bilateral reticular-nodular opacities and/or ground glass pulmonary infiltrates.

Cytologic and histologic features of human parainfluenza virus lung infection

Like other *paramyxoviruses*, PIV infection produces a typical but not pathognomonic VCE which is commonly seen in patients with severe immunodeficiency and rarely found in immunocompetent patients. The virus infects primarily respiratory epithelial cells that will only show mild increase in cytoplasm and enlarged nucleus in early stages of infection[101] and are only recognized by IHC. Later, the infected cells fuse and show abundant eosinophilic cytoplasm and multiple nuclei (syncytial cells). Multinucleated giant cells may exhibit cilia and show several small eosinophilic cytoplasmic inclusions (viral nucleocapsids) as well as focal to diffuse vacuolization of the cytoplasm. Although PIV-infected giant cells usually contain <10 round nuclei,[101] they tend to be larger than those seen in measles and RSV infection.

No definitive nuclear inclusions have been described. PIV pneumonia shows a pattern similar to RSV infection with bronchiolitis, peribronchiolar reactive lymphoid hyperplasia, squamous metaplasia, abundant mucus, and obstruction of the small airways by edema, inflammatory and epithelial cell debris. The lung parenchyma may show focal or minimal damage and fibrosis. On the other hand, immunocompromised patients with PIV pneumonia usually progress to a giant cell interstitial pneumonia, sometimes with organizing pneumonia and less *commonly* with DAD. One case report has shown association of PIV pneumonia with alveolar proteinosis in a 2 year old, following cord blood transplantation.[108] PIV syncytial cells may be observed in BAL.[109] Detection of viral antigens in infected epithelial cells can be done by IHC or IF to confirm the diagnosis. IHC studies performed on PIV-3 infected caprine lungs demonstrates the presence of PIV antigens in the cytoplasm of bronchiolar epithelial cells, syncytial cells, type II pneumocytes, and less frequently in alveolar macrophages, peribronchiolar lymphocytes, and plasma cells.[110]

Laboratory diagnosis of human parainfluenza viruses

Laboratory detection of PIV-3 can be performed by viral antigen detection via IF on nasopharyngeal secretions, BAL samples, or lung tissue. Shell vial cultures with antigen detection by IF will show positive results within 5 days of inoculation.[101] Serology is usually not performed for diagnosis. PCR is a more sensitive and rapid method to detect PIV-3 and can be performed on BAL fluid samples or lung biopsy tissue. Multiplex RT-PCR has high sensitivity (91%) and specificity (100%) for the detection of PIV-3[1,27] as well as other respiratory viruses.

Treatment of human parainfluenza virus lung infection

Treatment of PIV-induced bronchiolitis include supportive measures, use of bronchodilators and in severe cases, mechanical ventilation. Corticosteroids show no benefit. Treatment of pneumonia includes supportive care and use of aerosolized or oral ribavirin, which has shown reduction of PIV shedding and clinical improvement in immunocompromised patients.[66] Combinations of ribavirin and steroids has also shown positive results.[111] No vaccine to protect for PIV is available hitherto.

Prognosis of human parainfluenza virus lung infection

In allogeneic HSCT patients, mid- to long-term complications of PIV infection include constrictive bronchiolitis (bronchiolitis obliterans syndrome) and airflow decline, which may develop within 3 months of transplantation and persist for as long as 1 year after transplantation.[40] In a series of 32 lung transplant recipients with PIV infection, 82% of patients developed acute allograft rejection and 32% subsequently showed bronchiolitis obliterans.[107]

Other Viruses

Parvoviruses (human bocaviruses)

The family *Parvoviridae* (Latin word "parvum" or "small") is composed of small (18-25 nm) icosahedral, nonenveloped, linear single-stranded DNA viruses. Four types of the subfamily *Parvoviridae* are known to infect humans, the two most common being parvovirus B19 and the newly discovered human bocaviruses (HBoV). These viruses were originally detected in respiratory samples of children with lower respiratory tract infection in Sweden in 2005 by novel molecular methods.[112] Four subtypes have been recognized (HBoV1-4) with HBoV1 being the predominant subtype recovered from respiratory secretions.[113] HBoV1 may produce up to 5% of community-acquired pneumonia in children worldwide and is an uncommon cause of pneumonia in adults (reviewed in.[66] There is controversy regarding HBoV-1 pathogenicity since the virus is frequently codetected with other viral pathogens, including rhinovirus, influenza, and RSV. However, children coinfected with HBoV and other viruses develop wheezing more frequently than seen in viral pneumonia caused by a single pathogen.[66] Seroconversion occurs in early childhood.[114] The frequency of detection of HBoV ranges from 0% to 3% in BAL samples from adult patients.[40] Associated radiological findings include nonspecific bilateral patchy interstitial infiltrates, lung hyperinflation, peribronchial cuffing, and atelectasis (reviewed in.[113] HBoV-1 has been detected in HSCT recipients but data are missing regarding risk factors associated with the disease as well as for any associated histopathologic changes.[40] Human bocaviruses can only be detected by PCR in blood, respiratory secretions (HBoV-1), and stools (HBoV2-4). Antibody titers can be detected in blood. Currently, there is no treatment available for HBoV infection.

Human metapneumovirus

Human metapneumovirus (HMPV) is a member of the *Paramyxoviridae* family, subfamily *Pneumovirus,* genus *Metapneumovirus.* It was originally isolated in 2001 from 28 children with symptoms similar to RSV infection with bronchiolitis and pneumonia in the Netherlands.[115] HMPV is a leading cause of acute respiratory disease in children and adults.[116-118] A population-based incidence study in the United States demonstrated that HMPV is detected in ~4% of hospitalized children with acute respiratory disease or fever.[116] Similar rates have been detected in China with pneumonia found in one-third of patients.[119] Children with cardiopulmonary dysplasia may be at higher risk for HMPV than for RSV infection.[120] Asymptomatic HMPV infection has been detected in ~40% of adults in the United States and in 8.5% of 1386 hospitalized patients, with similar rates of intensive care admission as RSV and influenza.[117] Up to 10.6% of HSCT recipients were positive for HPMV by PCR in a recent study,[121] and this population usually shows coinfection with other pathogens. In lung transplant recipients, HMPV is detected at a rate equivalent to RSV, showing similar clinical symptoms but with higher risk of chronic rejection.[122]

Symptoms of HPMV pneumonia in the pediatric population include cough, coryza, rhinorrhea, fever, dyspnea, and wheezing. Adults present with fatigue, hoarseness, severe cough, dyspnea, and wheezing, which are more common in patients >65 years of age. Fever may or not be present. Immunocompromised patients can develop respiratory failure with mortality rates close to 50%. In children, chest radiographs show perihilar and peribronchial cuffing, perihilar patchy consolidation, and hyperinflation.[119] Chest radiographs of infected adults show variable findings, ranging from single to multilobar infiltrates with peribronchial cuffing, and less commonly with bilateral lung involvement.[118] On CT scan, HSCT recipients may show bilateral nodular infiltrates and pleural effusions. In transbronchial biopsies, mixed acute and chronic peribronchial and peribronchiolar inflammation with features of obstruction (foamy macrophages and organizing pneumonia) may be observed.[122] A pattern of acute lung injury with hyaline membrane formation and presence of smudge cells similar to those seen in adenoviral infection can be seen.[123] Although HMPV may be isolated by viral culture from respiratory secretions or detected in tissue by ISH, RT-PCR is the preferred method of detection. Successful treatment of HMPV pneumonia with systemic ribavirin and IV immunoglobulin has been reported.[66]

Henipavirus (Hendra and Nipah viruses)

Hendra and Nipah viruses are paramyxoviruses of the subfamily *Paramyxoviridae*, genus *Henipavirus*. They are zoonotic viruses that can produce lethal encephalitis (Nipah virus) and pneumonitis in humans and domestic animals (Hendra virus). Pteropid bats (fruit bats or flying foxes) are the known reservoirs.[124,125] Individuals at risk of infection include those in close contact with infected animals (horses and pigs) or those who have been in contact with bat urine or ingested contaminated raw date palm sap.[126] Human-to-human transmission may occur. Hendra virus was originally identified in Australia in 1994 and Nipah virus in South East Asia in 1999.[124-126] In 2009, detection of *Henipavirus* was also confirmed in bats from Ghana, Africa.[127] The

infection usually starts with flu-like symptoms, headache, sore throat, and myalgias and rapidly progresses to encephalitis or severe acute respiratory failure and death (mortality ~60%).[124] Both viruses demonstrate similar histopathologic findings in the lungs including the presence of necrotizing alveolitis with hemorrhage and vasculitis with thrombosis and microinfarcts, but with minimal involvement of the tracheobronchial tree.[124,128] Multinucleated giant endothelial cells with viral inclusions are seen at the periphery of necrotic areas.[128] IHC for Nipah virus antigen has been detected in bronchial epithelial cells, type II pneumocytes, and pulmonary capillary endothelium.[128] The mechanism of pathogenesis is unknown and no treatment is currently available. Preventive measures are the best way to decrease risk of infection.

Hemorrhagic fever viruses

Hemorrhagic fever (HF) is a zoonotic infection caused by four families of viruses: *Arenaviridae, Bunyaviridae, Flaviviridae,* and *Filoviridae*. Common features among them are: all are enveloped RNA viruses; a rodent or arthropod (tick, mosquito) serves as a reservoir; and infection occurs in the geographic area restricted to the host species.[129] Humans become infected after contact with the primary reservoir or infected animals. Human-to-human transmission may occur. HF viruses are distributed worldwide and are named after the region where they were originally identified (Lassa HF, Marburg HF, Crimean-Congo HF, Ebola HF, Venezuelan HF, Omsk HF, etc). Older viruses that belong to this group include the yellow fever and dengue viruses. Clinical findings of HF can be classified as prehemorrhagic and hemorrhagic.[130] Initial clinical symptoms (prehemorrhagic) include the onset of fever, fatigue, and myalgias. In severe cases, infected patients develop petechial rashes that coalesce and form large ecchymoses of the skin and mucous membranes. There is internal organ bleeding, multiorgan failure, shock, and death. Histopathologic findings in the lung include diffuse intra-alveolar hemorrhage, alveolar edema, capillary congestion, and mild interstitial pneumonia[131] that progresses to DAD (*Figure 14-18*). There is no specific VCE. Since all HF viruses share these findings, IHC is needed to confirm a particular virus as a causative agent. IHC for Crimean-Congo HF virus is positive in monocytes and endothelial cells.[132] Diagnosis of HF is suspected in patients who present with the aforementioned symptoms and have traveled recently to an endemic region. However, a negative travel history does not exclude exposure to HF viruses. Diagnosis is established by serologic tests (ELISA), IHC, viral culture, or RT-PCR.[130] Ribavirin has been used in patients with Lassa and Crimean-Congo HF with good outcomes (reviewed in[130]).

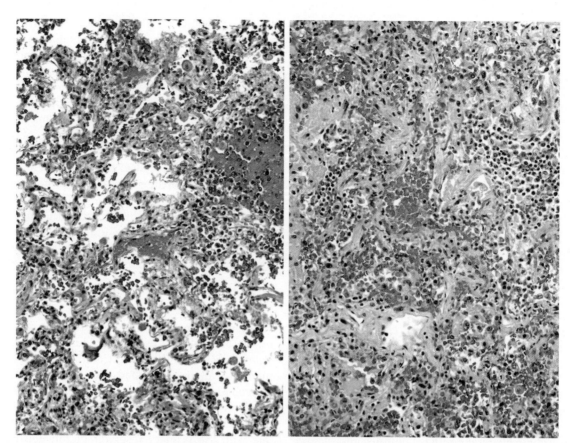

FIGURE 14-18 Hemorrhagic fever virus pneumonia. The histopathologic findings include diffuse intra-alveolar hemorrhage and alveolar edema with variable degree of capillary congestion, interstitial pneumonia (left). Diffuse alveolar damage with hyaline membrane formation may develop (right). No viral cytopathic effect has been described (H&E).

MYCOPLASMA, CHLAMYDIAL, AND RICKETTSIAL PNEUMONIAS

Mycoplasma pneumoniae

Risk factors of Mycoplasma pneumoniae pneumonia

Mycoplasmas and ureaplasmas are bacteria that lack a rigid cell wall and belong to the class *Mollicutes* (which means "soft skin"). They are the smallest known-free living microorganisms (<2 μm). There are three known species that produce disease in humans: *Mycoplasma pneumoniae, M hominis,* and *Ureaplasma urealyticum. M pneumoniae* is a common cause of atypical pneumonia,[133] whereas *M hominis* and *Ureaplasma* produce urinary tract infection and rarely pneumonia (see below). *M pneumoniae,* at that time thought to be a filterable virus, was recovered from patients with atypical pneumonia by Monroe Eaton and colleagues in 1944, hence the old name "Eaton agent."[134] *M pneumoniae* is one of the most common causes (12% globally) of community-acquired pneumonia in individuals <40 years, with the highest rate of infection in the first and second decades

of life (2-20 years).[133,135,136] Children younger than 4 years are at higher risk of coinfection with other pathogens.[136] Although respiratory illness can occur at any season, significant outbreaks occur in the late summer and fall. Pneumonia spreads rapidly in closed environments such as college dormitories and military academies. In the late fall-early winter of 2012, a large outbreak of *M pneumoniae* pneumonia (83 students) occurred in a university in Georgia, considered the largest reported outbreak in a US university in 35 years.[137]

Clinical features of Mycoplasma pneumoniae pneumonia

Approximately 5% to 15% of patients infected with *M pneumoniae* will develop pneumonia. The incubation period may extend up to 3 weeks. Usually pneumonia develops after a gradual onset of malaise, headache, dry cough, and sore throat, although some patients may remain asymptomatic or with only mild symptomatology. Clinical symptoms differ from those of typical bacterial (pneumococcal) pneumonia (high-grade fever, dyspnea, productive cough) and may be difficult to differentiate from other bacterial (*Chlamydophila pneumoniae*) or viral infections, thus the term "atypical" pneumonia.[138] In addition, patients may develop tracheobronchitis. Mycoplasmal infection may be accompanied by extrapulmonary symptoms including erythema multiforme, erythema nodosum, Stevens-Johnson syndrome, bullous myringitis (rare), and acquired hemolytic anemia secondary to cryoglobulins. Serum cold agglutination is seen in 50% to 70% of patients. Development of pleural effusion has been associated with young age and longer hospital stay in a short case series.[139] On the other hand, clinical symptoms and signs may not be reliable to diagnose *M pneumoniae* infection, according to a Cochrane Review done in 2012.[140] Most cases of pneumonia resolve after several weeks (usually <6 weeks) without serious complications.

Imaging features of *Mycoplasma pneumoniae* pneumonia

The radiologic findings are far more concerning than the clinical symptoms and easier to identify on HR-CT scans. Chest radiographs may show the presence of segmental or nonsegmental patchy bronchopneumonia, peribronchial thickening, subsegmental atelectasis, and interstitial infiltrates with rare consolidation. HR-CT shows centrilobular nodules (<1 cm), unilateral or bilateral consolidation in a lobular distribution, and thickening of the peribronchovascular and interlobular septal interstitium.[141]

Cytologic and histologic features of *Mycoplasma pneumoniae* pneumonia

M pneumoniae adheres to the surface of respiratory epithelial cells by the terminal attachment organelle that mainly contains protein P1.[142] Once attached to respiratory cells, the organism divides extracellularly and causes disarrangement and loss of cilia and local cellular damage.[143] Due to the benign nature of *M pneumoniae* pneumonia (mortality <1%), there is minimal knowledge of its gross and microscopic features, with most descriptions coming from autopsy studies. An analysis of lung wedge biopsies showed that common histopathologic findings included neutrophil-rich exudates, mucus and sloughed epithelium in the bronchial lumina, squamous metaplasia of the bronchiolar epithelium, peribronchiolar lymphoplasmacytic inflammation, peribronchiolar septal widening, and hyperplasia of type II pneumocytes. Less common findings include DAD and organizing pneumonia superimposed upon the bronchiolar reactive changes.[144] The presence of interstitial pneumonia and acute bronchiolitis with necrosis and sloughing of respiratory epithelium into the lumen may eventually produce bronchiolitis obliterans.

Laboratory diagnosis of *Mycoplasma pneumoniae*

Diagnosis of *M pneumoniae* is based on serologic methods by detection of IgM titers. However, recent studies have shown that PCR and RT-PCR are more sensitive and timely than serum antibodies. Using PCR as the gold standard, the *M pneumoniae* IgM assay has been found to show a sensitivity and specificity of 62% and 85%, respectively, in a study of pediatric patients.[145] *Mycoplasma* is fastidious and culture results may not be available before 6 weeks. RT-PCR can be performed on blood, nasal, and oropharyngeal secretions, BAL, and lung tissue and may be useful in cases when mycoplasmal respiratory infection is not obvious and/or extrapulmonary symptoms are the only findings.[142] Fluorescence quantitative-PCR has a higher sensitivity and specificity when compared with IgM serology.[146]

Treatment of *Mycoplasma pneumoniae* pneumonia

Treatment of *M pneumoniae* pneumonia requires the use supportive measures and antibiotics. Oral or systemic tetracyclins (doxycycline) and macrolides (erythromycin, azithromycin, clarithromycin) are effective against *M pneumoniae*. Use of fluoroquinolones (levofloxacin, moxifloxacin) may be used as a second line of treatment. Tetracyclines and fluoroquinolones should be avoided in children less than 9 and 18 years, respectively. Penicillins and their derivatives have no role in treatment.

Prognosis of *Mycoplasma pneumoniae* pneumonia

The complications associated with mycoplasmal pneumonia include lobar consolidation, pulmonary abscess, and bronchiolitis obliterans. Necrotizing pneumonitis is an extremely rare event.

M hominis and U urealyticum are infrequent causes of genitourinary tract infection and neonatal pneumonia.[147] One study showed that carriage of *U urealyticum* is high in infants with bronchopulmonary dysplasia.[148] However, the pathogenic role of these organisms in lung infection needs further investigation.

Chlamydiae

The genus *Chlamydiaceae* is composed of several species of small, obligate intracellular prokaryotic organisms (<1 μm) that can produce disease in animals (birds, marsupials, and reptiles) and/or humans. They are transmitted by human-to-human contact or zoonosis. Three species, *Chlamydophila pneumoniae, Chlamydophila psittaci* (formerly *Chlamydia*), and *Chlamydia trachomatis* can cause pneumonia. *Chlamydiae* have a unique life cycle which depends on the two distinct forms of the organism: the extracellular elementary body and the intracellular reticulate body. The elementary body represents the infectious form, whereas the reticulate body is metabolically active and adapted for multiplication. Elementary bodies become internalized by a mammalian cell into non-acidic phagosomes, the site where they reorganize as reticulate bodies. After several cycles of replication and division, reticulate bodies condense into several elementary bodies that are released after lysis of the host cell and are capable of infecting the neighboring cells (reviewed in[149]). The three species associated with chlamydial pneumonia are discussed.

Chlamydophila pneumoniae

Risk factors of *Chlamydophila pneumoniae* pneumonia

C pneumoniae is widespread in the human population and is responsible for approximately 7% of cases of atypical pneumonia worldwide.[133,150,151] *C pneumoniae* is the second most common atypical pathogen to cause community-acquired pneumonia in North and South America, after *M pneumoniae*.[133] However, accordingly to a study from Poland, the incidence of *C pneumoniae* pneumonia has decreased in pediatric patients since 2007.[152] The prevalence is low in children and increases with older age.

Clinical features of *Chlamydophila pneumoniae* pneumonia

Clinical symptoms in adolescents and young individuals produced by *C pneumoniae* include bronchitis and so-called atypical pneumonia. In a study of community-acquired pneumonia from Canada, patients with *C pneumoniae* pneumonia were older, had a lower leukocyte count, and were more likely to have congestive heart failure than patients with *S pneumoniae* pneumonia.[151] Pneumonia is reported more common in males than females. The incubation period is 3 to 4 weeks. The majority of patients remain asymptomatic (80%-90%). However, bronchitis or pneumonia develops after a gradual onset—from days to 1 week—of upper respiratory tract symptoms, including rhinitis, pharyngitis, sinusitis, otitis media, and laryngitis; fever is not commonly seen unless coinfection with other bacterial organism (*S pneumoniae*) exists. Eventually patients complain of malaise, headaches, and develop persistent dry cough and hoarseness, with rhonchi and rales. Most cases will resolve after several weeks without serious complications, but infection may recur, particularly in older individuals. Rarely pneumonia may be fatal.

Imaging features of *Chlamydophila pneumoniae* pneumonia

The radiologic findings are nonspecific. Chests roentgenograms show single homogeneous, subsegmental, or patchy alveolar or interstitial infiltrates mainly located in the lower lobes. Ground glass opacities or diffuse consolidations are uncommon. Pleural effusion may be seen in 25% to 50% of cases. A presentation with pulmonary migratory infiltrates has been reported.[153]

Cytologic and histologic features of *Chlamydophila pneumoniae* pneumonia

Pneumonia secondary to *C pneumoniae* rarely causes fatal disease in humans, so there is minimal knowledge of its gross and microscopic features. Experimental infection of animals has been done to assess the histopathologic changes of *C pneumoniae* in the lung. Primary infection of mice with *C pneumoniae* is characterized by prominent peribronchial and perivascular lymphoplasmacytic infiltrate that becomes more neutrophilic after passive immunization.[154] Chlamydial inclusions are found by electron microscopy in bronchial respiratory epithelium and less frequently in interstitial macrophages.[155] Lungs of rabbits inoculated with *C pneumoniae* demonstrate infiltration of bronchioles and surrounding alveolar ducts and alveoli by macrophages, lymphocytes, and plasma cells at 7 to 14 days, with occasional multinucleated giant cells and no neutrophils. At 21 days, most rabbit lungs show no pathology, besides the presence of mild lymphocytic interstitial and peribronchiolar infiltrate.[156]

Laboratory diagnosis of *Chlamydophila pneumoniae*

Serological methods are commonly used method for diagnosis of *C pneumoniae* infection. High titers of IgM are diagnostic, but they may take up to 6 weeks to become elevated. Thus, acute infection cannot be detected timely. The gold standard method for diagnosis is chlamydial serology microimmunofluorescence (MIF), which uses genus- and species-specific antigens to measure antibody titers for each chlamydial species. Fourfold increases of *C pneumoniae* IgG are diagnostic. Acute and convalescent sera samples should be analyzed since persistent elevated IgG levels are seen in recurrent infection. In contrast to MIF, complement fixation methods do not discern between the chlamydial species. Molecular methods are more sensitive and faster than serologic tests. A multiplex RT-PCR assay is available to detect *C pneumoniae*, *M pneumoniae*, and *Legionella pneumophila*.[157] In May 2012, the US Food and Drug Administration expanded the use for the test FilmArray Respiratory Panel that can detect viral and bacterial causes of respiratory infection in a single sample. This expanded panel included *C pneumoniae* and reports high sensitivity and specificity.[158]

Treatment of *Chlamydophila pneumoniae* pneumonia

Like *M pneumoniae* infection, the treatment of chlamydial pneumonias requires the use supportive measures and tetracycline and macrolide antibiotics. First-line antibiotics for *C pneumoniae* pneumonia include IV or oral doxycycline, or oral azithromycin and clarithromycin. Alternative medications include IV or oral levofloxacin or moxifloxacin, or telithromycin, a ketolide antibiotic with a mechanism of action similar to macrolides.

Prognosis of *Chlamydophila pneumoniae* pneumonia

Most cases of pneumonia resolve after several weeks. Infrequent serious complications include asthma exacerbation, chronic obstructive pulmonary disease, endocarditis, Guillain-Barre syndrome, and encephalitis. High titers of *C pneumoniae* are associated with high risk for bronchiolitis obliterans in lung transplant recipients (reviewed in[159]).

C pneumoniae is known to remain latent in the host and produce a chronic subclinical infection in the airways and possibly in the vascular system.[149] The pathogenesis of this mechanism is not well understood but may depend on interactions between the organism and leukocytes.[160] Pulmonary complications, such as asthma, COPD, and bronchiolitis obliterans syndrome, could be associated with persistent chlamydial infection (reviewed in[149,159]). Seroepidemiologic studies have demonstrated an association between *C pneumoniae* and coronary artery disease.[161]

Although not considered a zoonotic infection, genomic and phylogenetic evidence has shown that humans may have originally been infected via zoonosis with *C pneumoniae* by marsupials.[162]

Chlamydia trachomatis

Risk factors of *Chlamydia trachomatis* pneumonia

C trachomatis (from the Greek word "trachoma" which means "roughness") is an important cause of sexually transmitted disease and genitourinary tract infections in women and men (urethritis, epididymitis, mucopurulent cervicitis, and pelvic inflammatory disease).[163] It is also an important cause of conjunctivitis and pneumonia in infants. *C trachomatis* was recognized in 1911 as cytoplasmic inclusions in conjunctival cells from infants (neonatal inclusion conjunctivitis) whose mothers also had inclusions in their cervical epithelial cells.[164] Infants acquire the infection during birth by direct contact with infected endocervical cells. Approximately 100,000 cases of neonatal infection occur every year in the United States. In addition to conjunctival infection, respiratory tract colonization commonly occurs with progression to pneumonia in approximately 10% to 20% of cases. *C trachomatis* is the cause of pneumonia in 25% to 30% of infants. Pneumonia in adults is uncommon but has been reported in immunocompromised patients.[165]

Clinical features of *Chlamydia trachomatis* pneumonia

Clinically, infants who have been infected with *C trachomatis* during delivery will remain asymptomatic for about 3 weeks with onset of symptoms before 8 weeks of age.[166] Low birth weight neonates may develop pneumonia shortly after birth. Patients develop nasal obstruction and discharge, cough, tachypnea, and rales but symptoms usually remain mild. Typically, patients do not have fever or develop wheezing. Conjunctivitis and otitis media are seen in half of infants with pneumonia. When coinfection occurs (mainly with CMV or RSV) the infants may develop severe or fatal disease. Otherwise, *C trachomatis* pneumonia is usually self-limited. If untreated, chronic persistent infection may occur, similar to *C pneumoniae* infection.

Imaging features of *Chlamydia trachomatis* pneumonia

Radiologically, chest films show bilateral, symmetrical, and diffuse interstitial infiltrates with hyperexpansion of the lungs. Multilobar involvement or consolidations are not seen.[167] On laboratory findings, patients characteristically show mild peripheral blood eosinophilia and increased levels of serum immunoglobulins.[166]

Cytologic and histologic features of *Chlamydia trachomatis* pneumonia

The histopathologic findings of *C trachomatis* pneumonia in infants have not been well portrayed. There is a mixture of interstitial and alveolar inflammation with bronchiolitis. The inflammatory infiltrate is mostly lymphoplasmacytic but accompanied by eosinophils, neutrophils, and alveolar macrophages. On the other hand, in a case report of an immunocompromised adult, the histopathologic findings seen in the lung biopsy showed discrete nodular foci of interstitial and alveolar inflammation adjacent to and involving the bronchioles. The alveolar spaces contained hemosiderin-laden macrophages and prominent type II pneumocyte hyperplasia with lack of neutrophils or multinucleated cells.[165] Experimental infection of baboons and mice has been done to assess the histopathologic changes of *C trachomatis* in the lung. Baboons infected with the isolate from a human infant with chlamydial pneumonitis develop infection of the upper and lower respiratory tract with epithelial inclusions of *C trachomatis* identified morphologically and by IF. Lung parenchymal changes included patchy atelectasis, mucus plugging, and peribronchiolar and perivascular infiltrates of lymphocytes, plasma cells, and macrophages.[168] In contrast to the previous findings, lungs of infected mice with *C trachomatis* showed abundant early neutrophilic infiltrates in alveoli and alveolvar ducts that gradually changed peribronchiolar and alveolar inflammation composed of lymphocytes, plasma cells, and macrophages. Ultrastructurally, elementary and reticulate bodies were seen in bronchial respiratory cells.[169]

Laboratory diagnosis of *Chlamydia trachomatis*

The diagnosis of *C trachomatis* pneumonia is usually established by clinical suspicion. Traditional methods of diagnosis included the detection of chlamydial cytoplasmic inclusions (elementary bodies) on smears from conjunctivae or nasopharynx stained with Giemsa—also PAS-positive—or culture of respiratory secretions on McCoy cells with detection of chlamydial antigens by IF or ELISA. Serologic tests, MIF, and other methods are described under *C pneumoniae* pneumonia. Serologic test can increase the sensitivity of *C trachomatis* infection.[170] PCR amplification is the preferred method of detection and can be performed in respiratory secretions for rapid diagnosis.

Treatment of *Chlamydia trachomatis* pneumonia

The treatment of chlamydial pneumonia is the same for the different species (see *C pneumoniae* pneumonia). Important preventive methods to decrease transmission of *C trachomatis* include screening of mothers and sexually active partners for infections and administer antibiotic treatment as needed. Pulmonary complications may be similar as those described for *C pneumoniae* infection.

Prognosis of *Chlamydia trachomatis* pneumonia

C trachomatis pneumonia is usually self-limited in healthy neonates, although chronic infection may occur. Coinfection with other respiratory viruses may cause severe infection or death.

Chlamydophila psittaci

Risk factors of *Chlamydophila psittaci* pneumonia

C psittaci primarily produces disease in birds (avian chlamydiosis), rarely in cattle, pigs, and cats, and causes a zoonotic pneumonia in humans. The word *psittaci* derives from the Greek *psittakos* which means parrot. The disease is called psittacosis if acquired from psittacine birds (parrots, parakeets) or ornithosis if acquired from nonpsittacine birds (pigeons, chickens, turkeys, and ducks). It was originally recognized in 1879 in Ulster, Switzerland, by J. Ritter who described the presence of fever, pneumonia, and stupor in seven individuals exposed to sick birds. Three of the seven patients died of the disease. The term psittacosis was first coined in 1985.[171] Individuals who are exposed to feces, secretions, plumage, and tissues of infected birds, that is, bird breeders, poultry farmers, pet shop employees, and laboratory workers, are at risk for infection. A single exposure may be enough to become infected, which is why many patients with the disease cannot recall previous contact with birds. It is uncertain if human-to-human transmission occurs. After introduction of preventive measures, that is, quarantine periods for imported birds and use of antibiotics in bird food, the frequency of psittacosis has decreased in developed countries. From 2005 to 2009, 66 cases of psittacosis were reported in the United States, but milder cases of the disease may go unrecognized.[172] *C psittaci* is an uncommon cause of community-acquired pneumonia in adults and most cases are sporadic. In one study, the pathogen was detected in 2 of 700 adults.[150] Similarly, in another study of 539 patients with community-acquired pneumonia, only two patients had infection with the feline variant of *C psittaci*.[151]

Clinical features of *Chlamydophila psittaci* pneumonia

Clinically, infection with *C psittaci* may range from asymptomatic to severe pneumonia, or rarely, to systemic disease. The incubation period is approximately 5 to 14 days. Patients with pneumonia usually develop high fever, flu-like symptoms, nonproductive cough, malaise, headache, dyspnea, and chest pain. Many patients present with fever of unknown origin. Half of the patients with pneumonia develop nausea, vomiting, diarrhea, photophobia, acrocyanosis, and a blanching maculopapular rash, known as Horder spots (very rare).[173,174] Pulse-temperature dissociation and splenomegaly may be present. If treated on time, the disease is usually limited and resolves in few weeks, but relapses may occur. Rare cases may progress to severe respiratory failure and death.[175] Extrapulmonary symptoms include culture-negative endocarditis, hepatitis, arthritis, encephalitis, and disseminated intravascular coagulation (DIC).[173,174] A history of exposure to birds is crucial to establish a correct diagnosis since the clinical findings of *C psittaci* pneumonia are nonspecific and mimic atypical pneumonia caused by other pathogens.

Imaging features of *Chlamydophila psittaci* pneumonia

Chest radiographs in *C psittaci* pneumonia feature a wide range of patterns including segmental and lobar consolidation (most common), bilateral interstitial infiltrates in the lower lobes, small nodular densities (miliary pattern), and pleural effusion.[174]

Cytologic and histologic features of *Chlamydophila psittaci* pneumonia

Likewise *C pneumoniae* infection, *C psittaci* pneumonia rarely causes fatal disease in humans and few reports on the histopathology of the disease are available. Some of the reported findings from lung wedge biopsies include the presence of acute purulent bronchiolitis with erosion of respiratory epithelium and bronchopneumonia.[173,174,176] The latter is characterized by relatively well-circumscribed inflammatory nodules (2-5 mm) that are separated by normal lung parenchyma.[176] These inflammatory nodules are composed of lymphocytes and macrophages with abundant intra-alveolar fibrin at the edges; capillary thrombosis may be observed. Bronchiolitis is characterized by focal necrosis of the respiratory epithelium and filling of the bronchiolar lumen by neutrophils and macrophages. Chlamydial inclusions may be seen in the cytoplasm of pneumocytes and macrophages, which are better highlighted with Giemsa stain. In contrast to *C trachomatis* inclusions, the inclusions found in psittacosis are PAS negative. The resolution phase is characterized by organizing bronchiolitis or interstitial pneumonitis.[173,176] In fatal cases, confluent and extensive acute bronchopneumonia, massive intra-alveolar hemorrhage, and DAD are observed.[175]

In 2012, a bovine model of respiratory infection with *C psittaci* was reported.[177] The histopathologic findings included development of purulent bronchopneumonia and small fibrinous exudates and necrosis at day 3 postinoculation (p.i.), with few chlamydial inclusions in alveolar epithelium, as detected by IHC. With higher bacterial inocula, fibrinopurulent bronchopneumonia, multifocal necrosis, pleuritis, and abundant chlamydial inclusions associated with neutrophils and macrophages were seen. At day 7 p.i., organization of the areas of pneumonia with alveolar macrophages and mild lymphohistiocytic infiltrates was observed. Inclusions of *C psittaci* were abundant in areas of necrosis but not

in areas of organization. Resolution of pneumonia was seen by day 14 p.i., characterized by thickened alveolar septae, type II pneumocyte hyperplasia, and lymphocytic infiltrates with few chlamydial inclusions within alveolar macrophages.[177]

Laboratory diagnosis of *Chlamydophila psittaci*

The serologic tests for diagnosis of *C psittaci* infection are the same as for other types of *Chlamydiae* (see above). Molecular methods such as PCR amplification of *C psittaci* DNA can be performed on sputum, pleural fluid, BAL, or lung tissue. RT-PCR for the *ompA* gene is a rapid method of *C psittaci* DNA detection and has the advantage of distinguish different genotypes of the organism; however, it has not been approved for use on human samples.[178]

Treatment of *Chlamydophila psittaci* pneumonia

The antibiotic treatment of psittacosis is identical to that for *C pneumoniae* and *C trachomatis*, which include oral or IV tetracyclines (doxycycline) as first-line treatment, and macrolides as an alternative. Typically, the infection responds to antibiotics within 1 to 2 days. Patients with severe symptoms may require intensive care and ventilatory support.

Prognosis of *Chlamydophila psittaci* pneumonia

Severe but rare complications of *C psittaci* infection include endocarditis, thrombophlebitis, myocarditis, hepatitis, and DIC. Prevention is the most important way to avoid infection and transmission of the disease. People at risk should minimize their exposure to birds or use protective equipment. For pathologists, it is important to be aware of autopsy cases of suspected or confirmed psittacosis to avoid airborne transmission.[173]

Rickettsiae

Risk factors of rickettsial pulmonary infection

Rickettsia are obligated intracellular gram-negative, nonmotile bacteria with a pleomorphic coccobacillary morphology (range size <1-10 μm). In contrast to *Mycoplasma*, they do contain cell walls. The order *Rickettsiales* is divided into the *Rickettsiaceae* and *Anaplasmataceae* families (the latter discussed in the next section). The *Rickettsiaceae* family is composed of several species of the genus *Rickettsia*, including *R rickettsii*, *R conorii*, *R prowazekii*, and *R typhi*, among others. The name *Rickettsia* was established in honor to the physician Howard T. Ricketts, whose investigations in the Bitterroot Valley of western Montana in 1906 led to the understanding of important principles related to these organisms and to the pathogenesis of Rocky Mountain spotted fever (RMSF).[179] Rickettsiae are carried by arthropod vectors (ticks, fleas, mites, and lice) and produce an accidental infection in humans that travel to endemic areas. When a vector bites a human, rickettsial organisms multiply at the bite site, invade the circulation, and infect the endothelial cells of several organs, including the lungs, and produce life-threatening pneumonitis.

Pulmonary vascular endothelial infection by rickettsia

Rickettsiae bind to endothelial cells via adhesins and become internalized into cytoplasmic endosomes that the bacteria later disrupts using a rickettsial phospholipase.[180] The organisms replicate in the cytoplasm and may follow two routes: extracellular release into the circulation or cell-to-cell spread mediated by rickettsial-induced actin polymerization (reviewed in[180]). The latter mechanism may not be the same in all species. Damage of endothelial cells produces increased microvascular permeability.

Clinical features of rickettsial pneumonia

R rickettsii is the causative agent of RMSF. Although considered a rare disease, its incidence has increased from 345 cases reported in 1993 to approximately 2000 cases in the year 2010, with an annual incidence of 6 cases per million persons.[181] A major number of cases are found in Arkansas, Delaware, Missouri, North Carolina, Oklahoma, and Tennessee.[181] The incubation period is 3 to 14 days. Patients present with high fever, chills, malaise, headaches, myalgias, flu-like illness, and gastrointestinal symptoms. Approximately 3 to 12 days after the *Dermacentor* tick bite, a centripetal maculopapular rash develops. The rash later becomes petechial and does not spare the palms and soles. Encephalitis and hepatitis may occur. Pneumonia is characterized by nonproductive cough, rales, dyspnea, tachypnea, and respiratory failure needing intensive care and ventilator support. The acute respiratory failure is secondary to noncardiogenic pulmonary edema due to rickettsial-induced damage of the lung microvasculature.

Mediterranean spotted fever (MSF), or Boutonneuse fever, is caused by *R conorii*, and is seen in several regions of the world including South Africa, Northeastern Australia, and Siberia, just to mention a few. These illnesses are associated with a necrotic eschar at the site of tick bite (*tache noire*) and regional lymphadenopathy. Patients present with similar symptoms as RMSF and those with pneumonia usually have

fever, headache, malaise, arthralgias, cough, and dyspnea. It is a common misbelief that patients with RMSF and MSF progress to DIC; life-threatening hemorrhage and vaso-occlusive disease with infarction have been reported only rarely in these illnesses.[180]

Murine typhus, caused by *R typhi*, is endemic in regions with a high population of rats and opposums that are infested with fleas (*Xenopsylla cheopis*), such as big cities and ports. *R felis*, not *R typhi*, has been characterized as a cause of endemic typhus in southern California and Texas. The disease is found throughout the year with peak prevalence in the summer and early fall. The incubation period is 6 to 14 days. Initial symptoms after contact with infected flea feces include headache, chills, malaise, and back pain. After 10 to 14 days, a centripetal maculopapular rash with sparing of palms and soles develops. Pulmonary symptoms are common, particularly nonproductive cough and rales.

Epidemic (louse-born) typhus is caused by *R prowazekii*. In the 19th century, typhus was responsible for millions of deaths during World War I and II. It is now still found around the globe but the majority of cases are identified in central Africa, Asia, and the Americas. Infection occurs after scratching a site where a louse (*Pediculus humanus*) had defecated feces contaminated with rickettsial organisms. After 7 days, patients present with severe acute disease with high fever, severe headache, a centripetal maculopapular rash with sparing of palms and soles, conjunctival injection, and diffuse vascular lesions. A relapsing and milder form is known as Brill-Zinsser disease.

Scrub typhus, or tsutsugamushi disease (from the Japanese *tsutsuga* small and dangerous, and *mushi* creature), is endemic in the Southeast Asia, India, and Northeastern Australia.[182,183] It is caused by *Orientia tsutsugamushi*, a bacterium from a separate genus of *Rickettsiaceae*. The vector is a larval form of *Leptotrombidium* mites (chiggers) that live and breed in the soil and scrub vegetation. After 5 days, patients will develop a necrotic eschar at the site of the mite bite and regional lymphadenopathy. Central nervous system involvement is common. Pulmonary manifestations include interstitial pneumonia, interstitial edema, and lung hemorrhage secondary to vasculitis.[182]

Imaging features of rickettsial pneumonia

Radiologic findings for all rickettsial diseases are shared and are nonspecific. The lungs may show ground glass opacities, peribronchial cuffing, pulmonary edema, and bilateral pleural effusions. Consolidations are rare. Common HRCT findings are interlobular septal thickening, interstitial thickening, mediastinal lymphadenopathy, ground glass opacity and centrilobular nodules.[182]

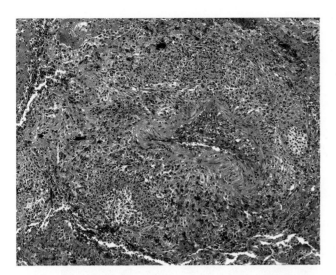

FIGURE 14-19 Rickettsial pneumonia. Wedge lung resection shows severe lymphohistiocytic vasculitis with hemorrhage, necrosis, and marked congestion. Case of a 45-year-old immunocompetent male who developed fever, arthralgias, dry cough, headache, leukopenia, and thrombocytopenia after a trip to the Caribbean. Chest x-ray revealed several small nodularities in the lungs. The serology confirmed high titers of *R rickettsi* and *R typhi* anti-IgM and anti-IgG. (Clinical history and image provided by Dr Diego Jorge-Buys, Hospital Angeles Interlomas, Mexico City, Mexico.)

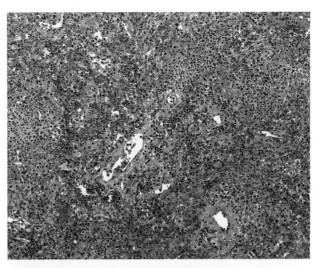

FIGURE 14-20 Rickettsial pneumonia (same case as Figure 14-19). Prominent lymphohistiocytic vasculitis with prominent fibrinoid necrosis and massive parenchymal hemorrhage. (Used with permission of Dr Diego Jorge-Buys, Hospital Angeles Interlomas, Mexico City, Mexico.)

Cytologic and histologic features of rickettsial pneumonia

The histopathologic changes seen in rickettsial diseases confirm the pathophysiology of the disease. In a study of 10 cases of fatal RMSF, lung involvement was characterized by vasculitis with hemorrhage and interstitial pneumonia with alveolar septal congestion, interstitial and alveolar edema, fibrin deposition, and abundant macrophages (*Figures 14-19 and 14-21*). The areas of vasculitis show lymphohistiocytic infiltrates and contain the most *R rickettsii* organisms by IF.[184] Similar findings are seen in the lungs in patients with MSF, with perivascular lymphohistiocytic infiltrates, interstitial pneumonia, and edema (*Figures 14-19 and 14-21*). In epidemic typhus there is interstitial pneumonia with or without DAD (reviewed in[185]). Rickettsial organisms can be detected by IHC in pulmonary endothelial cells and in alveolar macrophages.

In scrub typhus, the vasculature within the interlobular septa and alveolar walls is congested and surrounded by macrophages and lymphocytes; vasculitis may or may not be present. Macrophages and lymphocytes are also found within the edematous interstitium and alveolar septae. Hyaline membranes and intraalveolar hemorrhage may be seen. By IHC, *O tsutsugamushi* localizes to endothelial cells and alveolar macrophages.[186]

Laboratory diagnosis of rickettsia

Although half of infected patients have thrombocytopenia (<100,000 cells/µL), rickettsial organisms cannot be identified on peripheral blood smears, in contrast to *Ehrlichia*. Serologic methods to detect rickettsial antigens are available for diagnosis. These tests include IF, complement fixation, indirect hemagglutination, latex fixation, ELISA, and microagglutination. Of all these tests, IF is the most sensitive and specific. Serology is no longer considered adequate for diagnosis of acute infection since positive results are only seen after 7 to 14 days and persistent antibodies may be found at any time in patients who have been previously infected. The Weil-Felix test (serum agglutination to strains of *Proteus vulgaris*) is nonspecific for diagnosis. Rickettsial culture is difficult and hazardous for laboratory personnel. Quantitative-PCR can be performed on whole blood or skin samples to confirm diagnosis.[187] RT-PCR is the most sensitive, specific, and fastest method to detect rickettsial infections from the spotted fever and typhus groups.[188]

Treatment of rickettsial pneumonia

Treatment for rickettsial infections includes the use of supportive measures and in cases with severe acute respiratory failure intensive care and ventilatory support. Antibiotic treatment should be initiated during the first week of the onset of disease for better outcome and higher chance of recovery.

Characteristically, fever disappears 1 to 3 days after initiation of antibiotic treatment with doxycycline or chloramphenicol. Fluoroquinolones (ciprofloxacin

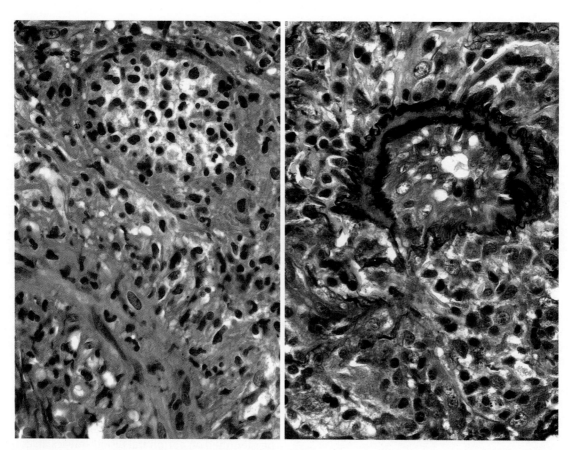

FIGURE 14-21 Rickettsial pneumonia (same case as Figure 14-19). The vasculitic process shows prominent lymphohistiocytic infiltrate with obliteration of blood vessels (left, H&E). The disruption of the arteriole wall and elastic lamina is confirmed by the Movat pentachrome stain (right). (Used with permission of Dr Diego Jorge-Buys, Hospital Angeles Interlomas, Mexico City, Mexico.)

and ofloxacin) are also effective for rickettsiosis. Sulfonamides are contraindicated.

Prognosis of rickettsial pneumonia

The reported case fatality rate of RMSF is <0.5% in the United States.[181] Risk factors for severity of illness include older age, glucose-6-phosphate dehydrogenase deficiency, sulfonamide treatment, diabetes mellitus, and male sex.[180] MSF has only rare complications. The mortality of epidemic typhus is higher in individuals >50 years old (70%) compared to younger adults (10%). Endemic typhus rarely causes complications. Scrub typhus is self-limited but patients may develop meningoencephalitis or renal failure, with a variable rate of mortality.

Ehrlichia and Anaplasma

The family *Anaplasmataceae* includes pathogenic and nonpathogenic species. *Ehrlichia chaffeensis* and *Anaplasma phagocytophilum* are the cause of the zoonotic diseases human monocytic ehrlichiosis (HME)

and human granulocytic anaplasmosis (HGA), respectively.[189] HME is frequently associated with respiratory symptoms, whereas pulmonary manifestations are rare in HGA. Both diseases are life-threatening tick-borne zoonoses found particularly in the Northeast United States, and are less common seen in other countries.[190] Using serologic data from children, one study suggests that most infections of *E chaffeensis* may be asymptomatic and self-limited.[191] *E chaffeensis* is transmitted by *Amblyomma americanum* (the lone-star tick) and its reservoir is the white-tailed deer. *A phagocytophilum* is transmitted by *Ixodes scapularis* (black-legged tick) and *I pacificus* in the United States and its reservoir is the white-footed mouse. *E chaffeensis* infects monocytes and macrophages while *A phagocytophilum* infects neutrophils and endothelial cells. Their intracellular development is different from that of the *Rickettsiaceae* family.[189]

Clinical symptoms include fever, myalgias, anorexia and chills, leukopenia (<2500 cells/μL), thrombocytopenia (<100,000 cells/μL), anemia, and elevated liver enzymes.[192] Approximately half of the patients with HME or HGA will require hospitalization and

7% require admission to an intensive care unit. The case fatality rate for HME is 3% and 0.5% for HGA.[192] Pulmonary symptoms are frequently seen in HME (up to 40% of cases). These patients present with dry cough and progress to interstitial pneumonitis and noncardiogenic pulmonary edema.[192] ARDS is seen in approximately 15% of cases of HME. In contrast, HGA manifests more commonly with ARDS and atypical pneumonitis.[192] Fatal cases have been reported in immunocompromised patients. On chest roentgenograms, bilateral interstitial opacities are common.

The histopathologic changes seen in the lungs vary from a mild interstitial pneumonitis to a diffuse interstitial lymphocytic pneumonitis with organizing pneumonia and abundant intra-alveolar macrophages[192,193]). DAD may be observed if a patient develops ARDS. Microorganisms may be seen within cytoplasmic vacuoles in macrophages (*Ehrlichia* morules) on routine stains, but are more easily identified with the Brown-Hopps stain. Similarly to *Ehrlichia* infection, *Anaplasma* will demonstrate interstitial pulmonary infiltrates composed of macrophages and lymphocytes with DAD. IHC is a better method for confirmation of *Ehrlichia* and *Anaplasma* in paraffin-embedded tissues.

Review of peripheral blood smears for cytoplasmic morules in leukocytes is less sensitive for HME than for HGA and is also quite time consuming. Detection of *Anaplasmataceae* is done by serologic methods which are basically the same as those used for rickettsial antigen detection. PCR has a higher specificity and sensitivity for detection of both *E chaffeensis* and *A phagocytophilum*. PCR also has a rapid turnaround time and is the test of choice for confirming serology that indicates HME or HGA.[194]

Similar to treatment for rickettsial infections, antibiotic treatment with doxycycline for HME and HGA should be initiated during the first week of the onset of disease for better outcome and higher chance of recovery.[190,194]

Q Fever

Q fever is a zoonotic disease caused by the bacterium *Coxiella burnetii*. The term Q—for "query"—fever was coined by the physician Edward H. Derrick in Australia in 1936 who studied an outbreak of febrile illness in abattoir workers that was negative by culture and serology for typhus, leptospirosis, typhoid, and paratyphoid.[195] *C burnetii* is a gram-negative bacterium that shares biological features with *Legionella* spp and differs from *Rickettsiaceae*. Reservoirs of *C burnetii* include cattle, sheep, goats, cats, and rabbits; the organism is excreted in milk, urine, and feces and is present in placental tissue. *C burnetii* can form spores that are resistant to extreme heat, desiccation, and many common disinfectants. For this reason the organisms can survive

in the environment for longer periods of time (weeks to several months). Humans become infected after inhalation of organisms from dried or particulate tissues, or fluids and excreta from infected reservoirs. Although Q fever is considered rare, its incidence has increased from 17 cases reported in 2000 to 167 cases in the year 2008.[196] *C burnetii* was the second most common isolated organism in a cohort of patients with community-acquired pneumonia in Spain.[150] The infection is usually asymptomatic with an incubation period of 2 to 3 weeks. Q fever is divided into acute (95% of cases) or chronic (5%). Pneumonia is one of the major manifestations of acute infection. Acute Q fever starts with chills, fever, a characteristic intense retrobulbar headache, fatigue, relative bradycardia, nausea, vomiting, and diarrhea.[195] About half of the patients develop hepatosplenomegaly. Patients with pneumonia frequently have either productive or nonproductive cough, but rarely complain of pleuritic pain. Chronic Q fever manifests as endocarditis, osteomyelitis, and hepatitis, and may develop after pregnancy.[195] *C burnetii* is an opportunistic pathogen in immunocompromised patients.

Radiologically, there may be no evidence of pneumonia in the early stages of Q fever. Later nonspecific findings include the presence of multiple rounded opacities (the so-called round pneumonia), increased reticular markings, atelectasis, segmental lobar consolidation, and bilateral hilar adenopathy.[195] Patchy lung infiltrates are uncommon and pleural effusions are usually small.[196] On chest CT scan, segmental or lobar airspace involvement and segmental consolidation can be seen.

The primary cells infected by *C burnetii* are monocytes and macrophages. The organisms reside and multiply within the phagolysosomes of these cells. Pathologic evaluation of one case of fatal Q fever pneumonia showed marked infiltration of alveolar septae by macrophages with numerous macrophages, lymphocytes, and plasma cells in the alveolar spaces with focal necrosis, but without neutrophils.[197] Immunofluorescence and electron microscopic studies performed after nasal inoculation of *C burnetii* into mice have shown organisms in type I and type II pneumocytes, pulmonary fibroblasts, and alveolar macrophages.[198] Another study in guinea pigs that received aerosolized *C burnetii* showed coalescing bronchointerstitial pneumonia composed of polymorphous leukocytic infiltrate at 7 days p.i. and multifocal lymphohistiocytic interstitial pneumonia at 28 days.[199] IHC for *C burnetii* is available and can be used to confirm the diagnosis in paraffin embedded tissues.[196]

Serologic tests have the similar advantages and disadvantages as for diagnosis of rickettsial infections. They include a complement fixation test and IF, since most laboratories do not have the capability to isolate *C burnetii*. A fourfold rise in antibody titers between acute and convalescent serum samples is considered diagnostic. Immunofluorescence is the preferred serologic method for detection. PCR of whole blood or serum samples provides rapid results and can be used to diagnose acute Q fever in the first 2 weeks after the onset of symptoms.[196]

The majority of patients with acute Q fever improve within few weeks even without antibiotic treatment. However, antibiotics are needed to diminish the risk of chronic Q fever complications, particularly endocarditis. The first line of treatment includes doxycycline; macrolides can be used as a second option. Hydroxychloroquine may be used in cases of Q fever endocarditis.

PARASITIC INFECTIONS

Malaria

Plasmodium species are obligate intracellular protozoans infecting red blood cells and hepatocytes. Five species infect humans (*P falciparum, P vivax, P ovale, P malariae,* and *P knowlesi*), but only *P falciparum* and *P vivax* are reported to cause pulmonary disease. *P falciparum* infects red cells of all ages, while *P vivax* prefers reticulocytes and younger red cells. Malaria is transmitted by the bite of an infected *Anopheles* mosquito, which deposits infective sporozoites into the host. The sporozoites travel to the liver and invade hepatocytes for several days of maturation to become liver schizonts. After further maturation, the schizont ruptures, releasing merozoites into the peripheral circulation where they infect erythrocytes. Once inside erythrocytes, the merozoites mature into ring forms, then trophozoites, and finally into schizonts which will release more merozoites (*Figure 14-22*). Some merozoites develop into gametocytes to complete the sexual cycle of *Plasmodium*, which occurs within the mosquito's gut. In the mosquito's stomach the microgametocyte exflagellates within minutes to form several microgametes, which fertilize the nearest macrogamete. After fertilization, the zygotes become motile ookinetes, which traverse the mosquito's gut wall and encyst on its outer surface. After encysting, the oocyst forms sporoblasts, which mature into sporozoites. Rupture of the oocysts releases sporozoites,

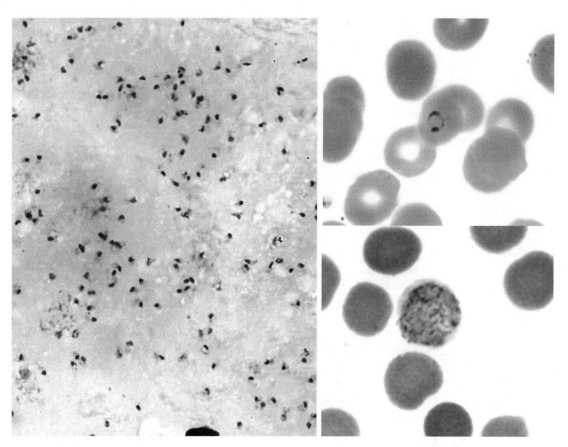

FIGURE 14-22 Malaria. Innumerable trophozoites are seen in a thick blood smear (left), the best screening test for malaria. Peripheral blood smear with *Plasmodium falciparum* in ring form (top right) and amoeboid form (bottom right) (Giemsa stain). Alveolar capillaries in the lung may get clogged with infected red blood cells and induce diffuse alveolar damage and ARDS.

which migrate to the mosquito's salivary glands, poised to infect the next host.[200,201]

Clinical features

The characteristic febrile episodes of malaria begin approximately 7 to 10 days after the bite of an infected mosquito.[202] Pulmonary involvement manifests with a variety of symptoms, ranging from cough to pulmonary edema to fatal ARDS and may occur in either uncomplicated malaria (fever, night sweats, malaise) or severe malaria (organ failure, cerebral malaria, anemia).[203] For adults with severe *P falciparum* malaria, reported rates of ARDS range from 5% to 25%. Patients with ARDS usually present with increased respiratory rate and dyspnea, followed by sweating, labored breathing, and cyanosis.[204] Patients may present with ARDS earlier in the disease, when parasitemia is at its highest, or may develop ARDS several days later, after initiation of treatment, when parasitemia has reached a relative nadir.[205] Patients with ARDS secondary to malaria have an overall poor prognosis, even with invasive mechanical ventilation.[204] Patients with less severe pulmonary symptoms usually show improvement with antimalarial therapy. Currently, Taylor et al advocate for the use of IV artesunate for therapy of severe malaria.[204]

Examination of patients with uncomplicated malaria lacking overt pulmonary symptoms shows that many have impairment of lung function characterized by small airway obstruction, impaired alveolar ventilation, reduced gas transfer, and increased pulmonary phagocytic activity.[205] The pulmonary consequences of *P falciparum* are more commonly significant (and deadly) than those associated with *P vivax*, although poor outcomes have been reported in association with both species.[206]

P falciparum causes infected red blood cells to adhere to the endothelium of the microvasculature, leading to sluggish flow of blood and sequestration of infected red cells. This impairs oxygen exchange and causes end-organ hypoxia. Postmortem studies have demonstrated sequestration of *P falciparum*—infected red blood cells in pulmonary microvasculature.[207] The mechanism by which *P vivax* causes pulmonary disease is less clear, although in vitro studies have shown that *P vivax* is capable of adhering to some molecules present on endothelial cells within the lung.[206] Both *P falciparum* and *P vivax* related lung disease may be mediated in part by a post-therapeutic inflammatory response to the dead parasites coupled with reperfusion injury.[204,206]

Imaging features

Radiologic features usually become appreciable between 6 and 24 hours after the onset of dyspnea.[208] Chest x-ray may show lobar consolidation, diffuse interstitial edema, and pleural effusion.[203] Diffuse bilateral infiltrates, as seen in ARDS, have also been described.[204,206] Less commonly, only interstitial infiltrates or thickening of lung fissures may be seen.[208]

Histologic features

Postmortem studies have documented pulmonary edema with increased gross lung weights and punctate hemorrhages.[204,207,209] Histologically, the alveolar capillaries are congested, filled with infected red blood cells. Increased alveolar macrophages are also seen, some of which contain malarial hemozoin pigment. In patients with DAD/ARDS, hyaline membranes are seen. Some patients may also have superimposed acute or organizing pneumonia.[208,210]

Laboratory diagnosis

Examination of thick blood films is the gold standard to diagnose the presence of malaria. Examination of thin films is required to determine the species (*Figure 14-22*). To exclude malaria on the basis of peripheral blood smears, sets of smears should be examined every 12 hours for 40 hours.[208] PCR-based tests, which can also speciate the parasites, are available, although are not currently FDA approved.[211]

Pulmonary Dirofilariasis

Clinical features

Pulmonary dirofilariasis is infection of the lung with the filarial nematode *Dirofilaria immitis*. Humans are accidental hosts in the life cycle of *D immitis* and other similar zoonotic filarial nematodes (*D repens, D tenuis, D ursi*). *D immitis* primarily infects canines and is better known as the dog heartworm, although other animals may also be infected. In the United States, the prevalence of *D immitis* is highest surrounding the East and Gulf coasts, where the mosquito population is most robust.[200,212]

Hosts are infected by the bite of an infected mosquito, which deposits the filariform juveniles into the host's skin. The worms molt and enter the circulation to reach the right heart (*Figure 14-23*). In dogs, the worms reach maturity after 5 months, but in humans, the worms die as juveniles and eventually lodge in the small pulmonary arteries. In addition to embolizing small pulmonary arteries and causing infarction, the worms are antigenic and evoke an inflammatory response from the host, leading to granulomatous inflammation and an eosinophilic infiltrate.[213]

Most patients are asymptomatic, but chest pain, shortness of breath, hemoptysis, cough, and fever have all been reported in infected individuals.[214]

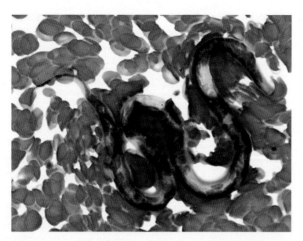

FIGURE 14-23 *Dirofilaria immitis*. **Peripheral blood smear from a dog with dirofilariasis. (Used with permission of Dr Javier Baquera Heredia, Hospital ABC, Mexico City, Mexico.)**

Imaging features

Dirofilariasis most commonly presents as a solitary coin lesion on chest x-ray.[215] The coin lesions are well defined, range in size from 1 cm to 3 cm, and are usually located at the periphery of the lung, frequently in a subpleural distribution. In older lesions, the worms may calcify. CT scan shows a well-defined subpleural nodule with a smooth margin that is usually attached to a branch of the pulmonary artery.[216] Rarely, dirofilariasis can mimic aggressive malignancy, with invasion of the mediastinum and chest wall.[217] Dirofilariasis has also been reported in concurrence with lung cancer.[218]

Histologic features

Sections of human lung will show immature worms lodged in pulmonary vessels, which can be demonstrated with elastin stains if necessary (*Figure 14-24*).

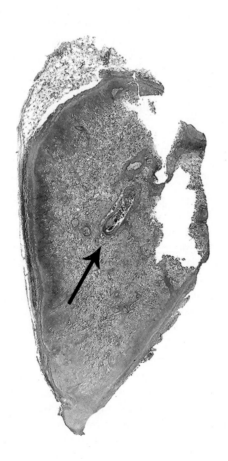

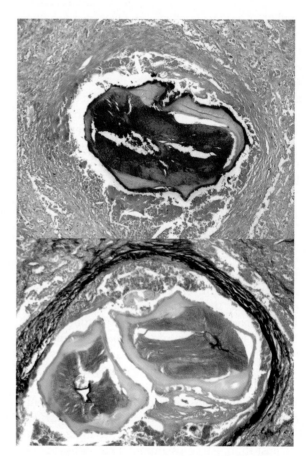

FIGURE 14-24 **Dirofilariasis. Full montage of a wedge resection in a patient with a pleural-based lung nodule. The arrow points to a blood vessel containing a worm of *D immitis* in the lumen. The surrounding tissue showed extensive fibrosis and focal necrosis (left, Masson trichrome stain). The parasite lodges into a pulmonary vessel and dies within the lumen producing obstruction and necrosis of the surrounding tissue (top right, H&E). In this particular case, an elastic special stain highlights the elastic fibers from the arterial wall (bottom right). (Used with permission of Dr Cecilia Gallegos, Hospital Angeles and Dr Javier Baquera Heredia, Hospital ABC, Mexico City, Mexico.)**

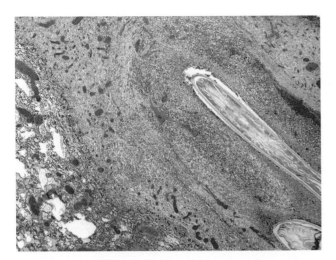

FIGURE 14-25 Dirofilariasis. The parasite (right) is surrounded by extensive granulomatous reaction, necrosis, inflammation and fibrosis (H&E). The uninvolved lung parenchyma shows marked vascular congestion (left).

The worms have a smooth cuticle and measure about 100 to 359 μm in diameter.[219] The worms are surrounded by necrosis, inflammatory cells, epithelioid histiocytes, and fibrosis. Foreign body giant cells may also be seen (*Figures 14-25 and 14-26*). The surrounding lung parenchyma may show nonspecific alveolitis or organizing pneumonia. Hemosiderin laden macrophages may also be present.[213]

Laboratory diagnosis

Serologic studies for antigens of *D immitis* lack sensitivity and specificity, so diagnosis is generally made upon excision of the pulmonary nodule. Microfilaremia does not occur in humans, so peripheral smears are not

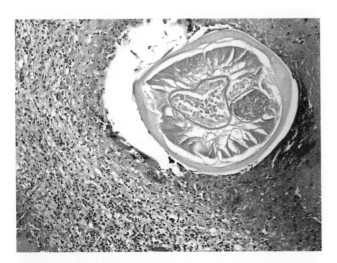

FIGURE 14-26 Dirofilariasis. Worm surrounded by inflammation and foreign-body-type giant cells (H&E).

helpful. The worms may show marked degenerative changes, so histologic examination of multiple levels and blocks may be necessary to reach a diagnosis.

Pulmonary Trichomoniasis

Trichomonas tenax is a flagellate protozoan with worldwide distribution. The organism colonizes the oral cavity, particularly of those with suboptimal dental hygiene, but may also infect the respiratory tract. Newborns and very rarely adults may suffer from pulmonary infection with *Trichomonas vaginalis*.[220,221]

Clinical and imaging features

Pulmonary trichomoniasis usually affects patients with preexisting pulmonary disease, so it is uncertain if there are any specific associated signs or symptoms that are directly related to the organism. Trichomonosis has been observed in patients with preexisting pneumonia, bronchitis, bronchiectasis, bronchogenic carcinoma, *Pneumocystis* pneumonia, and acute respiratory distress syndrome.[222,223] The organism feeds on the necrotic debris and bacteria resulting from the preceding condition.[219,222] The organism may also reside within pleural effusions.[224,225]

Histologic features

Although the organism is frequently found in necrotic lesions, no specific histologic features have been described.

Laboratory diagnosis

Pulmonary trichomoniasis is usually diagnosed by finding trichomonads in BAL or sputum samples. In BAL samples, the trichomonads may assume an amoeboid shape, rather than their more familiar pear shape. The amoeboid trichomonads lose their flagella and axostyle, making them more difficult to identify.[223] When in their well-known form, *T tenax* ranges in length from 5 to 12 μm by 4 to 10 μm in width. *T vaginalis* is larger, measuring up to 19 μm in length and 13 μm in width. On Papanicolaou stain, the organism has diaphanous gray-blue cytoplasm, a small pale basophilic oval nucleus, and red cytoplasmic granules. PCR can be used for speciation.[224]

American Trypanosomiasis (Chagas Disease)

Trypanosoma cruzi is a protozoan hemoflagellate endemic to the Americas. *T cruzi* is transmitted via the feces of the reduviid bug, which ingests trypomastigotes by taking a blood meal from an infected reservoir mammal (raccoons, armadillos). The trypomastigotes transform into epimastigotes in the bug's midgut and then become infective metacyclic trypomastigotes after about 1 week. After feeding, the insect defecates, leaving trypanosome-laden feces near the bite wound. The trypanosomes enter the host when the bug's feces come in contact with the bite wound or any mucosal surface. Once in the host, the trypomastigotes enter the blood stream and infect host cells, primarily reticuloendothelial and muscle cells. Upon entering the host cell, the trypomastigote loses its flagellum and undulating membrane and becomes an amastigote. Amastigotes reproduce until the host cell bursts, causing tissue damage and releasing more trypomastigotes into the blood stream.[200,226] T cruzi may also be congenital, acquired through blood transfusion, orally, or organ transplantation.

Clinical features

Pulmonary consequences of Chagas disease arise due to either congenital infection or secondary to megaesophagus. Patients with megaesophagus are prone to aspiration pneumonia, pulmonary abscess, and bronchiectasis. Other complications include pulmonary thromboembolism, which may be accompanied by pulmonary infarction.[227] Mothers with Chagas disease may transmit the organism to the fetus in either the acute or chronic phase of disease. The rate of vertical transmission of Chagas disease in Latin America has been reported to be as high as 18.2%.[228] Infected infants may be asymptomatic or have neurological, cardiovascular, respiratory, or gastrointestinal impairments.[228] Treatment of pulmonary trypanosomiasis includes use of nifurtimox or beznidazole.[229]

Imaging features

Imaging features of pulmonary involvement by American trypanosomiasis would reflect the extent of pulmonary involvement, but are overall nonspecific.

Histologic features

In the setting of megaesophagus, pneumonia, abscess formation, and subsequent interstitial fibrosis may occur.[227] Interstitial edema and histiocytic infiltration of the alveolar walls may occur. Amastigotes accumulate within alveolar macrophages, either expanding the alveolar septae to compress the airspaces or filling alveoli directly. Peribronchial chronic inflammation has also been observed.[230]

Laboratory diagnosis

Only the trypomastigote and amastigote stages are present in the human host. These stages are diagnostic. Peripheral blood, saliva, tissue biopsy, and fine needle aspiration samples may all be used to reach the diagnosis. On Giemsa-stained blood films, the trypomastigotes are usually shaped like a question mark or the letter C, with blue cytoplasm and violet nucleus, flagella, and kinetoplast.[226] Trypomastigotes may be found in the blood approximately 10 days after the onset of infection and throughout the rest of the acute phase of the disease. In the chronic phase of the disease, trypomastigotes may not be easily demonstrated in peripheral blood.

The amastigote is intracellular and usually infects muscle and reticuloendothelial cells. Amastigotes are visible on H and E stain and are round, ranging in diameter from 2 to 6 μm, with a basophilic nucleus. The intracellular amastigotes may also be visualized on fine needle aspiration samples from chagomas.

Other methods for diagnosis include ELISA, PCR, serology, and complement fixation. These tests may be performed on blood or saliva.[226]

The differential diagnosis includes infection with Leishmania donovani, whose amastigotes are very similar in appearance to those of T cruzi. However, T cruzi amastigotes are slightly larger than the amastigotes of L donovani.[219] L donovani pneumonitis has also been reported to cause a prominent plasma cell infiltrate, which has not been observed in chagastic pneumonitis. Notably, vertical transmission of L donovani has not been reported.[230]

Pulmonary Ascariasis

Ascaris lumbricoides is one of the most common nematodes to infect the gastrointestinal tract and is found all over the world. Humans are infected by the fecal-oral route, after ingestion of contaminated food or water. Fertilized eggs become infective in the soil, are ingested, mature over 1 to 2 weeks, and hatch in the duodenum. After hatching, the juvenile worms access vessels and lymphatics via the duodenal mucosa and are transported via the portal system through the liver, right heart, and to the lungs. Once in the lungs, the worms mature for about another week, and are then free to move up the respiratory tract, where they are coughed up and swallowed. Maturation is completed in the duodenum. After spending about 2 months within the host, the worms are finally mature enough to begin producing eggs, which are passed in the stool. Ascaris suum, a parasite of pigs, may also infect humans.

Clinical features

Although there are many nematodes that pass through the lungs and cause pulmonary eosinophilia (Loeffler syndrome), A lumbricoides is one of the most common offenders.[231] A lumbricoides–related pulmonary eosinophilia is usually self-limited and only 8% to 15%

of infected individuals experience symptoms.[232] The symptoms are transient and include wheezing, dyspnea, cough, and hemoptysis.[214,219] Treatment consists of either albendazole or menbendazole.[232]

Imaging features

Ascaris infections of the lung show patchy migratory airspace opacities which may become confluent in more severe cases.[214,232]

Histologic features

Larvae can be seen within alveolar spaces and walls, bronchioles, and bronchi. Small alveolar hemorrhages occur when the worms escape into the airspaces. Fibrin deposition and an eosinophil-rich inflammatory infiltrate occur within bronchioles and surrounding the worms. The larvae may also be surrounded by epithelioid histiocytes and macrophages. Interstitial inflammation and bronchopneumonia have also been observed.[219]

Laboratory diagnosis

After passing through the lungs, it takes several weeks for the larvae to become mature enough to produce eggs. Therefore, pulmonary symptoms usually precede the detection of eggs in stool samples.[231] Patients will have absolute peripheral eosinophilia and sputum samples also demonstrate eosinophilia, often with many Charcot-Leyden crystals.[232] Larvae may be found in sputum, BAL, bronchial wash, bronchial brush, or gastric aspirate specimens. While in the lungs, the larvae are usually in their third stage of development and range in length from 1.4 to 1.8 mm.[200] Adult male worms range in length from 15 to 30 cm and measure up to 4 mm in diameter while females are generally 20 to 49 cm in length and up to 6 mm in diameter. Male worms have ventrally curled tails while females have straight tails. Both genders have three prominent lips. Although adults of *Ascaris suum* are morphologically identical to those of *A lumbricoides*, *A suum* does not reach maturity in the human host, so the presence of an adult worm in a human sample is essentially diagnostic of *A lumbricoides*. In fecal specimens, eggs of *Ascaris lumbricoides* are bile stained. Fertilized eggs are oval, with a unicellular ovum, and range in size from 45 to 75 μm in length by 35 to 50 μm in width. The eggs usually have a thick bumpy capsule. Unfertilized eggs may also be seen in stool and are longer and thinner.[200,233]

Pulmonary Amoebiasis

Entamoeba histolytica is a protozoan with worldwide distribution, but most commonly found in tropical and subtropical climes, especially those with suboptimal

sanitation services. It is spread via the fecal-oral route, often with the assistance of flies and cockroaches. Patients are infected by ingesting mature amoebic cysts. Trophozoites excyst in the small bowel and travel to the large bowel, where they reside in the intestinal crypts. When stool dehydrates in the distal portions of the large bowel, the amoeba encyst. Thus, cysts are passed in formed stool into the environment.

Although the trophozoites could exist in the crypts without causing harm, they often hydrolyze enterocytes for additional nutrition, leading to ulceration of the colonic mucosa and invasion into the host's circulatory system. Once blood borne, the amoebae are free to travel throughout the body. The most common site for secondary amoebic lesions is the liver, followed by the lung. The lung may become involved in several ways. Most commonly, this occurs via direct extension from the liver. Should an amoebic abscess become large enough, a hepatopulmonary fistula ensues.[219,229] Therefore, the right lower lobe is the most commonly affected portion of the lungs due to its proximity to the dome of the liver. Amoebic abscesses may also be found in the left lower lobe and lingua. The lung may also become involved through hematogenous spread or through inhalation of dust containing mature cysts, although the latter situation is quite rare.[234,235]

Clinical features

Most patients infected with *Entamoeba histolytica* are asymptomatic. When symptoms do occur, as in the setting of invasive disease, they are gastrointestinal, with abdominal pain and bloody diarrhea. Patients with pulmonary amoebiasis present with fever, pleuritic pain, cough, hemoptysis, and tender hepatomegaly.[203,229] The presentation of pulmonary amoebiasis may not be straightforward. Patients presenting with superior vena cava syndrome and mass lesions mimicking malignancy have been reported.[236,237]

Draining of amoebic abscesses, regardless of their location, yields purulent material dysphemistically likened to anchovy paste. Should a liver abscess erode into a bronchus, expectoration of said material occurs. Pleural involvement carries a worse prognosis, leading to empyema and occasionally to sepsis.[219]

Pulmonary amoebiasis is most common in men (male to female ratio 10:1) between the ages of 30 and 40 years and rarely affects children.[234] Mortality depends on the patient's comorbidities, but rates ranging from 5.4% to 16.5% have been reported.[234]

Imaging features

Radiographic features of pulmonary amoebiasis are variable, depending on the extent of disease, and may range from minimal findings to extensive bilateral infiltrates.[229] In the setting of pulmonary involvement secondary to hepatic abscess, chest x-ray shows elevation of the right hemidiaphragm with infiltrates or opacification of the right lower lobe. An air-fluid level may be observed in the liver if erosion of the abscess into a bronchus has occurred. Opacification of the entire lung field may occur with rupture of the abscess into the pleural space. Amoebic empyema usually does not cause a loculated effusion, as seen in bacterial empyema.[234] The therapeutic effects of drainage and appropriate antimicrobial therapy (metronidazole) should be appreciable by imaging.[235]

Histologic features

Amoebic abscesses have a central necrotic zone containing debris. Occasionally inflammatory cells and trophozoites are identified within the necrotic center, but they are more likely to be encountered within the viable rim of tissue surrounding the abscess (*Figure 14-27*). The adjacent viable lung parenchyma shows edema and a mixed inflammatory infiltrate.[219]

Laboratory diagnosis

Patients generally have leukocytosis and elevation of acute phase reactants. Eosinophilia is generally not a feature of amoebiasis.[215] Elevated serum antibody titers may be detected, but these do not discriminate between active and prior infections. Additionally, serologic tests may remain positive for up to 2 years after treatment and eradication of the parasite.[231]

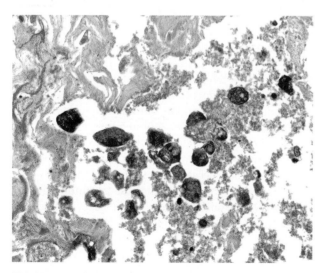

FIGURE 14-27 Amebiasis. Trophozoites of *Entamoeba histolytica* in a background of necrosis. Lung biopsy from a patient with a liver abscess. The PAS stain highlights the parasites and leaves a negative image for the nucleus and phagocytosed red blood cells seen within the trophozoite's cytoplasm.

Trophozoites may be found in sputum samples and, in the case of abscess rupture into the pleural space, the pleural fluid. In sputum samples, caution must be taken to distinguish *E histolytica* from *E gingivalis*, a nonpathogenic species found in the oral cavity.[229] *E histolytica* will engulf only red blood cells while the less discriminating *E gingivalis* engulfs white and red blood cells.[234]

E histolytica may be detected by light microscopy. On wet preparations, *E histolytica* trophozoites move rapidly and measure between 12 and 60 μm, although invasive forms may be larger. Upon fixation, the trophozoites and cysts may appear several micrometers smaller. There is one nucleus with evenly distributed peripheral chromatin and a small central karyosome. The cytoplasm is finely granular. The cysts are 10 to 20 μm. Mature cysts have four nuclei with a single small central karyosome while immature cysts have one or two nuclei. The chromatin is fine. Some cysts have chromatoidal bodies, which are elongated with rounded edges.[238] Cysts are strongly positive for PAS, which helps identify them in tissue sections or on smears (*Figure 14-27*). Staining with PAS may obscure nuclear and cytoplasmic details, so examination of the trophozoites' morphology is best performed on H and E stains for tissue and Papanicolaou stain for cytologic material.[219]

Culture and serology will both detect *E histolytica*. PCR may be used to detect both cyst and trophozoite DNA in stool samples and aspirates of abscesses. ELISA is also available.

Pulmonary Strongyloidiasis

Strongyloides stercoralis is a versatile nematode with both free living and parasitic life cycles. Parasitic adult females embed their anterior ends in the submucosa of the small intestine and release partially embryonated eggs which hatch in the gut to become rhabditiform larvae which are then passed with feces. Once in the environment, the rhabditiform larvae mature into filariform larvae which must gain entry into a host, by either ingestion or penetration of the skin, in order to mature further.

The larvae cause dermatitis when penetrating the skin and after navigating into a blood vessel, the larvae are transported to the lungs where they exit into the alveoli. At this point, larvae may be seen in BAL, bronchial wash, or sputum samples (*Figure 14-28*). Once in the alveoli, and after several rounds of molting, the larvae are coughed up, swallowed, and delivered to the intestine to mature to adulthood. Alternatively, after hatching, the rhabditiform larvae may directly penetrate the intestine and renew the cycle of infection without exiting the host (autoinfection).[200] If the host is immunocompromised, and especially in the setting of chronic steroid therapy (chronic illness, advanced age, status post organ transplant, hematologic malignancies), the host-parasite relationship that governs autoinfection is skewed and

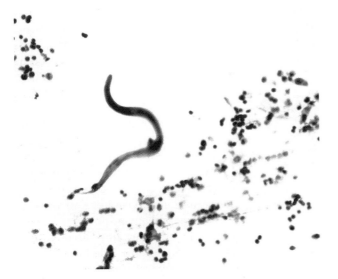

FIGURE 14-28 Strongyloidiasis. *Strongyloides stercoralis* rhabditiform larvae may be detected in **BAL**, bronchial wash or sputum samples (Diff-Quik stain).

hyperinfection results. Other patients at risk for developing hyperinfection include those with protein calorie malnutrition, chronic illnesses, hematologic malignancies, solid organ transplants, and HSCT transplant recipients.[239,240] In the setting of hyperinfection, mortality rates of up to 87% have been reported in patients on chronic corticosteroid therapy, although much lower rates (26%) have been reported in other patients.[241,242]

Clinical features

The degree of symptoms is directly related to the patient's worm burden. Patients may have asthma-like symptoms with coughing, wheezing, and shortness of breath. Patients may also develop hemoptysis and ARDS.[239,240] Patients are also at risk of gram-negative bacterial pneumonia as bacteria adhere to the worms as they leave the gut lumen.[203] Treatment regimens may include ivermectin, albendazole, or thiabendazole, although thiabendazole is currently the preferred agent. Steroids are contraindicated as they hamper the host's ability to fend off the worms and may even promote their growth and maturation.[243]

Imaging features

On chest x-ray, patients usually present with alveolar infiltrates which may be segmental or diffuse and bilateral. Initially, miliary nodules or reticular interstitial opacities are present.[215,239,240] With increasing worm burden, patchy bronchopneumonia and segmental and/or lobar opacities may occur in addition to abscess and pleural effusion. Serial radiographs may even show migration of opacities.[239,240]

Histologic features

The larvae penetrating the alveolar capillaries and alveoli cause hemorrhage. Cavitation and abscess formation may also occur, due in part to the hitchhiking gram-negative bacteria from the gut lumen. In the setting of hyperinfection, adult worms embed themselves in the bronchial epithelium.[219]

One case report describes predominantly granulomatous inflammation with associated interlobular septal fibrosis.[244]

Larvae may be detected on pulmonary cytologic specimens and are easily visualized on Papanicolaou, Romanowsky, Gram, and GMS stains[245] (*Figures 14-29 and 14-30*). The rhabditiform larvae have short buccal

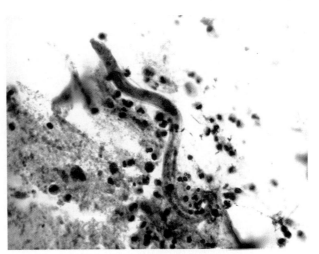

FIGURE 14-29 *Strongyloides stercoralis* detected in a **BAL**. Filariform larvae and necrotic debris (Diff-Quik stain).

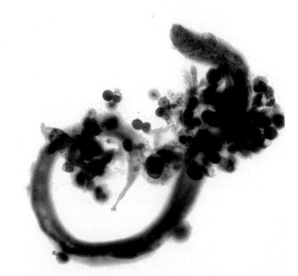

FIGURE 14-30 *Strongyloides stercoralis* detected in a **BAL**. Filariform larvae with attached degenerated red blood cells and mononuclear cells (Diff-Quik stain).

cavity and a prominent genital primordium and measure 380 × 20 μm.[202,219]

Laboratory diagnosis

Patients usually have some degree of peripheral eosinophilia, although immunocompromised patients and patients with disseminated disease or hyperinfection may lack this finding.[214] Elevated serum IgE is another frequent finding. Pulmonary strongyloidiasis is diagnosed when larvae are identified within sputum, BAL, bronchial brush, bronchial wash, or lung biopsy specimens. Hyperinfection may be diagnosed if adult worms are found in the lung or if rhabditiform larvae are present in the sputum and disseminated disease is diagnosed when larvae are found in extrapulmonary, extraintestinal sites.[219,242] The disease is easier to diagnose in the setting of hyperinfection, as the worm burden is usually profound. A serum antibody test for *Strongyloides* is available, but specificity is hindered by cross reactivity for other helminthic antigens, such as *Ascaris lumbricoides*. An ELISA test for serum IgG against *Strongyloides* antigens is also available.[242]

Pulmonary Cryptosporidiosis

Cryptosporidium is an intracellular spore-forming protozoan parasite with worldwide distribution. It is usually acquired through contaminated water and encountered in the context of gastrointestinal disease, but pulmonary infection is also known to occur. Respiratory transmission of the parasite has also been postulated to account for pulmonary disease, as has hematogenous spread.[246-248] Most patients with respiratory cryptosporidiosis present with productive cough, fever, and shortness of breath in addition to typical gastrointestinal symptoms (diarrhea). Respiratory cryptosporidiosis is most commonly reported in patients with AIDS and other immunosuppressed patients, such as those with hematologic malignancies or after bone marrow transplant.[229] It is also reported in HIV seronegative individuals.[248] *C parvum*, *C hominis*, and *C meleagridis* have all been reported as etiologic agents of pulmonary cryptosporidiosis.[249] The preferred treatment is nitazoxanide.[229]

Chest radiographs frequently show features of interstitial pneumonia, such as interstitial opacities, but no additional specific findings have been reported.[229,246] Alternatively, some patients may have a normal chest x-ray.[246]

Nonspecific histologic changes have been described, including diffuse alveolar damage with hyperplasia and reactive changes of type II pneumocytes. Intra-alveolar and interstitial inflammation, composed predominantly of lymphocytes and macrophages, in addition to interstitial fibrosis has also been reported.[229] The

organisms may be identified within the apical aspect of bronchial epithelial cells, within bronchial mucus glands, and within alveolar macrophages. Organisms may be easier to visualize with special stains, including Giemsa, PAS, GMS, or modified Kinyoun. Organisms may be rare and may be easier to visualize on sputum or BAL specimens. Aforementioned special stains can all be applied to cytologic preparations. Oocysts are thick walled and measure 4 to 6 μm in diameter.[250] After maturation within the oocysts, sporozoites exit and infect host cells, eventually residing in the apical aspect of respiratory epithelial cells. Merozoites are also infectious. These invasive forms (sporozoites and merozoites) are small comma-shaped organisms.[251]

Light microscopy with special stains, direct fluorescent antibody assays, and real-time PCR have all been employed to diagnose *Cryptosporidium*. Recently, a real-time PCR assay has been developed to quantify and identify *C parvum* and *C hominis* in stool samples.[252]

Pulmonary Capillariasis

Capillaria aerophila is a nematode that infects the tracheobronchial mucosa of carnivorous mammals including domestic cats and dogs, as well as wild animals like foxes, opossums, and wolves. After mating, females release unembryonated eggs into the respiratory tract that are coughed up, swallowed, and deposited into the environment with passage of feces. After further development in the soil, the embryonated eggs become infectious. Humans are very rarely infected, but become so by ingesting embryonated eggs. Infection in humans may cause cough, bronchitis, fever, and shortness of breath. One author reports mucosal abscesses which became mass forming, mimicking an endobronchial tumor.[253] Although experience is limited to isolated case reports, the worms have been observed in bronchioles, causing a marked eosinophilic infiltrate.[219] Diagnosis rests upon demonstration of the eggs in feces, sputum, or lung or bronchial biopsy. The eggs are ovoid with a double-layered shell and asymmetric mucoid polar plugs. Scanning electron microscopy shows that the outer shell has striated surface with anastomosing ridges and pits.[254] The eggs measure approximately 64 × 35 μm.[253,254] A PCR assay to detect amplicons of the organism's *cox1* gene has proved to be both sensitive and specific for diagnosis of capillariasis in the stool samples of cats and dogs.[255] Mebendazole or albendazole have been used in the rare cases of human infection.[253]

Tropical Pulmonary Eosinophilia

Although infection with filarial worms may be asymptomatic, patients infected with *Wuchereria bancrofti* and *Brugia malayi* may also suffer from tropical pulmonary eosinophilia (TPE), which is reported in less than

1% of all filarial infections worldwide.[25] Mosquitoes of *Anopheles*, *Culex*, and *Aedes* mosquitoes serve as vectors. Adult filarial worms reside and reproduce in the lymphatics, releasing microfilariae which are distributed systemically via the lymphatic system. The syndrome of TPE results from microfilariae becoming entrapped in the pulmonary circulation and degenerating, thus releasing antigens and causing a local inflammatory response.

Clinical features

Patients with TPE originate from or provide history of travel to endemic areas (most commonly India and Southeast Asia) and frequently present with asthmatic symptoms including wheezing and shortness of breath.[256] Other symptoms include paroxysmal cough, fever, weight loss, and fatigue. Most patients are young adult (30-40 year old) males.[231] Treatment with diethylcarbamazine citrate is the standard of care and many patients show clinical improvement within the first month of treatment.[256,257] Steroids may also be used in conjunction with diethylcarbamazine to prevent reaction to the dying worms.[231] Pulmonary function studies show an obstructive pattern initially, then a restrictive pattern as the disease progresses.[214] Acquired α-1 antitrypsin deficiency in the setting of TPE has also been reported.[258] Due to its relative rarity, TPE is frequently misdiagnosed as asthma. However, patients do not respond to treatment for asthma, leading to further clinical workup.[259] Untreated disease progresses to irreversible interstitial pulmonary fibrosis, but even patients who receive appropriate treatment may suffer from persistent symptoms and relapses of disease.[214,256,257]

Imaging features

Radiographic features of TPE include reticulonodular infiltrates of the middle and lower lobes, which may mimic miliary tuberculosis.[214,256,257,260] Increased bronchovascular markings are often seen, but hilar lymphadenopathy and pleural effusions are rare.[231,257] Up to 20% of patients have normal chest radiographs.[259]

Histologic features

Initially, TPE is characterized by an infiltrate of macrophages, but eosinophils arrive shortly thereafter, filling the alveoli, then infiltrating the interstitium and bronchioles. Eosinophilic abscesses may occur, in addition to eosinophilic granulomata. The lesions are not bronchocentric, but are closer to pulmonary venules.[219] Hyperplasia and reactive changes of type II pneumocytes are often seen.[231] With time, the inflammatory infiltrate within airspaces becomes predominantly histiocytic with lesser numbers of eosinophils and lymphocytes. Patchy areas of organization may be seen. Late stage disease is characterized by interstitial fibrosis.

Laboratory diagnosis

Patients with TPE have peripheral leukocytosis with persistent absolute eosinophilia, usually greater than 3000 cells/μL.[257] Patients also have marked elevation of parasite-specific IgE and IgG antibodies in serum as well as overall elevation of serum IgE.[257,259] Total serum IgE above 1000 U/mL is supportive of a diagnosis of TPE.[258] A rapid ELISA for *W bancrofti* antigens is also available. An ELISA for detecting antigens of *B malayi* is also available. This test has the advantage of being specific for *W bancrofti*, as other assays may cross-react with antigens from other filarial worms.[261] Microfilariae are usually not found in peripheral blood smears.[214,231,256] BAL samples from affected patients show marked eosinophilia in addition to elevated levels of IgE, IgG, IgM, and IgA.[231] Microfilaria may also be identified in BAL specimens.[231,262] Workup should also include examination of stool samples and serologic testing to rule out infection with *Ascaris* or *Strongyloides*, which would require different therapy.[259] Clinical response to treatment with diethylcarbamazine may help confirm the diagnosis.[260]

REFERENCES

1. Osiowy C. Direct detection of respiratory syncytial virus, parainfluenza virus, and adenovirus in clinical respiratory specimens by a multiplex reverse transcription-PCR assay. *J Clin Microbiol.* November 1998;36(11):3149-3154.
2. Ghoneim HE, Thomas PG, McCullers JA. Depletion of alveolar macrophages during influenza infection facilitates bacterial superinfections. *J Immunol.* August 1, 2013;191(3):1250-1259.
3. Cytomegalovirus (CMV) and congenital CMV infection. December 6, 2010. http://www.cdc.gov/cmv/overview.html. Accessed July 20, 2013.
4. Zamora MR. Cytomegalovirus and lung transplantation. *Am J Transplant.* August 2004;4(8):1219-1226.
5. Boeckh M. Complications, diagnosis, management, and prevention of CMV infections: current and future. *Hematology Am Soc Hematol Educ Program.* 2011;2011:305-309.
6. Chiche L, Forel JM, Papazian L. The role of viruses in nosocomial pneumonia. *Curr Opin Infect Dis.* April 2011;24(2):152-156.
7. Cunha BA. Cytomegalovirus pneumonia: community-acquired pneumonia in immunocompetent hosts. *Infect Dis Clin North Am.* March 2010;24(1):147-158.
8. Kim EA, Lee KS, Primack SL, et al. Viral pneumonias in adults: radiologic and pathologic findings. *Radiographics.* October 2002;22 Spec No:S137-S149.
9. Suster S, Moran CA. Viral lung infections. In: Epstein JI, ed. *Biopsy interpretation of the lung.* Philadelphia, PA: Lippincott Williams & Wilkins; 2013:155-174.
10. Strickler JG, Manivel JC, Copenhaver CM, Kubic VL. Comparison of in situ hybridization and immunohistochemistry for detection of cytomegalovirus and herpes simplex virus. *Hum Pathol.* April 1990;21(4):443-448.
11. Weinberg A, Hodges TN, Li S, Cai G, Zamora MR. Comparison of PCR, antigenemia assay, and rapid blood culture for detection and prevention of cytomegalovirus disease after lung transplantation. *J Clin Microbiol.* February 2000;38(2):768-772.
12. Bewig B, Haacke TC, Tiroke A, et al. Detection of CMV pneumonitis after lung transplantation using PCR of DNA from bronchoalveolar lavage cells. *Respiration.* 2000;67(2):166-172.

13. Kadmon G, Levy I, Mandelboim M, et al. Polymerase-chain-reaction-based diagnosis of viral pulmonary infections in immunocompromised children. *Acta Paediatr.* June 2013;102(6):e263-e268.

14. Ramsey PG, Fife KH, Hackman RC, Meyers JD, Corey L. Herpes simplex virus pneumonia: clinical, virologic, and pathologic features in 20 patients. *Ann Intern Med.* December 1982;97(6):813-820.

15. Engelmann I, Gottlieb J, Meier A, et al. Clinical relevance of and risk factors for HSV-related tracheobronchitis or pneumonia: results of an outbreak investigation. *Crit Care.* 2007;11(6):R119.

16. Cesario TC. Viruses associated with pneumonia in adults. *Clin Infect Dis.* July 2012;55(1):107-113.

17. Chong S, Kim TS, Cho EY. Herpes simplex virus pneumonia: high-resolution CT findings. *Br J Radiol.* July 2010;83(991):585-589.

18. Brodoefel H, Vogel M, Spira D, et al. Herpes-Simplex-Virus 1 pneumonia in the immunocompromised host: high-resolution CT patterns in correlation to outcome and follow-up. *Eur J Radiol.* April 2012;81(4):e415-e420.

19. Jouneau S, Poineuf JS, Minjolle S, et al. Which patients should be tested for viruses on bronchoalveolar lavage fluid? *Eur J Clin Microbiol Infect Dis.* May 2013;32(5):671-677.

20. Piret J, Boivin G. Resistance of herpes simplex viruses to nucleoside analogues: mechanisms, prevalence, and management. *Antimicrob Agents Chemother.* February 2011;55(2):459-472.

21. Scheithauer S, Manemann AK, Kruger S, et al. Impact of herpes simplex virus detection in respiratory specimens of patients with suspected viral pneumonia. *Infection.* October 2010;38(5):401-405.

22. Linssen CF, Jacobs JA, Stelma FF, et al. Herpes simplex virus load in bronchoalveolar lavage fluid is related to poor outcome in critically ill patients. *Intensive Care Med.* December 2008;34(12):2202-2209.

23. Costa C, Sidoti F, Saldan A, et al. Clinical impact of HSV-1 detection in the lower respiratory tract from hospitalized adult patients. *Clin Microbiol Infect.* August 2012;18(8):E305-E307.

24. Lasithiotaki I, Antoniou KM, Vlahava VM, et al. Detection of herpes simplex virus type-1 in patients with fibrotic lung diseases. *PLoS One.* 2011;6(12):e27800.

25. Luksic I, Kearns PK, Scott F, Rudan I, Campbell H, Nair H. Viral etiology of hospitalized acute lower respiratory infections in children under 5 years of age—a systematic review and meta-analysis. *Croat Med J.* April 2013;54(2):122-134.

26. Marcone DN, Ellis A, Videla C, et al. Viral etiology of acute respiratory infections in hospitalized and outpatient children in Buenos Aires, Argentina. *Pediatr Infect Dis J.* March 2013;32(3):e105-e110.

27. Pretorius MA, Madhi SA, Cohen C, et al. Respiratory viral coinfections identified by a 10-plex real-time reverse-transcription polymerase chain reaction assay in patients hospitalized with severe acute respiratory illness–South Africa, 2009-2010. *J Infect Dis.* December 15, 2012;206(suppl 1):S159-S165.

28. Chen SP, Huang YC, Chiu CH, et al. Clinical features of radiologically confirmed pneumonia due to adenovirus in children. *J Clin Virol.* January 2013;56(1):7-12.

29. Lai CY, Lee CJ, Lu CY, et al. Adenovirus serotype 3 and 7 infection with acute respiratory failure in children in Taiwan, 2010-2011. *PLoS One.* 2013;8(1):e53614.

30. Incidence of acute respiratory illnesses among enlisted service members during their first year of military service: did the 2011 resumption of adenovirus vaccination of basic trainees have an effect? *MSMR.* May 2013;20(5):14-18.

31. Acute respiratory disease associated with adenovirus serotype 14—four states, 2006-2007. *MMWR Morb Mortal Wkly Rep.* November 16, 2007;56(45):1181-1184.

32. Louie JK, Kajon AE, Holodniy M, et al. Severe pneumonia due to adenovirus serotype 14: a new respiratory threat? *Clin Infect Dis.* February 1, 2008;46(3):421-425.

33. Metzgar D, Osuna M, Kajon AE, Hawksworth AW, Irvine M, Russell KL. Abrupt emergence of diverse species B adenoviruses at US military recruit training centers. *J Infect Dis.* November 15, 2007;196(10):1465-1473.

34. Yilmaz M, Chemaly RF, Han XY, et al. Adenoviral infections in adult allogeneic hematopoietic SCT recipients: a single center experience. *Bone Marrow Transplant.* 2013;48(9):1218-1223.

35. Guo W, Wang J, Sheng M, Zhou M, Fang L. Radiological findings in 210 paediatric patients with viral pneumonia: a retrospective case study. *Br J Radiol.* October 2012;85(1018):1385-1389.

36. Erard V, Huang ML, Ferrenberg J, et al. Quantitative real-time polymerase chain reaction for detection of adenovirus after T cell-replete hematopoietic cell transplantation: viral load as a marker for invasive disease. *Clin Infect Dis.* October 15, 2007;45(8):958-965.

37. Taniguchi K, Yoshihara S, Tamaki H, et al. Incidence and treatment strategy for disseminated adenovirus disease after haploidentical stem cell transplantation. *Ann Hematol.* August 2012;91(8):1305-1312.

38. Bordigoni P, Carret AS, Venard V, Witz F, Le Faou A. Treatment of adenovirus infections in patients undergoing allogeneic hematopoietic stem cell transplantation. *Clin Infect Dis.* May 1, 2001;32(9):1290-1297.

39. Rudan I, O'Brien KL, Nair H, et al. Epidemiology and etiology of childhood pneumonia in 2010: estimates of incidence, severe morbidity, mortality, underlying risk factors and causative pathogens for 192 countries. *J Glob Health.* June 2013;3(1):10401.

40. Hirsch HH, Martino R, Ward KN, Boeckh M, Einsele H, Ljungman P. Fourth European Conference on Infections in Leukaemia (ECIL-4): guidelines for diagnosis and treatment of human respiratory syncytial virus, parainfluenza virus, metapneumovirus, rhinovirus, and coronavirus. *Clin Infect Dis.* January 2013;56(2):258-266.

41. Johnson JE, Gonzales RA, Olson SJ, Wright PF, Graham BS. The histopathology of fatal untreated human respiratory syncytial virus infection. *Mod Pathol.* January 2007;20(1):108-119.

42. Kotelkin A, Prikhod'ko EA, Cohen JI, Collins PL, Bukreyev A. Respiratory syncytial virus infection sensitizes cells to apoptosis mediated by tumor necrosis factor-related apoptosis-inducing ligand. *J Virol.* September 2003;77(17):9156-9172.

43. Lee N, Lui GC, Wong KT, et al. High morbidity and mortality in adults hospitalized for respiratory syncytial virus infections. *Clin Infect Dis.* 2013;57(8):1069-1077.

44. Chiner E, Ballester I, Betlloch I, et al. Varicella-zoster virus pneumonia in an adult population: has mortality decreased? *Scand J Infect Dis.* March 2010;42(3):215-221.

45. Feldman S. Varicella-zoster virus pneumonitis. *Chest.* July 1994;106(1 suppl):22S-27S.

46. Lamont RF, Sobel JD, Carrington D, et al. Varicella-zoster virus (chickenpox) infection in pregnancy. *BJOG.* September 2011;118(10):1155-1162.

47. Frangides CY, Pneumatikos I. Varicella-zoster virus pneumonia in adults: report of 14 cases and review of the literature. *Eur J Intern Med.* October 2004;15(6):364-370.

48. Inokuchi R, Nakamura K, Sato H, et al. Bronchial ulceration as a prognostic indicator for varicella pneumonia: case report and systematic literature review. *J Clin Virol.* April 2013;56(4):360-364.

49. Floudas CS, Kanakis MA, Andreopoulos A, Vaiopoulos GA. Nodular lung calcifications following varicella zoster virus pneumonia. *QJM.* February 2008;101(2):159.

50. Kim JS, Ryu CW, Lee SI, Sung DW, Park CK. High-resolution CT findings of varicella-zoster pneumonia. *AJR Am J Roentgenol.* January 1999;172(1):113-116.

51. Sauerbrei A, Eichhorn U, Schacke M, Wutzler P. Laboratory diagnosis of herpes zoster. *J Clin Virol.* September 1999;14(1):31-36.

52. Cohen JI. Clinical practice: herpes zoster. *N Engl J Med.* July 18, 2013;369(3):255-263.

53. Winn WC, Allen S, Janda WM, et al. Diagnosis of infections caused by viruses, Chlamydia, Rickettsia, and related organisms. *Koneman's Color Atlas and Textbook of Diagnostic Microbiology.* 6th ed. Philadelphia, PA: Lippincott Williams & Wilkins; 2006:1327-1419.

54. Watson DC, Sargianou M, Papa A, Chra P, Starakis I, Panos G. Epidemiology of Hantavirus infections in humans: a comprehensive, global overview. *Crit Rev Microbiol.* April 22, 2013.

55. Nolte KB, Feddersen RM, Foucar K, et al. Hantavirus pulmonary syndrome in the United States: a pathological description of a disease caused by a new agent. *Hum Pathol.* January 1995;26(1):110-120.

56. Firth C, Tokarz R, Simith DB, et al. Diversity and distribution of hantaviruses in South America. *J Virol.* December 2012;86(24):13756-13766.

57. Hantavirus pulmonary syndrome in visitors to a national park—Yosemite Valley, California, 2012. *MMWR Morb Mortal Wkly Rep.* November 23, 2012;61(46):952.

58. Hartline J, Mierek C, Knutson T, Kang C. Hantavirus infection in North America: a clinical review. *Am J Emerg Med.* June 2013;31(6):978-982.

59. Knust B, Macneil A, Rollin PE. Hantavirus pulmonary syndrome clinical findings: evaluating a surveillance case definition. *Vector Borne Zoonotic Dis.* May 2012;12(5):393-399.

60. Sargianou M, Watson DC, Chra P, et al. Hantavirus infections for the clinician: from case presentation to diagnosis and treatment. *Crit Rev Microbiol.* November 2012;38(4):317-329.

61. Zaki SR, Greer PW, Coffield LM, et al. Hantavirus pulmonary syndrome. Pathogenesis of an emerging infectious disease. *Am J Pathol.* March 1995;146(3):552-579.

62. Colby TV, Zaki SR, Feddersen RM, Nolte KB. Hantavirus pulmonary syndrome is distinguishable from acute interstitial pneumonia. *Arch Pathol Lab Med.* October 2000;124(10):1463-1466.

63. Perez-Padilla R, de la Rosa-Zamboni D, Ponce de Leon S, et al. Pneumonia and respiratory failure from swine-origin influenza A (H1N1) in Mexico. *N Engl J Med.* August 13, 2009;361(7):680-689.

64. Pandemic (H1N1) 2009. Global alert and response. http://www.who.int/csr/disease/swineflu/en/. Accessed August 3, 2013.

65. Chowell G, Bertozzi SM, Colchero MA, et al. Severe respiratory disease concurrent with the circulation of H1N1 influenza. *N Engl J Med.* August 13, 2009;361(7):674-679.

66. Ruuskanen O, Lahti E, Jennings LC, Murdoch DR. Viral pneumonia. *Lancet.* April 9, 2011;377(9773):1264-1275.

67. Zhou J, Wang D, Gao R, et al. Biological features of novel avian influenza A (H7N9) virus. *Nature.* July 3, 2013.

68. Avian influenza A (H7N9) virus. Seasonal influenza (flu). September 13, 2013. http://www.cdc.gov/flu/avianflu/h7n9-virus.htm. Accessed September 15, 2013.

69. Almond MH, McAuley DF, Wise MP, Griffiths MJ. Influenza-related pneumonia. *Clin Med.* February 2012;12(1):67-70.

70. Janke BH. Clinicopathological features of Swine influenza. *Curr Top Microbiol Immunol.* 2013;370:69-83.

71. Wu C, Cheng X, Wang X, et al. Clinical and molecular characteristics of the 2009 pandemic influenza H1N1 infection with severe or fatal disease from 2009 to 2011 in Shenzhen, China. *J Med Virol.* March 2013;85(3):405-412.

72. Qureshi NR, Hien TT, Farrar J, Gleeson FV. The radiologic manifestations of H5N1 avian influenza. *J Thorac Imaging.* November 2006;21(4):259-264.

73. Jamieson AM, Pasman L, Yu S, et al. Role of tissue protection in lethal respiratory viral-bacterial coinfection. *Science.* June 7, 2013;340(6137):1230-1234.

74. McCullers JA. Do specific virus-bacteria pairings drive clinical outcomes of pneumonia? *Clin Microbiol Infect.* February 2013;19(2):113-118.

75. Nakajima N, Sato Y, Katano H, et al. Histopathological and immunohistochemical findings of 20 autopsy cases with 2009 H1N1 virus infection. *Mod Pathol.* January 2012;25(1):1-13.

76. Brooks EG, Bryce CH, Avery C, Smelser C, Thompson D, Nolte KB. 2009 H1N1 fatalities: the New Mexico experience. *J Forensic Sci.* November 2012;57(6):1512-1518.

77. Shieh WJ, Blau DM, Denison AM, et al. 2009 pandemic influenza A (H1N1): pathology and pathogenesis of 100 fatal cases in the United States. *Am J Pathol.* July 2010;177(1):166-175.

78. Guarner J, Falcon-Escobedo R. Comparison of the pathology caused by H1N1, H5N1, and H3N2 influenza viruses. *Arch Med Res.* November 2009;40(8):655-661.

79. Bal A, Suri V, Mishra B, et al. Pathology and virology findings in cases of fatal influenza A H1N1 virus infection in 2009-2010. *Histopathology.* January 2012;60(2):326-335.

80. Nakajima N, Van Tin N, Sato Y, et al. Pathological study of archival lung tissues from five fatal cases of avian H5N1 influenza in Vietnam. *Mod Pathol.* March 2013;26(3):357-369.

81. Mahony J, Chong S, Bulir D, Ruyter A, Mwawasi K, Waltho D. Multiplex loop-mediated isothermal amplification (M-LAMP) assay for the detection of influenza A/H1, A/H3 and influenza B can provide a specimen-to-result diagnosis in 40min with single genome copy sensitivity. *J Clin Virol.* September 2013;58(1):127-131.

82. Hayden FG, Atmar RL, Schilling M, et al. Use of the selective oral neuraminidase inhibitor oseltamivir to prevent influenza. *N Engl J Med.* October 28, 1999;341(18):1336-1343.

83. Hayden FG, Treanor JJ, Fritz RS, et al. Use of the oral neuraminidase inhibitor oseltamivir in experimental human influenza: randomized controlled trials for prevention and treatment. *JAMA.* October 6, 1999;282(13):1240-1246.

84. Perry RT, Halsey NA. The clinical significance of measles: a review. *J Infect Dis.* May 1, 2004;189(suppl 1):S4-S16.

85. Duke T, Mgone CS. Measles: not just another viral exanthem. *Lancet.* March 1, 2003;361(9359):763-773.

86. Yasunaga H, Shi Y, Takeuchi M, et al. Measles-related hospitalizations and complications in Japan, 2007-2008. *Intern Med.* 2010;49(18):1965-1970.

87. Hussain H, Omer SB, Khan AJ, Bhurgri A, Memon A, Halsey NA. Endemic measles in Karachi, Pakistan and validation of IMCI criteria for measles. *Acta Paediatr.* April 2009;98(4):720-724.

88. Measles: United States, January May 20, 2011. *MMWR Morb Mortal Wkly Rep.* May 27, 2011;60(20):666-668.

89. Yu X, Qian F, Sheng Y, et al. Clinical and genetic characterization of measles viruses isolated from adult patients in Shanghai in 2006. *J Clin Virol.* October 2007;40(2):146-151.

90. Arenz S, Fischer R, Wildner M. Measles outbreak in Germany: clinical presentation and outcome of children hospitalized for measles in 2006. *Pediatr Infect Dis J.* November 2009;28(11):1030-1032.

91. Monfort L, Munoz D, Trenchs V, et al. [Measles outbreak in Barcelona. Clinical and epidemiological characteristics]. *Enferm Infecc Microbiol Clin.* February 2010;28(2):82-86.

92. Becroft DM, Osborne DR. The lungs in fatal measles infection in childhood: pathological, radiological and immunological correlations. *Histopathology.* July 1980;4(4):401-412.

93. Radoycich GE, Zuppan CW, Weeks DA, Krous HF, Langston C. Patterns of measles pneumonitis. *Pediatr Pathol.* November-December 1992;12(6):773-786.

94. Rahman SM, Eto H, Morshed SA, Itakura H. Giant cell pneumonia: light microscopy, immunohistochemical, and ultrastructural study of an autopsy case. *Ultrastruct Pathol.* November-December 1996;20(6):585-591.

95. Vargas PA, Bernardi FD, Alves VA, et al. Uncommon histopathological findings in fatal measles infection: pancreatitis, sialoadenitis and thyroiditis. *Histopathology.* August 2000;37(2):141-146.

96. Harboldt SL, Dugan JM, Tronic BS. Cytologic diagnosis of measles pneumonia in a bronchoalveolar lavage specimen. A case report. *Acta Cytol.* May-June 1994;38(3):403-406.

97. Plaza JA, Nuovo GJ. Histologic and molecular correlates of fatal measles infection in children. *Diagn Mol Pathol.* June 2005;14(2):97-102.

98. Lemon K, de Vries RD, Mesman AW, et al. Early target cells of measles virus after aerosol infection of non-human primates. *PLoS Pathog.* 2011;7(1):e1001263.

99. Sata T, Kurata T, Aoyama Y, Sakaguchi M, Yamanouchi K, Takeda K. Analysis of viral antigens in giant cells of measles pneumonia by immunoperoxidase method. *Virchows Arch A Pathol Anat Histopathol.* 1986;410(2):133-138.

100. Koh YY, Jung da E, Koh JY, Kim JY, Yoo Y, Kim CK. Bronchoalveolar cellularity and interleukin-8 levels in measles bronchiolitis obliterans. *Chest.* May 2007;131(5):1454-1460.

101. Henrickson KJ. Parainfluenza viruses. *Clin Microbiol Rev.* April 2003;16(2):242-264.

102. Schomacker H, Schaap-Nutt A, Collins PL, Schmidt AC. Pathogenesis of acute respiratory illness caused by human parainfluenza viruses. *Curr Opin Virol.* June 2012;2(3):294-299.

103. Lewis VA, Champlin R, Englund J, et al. Respiratory disease due to parainfluenza virus in adult bone marrow transplant recipients. *Clin Infect Dis.* November 1996;23(5):1033-1037.

104. Teo WY, Rajadurai VS, Sriram B. Morbidity of parainfluenza 3 outbreak in preterm infants in a neonatal unit. *Ann Acad Med Singapore.* November 2010;39(11):837-836.

105. Cunha BA, Mickail N, Schoch P. Human parainfluenza virus type 3 (HPIV 3) community-acquired pneumonia (CAP) mimicking pertussis in an adult: the diagnostic importance of hoarseness and monocytosis. *Heart Lung.* November-December 2011;40(6):569-573.

106. Rubinas TC, Carey RB, Kampert MC, Alkan S, Lednicky JA. Fatal hemorrhagic pneumonia concomitant with Chlamydia pneumoniae and parainfluenza virus 4 infection. *Arch Pathol Lab Med.* June 2004;128(6):640-644.

107. Vilchez RA, McCurry K, Dauber J, et al. The epidemiology of parainfluenza virus infection in lung transplant recipients. *Clin Infect Dis.* December 15, 2001;33(12):2004-2008.

108. Butnor KJ, Sporn TA. Human parainfluenza virus giant cell pneumonia following cord blood transplant associated with pulmonary alveolar proteinosis. *Arch Pathol Lab Med.* February 2003;127(2):235-238.

109. Pokharel S, Merickel CR, Alatassi H. Parainfluenza virus-3-induced cytopathic effects on lung tissue and bronchoalveolar lavage fluid in a bone marrow transplant recipient: a case report. *Diagn Cytopathol.* 2014;42(6):521-524.

110. Yener Z, Saglam YS, Timurkaan N, Ilhan F. Immunohistochemical detection of parainfluenza type 3 virus antigens in paraffin sections of pneumonic caprine lungs. *J Vet Med A Physiol Pathol Clin Med.* August 2005;52(6):268-271.

111. Shima T, Yoshimoto G, Nonami A, et al. Successful treatment of parainfluenza virus 3 pneumonia with oral ribavirin and methylprednisolone in a bone marrow transplant recipient. *Int J Hematol.* October 2008;88(3):336-340.

112. Allander T, Tammi MT, Eriksson M, Bjerkner A, Tiveljung-Lindell A, Andersson B. Cloning of a human parvovirus by molecular screening of respiratory tract samples. *Proc Natl Acad Sci U S A.* September 6, 2005;102(36):12891-12896.

113. Jartti T, Hedman K, Jartti L, Ruuskanen O, Allander T, Soderlund-Venermo M. Human bocavirus-the first 5 years. *Rev Med Virol.* January 2012;22(1):46-64.

114. Don M, Soderlund-Venermo M, Valent F, et al. Serologically verified human bocavirus pneumonia in children. *Pediatr Pulmonol.* February 2010;45(2):120-126.

115. van den Hoogen BG, de Jong JC, Groen J, et al. A newly discovered human pneumovirus isolated from young children with respiratory tract disease. *Nat Med.* June 2001;7(6):719-724.

116. Williams JV, Edwards KM, Weinberg GA, et al. Population-based incidence of human metapneumovirus infection among hospitalized children. *J Infect Dis.* June 15, 2010;201(12):1890-1898.

117. Walsh EE, Peterson DR, Falsey AR. Human metapneumovirus infections in adults: another piece of the puzzle. *Arch Intern Med.* December 8, 2008;168(22):2489-2496.

118. Johnstone J, Majumdar SR, Fox JD, Marrie TJ. Human metapneumovirus pneumonia in adults: results of a prospective study. *Clin Infect Dis.* February 15, 2008;46(4):571-574.

119. Peiris JS, Tang WH, Chan KH, et al. Children with respiratory disease associated with metapneumovirus in Hong Kong. *Emerg Infect Dis.* June 2003;9(6):628-633.

120. Zhang SX, Tellier R, Zafar R, Cheung R, Adachi D, Richardson SE. Comparison of human metapneumovirus infection with respiratory syncytial virus infection in children. *Pediatr Infect Dis J.* November 2009;28(11):1022-1024.

121. Souza JS, Watanabe A, Carraro E, Granato C, Bellei N. Severe metapneumovirus infections among immunocompetent and immunocompromised patients admitted to hospital with respiratory infection. *J Med Virol.* March 2013;85(3):530-536.

122. Hopkins P, McNeil K, Kermeen F, et al. Human metapneumovirus in lung transplant recipients and comparison to respiratory syncytial virus. *Am J Respir Crit Care Med.* October 15, 2008;178(8):876-881.

123. Sumino KC, Agapov E, Pierce RA, et al. Detection of severe human metapneumovirus infection by real-time polymerase chain reaction and histopathological assessment. *J Infect Dis.* September 15, 2005;192(6):1052-1060.

124. Escaffre O, Borisevich V, Rockx B. Pathogenesis of Hendra and Nipah virus infection in humans. *J Infect Dev Ctries.* April 2013;7(4):308-311.

125. Aljofan M. Hendra and Nipah infection: emerging paramyxoviruses. *Virus Res.* 2013;177(2):119-126.

126. Luby SP, Gurley ES. Epidemiology of henipavirus disease in humans. *Curr Top Microbiol Immunol.* 2012;359:25-40.

127. Drexler JF, Corman VM, Gloza-Rausch F, et al. Henipavirus RNA in African bats. *PLoS One.* 2009;4(7):e6367.

128. Wong KT, Tan CT. Clinical and pathological manifestations of human henipavirus infection. *Curr Top Microbiol Immunol.* 2012;359:95-104.

129. Viral hemorrhagic fevers. Special Pathogens Branch. June 19, 2013. http://www.cdc.gov/ncidod/dvrd/spb/mnpages/dispages/vhf.htm. Accessed 8/10/ 2013.

130. Bente DA, Forester NL, Watts DM, McAuley AJ, Whitehouse CA, Bray M. Crimean-Congo hemorrhagic fever: history, epidemiology, pathogenesis, clinical syndrome and genetic diversity. *Antiviral Res.* 2013;100(1):159-189.

131. Walker DH, McCormick JB, Johnson KM, et al. Pathologic and virologic study of fatal Lassa fever in man. *Am J Pathol.* June 1982;107(3):349-356.

132. Burt FJ, Swanepoel R, Shieh WJ, et al. Immunohistochemical and in situ localization of Crimean-Congo hemorrhagic fever (CCHF) virus in human tissues and implications for CCHF pathogenesis. *Arch Pathol Lab Med.* August 1997;121(8):839-846.

133. Arnold FW, Summersgill JT, Lajoie AS, et al. A worldwide perspective of atypical pathogens in community-acquired pneumonia. *Am J Respir Crit Care Med.* May 15, 2007;175(10):1086-1093.

134. Cunha CB. The first atypical pneumonia: the history of the discovery of Mycoplasma pneumoniae. *Infect Dis Clin North Am.* March 2010;24(1):1-5.

135. Ishiguro T, Takayanagi N, Yamaguchi S, et al. Etiology and factors contributing to the severity and mortality of community-acquired pneumonia. *Intern Med.* 2013;52(3):317-324.

136. Sorensen CM, Schonning K, Rosenfeldt V. Clinical characteristics of children with Mycoplasma pneumoniae infection hospitalized during the Danish 2010-2012 epidemic. *Dan Med J.* May 2013;60(5):A4632.

137. Centers for Disease Control and Prevention (CDC). Mycoplasma pneumoniae Outbreak at a University—Georgia, 2012. *Morb Mortal Wkly Rep.* August 2, 2013;62(30):603-606.

138. Marrie TJ, Costain N, La Scola B, et al. The role of atypical pathogens in community-acquired pneumonia. *Semin Respir Crit Care Med.* June 2012;33(3):244-256.

139. Cha SI, Shin KM, Jeon KN, et al. Clinical relevance and characteristics of pleural effusion in patients with Mycoplasma pneumoniae pneumonia. *Scand J Infect Dis.* October 2012;44(10): 793-797.

140. Wang K, Gill P, Perera R, Thomson A, Mant D, Harnden A. Clinical symptoms and signs for the diagnosis of Mycoplasma pneumoniae in children and adolescents with community-acquired pneumonia. *Cochrane Database Syst Rev.* 2012;10:CD009175.

141. Reittner P, Muller NL, Heyneman L, et al. Mycoplasma pneumoniae pneumonia: radiographic and high-resolution CT features in 28 patients. *AJR Am J Roentgenol.* January 2000;174(1):37-41.

142. Waites KB, Balish MF, Atkinson TP. New insights into the pathogenesis and detection of Mycoplasma pneumoniae infections. *Future Microbiol.* December 2008;3(6):635-648.

143. Liang H, Jiang W, Han Q, Liu F, Zhao D. Ciliary ultrastructural abnormalities in Mycoplasma pneumoniae pneumonia in 22 pediatric patients. *Eur J Pediatr.* March 2012;171(3):559-563.

144. Rollins S, Colby T, Clayton F. Open lung biopsy in Mycoplasma pneumoniae pneumonia. *Arch Pathol Lab Med.* January 1986;110(1):34-41.

145. Chang HY, Chang LY, Shao PL, et al. Comparison of real-time polymerase chain reaction and serological tests for the confirmation of Mycoplasma pneumoniae infection in children with clinical diagnosis of atypical pneumonia. *J Microbiol Immunol Infect.* 2014;47(2):137-144.

146. Qu J, Gu L, Wu J, et al. Accuracy of IgM antibody testing, FQ-PCR and culture in laboratory diagnosis of acute infection by Mycoplasma pneumoniae in adults and adolescents with community-acquired pneumonia. *BMC Infect Dis.* April 11, 2013;13(1):172.

147. Pinna GS, Skevaki CL, Kafetzis DA. The significance of Ureaplasma urealyticum as a pathogenic agent in the paediatric population. *Curr Opin Infect Dis.* June 2006;19(3):283-289.

148. Garland SM, Bowman ED. Role of Ureaplasma urealyticum and Chlamydia trachomatis in lung disease in low birth weight infants. *Pathology.* August 1996;28(3):266-269.

149. Hammerschlag MR. The intracellular life of chlamydiae. *Semin Pediatr Infect Dis.* October 2002;13(4):239-248.

150. Capelastegui A, Espana PP, Bilbao A, et al. Etiology of community-acquired pneumonia in a population-based study: link between etiology and patients characteristics, process-of-care, clinical evolution and outcomes. *BMC Infect Dis.* 2012;12:134.

151. Marrie TJ, Peeling RW, Reid T, De Carolis E. Chlamydia species as a cause of community-acquired pneumonia in Canada. *Eur Respir J.* May 2003;21(5):779-784.

152. Choroszy-Krol I, Frej-Madrzak M, Jama-Kmiecik A, Sarowska J, Gosciniak G, Pirogowicz I. Incidence of chlamydophila pneumoniae infection in children during 2007-2010. *Adv Exp Med Biol.* 2013;788:83-87.

153. Imokawa S, Yasuda K, Uchiyama H, et al. Chlamydial infection showing migratory pulmonary infiltrates. *Intern Med.* 2007;46(20):1735-1738.

154. Kaukoranta-Tolvanen SE, Laurila AL, Saikku P, Leinonen M, Laitinen K. Experimental Chlamydia pneumoniae infection in mice: effect of reinfection and passive immunization. *Microb Pathog.* April 1995;18(4):279-288.

155. Yang ZP, Cummings PK, Patton DL, Kuo CC. Ultrastructural lung pathology of experimental Chlamydia pneumoniae pneumonitis in mice. *J Infect Dis.* August 1994;170(2):464-467.

156. Fong IW, Chiu B, Viira E, Fong MW, Jang D, Mahony J. Rabbit model for Chlamydia pneumoniae infection. *J Clin Microbiol.* January 1997;35(1):48-52.

157. Welti M, Jaton K, Altwegg M, Sahli R, Wenger A, Bille J. Development of a multiplex real-time quantitative PCR assay to detect Chlamydia pneumoniae, Legionella pneumophila and Mycoplasma pneumoniae in respiratory tract secretions. *Diagn Microbiol Infect Dis.* February 2003;45(2):85-95.

158. FDA expands use for FilmArray Respiratory Panel. May 15, 2012. http://www.fda.gov/NewsEvents/Newsroom/PressAnnouncements/ucm304177.htm. Accessed August 17, 2013.

159. Stewart S. Pulmonary infections in transplantation pathology. *Arch Pathol Lab Med.* August 2007;131(8):1219-1231.

160. Rupp J, Pfleiderer L, Jugert C, et al. Chlamydia pneumoniae hides inside apoptotic neutrophils to silently infect and propagate in macrophages. *PLoS One.* 2009;4(6):e6020.

161. Kuo CC, Shor A, Campbell LA, Fukushi H, Patton DL, Grayston JT. Demonstration of Chlamydia pneumoniae in atherosclerotic lesions of coronary arteries. *J Infect Dis.* April 1993;167(4):841-849.

162. Myers GS, Mathews SA, Eppinger M, et al. Evidence that human Chlamydia pneumoniae was zoonotically acquired. *J Bacteriol.* December 2009;191(23):7225-7233.

163. Mishori R, McClaskey EL, WinklerPrins VJ. Chlamydia trachomatis infections: screening, diagnosis, and management. *Am Fam Physician.* December 15, 2012;86(12):1127-1132.

164. Darville T. Chlamydia trachomatis infections in neonates and young children. *Semin Pediatr Infect Dis.* October 2005;16(4):235-244.

165. Ito JI Jr, Comess KA, Alexander ER, et al. Pneumonia due to chlamydia trachomatis in an immunocompromised adult. *N Engl J Med.* July 8, 1982;307(2):95-98.

166. Tipple MA, Beem MO, Saxon EM. Clinical characteristics of the afebrile pneumonia associated with Chlamydia trachomatis infection in infants less than 6 months of age. *Pediatrics.* February 1979;63(2):192-197.

167. Edelman RR, Hann LE, Simon M. Chlamydia trachomatis pneumonia in adults: radiographic appearance. *Radiology.* August 1984;152(2):279-282.

168. Harrison HR, Alexander ER, Chiang WT, et al. Experimental nasopharyngitis and pneumonia caused by Chlamydia trachomatis in infant baboons: histopathologic comparison with a case in a human infant. *J Infect Dis.* February 1979;139(2):141-146.

169. Chen W, Kuo C. A mouse model of pneumonitis induced by Chlamydia trachomatis. morphologic, microbiologic, and immunologic studies. *Am J Pathol.* August 1980;100(2): 365-382.

170. She RC, Welch R, Wilson AR, Davis D, Litwin CM. Correlation of Chlamydia and Chlamydophila spp. IgG and IgM antibodies by microimmunofluorescence with antigen detection methods. *J Clin Lab Anal.* 2011;25(4):305-308.

171. Pospischil A. From disease to etiology: historical aspects of Chlamydia-related diseases in animals and humans. *Drugs Today (Barc).* November 2009;45(suppl B):141-146.

172. Smith KA, Campbell CT, Murphy J, Stobierski MG, Tengelsen LA. Compendium of measures to control Chlamydophila psittaci infection among humans (psittacosis) and pet birds (avian Chlamydiosis), 2010. www.nasphv.org/Documents/Psittacosis. Accessed 9/22/2013.

173. Case Records of the Massachusetts General Hospital. Weekly clinicopathologic exercises. Case 16-1998. Pneumonia and the acute respiratory distress syndrome in a 24-year-old man. *N Engl J Med.* May 21, 1998;338(21):1527-1535.

174. McPhee SJ, Erb B, Harrington W. Psittacosis. *West J Med.* January 1987;146(1):91-96.

175. Petrovay F, Balla E. Two fatal cases of psittacosis caused by Chlamydophila psittaci. *J Med Microbiol.* October 2008;57(pt 10):1296-1298.

176. Case Records of the Massachusetts General Hospital. Weekly clinicopathologic exercises. Case 48-1990. A 65-year-old man with pulmonary infiltrates after treatment for Wegener's granulomatosis. *N Engl J Med.* November 29, 1990;323(22): 1546-1555.

177. Reinhold P, Ostermann C, Liebler-Tenorio E, et al. A bovine model of respiratory Chlamydia psittaci infection: challenge dose titration. *PLoS One.* 2012;7(1):e30125.

178. Mitchell SL, Wolff BJ, Thacker WL, et al. Genotyping of Chlamydophila psittaci by real-time PCR and high-resolution melt analysis. *J Clin Microbiol.* January 2009;47(1):175-181.

179. Walker DH. Ricketts creates rickettsiology, the study of vector-borne obligately intracellular bacteria. *J Infect Dis.* March 1, 2004;189(5):938-955.

180. Walker DH. Rickettsiae and rickettsial infections: the current state of knowledge. *Clin Infect Dis.* July 15, 2007;45(suppl 1): S39-S44.

181. Rocky Mountain Spotted Fever (RMSF). September 5, 2013. http://www.cdc.gov/rmsf/stats/index.html. Accessed August 20, 2013.

182. Jeong YJ, Kim S, Wook YD, Lee JW, Kim KI, Lee SH. Scrub typhus: clinical, pathologic, and imaging findings. *Radiographics.* January-February 2007;27(1):161-172.

183. Premaratna R, Loftis AD, Chandrasena TG, Dasch GA, de Silva HJ. Rickettsial infections and their clinical presentations in the Western Province of Sri Lanka: a hospital-based study. *Int J Infect Dis.* March 2008;12(2):198-202.

184. Walker DH, Crawford CG, Cain BG. Rickettsial infection of the pulmonary microcirculation: the basis for interstitial pneumonitis in Rocky Mountain spotted fever. *Hum Pathol.* May 1980;11(3):263-272.

185. Walker DH. Mycoplasmal, chlamydial, rickettsial, and ehrlichial pneumonias. In: Tomashefski JFJ, Cagle PT, Farver CF, Fraire AE, eds. *Dail and Hammar's Pulmonary Pathology.* Vol I. 3rd ed. New York, NY: Springer; 2008:476-486.

186. Moron CG, Popov VL, Feng HM, Wear D, Walker DH. Identification of the target cells of Orientia tsutsugamushi in human cases of scrub typhus. *Mod Pathol.* August 2001;14(8):752-759.

187. Eremeeva ME, Dasch GA, Silverman DJ. Evaluation of a PCR assay for quantitation of Rickettsia rickettsii and closely related spotted fever group rickettsiae. *J Clin Microbiol.* December 2003;41(12):5466-5472.

188. Stenos J, Graves SR, Unsworth NB. A highly sensitive and specific real-time PCR assay for the detection of spotted fever and typhus group Rickettsiae. *Am J Trop Med Hyg.* December 2005;73(6):1083-1085.

189. Rikihisa Y. Anaplasma phagocytophilum and Ehrlichia chaffeensis: subversive manipulators of host cells. *Nat Rev Microbiol.* May 2010;8(5):328-339.

190. Dumler JS, Madigan JE, Pusterla N, Bakken JS. Ehrlichioses in humans: epidemiology, clinical presentation, diagnosis, and treatment. *Clin Infect Dis.* July 15, 2007;45(suppl 1):S45-S51.

191. Schutze GE, Buckingham SC, Marshall GS, et al. Human monocytic ehrlichiosis in children. *Pediatr Infect Dis J.* June 2007;26(6):475-479.

192. Dumler JS. Anaplasma and Ehrlichia infection. *Ann N Y Acad Sci.* December 2005;1063:361-373.

193. Case Records of the Massachusetts General Hospital. Weekly clinicopathological exercises. Case 37-2001. A 76-year-old man with fever, dyspnea, pulmonary infiltrates, pleural effusions, and confusion. *N Engl J Med.* November 29, 2001;345(22):1627-1634.

194. Ismail N, Bloch KC, McBride JW. Human ehrlichiosis and anaplasmosis. *Clin Lab Med.* March 2010;30(1):261-292.

195. Marrie TJ. Q fever pneumonia. *Infect Dis Clin North Am.* March 2010;24(1):27-41.

196. Anderson A, Bijlmer H, Fournier PE, et al. Diagnosis and management of Q fever—United States, 2013: recommendations from CDC and the Q Fever Working Group. *MMWR Recomm Rep.* March 29, 2013;62(RR-03):1-30.

197. Urso FP. The pathologic findings in rickettsial pneumonia. *Am J Clin Pathol.* September 1975;64(3):335-342.

198. Khavkin T, Tabibzadeh SS. Histologic, immunofluorescence, and electron microscopic study of infectious process in mouse lung after intranasal challenge with Coxiella burnetii. *Infect Immun.* July 1988;56(7):1792-1799.

199. Russell-Lodrigue KE, Zhang GQ, McMurray DN, Samuel JE. Clinical and pathologic changes in a guinea pig aerosol challenge model of acute Q fever. *Infect Immun.* November 2006;74(11):6085-6091.

200. Roberts LS, Janovy JJ. *Gerald D. Schmidt and Larry S. Roberts' Foundations of Parasitology.* 6th ed. Boston, MA: McGraw Hill; 2000.

201. Rogers WO. Plasmodium and Babesia. In: Murray PR, Baron EJ, Jorgensen JH, Pfaller MA, Yolken RH, eds. *Manual of Clinical Microbiology.* 8th ed. Washington, DC: ASM Press; 2003:1944-1959.

202. Winn WJ, Allen S, Janda W, et al. *Koneman's Color Atlas and Textbook of Diagnostic Microbiology.* 6th ed. Philadelphia, PA: Lippincott Williams and Wilkins; 2006.

203. Vijayan VK, Kilani T. Emerging and established parasitic lung infestations. *Infect Dis Clin North Am.* September 2010;24(3):579-602.

204. Taylor WR, Hanson J, Turner GD, White NJ, Dondorp AM. Respiratory manifestations of malaria. *Chest.* August 2012;142(2):492-505.

205. Anstey NM, Jacups SP, Cain T, et al. Pulmonary manifestations of uncomplicated falciparum and vivax malaria: cough, small airways obstruction, impaired gas transfer, and increased pulmonary phagocytic activity. *J Infect Dis.* May 1, 2002;185(9): 1326-1334.

206. Tan LK, Yacoub S, Scott S, Bhagani S, Jacobs M. Acute lung injury and other serious complications of Plasmodium vivax malaria. *Lancet Infect Dis.* July 2008;8(7):449-454.

207. Menezes RG, Kanchan T, Rai S, et al. An autopsy case of sudden unexplained death caused by malaria. *J Forensic Sci.* May 2010;55(3):835-838.

208. Taylor WR, Canon V, White NJ. Pulmonary manifestations of malaria: recognition and management. *Treat Respir Med.* 2006;5(6):419-428.

209. Valecha N, Pinto RG, Turner GD, et al. Histopathology of fatal respiratory distress caused by Plasmodium vivax malaria. *Am J Trop Med Hyg.* November 2009;81(5):758-762.

210. Lacerda MV, Fragoso SC, Alecrim MG, et al. Postmortem characterization of patients with clinical diagnosis of Plasmodium vivax malaria: to what extent does this parasite kill? *Clin Infect Dis.* October 2012;55(8):e67-e74.

211. Vasoo S, Pritt BS. Molecular diagnostics and parasitic disease. *Clin Lab Med.* September 2013;33(3):461-503.

212. Orihel TC, Ash LR. Tissue helminths. In: Murray PR, Baron EJ, Jorgensen JH, Pfaller MA, Yolken RH, ed. *Manual of Clinical Microbiology.* 8th ed. Washington, DC: ASM Press; 2003:2047-2060.

213. Araya J, Kawabata Y, Tomichi N, et al. Allergic inflammatory reaction is involved in necrosis of human pulmonary dirofilariasis. *Histopathology.* October 2007;51(4):484-490.

214. Kuzucu A. Parasitic diseases of the respiratory tract. *Curr Opin Pulm Med.* May 2006;12(3):212-221.

215. Kunst H, Mack D, Kon OM, Banerjee AK, Chiodini P, Grant A. Parasitic infections of the lung: a guide for the respiratory physician. *Thorax.* June 2011;66(6):528-536.

216. Oshiro Y, Murayama S, Sunagawa U, et al. Pulmonary dirofilariasis: computed tomography findings and correlation with pathologic features. *J Comput Assist Tomogr.* November-December 2004;28(6):796-800.

217. Foroulis CN, Khaldi L, Desimonas N, Kalafati G. Pulmonary dirofilariasis mimicking lung tumor with chest wall and mediastinal invasion. *Thorac Cardiovasc Surg.* June 2005;53(3): 173-175.

218. Mulanovich EA, Mulanovich VE, Rolston KV. A case of Dirofilaria pulmonary infection coexisting with lung cancer. *J Infect*. April 2008;56(4):241-243.

219. Procop GW, Marty AM. Parasitic infections. In: Tomashefski JFJ, Cagle PT, Farver CF, Fraire AE, eds. *Dail and Hammar's Pulmonary Pathology*. 3rd ed. New York, NY: Springer; 2008:515-560.

220. Carter JE, Whithaus KC. Neonatal respiratory tract involvement by Trichomonas vaginalis: a case report and review of the literature. *Am J Trop Med Hyg*. January 2008;78(1):17-19.

221. Duboucher C, Noel C, Durand-Joly I, et al. Pulmonary coinfection by Trichomonas vaginalis and Pneumocystis sp. as a novel manifestation of AIDS. *Hum Pathol*. May 2003;34(5):508-511.

222. Duboucher C, Barbier C, Beltramini A, et al. Pulmonary superinfection by trichomonads in the course of acute respiratory distress syndrome. *Lung*. September-October 2007;185(5):295-301.

223. Duboucher C, Caby S, Pierce RJ, Capron M, Dei-Cas E, Viscogliosi E. Trichomonads as superinfecting agents in Pneumocystis pneumonia and acute respiratory distress syndrome. *J Eukaryot Microbiol*. 2006;53(suppl 1):S95-S97.

224. Leterrier M, Morio F, Renard BT, Poirier AS, Miegeville M, Chambreuil G. Trichomonads in pleural effusion: case report, literature review and utility of PCR for species identification. *New Microbiol*. January 2012;35(1):83-87.

225. Wang HK, Jerng JS, Su KE, Chang SC, Yang PC. Trichomonas empyema with respiratory failure. *Am J Trop Med Hyg*. December 2006;75(6):1234-1236.

226. Bruckner DA, Labarca JA. Leishmania and Trypanosoma. In: Murray PR, Baron EJ, Jorgensen JH, Pfaller MA, Yolken RH, eds. *Manual of Clinical Microbiology*. 8th ed. Washington, DC: ASM Press; 2003:1960-1969.

227. Camara EJ, Lima JA, Oliveira GB, Machado AS. Pulmonary findings in patients with chagasic megaesophagus. Study of autopsied cases. *Chest*. January 1983;83(1):87-91.

228. Murcia L, Carrilero B, Munoz-Davila MJ, Thomas MC, Lopez MC, Segovia M. Risk factors and primary prevention of congenital Chagas disease in a nonendemic country. *Clin Infect Dis*. February 2013;56(4):496-502.

229. Martinez-Giron R, Esteban JG, Ribas A, Doganci L. Protozoa in respiratory pathology: a review. *Eur Respir J*. November 2008;32(5):1354-1370.

230. Bittencourt AL, Rodrigues de Freitas LA, Galvao de Araujo MO, Jacomo K. Pneumonitis in congenital Chagas' disease. A study of ten cases. *Am J Trop Med Hyg*. January 1981;30(1):38-42.

231. Chitkara RK, Krishna G. Parasitic pulmonary eosinophilia. *Semin Respir Crit Care Med*. April 2006;27(2):171-184.

232. Akuthota P, Weller PF. Eosinophilic pneumonias. *Clin Microbiol Rev*. October 2012;25(4):649-660.

233. Ash LR, Orihel TC. Intestinal Helminths. In: Murray PR, Baron EJ, Jorgensen JH, Pfaller MA, Yolken RH, eds. *Manual of Clinical Microbiology*. 8th ed. Washington, DC: ASM Press; 2003:2031-2046.

234. Shamsuzzaman SM, Hashiguchi Y. Thoracic amebiasis. *Clin Chest Med*. June 2002;23(2):479-492.

235. Shrestha M, Shah A, Lettieri C. Dyspnea and dysentery: a case report of pleuropulmonary amebiasis. *South Med J*. February 2010;103(2):165-168.

236. Lichtenstein A, Kondo AT, Visvesvara GS, et al. Pulmonary amoebiasis presenting as superior vena cava syndrome. *Thorax*. April 2005;60(4):350-352.

237. Yapar AF, Reyhan M, Canpolat ET. Interesting image. Ameboma mimicking lung cancer on FDG PET/CT. *Clin Nucl Med*. January 2010;35(1):55-56.

238. Leber AL, Novak SM. Intestinal and urogenital Amebae, Flagellates, and Ciliates. In: Murray PR, Baron EJ, Jorgensen JH, Pfaller MA, Yolken RH, eds. *Manual of Clinical Microbiology*. 8th ed. Washington, DC: ASM Press; 2003:1990-2007.

239. Woodring JH, Halfhill H 2nd, Berger R, Reed JC, Moser N. Clinical and imaging features of pulmonary strongyloidiasis. *South Med J*. January 1996;89(1):10-19.

240. Woodring JH, Halfhill H 2nd, Reed JC. Pulmonary strongyloidiasis: clinical and imaging features. *AJR Am J Roentgenol*. March 1994;162(3):537-542.

241. Adedayo O, Grell G, Bellot P. Hyperinfective strongyloidiasis in the medical ward: review of 27 cases in 5 years. *South Med J*. July 2002;95(7):711-716.

242. Siddiqui AA, Berk SL. Diagnosis of Strongyloides stercoralis infection. *Clin Infect Dis*. October 1, 2001;33(7):1040-1047.

243. Genta RM. Dysregulation of strongyloidiasis: a new hypothesis. *Clin Microbiol Rev*. October 1992;5(4):345-355.

244. Lin AL, Kessimian N, Benditt JO. Restrictive pulmonary disease due to interlobular septal fibrosis associated with disseminated infection by Strongyloides stercoralis. *Am J Respir Crit Care Med*. January 1995;151(1):205-209.

245. Apewokin S, Stecluk M, Griffin S, Jhala D. Strongyloides hyperinfection diagnosed by bronchoalveolar lavage in an immunocompromised host. *Cytopathology*. October 2010;21(5):345-347.

246. Albuquerque YM, Silva MC, Lima AL, Magalhaes V. Pulmonary cryptosporidiosis in AIDS patients, an underdiagnosed disease. *J Bras Pneumol*. July-August 2012;38(4):530-532.

247. Collinet-Adler S, Ward HD. Cryptosporidiosis: environmental, therapeutic, and preventive challenges. *Eur J Clin Microbiol Infect Dis*. August 2010;29(8):927-935.

248. Mor SM, Tumwine JK, Ndeezi G, et al. Respiratory cryptosporidiosis in HIV-seronegative children in Uganda: potential for respiratory transmission. *Clin Infect Dis*. May 15, 2010;50(10):1366-1372.

249. Vijayan VK. Parasitic lung infections. *Curr Opin Pulm Med*. May 2009;15(3):274-282.

250. Fritsche TR, Selvarangan R. Medical parasitology. In: McPherson RA, Pincus MR, eds. *Henry's Clinical Diagnosis and Management by Laboratory Methods*. 21st ed. Philadelphia, PA: Saunders Elsevier; 2007:1119-1168.

251. Dupont C, Bougnoux ME, Turner L, Rouveix E, Dorra M. Microbiological findings about pulmonary cryptosporidiosis in two AIDS patients. *J Clin Microbiol*. January 1996;34(1):227-229.

252. Mary C, Chapey E, Dutoit E, et al. Multicentric evaluation of a new real-time PCR assay for quantification of Cryptosporidium spp. and identification of Cryptosporidium parvum and Cryptosporidium hominis. *J Clin Microbiol*. August 2013;51(8):2556-2563.

253. Lalosevic D, Lalosevic V, Klem I, Stanojev-Jovanovic D, Pozio E. Pulmonary capillariasis miming bronchial carcinoma. *Am J Trop Med Hyg*. January 2008;78(1):14-16.

254. Traversa D, Di Cesare A, Lia RP, et al. New insights into morphological and biological features of Capillaria aerophila (Trichocephalida, Trichuridae). *Parasitol Res*. August 2011;109(suppl 1):S97-S104.

255. Di Cesare A, Castagna G, Otranto D, et al. Molecular detection of Capillaria aerophila, an agent of canine and feline pulmonary capillariosis. *J Clin Microbiol*. June 2012;50(6):1958-1963.

256. Vijayan VK. Tropical pulmonary eosinophilia: pathogenesis, diagnosis and management. *Curr Opin Pulm Med*. September 2007;13(5):428-433.

257. Ottesen EA, Nutman TB. Tropical pulmonary eosinophilia. *Annu Rev Med*. 1992;43:417-424.

258. Ray D, Harikrishna S, Immanuel C, Victor L, Subramanyam S, Kumaraswami V. Acquired alpha 1-antitrypsin deficiency in tropical pulmonary eosinophilia. *Indian J Med Res*. July 2011;134:79-82.

259. Boggild AK, Keystone JS, Kain KC. Tropical pulmonary eosinophilia: a case series in a setting of nonendemicity. *Clin Infect Dis*. October 15, 2004;39(8):1123-1128.

CHAPTER 14

260. Ray S, Kundu S, Goswami M, Maitra S. Tropical pulmonary eosinophilia misdiagnosed as miliary tuberculosis: a case report and literature review. *Parasitol Int*. June 2012;61(2): 381-384.

261. Steel C, Golden A, Kubofcik J, et al. Rapid Wuchereria bancrofti-specific antigen Wb123-based IgG4 immunoassays as tools for surveillance following mass drug administration programs on lymphatic filariasis. *Clin Vaccine Immunol*. August 2013;20(8):1155-1161.

262. Marshall BG, Wilkinson RJ, Davidson RN. Pathogenesis of tropical pulmonary eosinophilia: parasitic alveolitis and parallels with asthma. *Respir Med*. January 1998;92(1):1-3.

15 Pulmonary Hypertension, Emboli, and Other Vascular Diseases

Abida K. Haque and Alexander G. Duarte

TAKE HOME PEARLS

- Pulmonary arterial hypertension (PAH) is a progressive pulmonary vascular disease that leads to right ventricular failure and early death.
- PAH encompasses a group of conditions including idiopathic and hereditary pulmonary hypertension, and pulmonary hypertension associated with connective tissue disorders, congenital heart disease, portal hypertension, HIV infection, medications, and illicit drugs.
- Idiopathic PAH represents pulmonary hypertension in which neither a recognizable cause nor a family history can be identified. The term idiopathic PAH identifies the anatomical location of the vascular disease state to the arterial or precapillary pulmonary vascular bed, and has replaced the term primary pulmonary hypertension.
- Demographic and clinical information from various patient registries regarding heritable PAH indicates that the clinical and pathological features between sporadic and heritable forms of PAH are indistinguishable.
- PAH associated with connective tissue disorder is identified most frequently in patients with systemic sclerosis, particularly in patients with limited cutaneous systemic sclerosis.
- Patients with systemic to pulmonary shunts (left to right) are likely to develop PAH.

- Medial proliferation is the most common lesion in pulmonary hypertension.
- Plexiform lesions are most commonly seen in primary pulmonary hypertension, portopulmonary hypertension, and congenital cardiac left to right shunt.
- Pulmonary veno-occlusive disease is a rare condition that accounts for a small number of cases of pulmonary hypertension.
- Pulmonary capillary hemangiomatosis (PCH) is considered a subgroup of PAH.
- Pulmonary hypertension secondary to left ventricular dysfunction or valvular heart disease is more common than pulmonary arterial hypertension.
- Pulmonary hypertension owing to lung diseases and/or hypoxia includes chronic obstructive pulmonary disease, interstitial lung disease, sleep disordered breathing, alveolar hypoventilation disorders, residence at high altitude, and developmental abnormalities.
- Chronic thromboembolic pulmonary hypertension (CTEPH) is characterized by single or multiple pulmonary thromboemboli that organize to obstruct the pulmonary vascular bed.
- Although the majority of pulmonary emboli originate in the deep veins of the lower extremities, they can also originate from renal, pelvic, ovarian, upper extremity, or right heart chambers.
- Clinical conditions that predispose to pulmonary embolism include immobilization, surgery and

trauma, pregnancy, oral contraceptives and estrogen replacement therapy, malignancy, hypercoagulable states, and HIV infection.

- Tumor emboli in pulmonary vasculature are commonly seen from primary carcinomas of breast, lung, liver, stomach, pancreas, and prostate.
- Pulmonary infarcts occur in a setting of pulmonary embolism, in a background of preexisting pulmonary or cardiac disease with a low flow state, and more often in the lower lobes.
- A healed infarct manifests as a fibroelastic scar.

PULMONARY HYPERTENSION

Definition

Pulmonary arterial hypertension (PAH) is a progressive pulmonary vascular disease that leads to right ventricular failure and early death. PAH is defined by a mean pulmonary artery pressure ≥25 mm Hg and a pulmonary capillary wedge pressure <15 mm Hg. PAH encompasses a group of conditions including idiopathic and hereditary pulmonary hypertension, and pulmonary hypertension associated with connective tissue disorders, congenital heart disease, portal hypertension, HIV infection, medications, and illicit drugs.

Clinical Classification of Pulmonary Hypertension

The classification of PAH was first attempted in 1973, and has since gone through several changes.[1-4] During the fourth World Symposium on Pulmonary Hypertension (PH) held in 2008 in Dana Point, California, it was decided to update the Evian-Venice classification (*Table 15-1*), and to classify pulmonary hypertension into five categories.[5] There are important critical implications for treatment in this classification. Although there are many similar features, there are some histologic features that are characteristic of different clinical groups. Cardiac catheterization and imaging of cardiopulmonary structures, including heart, and lung parenchyma and pulmonary vasculature are critical in diagnosing a patient with a particular form of pulmonary hypertension.

Pulmonary arterial hypertension (PAH)

This group is diverse, with the unifying feature being the hemodynamic profile (mean pulmonary artery pressure ≥25 mm Hg and a pulmonary capillary wedge pressure <15 mm Hg), and closely similar histologic findings. The chest radiograph shows enlarged cardiac silhouette and enlarged pulmonary arteries (*Figure 15-1*). Chest CT may show aneurysmal dilatation of the

Table 15-1 Updated Clinical Classification of Pulmonary Hypertension (Dana Point, 2008)

1. Pulmonary Arterial Hypertension (PAH)
   1.1. Idiopathic PAH
   1.2. Heritable; *BMPR2*, Alk 1, endoglin (with or without hereditary hemorrhagic telangiectasia)
   1.3. Drugs and toxins induced
   1.4. Associated with
       1.4.1. Connective tissue diseases
       1.4.2. HIV infection
       1.4.3. Portal hypertension
       1.4.4. Congenital heart disease
       1.4.5. Schistosomiasis
       1.4.6. Chronic hemolytic anemia
   1.5. Persistent pulmonary hypertension of the newborn
   1.6. Pulmonary veno-occlusive disease (PVOD) and/or pulmonary capillary hemangiomatosis (PCH)
2. Pulmonary hypertension due to left heart disease
   2.1. Systolic dysfunction
   2.2. Diastolic dysfunction
   2.3. Valvular disease
3. Pulmonary hypertension due to lung disease and/or hypoxia
   3.1. Chronic obstructive pulmonary disease
   3.2. Interstitial lung disease
   3.3. Other pulmonary diseases with mixed restrictive and obstructive pattern
   3.4. Sleep-disordered breathing
   3.5. Alveolar hypoventilation disorders
   3.6. Chronic exposure to high altitude
   3.7. Developmental abnormalities
4. Chronic thromboembolic pulmonary hypertension (CTEPH)
5. Pulmonary hypertension with unclear multifactorial mechanisms
   5.1. Hematologic disorders: myeloproliferative disorders, splenectomy
   5.2. Systemic disorders: Sarcoidosis, pulmonary Langerhans cell histiocytosis, lymphangioleiomyomatosis, neurofibromatosis, vasculitis
   5.3. Metabolic disorders: glycogen storage disorders, Gaucher disease, thyroid disorders
   5.4. Others: tumoral obstruction, fibrosing mediastinitis, chronic renal failure on dialysis

Source: Simonneau G, Galie N, Rubin LJ, et al. Clinical classification of pulmonary hypertension. *J Am Coll Cardiol*. 2004;43(12 suppl S): 5S-12S.

pulmonary artery, enlarged cardiac chambers, particularly an enlarged right ventricle, and pericardial effusion (*Figures 15-2* to *15-4*). An echocardiogram reveals enlarged right atrium and ventricle, with bowing of the septum towards the left ventricle (*Figures 15-5* and *15-6*). A diagnosis of PAH is largely based on exclusion of the other categories of pulmonary hypertension using clinical history, hemodynamics, and cardiopulmonary imaging techniques.

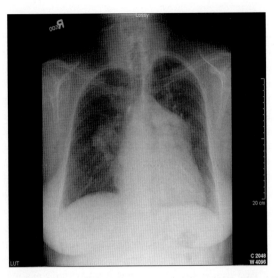

FIGURE 15-1 Chest radiograph of a patient with idiopathic pulmonary arterial hypertension demonstrating enlarged cardiac silhouette and bilaterally enlarged pulmonary arteries.

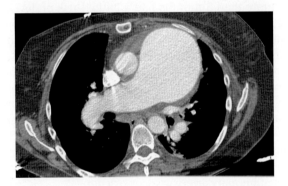

FIGURE 15-2 Chest CT of a female patient with idiopathic pulmonary arterial hypertension. Aneurysmal dilatation of the left pulmonary artery is noted when compared with ascending aorta.

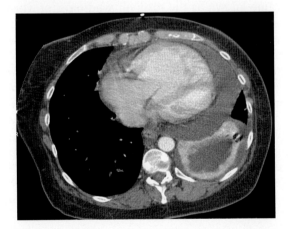

FIGURE 15-3 Chest CT revealing enlarged cardiac chambers with a dilated right ventricle and a pericardial effusion. A line traverses the right ventricle that is twice as long as the line traversing the left ventricle, indicating significant right ventricular dilation. Under normal circumstances, the ratio of RV to LV diameter is less than 1.

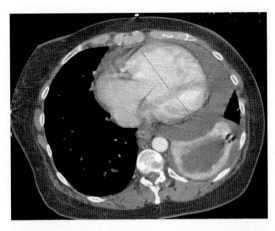

FIGURE 15-4 Chest CT revealing enlarged cardiac chambers with a dilated right ventricle and a pericardial effusion.

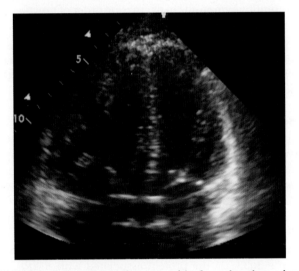

FIGURE 15-5 Echocardiogram with four-chamber view revealing enlargement of right ventricle with bowing of the septum towards the left ventricle.

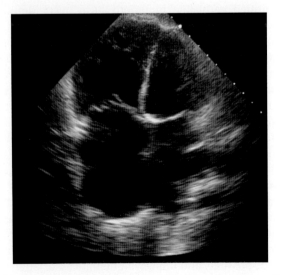

FIGURE 15-6 Echocardiogram with four-chamber view demonstrating enlargement of right ventricle and dilatation of right atrium.

CHAPTER 15

Idiopathic PAH

Idiopathic PAH represents pulmonary hypertension in which neither a recognizable cause nor a family history can be identified. The term idiopathic PAH identifies the anatomical location of the vascular disease state to the arterial or precapillary pulmonary vascular bed, and has replaced the term primary pulmonary hypertension.[3] Individuals with idiopathic PAH usually do not have an identified first-degree family member with the condition, therefore the term "sporadic" disease has been also applied to this group. Idiopathic PAH is a rare disease, with a reported incidence of 1 to 3 per million and prevalence of 6 to 12 per million.[6,7] While not well understood, women are affected two to three times more often than men.[6,8] The mean age at diagnosis, based on two large registries is 53 years.[6,9] Common presenting symptoms in decreasing order of prevalence are dyspnea, fatigue, chest pain, syncope, and lower extremity edema.[9] However, due to the nonspecific nature of these symptoms, diagnosis is often delayed, with the time of initial symptom to diagnosis by right heart catheterization being more than 2 years.

Heritable PAH

This category includes *BMPR2*, ALK 1, endoglin related (with or without hereditary hemorrhagic telangiectasia), and unknown cases. That PAH is inherited has been recognized for decades, as initially reported by Dresdale.[10] Genetic studies of familial cases of PAH have been identified in 6% of individuals.[11] A genetic link has been identified with idiopathic PAH and bone morphogenetic protein (*BMPR2*) located on chromosome 2q33.[12,13] The protein associated with *BMPR2* is a member of the transforming growth factor β (TGF β) family.[14] Subsequently, germ-line mutations in *BMPR2* gene have been reported in 80% of patients.[11] Other identified germ-line mutations have been identified in caveolin, SMAD protein and potassium channel.[15-17] Consequently, to account for individuals without a recognized family member with PAH but with a genetic marker, the term "familial PAH" has been changed to "heritable PAH." Demographic and clinical information from various patient registries regarding heritable PAH indicates that the clinical and pathological features between sporadic and heritable forms of PAH are indistinguishable.

Drug- and toxin-induced PAH

Risk factors associated with development of PAH include prescribed and illicit drugs. The strength of association for a given agent has been determined through consensus and classified into four categories: definite, likely, possible, and unlikely. A definite association was based on epidemiologic studies indicating a link between the drug and development of PAH. A "likely" association arises from single center case-control study or multiple case series. A "possible" association indicates agents that have not been studied but have a similar mechanism of action as the previous categories. Lastly, the "unlikely" category refers to agents that have been proposed but an association has not been established through use of epidemiologic studies. Two epidemics of pulmonary hypertension were recorded through epidemiologic studies that associated the use of medically prescribed anorexigens and the development of PAH. The initial description of drug-induced PAH occurred in the late 1960s, with a 20-fold rise of pulmonary hypertension in Switzerland, Austria, and West Germany.[18] More than 500 cases were documented and approximately 2% of patients taking Aminorex developed pulmonary hypertension.[19] Following the ban of Aminorex, the number of cases of PAH declined. Fenfluramine and dexfenfluramine were two medically prescribed anorexigens associated with PAH as early as 1981.[20-22] Subsequently, an international prospective case control study reported that obese individuals who had used these anorexic medications for more than 3 months had a 30-fold risk of developing PAH.[23] Compared to idiopathic PAH, patients with fenfluramine-induced PAH demonstrated similar symptoms, hemodynamic profile, pathologic findings, and outcomes.[24,25] Notably, after being banned, the number of new cases of PAH declined. Although, the mechanism for development of PAH with anorexigens is unknown, investigators have proposed that fenfluramine increased serum serotonin, an inducer of smooth muscle proliferation and vasoconstriction, via platelet release that produced pulmonary vascular smooth muscle proliferation and pulmonary artery vasoconstriction.[26,27]

In 1981, following intake of rapeseed cooking oil, a large number of individuals developed a syndrome of noncardiogenic pulmonary edema, myalgias, scleroderma, and pulmonary hypertension.[28] This disorder became known as the toxic oil syndrome, of which a group of patients developed progressive, fatal pulmonary hypertension. Clinicopathological features were similar to those observed in patients with PAH.[29] The etiology of this outbreak was associated with the sale of contaminated bulk cooking oil, and once removed from the market place, the incidence of this disorder declined. Another group of agents associated with development of PAH are the stimulants such as cocaine, amphetamines, and methamphetamines. A retrospective study of 340 patients found that stimulant use was a significant risk factor for development of PAH.[30] Other medications associated with PAH include benfluorex, dasatinib, and interferon.[31]

PAH associated with

Connective tissue diseases. PAH associated with connective tissue disorder is identified most frequently in patients with systemic sclerosis, particularly in patients with limited cutaneous systemic sclerosis, formerly referred to as CREST (calcinosis, Raynaud, esophageal dysfunction, sclerodactyly, and telangiectasia). The prevalence of systemic sclerosis ranges from 30 to 70 cases per million in Japan and Europe,[32-34] and 240 cases per million in the United States.[35] While, the prevalence of PAH associated with systemic sclerosis, based on right heart catheterization, is in the range of 8% to 14%.[36,37] Individuals afflicted by PAH associated with systemic sclerosis are more frequently older females with limited cutaneous sclerosis and serum anticentromere antibodies.[38] PAH has also been associated with other connective tissue diseases including systemic lupus erythematosus (SLE), mixed connective tissue disorder, rheumatoid arthritis, and Sjögren syndrome. The prevalence of SLE is not well established, but is less than systemic sclerosis, estimated at 0.5% to 14%.[38] With regard to PAH-associated mixed connective tissue disorders, the clinical features overlap with systemic sclerosis and SLE. Rheumatoid arthritis infrequently leads to PAH and the clinical characteristics are not well defined as they are for systemic sclerosis. Sjögren syndrome is rarely complicated by PAH and primarily afflicts women, with a mean age of 50 ± 11 years (range 23-68 years). Patients with Sjögren syndrome associated PAH frequently have Raynaud disease, interstitial lung disease, cutaneous vasculitis, antinuclear, anti-Ro/SSA, and anti-RNP antibodies and hypergammaglobulinemia.[39]

Associated with HIV infection. In 1987, the first report of pulmonary hypertension associated with HIV was described in a 40-year-old male with dyspnea who on right heart catheterization was noted to have pulmonary hypertension, and postmortem examination revealed plexogenic arteriopathy.[40] Several years later, a case series of 1200 HIV infected patients found an estimated prevalence of 0.5%.[41] The prevalence of PAH in the era of ART in a prospective multicenter study of 7648 patients was reported to be 0.46%.[42] In this study, patients with HIV-associated PAH were noted to be predominantly males, mean duration of HIV infection of 10 years, with a mean age of 41.5 ± 8 years, who had acquired HIV through IV drug use. In a later study, it was observed that well-controlled HIV infection and HAART were unable to prevent onset of PAH in HIV-infected patients.[43] The symptoms, hemodynamic profile, and survival for patients with PAH-associated HIV are similar compared to those with idiopathic PAH.[44] The etiology of PAH-associated HIV is unclear. Evidence to suggest direct HIV infection of the endothelium or pulmonary vascular smooth muscle has not been demonstrated.[45] However, HIV-viral proteins, specifically HIV-1 nef, has been linked with development of pulmonary plexogenic vascular lesions using chimeric simian (human) immunodeficiency virus–infected macaques.[46,47] A complex host-viral interaction producing endothelial cell injury with further vascular insult in the form of intravenous injection of illicit opioids and stimulants,[48] infectious agents,[49] or autoimmune mechanisms[50] has been proposed.[51]

Associated with portal hypertension. Initially described in a patient with portal vein stenosis and thrombosis of a portacaval shunt, portopulmonary hypertension represents PAH associated with portal hypertension.[52] Subsequent reports have documented the presence of pulmonary hypertension in patients with chronic liver disease.[53-55] In an autopsy case series the incidence of portopulmonary hypertension was reported as 0.73%, while a more recent postmortem study has reported a prevalence of 4.5%. This value is within the range of reported prevalence values of 2% and 8.5% in which hemodynamics studies have been used.[56,57] Among patients with PAH, the Registry to Evaluate Early and Long-term Pulmonary Arterial Hypertension (REVEAL) found 136 subjects with portopulmonary hypertension of 2525 patients with PAH, with a prevalence of 10.6%.[9] The mean age for patients with portopulmonary hypertension was 53 ± 10 years and 52% were female. Notably, in retrospective analyses, neither the extent of liver disease nor severity of portal hypertension portends the presence or degree of portopulmonary hypertension. Proposed mechanisms of development of PAH in patients with portal hypertension involve a reduction in prostacyclin synthase within pulmonary arteries, alteration in endothelin expression, and genetic variants of aromatase and estrogen receptor alpha.[58] In general, prognosis of portopulmonary hypertension is poor; several reports have shown that if left untreated, 1-year survival is 35% to 46%.[59-61] Recent data from a multicenter, prospective US registry indicate that 2- and 5-year survival are worse for patients with portopulmonary hypertension compared to idiopathic PAH, 67% and 40% versus 85% and 64%, respectively.[62]

Associated with congenital heart diseases. PAH is a frequent complication of congenital heart disease. Notably, patients with systemic to pulmonary shunts (left to right) are likely to develop PAH. The risk associated with development of PAH is dependent on the size of the (defect) shunt and blood flow through the defect.[63] Chronic high blood flow induces endothelial injury with vascular remodeling and dysfunction. Consequently, this is associated with an elevation in pulmonary vascular resistance and shunt reversal, also referred to as Eisenmenger syndrome, and observed in patients with atrioventricular defects, tetralogy of Fallot, truncus arteriosus, and single ventricle lesions. Yet, PAH may also occur in "less complex" conditions such as atrial septal defect, ventricular septal defects, and patent ductus arteriosus.[64] The estimated prevalence of congenital heart disease is 6 to 8 per 1000 live births,[65,66] and 4% to 15% will develop PAH.[67] The likelihood of developing Eisenmenger syndrome depends on the underlying heart defect: 10% to 17%[68-70] for an ASD (pretricuspid), ~50% VSD (posttricuspid), 90% with unrepaired atrioventricular septal defect, and 100% with truncus arteriosus.[67,71,72] As previously noted, compared to patients with idiopathic or connective tissue disease associated PAH, individuals with congenital heart disease associated PAH are reported to have better long-term survival.[73,74]

Associated with schistosomiasis. Previously included in Group 4, this category is now included in Group 1, since some recent publications suggest that this disease can have clinical and histologic features similar to idiopathic PAH.[68-70] Although uncommon in the United States, PAH associated with schistosomiasis is common in countries where this infection is endemic. It is estimated that more than 200 million people are infected in these endemic areas, with a 4.6% prevalence of PAH. The mechanism of PAH in schistosomiasis may be multifactorial, including development of portopulmonary hypertension and vascular inflammation.

Associated with chronic hemolytic anemia. Pulmonary hypertension has become a frequently recognized complication of sickle cell disease, as well as other hereditary and acquired hemolytic anemias.[75] The pathology of the pulmonary vasculature has been described in patients with advanced sickle cell disease undergoing postmortem examination and the presence of medical hypertrophy with intimal changes and plexiform lesions is similar to the changes seen in patients with idiopathic PAH.[76] Using Doppler echocardiography to assess for pulmonary hypertension, defined as a tricuspid regurgitant velocity ≥2.5 m/s, the prevalence in patients with sickle cell disease has been reported to be 30% to 40%.[77-79] Pulmonary vascular disease in this group of patients may develop from chronic left ventricular (postcapillary) or pulmonary arterial hypertension (precapillary). Therefore, a right heart catheterization is required to establish a diagnosis of PAH. A recent NIH registry screened 529 patients, and identified 84 patients that underwent right heart catheterization. Their mean age was 41 ± 13 years with predominantly hemoglobin SS disease. These investigators found a prevalence of precapillary pulmonary hypertension to be 6% (31/529). Compared to other patients with pulmonary hypertension, patients with sickle cell disease and pulmonary hypertension have a relatively low PVR and this is likely related to low viscosity due to anemia and elevated cardiac output.[75] Similarly, investigators in France and Brazil undertook echocardiography and right heart catheterization in adults with sickle cell disease and reported a prevalence of precapillary pulmonary hypertension between 6% and 10%.[78,80] Furthermore, these investigators confirmed earlier findings of risk factors for pulmonary hypertension to be renal insufficiency, hemolytic anemia, and liver dysfunction. They also noted an association between pulmonary hypertension and lower extremity skin ulcerations, poor exercise tolerance and an increased risk of death.

Pathologic features of group I PAH

The characteristic changes seen in group I pulmonary arterial hypertension affect the distal pulmonary arteries, particularly those less than 500 μm in diameter. The arteries show medial hypertrophy, intimal thickening and fibrosis (concentric or laminar), adventitial thickening, and perivascular chronic inflammation. With more severe pulmonary hypertension complex lesions such as plexiform and dilated lesions, and vascular thrombosis may be seen. The pulmonary veins do not show hypertensive changes.

Medial hypertrophy and muscularization of arterioles. Medial proliferation is the most common lesion in pulmonary hypertension. It is also designated grade 1 in Heath-Edward scheme.[81] The media shows an increase in size and number of smooth muscle cells. The degree of hypertrophy is roughly proportional to the severity of pulmonary hypertension, as measured by the ratio of medial thickness to the outside diameter of the artery (*Figures 15-7* to *15-9*). A value greater than 15% signifies severe hypertrophy.[81] Muscularization of the arterioles is also an early manifestation of pulmonary hypertension (*Figure 15-10*). In a normal arteriole, no smooth muscle is seen in vessels 70 to 100 μm in diameter, but in pulmonary hypertension, the muscular layer may be seen in arterioles as small as 20 to 30 μm in diameter, with recognizable internal and external elastic lamina.[18]

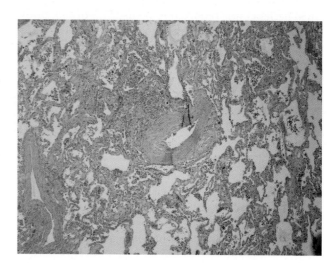

FIGURE 15-7 A small pulmonary artery branch shows medial thickening.

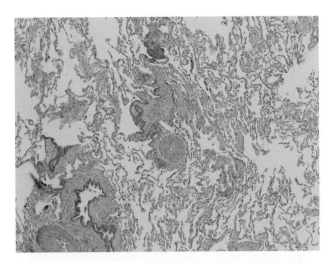

FIGURE 15-8 Low-magnification photomicrograph shows a small pulmonary artery branch in the center of the field and another at the lower left corner, with intimal thickening and mild medial thickening.

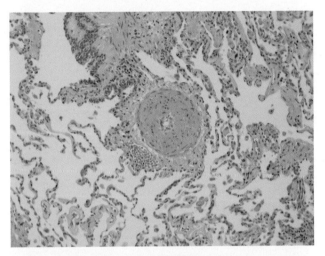

FIGURE 15-9 Higher magnification of the pulmonary artery branch with accompanying small airway.

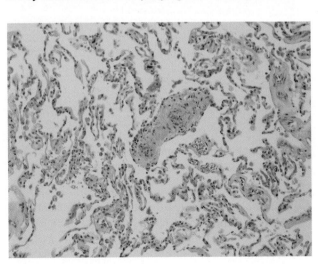

FIGURE 15-10 Lung section shows a small arteriole with muscularization of the wall.

Intimal cellular proliferation. Intimal cellular proliferation is seen most commonly in vessels of 100 to 150 µm diameter, and classified as Heath-Edward grade 2. It is characterized by migration of medial myofibroblasts and smooth muscle cells into the intima between the internal elastic lamina and endothelium with a radial orientation (*Figures 15-11A* and *B*).

Concentric laminar intimal fibrosis. Concentric laminar intimal fibrosis follows cellular intimal proliferation, when the migrated medial smooth muscle cells convert into myofibroblasts and form a collagen and proteoglycan matrix, which is deposited to form lamellar or "onionskin" layers of circumferential spindle cell within a fibrous and hyalinized stroma (*Figures 15-12A* and *B*). At a later stage, the intima may have elastic fibrils and thickening and reduplication of internal elastic lamina. Any of these features are considered grade 3 in the Heath-Edward classification.

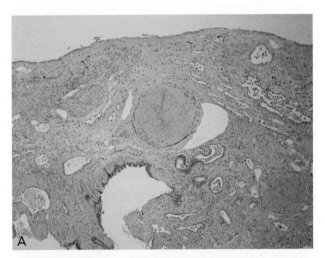

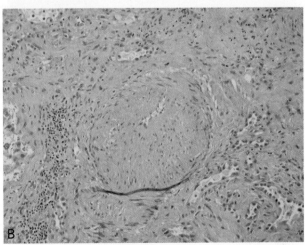

FIGURE 15-11 Low and higher magnification of a small pulmonary artery branch with marked cellular intimal proliferation and narrowing of the lumen, in a patient with usual interstitial pneumonia (UIP). Pleural surface is seen at the top of the field in A.

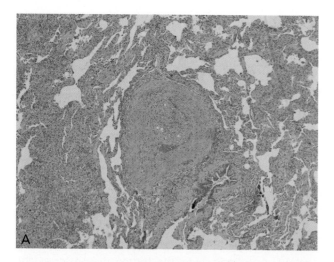
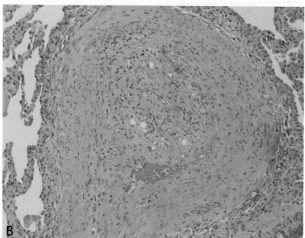

FIGURE 15-12 **Low and higher magnification of a small pulmonary artery branch with marked cellular intimal proliferation and early fibrosis.**

Plexiform lesions. Plexiform lesions are most commonly seen in primary pulmonary hypertension, portopulmonary hypertension, and congenital cardiac left to right shunt. It is designated as Heath-Edwards grade 4. Although it is considered a characteristic lesion of primary pulmonary hypertension, its presence is not required for the diagnosis. The presence of plexiform lesion signifies severe pulmonary hypertension.

Histologically, the plexiform lesion consists of intraluminal proliferation of slit-like vascular channels separated by connective tissue septa containing smooth muscle, myofibroblasts, and fibrillary cells.[82] *Figures 15-13A, B* and *15-14* show the histologic features of the plexiform lesions. The cells lining the vascular channels are plump and stain positive for factor VIII antigen; however, they do not have a basement membrane, pinocytotic vesicles, or Weibel-Palade bodies.[81] The older plexiform lesions show thickened, fibrous, and less cellular septa, with enlarged and rounded vascular spaces, resembling the recanalized lesions of thrombotic vasculopathy (*Figure 15-15*).

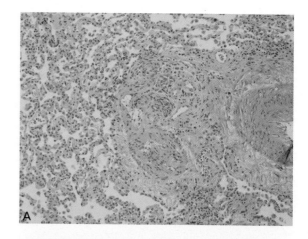
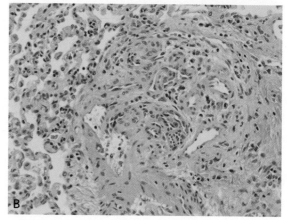

FIGURE 15-13 **Low and higher magnification of a plexiform lesion showing intraluminal proliferation of slit-like vascular spaces lined by plump cells.**

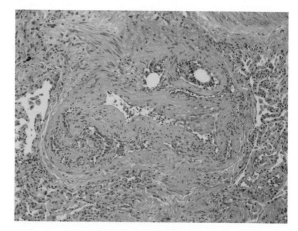

FIGURE 15-14 **High magnification of a plexiform lesion, and the accompanying thickened pulmonary artery branch.**

Dilation lesions. The dilation lesion may be seen as a component of plexiform lesion, with the dilated thin-walled vessels surrounding the proliferative plexiform lesion (*Figures 15-16A* and *B*). In this scenario, the dilation is most likely secondary to weakening of the arterial wall secondary to fibrinoid degeneration, and still

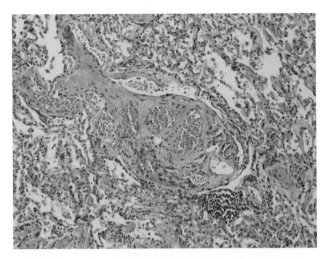

FIGURE 15-15 An older plexiform lesion showing less cellular septa with focal fibrosis, and a few enlarged vascular spaces.

considered a Heath-Edward grade 4 lesion. According to Heath these changes antedate the cellular form of the plexiform lesion, and that deposition of the fibrinoid material may initiate the formation of plexiform lesion.

Another form of dilation lesion is seen in long-standing pulmonary hypertension, as there is maturation of the angiomatoid lesion with thinning of the wall surrounding the cellular tuft of the plexiform lesion and virtual loss of the media, giving rise to the characteristic vein-like branches. These dilated vessels may become clustered together to form "angiomatoid lesions." Examples of the dilation lesion are seen in *Figures 15-17A* and *B*. Another form of dilation lesion may be seen proximal to a thickened arterial segment, probably forming a bypass channel around the obstructed artery. The term "cavernous lesion" is used to describe an intermediate stage between the vein-like branches and the angiomatoid lesion. All these forms of dilated lesions are considered Heath-Edward grade 5.

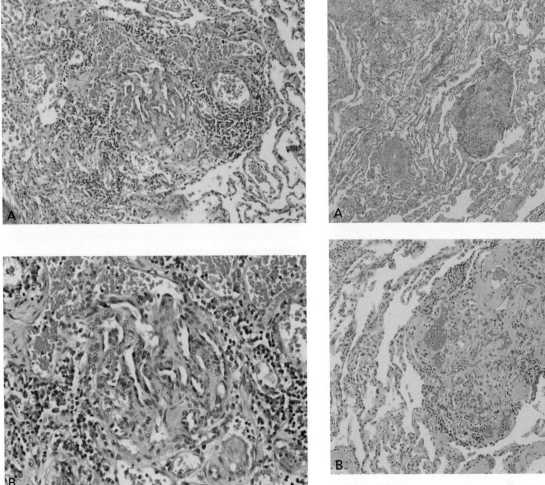

FIGURE 15-16 Low and higher magnification of dilation lesion with an accompanying plexiform lesion.

FIGURE 15-17 Low and higher magnification of another dilation lesion, with a cluster of dilated vessels resulting in an "angiomatoid lesion."

CHAPTER 15

Fibrinoid necrosis/vasculitis. Fibrinoid necrosis of pulmonary arteries in pulmonary hypertension is an uncommon lesion, considered a grade 6 lesion in the Heath-Edward classification scheme. It is characterized by replacement of the medial smooth muscles with an eosinophilic fibrinoid material (*Figures 15-18A, B* and *15-19*). The change is the result of insudation of fibrin through the intima into the media, with degeneration of the medial smooth muscle cells progressing to frank necrosis. Some cases may show focal, segmental frank necrotizing arteritis with neutrophil infiltrate, and healing with granulation tissue formation in the media.[82] It should be pointed out that this full spectrum of necrotizing arteritis must be distinguished from the focal fibrinoid degeneration that may be seen as a component of the plexiform lesion.

The large pulmonary artery branches and the elastic pulmonary arteries may show atherosclerosis in severe pulmonary hypertension with formation of typical plaques within the intima, containing amorphous

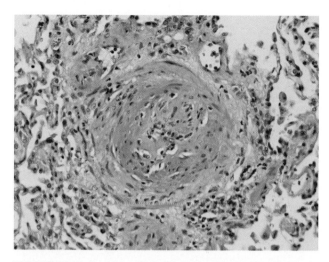

FIGURE 15-19 Another area of the same lung shows fibrinoid necrosis of the medial muscle. The lumen has a few vascular spaces that may represent an early plexiform lesion.

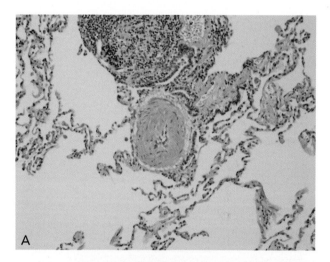

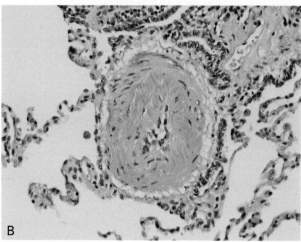

FIGURE 15-18 Low and higher magnification of a small pulmonary artery branch with fibrinoid necrosis of the medial muscle.

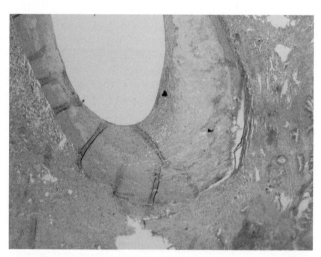

FIGURE 15-20 Large pulmonary artery branches in patients with **PAH** may show atherosclerosis, with the atherosclerotic plaque containing fatty material, foamy macrophages, cholesterol clefts, and focal lymphocytic infiltrates.

atheromatous material, foamy macrophages, cholesterol clefts, and inflammatory cells (*Figure 15-20*).

Pulmonary veno-occlusive disease and pulmonary capillary hemangiomatosis

Pulmonary veno-occlusive disease (PVOD) and pulmonary capillary hemangiomatosis (PCH) are considered within the subgroup of PAH. While there are differences between PVOD/PCH and PAH, a hypothesis has been put forth that these represent different forms of the same disease spectrum.[83]

PVOD is a rare condition that accounts for a small number of cases of pulmonary hypertension. The term PVOD was coined by Heath in which he described an extensive fibrotic and obliterative condition predominantly involving the small pulmonary veins in a 45-year-old woman.[84] The incidence and prevalence are not known, as many cases are misclassified as idiopathic PAH.[85] The clinical features and hemodynamic profile are very similar to patients with idiopathic PAH. However, PVOD affects men and women equally; unlike PAH that disproportionately affects women. Common symptoms include exertional dyspnea, fatigue, and syncope and the nonspecific nature of symptoms frequently leads to a delay in diagnosis.[86] The hemodynamics assessed by right heart catheterization reveal a mean pulmonary artery ≥25 mm Hg and a pulmonary capillary wedge pressure ≤15 mm Hg. The radiographic features are useful in the diagnosis and chest radiographs reveal enlarged pulmonary arteries, Kerley B lines, and patchy opacities.[85] Chest computed tomography (CT) reveals enlarged pulmonary arteries, thickened interlobular septa, and patchy opacities in a diffuse, mosaic, or centrilobular distribution and occasionally mediastinal lymphadenopathy or pleural effusions.[87] The radiographic features are helpful in distinguishing PVOD from PAH. Moreover, the features of pulmonary arterial hypertension with normal pulmonary capillary wedge pressure and radiographic findings of pulmonary edema are very helpful in establishing a diagnosis of PVOD. The prognosis is poor, as this is a progressive condition with limited medical therapies. Lung transplantation offers the best opportunity for an effective therapy.[87]

Pulmonary capillary hemangiomatosis (PCH) is considered a subgroup of PAH. The first case of PCH described several decades ago, by Wagenvoort, involved a 71-year-old woman with progressive dyspnea, hemoptysis, and hemorrhagic effusions that upon examination of the lung revealed proliferation of capillary channels in lung tissue.[88] Subsequent authors have reported this condition in children and adults with an equal sex distribution.[89,90] Patients present with signs and symptoms of right heart failure and hemoptysis. The hemodynamic profile is similar to PAH in that the mean pulmonary artery pressure is greater than 25 mm Hg and the pulmonary capillary wedge pressure is less than 15 mm Hg.[91] Chest CT imaging reveals enlargement of the main pulmonary arteries and diffuse bibasilar centrilobular nodules.[92] Prognosis is poor, with lung transplantation being the most effective treatment.

Pathologic features of PVOD consist of involvement of septal veins and preseptal venules. There is associated fibrotic occlusion of the veins, muscularization of veins, and patchy capillary proliferation. In addition, the lung parenchyma may show edema, congestion, hemorrhage, dilated lymphatics, and chronic inflammatory infiltrates. The draining lymph nodes may be enlarged and show vascular transformation of sinuses. The small pulmonary arteries may show mild hypertensive changes of medial hypertrophy and intimal fibrosis. Complex arterial hypertensive changes are usually not seen.

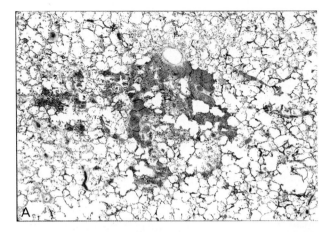
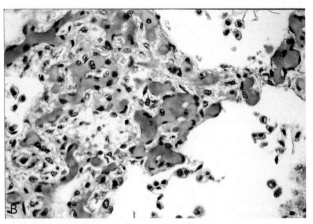

FIGURE 15-21 Low and higher magnifications of lung section showing capillary hemangiomatosis with focal clusters of dilated and congested capillaries. The alveolar septa usually have two or more lines of the capillaries, and sometimes clusters that protrude into the alveolar spaces. Similar proliferation may be seen in the small airway walls.

Histologic features of capillary hemangiomatosis consist of proliferation of capillaries within the alveolar septa and the walls of small airways and pulmonary arteries. The capillaries often line the alveolar walls in two or more layers, with focal protrusion into the alveolar spaces. Focal clusters of the proliferating capillaries may be seen extending from the alveolar septa into the alveolar spaces (*Figures 15-21A* and *B*).

Pulmonary hypertension owing to left heart disease
Pulmonary hypertension secondary to left ventricular dysfunction or valvular heart disease is more common than pulmonary arterial hypertension.[93] Mitral stenosis was the most common cause of pulmonary hypertension; however, conditions such as systemic hypertension and ischemic heart disease that lead to impaired left ventricular diastolic function result in an elevation of left ventricular diastolic, left atrial, and pulmonary venous pressure.[94,95] The mechanism of pulmonary hypertension arising from left heart disease has been

described early as an increase in left atrial pressure transmitted to the pulmonary vasculature, resulting in elevation of the pulmonary capillary wedge pressure and pulmonary artery pressure.[95] A hemodynamic definition of pulmonary venous hypertension is a mean pulmonary artery pressure ≥25 mm Hg and a mean pulmonary capillary wedge pressure >15 mm Hg. This has also been termed postcapillary pulmonary hypertension arising from elevated left atrial or left ventricular filling pressures.[96]

Diagnosis of postcapillary pulmonary hypertension using echocardiography allows identification of features associated with this condition including left atrial enlargement, left ventricular (LV) hypertrophy, impaired LV relaxation, reduced LV ejection fraction, and mitral or aortic valve disease.[97] Right heart catheterization is important in distinguishing pulmonary arterial hypertension (PAH) and pulmonary venous hypertension, especially when the latter is caused by preserved ejection fraction heart failure. Clinical characteristics associated with preserved EF heart failure and pulmonary venous hypertension include older age, systemic hypertension, atrial fibrillation, and coronary artery disease.[98]

Histologic findings. Chronic elevation of pulmonary venous pressures leads to histologic changes of the pulmonary veins and arteries that produce thickening of the intima and media. The pulmonary veins have been observed to become dilated and develop medial hypertrophy (*Figures 15-22A* and *B*). Thickening of the intima of the pulmonary arteriole is observed. Changes to the pulmonary arteriolar media consist of smooth muscle hypertrophy and hyperplasia. Also seen are chronic congestion, hemorrhage, and hemosiderin-laden macrophages in the lung parenchyma (*Figure 15-23*). Notably absent are plexiform lesions.[93]

Pulmonary hypertension owing to lung diseases and/or hypoxia

This category of pulmonary hypertension includes chronic obstructive pulmonary disease, interstitial lung disease, sleep disordered breathing, alveolar hypoventilation disorders, residence at high altitude, and developmental abnormalities.[3] Pulmonary hypertension in these categories is often associated with hypoxia, and has been defined as a mean pulmonary pressure ≥25 mm Hg and a PCWP <15 mm Hg. The prevalence of pulmonary hypertension in COPD ranges from 20% to 50%.[99-101] In general, patients with COPD with pulmonary hypertension demonstrate a mean PAP between 25 and 30 mm Hg and preserved right ventricular function.[101,102] Severe pulmonary hypertension in COPD is rare. In patients with pulmonary fibrosis, the prevalence of pulmonary hypertension, as assessed by right heart catheterization ranges from 32% to 46%.[103-105]

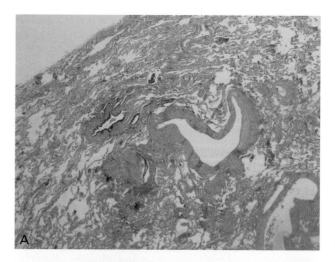
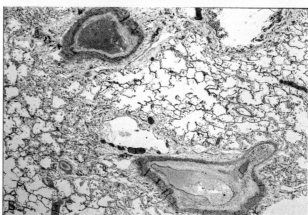

FIGURE 15-22 Pulmonary hypertension owing to left heart disease produces changes in both arteries and veins with thickening and dilation of the vessels, as seen in A. The vascular changes are better visualized with the use of a special stain, (such as pentachrome stain MOVAT used in B), or an elastic stain.

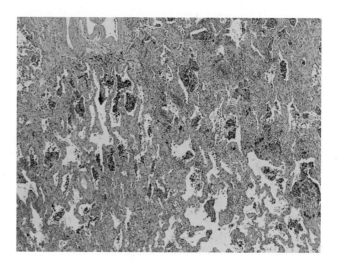

FIGURE 15-23 Chronic left ventricular failure may result in chronic congestion and hemosiderin-laden macrophages within the lung, as seen in this figure.

Sleep disordered breathing, obstructive sleep apnea, and obesity hypoventilation syndrome are associated with intermittent hypoxia and mild pulmonary hypertension.[106] The prevalence of pulmonary hypertension associated with obstructive sleep apnea has been reported at 20%.[107] A greater body mass index and severe nocturnal desaturations have been associated with pulmonary hypertension in obstructive sleep apnea.[108]

Pathologic features. The changes in the pulmonary vasculature have been reported to correlate with the degree of pulmonary hypertension in patients with COPD. Most patients demonstrate mild hypertensive changes including intimal thickening as well as medial hypertrophy.[99] The pulmonary vascular changes in patients with pulmonary fibrosis consist of intimal thickening and medial hypertrophy similar to the pathology observed in patients with COPD (*Figure 15-24*).

Chronic thromboembolic pulmonary hypertension (CTEPH)

CTEPH is characterized by single or multiple pulmonary thromboemboli that organize to obstruct the pulmonary vascular bed. Chronic obstruction of the pulmonary vascular bed leads to elevation of pulmonary vascular resistance and subsequent development of right heart failure. Symptoms of CTEPH include progressive exertional dyspnea, fatigue, syncope, and hemoptysis that frequently coincide with the degree of right ventricular dysfunction.[109] Chest discomfort may also be reported and is pleuritic in nature, presumably due to infarction of the lung. The nonspecific nature of these symptoms frequently leads to misdiagnosis of other conditions such as COPD or congestive heart

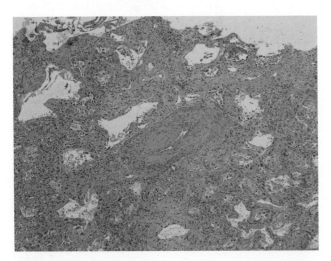

FIGURE 15-24 Lung section shows the vascular changes in a patient with pulmonary fibrosis. There is intimal thickening and fibrosis and medial hypertrophy of small pulmonary artery branches. The surrounding lung parenchyma shows histologic changes of pulmonary fibrosis.

failure.[110] An international registry reported findings and outcomes in 679 patients diagnosed with CTEPH. The median age was 63 years, 50% were men, and dyspnea was the most common diagnosis (99%), followed by edema (40.5%), fatigue (31.5%), chest pain (15%), and syncope (13.7%). At time of diagnosis 14 months had passed since the first symptoms were observed. Right heart catheterization findings revealed median pulmonary artery pressure 47 mm Hg (interquartile range 38-55 mm Hg). The most frequent cause of death was perioperative complications related to pulmonary thromboendarterectomy and right heart failure.

Current evidence suggests that CTEPH is an extension of the natural history of acute pulmonary embolism arising from the lower extremities.[111] Thus, patients with prior pulmonary emboli or deep vein thrombosis would be high-risk individuals for CTEPH. However, only a minority of patients experiencing acute pulmonary embolism go on to develop CTEPH. Early estimates indicated that 0.1% to 0.5% of patients surviving an acute pulmonary embolism would develop CTEPH[112,113]; however, a prospective, longitudinal report by Pengo and colleagues described a cumulative incidence of symptomatic CTEPH at 2 years to be 3.8%.[114] These authors also reported previous pulmonary embolism, younger age, and idiopathic pulmonary embolism at time of presentation as risk factors for development of CTEPH. Other risk factors include prior splenectomy, ventriculoatrial shunt and chronic inflammatory states, and thyroid diseases.[115,116] The frequency of antithrombin, protein C, protein S, and factor V Leiden mutations have not been found to be greater than in the general population.[117] However, the antiphospholipid antibody syndrome has been noted to occur in up to 20% of patients.[118]

A diagnosis of CTEPH may be established in a symptomatic patient with hemodynamic evidence of mean pulmonary artery pressure ≥25 mm Hg and PCWP <15 mm Hg, with imaging studies indicative of a pulmonary vascular filling defect. The most frequently used imaging studies are ventilation/perfusion scintigraphy or chest CT.[113] Both of these imaging studies correlate with the distribution of the pulmonary vascular occlusion. Ventilation-perfusion scintigraphy has been used for clinical purposes to assess for presence and extent of perfusion defects. Chest CT imaging has also been demonstrated to be of clinical utility in identification of patients with chronic thromboemboli (*Figures 15-25 to 15-27*). However, neither of these imaging techniques is sufficiently adequate to determine the amount of thromboemboli. Pulmonary angiography is required to accurately assess the amount and distribution of pulmonary vascular occlusions.[113]

Pathologic findings in CTEPH. Pathologic examination of the heart reveals right ventricular enlargement with hypertrophy of right ventricular myocytes. Lung tissue

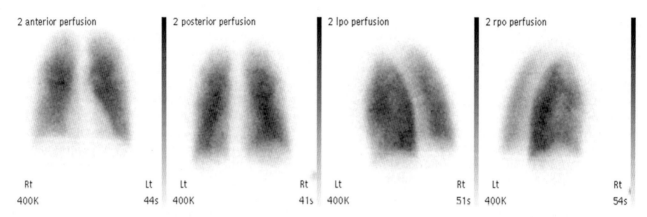

FIGURE 15-25 Technetium radionuclide scan with normal pulmonary perfusion. The four views represented are anterior, posterior, left posterior oblique (LPO), and right posterior oblique.

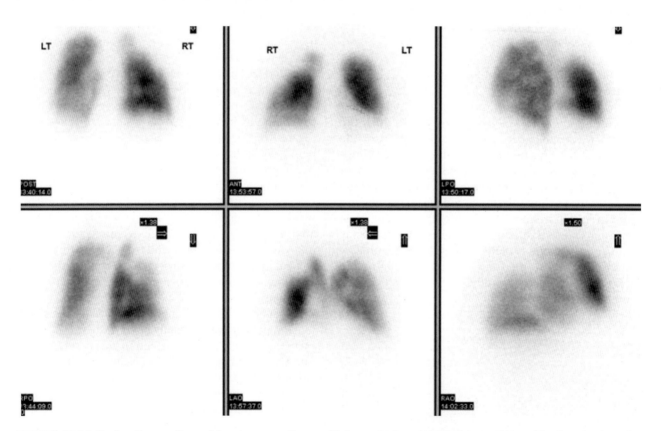

FIGURE 15-26 Technetium radionuclide scan revealing multiple perfusion defects in a patient with chronic thromboembolic pulmonary hypertension (CTEPH). Six views are represented from right to left, starting in left upper corner as posterior, anterior, left posterior oblique (LPO), right posterior oblique (RPO), left anterior oblique (LAO), and right anterior oblique (RAO).

obtained from pulmonary thromboendarterectomy or postmortem examination shows organizing thrombi present in the large, segmental, and distal pulmonary arteries. The thrombi are adherent to the pulmonary arterial wall and may partially or completely occlude the lumen.[119] Recanalized thrombi may also be seen, with bands and webs stretched across the nonoccluded vascular lumen. The small pulmonary arteries with CTEPH demonstrates smooth muscle hypertrophy,

intimal proliferation, and rarely plexogenic lesions similar to those observed in the pulmonary vasculature of patients with idiopathic PAH and PAH associated with congenital heart disease.[120]

PAH with unclear or multifactorial mechanisms
This group of PAH comprises disorders of hematologic, systemic, and metabolic nature, and other entities for which the etiology is either unclear or multifactorial.

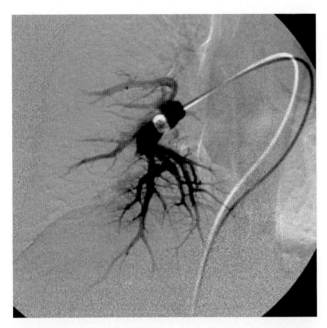

FIGURE 15-27 Pulmonary arteriogram of the patient with chronic thromboembolic pulmonary hypertension (CTEPH). Absent perfusion of right lower lobe is demonstrated.

Hematologic disorders. PAH has been reported in chronic myeloproliferative diseases such as polycythemia vera, chronic myeloid leukemia, and essential thrombocythemia.[121] Possible mechanisms of development of PAH include high cardiac output, asplenia, obstruction of pulmonary vasculature by circulating megakaryocytes, CTEPH, POPH, and congestive heart failure. Splenectomy by itself may increase the risk of PAH, with pulmonary vasculature showing medial hypertrophy, intimal fibrosis, and plexiform lesions.[122]

Systemic disorders. Systemic diseases including sarcoidosis, pulmonary Langerhans cell histiocytosis, lymphangioleiomyomatosis, neurofibromatosis, and rarely antineutrophil cytoplasmic antibodies-associated vasculitis have been reported to be associated with PAH. Prevalence of PAH in sarcoidosis is reported to be 1% to 28%.[104] Possible pathogenetic factors are destruction of capillary bed by fibrosis, extrinsic compression of pulmonary arteries by thoracic lymphadenopathy, and direct granulomatous infiltration of pulmonary arteries and veins.[123]

Although an uncommon disease, patients with end-stage pulmonary Langerhans cell histiocytosis can develop severe PAH. Chronic hypoxemia, abnormal pulmonary mechanics, and pulmonary vasculopathy are possible pathogenetic factors. Severe diffuse medial hypertrophy and intimal fibrosis involving predominantly intralobar veins and muscular pulmonary arteries has been reported by one author. PAH is an uncommon occurrence in patients with lymphangioleiomyomatosis, and may develop secondary to hypoxemia or destruction of capillary bed from the cystic lesions.[124] PAH has been reported in another systemic disorder, neurofibromatosis type 1 or von Recklinghausen disease. The mechanism of PAH is not clear; however, pulmonary fibrosis and CTEPH are believed to play a role.[125] Histologic examination in some cases found medial hypertrophy and intimal hypertrophy or fibrosis.[126]

Metabolic disorders. The third subgroup includes metabolic disorders, that is, type Ia and type II glycogen storage diseases and Gaucher disease. PAH is an uncommon complication in these diseases. Possible mechanisms include restrictive pulmonary function with hypoxia, portocaval shunt, or atrial septal defect in type Ia disease, and additionally capillary plugging by Gaucher cells.[127,128] PAH has been reported with thyroid diseases, both hypo- and hyperthyroidism. One echocardiographic study reports PAH in 40% of patients with thyroid disease, while another study of 63 patients with PAH found a 49% prevalence of autoimmune thyroid disease, suggesting a possible common immunogenetic susceptibility.[129]

Others. This subgroup includes miscellaneous conditions including tumoral obstruction, fibrosing mediastinitis, and chronic renal failure on dialysis. Tumoral obstruction may be the result of a tumor such as sarcoma growing into the major pulmonary arteries, as well as occlusion of the microvasculature by metastatic tumor emboli.[130] Mediastinal fibrosis may cause PAH by compression of pulmonary arteries and veins. Almost 40% of patients with end-stage renal failure maintained on long-term hemodialysis are reported to develop PAH.[131] There are several possible reasons for the development of PAH in these patients. Hormonal and metabolic abnormalities resulting in pulmonary vascular constriction, high cardiac output from arteriovenous shunt and anemia, and fluid overload are all possible culprits in development of PAH.[131,132]

PULMONARY EMBOLI

Pulmonary embolism is a common and potentially lethal complication of deep vein thrombosis. Although majority of pulmonary emboli originate in the deep veins of the lower extremities, they can also originate from renal, pelvic, ovarian, upper extremity, or right heart chambers. The incidence of pulmonary embolism in the United States is estimated to be 117 cases per 100,000 persons per year, with 250,000 cases occurring per year.[133] The age-adjusted death rate for pulmonary embolism in the United States decreased from 191 deaths/million to 94 deaths/million population from 1979 to 1998.[133] Studies suggest that the increasing use of CT scanning has led to an increased reported incidence of pulmonary embolism.[134,135] Pulmonary embolism may be seen in 60% to 80% of patients with DVT, even in the absence of symptoms. It is the third most common cause of death in hospitalized patients, and approximately 60% of hospital deaths have pulmonary emboli, most of these often missed clinically. Pulmonary embolism is more frequent in elderly males, and African Americans.[133,136] There is an increased incidence of DVT and pulmonary embolism in women with pregnancy, and postpartum, at 199.7 incidents/100,000 women.[137]

Factors that predispose to the development of pulmonary emboli include endothelial injury, stasis or turbulent blood flow, and hypercoagulability. Clinical conditions that predispose to pulmonary embolism include immobilization, surgery and trauma, pregnancy, oral contraceptives and estrogen replacement therapy, malignancy, hypercoagulable states, and HIV infection.[138]

Deep venous thrombi can break off, and travel to the lung, lodging in the pulmonary arteries. A large thrombus can lodge at the bifurcation of the main pulmonary artery or the lobar branches and cause sudden death or severe hemodynamic compromise. Smaller thrombi travel more distally and may produce pleuritic chest pain. The lower lobes are more commonly affected than the upper lobe. Approximately 10% of subjects who develop pulmonary embolism die within the first hour, and 30% die subsequently from recurrent embolism.

Clinical Features of Thromboemboli

The classic presenting symptoms of pulmonary thromboemboli are sudden onset of pleuritic chest pain, shortness of breath, and hypoxia. Massive thrombolus results in sudden hemodynamic collapse, whereas small recurrent emboli result in gradually progressive dyspnea. Atypical presentation with syncope, seizures, wheezing, hemoptysis, and fever with productive cough may be seen.

Imaging features

Computed tomography angiography (CTA) is the criterion standard for diagnosis of pulmonary emboli (*Figure 15-28*). Other diagnostic tests include pulmonary angiography, chest radiography, V/Q scanning, MRI, and duplex ultrasonography. CTA can show intraluminal filling defect occluding the pulmonary artery branch, and corresponding infarct that may be seen as a triangular, pleural-based consolidation.

Pathologic features

Grossly, the large acute thromboemboli in the main pulmonary artery or its lobar branches distend the vessel, are firm, and have a laminated granular appearance,

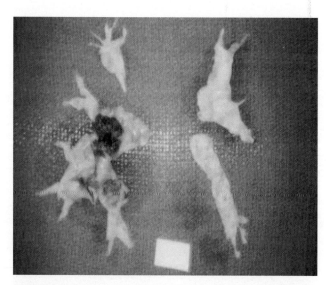

FIGURE 15-28 Surgical specimens of chronic thromboemboli. White appearing thrombi represent old emboli while red appearing thrombi represent more recent emboli.

and are not attached to the vessel wall. These usually do not confirm to the shape of the surrounding vessel, and appear fibrotic and tan white (*Figure 15-29*). In case of a massive thromboembolus, usually from the leg veins, it may lodge in the main pulmonary artery at its bifurcation, completely occluding the lumen and resulting in sudden death (*Figures 15-30* and *15-31*). Careful examination may reveal the impressions of the leg vein valves on the surface of the thromboembolus. In contrast, the postmortem clots are soft, with components that look like red currant jelly and chicken fat. The recanalized thromboembolus in larger arteries may be seen as pulmonary webs, with attenuated fibrous strands across the vascular lumen (*Figure 15-32*).

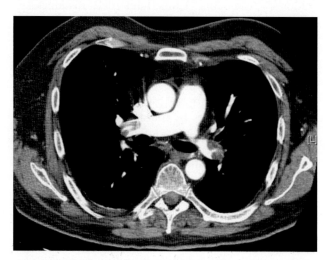

FIGURE 15-29 Chest CT obtained from a patient with chronic dyspnea and syncope that reveals the presence of bilateral pulmonary emboli represented as filling defects in the main pulmonary arteries.

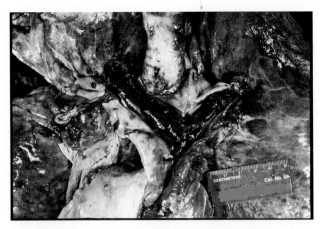

FIGURE 15-30 Gross photograph of the main pulmonary artery at bifurcation site, showing a large recent red thromboembolus (with impressions of the vein valves), occluding both branches, so-called saddle embolus.

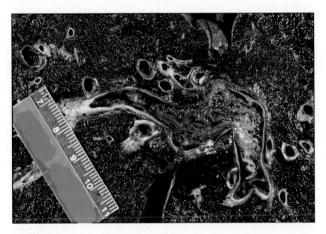

FIGURE 15-31 Gross photograph of a lobar branch of pulmonary artery, showing an organizing tan to red thrombus with a granular appearance.

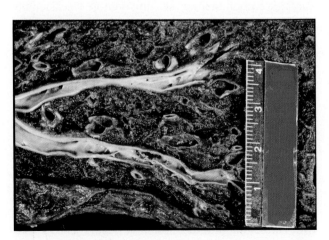

FIGURE 15-32 Gross photograph of pulmonary artery branches with delicate pulmonary webs within the lumen, as a result of old organized thrombi.

Histologically, lines of Zahn may be seen, with alternating layers of fibrin and platelets, and erythrocytes and leucocytes. In the large thromboemboli, features of organization, including neutrophil infiltrates in the vessel wall, and adjacent thrombus, as well as fibroblast proliferation are seen at approximately 1 week. Later, there is deposition of fibroelastic tissue with recanalization of some vessels. In the small arterial branches, the organizational phases are the same as in the larger thromboemboli. However, the residual thrombi can get incorporated in the small vessels as eccentric intimal plaques. Occasionally, the thrombus can develop a collagen matrix, with rounded punched out rigid appearing recanalized lumens, the so-called "colander lesion."

Bone Marrow Emboli

Fragments of fat and bone marrow may be released in circulation following fractures, surgery, bone infarcts with sickle cell disease or following steroid therapy, or cardiopulmonary resuscitation.

Clinically, bone marrow emboli are incidental findings, except in patients with fat embolism syndrome, who may present with acute respiratory distress, petechial rash, and central nervous system symptoms.[139]

Pathologic features include distention of small to medium pulmonary arteries with myeloid and erythroid hematopoietic elements and adipose cells (*Figure 15-33*). Larger thromboemboli may also have megakaryocytes. With fat embolism, it is difficult to demonstrate intravascular lipid droplets, because of the organic solvents used in slide preparations. One histologic clue would be the expanded empty small vascular and capillary lumens. If fat embolism is suspected, frozen sections using oil red-o stain should be used. Alternately, osmium tetroxide may be used on fixed blocks.[140]

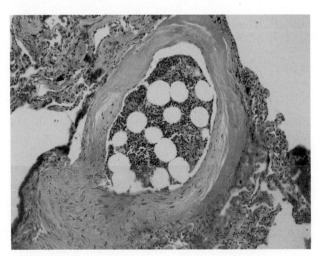

FIGURE 15-33 A bone marrow embolus is seen distending the lumen of a small pulmonary artery branch, as a result of resuscitation.

CHAPTER 15

Foreign Body Emboli

Most common foreign body emboli are seen in intravenous drug users, when oral tablets containing insoluble binding agents are used intravenously. Cardiovascular procedures may be associated with embolization of cotton woolor gauze fibers, silicone agents, and fragments of plastic tubing and catheters may also be seen in the pulmonary vasculature.[141]

Histologically, most commonly seen foreign body materials in intravenous drug users include talc (5-15 μm needle/plate like), microcrystalline cellulose (25-200 μm needle/rod like), and cornstarch (8-12 μm polyhedral), birefringent particles.

Tumor Emboli

Tumor emboli in pulmonary vasculature are commonly seen from primary carcinomas of breast, lung, liver, stomach, pancreas, and prostate.[142] Clinically, if extensive, the tumor emboli may be associated with microangiopathic hemolytic anemia and disseminated intravascular coagulation, the so-called "thrombotic microangiopathy."

Histologically, pulmonary small vessels and capillaries contain either pure malignant cell aggregates or mixed with thrombi. With extensive and recurrent tumor emboli, patients may develop hypertensive lesions including intimal and medial hyperplasia with vascular remodeling.[143]

Tissue Emboli

Tissue emboli are uncommon occurrence; however, these may be seen following trauma, with liver and brain laceration. Rarely, newborns with central nervous system malformations or severe head trauma during delivery may have brain tissue pulmonary emboli. Histologically, the damaged organ tissue is seen in the pulmonary artery branches, often at autopsy.

Amniotic Fluid Emboli

Amniotic fluid embolism is associated with difficult labor, therapeutic abortion, and rarely with cesarean section.[139,144] Clinically, the patient develops sudden cardiovascular collapse and pulmonary edema, and it can be fatal if massive embolism occurs.

Pathologic features include grossly edema, atelectasis, hyperinflation, and disseminated intravascular coagulation (DIC). Histologically, pulmonary small vessels contain aggregates of epithelial squames, lipid, mucus, meconium and bile, and lanugo hair (*Figure 15-34*).[144] Additional histochemical and immunohistochemical stains may be used for confirmation.[144]

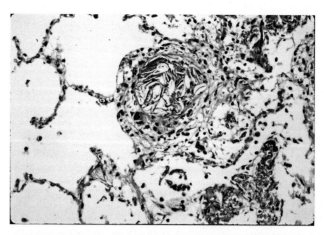

FIGURE 15-34 **A patient who sustained amniotic fluid embolism shows a small pulmonary vessel distended with collapsed and compressed squamous cells.**

Air Emboli

Air embolism can occur following trauma with laceration of veins, during surgery and intravenous injections. Other procedures associated with air embolism include therapeutic insufflation of fallopian tubes, ventilation therapy, and hyperbaric decompression. Patients with severe air embolism can develop cardiovascular collapse, pulmonary edema, and death.

Pathologic features include pulmonary edema and frothy blood in pulmonary vessels. If suspected antemortem, air in the pulmonary vessels may be demonstrated by opening the pulmonary artery under water. The right heart is dilated, and the left heart is contracted. Histologically, pulmonary arteries may show empty circular spaces within the column of blood.

Parasite Emboli

Parasitic emboli in lungs are uncommon. Occasionally parasites such as Wuchereria, Dirofilaria immitis, Strongyloides, Ascaris, and Schistosoma mansoni may be found in the lung vasculature and parenchyma. Dirofilaria infestation typically produces pulmonary infarct due to the large parasite occluding the small pulmonary arterial branch, and may present as a solitary nodule on chest radiograph or CT scan. The other parasites may produce pulmonary edema, hemoptysis, productive cough, and pleuritic chest pain. Chronic infection with Schistosoma mansoni may result in pulmonary hypertension and cor pulmonale.[145]

Histologically, pulmonary infarct with a central thrombosed vessel containing parts of the parasite may be seen with Dirofilaria immitis infestation (*Figure 15-35*). With the other parasite infections, granulomatous inflammation, vascular intimal and medial hyperplasia, small vessel thrombosis and recanalized lesions may be seen.

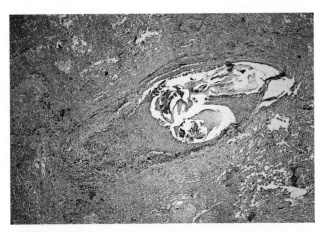

FIGURE 15-35 Lung shows organizing infarct with a pulmonary artery branch in the center containing fragments of the parasite, dog heartworm Dirofilaria immitis.

Pulmonary Infarct

Pulmonary infarcts occur in a setting of pulmonary embolism, in a background of preexisting pulmonary or cardiac disease with a low flow state, and more often in the lower lobes.[146,147] The average infarct is 3 cm, pleural based, and roughly triangular in shape. Chest CT shows a wedge-shaped pleural-based defect (*Figure 15-36*). If the infarct results from vascular thrombosis due to vasculitis from fungus infection or other causes, the infarct may be round and not pleural based.

Pathologic features

Grossly, an acute infarct is roughly triangular, pleural based, hemorrhagic, with fibrinous pleuritis of the overlying pleura, or round if associated with infectious vasculitis (*Figures 15-37* and *15-38*). An organizing infact is gray or tan and contracted. Histologically, an early/acute infarcted area has edema, congestion, hemorrhage, and loss of cellular detail as a result of coagulative necrosis (*Figure 15-39*). Within 24 to 48 hours, neutrophil

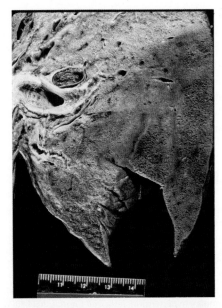

FIGURE 15-37 Gross photograph of a lung showing a triangular area of early infarction , and a thrombosed pulmonary artery branch close to the infarct.

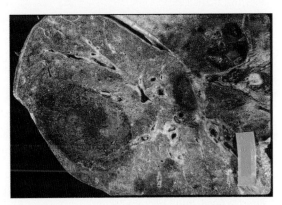

FIGURE 15-38 Gross photograph of the lung with multiple infarcts associated with thrombosed pulmonary artery branches, in a patient who had disseminated pulmonary aspergillosis with vasculitis and thrombosis. These infarcts are somewhat rounded in shape.

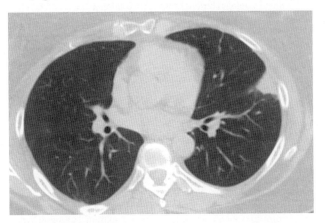

FIGURE 15-36 Chest CT obtained from a patient with pleuritic chest pain and dyspnea found to have a left pulmonary infarct represented as a wedge shaped defect.

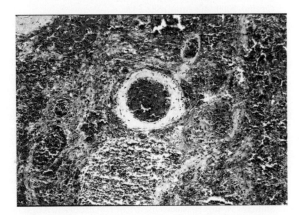

FIGURE 15-39 Photomicrograph of an infarct with hemorrhagic coagulative necrosis of pulmonary parenchyma. An infarcted small vessel may be seen in the center.

CHAPTER 15

infiltration may be seen at the periphery of the infarct, followed by macrophages and removal of necrotic debris, and hemosiderin deposition. Organization of the infarct follows with granulation tissue and remodeling starting from the periphery inward. A healed infarct manifests as a fibroelastic scar. The organization of an infarct depends on its size, with large infarcts taking several months to even 1 year for complete collagenization.

REFERENCES

1. Fishman AP. Clinical classification of pulmonary hypertension. *Clin Chest Med.* 2001;22(3):385-391, vii.
2. Hatano S, Strasser T. *Primary Pulmonary Hypertension : Report on a WHO Meeting, Geneva, 15-17 October 1973.* Geneva; Albany, NY: World Health Organization; distributed by Q Corporation; 1975.
3. Simonneau G, Galie N, Rubin LJ, et al. Clinical classification of pulmonary hypertension. *J Am Coll Cardiol.* 2004;43(12 suppl S): 5S-12S.
4. Rich S, Dantzker DR, Ayres SM, et al. Primary pulmonary hypertension. A national prospective study. *Ann Intern Med.* 1987;107(2):216-223.
5. Simonneau G, Robbins IM, Beghetti M, et al. Updated clinical classification of pulmonary hypertension. *J Am Coll Cardiol.* 2009;54(1 suppl):S43-S54.
6. Humbert M, Sitbon O, Chaouat A, et al. Pulmonary arterial hypertension in France: results from a national registry. *Am J Respir Crit Care Med.* 2006;173(9):1023-1030.
7. Peacock AJ, Murphy NF, McMurray JJ, Caballero L, Stewart S. An epidemiological study of pulmonary arterial hypertension. *Eur Respir J.* 2007;30(1):104-109.
8. D'Alonzo GE, Barst RJ, Ayres SM, et al. Survival in patients with primary pulmonary hypertension. Results from a national prospective registry. *Ann Intern Med.* 1991;115(5):343-349.
9. Badesch DB, Raskob GE, Elliott CG, et al. Pulmonary arterial hypertension: baseline characteristics from the REVEAL Registry. *Chest.* 2010;137(2):376-387.
10. Dresdale DT, Michtom RJ, Schultz M. Recent studies in primary pulmonary hypertension, including pharmacodynamic observations on pulmonary vascular resistance. *Bull N Y Acad Med.* 1954;30(3):195-207.
11. Machado RD, Eickelberg O, Elliott CG, et al. Genetics and genomics of pulmonary arterial hypertension. *J Am Coll Cardiol.* 2009;54(1 suppl):S32-S42.
12. Nichols WC, Koller DL, Slovis B, et al. Localization of the gene for familial primary pulmonary hypertension to chromosome 2q31-32. *Nat Genet.* 1997;15(3):277-280.
13. Morse JH, Jones AC, Barst RJ, Hodge SE, Wilhelmsen KC, Nygaard TG. Mapping of familial primary pulmonary hypertension locus (PPH1) to chromosome 2q31-q32. *Circulation.* 1997;95(12):2603-2606.
14. Austin ED, Ma L, LeDuc C, et al. Whole exome sequencing to identify a novel gene (caveolin-1) associated with human pulmonary arterial hypertension. *Circ Cardiovasc Genet.* 2012;5(3):336-343.
15. Nasim MT, Ogo T, Ahmed M, et al. Molecular genetic characterization of SMAD signaling molecules in pulmonary arterial hypertension. *Hum Mutat.* 2011;32(12):1385-1389.
16. Shintani M, Yagi H, Nakayama T, Saji T, Matsuoka R. A new nonsense mutation of SMAD8 associated with pulmonary arterial hypertension. *J Med Genet.* 2009;46(5):331-337.
17. Ma L, Roman-Campos D, Austin ED, et al. A novel channelopathy in pulmonary arterial hypertension. *N Engl J Med.* 2013;369(4):351-361.
18. Kay JM, Smith P, Heath D. Aminorex and the pulmonary circulation. *Thorax.* 1971;26(3):262-270.
19. Gurtner HP. Aminorex and pulmonary hypertension. A review. *Cor Vasa.* 1985;27(2-3):160-171.
20. Douglas JG, Munro JF, Kitchin AH, Muir AL, Proudfoot AT. Pulmonary hypertension and fenfluramine. *Br Med J (Clin Res Ed).* 1981;283(6296):881-883.
21. McMurray J, Bloomfield P, Miller HC. Irreversible pulmonary hypertension after treatment with fenfluramine. *Br Med J (Clin Res Ed).* 1986;293(6538):51 52.
22. Brenot F, Herve P, Petitpretz P, Parent F, Duroux P, Simonneau G. Primary pulmonary hypertension and fenfluramine use. *Br Heart J.* 1993;70(6):537-541.
23. Abenhaim L, Moride Y, Brenot F, et al. Appetite-suppressant drugs and the risk of primary pulmonary hypertension. International Primary Pulmonary Hypertension Study Group. *N Engl J Med.* 1996;335(9):609-616.
24. Mark EJ, Patalas ED, Chang HT, Evans RJ, Kessler SC. Fatal pulmonary hypertension associated with short-term use of fenfluramine and phentermine. *N Engl J Med.* 1997;337(9):602-606.
25. Souza R, Humbert M, Sztrymf B, et al. Pulmonary arterial hypertension associated with fenfluramine exposure: report of 109 cases. *Eur Respir J.* 2008;31(2):343-348.
26. Egermayer P, Town GI, Peacock AJ. Role of serotonin in the pathogenesis of acute and chronic pulmonary hypertension. *Thorax.* 1999;54(2):161-168.
27. Herve P, Drouet L, Dosquet C, et al. Primary pulmonary hypertension in a patient with a familial platelet storage pool disease: role of serotonin. *Am J Med.* 1990;89(1):117-120.
28. Alonso-Ruiz A, Calabozo M, Perez-Ruiz F, Mancebo L. Toxic oil syndrome. A long-term follow-up of a cohort of 332 patients. *Medicine (Baltimore).* 1993;72(5):285-295.
29. Gomez-Sanchez MA, Mestre de Juan MJ, Gomez-Pajuelo C, Lopez JI, Diaz de Atauri MJ, Martinez-Tello FJ. Pulmonary hypertension due to toxic oil syndrome. A clinicopathologic study. *Chest.* 1989;95(2):325-331.
30. Chin KM, Channick RN, Rubin LJ. Is methamphetamine use associated with idiopathic pulmonary arterial hypertension? *Chest.* 2006;130(6):1657-1663.
31. Montani D, Seferian A, Savale L, Simonneau G, Humbert M. Drug-induced pulmonary arterial hypertension: a recent outbreak. *Eur Respir Rev.* 2013;22(129):244-250.
32. Allcock RJ, Forrest I, Corris PA, Crook PR, Griffiths ID. A study of the prevalence of systemic sclerosis in northeast England. *Rheumatology (Oxford).* 2004;43(5):596-602.
33. Silman A, Akesson A, Newman J, et al. Assessment of functional ability in patients with scleroderma: a proposed new disability assessment instrument. *J Rheumatol.* 1998;25(1):79-83.
34. Tamaki T, Mori S, Takehara K. Epidemiological study of patients with systemic sclerosis in Tokyo. *Arch Dermatol Res.* 1991;283(6):366-371.
35. Mayes MD, Lacey JV Jr, Beebe-Dimmer J, et al. Prevalence, incidence, survival, and disease characteristics of systemic sclerosis in a large US population. *Arthritis Rheum.* 2003; 48(8):2246-2255.
36. Hachulla E, Gressin V, Guillevin L, et al. Early detection of pulmonary arterial hypertension in systemic sclerosis: a French nationwide prospective multicenter study. *Arthritis Rheum.* 2005;52(12):3792-3800.
37. Mukerjee D, St George D, Coleiro B, et al. Prevalence and outcome in systemic sclerosis associated pulmonary arterial hypertension: application of a registry approach. *Ann Rheum Dis.* 2003;62(11):1088-1093.

38. Fisher MR, Mathai SC, Champion HC, et al. Clinical differences between idiopathic and scleroderma-related pulmonary hypertension. *Arthritis Rheum.* 2006;54(9):3043-3050.

39. Launay D, Hachulla E, Hatron PY, Jais X, Simonneau G, Humbert M. Pulmonary arterial hypertension: a rare complication of primary Sjogren syndrome: report of 9 new cases and review of the literature. *Medicine (Baltimore).* 2007;86(5):299-315.

40. Kim KK, Factor SM. Membranoproliferative glomerulonephritis and plexogenic pulmonary arteriopathy in a homosexual man with acquired immunodeficiency syndrome. *Hum Pathol.* 1987;18(12):1293-1296.

41. Speich R, Jenni R, Opravil M, Pfab M, Russi EW. Primary pulmonary hypertension in HIV infection. *Chest.* 1991;100(5):1268-1271.

42. Sitbon O, Lascoux-Combe C, Delfraissy JF, et al. Prevalence of HIV-related pulmonary arterial hypertension in the current antiretroviral therapy era. *Am J Respir Crit Care Med.* 2008;177(1):108-113.

43. Degano B, Guillaume M, Savale L, et al. HIV-associated pulmonary arterial hypertension: survival and prognostic factors in the modern therapeutic era. *AIDS.* 2010;24(1):67-75.

44. Petitpretz P, Brenot F, Azarian R, et al. Pulmonary hypertension in patients with human immunodeficiency virus infection. Comparison with primary pulmonary hypertension. *Circulation.* 1994;89(6):2722-2727.

45. Mette SA, Palevsky HI, Pietra GG, et al. Primary pulmonary hypertension in association with human immunodeficiency virus infection. A possible viral etiology for some forms of hypertensive pulmonary arteriopathy. *Am Rev Respir Dis.* 1992;145(5):1196-1200.

46. Flores SC, Almodovar S. Human immunodeficiency virus, herpes virus infections, and pulmonary vascular disease. *Pulm Circ.* 2013;3(1):165-170.

47. Marecki JC, Cool CD, Parr JE, et al. HIV-1 Nef is associated with complex pulmonary vascular lesions in SHIV-nef-infected macaques. *Am J Respir Crit Care Med.* 2006;174(4):437-445.

48. Spikes L, Dalvi P, Tawfik O, et al. Enhanced pulmonary arteriopathy in simian immunodeficiency virus-infected macaques exposed to morphine. *Am J Respir Crit Care Med.* 2012;185(11):1235-1243.

49. Swain SD, Han S, Harmsen A, Shampeny K, Harmsen AG. Pulmonary hypertension can be a sequela of prior Pneumocystis pneumonia. *Am J Pathol.* 2007;171(3):790-799.

50. Morse JH, Barst RJ, Itescu S, et al. Primary pulmonary hypertension in HIV infection: an outcome determined by particular HLA class II alleles. *Am J Respir Crit Care Med.* 1996;153(4 pt 1):1299-1301.

51. George MP, Champion HC, Gladwin MT, Norris KA, Morris A. Injection drug use as a "second hit" in the pathogenesis of HIV-associated pulmonary hypertension. *Am J Respir Crit Care Med.* 2012;185(11):1144-1146.

52. Mantz FA Jr, Craige E. Portal axis thrombosis with spontaneous portacaval shunt and resultant cor pulmonale. *AMA Arch Pathol.* 1951;52(1):91-97.

53. Edwards BS, Weir EK, Edwards WD, Ludwig J, Dykoski RK, Edwards JE. Coexistent pulmonary and portal hypertension: morphologic and clinical features. *J Am Coll Cardiol.* 1987;10(6):1233-1238.

54. Hadengue A, Benhayoun MK, Lebrec D, Benhamou JP. Pulmonary hypertension complicating portal hypertension: prevalence and relation to splanchnic hemodynamics. *Gastroenterology.* 1991;100(2):520-528.

55. Le Pavec J, Souza R, Herve P, et al. Portopulmonary hypertension: survival and prognostic factors. *Am J Respir Crit Care Med.* 2008;178(6):637-643.

56. Budhiraja R, Hassoun PM. Portopulmonary hypertension: a tale of two circulations. *Chest.* 2003;123(2):562-576.

57. Ramsay MA, Simpson BR, Nguyen AT, Ramsay KJ, East C, Klintmalm GB. Severe pulmonary hypertension in liver transplant candidates. *Liver Transpl Surg.* 1997;3(5):494-500.

58. Fritz JS, Fallon MB, Kawut SM. Pulmonary vascular complications of liver disease. *Am J Respir Crit Care Med.* 2013;187(2):133-143.

59. Kawut SM, Taichman DB, Ahya VN, et al. Hemodynamics and survival of patients with portopulmonary hypertension. *Liver Transpl.* 2005;11(9):1107-1111.

60. Robalino BD, Moodie DS. Association between primary pulmonary hypertension and portal hypertension: analysis of its pathophysiology and clinical, laboratory and hemodynamic manifestations. *J Am Coll Cardiol.* 1991;17(2):492-498.

61. Swanson KL, Wiesner RH, Nyberg SL, Rosen CB, Krowka MJ. Survival in portopulmonary hypertension: Mayo Clinic experience categorized by treatment subgroups. *Am J Transplant.* 2008;8(11):2445-2453.

62. Krowka MJ, Miller DP, Barst RJ, et al. Portopulmonary hypertension: a report from the US-based REVEAL Registry. *Chest.* 2012;141(4):906-915.

63. Wood P. The Eisenmenger syndrome or pulmonary hypertension with reversed central shunt. *I Br Med J.* 1958;2(5098):701-709.

64. Galie N, Hoeper MM, Humbert M, et al. Guidelines for the diagnosis and treatment of pulmonary hypertension: the Task Force for the Diagnosis and Treatment of Pulmonary Hypertension of the European Society of Cardiology (ESC) and the European Respiratory Society (ERS), endorsed by the International Society of Heart and Lung Transplantation (ISHLT). *Eur Heart J.* 2009;30(20):2493-2537.

65. Friedman WF. Proceedings of National Heart, Lung, and Blood Institute pediatric cardiology workshop: pulmonary hypertension. *Pediatr Res.* 1986;20(9):811-824.

66. Marelli AJ, Mackie AS, Ionescu-Ittu R, Rahme E, Pilote L. Congenital heart disease in the general population: changing prevalence and age distribution. *Circulation.* 2007;115(2):163-172.

67. Duffels MG, Engelfriet PM, Berger RM, et al. Pulmonary arterial hypertension in congenital heart disease: an epidemiologic perspective from a Dutch registry. *Int J Cardiol.* 2007;120(2):198-204.

68. Chaves E. The pathology of the arterial pulmonary vasculature in manson's schistosomiasis. *Dis Chest.* 1966;50(1):72-77.

69. Lapa MS, Ferreira EV, Jardim C, Martins Bdo C, Arakaki JS, Souza R. [Clinical characteristics of pulmonary hypertension patients in two reference centers in the city of Sao Paulo]. *Rev Assoc Med Bras.* 2006;52(3):139-143.

70. Simonneau G. [A new clinical classification of pulmonary hypertension]. *Bull Acad Natl Med.* 2009;193(8):1897-1909.

71. Beghetti M, Galie N. Eisenmenger syndrome a clinical perspective in a new therapeutic era of pulmonary arterial hypertension. *J Am Coll Cardiol.* 2009;53(9):733-740.

72. Collins-Nakai RL, Rabinovitch M. Pulmonary vascular obstructive disease. *Cardiol Clin.* 1993;11(4):675-687.

73. Hopkins WE, Ochoa LL, Richardson GW, Trulock EP. Comparison of the hemodynamics and survival of adults with severe primary pulmonary hypertension or Eisenmenger syndrome. *J Heart Lung Transplant.* 1996;15(1 pt 1):100-105.

74. Manes A, Palazzini M, Leci E, Bacchi Reggiani ML, Branzi A, Galie N. Current era survival of patients with pulmonary arterial hypertension associated with congenital heart disease: a comparison between clinical subgroups. *Eur Heart J.* 2014;35(11):716-724.

75. Miller AC, Gladwin MT. Pulmonary complications of sickle cell disease. *Am J Respir Crit Care Med.* 2012;185(11):1154-1165.

76. Haque AK, Gokhale S, Rampy BA, Adegboyega P, Duarte A, Saldana MJ. Pulmonary hypertension in sickle cell hemoglobinopathy: a clinicopathologic study of 20 cases. *Hum Pathol.* 2002;33(10):1037-1043.

CHAPTER 15

77. Ataga KI, Moore CG, Jones S, et al. Pulmonary hypertension in patients with sickle cell disease: a longitudinal study. *Br J Haematol.* 2006;134(1):109-115.

78. Fonseca GH, Souza R, Salemi VM, Jardim CV, Gualandro SF. Pulmonary hypertension diagnosed by right heart catheterisation in sickle cell disease. *Eur Respir J.* 2012;39(1):112-118.

79. Gladwin MT, Sachdev V, Jison ML, et al. Pulmonary hypertension as a risk factor for death in patients with sickle cell disease. *N Engl J Med.* 2004;350(9):886-895.

80. Parent F, Bachir D, Inamo J, et al. A hemodynamic study of pulmonary hypertension in sickle cell disease. *N Engl J Med.* 2011;365(1):44-53.

81. Smith P, Heath D. Electron microscopy of the plexiform lesion. *Thorax.* 1979;34(2):177-186.

82. Heath D, Edwards JE. The pathology of hypertensive pulmonary vascular disease; a description of six grades of structural changes in the pulmonary arteries with special reference to congenital cardiac septal defects. *Circulation.* 1958;18(4 pt 1): 533-547.

83. Lantuejoul S, Sheppard MN, Corrin B, Burke MM, Nicholson AG. Pulmonary veno-occlusive disease and pulmonary capillary hemangiomatosis: a clinicopathologic study of 35 cases. *Am J Surg Pathol.* 2006;30(7):850-857.

84. Heath D, Segel N, Bishop J. Pulmonary veno-occlusive disease. *Circulation.* 1966;34(2):242-248.

85. Mandel J, Mark EJ, Hales CA. Pulmonary veno-occlusive disease. *Am J Respir Crit Care Med.* 2000;162(5):1964-1973.

86. Montani D, Achouh L, Dorfmuller P, et al. Pulmonary veno-occlusive disease: clinical, functional, radiologic, and hemodynamic characteristics and outcome of 24 cases confirmed by histology. *Medicine (Baltimore).* 2008;87(4):220-233.

87. Montani D, Price LC, Dorfmuller P, et al. Pulmonary veno-occlusive disease. *Eur Respir J.* 2009;33(1):189-200.

88. Wagenvoort CA, Beetstra A, Spijker J. Capillary haemangiomatosis of the lungs. *Histopathology.* 1978;2(6):401-406.

89. Eltorky MA, Headley AS, Winer-Muram H, Garrett HE Jr, Griffin JP. Pulmonary capillary hemangiomatosis: a clinicopathologic review. *Ann Thorac Surg.* 1994;57(3):772-776.

90. Tron V, Magee F, Wright JL, Colby T, Churg A. Pulmonary capillary hemangiomatosis. *Hum Pathol.* 1986;17(11):1144-1150.

91. Almagro P, Julia J, Sanjaume M, et al. Pulmonary capillary hemangiomatosis associated with primary pulmonary hypertension: report of 2 new cases and review of 35 cases from the literature. *Medicine (Baltimore).* 2002;81(6):417-424.

92. Frazier AA, Franks TJ, Mohammed TL, Ozbudak IH, Galvin JR. From the archives of the AFIP: pulmonary veno-occlusive disease and pulmonary capillary hemangiomatosis. *Radiographics.* 2007;27(3):867-882.

93. Guazzi M, Borlaug BA. Pulmonary hypertension due to left heart disease. *Circulation.* 2012;126(8):975-990.

94. Alexopoulos D, Lazzam C, Borrico S, Fiedler L, Ambrose JA. Isolated chronic mitral regurgitation with preserved systolic left ventricular function and severe pulmonary hypertension. *J Am Coll Cardiol.* 1989;14(2):319-322.

95. Aurigemma GP, Gaasch WH. Clinical practice. Diastolic heart failure. *N Engl J Med.* 2004;351(11):1097-1105.

96. Hoeper MM, Barbera JA, Channick RN, et al. Diagnosis, assessment, and treatment of non-pulmonary arterial hypertension pulmonary hypertension. *J Am Coll Cardiol.* 2009; 54(1 suppl):S85-S96.

97. Willens HJ, Chirinos JA, Gomez-Marin O, et al. Noninvasive differentiation of pulmonary arterial and venous hypertension using conventional and Doppler tissue imaging echocardiography. *J Am Soc Echocardiogr.* 2008;21(6):715-719.

98. Thenappan T, Shah SJ, Gomberg-Maitland M, et al. Clinical characteristics of pulmonary hypertension in patients with heart failure and preserved ejection fraction. *Circ Heart Fail.* 2011;4(3):257-265.

99. Andersen KH, Iversen M, Kjaergaard J, et al. Prevalence, predictors, and survival in pulmonary hypertension related to end-stage chronic obstructive pulmonary disease. *J Heart Lung Transplant.* 2012;31(4):373-380.

100. Minai OA, Chaouat A, Adnot S. Pulmonary hypertension in COPD: epidemiology, significance, and management: pulmonary vascular disease: the global perspective. *Chest.* 2010;137(6 suppl):39S-51S.

101. Thabut G, Dauriat G, Stern JB, et al. Pulmonary hemodynamics in advanced COPD candidates for lung volume reduction surgery or lung transplantation. *Chest.* 2005;127(5):1531-1536.

102. Chaouat A, Bugnet AS, Kadaoui N, et al. Severe pulmonary hypertension and chronic obstructive pulmonary disease. *Am J Respir Crit Care Med.* 2005;172(2):189-194.

103. Lettieri CJ, Nathan SD, Barnett SD, Ahmad S, Shorr AF. Prevalence and outcomes of pulmonary arterial hypertension in advanced idiopathic pulmonary fibrosis. *Chest.* 2006;129(3):746-752.

104. Shorr AF, Wainright JL, Cors CS, Lettieri CJ, Nathan SD. Pulmonary hypertension in patients with pulmonary fibrosis awaiting lung transplant. *Eur Respir J.* 2007;30(4):715-721.

105. Zisman DA, Ross DJ, Belperio JA, et al. Prediction of pulmonary hypertension in idiopathic pulmonary fibrosis. *Respir Med.* 2007;101(10):2153-2159.

106. Sajkov D, Cowie RJ, Thornton AT, Espinoza HA, McEvoy RD. Pulmonary hypertension and hypoxemia in obstructive sleep apnea syndrome. *Am J Respir Crit Care Med.* 1994;149(2 pt 1): 416-422.

107. Chaouat A, Weitzenblum E, Krieger J, Oswald M, Kessler R. Pulmonary hemodynamics in the obstructive sleep apnea syndrome. Results in 220 consecutive patients. *Chest.* 1996;109(2):380-386.

108. Bady E, Achkar A, Pascal S, Orvoen-Frija E, Laaban JP. Pulmonary arterial hypertension in patients with sleep apnoea syndrome. *Thorax.* 2000;55(11):934-939.

109. Fedullo PF, Auger WR, Kerr KM, Rubin LJ. Chronic thromboembolic pulmonary hypertension. *N Engl J Med.* 2001;345(20):1465-1472.

110. Pepke-Zaba J, Delcroix M, Lang I, et al. Chronic thromboembolic pulmonary hypertension (CTEPH): results from an international prospective registry. *Circulation.* 2011;124(18):1973-1981.

111. Tapson VF, Humbert M. Incidence and prevalence of chronic thromboembolic pulmonary hypertension: from acute to chronic pulmonary embolism. *Proc Am Thorac Soc.* 2006;3(7):564-567.

112. Dalen JE, Alpert JS. Natural history of pulmonary embolism. *Prog Cardiovasc Dis.* 1975;17(4):259-270.

113. Fedullo P, Kerr KM, Kim NH, Auger WR. Chronic thromboembolic pulmonary hypertension. *Am J Respir Crit Care Med.* 2011;183(12):1605-1613.

114. Pengo V, Lensing AW, Prins MH, et al. Incidence of chronic thromboembolic pulmonary hypertension after pulmonary embolism. *N Engl J Med.* 2004;350(22):2257-2264.

115. Bonderman D, Wilkens H, Wakounig S, et al. Risk factors for chronic thromboembolic pulmonary hypertension. *Eur Respir J.* 2009;33(2):325-331.

116. Jais X, Ioos V, Jardim C, et al. Splenectomy and chronic thromboembolic pulmonary hypertension. *Thorax.* 2005;60(12):1031-1034.

117. Lang I, Kerr K. Risk factors for chronic thromboembolic pulmonary hypertension. *Proc Am Thorac Soc.* 2006;3(7):568-570.

118. Wolf M, Boyer-Neumann C, Parent F, et al. Thrombotic risk factors in pulmonary hypertension. *Eur Respir J.* 2000;15(2):395-399.

119. Bernard J, Yi ES. Pulmonary thromboendarterectomy: a clinicopathologic study of 200 consecutive pulmonary

thromboendarterectomy cases in one institution. *Hum Pathol.* 2007;38(6):871-877.

120. Galie N, Kim NH. Pulmonary microvascular disease in chronic thromboembolic pulmonary hypertension. *Proc Am Thorac Soc.* 2006;3(7):571-576.

121. Dingli D, Utz JP, Krowka MJ, Oberg AL, Tefferi A. Unexplained pulmonary hypertension in chronic myeloproliferative disorders. *Chest.* 2001;120(3):801-808.

122. Guilpain P, Montani D, Damaj G, et al. Pulmonary hypertension associated with myeloproliferative disorders: a retrospective study of ten cases. *Respiration.* 2008;76(3):295-302.

123. Nunes H, Humbert M, Capron F, et al. Pulmonary hypertension associated with sarcoidosis: mechanisms, haemodynamics and prognosis. *Thorax.* 2006;61(1):68-74.

124. Taveira-DaSilva AM, Hathaway OM, Sachdev V, Shizukuda Y, Birdsall CW, Moss J. Pulmonary artery pressure in lymphangioleiomyomatosis: an echocardiographic study. *Chest.* 2007;132(5):1573-1578.

125. Engel PJ, Baughman RP, Menon SG, Kereiakes DJ, Taylor L, Scott M. Pulmonary hypertension in neurofibromatosis. *Am J Cardiol.* 2007;99(8):1177-1178.

126. Samuels N, Berkman N, Milgalter E, Bar-Ziv J, Amir G, Kramer MR. Pulmonary hypertension secondary to neurofibromatosis: intimal fibrosis versus thromboembolism. *Thorax.* 1999;54(9):858-859.

127. Theise ND, Ursell PC. Pulmonary hypertension and Gaucher's disease: logical association or mere coincidence? *Am J Pediatr Hematol Oncol.* 1990;12(1):74-76.

128. Hamaoka K, Nakagawa M, Furukawa N, Sawada T. Pulmonary hypertension in type I glycogen storage disease. *Pediatr Cardiol.* 1990;11(1):54-56.

129. Chu JW, Kao PN, Faul JL, Doyle RL. High prevalence of autoimmune thyroid disease in pulmonary arterial hypertension. *Chest.* 2002;122(5):1668-1673.

130. Dot JM, Sztrymf B, Yaici A, et al. [Pulmonary arterial hypertension due to tumor emboli]. *Rev Mal Respir.* 2007;24(3 pt 1):359-366.

131. Yigla M, Nakhoul F, Sabag A, et al. Pulmonary hypertension in patients with end-stage renal disease. *Chest.* 2003;123(5):1577-1582.

132. Nakhoul F, Yigla M, Gilman R, Reisner SA, Abassi Z. The pathogenesis of pulmonary hypertension in haemodialysis patients via arterio-venous access. *Nephrol Dial Transplant.* 2005;20(8):1686-1692.

133. Horlander KT, Mannino DM, Leeper KV. Pulmonary embolism mortality in the United States, 1979-1998: an analysis using multiple-cause mortality data. *Arch Intern Med.* 2003;163(14):1711-1717.

134. Burge AJ, Freeman KD, Klapper PJ, Haramati LB. Increased diagnosis of pulmonary embolism without a corresponding decline in mortality during the CT era. *Clin Radiol.* 2008;63(4):381-386.

135. DeMonaco NA, Dang Q, Kapoor WN, Ragni MV. Pulmonary embolism incidence is increasing with use of spiral computed tomography. *Am J Med.* 2008;121(7):611-617.

136. Silverstein MD, Heit JA, Mohr DN, Petterson TM, O'Fallon WM, Melton LJ 3rd. Trends in the incidence of deep vein thrombosis and pulmonary embolism: a 25-year population-based study. *Arch Intern Med.* 1998;158(6):585-593.

137. Heit JA. The epidemiology of venous thromboembolism in the community. *Arterioscler Thromb Vasc Biol.* 2008;28(3):370-372.

138. Malek J, Rogers R, Kufera J, Hirshon JM. Venous thromboembolic disease in the HIV-infected patient. *Am J Emerg Med.*;29(3):278-282.

139. Dudney TM, Elliott CG. Pulmonary embolism from amniotic fluid, fat, and air. *Prog Cardiovasc Dis.* 1994;36(6):447-474.

140. Abramowsky CR, Pickett JP, Goodfellow BC, Bradford WD. Comparative demonstration of pulmonary fat emboli by "en bloc" osmium tetroxide and oil red O methods. *Hum Pathol.* 1981;12(8):753-755.

141. Orenstein JM, Sato N, Aaron B, Buchholz B, Bloom S. Microemboli observed in deaths following cardiopulmonary bypass surgery: silicone antifoam agents and polyvinyl chloride tubing as sources of emboli. *Hum Pathol.* 1982;13(12):1082-1090.

142. Soares FA, Pinto AP, Landell GA, de Oliveira JA. Pulmonary tumor embolism to arterial vessels and carcinomatous lymphangitis. A comparative clinicopathological study. *Arch Pathol Lab Med.* 1993;117(8):827-831.

143. Roberts KE, Hamele-Bena D, Saqi A, Stein CA, Cole RP. Pulmonary tumor embolism: a review of the literature. *Am J Med.* 2003;115(3):228-232.

144. Marcus BJ, Collins KA, Harley RA. Ancillary studies in amniotic fluid embolism: a case report and review of the literature. *Am J Forensic Med Pathol.* 2005;26(1):92-95.

145. Frazier AA, Galvin JR, Franks TJ, Rosado-De-Christenson ML. From the archives of the AFIP: pulmonary vasculature: hypertension and infarction. *Radiographics.* 2000;20(2):491-524; quiz 30-31, 32.

146. Dalen JE, Haffajee CI, Alpert JS 3rd, Howe JP, Ockene IS, Paraskos JA. Pulmonary embolism, pulmonary hemorrhage and pulmonary infarction. *N Engl J Med.* 1977;296(25):1431-1435.

147. Tsao MS, Schraufnagel D, Wang NS. Pathogenesis of pulmonary infarction. *Am J Med.* 1982;72(4):599-606.

Hemorrhage and Vasculitis

Deepika Sirohi and Jaishree Jagirdar

TAKE HOME PEARLS

- Diffuse alveolar hemorrhage is a clinicopathologic syndrome with widespread bleeding into the alveoli derived from alveolar capillaries and venules.
- Pulmonary hemorrhage may be a part of diffuse alveolar injury due to any cause or may be secondary to capillaritis.
- Diffuse alveolar damage is a histologic pattern of acute lung injury most often encountered in acute respiratory distress syndrome that may occur secondary to a variety of etiologies including infections, sepsis, trauma, aspiration, inhalational injury, drug reaction, and metabolic disorders.
- Congestive vasculopathy refers to elevated pulmonary venous pressure, often secondary to elevated left atrial pressure, which results in rupture of small capillaries with local hemorrhage with hemosiderin deposition. Over time, fibrosis of alveolar septa along with hemosiderin deposition, also known as "brown induration" of the lung occurs.
- Hemosiderin-laden macrophages ("heart-failure cells") provide evidence of chronic hemorrhage within the alveolar spaces in congestive vasculopathy.
- Idiopathic pulmonary hemosiderosis is a very rare disease mostly affecting children and causing recurrent episodes of diffuse alveolar hemorrhage leading to pulmonary fibrosis in the absence of vasculitis or capillaritis.
- The underlying anomaly in arteriovenous malformations is an abnormal and direct communication between pulmonary arteries and veins through small aneurysms resulting in right-to-left shunt.

Approximately 95% of AVMs originate from the pulmonary arteries.
- Pulmonary vasculitis may present in a number of ways including recurrent alveolar hemorrhage, pulmonary nodules, cavitating lesions, or airway disease depending on the disease process and patient-related factors. The disease process may be centered on small, medium, or less commonly large vessels and may be either immune mediated or not.
- Diffuse pulmonary hemorrhage has been reported in systemic lupus erythematosus, rheumatoid arthritis, and juvenile rheumatoid arthritis, but can probably occur in any of the collagen vascular diseases.
- Granulomatosis with polyangiitis (GPA), formerly known as Wegener granulomatosis, is a multisystem disorder characterized by aseptic necrotizing granulomatous vasculitis predominantly involving the upper respiratory tract, lower respiratory tract, and the kidney.
- Pulmonary involvement occurs in 55% to 90% of patients with GPA.
- Antineutrophil cytoplasmic antibodies (ANCA) when positive are useful to establish of GPA and also monitor therapy. However, they should be interpreted in appropriate clinical context and are not absolute for diagnosis.
- The major histologic diagnostic criteria for GPA include vasculitis, granulomatous inflammation, and parenchymal necrosis.
- Most patients with antiglomerular basement membrane antibody disease or Goodpasture syndrome have both diffuse alveolar hemorrhage and glomerulonephritis.

- Eosinophilic granulomatosis with polyangiitis or Churg-Strauss syndrome is a rare systemic vasculitis of small and medium-sized vessels associated with severe asthma and blood and tissue eosinophilia.
- Microscopic polyangiitis is a systemic necrotizing small vessel vasculitis involving the arterioles, venules, and capillaries and is characterized by few or no immune deposits.
- Necrotizing glomerulonephritis is present in almost all patients with microscopic polyangiitis and the characteristic pulmonary manifestation when present is diffuse pulmonary hemorrhage resulting from small vessel vasculitis (capillaritis).
- Behcet disease is a vasculitis affecting vessels of any size characterized by relapsing uveitis (iridocyclitis), oral and genital ulcers. Pulmonary artery aneurysm is the most common pulmonary manifestation.
- Henoch-Schonlein purpura is an acute self-limited systemic small vessel vasculitis presenting with a tetrad of palpable purpura, abdominal pain, arthralgias, and nephritis that rarely causes pulmonary hemorrhage secondary to small vessel vasculitis.
- Polyarteritis nodosa is a systemic necrotizing vasculitis that can involve medium-sized and small arteries of any organ, but only rarely involves the lungs.
- Pulmonary involvement is common as interstitial lung disease in cryoglobulinemia and leukocytoclastic vasculitis of medium-sized arteries and small vessel vasculitis with pulmonary hemorrhage have been reported.
- Pulmonary involvement in Takayasu arteritis occurs in 12% to 86% of cases by angiography. Arteritis is histologically seen as an infiltrate of lymphocytes, macrophages, giant cells predominantly in the outer two-thirds of the vessel wall, sometimes with a thrombus, leading to stenosis and aneurysm.
- Giant cell arteritis (GCA) is a disease most common to the temporal arteries and rarely both the main pulmonary artery (rare) and the trunk can be affected by a giant cell infiltrate, resulting in destruction of the elastic fibers and fibrinoid necrosis.
- Systemic conditions that may be associated with pulmonary vasculitis include inflammatory bowel disease, malignant neoplasm, and sarcoidosis.
- Localized vasculitis and secondary vasculitis may be due to drugs and toxins, interstitial lung diseases, emboli, infection, pulmonary hypertension, transplantation, and radiation.

DEFINITION OF PULMONARY HEMORRHAGE

Diffuse alveolar hemorrhage is a clinicopathologic syndrome with widespread bleeding into the alveoli derived from alveolar capillaries and venules.

Pulmonary hemorrhage may be a part of diffuse alveolar injury due to any cause or may be secondary to capillaritis. Clinically, DAH is recognized by hemoptysis, anemia, diffuse radiographic pulmonary infiltrates, and hypoxemic respiratory failure. Pulmonary hemorrhage is hard to diagnose solely based on morphology, unless there are hemosiderin-laden macrophages in the tissue in association with the appropriate clinical findings, since fresh blood can be present in alveolar spaces as part of the procedure.

ACUTE HEMORRHAGE

Diffuse Alveolar Damage

Acute respiratory distress syndrome (ARDS) was first reported by Ashbaugh et al in 1967 to define rapid onset of tachypnea and hypoxemia with loss of lung compliance and bilateral lung infiltrates on chest radiographs in otherwise healthy individuals.[1] Clinically, a screening criterion was defined by the American-European Consensus Conference to identify patients with ARDS. These include the presence of acute severe hypoxemia (defined as a ratio of arterial oxygen tension over fractional inspired oxygen (PaO_2/FiO_2) <200 mm Hg (26.7 kpa)), bilateral infiltrates on chest radiography (CXR), and the absence of raised pulmonary artery wedge.[2] The estimated incidence of ARDS and acute lung injury varies due to the limitations of the diagnostic criteria. A study of critical care units in the USA in 2005 estimated the incidence of ARDS to be 58/100,000 person-years with 141,500 new cases per year and an annual death rate of 59,000 per year.[3]

Diffuse alveolar damage (DAD) is a histologic pattern of acute lung injury most often encountered in ARDS that may occur secondary to a variety of etiologies. Common etiologies include infections, sepsis, trauma, aspiration, inhalational injury, drug reaction, and metabolic disorders. Outcome of the disease varies with underlying etiology; patients with DAD secondary to trauma do better than patients with sepsis.[3] Genetic predisposition,[4] chronic alcohol abuse,[5] age, chronic liver disease, immunosuppression,[6] and obesity[7] are all associated with the development of acute lung injury, whereas diabetes mellitus appears to be protective.[8]

On occasion, no underlying cause is determined and for such idiopathic cases, the term "acute interstitial pneumonia" (AIP) is applied. Correlation of clinical and laboratory data is helpful to ascertain the etiology.

Clinical features

Patients with ARDS characteristically presents with rapidly progressive respiratory failure developing within 24 to 48 hours following an initiating event. Respiratory failure manifests as dyspnea, tachypnea, and profound hypoxemia unresponsive to oxygen therapy with nearly all patients requiring mechanical ventilation.

Radiologic features

X-rays of chest classically demonstrate patchy air space consolidation that rapidly progresses to diffuse bilateral infiltrates ("white out"). The findings may mimic acute cardiogenic pulmonary edema. Additionally, air bronchogram and occasionally pleural effusions may be present. The findings on computed tomography parallel the chest x-rays with patchy consolidation more pronounced in dependent regions. As the disease progresses, areas of consolidation are replaced by fibrosis that are seen as linear opacities.

Pathologic features

A temporally homogeneous pattern of changes are seen in the lungs as the disease progresses from the acute edema phase to the phase of organization and fibrosis.

Gross

In the acute phase the lungs are dark, red, heavy, and consolidated. As the disease progresses, they become more fibrotic with firm yellowish-gray cut surface. The end-stage fibrotic phase has a cobble stone appearance with areas of scarring and microcystic change.

Microscopic

Histologically the evolution of DAD can be divided into two phases: the acute or exudative phase and the organizing or proliferative phase. These two phases are not separate and instead represent a continuum of changes. The changes in lungs are diffuse and temporally uniform.

The acute or exudative phase begins 1 to 2 days following initial pulmonary insult. The earliest changes occur at the ultrastructural level and include injury to the type 1 pneumocytes and capillary endothelial cells, which are the critical initiating events of DAD. On light microscopy these are seen as capillary congestion and intra-alveolar edema that develop over the next few hours (*Figure 16-1*). The defining feature of DAD, "hyaline membranes" begin to appear by day 2, peaking by day 4 or 5. The hyaline membranes are composed of necrotic alveolar epithelial cells and serum proteins extruded from the damaged capillaries. The hyaline membranes appear as dense glassy eosinophilic membranes lining the alveolar septa with accentuation along the alveolar ducts. Inflammation is characteristically sparse in absence of acute pneumonia.

Within 5 to 7 days following injury the disease evolves to the organizing (proliferative) phase centered on the interstitium. During this phase the hyaline

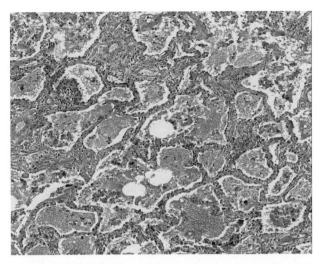

FIGURE 16-1 **Diffuse alveolar damage in a patient with systemic lupus erythematosus (SLE): alveolar spaces filled with eosinophilic edema fluid (H&E, 100×).**

membranes are phagocytosed by macrophages or transformed into granulation tissue by myofibroblasts. Loose expansile myxoid fibroblastic tissue and proliferating small blood vessels expand the interstitium. These areas of organization have a distinct pale blue-gray appearance in contrast to eosinophilic collagen fibrosis. Reactive type 2 pneumocyte and fibroblast hyperplasia usually accompanies the reparative phase and may be quite pronounced with focal atypical features. Over time alveolar collapse, organization and type II pneumocyte proliferation give the appearance of alveolar thickening. Alveolar collapse, interstitial edema, and squamous metaplasia may be present. Thrombi may be present in both phases. Ischemic changes may occur secondary to thrombi or vascular remodeling.

An end-stage, infrequent, fibrotic phase has been described by some authors. Dense collagenous fibrosis replaces foci of organization. Like other end-stage lung disease, honeycomb changes may be seen infrequently, accompanied by traction bronchiectasis.

Pathologic consideration

DAD may be difficult to diagnose on small biopsy and often requires a wedge biopsy for precise classification. A careful correlation of clinical and laboratory data is useful to ascertain the underlying cause. It is recommended that all cases should be routinely stained for fungi, mycobacteria, and bacteria. A diligent search for granulomas and viral inclusions should be done and immunohistochemical staining for cytomegalovirus, herpes simplex virus, and respiratory viruses should be considered especially in immunocompromised hosts, particularly in the presence of an equivocal viral cytopathic morphology.

Differential diagnosis

Acute eosinophilic pneumonia
Histologically, hyaline membranes similar to DAD may be seen in acute eosinophilic pneumonia, but additionally they have a prominent eosinophilic infiltrate. Intra-alveolar fibrin and macrophages are seen in the chronic phase. Since acute eosinophilic pneumonia has a good response to corticosteroid therapy, it is important to differentiate the two.

Nonspecific interstitial pneumonia fibrosing variant
The fibrosis in nonspecific interstitial pneumonia (NSIP) is characteristically diffuse established collagenous fibrosis rather than the loose myxoid fibrosis of DAD. NSIP lacks pronounced type II pneumocyte hyperplasia. On careful search hyaline membranes are often identified in DAD. Occasionally it may be impossible to separate the two.

Usual interstitial pneumonia
The fibrosis in usual interstitial pneumonia (UIP) is characteristically patchy and temporally heterogeneous in contrast to diffuse and uniform fibrosis of DAD. DAD may be superimposed on UIP and in these instances; close attention to the background pattern of injury may be helpful.

Organizing pneumonia/cryptogenic organizing pneumonia
The fibrosis in organizing pneumonia (OP) is patchy and intraluminal fibrosis as opposed to predominantly interstitial fibrosis in DAD. Type 2 pneumocyte hyperplasia is subtle and hyaline membranes are not seen.

Diffuse alveolar hemorrhage
Blood, fibrin, and macrophages fill the alveolar spaces in diffuse alveolar hemorrhage with lack of hyaline membranes. With organization the fibrosis is intraluminal and not interstitial as in DAD. Necrosis of alveolar septa may be accompanied by neutrophilic capillaritis. This should be differentiated from neutrophilic sequestration in DAD.

Acute fibrinous and organizing pneumonia
Intra-alveolar fibrin with absence of hyaline membranes defines acute fibrinous and organizing pneumonia. The disease is often patchy unlike DAD.

Therapy
The mainstay of treatment of ARDS involves general supportive measures necessary combined with focused ventilatory strategies and appropriate treatment of the underlying conditions.[9] Despite advances in mechanical ventilation mortality rate from DAD continues to be high at around 36% to 44%.[10] In patients who survive, radiographs improve and pulmonary function returns to normal in 6 months to a year, although patients with significant fibrosis may retain some restrictive deficit.[11]

Congestive Vasculopathy

Congestive vasculopathy refers to elevated pulmonary venous pressure, often secondary to elevated left atrial pressure. This is a passive process resulting in locally increased blood volume within the pulmonary vasculature with consequent edema and congestion. Long-standing chronic passive venous congestion causes chronic hypoxia with ischemic tissue injury and scarring. Rupture of small capillaries results in local hemorrhage with hemosiderin deposition. Over time, these events lead to fibrosis of alveolar septa along with hemosiderin deposition, also known as "brown induration" of the lung. Additionally pulmonary arteries, veins, and arterioles can be remodeled.

Clinical features

The most common cause of pulmonary hypertension and congestive vasculopathy is chronic congestive heart failure with elevated left atrial pressure. Clinically orthopnea and paroxysmal nocturnal dyspnea are the presenting features that gradually progress to exertional dyspnea. With long-standing disease, the pulmonary artery pressures are elevated and eventually result in right-sided heart failure. On chest x-rays, there is an increase in size of the major vessels in upper lobes as compared to the lower lobes. Other findings include cardiomegaly and pulmonary edema. In mitral stenosis there may be prominence of left atrial appendage.

Pathologic features:

Gross
The gross changes in lung include fibrosis and discoloration due to hemosiderin deposition, also known as "brown induration" of lung.

Microscopic
The histologic findings are characterized by changes most conspicuous in the vasculature including the pulmonary veins, arteries, and arterioles which are obviously remodeled. The pulmonary veins undergo "arterialization" and become thickened due to smooth muscle hypertrophy of the media. They acquire an external elastic lamina that can be better appreciated on elastic stains. The venous adventitia becomes fibrotic. Medial hypertrophy is also seen in the arteries that become thickened and there is acquisition of a *muscular* layer in the arterioles. With increase in the venous pressure, the lymphatics within interlobular septa become

dilated. Hemosiderin-laden macrophages ("heart-failure cells") provide evidence of chronic hemorrhage within the alveolar spaces. Iron and calcium deposits with foreign body–type giant cells may be seen if there is excessive hemosiderin deposition. This phenomenon has been called as "endogenous pneumoconiosis".

Differential diagnosis

Both alveolar hemorrhage syndrome and pulmonary venous hypertension may have excessive hemosiderin deposition. However, marked abnormalities of vessels are present in pulmonary hypertension.

Pulmonary veno-occlusive disease can also be associated with congestive vasculopathy and may be difficult to distinguish from passive venous congestion. Occlusion of veins in interlobular septa can be helpful to distinguish them.

Treatment is aimed at managing the underlying etiology. Pulmonary vascular findings may persist even after clinical cause of venous hypertension is resolved.

Idiopathic Pulmonary Hemosiderosis

Idiopathic pulmonary hemosiderosis (IPH) is a very rare disease mostly affecting children and causing recurrent episodes of diffuse alveolar hemorrhage leading to pulmonary fibrosis in the absence of vasculitis or capillaritis.

Clinical features

Over 80% of cases occur in children, mostly in the first decade of life. Most children are between 3 and 6 years of age, but it can occur as early as 4 to 6 months of age.[12] Of the 20% with adult onset disease, most are diagnosed before 30 years of age. There is no sex predilection. IPH has been linked with certain pathogenic household molds and decreased levels of von Willebrand factor, suggesting an environmental trigger in genetically predisposed individuals.[13,14] Consanguinity and environmental factors may appear to play a role.[15]

Clinically, patients present with *recurrent* hemoptysis, which can vary from life-threatening episodes to intermittent blood streaked sputum; iron deficiency anemia; dyspnea; and hypoxemia. Less specific features may include fever, lymphadenopathy, hepatomegaly, and splenomegaly. The disease appears to be limited to the lungs without renal or systemic involvement. In chronic phase patients have nonspecific symptoms of fatigue, chronic cough, and asymptomatic microcytic anemia. In addition, there may be failure to thrive, emaciation, and pallor. Pulmonary fibrosis can develop, and if so, physical examination may reveal bilateral crackles and clubbing.

Microcytic hypochromic anemia due to blood loss is seen in virtually all cases and eosinophilia in 12% to 15% of patients.[14] Association with celiac disease,[16] juvenile idiopathic arthritis,[17] cardiomyopathy,[18] and ANCA antibodies[19] have been reported.

Radiologic features vary with the phase of disease. In the acute phase, patchy or diffuse ground glass infiltrates or massive confluent shadows are seen predominantly in the lower lobes that may clear rapidly. These resolve over time and perihilar reticulonodular infiltrates appear with diffuse interstitial fibrosis. The apices and costophrenic angles are spared. Radionuclide imaging can be helpful in detecting active bleeding. The clinical triad of hemoptysis, iron deficiency anemia, and diffuse parenchymal infiltrates is strongly suggestive of IPH.

Pathologic features

Gross
The gross features are nonspecific and reflect recurrent hemorrhage. The lungs show brown induration secondary to hemosiderin deposition and fibrosis.

Microscopic features
Hemosiderin-laden macrophages are seen in large numbers in bronchoalveolar lavage that provide evidence of recent hemorrhage. Biopsies are generally not indicated. Histologically, there is evidence of alveolar hemorrhage, including alveolar red blood cells and alveolar hemosiderin-laden macrophages (*Figures 16-2A* and *B*). Interstitial fibrosis with focal areas of organization of alveolar spaces may be seen. Secondary changes may include type 2 pneumocyte hyperplasia, peribronchial lymphoid hyperplasia, and alveolar septal mastocytosis. No immunoglobulin deposits are seen on immunofluorescence.

Differential diagnosis includes ABMA (antibasement membrane antibody), ANCA (antineutrophil cytoplasmic antibody) associated vasculitis, other immunologic and nonimmunologic causes of pulmonary hemorrhage. IPH is characterized by absence of small vessel vasculitis or immunoglobulin deposits. Moreover, it occurs predominantly in a younger population as compared to other causes.

Therapy
Corticosteroids are main therapy; however, the response is variable. While some children may die of massive hemorrhage shortly after presentation, others have a history of progressive respiratory insufficiency leading to death 2 to 5 years after diagnosis. Recurrence has been reported after bilateral lung transplantation.[20]

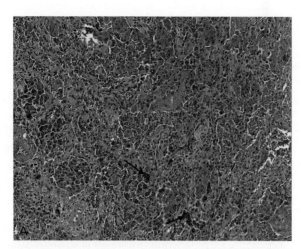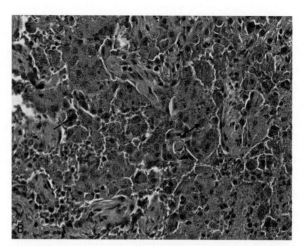

FIGURE 16-2 **A, B: Idiopathic pulmonary hemosiderosis: extensive alveolar hemorrhage with refractile coarse hemosiderin-laden macrophages (arrow) (H&E, A-100×, B-200×).**

Arteriovenous Malformations

Arteriovenous malformations (AVMs) are congenital vascular malformations due to abnormal development of the blood vessels. The mean age at diagnosis is approximately 41 years,[21] with an incidence of two to three cases per 100,000 population.[22] Most patients are clinically asymptomatic. When symptomatic, the clinical features include cyanosis, clubbing, dyspnea, fatigue, and polycythemia.[22] AVMs are bilateral in 8%, and multiple in 33% to 50% of patients, the incidence being higher in the middle and left lower lobes.[21,22]

Complications of AVMs are related to connections of the pulmonary capillary bed, with loss of the filtering function of the lung; this allows emboli and bacteria to directly exit the systemic circulation, which results in embolism or brain abscesses. It can also result in bleeding of these abnormal vessels, leading to hemoptysis or hemothorax.[23]

The underlying anomaly in AVM is an abnormal and direct communication between pulmonary arteries and veins through small aneurysms resulting in right-to-left shunt. Patients with AVM generally present with a normal echocardiogram, and chest x-rays reveal one or more nodules in the affected area.[22] CT imaging (*Figure 16-3A*) can identify AVMs by presence of feeding artery and a draining vein.[24] Pulmonary angiography is the method of choice for the diagnosis of AVM, as well as for the delineation of the arterial supply and venous drainage of AVM.[22,25] More recently, three-dimensional magnetic resonance imaging has been shown to be effective and accurate in diagnosing AVM, with the advantage of being a noninvasive test.

Grossly, AVMs appear as single or multiple nodules consisting of tangled networks of dilated, wormlike channels that vary in size. Thrombi may be present. Histologically, they range from diffuse telangiectasia to complex structures consisting of an aneurysmal sac dilated by the confluence of arteries and veins (*Figure 16-3B, C*). The walls are thickened to varying degrees and the lumen often contains blood clots.

Approximately 95% of AVMs originate from the pulmonary arteries. However, various other arterial origins have been diagnosed, the most common being those that originate from the bronchial arteries, internal mammary artery, or descending aorta. Such malformations tend to increase in size, especially when there is more than one, and rarely resolve spontaneously.[25]

Of the patients with hereditary hemorrhagic telangiectasia (Osler-Weber-Rendu syndrome), 45% to 88% present with pulmonary AVMs.[22] These patients have abnormal blood vessel development in the body, including the lungs, brain, nasal passages, liver, and gastrointestinal organs.

Embolization and surgical resection are the principal methods for the treatment of AVM.[25]

DEFINITION OF VASCULITIS

A diverse group of disease entities with inflammation of the vessel wall resulting in vascular necrosis and tissue injury.

APPROACH TO VASCULITIS

Pulmonary vasculitis may present in a number of ways including recurrent alveolar hemorrhage, pulmonary nodules, cavitating lesions, or airway disease depending on the disease process and patient-related factors. The disease process may be centered on small, medium, or less commonly large vessels and may be either immune mediated or not. However, the small vessel ANCA-associated vasculitides most commonly affects the lung. They are listed in order of occurrence in

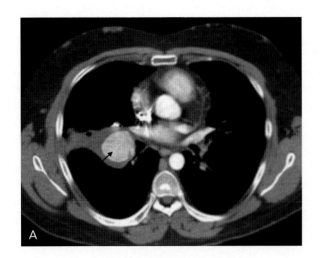

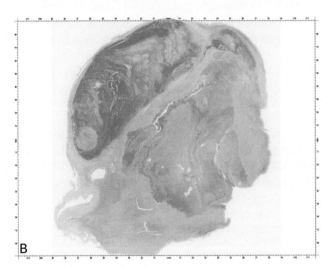

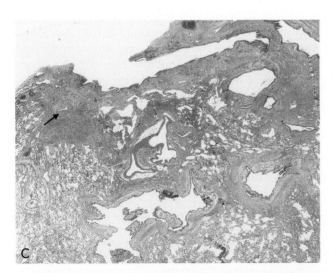

FIGURE 16-3 **A:** Contrast-enhanced CT of the chest demonstrating a large pulmonary artery aneurysm (arrow) in the right lower lobe. **B:** Arteriovenous aneurysm: aneurysmal dilatation of a vascular channel with thrombus formation (H&E, 40×). **C:** Arteriovenous malformation: anastomosing, tortuous arterial (black arrow) and venous channels (green arrow).

North America: granulomatosis with polyangiitis (GPA, formerly Wegener granulomatosis), Churg-Strauss syndrome (CSS), microscopic polyangiitis (MPA), and idiopathic pauci-immune pulmonary capillaritis (IPIPC). In Asia, particularly China MPA is more common than GPA. Nevertheless, all ANCA associated vasculitides are rare on the whole with an incidence of 90 to 300/million. Poor prognostic factors include older age, higher disease activity, pulmonary hemorrhage, cardiac involvement, and proteinase-3 positivity.[26]

VASCULITIS ASSOCIATED WITH HEMORRHAGE

Collagen Vascular Diseases

Immune-mediated vascular injury is a pattern common to collagen vascular diseases. Being systemic disorders, the pulmonary vascular bed is a frequent target of the immune injury. The vascular injury is accompanied by an inflammatory response resulting in vasculitis. The patterns of vascular injury vary and can take several forms including vasculitis of medium-sized vessels, pulmonary hypertension, or capillaritis with pulmonary hemorrhage.

The most common form of vascular injury in collagen vascular disease is vasculitis. It is most often seen in systemic lupus erythematosus (SLE) and rheumatoid arthritis. However, any collagen vascular disease, including scleroderma, idiopathic inflammatory myopathy, and mixed connective tissue disease may result in vasculitis. Certain histologic patterns are characteristic of particular disease entities. In scleroderma, pulmonary hypertensive vasculopathy and focal endothelialitis are more common. The vasculitis is nonnecrotizing and fibrinoid necrosis and acute vasculitis are uncommon. In rheumatoid arthritis, vasculitis is commonly localized adjacent to foci of rheumatoid nodules. Vasculitis affecting medium-sized vessels can occur, but is uncommon.

Diffuse pulmonary hemorrhage has been reported in SLE, rheumatoid arthritis, and juvenile rheumatoid arthritis, but can probably occur in any of the collagen vascular diseases. Like other pulmonary hemorrhage syndromes it has a fulminant clinical presentation and acute renal failure.

Pulmonary hypertension can also occur in SLE, rheumatoid arthritis, and idiopathic inflammatory myopathy. In some cases, it appears to be a complication of pulmonary vasculitis. In patients with rheumatoid arthritis, pulmonary hypertension should be considered, especially when Raynaud phenomenon is present.

Granulomatosis with Polyangiitis

Granulomatosis with polyangiitis (GPA) is a multisystem disorder characterized by aseptic necrotizing granulomatous vasculitis predominantly involving the upper respiratory tract, lower respiratory tract, and the kidney. The term granulomatosis with polyangiitis was proposed to gradually replace Wegener granulomatosis by the boards of directors of the American College of Rheumatology (ACR), American Society of Nephrology (ASN), and the European League Against Rheumatism (EURL) in November 2010.[27]

Clinical features of GPA

The peak incidence of the disease is in the fourth to sixth decades of life[28] with no gender predilection.[29] The annual incidence has been steadily increasing from less than 1/100,000 in 1970s to current incidence of 4 to 12 cases per million.[30,31]

Primary sites of involvement include the head and neck region, followed by the lungs, kidney, and the eye. The classic triad of sinusitis, pneumonia, and glomerulonephritis defines the clinical picture of GPA. The clinical features of GPA are varied depending on the sites of involvement.

Upper respiratory tract involvement is the most common presentation seen in more than 90% of the patients.[32,33] Head and neck lesions present as sinusitis, nasal disease, otitis media, hearing loss, subglottic stenosis, ear pain, cough, and oral lesions.[34,35] Nasopharynx involvement can present with nasal septal perforation, mucosal ulcers, and saddle nose deformity.[27]

Lower respiratory tract involvement manifests as cough, chest pain, dyspnea, wheezing, and hemoptysis. Stenosis of the trachea or bronchi may occur.[36] Pulmonary involvement occurs in 55% to 90% of patients with GPA.[28,36,37]

Pauci-immune glomerulonephritis occurs in 70% to 85% of patients with GPA during the course of the disease.[28] Hematuria, red blood cell casts, proteinuria, and azotemia suggest renal involvement.

Systemic symptoms commonly accompany the disease and patients often present with fever, skin lesions, weight loss, peripheral neuropathy, central nervous system abnormalities, and pericarditis. The skin lesions may include purpura, petechiae, nodules, hemorrhagic bullae, and pyoderma gangrenosum-like lesions. Unusual sites of involvement include breast, salivary gland, intestine, prostate, ureter, urethra, cervix, vagina, perianal region.

Laboratory workup is consistent with a chronic process. Findings include normocytic normochromic anemia, elevated erythrocyte sedimentation rates, elevated C-reactive protein, and occasionally elevated rheumatoid factor titers.

Microhematuria and proteinuria (active sediment) on urine analysis suggest renal involvement.

Antineutrophil cytoplasmic antibodies (ANCA) when positive are useful to establish and also monitor therapy. However, they should be interpreted in appropriate clinical context and are not absolute for diagnosis.

The cytoplasmic staining pattern (c-ANCA): c-ANCA reacts in 95% of cases with proteinase 3 (PR3 or myeloblastin) which is a 29 k-Da serine protease found in lysosomal granules and on plasma membranes of neutrophils and monocytes. The specificity is 84% to 99% in patients with active disease, 50% to 71% in partial remission, and 30% to 40% in complete remission.

The perinuclear staining pattern (p-ANCA): p-ANCA has 90% specificity for myeloperoxidase. It may also be detected against elastase and lactoferrin found in primary and secondary granules, respectively. p-ANCA pattern is found in patients with idiopathic necrotizing and crescentic glomerulonephritis. Elevated levels are seen in CSS, systemic polyarteritis nodosa, small vessel vasculitis, giant cell arteritis. Positivity may also be present in few nonvasculitis conditions like Felty syndrome, ABMA, atypical pneumonia and Legionnaire disease, poststreptococcal glomerulonephritis, SLE, and inflammatory bowel disease. Unfortunately, the p-ANCA does not have the desired sensitivity either, with only 50% of CSS cases being positive.

Cases with positive p-ANCA (10%) or even negative ANCA may occur and are more common in indolent, previously treated, or limited disease.

For patients with apparent clinical reactivation of disease, negative c-ANCA may raise concern about opportunistic infection.

Imaging features of GPA

On imaging the lesions are characteristically multiple, bilateral, subpleural well-marginated nodules with or without cavitation and predominant in the lower lobes. Radiologically, the thick walls, irregular margins, and cavitation may mimic a neoplasm (*Figure 16-4*). Lesions can wax and wane over time. Pulmonary hemorrhage appears as diffuse infiltrates or air space opacities. Solitary cavitary nodules are rare and more likely to be infectious. Rarely, there may be associated mediastinal or hilar lymph node enlargement and pleural effusions. Chronic fibrotic changes and bronchiectasis are common after therapy.

Gross and histologic features of GPA

Open lung biopsies are optimal tissue specimens for diagnosis.

Grossly, the lesions of GPA are multiple bilateral nodular masses with an average diameter of 2.4 cm. The nodules have irregular borders with a tan-brown cut-surface that may be solid or cavitated.[38] Central necrosis is common. Surrounding parenchyma is unremarkable, may be red/ hemorrhagic or yellow and consolidated. Solitary lesions are rare, and more likely to be infectious.[39]

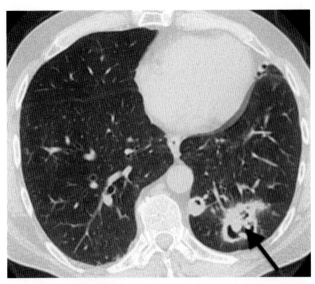

FIGURE 16-4 Granulomatosis with polyangiitis: CT scan with spiculated cavitary lesion (arrow).

Other associate findings may include diffuse pulmonary hemorrhage, interstitial fibrosis with firm tan fibrotic parenchyma, and lipoid pneumonia with diffuse yellow consolidation. Rarely, GPA may have a bronchocentric/bronchiolocentric pattern and be associated with bronchopneumonia with 1 to 2 mm nodules centered on bronchi and bronchioles and bronchial stenosis may be seen.

The major histologic diagnostic criteria for GPA include vasculitis, granulomatous inflammation, and parenchymal necrosis.

The medium-sized vessels, small veins and arteries, and capillaries are most often affected by vasculitis (*Figure 16-5A, B*). It is best appreciated in parenchyma away from other inflammatory lesions, since vasculitis may be seen within the inflammatory foci from other causes. Vasculitis may be focal or eccentric and can be limited to endothelium and subendothelial spaces. Inflammatory cells in vasculitis can vary and lymphocytes, macrophages, plasma cells, and occasional eosinophils may be seen. Granulomatous reaction may obscure and destroy the vessel wall. Elastic stain can be helpful for identification of vessel wall in granulomatous inflammation (*Figure 16-5C*). Inflammation may have one of many different patterns: chronic, acute, necrotizing granulomatous, nonnecrotizing granulomatous, and fibrinoid necrosis (*Figure 16-5D*). Cicatricial changes (medial scarring or intimal proliferation) may represent effects of therapy.

The granulomas are usually poorly formed with palisading histiocytes. Importantly, the granulomas in GPA do not have a clear demarcation from adjacent uninvolved parenchyma. Well-formed granulomas (sarcoid like) are uncommon and when present should alert one to consider other infectious diagnosis

or necrotizing sarcoidosis. Rarely, the granulomas may appear as scattered clusters of giant cells lining the microabscesses.

The necrosis in GPA may be geographic or appear as neutrophilic microabscesses centered on septal capillaries (*Figure 16-5E*). The parenchymal necrosis is geographic and basophilic, rich in cellular debris with neutrophils imparting a dirty appearance. The necrosis is not confined to the center of granulomas. Small foci of collagen necrosis around blood vessels or within pulmonary parenchyma may be present. There may be a small collection of neutrophils or microabscess around an area of dense eosinophilic collagen fibers.

The background comprises scattered multinucleated giant cells within the vasculitic process or within the background inflammatory infiltrate. Areas of organizing pneumonia hemosiderin-laden macrophages may be present (*Figure 16-5F*). Adjacent areas may show evidence of bronchitis, bronchiolitis, or even endogenous lipoid pneumonia.

Additionally minor histologic features may be seen along the periphery of typical nodules. These include dense interstitial fibrosis, diffuse pulmonary hemorrhage, lipoid pneumonia, acute bronchopneumonia, tissue eosinophils, xanthogranulomatous lesions. Chronic fibrosing pleuritis, acute and fibrinous pleuritis, and granulomatous pleuritis may be seen overlying nodular inflammatory lesions. Therefore, sampling issues exist if only the periphery is biopsied. Here the absence of positive cultures with other clinical features and serologic evidence of GPA clinches the diagnosis despite the misleading morphology.

Rare forms described are limited or localized form of GPA, bronchocentric variant, eosinophilic variant, and small vessel vasculitis and capillaritis.[40-43] Furthermore, biopsy may not show all features if taken early in disease or following treatment. Interstitial fibrosis, sometimes scattered giant cells, bronchial or bronchiolar scarring, and cicatricial vascular changes are frequently present in posttreatment biopsies.

Differential diagnosis

Lymphomatoid granulomatosis (LYG) has similar clinical and demographic features as GPA. The infiltrate in LYG is typically vasocentric and vasodestructive comprised of a polymorphic (CD20 positive) population of small and large atypical lymphocytes in varying proportions. LYG represents an EBV-infected, T-cell rich, B-cell lymphoma with prominent vascular infiltration. Granulomas are comparatively rare, and their presence should suggest an alternate diagnosis. ANCA is not characteristically elevated. In GPA the infiltrate is mixture of *acute* and chronic inflammatory cells with necrosis of the vessel wall.

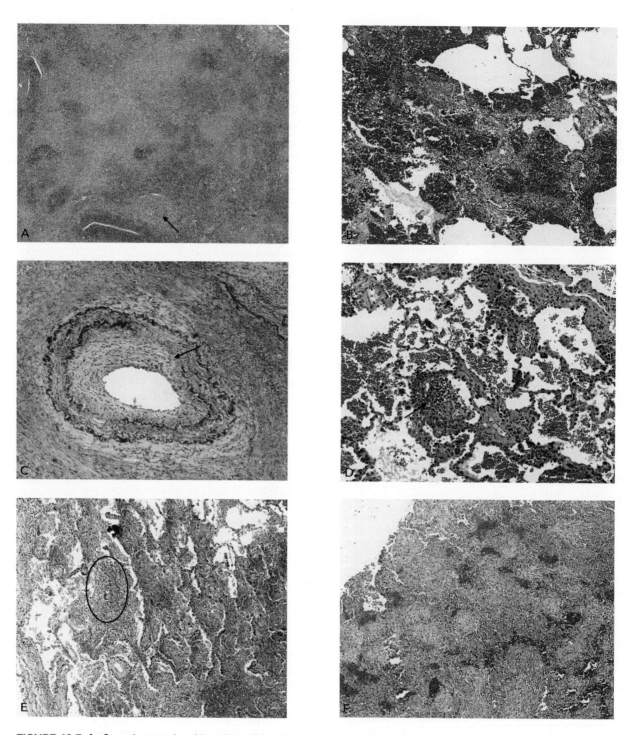

FIGURE 16-5 A: Granulomatosis with polyangiitis with geographic areas of necrosis, giant cells (arrow) and large vessel vasculitis (arrow) (H&E, 100×). **B:** Granulomatosis with polyangiitis with hemorrhage and focal capillaritis (arrows) (H&E, 100×). **C:** Granulomatosis with polyangiitis. Elastic Von Geissa stain demonstrating disruption of elastic laminae (arrow) of a medium-sized muscular artery with intimal inflammation (200×). **D:** Granulomatosis with polyangiitis with microabscesses with capillaritis (arrow) (H&E, 200×). **E:** Granulomatosis with polyangiitis with septal necrosis, microabscesses, giant cells, and hemorrhage (circle) (H&E, 100×). **F:** Granulomatosis with polyangiitis, organizing pattern with giant cell (arrow) (H&E, 100×).

Churg-Strauss syndrome

Patients with Churg-Strauss syndrome (CSS) have history of asthma, peripheral eosinophilia, and systemic vasculitis. Peripheral eosinophilia is absent in GPA. Destructive upper airway disease, tracheal stenosis and severe renal disease, or cavitating pulmonary disease is less likely to be seen in CSS. ANCA tends to be perinuclear rather than cytoplasmic.

Microscopic polyangiitis (MPA) differ in clinical and lab features. Early lesions of GPA or a limited specimen may lack granulomatous inflammation and mimic MPA. Clinical correlation and ANCA may be of diagnostic aid. Upper airway involvement is absent in MPA. *Table 16-1* compares and contrasts clinical manifestations of major vasculitides.

Bronchocentric granulomatosis

GPA may have a bronchocentric pattern of lung involvement and bronchocentric granulomatosis (BCG) may show secondary involvement of blood vessels. However, GPA is a systemic disease unlike BCG and a positive ANCA strongly favors its diagnosis.

Necrotizing sarcoid granulomas

Confluent areas of nonnecrotizing granulomas with extensive coagulative necrosis are seen in necrotizing sarcoid granulomas (NSG). The granulomas are well formed, sarcoid like with clear demarcation between granulomatous and normal pulmonary parenchyma. ANCA is negative.

Granulomatous infections always need to be excluded. Vasculitis may be seen adjacent to necrotizing granulomas of mycobacterial or fungal infections. Special stains are more sensitive than cultures for fungal infections in this instance. Solitary necrotizing granulomas especially at the apex are more likely to be infectious.

Table 16-1 Clinical Manifestations of Pulmonary Vasculitis

Manifestations	GPA	MPA	CSS	IPIPC
Upper airway	Common. May include destructive and ulcerating lesions	Uncommon	Rhinitis and sinusitis	N/A
Asthma and airway	No asthma. Subglottic or tracheal stenosis, airway narrowing, and ulcerations are common	Uncommon	Present with asthma. Variable severity, but commonly steroid-requiring	N/A
Nodules, cavities, and infiltrates	Common will have focal consolidation, infiltrates, atelectasis, nodules, cavities, or other abnormalities Easily confused with infection or malignancy	Less common than GPA and CSS will have diffuse infiltrates, consistent with alveolar hemorrhage	Common by plain film and up to 90% by HRCT. Commonly appears as patchy, bilateral, heterogeneous disease with areas of ground glass appearance and consolidation	Infiltrates consistent with alveolar hemorrhage
Alveolar hemorrhage Thromboembolic disease	Unusual. Comparable to patients with a known history of VTE	Less common than IPIPC. Unknown incidence	Rare Unknown incidence	Common Unknown incidence
Infection	Common cause of morbidity and mortality	See GPA	See GPA	See GPA
Drug toxicity	Pulmonary Toxicity most commonly with methotrexate	See GPA	See GPA	See GPA
Extrapulmonary disease	Constitutional symptoms, common	Constitutional symptoms, very common	Constitutional symptoms, Common	
	GN common	Musculoskeletal disease, common	Musculoskeletal disease, common	
	Cutaneous disease, common	PNS 10%–50%	Cutaneous disease, common	
	Musculoskeletal disease, common	GI disease 35%–45%	PNS > common	
	Ocular involvement, common	Cardiac involvement 10%–20%	GI disease, common	
	Cardiac involvement, uncommon		Cardiac involvement, common	

CSS, Churg-Strauss syndrome; GI, gastrointestinal; GN, glomerulonephritis; GPA, granulomatosis with polyangiitis; IPIPC, idiopathic pauci-immune pulmonary capillaritis; MPA, microscopic polyangiitis; PNS, peripheral nervous system; VTE, venous thromboembolic disease.

Rheumatoid nodules

The nodules of RA lack geographic necrosis and micro-abscess formation. Most patients have rheumatoid arthritis and do not have upper airway and renal disease. There is fibrinoid necrosis.

Other conditions that may mimic GPA are drug-induced vasculitis, collagen vascular disease–associated vasculitis, cryoglobulinemia, antiphospholipid antibody syndrome. Careful interpretation of the clinical, radiological, and laboratory data is often helpful in narrowing the diagnosis.

Therapy

Steroids and cyclophosphamide are the mainstay of treatment. Ninety percent of patients respond to therapy and 75% experience complete remission within a year of therapy. Most patients have a high relapse rate and approximately 50% of patients require a second line of therapy. Addition of trimethoprim-sulfamethoxazole has been suggested to reduce relapse rate. Other forms of therapy include pulse cyclophosphamide and methotrexate and rituximab. Morbidity during the disease course is related to due to disease or therapy or both. Infections are common due to immunosuppression.

Antiglomerular Basement Membrane Antibody Disease (Goodpasture Syndrome)

Antiglomerular basement membrane antibody (ABMA) disease is a disorder of circulating antibodies directed against the NCI domain of the α_3 chain of the basement membrane collagen type 4 of both the lung and the kidneys, resulting in vascular damage. Most patients have Goodpasture syndrome that is defined by presence of both diffuse alveolar hemorrhage and glomerulonephritis. Less than a third of the patients will have glomerulonephritis alone.[44]

Clinical features of antiglomerular basement membrane antibody disease

ABMA disease shows a bimodal age distribution with peaks at 30 and 60 years, the average age being 35. It is more common in men who smoke.[45]

Clinical features reflect development of pulmonary hemorrhage and proliferative glomerulonephritis, with most patients having both features. Rarely, the disease is restricted to kidney or lung.

Patients present with hemoptysis, cough, dyspnea, and rhonchi or crackles on auscultation. Systemic symptoms including fever, weight loss, and arthralgias are frequently present.

Renal involvement manifests as hematuria, granular casts, and proteinuria. The constant immunological

hallmark of the disease is the occurrence of circulating anti-GBM antibodies, whose titer is directly related to the clinical severity of GD. The antibodies are associated with serum ANCAs in 10% to almost 40% of GD patients, with double positivity indicative of a worse renal prognosis. The target antigen of anti-GBM antibodies is a component of the non-collagenous-1 (NC1) domain of the α3 chain of type IV collagen, α345NC1. The prevalent expression of this hexamer on the basement membrane of both the glomeruli and the pulmonary alveoli accounts for the frequently combined renal and pulmonary involvement. A strong positive association of GD with the HLA-DRB1*15:01 allele has been described, but the factor(s) responsible for the loss of self-tolerance to NC1 autoantigen has not yet been identified. A conformational change in the quaternary structure of the α345NC1 likely plays a crucial role in triggering an immune response and justifies the proposed description of GD as an autoimmune "conformeropathy." The function of autoreactive T cells in GD is poorly defined but may involve a shift from TH2 to TH1 cytokine regulation, such that affinity maturation and the antigen specificity of the antibody response are enhanced.[46]

Imaging features of antiglomerular basement membrane antibody disease

Alveolar hemorrhage is seen as bilateral consolidation on chest x-rays. The infiltrates may disappear in patients during quiescent phase (Figure 16-6A).

Gross and histologic features of antiglomerular basement membrane antibody disease

Grossly, the lungs have a dense, firm, and red homogeneous appearance without any mass lesions or nodules.

Diffuse pulmonary hemorrhage with alveolar red blood cells and hemosiderin-laden macrophages are seen histologically (Figure 16-6B). With time the hemorrhage resolves and is replaced by iron deposition on the elastic fibers in the alveolar septa. Small vessel vasculitis with fibrin thrombi are frequently present. Type 2 pneumocyte hyperplasia and organizing fibrosis result in thickened alveolar septa. Hyaline membranes may be present in active disease. Immunofluorescence and ultrastructural analysis reveal linear deposition of IgG and complement along the capillaries in the alveolar septa and glomeruli.

Differential diagnosis

Other causes of small vessel vasculitis and nonimmunologic causes of pulmonary hemorrhage.

Plasmapheresis is the choice of treatment aimed at removing the circulating antibodies, supplemented

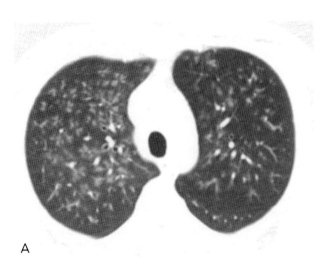
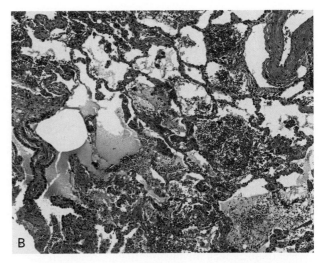

FIGURE 16-6 **A: CT chest demonstrates centrilobular ground glass opacities scattered throughout the bilateral lungs in a 30-year-old female with pANCA-positive renal-pulmonary syndrome. B: Goodpasture syndrome with diffuse alveolar damage (H&E, 100×).**

with corticosteroids, and in some cases cytotoxic drugs like cyclophosphamide. One-year survival with the triple therapy is up to 90%.

Renal transplantation extends survival for patients with end stage kidney disease.

Churg-Strauss Syndrome

CSS is a rare systemic vasculitis of small and medium-sized vessels. It differs from other small vessel vasculitis by its association with severe asthma and blood and tissue eosinophilia. It is a peculiar hybrid of a primary often ANCA associated vasculitis and a hypereosinophilic disorder. The clinical diagnosis is suggested by the presence of four of six criteria proposed by the American College of Rheumatology (1990 criteria): (1) Asthma or history of allergy; (2) peripheral eosinophilia greater than 10% of the white blood cell count; (3) neuropathy; (4) nonfixed radiographic pulmonary infiltrates; (5) sinusitis; (6) biopsy containing extravascular eosinophils. The presence of any four is sufficient for clinical diagnosis. The above carries a sensitivity of 85% and a specificity of 99.7%. The 2012 Chapel Hill Consensus Conference defined Churg-Strauss (eosinophilic granulomatosis with polyangiitis, EGPA) as "eosinophil-rich and necrotizing granulomatous inflammation often involving the respiratory tract and necrotizing vasculitis involving small and medium-sized vessels, and associated with asthma and eosinophilic pneumonia." Candidate gene association studies from Germany and Italy provided evidence for a genetic background in EGPA. Positive associations were found with human leukocyte antigen (HLA)-DRB1_04 and HLA-DRB1_07 genotypes and a protective effect for HLA-DRB3.[47]

Clinical features of Churg-Strauss syndrome

CSS is the rarest of the major vasculitis syndromes with a prevalence of 10.4 to 13 per million in adults.[47-49] The incidence is higher in patients with asthma ranging from 34.6 to 64.4 cases per million patient-years.[50,51] CSS can occur in all ages with a mean age of 48 years at diagnosis.[52] Occurrence in children is rare. It is usually seen in patients with asthma, some of whom have inadequate use of corticosteroids or history of corticosteroid tapering. Association between patients taking leukotriene receptor antagonists and development of CSS has been reported. CSS is thought to be mediated through hypersensitivity drug reaction.

The disease progresses through three clinical phases in order: prodromal phase of allergic rhinitis, asthma, peripheral blood eosinophilia, and infiltration of eosinophils in tissues. The tissue eosinophilia is seen as eosinophilic pneumonia or eosinophils in alveolar spaces. Eosinophils may be present in the gastrointestinal tract. Nasal polyposis is the most common initial manifestation and may last for years with multiple exacerbations.

This is followed by the vasculitis phase in which the patients develop systemic signs and symptoms like neuropathy and cutaneous leukocytoclastic vasculitis. Additionally other features of CSS are present, so it is only during this phase that diagnosis can be established.

In the post-vasculitis phase, patients develop neuropathy and hypertension. However, they may continue to have asthma and allergic rhinitis.

Limited CSS is said to be present when one of the primary diagnostic features, such as asthma or eosinophilia, is lacking. The vasculitis may not be systemic and pathologic features are restricted to a single organ.

Cardiac involvement is seen in approximately 47% of patients. Cardiac failure, pericarditis, hypertension, restrictive cardiomyopathy, acute myocardial infarction, and arrhythmias may occur.

Gastrointestinal involvement is suggested by abdominal pain, diarrhea, and gastrointestinal bleeding and carries a bad prognosis.[52] The small intestine, stomach, and colon are most commonly affected in that order. Mucosal ulceration may resemble ulcerative colitis. Perforation is an infrequent but life-threatening complication. Rarely the patients may present with acalculous cholecystitis.

Renal involvement is less frequent and less severe than GPA, and may be seen in 25% of patients.[53] Symptoms are mild or moderate.

Head and neck involvement can result in nasal obstruction or rhinorrhea, nasal polyps and crusting, abnormal sinus roentgenograms, septal perforations, and subcutaneous nodules involving the skin. On rare occasions, conjunctival involvement has been reported.

Cutaneous lesions are diverse and present in 40% to 70% of patients.[54] Cutaneous nodules, purpura, erythema, urticaria are common skin manifestations. Arthritis or arthralgias and myalgias are seen in 40% to 50% of patients.

Peripheral neuropathy can occur in CSS and presents as mononeuritis multiplex or central nervous system abnormalities ranging from hemiplegia to seizures and rare subarachnoid hemorrhages.

Laboratory tests are nonspecific. Peripheral blood eosinophilia, high IgE titers, and anti-MPO p-ANCA positivity are the three main laboratory anomalies found in CSS. Other findings may include chronic normocytic normochromic anemia, leukocytosis, thrombocytosis, and elevated sedimentation rate. CSS is associated with 40% of ANCA positive patients[52] usually with a p-ANCA pattern; though c-ANCA pattern has also been demonstrated. The clinical presentation differs significantly among ANCA positive and negative patients.[55] Serum rheumatoid factor may be weakly positive, complement may be increased, and most patients have elevated immunoglobulin E (Ig E) levels.

Imaging features of Churg-Strauss syndrome

The imaging findings are nonspecific. Multifocal migratory parenchymal consolidation or nodules may be seen (*Figure 16-7A*). Lesions are generally seen in the periphery of the lung, though it can be more widespread. High resolution CT may show enlarged, irregular, and stellate-shaped arteries with stenosis or rarely microaneurysms.

Histologic features of Churg-Strauss syndrome

Histologically, the three major features of CSS are necrotizing vasculitis predominantly affecting small to medium-sized arteries and veins; tissue infiltration by eosinophils; and extravascular granulomas.

The histologic picture depends on the phase of the disease and a single biopsy specimen is unlikely to exhibit all three features.[56]

In the prodromic phase, the lungs show a picture of eosinophilic pneumonia. Extravasation of eosinophils in other anatomic sites or eosinophilic bronchitis can be seen. Eosinophilic inflammation, subepithelial basement membrane thickening, submucosal gland hyperplasia, and smooth muscle hypertrophy are seen in asthmatic bronchitis.

During the vasculitis phase, fibrinoid necrosis of the media, and pleomorphic cellular infiltrates, predominantly eosinophils characterize the vascular lesions (*Figure 16-7B, C*). The inflammatory infiltrate can be comprised of lymphocytes, neutrophils, plasma cells, epithelioid macrophages in addition to eosinophils. Vasculitis predominantly affects the small and medium-sized muscular arteries or veins, but capillaries may be involved as well. Eosinophilic granulomas (allergic granulomas) and eosinophilic vasculitis can be seen besides eosinophilic pneumonia. Granulomas are extravascular with necrotic center and surrounded by palisading histiocytes. Multinucleated giant cells can be seen. Cicatricial changes represent features of healing.

Diffuse pulmonary hemorrhage can occur in association with eosinophilic capillaritis. Ischemia and infarction are frequent complications of vasculitis. Wall destruction can result in aneurysms formation.

Nasal biopsies may demonstrate allergic polyps, allergic granulomas, eosinophilic submucosal infiltrates with giant cells, and chronic inflammation.

Heart involvement is reflected by acute fibrinous pericarditis, pericardial fibrosis, eosinophilic and granulomatous myocarditis, and interstitial fibrosis. Thrombosis and acute myocardial infarction are complications of coronary arteritis. Endocarditis with mural thrombi are uncommon.

Eosinophils are very sensitive to corticosteroids. In treated patients, eosinophils can be absent, reduced, or fragmented, making histologic interpretation difficult. They may be misinterpreted as neutrophils. The large size of nuclear lobes and more eosinophilic appearance of background are helpful clues.

Differential diagnosis

Granulomatosis with polyangiitis

The clinical presentation, histopathology, and presence of c-ANCA are helpful in diagnosing GPA. Eosinophils may be seen in GPA but are not the predominant cell type. Renal involvement is much less common in CSS and are glomerular. Cavitating lesions are rare in CSS and peripheral eosinophilia greater than 5% is unusual for GPA.

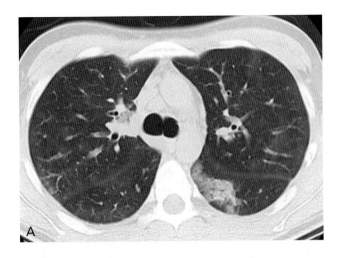

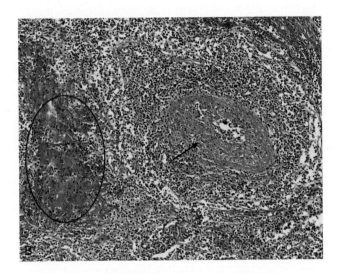

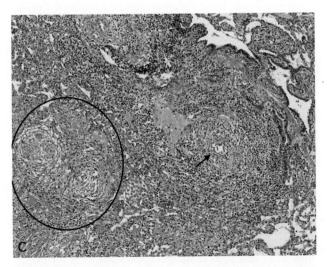

FIGURE 16-7 **A: Churg-Strauss syndrome: CT chest shows air-space consolidation in the superior segment of the left upper lobe with minimal areas of ground glass opacity in the bilateral lungs. B: Churg-Strauss vasculitis (arrow) with eosinophilic abscess (circle) (H&E, 200×). C: Churg-Strauss vasculitis with eosinophilic vasculitis (arrow) and granulomas (circle) (H&E, 100×).**

Eosinophilic pneumonia (parasitic infections, drugs)

A systemic disease pattern with observation of vasculitis favor a diagnosis of CSS. Diagnosis of CSS should only be made after careful exclusion of parasites in stool, sputum, pleural fluid, and tissue biopsies.

Allergic bronchopulmonary aspergillosis can show bronchocentric granulomas and eosinophilic pneumonia; however, signs and symptoms of systemic vasculitis are absent (*Figure 16-7B*).

Therapy

The disease responds very well to corticosteroids. Other immunosuppressive drugs like cyclophosphamide can be used to prevent irreversible organ injury in patients unresponsive to corticosteroids. Since significant number of patients may develop irreversible organ injury, current recommendation is to use immunosuppressive medication like cyclophosphamide, azathioprine, or chlorambucil from the beginning. Untreated it is fatal, most patients dying of cardiac complications. Other less common causes of death include renal failure, cerebral hemorrhage, respiratory failure, and gastrointestinal perforation. Higher 5-year mortality is associated independently with the following five criteria: (1) age over 65 years; (2) cardiac symptoms; (3) gastrointestinal involvement; (4) renal insufficiency characterized by serum creatinine >150 μmol/L; and (5) absence of ear, nose, and throat manifestations.[57]

Microscopic Polyangiitis

Microscopic polyangiitis is a systemic necrotizing small vessel vasculitis involving the arterioles, venules, and capillaries and is characterized by few or no immune deposits. The characteristic pulmonary manifestation when present is diffuse pulmonary hemorrhage resulting from small vessel vasculitis (capillaritis). Necrotizing glomerulonephritis is present in almost all patients.

Clinical features of microscopic polyangiitis

MPA occurs mostly between the fourth and fifth decades of life with a slight female predominance (1.5:1). Rarely, it can also occur in children. The incidence is about 1 in 100,000. Lungs are affected in 50% of patients.

In most patients there is rapid progression of the disease, but indolent forms with symptoms over 1 year have been reported.

MPA is the most common cause of pulmonary renal syndrome[58] and may occur with predominant or exclusive involvement of either the kidney or the lung. Most common clinical manifestation is glomerulonephritis, followed by nonspecific systemic symptoms like fever, weight loss, myalgias, and arthralgias. The lungs are involved in 50%, upper respiratory tract in 30%, and skin in 20% of the patients. p-ANCA is positive in 80%. Ear, nose, and throat symptoms, skin involvement, ocular involvement, and peripheral neuropathy may occur.[59] Nearly all patients have pulmonary signs or symptoms of cough, dyspnea, chest pain, or crackles.

Bronchoalveolar lavage fluid shows acute inflammation and hemosiderin-laden macrophages but is a nonspecific finding.

Imaging features of microscopic polyangiitis

The imaging features of MPA reflect diffuse pattern of pulmonary hemorrhage seen as bilateral alveolar opacities without nodules diffusely in upper and lower lobes. Less often, consolidation, ground glass opacities, and dense small nodules or pleural effusions may be seen.

Histologic features of microscopic polyangiitis

The hallmark histologic feature of MPA is neutrophilic small vessel vasculitis (capillaritis) in a background of pulmonary hemorrhage.

Neutrophilic capillaritis may be difficult to appreciate in a background of hemorrhage. In such cases, findings of patchy foci of acute inflammation focused on alveolar wall, which is distended and thickened by the neutrophilic infiltrate may be a clue to capillaritis. Moreover, recognizing that process is centered on alveolar wall and presence of pulmonary hemorrhage is helpful. Extravasation of neutrophils in alveolar spaces in severe cases resembles acute pneumonia. Neutrophils often show karyorrhexis. Nonspecific changes such as interstitial thickening, hemosiderosis, and organizing pneumonia may be present. Hyaline membranes giving the pattern of DAD may be seen. Pulmonary fibrosis and progressive obstructive airway disease with emphysematous features have been reported.

Differential diagnosis

GPA

Granulomatous inflammation is absent in MPA. It may also be absent in GPA early in disease or due to sampling error. Clinical correlation and ANCA may be of diagnostic aid. Upper airway involvement is absent.

In Goodpasture syndrome antibodies to glomerular basement membrane demonstrable are serologically or by immunofluorescence.

Polyarteritis nodosa rarely affects lungs and preferentially affects the bronchial arteries. Patients may have a positive p-ANCA. In MPA, the vessels affected are smaller than medium sized.

Vasculitis due to hypersensitivity reactions to drugs, collagen vascular diseases, cryoglobulinemic vasculitis, serum sickness disease may mimic MPA. In MPA there are minimal or no immune complex deposits.

Therapy

Good response is seen with cyclophosphamide and prednisone. Relapses are seen in 35% to 40% patients. Plasmapheresis may be helpful in some.

Behcet Disease

Behcet disease (BD) is a vasculitis affecting vessels of any size. It is characterized by a clinical triad of relapsing uveitis (iridocyclitis), oral and genital ulcers. Other sites like gastrointestinal tract, central nervous system, skin, and lung may also be involved.

Clinical features of Behcet disease

BD is a disease of young men distributed throughout the world, though majority of the cases are seen in eastern Asia, the Mediterranean basin, and Japan.

Diagnostic criteria include presence of recurrent oral ulceration and at least two of the following: recurrent genital ulceration, typical defined eye lesions (uveitis), typical defined skin lesions (leukocytoclastic vasculitis), and a positive pathergy test. Other criteria that may be helpful in diagnosis are synovitis, meningoencephalitis, absence of inflammatory bowel disease, or other collagen vascular disease.

Pulmonary involvement occurs in 1.8% of cases and patients often have dyspnea, cough, chest pain, or hemoptysis at presentation. Hemoptysis may occur due to rupture of aneurysm with erosion into a bronchus or active vasculitis and can be life threatening or fatal.

Imaging features of Behcet disease

Imaging shows hilar enlargement or lobulated masses on chest radiographs secondary to pulmonary artery aneurysms. The aneurysm can be located in the main, segmental, or lobar pulmonary arteries. Chest helical CT scan and magnetic resonance imaging can define saccular or fusiform dilatations in proximal arteries. The aneurysms may be accompanied by atelectasis, volume loss, wedge-shaped or linear shadows, and ill-defined or reticular opacities.

Histologic features of Behcet disease

The vasculitis in BD can involve arteries and veins of all sizes or capillaries. The inflammation is necrotizing with perivascular inflammatory infiltrate that may be neutrophilic, mononuclear, or mixed. Elastic destruction in vessel wall is better appreciated on an elastic stain. Pulmonary artery aneurysm is the most common pulmonary manifestation. Thrombus formation occurs frequently. Pulmonary infarction, bronchial erosion, and arteriobronchial fistulas are complications of long-standing disease. Collateral vessels commonly develop in periadventitial fibrosis surrounding the large affected vessels. Presence of eccentric intimal fibrosis may mimic pulmonary thrombotic arteriopathy.

Therapy

Corticosteroids to control vasculitis and anticoagulants to prevent thrombosis are commonly used therapeutic agents. With progression of disease, cyclophosphamide and azathioprine are useful adjuncts. Surgical resection (lobectomy or pneumonectomy) may be required to control massive hemoptysis. The disease has a chronic course, with exacerbations and remissions. It is most severe in young patients and 30% of patients with pulmonary artery aneurysms die within 2 years.

OTHER VASCULITIS SYNDROMES INFREQUENTLY INVOLVING THE LUNG

Henoch-Schonlein Purpura

HSP is an acute self-limited systemic small vessel vasculitis presenting with a tetrad of palpable purpura, abdominal pain, arthralgias, and nephritis.

The diagnostic criteria proposed by ACR include age ≤20 years at onset of disease, palpable purpura, acute abdominal pain, biopsy showing granulocytes in walls of small arterioles or venules. Presence of two or more criteria has a sensitivity of 87.1% and specificity of 87.7%.

Lung involvement is rare and present with hemoptysis due to pulmonary hemorrhage secondary to small vessel vasculitis.

Clinical features of Henoch-Schonlein purpura

HSP is mostly a disease of children and most often manifests between 4 and 7 years, but it may occur in adults.[60] Pulmonary involvement is uncommon, reported in 2.4% to 6.5% of adult cases. Patients present with hemoptysis, dyspnea, and pleuritic chest pain. Intra-alveolar hemorrhage due to vasculitis can be fatal. Patients with pulmonary hemorrhage often also have acute renal failure.

Imaging features of Henoch-Schonlein purpura

HRCT findings are nonspecific with ground glass infiltrates in patients with pulmonary hemorrhage.

Histologic features of Henoch-Schonlein purpura

Capillaritis and perivascular infiltrates are commonly seen in HSP. The vasculitis is associated with immunoglobulin A (IgA) deposits. Nonspecific findings include pulmonary edema and usual interstitial pneumonia.

Polyarteritis Nodosa

PAN is a systemic necrotizing vasculitis that can involve medium-sized and small arteries of any organ. Lungs are rarely involved.[61] Arterioles, capillaries, and venules are spared unlike MPA.[62] Like MPA, granulomatous and eosinophilic inflammation is absent. There is a considerable overlap in histologic features with MPA. Bronchial arteries are characteristically involved with sparing of the pulmonary arteries[63] (*Figure 16-8A, B*).

Cryoglobulinemic Vasculitis

Cryoglobulinemia can be idiopathic or secondary to lymphoproliferative disorders, infections, or collagen vascular diseases. The patients have serum immunoglobulins that reversibly precipitate in cold temperatures.

Pulmonary involvement is common as interstitial lung disease. Leukocytoclastic vasculitis of medium-sized arteries and small vessel vasculitis with pulmonary hemorrhage have been reported.

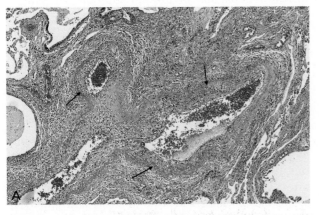
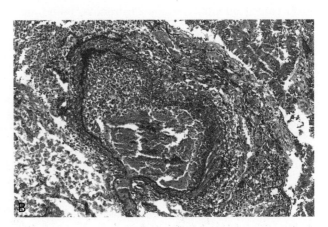

FIGURE 16-8 A: Polyarteritis. Medium-sized artery with fibrinoid necrosis and inflammation (arrow). (H&E, 100×) B: Polyarteritis. Artery with transmural inflammation. EVG stain (200×).

Clinical features of cryoglobulinemic vasculitis

Cutaneous purpuras, arthralgias, hypocomplement-emia, glomerulonephritis with or without vasculi-tis. Pulmonary symptoms: dyspnea, cough, asthma, pleurisy, hemoptysis.

Imaging features of cryoglobulinemic vasculitis

Interstitial lung involvement is seen in up to 78% of patients.

Histologic features of cryoglobulinemic vasculitis

Vasculitis: usually leukocytoclastic, but can involve medium-sized arteries. Lungs: infiltration of alveolar septa and small vessel walls by a mixture of neutrophils, lymphocytes, and plasma cells. One may see pulmo-nary hemorrhage and fibrosis.

Hypocomplementemic Vasculitis

Hypocomplementemic vasculitis (HV) was defined by McDuffie et al in 1973 as a syndrome characterized by hypocomplementemia, cutaneous vasculitis, and arthri-tis. Subsequently the following diagnostic criteria were established: (1) chronic urticaria of more than 6 months' duration, (2) hypocomplementemia, and (3) two of the following: biopsy confirmed dermal venulitis, arthralgias or arthritis, glomerulonephritis, uveitis or episcleritis, recurrent abdominal pain, and a positive C1q precipitin test. Diagnosis requires exclusion of the presence of sig-nificant cryoglobulinemia, elevated anti-DNA titers (>1:32), hepatitis B antigenemia, decreased blood C1-esterase inhibitor, or a hereditary complement deficiency.

Pulmonary involvement is uncommon though pleu-ritic chest pain and transient lung infiltrates have been observed. Often patients have asthmatic symptoms, due to laryngeal edema. Chronic obstructive pulmonary disease may be seen in up to 50% of patients. Although small vessel vasculitis of lung has been postulated, his-tologic confirmation has not been documented. It may represent a manifestation of collagen vascular disease.

Therapy

Low-dose corticosteroids may be effective. With renal dis-ease cyclophosphamide or azathioprine may be required.

Takayasu Arteritis

Takayasu arteritis is a large vessel vasculitis, most com-monly affecting the aorta and its proximal branches. It is usually seen in women less than 40 years of age.

Pulmonary involvement occurs in 12% to 86% of cases by angiography. Lung involvement has been linked to Bw52/Dw12 haplotype.[64] Histologically, lym-phocytic or giant cell arteritis with elastic destruction, fibrosis, narrowing, and occlusion of the affected ves-sels are seen. The disease is on most occasions, diag-nosed by angiography.

ACR proposed the following six criteria for diagno-sis: onset at age less than 40 years, claudication of an extremity, decreased brachial artery pulse, greater than 10 mm Hg difference in systolic blood pressure between arms, a bruit over the subclavian arteries or the aorta, and arteriographic evidence of narrowing or occlusion of the entire aorta, its primary branches, or large arter-ies in the proximal upper or lower extremities. The pres-ence of three of these had a sensitivity of 90.5% and a specificity of 97.8%.

Clinical features of Takayasu arteritis

The disease progresses through three clinical phases:

Inflammatory phase: fever, malaise, weight loss, arthralgias, elevated ESR.

Vascular inflammation: localized pain, vascular ste-nosis, formation of aneurysms.

Ischemia due to vascular narrowing or occlusion: pulseless disease.

Respiratory symptoms are uncommon and include dyspnea, pleuritic chest pain, and pulmonary hypertension.

Rarely, there can have cerebral manifestations, aortic insufficiency, aortic aneurysms, renovascular hypertension.

Imaging features of Takayasu arteritis

Pulmonary artery angiography shows characteristic features of vessel stenosis, irregular narrowing, and occlusion. Abnormal ventilation perfusion scans in up to 76% of cases may be present. Multiple, bilateral, or unilateral defects can be present. Fistula may develop between pulmonary arteries and bronchial or coronary arteries and systemic arteries.

Histologic features of Takayasu arteritis

Large pulmonary arteries are affected. Arteritis is histologically seen as an infiltrate of lymphocytes, macrophages, giant cells predominantly in the outer two-thirds of the vessel wall, sometimes with a throm-bus. It can progress to diffuse or nodular fibrosis of the artery wall with disintegration or loss of elastic fibers. Major complications include stenosis and aneurysm formation.[65,66] Fistula formation is a rare but deadly complication.[65]

Corticosteroid therapy is often successful; cyclophosphamide may be necessary in some cases. Vascular surgery may be required to reverse ischemia.

Giant Cell Arteritis

Giant cell arteritis (GCA) is a disease most common to the temporal arteries and rarely involves the lungs. Rarely, the disease is isolated to pulmonary arteries.

Patients may have respiratory tract symptoms in up to 6% of cases. In reported cases, both the main pulmonary artery (rare) and the trunk can be affected by a giant cell infiltrate, resulting in destruction of the elastic fibers and fibrinoid necrosis.

Differential diagnosis

Takayasu arteritis involves cranial arteries and occurs in a younger age as compared to GCA.

Clinical features of giant cell arteritis

Cough, sore throat, hoarseness, and chest pain.

Histologic features of giant cell arteritis

Histologically, the lesions of GCA show medial and adventitial mononuclear inflammation with giant cells and disruption of elastic laminae (*Figure 16-9*). Focal fibrinoid necrosis of media may be seen. Rarely, granulomatous inflammation of pulmonary arteries may be seen.

Differential diagnosis

Other granulomatous vasculitis: extravascular granulomas are absent in GCA.

Takayasu arteritis: prominent involvement of temporal artery, older age, histologic features.

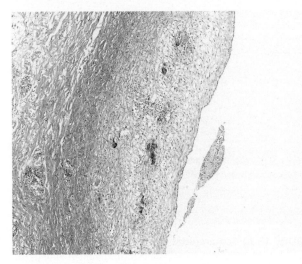

FIGURE 16-9 Giant cell arteritis: multinucleate giant cells in intima of large muscular artery (H&E, 100×).

Disseminated visceral giant cell angiitis

Disseminated visceral giant cell angiitis is a disease of males that is usually clinically unsuspected and mostly discovered incidentally at autopsy. Extracranial small arteries and arterioles typically involve at least three of the following: heart, lung, kidneys, liver, pancreas, and stomach. The inflammation is characteristically chronic with histiocytes, lymphocytes, plasma cells, or multinucleated giant cells, both foreign body type and Langhans type.

SYSTEMIC CONDITIONS THAT MAY BE ASSOCIATED WITH PULMONARY VASCULITIS

Inflammatory Bowel Disease

Pulmonary vasculitis has been reported in patients with inflammatory bowel disease, especially ulcerative colitis. Since these patients are treated with sulfonamides, a known cause of pulmonary vasculitis, a drug reaction should be excluded before attributing pulmonary vasculitis to IBD. Although p-ANCA can be found in patients with IBD, in particular UC, it does not correlate with activity of disease or evidence of systemic or pulmonary vasculitis. A GPA-like syndrome with pulmonary nodular infiltrates, vasculitis, and positive c-ANCA can occur in patients with UC.

Malignant Neoplasms

Rarely malignancy may result in vasculitis involving the lung. In most cases, patients present with cutaneous small vessel vasculitis, and the lung is only one of the several sites involved. Vasculitis as a paraneoplastic syndrome occurs most often in association with lympho- or myeloproliferative disorders. Pulmonary involvement by a microscopic polyangiitis–like syndrome can occur in hairy cell leukemia, acute promyelocytic leukemia with retinoic acid syndrome, and prostate cancer. Churg-Strauss syndrome has also been reported in a patient with malignant melanoma. Pulmonary vasculitis has been reported in a patient with cholangiocarcinoma. Lung cancer may be associated with systemic vasculitis in the form of microvasculitis of the vasa nervosum or Henoch-Schonlein purpura.

Vasculitis can also occur as a local phenomenon when there is prominent intra-arterial or lymphangitic spread of metastatic tumor.

Sarcoidosis

Sarcoidosis is a multisystem granulomatous disorder with frequent lung involvement. Vasculitis is frequently seen in both open lung biopsy specimens and transbronchial specimens of classic sarcoidosis. The vascular lesions can be granulomatous or may consist of lymphocytes and plasma cells with or without necrosis. Venous involvement is more common than combined venous and arterial or arterial involvement. Additionally, patients may develop systemic vasculitis.

Clinical features of sarcoidosis-related vasculitis

Sarcoid-related vasculitis is more common in women (2.2:1) with a mean age of 49 (range: 11–75 years). The peak incidence is in the third and seventh decades.

Fifteen to twenty-five percent of patients are asymptomatic. Symptoms occur in setting of extensive bilateral infiltrates or nodules and include cough, fever, chest pain, dyspnea, malaise, and weight loss.

Extrapulmonary features are present in 13% of cases and commonly include leg weakness and numbness due to spinal cord involvement. Other manifestations are diabetes insipidus due to hypothalamic insufficiency, and iritis, uveitis, or unilateral loss of vision due to retinal involvement.

Elevated sedimentation rate and hypergammaglobulinemia are usually associated.

Imaging features of sarcoidosis-related vasculitis

Diffuse bilateral nodules, unilateral nodules, nodular infiltrates or infiltrates are the common presentations of sarcoidosis with bilateral nodules or nodular infiltrates being most common. Nodules can range from several millimeters up to 5 cm in diameter. They are common in lower lobes and can disappear spontaneously. Cavitation is seen in one-fourth of cases in the nodules or ill-defined infiltrates. Pleural effusion may be present with diffuse disease. Localized lesions may occur, and in such cases may mimic carcinoma or granulomatous lesions. Bilateral hilar adenopathy is uncommon.

Histologic features of sarcoidosis-related vasculitis

Grossly nodular lesions are characteristic. The lesions are less widespread and necrotic than GPA.

Microscopically: Three distinct elements are identified.

Nodular granulomatous pneumonitis with many confluent sarcoid-like granulomas that are discrete and distributed along the pleura, bronchovascular bundles, interlobular septa, and submucosal areas. Hyalinizing granulomas may be seen.

Necrosis: is of variable extent ranging from small central foci of coagulative necrosis to larger geographic zones of infarct-like necrosis.

Vasculitis: Commonly involves muscular pulmonary arteries and veins (*Figure 16-10A, B*). Three types of vascular lesions usually occur: necrotizing granulomas, giant cell vasculitis, or infiltration by mononuclear cells including lymphocytes and macrophages.

Secondary changes like bronchiolitis obliterans, sometimes granulomatous, intra-alveolar foamy macrophages (postobstructive pneumonia) may be seen.

Differential diagnosis

Granulomatous infections: Exclusion of infectious etiology with cultures or special stains.

GPA

Extrapulmonary involvement in NSG is rare and neutrophilic microabscesses and capillaritis are not seen.

Etiology of NSG is uncertain. It is thought that it may be a hypersensitivity reaction to fungal antigens.

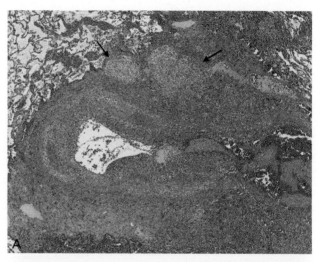

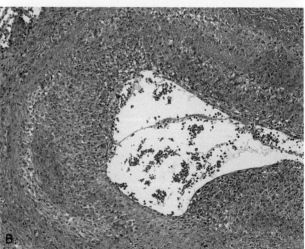

FIGURE 16-10 **A: Sarcoidal vasculitis, epithelioid granulomas (arrow) infiltrating and surrounding vessel wall (H&E, 100×). B: Sarcoidal vasculitis, epithelioid histiocytes infiltrating vessel wall (H&E, 200×).**

Elevated ANCA titers have not been reported and it is uncertain if the vasculitis represents a primary underlying event.

Therapy

NSG has an excellent prognosis and responds well to corticosteroids, with clearing or diminution of infiltrates within 1 week to 10 months after starting therapy. Radiographic infiltrates persist in minority of cases. If the disease relapses, low-dose chlorambucil may be effective. Resection can be performed for localized lesions.

LOCALIZED VASCULITIS AND SECONDARY VASCULITIS

Drugs and Toxins

Pulmonary vasculitis associated with drug or toxic exposure typically causes a small vessel vasculitis. Cases were previously often classified as hypersensitivity vasculitis, which was originally described in 1948 as a leukocytoclastic vasculitis of small blood vessels with prominent cutaneous involvement and frequent association with drug exposure. Zeek et al differentiated hypersensitivity vasculitis, which affected small vessels, from polyarteritis nodosa, which affects larger arteries. The terms microscopic polyarteritis and leukocytoclastic vasculitis have also been used for hypersensitivity vasculitis. The ACR proposed five criteria for a traditional format classification of hypersensitivity vasculitis: (1) age >16 years at onset of disease, (2) history of ingestion of a drug that could have been a precipitating factor, (3) palpable purpura, (4) a maculopapular rash, and (5) a biopsy demonstrating neutrophils around an arteriole or venule.

Pulmonary vasculitis induced by drugs is uncommon. It may reflect a localized pulmonary reaction or be a part of a systemic vasculitis. Since patients with drug-induced vasculitis often have a complex clinical picture, it can be difficult to prove that a given drug was the sole cause of the vasculitis. Careful correlation with the history of drug intake, clinical presentation, and the response to withdrawal of drug is essential before implicating the drug as a cause. Commonly implicated drugs implicated include α-adrenergic nasal sprays, carbamazepine, diphenylhydantoin, allopurinol, cromoglycate, penicillin, nitrofurantoin, propylthiouracil, sulfonamides, procainamide, oral contraceptives, and anti-Tac antibodies. An exhaustive list of drugs that may cause diffuse alveolar hemorrhage is available on www. pneumotox.com.

The lesions of drug-induced vasculitis can have a spectrum of changes. Medium-sized or small arteries or veins, or capillaries can be involved. The infiltrate comprises mononuclear cells, giant cells, or eosinophils.

Surrounding lung may show an interstitial pneumonia consisting of chronic inflammatory cells, lymphoid aggregates, granulomas, cavitary lung nodules, or eosinophils. Thus, it may resemble polyarteritis nodosa, small vessel vasculitis, Churg-Strauss syndrome, and giant cell arteritis.

Pulmonary vasculitis has been described in association with ingestion of specific dietary toxic substances contaminating products such as L-tryptophan and Spanish rapeseed oil.

Drug-induced vasculitis can closely resemble an idiopathic vasculitis syndrome. The clinical severity may vary from mild to severe disease and may be fatal. Some may be self-limited; others may have a prolonged course. Treatment includes discontinuation of the offending drug supplemented with steroids or other immunosuppressive medication when indicated.

Interstitial lung diseases

Vasculitis can be observed in lung biopsies from patients with ILD such as chronic eosinophilic pneumonia or histiocytosis X; however, it is relatively uncommon and is usually inconspicuous. Histologically, the vascular lesions of chronic eosinophilic pneumonia typically show few lymphocytes infiltrating the wall of a small artery or a vein. In histiocytosis X, vasculitis is very rare and may consist of eosinophils or lymphocytes infiltrating the wall of a blood vessel adjacent to an active inflammatory lesion.

Emboli

A foreign body type of granulomatous vasculitis can occur in association with pulmonary lipid accumulations in patients who received intralipid infusions as a part of total parenteral nutritional support.

Vasculitis can be observed in lungs from intravenous drug abusers (*Figure 16-11A*). These individuals develop a foreign body–type granulomatous reaction to embolic talc (*Figure 16-11B, C*) that migrates into tissues surrounding pulmonary arteries.

Infection

Vasculitis can be seen as a part of the disease process in a variety of infections. Invasion and necrosis of blood vessels is characteristic of bacterial infections like *Pseudomonas aeruginosa* and *Legionella pneumatophila* resulting in hemorrhagic pneumonia (*Figure 16-12A*). Syphilis and rickettsial disease are usually associated with vasculitis. Vasculitis can be seen in areas adjacent to fungal or mycobacterial organisms (*Figure 16-12B*) and can mimic GPA. *Malassezia furfur* a fungus that commonly infects skin has been reported to cause vasculitis in infants who developed pulmonary artery lipid deposits associated with Intralipid therapy.

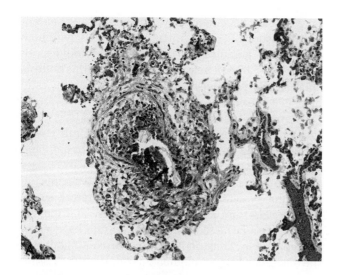

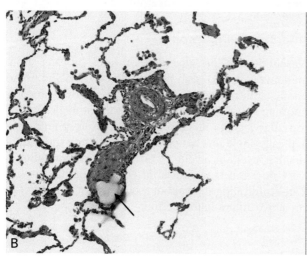

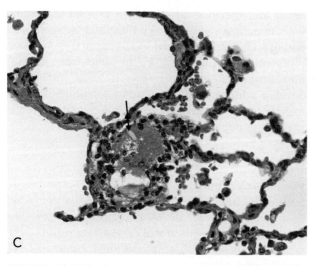

FIGURE 16-11 A: Intravenous drug use, foreign body giant cells around intraluminal foreign body (arrow) (H&E, 200×). **B:** Intravenous drug use, foreign material within vascular lumen (arrow), and intimal and muscular thickening consistent with hypertensive vasculopathy (H&E, 200×). **C:** Talcosis, foreign material (arrow) within a giant cell (H&E, 200×).

Fungi such as *Aspergillus* (*Figure 16-12C*) and *Mucor* (*Figure 16-12D*) are angioinvasive and associated with pulmonary infarctions. Vasculitis has been reported as a rare complication of *Pneumocystis jiroveci* pneumonia in HIV-infected patients. The vasculitis may be observed adjacent to cavitary nodular lesions or in association with disseminated extrapulmonary infections.

Vasculitis can also be seen in association with pulmonary infection caused by certain parasites such as *Dirofilaria immitis* (*Figure 16-12E, F*), *Schistoma*, and *Wuchereria*. In pulmonary dirofilariasis, the adult worm embolizes to a pulmonary artery, occluding the lumen, and resulting in an infarct that may be surrounded by granulomatous reaction and eosinophilia. The affected pulmonary artery is often situated in the center of the infarct and may have inflammatory changes in the wall with infiltration by chronic inflammatory cells or eosinophils.

Many viruses can cause vasculitis, hepatitis B virus–related polyarteritis nodosa being the most common. Mixed cryoglobulinemia associated with more than 80% hepatitis C virus infection can result in a vasculitis in few cases. Other viral infections that can cause vasculitis are human immunodeficiency virus (HIV), erythrovirus B19, cytomegalovirus, varicella-zoster virus, and human T-cell lymphotropic virus (HTLV-1).[67]

Pulmonary hypertension

Pulmonary arterial hypertension can occur secondary to a variety of causes including idiopathic plexogenic pulmonary arteriopathy, congenital heart disease, toxins, collagen vascular disease, and liver disease. Vasculitis may be seen in these conditions. However, arteritis occurs only in severe pulmonary hypertension, and necrotizing arteritis is a characteristic feature of grade 6 pulmonary hypertension. Necrotizing arteritis in pulmonary hypertension can be acute, consisting of necrosis of the media and infiltration by neutrophils, or it may be subacute with granulomatous changes in the arterial walls (*Figure 16-13*). The underlying events that contribute to vascular injury are varied and can include chronic vasospasm, or dietary toxins such as crotalaria, aminorex, and Spanish rapeseed oil.

Vasculitis is not a characteristic of pulmonary veno-occlusive disease, but fibrinoid necrosis of arteries has been described in rare cases. Granulomatous venulitis is a rare potential cause of pulmonary veno-occlusive disease; granulomatous vasculitis causing veno-occlusive disease has also been reported in sarcoidosis.

Transplantation

Periarteriolar and perivenular mononuclear inflammation with intimal hyperplasia and mild muscular hypertrophy can be seen in recipients of heart-lung

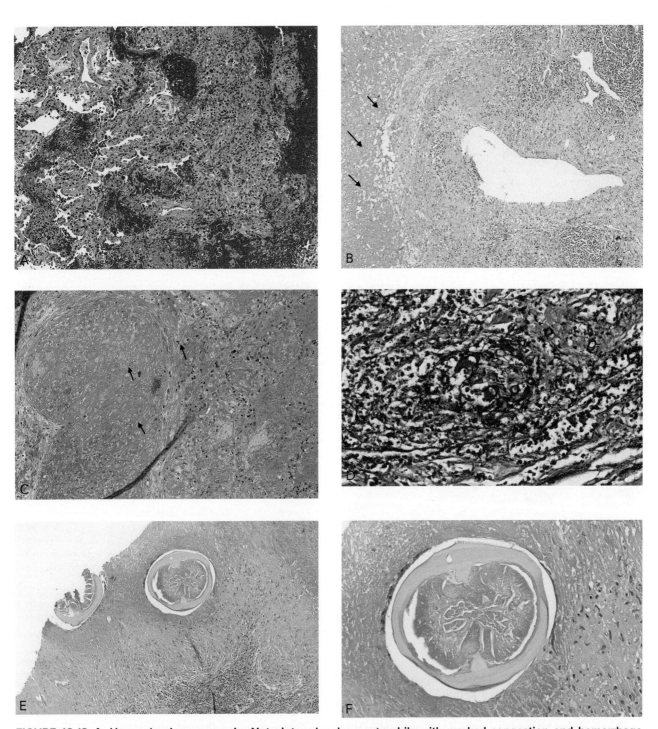

FIGURE 16-12 A: Hemorrhagic pneumonia. Note intra-alveolar neutrophils with marked congestion and hemorrhage (H&E, 100×). B: Tuberculosis vasculitis, caseating granulomas (arrow) involving a medium-sized vessel (H&E, 100×). C: Aspergillus vasculitis, septate hyaline fungal hyphae (arrow) occluding a vessel and infiltrating through the wall (H&E, 200×). D: Mucor vasculitis. Hyaline ribbon–like fungal hyphae (arrow) infiltrating a blood vessel (H&E, 200×). E,F: Dirofilariasis, cross section of the parasite in possible vascular lumen (H&E, e-100×, f-200×).

transplants. A necrotizing, pauci-inflammatory septal capillary injury is a morphologic marker for acute rejection (*Figure 16-14*). Acute vasculitis can be found in 5% to 9% of the lung biopsies from lung transplant recipients. Pulmonary capillaritis is a very rare manifestation of

acute pulmonary allograft rejection.[68] Arteriosclerosis of pulmonary arteries can occur in long-term survivors of heart-lung transplantation.

A long-term survivor of bone marrow transplantation has been reported to have developed a vasculitis with

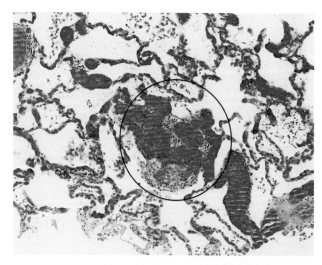

FIGURE 16-13 Pulmonary hypertensive vasculopathy with cavernous lesions (circle) (H&E, 100×).

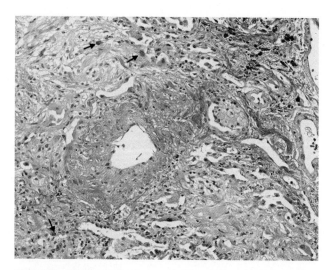

FIGURE 16-15 Radiation vasculopathy demonstrating thick-walled hyalinized vessel with stromal nuclear atypia (arrow) (H&E, 100×).

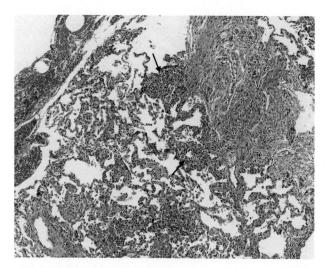

FIGURE 16-14 Acute cellular rejection, moderate grade with a mononuclear perivascular (arrow) and interstitial inflammatory infiltrate (H&E, 100×).

recurrent pulmonary hemorrhage, clinical and pathologic evidence of cutaneous and pulmonary leukocytoclastic vasculitis, and an elevated serum ANCA. It is not certain whether pulmonary vasculitis syndrome in this patient was a coincidental phenomenon or whether it represented a newly recognized complication of bone marrow transplantation. The vasculitis in this patient responded to treatment with cyclophosphamide and prednisone.

Radiation

Vasculitis may occur as a complication of radiation exposure. Early vascular injury in radiation damage to the lungs consists of edema of the walls of small arteries and arterioles followed by intimal proliferation and

medial injury (*Figure 16-15*). Fibrinoid necrosis can affect the small arteries and hyaline thickening can occur in vessel wall. Foam cell plaques are highly suggestive of radiation vasculitis and consist of subintimal deposition of macrophages with foamy cytoplasm in arterial walls.

REFERENCES

1. Ashbaugh DG, Bigelow DB, Petty TL, et al. Acute respiratory distress in adults. *Lancet*. 1967;2:319-323.
2. Bernard GR, Artigas A, Brigham KL, et al. The American-European Consensus Conference on ARDS. Definitions, mechanisms, relevant outcomes, and clinical trial coordination. *Am J Respir Crit Care Med*. 1994;149(3 pt 1):818-824.
3. Rubenfeld GD, Caldwell E, Peabody E, et al. Incidence and outcomes of acute lung injury. *N Engl J Med*. 2005;353:1685-1693.
4. Gao L, Barnes KC. Recent advances in genetic predisposition to clinical acute lung injury. *Am J Physiol Lung Cell Mol Physiol*. 2009;296:713-725.
5. Berkowitz DM, Danai PA, Eaton S, et al. Alcohol abuse enhances pulmonary edema in acute respiratory distress syndrome. *Alcohol Clin Exp Res*. 2009;33:1690-1696.
6. Luhr OR, Antonsen K, Karlsson M, et al. Incidence and mortality after acute respiratory failure and acute respiratory distress syndrome in Sweden, Denmark, and Iceland. The ARF Study Group. *Am J Respir Crit Care Med*. 1999;159:1849-1861.
7. Gajic O, Dabbagh O, Park PK, et al. Early identification of patients at risk of acute lung injury: evaluation of lung injury prediction score in a multicenter cohort study. *Am J Respir Crit Care Med*. 2010;183:462-470.
8. Moss M, Guidot DM, Steinberg KP, et al. Diabetic patients have a decreased incidence of acute respiratory distress syndrome. *Crit Care Med*. 2000;28:2187-2192.
9. Dushianthan A, Grocott MP, Postle AD, Cusack R. Acute respiratory distress syndrome and acute lung injury. *Postgrad Med J*. 2011;87(1031):612-622.
10. Phua J, Badia JR, Adhikari NK, et al. Has mortality from acute respiratory distress syndrome decreased over time? A systematic review. *Am J Respir Crit Care Med*. 2009;179:220-227.

11. Avecillas JF, Freire AX, Arroliga AC. Clinical epidemiology of acute lung injury and acute respiratory distress syndrome: incidence, diagnosis, and outcomes. *Clin Chest Med.* 2006;27(4):549-557.

12. Saeed MM, et al. Prognosis in pediatric idiopathic pulmonary hemosiderosis, *Chest.* 1999;116(3):721-725.

13. Nuesslein TG, Teig N, Rieger CHL. Pulmonary hemosiderosis in infants and children. *Paediatr Respir Rev.* 2006;7(1):45-48.

14. Gordon IO, Cipriani N, Quidsia A, Craig M, Husain A. Update in nonneoplastic lung diseases. *Arch Pathol Lab Med.* 2009;133:1096-1105.

15. Kiper N, et al. Long-term clinical course of patients with idiopathic pulmonary hemosiderosis (1979-1994): prolonged survival with low-dose corticosteroid therapy. *Pediatr Pulmonol.* 1999;27(3):180-184.

16. Khemiri M, Ouederni M, Khaldi F, Barsaoui S. Screening for celiac disease in idiopathic pulmonary hemosiderosis. *Gastroenterol Clin Biol.* 2008;32(8-9):745–748

17. Chu SH, et al. Juvenile idiopathic arthritis with pulmonary hemosiderosis: a case report. *J Microbiol Immunol Infect.* 2002;35(2):133-135.

18. Yacoub M, et al. Idiopathic pulmonary hemosiderosis, celiac disease and cardiomyopathy. *Arch Pediatr.* 1994;1(6):587-590.

19. Attia S, et al. Antineutrophilic cytoplasmic antibodies positivity in a case of idiopathic pulmonary hemosiderosis. *Ann Biol Clin (Paris).* 2005;63(2):209-212.

20. Calbrese F, et al. Recurrence of idiopathic pulmonary hemosiderosis in a young adult patient after bilateral single-lung transplantation. *Transplantation.* 2002;74(11):1643-1645.

21. Butter A, Emran M, Al-Jazaeri A, Bouron-Dal Soglio D, Bouchard S. Pulmonary arteriovenous malformation mimicking congenital cystic adenomatoid malformation in a newborn. *J Pediatr Surg.* 2006;41(5):9-11.

22. Fraga JC, Favero E, Contelli F, Canani F. Surgical treatment of congenital pulmonary arteriovenous fistula in children. *J Pediatr Surg.* 2008;43(7):1365-1367.

23. Mitchell RO, Austin EH 3rd. Pulmonary arteriovenous malformation in the neonate. *J Pediatr Surg.* 1993;28(12):1536-1538.

24. Marianeschi SM, McElhinney DB, Reddy VM, Pulmonary arteriovenous malformations in and out of the setting of congenital heart disease. *Ann Thorac Surg.* 1998;66(2):688-691.

25. Thung KH, Sihoe AD, Wan IY, Lee TW, Wong R, Yim AP. Hemoptysis from an unusual pulmonary arteriovenous malformation. *Ann Thorac Surg.* 2003;76(5):1730-1733.

26. Frankel, SK, Schwarz, MI. The pulmonary vasculitides. *Am J Respir Crit Care Med.* 2012;86(3):216-224.

27. Falk RJ, Gross WL, Guillevin L, et al. Granulomatosis with polyangiitis (Wegener's): an alternative name for Wegener's granulomatosis. *Ann Rheum Dis.* 2011;70(4):704.

28. Hoffman GS, Kerr GS, Leavitt RY, et al. Wegener granulomatosis: an analysis of 158 patients. *Ann Intern Med.* 1992;116(6):488-498.

29. Watts RA, Al-Taiar A, Scott DG, Macgregor AJ. Prevalence and incidence of Wegener's granulomatosis in the UK general practice research database. *Arthritis Rheum.* 2009;61(10):1412-1416.

30. Watts RA, Scott DG. Epidemiology of the vasculitides. *Semin Respir Crit Care Med.* 2004;25(5):455-464.

31. Koldingsnes W, Nossent H. Epidemiology of Wegener's granulomatosis in northern Norway. *Arthritis Rheum.* 2000;43(11):2481-2487.

32. Lynch JP III, Tazelaar H. Wegener granulomatosis (granulomatosis with polyangiitis): evolving concepts in treatment. *Semin Respir Crit Care Med.* 2011;32:274-297.

33. Gubbels SP, Barkhuizen A, Hwang PH. Head and neck manifestations of Wegener's granulomatosis. *Otolaryngol Clin North Am.* 2003;36(4):685-705.

34. Cannady SB, Batra PS, Koening C, et al. Sinonasal Wegener granulomatosis: a single-institution experience with 120 cases. *Laryngoscope.* 2009;119(4):757-761.

35. Lynch JP III, White E, Tazelaar H, Langford CA. Wegener's granulomatosis: evolving concepts in treatment. *Semin Respir Crit Care Med.* 2004;25(5):491-521.

36. Hoffman GS, Thomas-Golbanov CK, Chan J, Akst LM, Eliachar I. Treatment of subglottic stenosis, due to Wegener's granulomatosis, with intralesional corticosteroids and dilation. *J Rheumatol.* 2003;30(5):1017-1021.

37. Reinhold-Keller E, Beuge N, Latza U, et al. An interdisciplinary approach to the care of patients with Wegener's granulomatosis: long-term outcome in 155 patients. *Arthritis Rheum.* 2000;43(5):1021-1032.

38. Travis WD, Hoffman GS, Leavitt RY, Pass HI, Fauci AS. Surgical pathology of the lung in Wegener's granulomatosis: review of 87 open-lung biopsies from 67 patients. *Am J Surg Pathol* 1991;15:315-333.

39. Ulbright TM, Katzenstein AL. Solitary necrotizing granulomas of the lung: differentiating features and etiology. *Am J Surg Pathol.* 1980;4:13-28.

40. Myers JL, Katzenstein A-LA. Wegener's granulomatosis presenting with massive pulmonary hemorrhage and capillaritis. *Am J Surg Pathol.* 1987;11:895-898.

11. Yousem SA. Bronchocentric injury in Wegener's granulomatosis: a case report of five cases. *Hum Pathol.* 1991;22:535-540.

42. Yousen SA, Lombard CM. The eosinophilic variant of Wegener's granulomatosis. *Hum Pathol.* 1988;19:682-688.

43. Katzenstein A-LA, Locke KW. Solitary lung lesions in Wegener's granulomatosis. *Am J Surg Pathol.* 1995;19(5):545-552.

44. Ramsey J, Amari M, Kantrow SP. Pulmonary vasculitis: clinical presentation, differential diagnosis, and management. *Curr Rheumatol Rep.* 2010;12:420-428.

45. Donaghy M, Rees AJ. Cigarette smoking and lung haemorrhage in glomerulonephritis caused by autoantibodies to glomerular basement membrane . *Lancet.* 1983;2(8364):1390-1393.

46. Dammacco F, Battaglia S, Gesualdo L, Racanelli V. Goodpasture's disease: a report of ten cases and a review of literature. *Autoimmun Rev.* 2013;12(11):1101-1106.

47. Mahra A, Moosigb F, Neumannc T, et al. Eosinophilic granulomatosis with polyangiitis (Churg–Strauss): evolutions in classification, etiopathogenesis, assessment and management. www.co-rheumatology.com. 2014:26(1).

48. Mahr A, Guillevin L, Poissonnet M, Aymé S. Prevalences of polyarteritis nodosa, microscopic polyangiitis, Wegener's granulomatosis, and Churg-Strauss syndrome in a French urban multiethnic population in 2000: a capture-recapture estimate. *Arthritis Rheum.* 2004;51(1):92-99.

49. Haugeberg G, Bie R, Bendvold A, Larsen AS, Johnsen V. Primary vasculitis in a Norwegian community hospital: a retrospective study. *Clin Rheumatol.* 1998;17(5):364-368.

50. Harrold LR, Andrade SE, Go AS, et al. Incidence of Churg-Strauss syndrome in asthma drug users: a population-based perspective. *J Rheumatol.* 2005;32(6):1076-1080.

51. Martin RM, Wilton LV, Mann RD. Prevalence of Churg-Strauss syndrome, vasculitis, eosinophilia and associated conditions: retrospective analysis of 58 prescription-event monitoring cohort studies. *Pharmacoepidemiol Drug Saf.* 1999;8(3):179-189.

52. Guillevin L, Cohen P, Gayraud M, Lhote F, Jarrousse B, Casassus P. Churg-Strauss syndrome: clinical study and long-term follow-up of 96 patients. *Medicine (Baltimore).* 1999;78(1):26-37.

53. Sinico R, Di Toma L, Maggiore U, et al. Renal involvement in Churg-Strauss syndrome. *Am J Kidney Dis.* 2006;47(5): 770-779.

54. Dunogué B, Pagnoux C, Guillevin L. Churg-Strauss syndrome: clinical symptoms, complementary investigations, prognosis and outcome, and treatment. *Semin Respir Crit Care Med.* 2011;32:298-309.

55. Sinico RA, Di Toma L, Maggiore U, et al. Prevalence and clinical significance of antineutrophil cytoplasmic antibodies in Churg-Strauss syndrome. *Arthritis Rheum.* 2005;52(9):2926-2935.

56. Roufosse F, Cogan E, Goldman M. The hypereosinophilic syndrome revisited. *Annu Rev Med*. 2003;54:169-184.

57. Guillevin L, Pagnoux C, Seror R, et al. The Five-Factor Score revisited: assessment of prognoses of systemic necrotizing vasculitides based on the French Vasculitis Study Group (FVSG) cohort. *Medicine (Baltimore)*. 2011;90(1):19-27.

58. Niles J, Bottinger E, Saurina G, et al. The syndrome of lung hemorrhage and nephritis is usually an ANCA-associated condition. *Arch Intern Med*. 1996;156(4):440-445.

59. Jennette J, Falk R. Small-vessel vasculitis. *N Engl J Med*. 1997;337(21):1512-1523.

60. Saulsbury FT. Henoch-Schönlein purpura. *Curr Opin Rheumatol*. 2001;13:35-40.

61. Matsumoto T, Homma S, Okada M, et al. The lung in polyarteritis nodosa: a pathologic study of 10 cases. *Hum Pathol*. 1993;24(7):717-724.

62. Jennette J, Falk R, Andrassy K, et al. Nomenclature of systemic vasculitides. *Arthritis Rheum*. 1994;37(2):187-192.

63. Fishbein GA, Fishbein MC. Lung vasculitis and alveolar hemorrhage. *Pathology Semin Respir Crit Care Med*. 2011;32: 254-263.

64. Numano F, Ohta N, Sasazuki T. HLA and clinical manifestations in Takayasu disease. *Jpn Circ J*. 1982;46(2):184-189.

65. Kerr G, Hallahan C, Giordano J, et al. Takayasu arteritis. *Ann Intern Med*. 1994;120(11):919-929.

66. Endo M, Tomizawa Y, Nishida H, et al. Angiographic findings and surgical treatments of coronary artery involvement in Takayasu arteritis. *J Thorac Cardiovasc Surg*. 2003;125(3):570-577.

67. Pagnoux C. Vasculitides secondary to infections. *Clin Exper Rheum*. 2006;24(2):71-81.

68. Astor TL, Weill D, Cool C, Teitelbaum I, Schwarz MI, Zamora MR. Pulmonary capillaritis in lung transplant recipients: treatment and effect on allograft function. *J Heart Lung Transplant*. 2005;24(12):2091-2097.

17 Transplant-Related Conditions

Yimin Ge, Haijun Zhou and Eunice K. Choi

TAKE HOME PEARLS

- Interpreting pathologic findings of lung transplant biopsies within the context of the clinical situation and communicating with the treating physicians is critical to ensure accurate diagnosis and appropriate treatment.
- The clinical history can be very helpful in histology interpretation, including patient's age, primary lung disease, time of transplant, previous biopsy findings, current clinical issues, laboratory data, and compliance with treatment.
- Knowledge about the time sequence of common conditions involving lung transplant is valuable during histology evaluation. For example, hyperacute rejection and primary graft dysfunction may occur during or shortly after the transplant procedure, while acute cellular rejection usually takes more than 2 weeks to develop and chronic rejection is not seen until 6 months or more after transplant.
- Most of the posttransplant lung infections occur in the first 6 months after transplant, with bacterial infections mostly in the first month and viral, fungal, and other opportunistic infections in the following months.
- The common conditions involving lung transplant recipients often have significant overlapping histologic features and they may coexist. Communication with the treating physician and correlation with clinical, radiographic, microbiologic, and serologic findings are valuable for accurate diagnosis.

- Lung transplant rejection is usually evaluated by transbronchial biopsies which often provide limited tissue. Both the pulmonologists and the pathologists should be aware of the sampling limitation and clinicopathological correlation is essential.
- Diagnosis of acute cellular rejection requires a circumferential lymphocytic cuffing around blood vessels in the lung parenchyma, preferably away from airways. The reason is that the bronchial associated lymphoid tissue (BALT) can simulate acute rejection on tangential sections. Deeper sections may be helpful if there is uncertainty about the diagnosis.
- BALT can also be misinterpreted as airway inflammation in poorly oriented tissue sections. Airway inflammation often has a variety of types of inflammatory cells infiltrating the mucosa or submucosa, or dissecting smooth muscle with associated edema and stromal reactive change. Epithelial damage can be seen in severe inflammation. In contrast, BALT is a relatively confined cluster of lymphoid tissue often with a clean background and absence of epithelial damage. Deeper sections may be helpful if there is uncertainty about the diagnosis.
- Rarely, scant vessels with incomplete or almost complete lymphocytic cuffing are seen, giving rise to a differential diagnosis between minimal acute rejection (Grade A1) and nonspecific inflammatory change. The approach to such cases should be conservative and descriptive, and the equivocal findings should be communicated to the pulmonologist for clinical correlation.

INTRODUCTION

The first lung transplantation in a human was performed in 1963 by Dr James Hardy and the patient survived with the lung graft for 18 days.[1] However, lung transplantation did not become a meaningful treatment choice in clinical practice until the late 1980s, thanks to the improvement in immunosuppression drugs, especially by cyclosporine A, and enhanced surgical techniques. Through 2011, more than 40,000 lung transplant procedures have been performed worldwide.[2,3] In current medical practice, lung transplantation has become an accepted, if not routine, procedure for end-stage lung diseases in both adults and children.

The most common indications for lung transplantation in adults are chronic obstructive pulmonary disease (COPD)/emphysema, idiopathic pulmonary fibrosis (IPF), cystic fibrosis and α-1 antitrypsin deficiency. The indication for children varies by age: in infants and preschoolers, the most common indication is idiopathic pulmonary arterial hypertension, which is followed by congenital heart disease, idiopathic pulmonary fibrosis, and surfactant protein B deficiency, while cystic fibrosis is the most common indication in children 6 years and older.

This chapter will focus on pathology of post-lung transplantation complications, rejection, infection, and other related conditions. The native lung diseases will be discussed in other chapters in the book and readers need to refer to other books or literatures for issues related to allograft selection, donor match, or surgical procedures.

PRIMARY GRAFT DYSFUNCTION

Primary graft dysfunction (PGD) is a syndrome with a spectrum of mild to severe lung injury that occurs within the first 72 hours following lung transplantation in absence of secondary causes. Before the taxonomy was standardized in 2005 as PGD,[4] various terms have been used for the syndrome including ischemia-reperfusion injury, noncardiac pulmonary edema, early graft dysfunction, posttransplant ARDS, and primary graft failure. PGD is the leading cause of early morbidity and mortality of lung transplantation and affects 11% to 57% of all lung transplant recipients in early studies.[4-16] Since the International Society for Heart & Lung Transplantation (ISHLT) standardized definition and grading, the overall incidence of severe PGD (grade 3) has been reported at about 30% within the first 72 hours.[17-24] The 30-day mortality of patients with PGD is about 40%, which is sevenfold higher than that of recipients who do not develop PGD.[25] Furthermore, PGD is associated with impaired long-term graft function[9] and an increased risk for bronchiolitis obliterans syndrome (BOS).[19]

The central pathogenesis of PGD is believed to be initiated by ischemia-reperfusion injury after reestablishment of pulmonary circulation with subsequent generation of damaging reactive oxygen species (ROS). ROS are known to cause direct injury to pulmonary endothelium and epithelium, resulting in capillary and alveolar leakiness that manifests histologically as acute lung injury pattern including diffuse alveolar damage (DAD). Secondary activation of complex inflammatory cascade results in upregulation of chemokines and cytokines leading to the recruitment of recipient T cells and neutrophils, which further damages the graft function and may also simulate acute rejection or infection.

Patients with PGD commonly present with immediate impairment in lung function after transplantation accompanied by rapid development of pulmonary edema, increased pulmonary vascular resistance, and decreased airway compliance. PGD is usually diagnosed clinically based on PaO_2/FiO_2 (P/F) ratio and radiological infiltrates assessed at time points up to 72 hours after transplant, according to the grading system proposed by the ISHLT working group on PGD.[4] It is important to stress that the diagnosis of PGD requires exclusion of mechanical causes, pneumonia, aspiration, hyperacute rejection, cardiogenic pulmonary edema, and pulmonary venous anastomotic obstruction.

As mentioned above, the diagnosis of PGD is made based on clinical assessments, whereas histologic evaluation is usually unnecessary and often unfeasible due to critical clinical condition. However, transbronchial or wedge lung biopsies may occasionally be performed to rule out other etiologies that may mimic, modify, or confound the diagnosis and grading of PGD. The histologic features of PGD vary from mild to severe acute lung injury, with majority of those acquired biopsies being diffuse alveolar damage indistinguishable from those occurred in other conditions. Pulmonary edema, hyaline membranes, intravascular thrombi, intra-alveolar hemorrhage, infarction, reactive pneumocyte hyperplasia, and inflammatory infiltration can be seen (*Figure 17-1A–D*).

The important responsibility for pathologists in this clinical setting is not only to diagnose diffuse alveolar damage that may be compatible with PGD, but also to carefully assess the possibilities of other common and treatable etiologies such as rejection, infection, or aspiration. Hyperacute rejection may have similar histologic findings, but usually occurs even earlier than PGD and can be evaluated by detection of circulating specific antidonor antibody. Acute cellular rejection is uncommon in the first 72 hours after transplant and is characterized by perivascular lymphoplasmacytic infiltration which is not a standout feature in PGD. Pathologists should also diligently search for foreign material (such as vegetable matter), viral inclusions, granulomas and excessive acute inflammation, or abscesses that may

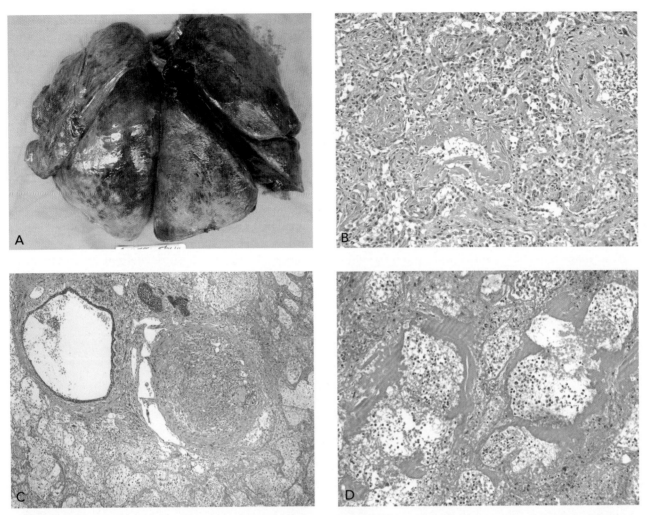

FIGURE 17-1 A: Lungs from a patient died of primary graft dysfunction demonstrate diffuse congestion, hemorrhage, and significant increase of weight (combined weight of bilateral lungs 1970 g). **B:** Histologically, severe acute lung injury is observed with hyaline membranes (diffuse alveolar damage), inflammatory infiltration, and reactive pneumocyte hyperplasia. **C:** Intravascular thrombi are common and often lead to infarction and hemorrhage. **D:** Advanced acute lung injury can be seen with extensive necrosis, intra-alveolar hemorrhage, and residual hyaline membranes.

indicate aspiration or infection. Special stains such as GMS, Gram, or AFB should be performed, and microbiology cultures may be submitted if extra tissue is available. It is worth to point out that these conditions have significant overlapping features with PGD or coexist with PGD, and clinical and radiographic correlation is essential during histologic evaluation.

The risk factors for development of PGD can be donor related (female, old age, African-American race, smoker, low PaO_2/FIO_2 ratio),[8,26-28] recipient related (idiopathic pulmonary arterial hypertension, idiopathic pulmonary fibrosis, sarcoidosis, high body mass index),[8,20,27-32] or operative related (single lung transplant, prolonged ischemia, intracellular preservation solutions, blood transfusion).[20,30,33,34] Understanding the risk factors is critical for development of strategy to safely expand the donor lung pool. Strategies aimed

to prevent and minimize the development and severity of PGD include optimizing selection and matching of donors and recipients, improving lung preservation and storage methods, and improving lung implantation and reperfusion techniques. Utilizing molecular and genetic markers for prediction, diagnosis, and prognosis of PGD are currently under investigation.

LUNG TRANSPLANT ANASTOMOSIS COMPLICATIONS

Lung transplant anastomosis complications include vascular and bronchial anastomotic complications. Vascular complication is rare and occurs in about 1.75% of vascular anastomoses.[35] However, the incidence of airway complications following lung transplantation ranges from 7% to 18% with mortality approximating 2% to 5%.[36,37] Patients are predisposed to anastomotic site ischemia and resultant infection since no attempt is routinely made to reestablish systemic blood flow via bronchial artery circulation.[38] Bronchial arteries often fail to regrow distally to the bronchial anastomosis and mucosal oxygen saturation distal to the anastomosis is lower than that in the native airways.[39] Ischemic injury generally causes ulceration and necrosis as well as the formation of granulation tissue and fibrosis, eventually leading to airway narrowing and potentially obstruction at the anastomotic site.

Airway Dehiscence

Airway anastomotic site dehiscence, caused by donor bronchus ischemia, is a significant complication and used to be a common cause of early death in the first 15 years of lung transplantation.[40] With improved surgical techniques, the frequency of airway dehiscence has recently decreased dramatically to less than 1%.[36,41,42] In addition to ischemia, several other factors can compromise airway healing, including inadequate organ preservation, infection, intensive immunosuppressive therapy,[43] and rejection.

Histologically, the airway ischemia typically shows mural or transmural ulceration and necrosis of bronchial mucosa, submucosa (*Figure 17-2A, B*), and underlying cartilage (*Figure 17-2C*). Superficially, acute inflammatory and fibrinous exudative material may be deposited, and a variable neutrophilic infiltrate may involve mucosa, submucosa, and underlying cartilage (*Figure 17-2C, D*). These devitalized areas can serve as a nidus for subsequent bacterial or fungal infection

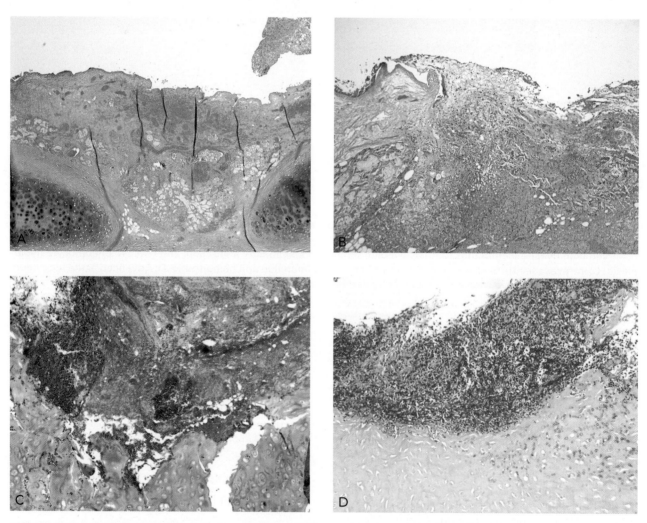

FIGURE 17-2 A: Endobronchial biopsy of anastomotic site from a post-lung transplant patient shows prominent mucosal ulceration, congestion, and hemorrhage. The cartilage and deeper tissue are viable. **B:** The anastomotic site shows ulceration and ischemic necrosis involving bronchial mucosa and submucosa. **C:** Transmural ischemic necrosis and inflammation involves full thickness of bronchial wall including cartilage. Abundant inflammatory exudate is observed on the ulcerated surface. **D:** Severe ischemic necrosis is associated with abundant inflammatory exudates and invasive fungal infection deep into the cartilage.

(*Figure 17-2D*). Special stains for fungal organisms may be helpful in determining a fungal etiology; however, fungal hyphae or yeasts are usually obvious in biopsy tissue with H&E stain. With the progression of the ischemia and/or infection, frank dehiscence may happen eventually, which can lead to mediastinitis, pneumothorax, hemorrhage, and death. However, improved surgical techniques, organ preservation technique, and immunosuppressive agents have dramatically reduced its incidence and mortality.

Airway Stenosis

Bronchial stenosis is the most common airway complication, which may occur at or distal to the anastomotic site and represents the collective results of initial ischemic insult, infection, and rejection.[36,44,45] Airway narrowing typically develops several weeks to months after transplantation. Patients with airway stenosis may be clinically silent or marked by focal wheezing, recurrent bouts of pneumonia or purulent bronchitis, retain secretions, and exhibit worsening pulmonary function test. Narrowing is most commonly due to fibrotic stricture, excessive formation of airway granulation tissue, bronchial fistulas, endobronchial infection, or tracheobronchomalacia.

Histologically, patients with airway stenosis often exhibit variable amounts of granulation tissue (*Figure 17-3A*) and fibrosis, with associated squamous metaplasia in affected site. Biopsies performed later in the course may exhibit variable amounts of granulation tissue, increased areas of fibrosis (*Figure 17-3B*), and foci of calcification. Tracheobronchomalacia is typically a bronchoscopic and radiologic diagnosis and is usually not biopsied. Bronchoscopy is the diagnostic modality and permits therapeutic interventions, including stenting, laser ablation, cryotherapy, electrocautery, or balloon dilation. Treatment of the underlying cause, such as fungal infection is also required. In cases of severe or recurrent narrowing or obstruction compromising functional outcomes, a surgical approach may be necessary.

Vascular Anastomotic Complications

Vascular anastomotic complications are less common and occur within the first week after transplant. Arterial anastomotic obstruction is usually due to suboptimal surgical anastomosis or excessive length of donor or recipient pulmonary artery.[46] Affected patients may present with dyspnea, hypoxemia, or elevated pulmonary arterial pressure. Venous anastomotic obstruction is usually associated with thromboembolism and manifested by unilateral pulmonary edema and sign of outflow obstruction.[47,48] Diagnosis of vascular anastomotic complications is typically

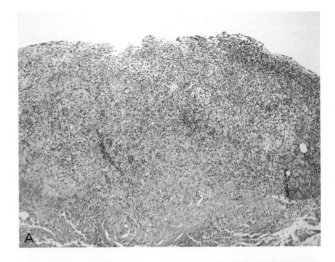

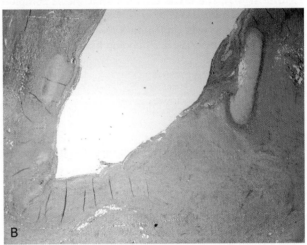

FIGURE 17-3 A: Overgrowth of granulation tissue is often associated with mucosal ulceration and inflammation at the anastomotic site leading to luminal stenosis. **B:** Marked fibrosis of anastomotic site with narrowed bronchus is seen in this patient with posttransplant airway stenosis.

made clinically and radiographically, and in some cases may be difficult to distinguish from reperfusion injury or myocardial dysfunction. Patients may have abnormalities on ventilation-perfusion scan or pulmonary arteriography.

Lung biopsy is usually not performed except for excluding other etiologies. Histologically, the lung tissue shows variable amounts of edema, pulmonary hemorrhage, congestion, and thrombi (*Figures 17-4A, B*). In some cases, thrombi may cause vascular stenosis or occlusion, which may lead to hemorrhagic infarction of lung parenchyma. Treatment with endovascular stents may be effective in selected patients. Emergency treatment is needed for venous obstruction by surgical revision of vascular anastomosis with removal of thrombus.[49]

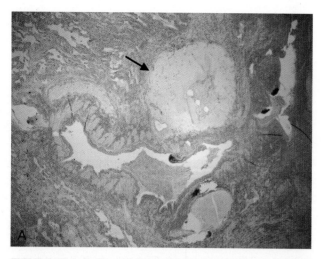
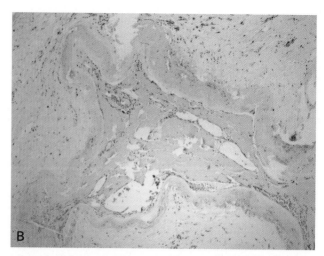

FIGURE 17-4 A: The explanted lung graft shows complete occlusion of a major branch of pulmonary artery by an organized thrombus (arrow) with nearby accompanying bronchus. The lung graft was found having no significant perfusion after surgery and was explanted a few years later. **B:** Higher magnification displays occluded vascular space with an organized thrombus. The surrounding tissue is fibrotic with hyalinization.

REJECTION

Overview

Rejection of allograft by recipient immune system occurs essentially in all solid organ transplantations except that between monozygotic twins. Rejection following lung transplantation is usually evaluated by transbronchial biopsy and, occasionally, by wedge biopsy. Posttransplant transbronchial biopsy is generally performed on a scheduled surveillance protocol, or when rejection, infection,

posttransplant lymphoproliferative disorder (PTLD) or recurrent disease is suspected. Recipients of lung transplantation may present with a wide range of rejection responses and resultant histologic changes depending on the nature and complexity of immunologic processes involved. The alloreactive injury to the donor lung affects both the vasculature and the airways.

In general, rejection of lung allograft is divided into hyperacute, acute, and chronic rejections according to the time of onset, the immunologic mechanisms, as well as the histologic features (*Table 17-1*). The lung rejection

Table 17-1 Clinical Features and Diagnostic Modalities of Lung Allograft Rejection

Type of Rejection	Posttransplant Onset Time	Pathogenesis	Diagnostic Modalities	Prognosis
Hyperacute rejection	Minutes to few hours	Type II hypersensitivity mediated by preexisting antibodies against donor ABO, HLA-I, or endothelium	Intraoperative findings; radiologic features; donor-specific antibody	Usually fatal
Antibody-mediated rejection	Days to weeks	Immune reaction thought to be mediated by preformed or de novo antibodies	Clinical/radiologic features; donor-specific antibody	Fair
Acute rejection	Days to weeks	Cell-mediated immune reaction against graft; development of antibodies to donor HLA-DR/B/A	Transbronchial biopsy; clinical features	Good
Small airway inflammation	Days to weeks	Believed due to donor-specific cellular and humoral immune reactions	Usually by wedge biopsy; transbronchial biopsy often inadequate	Good
Chronic airway rejection	Often after first year	Multifactorial: donor-specific cellular and humoral immune reactions; repeated acute rejection; infection	Clinical features; spirometric defect; transbronchial biopsy often inadequate	Poor
Chronic vascular rejection	Months to years	Unknown	Seen in wedge biopsy or larger specimens; transbronchial biopsy often inadequate	Fair

study group of ISHLT first introduced a "working formulation for the classification of pulmonary allograft rejection" in 1990,[50] which was further revised in 1996[51] and 2007.[52] The later revision simplified the grading scales for small airway inflammation (B category) and chronic airway rejection (C category), and has been generally accepted as a scheme for grading pulmonary allograft rejection. It is important to remember that the grading scheme is strictly based on histology with no clinical parameters included, and an accurate diagnosis relies on absence of current infection due to significant overlapping histologic features. The *Table 17-2* shows the 2007 revision of ISHLT consensus classifications of lung allograft rejection with minor expansion to include hyperacute and antibody-mediated rejections.

Hyperacute Rejection

Hyperacute rejection occurs within minutes to a few hours following perfusion of implanted lung, which is a type II hypersensitivity reaction mediated by preexisting antibodies to donor ABO blood groups, human leukocyte antigens (HLA) class I or other graft endothelial antigens. The subsequent activation of complement

system and platelets causes extensive injury of endothelial cells and vascular thrombosis, leading to graft destruction. Rare cases of hyperacute rejection have been reported and are usually fatal.[53-57] False-negative pretransplant panel-reactive antibody (PRA) reportedly contributed to the hyperacute rejection occurred in these patients.

Hyperacute rejection is usually diagnosed clinically or even intraoperatively since lung graft becomes cyanotic and edematous often immediately after perfusion, and histologic evaluation is confirmatory and retrospective. The pathologic changes of hyperacute rejection include graft edema and cyanosis on gross examination, and microscopic evidence of platelet and fibrin thrombosis, neutrophil infiltration, vascular wall necrosis, and features of diffuse alveolar damage (*Figure 17-5A, B*).[55]

Acute Cellular Rejection (A grade)

Based on ISHLT data, as many as 34% adult lung recipients had at least one episode of acute cellular rejection between discharge and 1 year of follow-up.[2] Acute cellular rejection may be silent in up to 40% of recipients,

Table 17-2 Classifications of Lung Allograft Rejection

Category of Rejection	Grade		Histological Features
Hyperacute rejection	No grading		Acute lung injury/diffuse alveolar damage
Antibody-mediated rejection	No grading		No consensus; capillaritis with perivascular C4d deposition were proposed features
Grade A: Acute rejection	0	None	Normal lung parenchyma
	1	Minimal	Scattered vessels with two to three layers of perivascular mononuclear infiltrates
	2	Mild	More frequent perivascular infiltrates often more than three layers; eosinophils may be present
	3	Moderate	Dense perivascular infiltrates with extension into alveolar septa with or without endotheliitis, eosinophils, and neutrophils
	4	Severe	Diffuse perivascular, interstitial, and air-space infiltrates with prominent pneumocyte damage and endotheliitis
Grade B: Small airway inflammation	0	None	No bronchiolar inflammation
	1R	Low grade	Scattered mononuclear cells in bronchiolar submucosa; no epithelial damage
	2R	High grade	Infiltration of lager activated lymphocytes in bronchiolar epithelium and submucosa with epithelial damage
	X	Ungradable	Small airway inflammation cannot be accurately assessed.
Grade C: Chronic airway rejection-bronchiolitis obliterans	0	Absent	No features of bronchiolitis obliterans
	1	Present	Subepithelial fibrosis with bronchiolar narrowing or obliteration
Grade D: Chronic vascular rejection—accelerated graft vascular sclerosis	0	Absent	No features of chronic vascular rejection
	1	Present	Fibrointimal thickening and hyaline sclerosis of arteries and veins

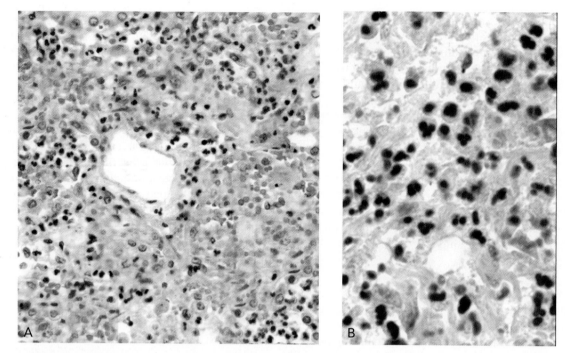

FIGURE 17-5 A, B: Microscopic examination of a postmortem lung graft with hyperacute rejection shows marked congestion, edema, and inflammatory infiltration including abundant neutrophils. Vascular wall necrosis is observed in the microphotographs.

which is the main evidence supporting the surveillance strategy with transbronchial biopsy. Acute cellular rejection is most common in the first year after lung transplantation and reduces markedly thereafter. Multiple episodes of acute cellular rejection and severe lymphocytic bronchiolitis have been associated with increased risk for BOS.[58,59]

Acute cellular rejection is a cell-mediated immune reaction to lung allograft. The hallmark of acute cellular rejection is the presence of perivascular infiltration of mononuclear cells which may or may be accompanied with endotheliitis. The infiltrates may spread into the alveolar septa and then the alveoli with the progression of rejection. The infiltrating cells are mainly T lymphocytes, although a few B lymphocytes and eosinophils may also present.

Grade A0: no acute cellular rejection

Normal lung parenchyma is present without perivascular mononuclear inflammation, hemorrhage, or necrosis.

Grade A1: minimal acute cellular rejection

There are scattered blood vessels in alveolated parenchyma with perivascular mononuclear infiltrates. Blood vessels, particularly venules, are cuffed by small round, plasmacytoid, and transformed lymphocytes forming a ring of two to three cells thick in the perivascular adventitia (*Figure 17-6A, B*). The cellular cuffing is loose

or compact but generally circumferential. Eosinophils and endotheliitis are absent.

Grade A2: mild acute cellular rejection

Circumferential lymphocytic infiltration is essentially confined to the perivascular adventitia with more layers of lymphocytes that are often greater than 3 cells thick (*Figure 17-7A, B*). It can be readily recognized at low magnification and eosinophils and macrophages may be present. Concurrent endotheliitis and lymphocytic bronchiolitis may also be observed.

Grade A3: moderate acute cellular rejection

Apparent perivascular cuffs around pulmonary venules and arterioles are composed of dense mononuclear cell infiltrates that commonly associated with endotheliitis, eosinophils, and occasional neutrophils. The hallmark to define a moderate acute cellular rejection is the inflammatory cell infiltrate extends into the interalveolar septa (*Figure 17-8A, B*). The associated changes include intra-alveolar macrophage collection, type II pneumocyte hyperplasia, and features of acute lung injury.

Grade A4: severe acute cellular rejection

Diffuse mononuclear cell infiltration is seen in perivascular space, interstitial, and air space with prominent

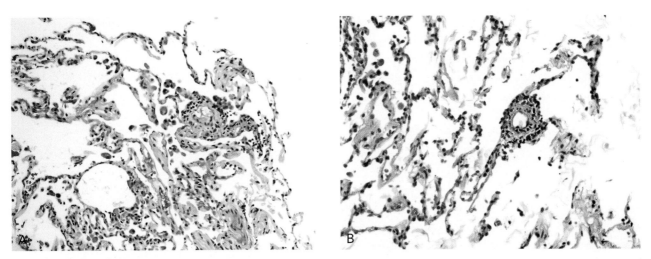

FIGURE 17-6 A, B: Minimal acute rejection (Grade A1) shows a few parenchymal blood vessels cuffed by lymphocytic infiltrates forming a ring of two to three cells thick in the perivascular adventitia. There are no features of aspiration pneumonia or infection present.

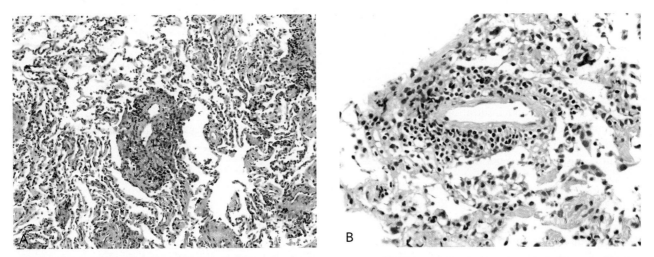

FIGURE 17-7 A, B: Mild acute rejection (Grade A2) shows more prominent perivascular lymphocytic infiltrates that are essentially confined to the perivascular adventitia.

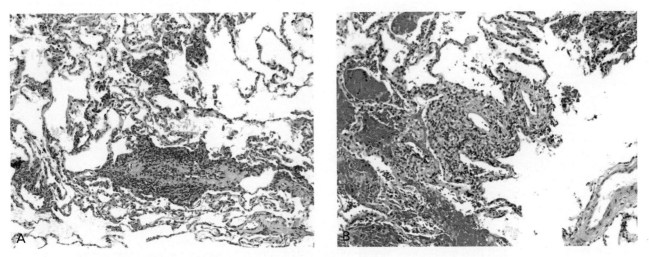

FIGURE 17-8 A, B: Moderate acute rejection (Grade A3) shows dense mononuclear cell infiltrates associated with rare neutrophils and endotheliitis. The inflammatory infiltrate extends into the widened interalveolar septa.

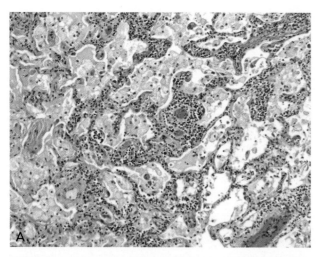
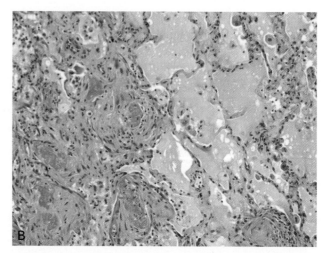

FIGURE 17-9 A, B: Severe acute rejection (Grade A4) shows diffuse inflammatory infiltration in perivascular space, interstitial, and air space with prominent pneumocyte damage, endotheliitis, and intra-alveolar edema. Fibrinoid exudates and hyaline membranes are observed with organization.

pneumocyte damage and endotheliitis (*Figure 17-9A*). Intra-alveolar hemorrhage, eosinophils, neutrophils. as well as necrotic epithelial cells may be present. Acute lung injury is often identified with hyaline membranes and organizing pneumonia (*Figure 17-9B*). As inflammatory cells extend into the alveolar septa and air spaces, the perivascular infiltration may paradoxically attenuate. The mimickers of severe acute rejection include infection, drug toxicity, antibody-mediated rejection, and harvest/reperfusion injury (discussed in the Primary Graft Dysfunction section).

Small Airway Inflammation (B Grade)

The small airways include terminal or respiratory bronchioles. The presence and intensity of combined large and small airway inflammation should be recognized as lymphocytic inflammation of the airways, which may be a harbinger of bronchiolitis obliterans. The airway inflammation is listed as a "B" category with four grades with the R behind grade 1 and 2 denoting the 2007 revision.

Grade B0: no airway inflammation

No inflammation is identified in small airways.

Grade B1R: low-grade small airway inflammation

The mononuclear infiltrates are confined in the submucosa of small airways with scattered or band-like distribution. Occasional eosinophils may or may not present. Epithelial damage or intraepithelial lymphocytic infiltration is not present (*Figure 17-10A*).

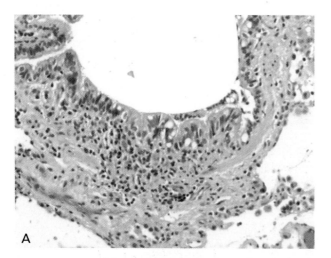
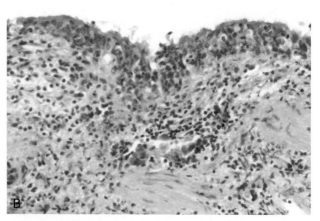

FIGURE 17-10 A: Grade B1R (low-grade small airway inflammation) shows scattered mononuclear infiltrates confined in the submucosa of small airways. Epithelial damage or intraepithelial lymphocytic infiltration is not present. **B: Grade B2R (high-grade small airway inflammation)** shows more severe small airway inflammation with prominent intraepithelial lymphocytic infiltration and epithelial damage.

Grade B2R: high-grade small airway inflammation

Marked lymphocytic infiltration is present in small airways and the mononuclear cells become larger with more eosinophils. Epithelial damage is present with variable necrosis, metaplasia, and marked intraepithelial lymphocytic infiltration (*Figure 17-10B*). If disproportionately high number of neutrophils is present, infection is suggested and subject to further investigation before the diagnosis of rejection is rendered

Grade Bx: ungradable small airway inflammation

This category is reserved sometimes when accurate grading of the small airway inflammation is not possible due to sampling problems, infection, tangential cutting, or other artifacts. Absence of small airways in transbronchial biopsies is common and should be noted in the pathology report.

Chronic Airway Rejection

Chronic airway rejection is to describe the presence of bronchiolitis obliterans (BO) defined as submucosal and intraluminal scaring of membranous or respiratory bronchioles. The fibroproliferative process narrows and eventually obliterates the lumen of small airways, resulting in progressive and irreversible airflow obstruction. Chronic allograft dysfunction due to BO represents the major impediment to long-term survival of lung transplant recipients. Typical histologic features of BO are rarely present in transbronchial biopsies and therefore a clinical equivalent term bronchiolitis obliterans syndrome (BOS) was created based on functional test (FEV$_1$). Approximately 50% of lung transplant recipients develop BOS by 5 years and 75% by 10 years.[60] The development of BOS may represent the result of a wide array of insults to the airway epithelium such as acute cellular rejection and lymphocytic bronchiolitis.[61]

Grade C0: no chronic airway rejection

No obliterative bronchiolitis is present. The small airways appear normal without inflammation or fibrosis.

Grade C1: chronic airway rejection

Obliterative bronchiolitis is present, which is manifested with submucosal eosinophilic hyaline fibrosis in membranous and respiratory bronchioles with variable luminal narrowing/occlusion and inflammation (*Figure 17-11A*). Subsequent changes include injury to bronchiolar smooth muscle and elastica, squamous metaplasia, mucostasis, and foamy histiocyte collections (*Figure 17-11B*). In advanced stage, the occluded small airways may be structurally distorted by extensive fibrosis and become unrecognizable on routine H&E stain (*Figure 17-11C*). Trichrome stain is useful in this situation by highlighting the residual bronchiolar smooth muscle in red (*Figure 17-11D*).

Until recently, bronchiolitis obliterans has been recognized as an almost exclusive contributor to chronic lung allograft dysfunction (CLAD). However, recent studies found that a subgroup of patients with CLAD exhibited restrictive spirometric defect with fibrotic processes in peripheral lung tissue, rather than classic bronchiolitis obliterans.[62] Restrictive allograft syndrome (RAS) was therefore proposed for the newly described subtype that accounts for about 25% to 35% of lung recipients with CLAD and carries significantly worse prognosis.[62,63] Histologically, ROS was reportedly featured by various stages of diffuse alveolar damage and extensive fibrosis in the interstitium, visceral pleura, and interlobular septa, with or without BO.[62] Currently, the pathologic diagnostic criteria of RAS have not been well established.

Chronic Vascular Rejection

Chronic vascular rejection is also known as accelerated graft vascular sclerosis, which may be seen in wedge biopsies, explants or autopsy specimens and rarely in transbronchial biopsies where the vessels with sufficient caliber are usually not present.

Grade D0: no chronic vascular rejection

The pulmonary arteries are unremarkable with a similar size as the accompanying airway. The intima and media are not thickened.

Grade D1: chronic vascular rejection

Intimal fibrous proliferation with vascular wall thickening is typically seen in pulmonary arteries and veins (*Figure 17-12A*). Concurrent endotheliitis has been reported in half of the cases (*Figure 17-12B*). The internal elastic lamella is intact in the early stage (*Figure 17-12C*) and may subsequently become fragmented and discontinuous (*Figure 17-12D, arrow*). Interestingly, the chronic vascular rejection itself does not resulted in graft loss; however, pulmonary hypertension may develop in some patients with BOS.[64,65]

Antibody-Mediated (Humoral) Rejection

Antibody-mediated rejection (AMR) or humoral rejection in lung is not well established as that in other solid organ transplantation such as kidney. AMR is thought to be caused by donor-specific anti-HLA antibodies either generated before transplantation by pregnancy, blood transfusion, prior transplantation, or infection, or developed de novo after lung transplantation.

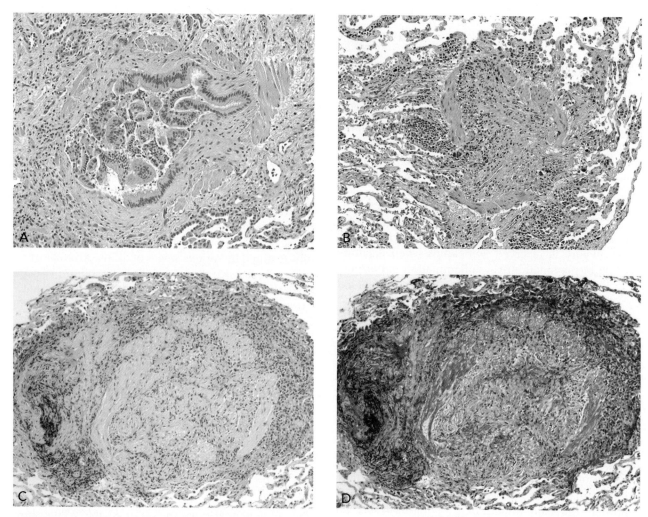

FIGURE 17-11 A-D: Chronic airway rejection (Grade C1) shows bronchiolar inflammation and submucosal fibrosis with luminal narrowing (A) or occlusion (B). Advanced obliterative bronchiolitis may have distorted architecture due to injury of bronchiole smooth muscle (C) and trichrome stain can be helpful by labeling the residual smooth muscle in red (D).

Donor-specific anti-HLA antibodies are associated with increased incidence of acute rejection[66] and BOS,[67] and worse overall survival after lung transplantation.[68]

No consensus has been reached on histopathologic criteria for AMR in lung transplantation. The clinical presentation is indistinguishable from acute cellular rejection and hemoptysis is seen in 25% of cases.[69] The diagnosis mainly relies on detection of circulating donor-specific anti-HLA antibodies in patients with allograft dysfunction. Whether there are specific histopathologic features associated with AMR remains controversial, although capillaritis and subendothelial deposition of immunoglobulin and complement fragments (Igs, C4d, C3d, C1q, and C5b-9) have been advocated by some authors as features of AMR. The histopathologic findings discovered in AMR are generally considered nonspecific and can be seen in number of conditions including high-grade acute rejection, primary graft dysfunction, drug reaction, and infection.[70]

Despite lack of histologic criteria for AMR, capillaritis and associated histologic changes (*Figure 17-13A, B*) should be communicated with clinicians for clinical correlation and further evaluation.

Recent studies questioned the correlation of complement and Ig staining with allograft rejection since the staining can occur in lung transplant recipients with nonalloimmune processes such as infection and primary graft dysfunction in absence of anti-HLA antibodies.[59,71,72] Inconsistency in published data regarding complement and Ig staining reflects the differences in staining techniques and lack of uniform interpretation criteria, that may further confused by high inherent autofluorescence and nonspecific binding of primary antibodies in lung tissue. In our practice, immunofluorescent stain for C4d has not been helpful in establishing a diagnosis of AMR. A recent study from our group demonstrated that the presence of anti-HLA donor-specific antibodies in lung allograft recipients does not

CHAPTER 17

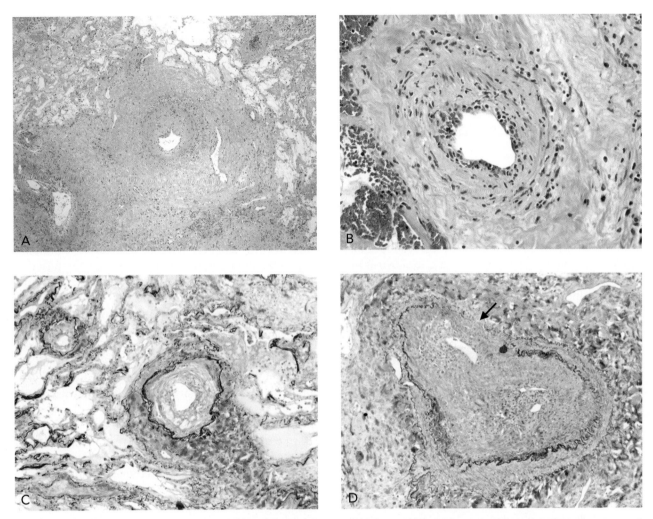

FIGURE 17-12 **A-D:** Chronic vascular rejection (Grade D1) is featured by intimal fibrous proliferation with vascular wall thickening in pulmonary arteries and veins **(A)**. Inflammatory infiltrate of vascular wall and endotheliitis can be seen **(B)**. MOVAT stain shows prominent intimal fibrosis with intact internal elastic lamella in the early stage **(C)**, which may progress to near occlusion of vascular lumen with fragmented and discontinuous internal elastic lamella **(D, arrow)**.

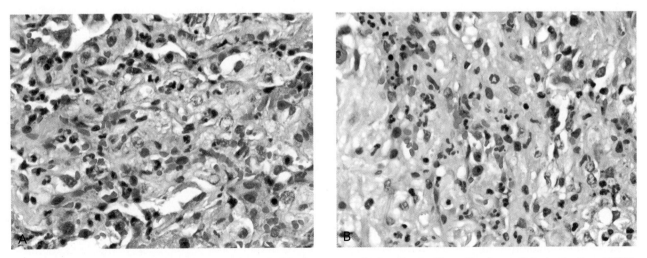

FIGURE 17-13 **A, B:** Capillaritis is observed in a double lung transplant patient with antibody-mediated rejection **(AMR)**. Although this is nondiagnostic for **AMR**, the finding should be reported to treating physician for clinical correlation.

correlate with C4d immunofluorescence in transbronchial biopsy specimens.[73] Multidisciplinary approach with integrating and analyzing clinical, serological, and histological findings is currently recommended by ISHLT for diagnosis of AMR.[70]

LUNG TRANSPLANT ASSOCIATED INFECTIONS

Lung transplant associated infections are common and contribute significantly to the morbidity and mortality in lung transplant recipients, with over 50% of patients experiencing one or more episodes of posttransplantation infection.[49] Lung transplant associated infections such as viral infections with cytomegalovirus and community-acquired respiratory viruses, are associated with increased incidence of chronic airway disease, specifically obstructive bronchiolitis syndrome (OBS).[74,75] Transplantation-related infection can occur initially in either the transplanted lung or native lung in patients with single lung transplantation. The remaining native lungs can be the source of infection due to pretransplantation colonization. It is important to remember that infection and rejection may coexist, and recognizing the two processes as they occur simultaneously may be difficult in limited biopsies.

Lung transplantation recipients are susceptible to infections due to a variety of risk factors. The lung allograft is different from other solid organ transplants in that it is constantly exposed to the environment and potential respiratory pathogens. Immunosuppression, denervation with resultant decrease of cough reflex and increase of gastroesophageal reflux and aspiration, reduced mucociliary clearance are major contributing factors for allograft infection. Bronchial artery blood flow interruption from surgery predisposes patients to anastomotic site ischemia, with resultant ulceration and necrosis, increases the risk of infection involving the anastomotic site. Furthermore, hypogammaglobulinemia, abnormal ciliary action in the donor epithelium and bronchial stenosis may also increase the risk of infection in post-lung transplantation patients.

Most of the lung transplant associated infections are caused by bacteria, which is followed by viruses and fungi. Parasitic infections are rarely reported.

Bacterial Infection

Bacterial pneumonias are the most common infections in lung transplantation recipients and occur in more than 35% of patients during the first year after transplantation.[76] Gram-negative organisms are predominant in bacterial infections and account for about 75% of the bacterial pneumonias.[77] *Pseudomonas aeruginosa* is most commonly isolated pathogen in bacterial pneumonia

Table 17-3 Primary Bacteria Organisms Causing Post-Lung Transplantation Infection

Pseudomonas aeruginosa
Klebsiella pneumonia
Staphylococcus aureus
Escherichia coli
Enterobacter cloacae

following lung transplantation,[78] especially in recipients with cystic fibrosis.[79] Although most of bacterial pneumonias arise in the first month after transplantation,[80] bacterial infections in the forms of bronchitis, bronchiectasis, and pneumonia reemerge as late complication that is associated with bronchiolitis obliterans syndrome (BOS) and graft failure.[61,81] *Table 17-3* lists the primary bacteria involved in post-lung transplant infection.

Histologically, bacterial infections may present with bronchopneumonia, acute bronchitis, microabscess or abscess formation, and, in severe cases, diffuse alveolar damage (*Figure 17-14A, B*). These histologic features can vary in intensity and distribution within lung parenchyma.

Mycobacteria tuberculosis infection is reported in 1% to 6% of lung transplantation recipients[82,83] due to reactivation, infection in remaining native lung, or acquired from donor lung. Pretransplantation screening for latent *M tuberculosis* infection is extremely important because the posttransplantation treatment for tuberculosis is challenging due to immunosuppression and complex drug interactions.

Fungal Infection

Post-lung transplantation fungal infections are less frequent than bacterial infections, and account between 15% and 35% of lung transplantation cases with an overall mortality of about 60%.[77] Fungal infection often arises 1 to 6 months posttransplantation[84] and may cause anastomotic site infections, localized disease, invasive pulmonary disease, or widely disseminated fungal infection. Up to 80% of fungal infections are caused by *Candida* and *Aspergillus* (*Figure 17-15A, B*); however, infections with *Pneumocystis jiroveci* (*Figures 17-15C, D*), *Histoplasma capsulatum* (*Figures 17-15E, F*), *Cryptococcus neoformans,* and *Coccidioides immitis* are not uncommon. *Pneumocystis jiroveci* infection has been significantly reduced in frequency due to the standard use of prophylaxis.

The cumulative rate of *Aspergillus* infection ranges from 20% to 60% after lung transplantation with mortality of 20% to 100%.[85] *Aspergillus fumigates* is the most commonly isolated species responsible for majority of the invasive disease. *Aspergillus* is commonly seen in a

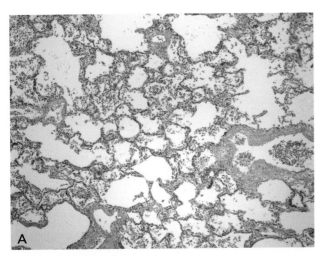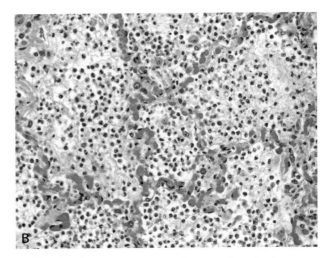

FIGURE 17-14 A, B: Sections of a lung graft from a patient died of bacterial pneumonia display diffuse and marked congestion and acute inflammation of the lung parenchyma. Microabscesses may be observed in severe cases as shown in **(B)**.

necrotic anastomosis and often invades the lung parenchyma with cavitation predominately in an upper lobe. Hemorrhagic infarction with scattered inflammatory cells is characteristic for *Aspergillus* pneumonia. The hyphae of *Aspergillus* species are regularly septated and branching dichotomously at 45° angle (*Figure 17-15B*), which may be seen invading blood vessels and alveolar septa. The *Candida* spp most often involves the upper tracheobronchial tree with occasional parenchymal invasion or disseminate disease. *Candida* infection is featured by intense acute inflammation and microabscesses with clusters of pseudohyphae and yeast forms in the center of necrosis.

Pneumocystis pneumonia may typically present with granular or "bubbly" eosinophilic intra-alveolar infiltrate in biopsy (*Figure 17-15C*). Moreover, *Pneumocystis jiroveci* infection is frequently diagnosed in bronchoalveolar lavage specimens with classic foamy exudate containing eosinophilic dotlike trophozoites on Papanicolaou stain and helmet-shaped pneumocystis cysts on GMS stain (*Figure 17-15D*).

Fungal organisms may be seen more or less on routine H&E stain in lung biopsy, particularly in areas of necrosis and granulation tissue, such as the anastomotic site. However, fungal organisms are often less obvious in bronchitis, bronchopneumonia, or diffuse alveolar damage. In those situations, special stains for fungal organisms should be performed to appropriately rule in or rule out the fungal infection.

Viral Infection

Viral pneumonias are less common than bacterial infections and develop in about 11% of lung transplantation recipients. Most of the viral infections arise between 2 weeks and 3 months post-lung transplantation but also can occur any other time following transplantation.[86] Viral infections not only pose a high risk of near-term mortality following lung transplantation, but also contribute to immunopathogenesis of BOS which eventually leading to graft failure in these patients. Acyclovir and Ganciclovir prophylaxis has significantly reduced morbidity and mortality from cytomegalovirus and herpes simplex virus infection; however, community-acquired respiratory virus (CARV) such as influenza virus, adenovirus, and respiratory syncytial virus are increasingly common infections in these patients.

Histologically, viral infections may present as mixed lymphocytic and neutrophilic interstitial infiltrate, zonal necrosis, microabscesses, inflammation and ulceration in the airways, or diffuse alveolar damage. Characteristic viral cytopathic effects are often observed on routine H&E stain. Immunohistochemical stains for specific viruses are frequently used to establish viral etiology when viral cytopathic effect is suspected on routine histology evaluation. In situ hybridization (ISH) and polymerase chain reaction (PCR) can be used to identify specific viral infection in difficult cases.

Cytomegalovirus (CMV) is the most commonly encountered viral infection despite of the standard viral prophylaxis that has reduced the incidence of CMV pneumonia from 83% to 55.6% in CMV seronegative recipients who acquired seropositive donor lungs.[87-89] It is obvious that CMV seronegative recipients acquiring seropositive donor organs are at greatest risk for CVM infection. A definite diagnosis of CMV pneumonia requires pathological characterization of viral infection in lung biopsy specimen or BAL samples.[90] CMV cytopathic changes include cytomegaly with a large intranuclear inclusion surrounded by a halo and multiple small basophilic cytoplasmic inclusions (*Figure 17-16A, B*).

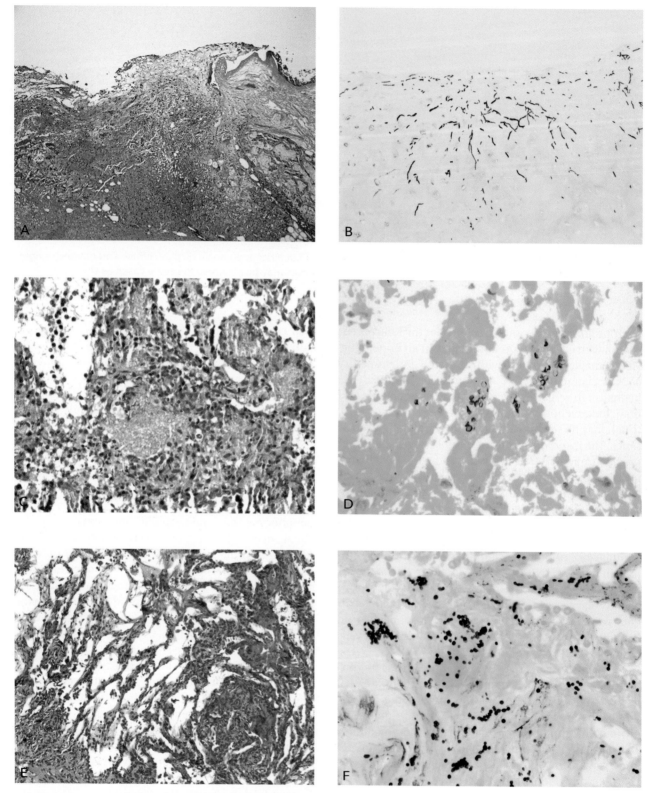

FIGURES 17-15 **A, B:** Aspergillus infection is extremely common at anastomotic site due to ischemia, mucosal ulceration, and tissue necrosis **(A)**. Invasive fungal hyphae are seen on **GMS** stain **(B)**. **C, D:** H&E stain displays classic *Pneumocystis jiroveci* pneumonia with abundant eosinophilic foamy material in the alveoli **(C)** which containing typical helmet-shaped pneumocystis cysts on **GMS** stains **(D)**. Histoplasma pneumonia usually shows acute or granulomatous inflammation at the early stage **(E)** when abundant *Histoplasma capsulatum* organisms can be detected by **GMS** stain **(F)**.

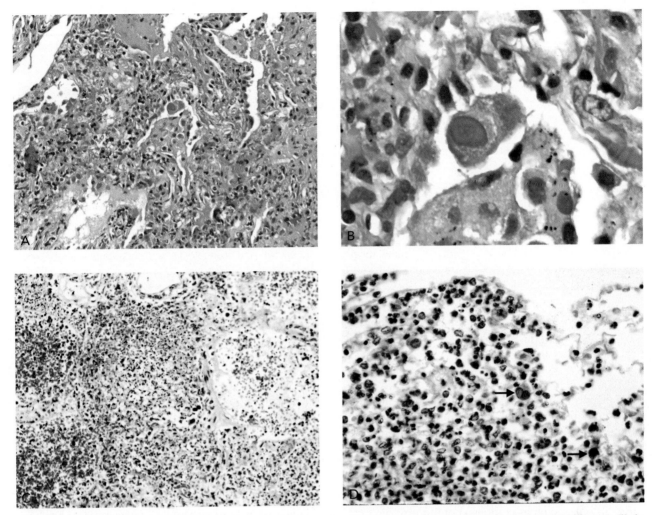

FIGURES 17-16 **A, B:** Cytomegalovirus pneumonia shows mixed lymphocytic and neutrophilic interstitial infiltrate, fibrin exudates, reactive type II pneumocyte hyperplasia, and large cells with viral inclusions (A). High magnification demonstrates characteristic viral cytopathic effect including cytomegaly, a large intranuclear inclusion surrounded by a halo, and multiple small basophilic cytoplasmic inclusions (B). **C, D:** Adenovirus pneumonia displays marked neutrophilic interstitial infiltrate with intra-alveolar hemorrhage and inflammatory exudates (C). High magnification (D, arrows) demonstrates large infected cells with smudgy chromatin (Used with permission of Abida Haque, MD).

Herpes simplex virus (HSV) infection is less common but can be a fatal complication. HSV infection usually starts with oral ulcer or tracheitis before development of pneumonia. The incidence of HSV infection is also reduced significantly with the routine antiviral prophylaxis. The histopathological changes of HSV infection are similar with it presentation in other places, including large multinucleated cells with chromatin margination and nuclear molding.

Other viral infections reported in lung transplantation recipients include adenovirus (*Figure 17-16C, D*), respiratory syncytial virus, varicella-zoster virus, influenza and parainfluenza virus. The cytopathic and histologic features of common viruses associated with post-lung transplantation infection are summarized in *Table 17-4*.

LUNG TRANSPLANT ASSOCIATED ORGANIZING PNEUMONIA

Organizing pneumonia or bronchiolitis obliterans organizing pneumonia is a common complication in lung transplantation recipients and can be caused by a broad range of insults to the lung graft.[91] The most common etiologies include posttransplant aspiration[92] due to surgery-related nerve injury, and lung infections caused by viral, bacterial, or fungal organisms. Organizing pneumonia can be associated with concurrent or resolving acute rejection and chronic rejection, which may result in diagnostic challenge or misinterpretation. The coexistence of organizing pneumonia with acute rejection in the first year posttransplantation

Table 17-4 Morphologic Features of Common Viral Infections in Lung Graft

Virus	Cytopathic effects	Histologic features
Cytomegalovirus	Marked cytomegaly, single large intranuclear inclusion with halo, multiple small cytoplasmic inclusions	Interstitial pneumonia ranging from subtle to extensive with microabscesses, zonal necrosis, granulomatous reaction, or DAD
Herpes simplex virus	Multinucleation, nuclear molding, chromatin margination with ground glass appearance	Usually florid pneumonia with extensive necrosis, abundant neutrophils, fibrinous exudates, hemorrhage, or DAD
Adenovirus	Cytomegaly, smudgy nucleus, ciliocytophthoria, multinucleation may be seen	Necrotizing bronchiolitis or bronchopneumonia with neutrophils, necrosis, karyorrhexis, hemorrhage, or DAD
Varicella-zoster virus	Multinucleation with eosinophilic nuclear inclusions (similar to HSV)	Usually military lesions with hemorrhagic necrosis; or DAD
Respiratory syncytial virus	Syncytial giant cells, round eosinophilic cytoplasmic inclusions with wide halos	Necrotizing bronchiolitis or bronchopneumonia, interstitial pneumonia, giant cell pneumonia, DAD
Influenza virus	No specific viral cytopathic changes, ciliocytophthoria can be seen	Necrotizing bronchiolitis, interstitial pneumonia, giant cell pneumonia, DAD
Parainfluenza virus	Syncytial giant cells, eosinophilic cytoplasmic inclusions, ciliocytophthoria	Bronchiolitis, interstitial pneumonia, giant cell pneumonia, rarely, DAD

is reportedly a strong predictive factor for development of bronchiolitis obliterans (BO) in future.[93] Organizing pneumonia has also been associated with drug reaction and ischemia-reperfusion injury. In some cases, no attributable etiologies can be identified clinically or histologically (so the term idiopathic or cryptogenic).

Histologically, organizing pneumonia present with large fibroblastic plugs composed of fibromyxoid granulation tissue occupying alveolar spaces and stretching into the respiratory bronchioles (*Figure 17-17A, B*). Portion of the fibroblastic plugs may be incorporated into the interstitium. Variable interstitial inflammation and foamy macrophages can be observed. It is important for a pathologist to remember the value of identifying any treatable etiologies such as viral inclusions, fungal organisms, aspirated material (*Figure 17-17C, arrows*), as well as acute rejection. Prompt and successful treatment of these conditions is critical for preservation of graft function in the near term as well as in the long term by preventing or slowing the development of BO.

A newly described entity of lung injury, acute fibrinoid organizing pneumonia (AFOP) was initially reported in 17 nontransplant patients[94] with organizing intra-alveolar fibrin and acute inflammation (*Figure 17-17D*). There is no hyaline membrane formation, eosinophils, or granulomatous inflammation observed in AFOP, which distinguish it from other patterns of lung injuries such as diffuse alveolar damage, eosinophilic pneumonia, hypersensitivity pneumonitis, and organizing pneumonia. AFOP was reportedly associated with collagen vascular diseases,[95] hematological malignancies,[94,96] and a number of infective

agents including *Haemophilus influenza, Acinetobacter baumannii,*[94] and severe acute respiratory syndrome (SARS).[97] Recently, AFOB was reported in a series of lung transplantation patients.[98] The pathological features of AFOB in transplanted lungs are similar to that described in the native lung without apparent predisposing factors. A lung transplant recipients developed AFOB in association within influenza A/H1N1 has been reported.[99] It has been proposed to consider AFOB as a novel form of chronic graft dysfunction that carries a significantly worse survival time than well-known BO.[98]

POSTTRANSPLANT LYMPHOPROLIFERATIVE DISORDERS

Posttransplant lymphoproliferative disorder (PTLD) is defined as a lymphoid or plasmacytic proliferation that develops as a consequence of immunosuppression in a transplant recipient.[100] The incidence of PTLD in lung transplant recipients varies from 1.8% to 20% with single center studies (most of the reports between 4% and 10%),[101-107] which is significantly higher than that in liver and kidney transplant recipients.[107] The variations may reflect the difference in the intensity of immunosuppression regimen used for individual organ transplantation, as well as that adapted by a given institution. PTLDs are the most commonly occur within the first year after lung transplantation in adults[2] and at any time in children.[108] More than 60% of the PTLDs in lung transplantation involve the allograft.[109] Compared to immunocompetent

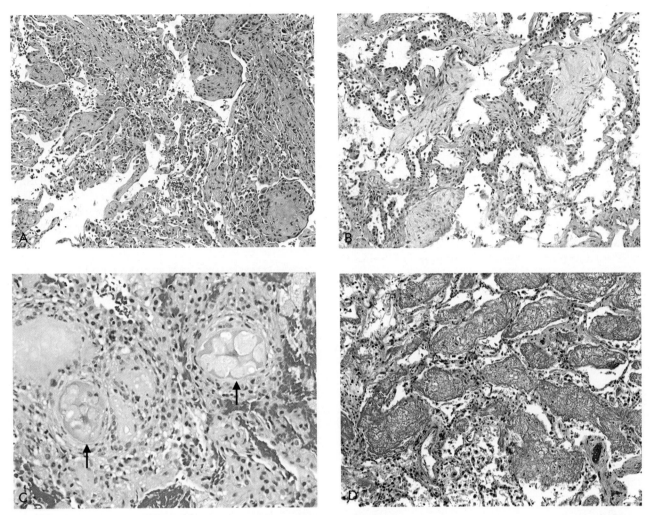

FIGURE 17-17 A, B: Transbronchial biopsy specimen shows organizing pneumonia. Intra-alveolar plug of fibromyxoid tissue is characteristic with incorporation into the interstitium. **C:** Aspiration is extremely common in patients with lung transplantation and is often associated with organizing pneumonia. The microphotograph shows vegetable matter (arrows) incorporated into the lung parenchyma with histiocytes and giant cells in an organizing pneumonia. **D:** A lung graft shows prominent deposition of intra-alveolar fibrin with organization. Inflammatory cells are seen in the background. Hyaline membrane, eosinophil, or granuloma is not a feature in this condition.

population, lung transplant patients have a 58.6-fold increase in non-Hodgkin lymphoma.[109]

EBV seronegativity is the most significant risk factor for PTLD after lung transplantation, although demographic factors such as age younger than 18 years and Caucasian race are also recognized risk factors.[107] In EBV-seronegative recipients, there is a 20-fold increase of risk for development of PTLD compared to those who were EBV seropositive before transplant.[102] Evidence of EBV infection is present in pathology samples in greater than 80% of cases.[110] Monitoring EBV viral load in peripheral blood has been proposed as a marker of impending PTLD.[111] However, EBV-negative PTLD has been reported in up to 30% of cases.[112,113] Greater than 80% of PTLDs originate from B cells, approximately 15% from T cells, and 1% from natural killer cells.

The clinical presentation of PTLD is nonspecific and depends on the site of involvement. The patients may have fever, sore throat, weight loss, or dyspnea. Solitary or multiple lung nodules are the most common pulmonary manifestation on radiologic examination.[114] Mediastinal and hilar adenopathy can be seen in 22% to 50% of patients with PTLD. Most of patients with PTLD have a rapid onset, an aggressive clinical curse, and poor prognosis.[106,115,116] Patients developed PTLD are at higher risk of graft rejection, posing further challenge on clinical management.[106,115]

The pathology of PTLD comprise a spectrum of lesions ranging from EBV-driven infectious mononucleosis-type polyclonal proliferations to EBV-positive or -negative lymphoid proliferations which are morphologically and immunophenotypically indistinguishable from lymphomas that occur in immunocompetent individuals.[100] Four categories of PTLD have been described by the World Health Organization,[100] including early lesions, polymorphic PTLD, monomorphic PTLD, and classical Hodgkin lymphoma. By definition, indolent B-cell lymphomas such as follicular and MALT lymphomas in allograft recipients are not considered a type of PTLD.

Early lesions of PTLD form mass lesion composed of plasmacytic hyperplasia and infectious mononucleosis-like (IM-like) lesion, with a polyclonal immunophenotype and preserved lymph node architecture. Early lesions more often involve lymph nodes or tonsils and often regress spontaneously of with reduction of immunosuppression. Polymorphic PTLD is characterized by a polymorphic proliferation composed of immunoblasts, plasma cells, and lymphocytes at various sizes, often with architectural effacement or destruction. B cell with light chain restriction may or may not be detected and EBER positive cells are usually numerous. Monomorphic PTLDs refers to clonal proliferations of B cells or T/NK cells that fulfill the criteria for conventional lymphomas. The most common types of monomorphic PTLD include diffuse large B-cell lymphoma, Burkitt lymphoma, plasma cell myeloma, and peripheral T-cell lymphoma. Classical Hodgkin lymphoma–type PTLD is least common and almost always EBV positive. Classical morphology of Hodgkin lymphoma and expressions of CD15 and CD30 are required for diagnosis because Reed-Sternberg-like cells can be present in early, polymorphous and monomorphous types of PTLD.

PTLD is a clinically, morphologically, and molecularly heterogeneous spectrum of lymphoproliferative disorders. Morphologic distinction between PTLD and more common conditions such as acute cellular rejection or infection can be very challenging based on small transbronchial biopsies. Currently, there is no consensus on the morphologic criteria for differentiation of these lesions. Identification of EBV by EBER in situ hybridization is in favor of, but not diagnostic of PTLD, especially when the EBV-positive cells are scant. Diligently search for infectious organisms with special stains is mandatory in cases suspected for PTLD. Flow cytometry study and standard lymphoma workup should be performed when fresh tissue is available from wedge biopsies or resections of suspected lesions. It is also important to remember that acute cellular rejection and PTLD can coexist in the same patient.

RECURRENCE OF PRIMARY DISEASES

Recurrence of primary disease in the allograft lung has been occasionally reported and account for about 1% of lung transplant cases.[117] Recurrent sarcoidosis (*Figure 17-18A, B*) is most common with a recurrent rate up to 35% in lung grafts.[117] Other reported recurrent diseases in allograft lungs include giant cell interstitial pneumonia (*Figure 17-18C, D*),[118] lymphangioleiomyomatosis,[119-121] Langerhans cell histiocytosis,[117] intravenous talc granulomatosis,[122] adenocarcinoma,[123,124] alveolar proteinosis,[117] and diffuse panbronchiolitis.[125] These recurrent diseases are often detected incidentally and are not the common indications for lung transplantation. Although recurrent diseases can occasionally become a serious complication, the impact on overall management strategy of lung transplant recipients is insignificant.

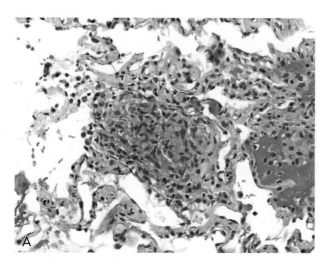
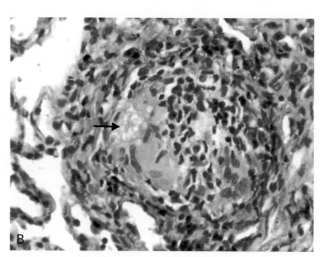

FIGURE 17-18 A, B: Recurrence of sarcoidosis occurred in this patient who had lung transplant 6 months prior due to advanced stage of sarcoidosis. The pictures show well-formed granulomas with epithelioid histiocytes and a few lymphocytes in the periphery **(A)**. Asteroid body can be seen in multinucleated giant cells **(B, arrow)**.

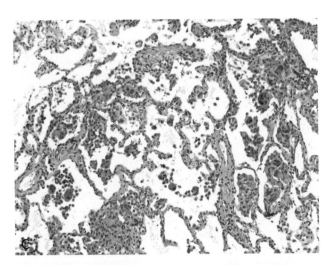
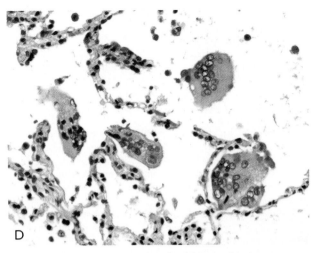

FIGURE 17-18 (*Continued*) **C, D. Giant cell interstitial pneumonia recurred in a patient who underwent double lung transplant 3.5 years ago. The low magnification shows interstitial lymphocytic infiltration with abundant macrophages and multinucleated giant cells within the alveoli (C). High magnification demonstrates osteoclast-like multinucleated giant cells filling the alveolar spaces (D).**

PULMONARY GRAFT VERSUS HOST DISEASE

Although graft versus host disease (GVHD) is a common complication of allogenic hematopoietic stem cell transplantation, it rarely occurs after lung transplantation. However, GVHD after lung transplantation is a highly fatal complication with no effective treatment. Scant reported cases, mostly grade 3 to 4 acute GVHD died within 7 months,[126] although rare patients reportedly survived of grade 3-4 acute GVHD after successful treatment with high dose of corticosteroids.[127] Secondary infection is the most common cause of death in patients with GVHD following lung transplantation.

The clinical presentation of GVHD in lung transplantation is similar to that in other solid organ transplants. Skin rush is the most common manifestation that may be accompanied by low-grade fever, diarrhea, leukopenia, anemia, or abnormal liver function tests. Histologically, a skin biopsy may show dermal inflammation, basal layer vacuolar degeneration, apoptosis, and cell necrosis. Intestinal crypts destruction and apoptosis of the epithelial cells may be observed in colon biopsies. Donor cell chimerism was reportedly detected in many of the patients with GVHD.[126-128]

REFERENCES

1. Hardy JD, et al. Lung homotransplantation in man. *JAMA.* 1963;186:1065-1074.
2. Christie JD, et al. The Registry of the International Society for Heart and Lung Transplantation: 29th adult lung and heart-lung transplant report-2012. *J Heart Lung Transplant.* 2012;31(10):1073-1086.
3. Kirk R, et al. The Registry of the International Society for Heart and Lung Transplantation: fifteenth pediatric heart transplantation report—2012. *J Heart Lung Transplant.* 2012;31(10):1065-1072.
4. Christie JD, et al. Report of the ISHLT Working Group on Primary Lung Graft Dysfunction part II: definition. A consensus statement of the International Society for Heart and Lung Transplantation. *J Heart Lung Transplant.* 2005;24(10):1454-1459.
5. Arcasoy SM, et al. Report of the ISHLT Working Group on Primary Lung Graft Dysfunction part V: predictors and outcomes. *J Heart Lung Transplant.* 2005;24(10):1483-1488.
6. Arcasoy SM, Kotloff RM. Lung transplantation. *N Engl J Med.* 1999;340(14):1081-91.
7. Christie JD, et al. Primary graft failure following lung transplantation. *Chest.* 1998;114(1):51-60.
8. Christie JD, et al. Clinical risk factors for primary graft failure following lung transplantation. *Chest.* 2003;124(4):1232-1241.
9. Christie JD, et al. Report of the ISHLT Working Group on Primary Lung Graft Dysfunction part I: introduction and methods. *J Heart Lung Transplant.* 2005;24(10):1451-1453.
10. King RC, et al. Reperfusion injury significantly impacts clinical outcome after pulmonary transplantation. *Ann Thorac Surg.* 2000;69(6):1681-1685.
11. Christie JD, et al. Impact of primary graft failure on outcomes following lung transplantation. *Chest.* 2005;127(1):161-165.
12. Chatila WM. Respiratory failure after lung transplantation. *Chest.* 2003;123(1):165-173.
13. Fiser SM, et al. Ischemia-reperfusion injury after lung transplantation increases risk of late bronchiolitis obliterans syndrome. *Ann Thorac Surg.* 2002;73(4):1041-1047; discussion 1047-1048.
14. Fisher AJ, et al. Non-immune acute graft injury after lung transplantation and the risk of subsequent bronchiolitis obliterans syndrome (BOS). *J Heart Lung Transplant.* 2002;21(11):1206-1212.
15. Khan SU, et al. Acute pulmonary edema after lung transplantation: the pulmonary reimplantation response. *Chest.* 1999;116(1):187-194.
16. Thabut G, et al. Primary graft failure following lung transplantation: predictive factors of mortality. *Chest.* 2002;121(6):1876-1882.
17. Christie JD, et al. Construct validity of the definition of primary graft dysfunction after lung transplantation. *J Heart Lung Transplant.* 2010;29(11):1231-1239.

CHAPTER 17

18. Christie JD, et al. The effect of primary graft dysfunction on survival after lung transplantation. *Am J Respir Crit Care Med.* 2005;171(11):1312-1316.

19. Daud SA, et al. Impact of immediate primary lung allograft dysfunction on bronchiolitis obliterans syndrome. *Am J Respir Crit Care Med.* 2007;175(5):507-513.

20. Diamond JM, et al. Clinical risk factors for primary graft dysfunction after lung transplantation. *Am J Respir Crit Care Med.* 187(5):527-534.

21. Huang HJ, et al. Late primary graft dysfunction after lung transplantation and bronchiolitis obliterans syndrome. *Am J Transplant.* 2008;8(11):2454-2462.

22. Kreisel D, et al. Short- and long-term outcomes of 1000 adult lung transplant recipients at a single center. *J Thorac Cardiovasc Surg.* 141(1):215-222.

23. Prekker ME, et al. Validation of the proposed International Society for Heart and Lung Transplantation grading system for primary graft dysfunction after lung transplantation. *J Heart Lung Transplant.* 2006;25(4):371-378.

24. Whitson BA, et al. Primary graft dysfunction and long-term pulmonary function after lung transplantation. *J Heart Lung Transplant.* 2007;26(10):1004-1011.

25. McGregor CG, et al. Evolving strategies in lung transplantation for emphysema. *Ann Thorac Surg.* 1994;57(6):1513-1520; discussion 1520-1521.

26. Oto T, et al. A donor history of smoking affects early but not late outcome in lung transplantation. *Transplantation.* 2004;78(4):599-606.

27. Pilcher DV, et al. High donor age, low donor oxygenation, and high recipient inotrope requirements predict early graft dysfunction in lung transplant recipients. *J Heart Lung Transplant.* 2005;24(11):1814-1820.

28. Whitson BA, et al. Risk factors for primary graft dysfunction after lung transplantation. *J Thorac Cardiovasc Surg.* 2006;131(1):73-80.

29. Barr ML, et al. Report of the ISHLT Working Group on Primary Lung Graft Dysfunction part IV: recipient-related risk factors and markers. *J Heart Lung Transplant.* 2005;24(10):1468-1482.

30. Kuntz CL, et al. Risk factors for early primary graft dysfunction after lung transplantation: a registry study. *Clin Transplant.* 2009;23(6):819-830.

31. Lederer DJ, et al. Obesity and primary graft dysfunction after lung transplantation: the Lung Transplant Outcomes Group Obesity Study. *Am J Respir Crit Care Med.* 2011;184(9):1055-1061.

32. Whelan TP, et al. Effect of preoperative pulmonary artery pressure on early survival after lung transplantation for idiopathic pulmonary fibrosis. *J Heart Lung Transplant.* 2005;24(9):1269-1274.

33. De Oliveira NC, et al. Lung transplant for interstitial lung disease: outcomes for single versus bilateral lung transplantation. *Interact Cardiovasc Thorac Surg.* 2012;14(3):263-267.

34. Oto T, et al. Definitions of primary graft dysfunction after lung transplantation: differences between bilateral and single lung transplantation. *J Thorac Cardiovasc Surg.* 2006;132(1):140-147.

35. Clark SC, et al. Vascular complications of lung transplantation. *Ann Thorac Surg.* 1996;61(4):1079-1082.

36. Wede W, et al. Airway complications after lung transplantation: risk factors, prevention and outcome. *Eur J Cardiothorac Surg.* 2009;35(2):293-298; discussion 298.

37. Santacruz JF, Mehta AC. Airway complications and management after lung transplantation: ischemia, dehiscence, and stenosis. *Proc Am Thorac Soc.* 2009;6(1):79-93.

38. Puchalski J, Lee HJ, Sterman DH. Airway complications following lung transplantation. *Clin Chest Med.* 32(2):357-366.

39. Dhillon GS, et al. Lung transplant airway hypoxia: a diathesis to fibrosis? *Am J Respir Crit Care Med.* 182(2):230-236.

40. Veith FJ, et al. Lung transplantation 1983. *Transplantation.* 1983;35(4):271-278.

41. Alvarez A, et al. Airway complications after lung transplantation: a review of 151 anastomoses. *Eur J Cardiothorac Surg.* 2001;19(4):381-387.

42. Fernandez-Bussy S, et al. Treatment of airway complications following lung transplantation. *Arch Bronconeumol.* 47(3):128-133.

43. King-Biggs MB, et al. Airway anastomotic dehiscence associated with use of sirolimus immediately after lung transplantation. *Transplantation.* 2003;75(9):1437-1443.

44. Dutau H, et al. A retrospective study of silicone stent placement for management of anastomotic airway complications in lung transplant recipients: short- and long-term outcomes. *J Heart Lung Transplant.* 2010;29(6):658-664.

45. Moreno P, et al. Incidence, management and clinical outcomes of patients with airway complications following lung transplantation. *Eur J Cardiothorac Surg.* 2008;34(6):1198-1205.

46. Griffith BP, et al. Anastomotic pitfalls in lung transplantation. *J Thorac Cardiovasc Surg.* 1994;107(3):743-753; discussion 753-754.

47. Leibowitz DW, et al. Incidence of pulmonary vein complications after lung transplantation: a prospective transesophageal echocardiographic study. *J Am Coll Cardiol.* 1994;24(3):671-675.

48. Schulman LL, et al. Four-year prospective study of pulmonary venous thrombosis after lung transplantation. *J Am Soc Echocardiogr.* 2001;14(8):806-812.

49. Nizami I, Frost AE. Clinical diagnosis of transplant-related problems. In: P Cagle, ed. *Diagnostic pulmonary pathology.* New York: Marcel Dekker;2000:485-499.

50. Berry GJ, et al. A working formulation for the standardization of nomenclature in the diagnosis of heart and lung rejection: Lung Rejection Study Group. The International Society for Heart Transplantation. *J Heart Transplant.* 1990;9(6):593-601.

51. Yousem SA, et al. Revision of the 1990 working formulation for the classification of pulmonary allograft rejection: Lung Rejection Study Group. *J Heart Lung Transplant.* 1996;15(1 pt 1):1-15.

52. Stewart S, et al. Revision of the 1996 working formulation for the standardization of nomenclature in the diagnosis of lung rejection. *J Heart Lung Transplant.* 2007;26(12):1229-1242.

53. Bittner HB, et al. Hyperacute rejection in single lung transplantation—case report of successful management by means of plasmapheresis and antithymocyte globulin treatment. *Transplantation.* 2001;71(5):649-651.

54. Choi JK, et al. Hyperacute rejection of a pulmonary allograft. Immediate clinical and pathologic findings. *Am J Respir Crit Care Med.* 1999;160(3):1015-1018.

55. de Jesus Peixoto Camargo J, et al. Hyperacute rejection after single lung transplantation: a case report. *Transplant Proc.* 2008;40(3):867-869.

56. Frost AE, Jammal CT, Cagle PT. Hyperacute rejection following lung transplantation. *Chest.* 1996;110(2):559-562.

57. Scornik JC, et al. Susceptibility of lung transplants to preformed donor-specific HLA antibodies as detected by flow cytometry. *Transplantation.* 1999;68(10):1542-1546.

58. Glanville AR, et al. Severity of lymphocytic bronchiolitis predicts long-term outcome after lung transplantation. *Am J Respir Crit Care Med.* 2008;177(9):1033-1040.

59. Saint Martin GA, et al. Humoral (antibody-mediated) rejection in lung transplantation. *J Heart Lung Transplant.* 1996;15(12):1217-1222.

60. Christie JD, et al. The Registry of the International Society for Heart and Lung Transplantation: twenty-seventh official adult lung and heart-lung transplant report—2010. *J Heart Lung Transplant.* 2010;29(10):1104-1118.

61. Sharples LD, et al. Risk factors for bronchiolitis obliterans: a systematic review of recent publications. *J Heart Lung Transplant.* 2002;21(2):271-281.

62. Sato M, et al. Restrictive allograft syndrome (RAS): a novel form of chronic lung allograft dysfunction. *J Heart Lung Transplant.* 2011;30(7):735-742.

63. Verleden SE, et al. Neutrophilic reversible allograft dysfunction (NRAD) and restrictive allograft syndrome (RAS). *Semin Respir Crit Care Med.* 2013;34(3):352-360.

64. Nathan SD, et al. Pulmonary hypertension in patients with bronchiolitis obliterans syndrome listed for retransplantation. *Am J Transplant.* 2008;8(7):1506-1511.

65. Saggar R, et al. Pulmonary hypertension associated with lung transplantation obliterative bronchiolitis and vascular remodeling of the allograft. *Am J Transplant.* 2008;8(9):1921-1930.

66. Girnita AL, et al. HLA-specific antibodies are associated with high-grade and persistent-recurrent lung allograft acute rejection. *J Heart Lung Transplant.* 2004;23(10):1135-1141.

67. Palmer SM, et al. Development of an antibody specific to major histocompatibility antigens detectable by flow cytometry after lung transplant is associated with bronchiolitis obliterans syndrome. *Transplantation.* 2002;74(6):799-804.

68. Hadjiliadis D, et al. Pre-transplant panel reactive antibody in lung transplant recipients is associated with significantly worse post-transplant survival in a multicenter study. *J Heart Lung Transplant.* 2005;24(7 suppl):S249-S254.

69. Astor TL, et al. Pulmonary capillaritis in lung transplant recipients: treatment and effect on allograft function. *J Heart Lung Transplant.* 2005;24(12):2091-2097.

70. Berry G, et al. Pathology of pulmonary antibody-mediated rejection: 2012 update from the Pathology Council of the ISHLT. *J Heart Lung Transplant,* 2013;32(1):14-21.

71. Westall GP, et al. C3d and C4d deposition early after lung transplantation. *J Heart Lung Transplant.* 2008;27(7):722-728.

72. Wallace WD, et al. C4d staining of pulmonary allograft biopsies: an immunoperoxidase study. *J Heart Lung Transplant.* 2005;24(10):1565-1570.

73. Roberts JA, et al. The presence of anti-HLA donor-specific antibodies in lung allograft recipients does not correlate with C4d immunofluorescence in transbronchial biopsy specimens. *Arch Pathol Lab Med.* 2014 Aug;138(8):1053-1058.

74. Keller CA, et al. Bronchiolitis obliterans in recipients of single, double, and heart-lung transplantation. *Chest.* 1995;107(4):973-980.

75. Husain S, Singh N. Bronchiolitis obliterans and lung transplantation: evidence for an infectious etiology. *Semin Respir Infect.* 2002;17(4):310-314.

76. Dauber JH, Paradis IL, Dummer JS. Infectious complications in pulmonary allograft recipients. *Clin Chest Med.* 1990;11(2):291-308.

77. Nakajima T, et al. Lung transplantation: infection, inflammation, and the microbiome. *Semin Immunopathol.* 2011;33(2):135-156.

78. Zeglen S, et al. Frequency of Pseudomonas aeruginosa colonizations/infections in lung transplant recipients. *Transplant Proc.* 2009;41(8):3222-3224.

79. Bonvillain RW, et al. Post-operative infections in cystic fibrosis and non-cystic fibrosis patients after lung transplantation. *J Heart Lung Transplant.* 2007;26(9):890-897.

80. Aguilar-Guisado M, et al. Pneumonia after lung transplantation in the RESITRA Cohort: a multicenter prospective study. *Am J Transplant.* 2007;7(8):1989-1996.

81. Gottlieb J, et al. Impact of graft colonization with gram-negative bacteria after lung transplantation on the development of bronchiolitis obliterans syndrome in recipients with cystic fibrosis. *Respir Med.* 2009;103(5):743-749.

82. Kesten S, Chaparro C. Mycobacterial infections in lung transplant recipients. *Chest.* 1999;115(3):741-745.

83. Malouf MA, Glanville AR. The spectrum of mycobacterial infection after lung transplantation. *Am J Respir Crit Care Med.* 1999;160(5 pt 1):1611-1616.

84. Mehrad B, et al. Spectrum of Aspergillus infection in lung transplant recipients: case series and review of the literature. *Chest.* 2001;119(1):169-175.

85. Kubak BM. Fungal infection in lung transplantation. *Transpl Infect Dis.* 2002;4(suppl 3):24-31.

86. Shah PD, McDyer JF. Viral infections in lung transplant recipients. *Semin Respir Crit Care Med.* 2010;31(2):243-254.

87. Gould FK, et al. Prophylaxis and management of cytomegalovirus pneumonitis after lung transplantation: a review of experience in one center. *J Heart Lung Transplant.* 1993;12(4):695-699.

88. Palmer SM, et al. Extended valganciclovir prophylaxis to prevent cytomegalovirus after lung transplantation: a randomized, controlled trial. *Ann Intern Med.* 2010;152(12):761-769.

89. Hodson EM, et al. Antiviral medications for preventing cytomegalovirus disease in solid organ transplant recipients. *Cochrane Database Syst Rev.* 2013 Feb 28;2:CD003774.

90. Kotton CN, et al. International consensus guidelines on the management of cytomegalovirus in solid organ transplantation. *Transplantation.* 2010;89(7):779-795.

91. Milne DS, et al. Organizing pneumonia following pulmonary transplantation and the development of obliterative bronchiolitis. *Transplantation.* 1994;57(12):1757-1762.

92. Miyagawa-Hayashino A, Wain JC, Mark EJ. Lung transplantation biopsy specimens with bronchiolitis obliterans or bronchiolitis obliterans organizing pneumonia due to aspiration. *Arch Pathol Lab Med.* 2005;129(2):223-226.

93. Chaparro C, et al. Bronchiolitis obliterans organizing pneumonia (BOOP) in lung transplant recipients. *Chest.* 1996;110(5):1150-1154.

94. Beasley MB, et al. Acute fibrinous and organizing pneumonia: a histological pattern of lung injury and possible variant of diffuse alveolar damage. *Arch Pathol Lab Med.* 2002;126(9):1064-1070.

95. Prahalad S, et al. Fatal acute fibrinous and organizing pneumonia in a child with juvenile dermatomyositis. *J Pediatr.* 2005;146(2):289-292.

96. Lee SM, et al. Acute fibrinous and organizing pneumonia following hematopoietic stem cell transplantation. *Korean J Intern Med.* 2009;24(2):156-159.

97. Hwang DM, et al. Pulmonary pathology of severe acute respiratory syndrome in Toronto. *Mod Pathol.* 2005;18(1):1-10.

98. Paraskeva M, et al. Acute fibrinoid organizing pneumonia after lung transplantation. *Am J Respir Crit Care Med.* 2013;187(12):1360-1368.

99. Otto C, et al. Acute fibrinous and organizing pneumonia associated with influenza A/H1N1 pneumonia after lung transplantation. *BMC Pulm Med.* 2013;13:30.

100. Swerdlow SH, Campo E, Harris NL, et al. Post-transplant lymphoproliferative disorders (PTLD). In: *Swerdlow SH, et al.: WHO Classification of Tumours of Haematopoietic and Lymphoid Tissue.* Lyon: World Health Organization; 2008:343-349.

101. Levine SM, et al. A low incidence of posttransplant lymphoproliferative disorder in 109 lung transplant recipients. *Chest.* 1999;116(5):1273-1277.

102. Aris RM, et al. Post-transplantation lymphoproliferative disorder in the Epstein-Barr virus-naive lung transplant recipient. *Am J Respir Crit Care Med.* 1996;154(6 pt 1):1712-1717.

103. Walker RC, et al. Pretransplantation seronegative Epstein-Barr virus status is the primary risk factor for posttransplantation lymphoproliferative disorder in adult heart, lung, and other solid organ transplantations. *J Heart Lung Transplant.* 1995;14(2):214-221.

104. Armitage JM, et al. Posttransplant lymphoproliferative disease in thoracic organ transplant patients: ten years of cyclosporine-based immunosuppression. *J Heart Lung Transplant.* 1991;10(6):877-886; discussion 886-7.

105. Montone KT, et al. Analysis of Epstein-Barr virus-associated posttransplantation lymphoproliferative disorder after lung transplantation. *Surgery.* 1996;119(5):544-551.

106. Reams BD, et al. Posttransplant lymphoproliferative disorder: incidence, presentation, and response to treatment in lung transplant recipients. *Chest.* 2003;124(4):1242-1249.

107. Dharnidharka VR, et al. Post-transplant lymphoproliferative disorder in the United States: young Caucasian males are at highest risk. *Am J Transplant.* 2002;2(10):993-998.

108. Benden C, et al. The Registry of the International Society for Heart and Lung Transplantation: fifteenth pediatric lung and heart-lung transplantation report—2012. *J Heart Lung Transplant.* 2012;31(10):1087-1095.

109. Opelz G, Dohler B. Lymphomas after solid organ transplantation: a collaborative transplant study report. *Am J Transplant.* 2004;4(2):222-230.

110. Mucha K, et al. Post-transplant lymphoproliferative disorder in view of the new WHO classification: a more rational approach to a protean disease? *Nephrol Dial Transplant.* 25(7):2089-2098.

111. Rogers BB, et al. Epstein-Barr virus polymerase chain reaction and serology in pediatric post-transplant lymphoproliferative disorder: three-year experience. *Pediatr Dev Pathol.* 1998;1(6):480-486.

112. Birkeland SA, Hamilton-Dutoit S. Is posttransplant lymphoproliferative disorder (PTLD) caused by any specific immunosuppressive drug or by the transplantation per se? *Transplantation.* 2003;76(6):984-988.

113. Nelson BP, et al. Epstein-Barr virus-negative post-transplant lymphoproliferative disorders: a distinct entity? *Am J Surg Pathol.* 2000;24(3):375-385.

114. Pickhardt PJ, et al. Chest radiography as a predictor of outcome in posttransplantation lymphoproliferative disorder in lung allograft recipients. *AJR Am J Roentgenol.* 1998;171(2):375-382.

115. Raj R, Frost AE. Lung retransplantation after posttransplantation lymphoproliferative disorder (PTLD): a single-center experience and review of literature of PTLD in lung transplant recipients. *J Heart Lung Transplant.* 2005;24(6):671-679.

116. Leblond V, et al. Identification of prognostic factors in 61 patients with posttransplantation lymphoproliferative disorders. *J Clin Oncol.* 2001;19(3):772-778.

117. Collins J, et al. Frequency and CT findings of recurrent disease after lung transplantation. *Radiology.* 2001;219(2):503-509.

118. Frost AE, et al. Giant cell interstitial pneumonitis. Disease recurrence in the transplanted lung. *Am Rev Respir Dis.* 1993;148(5):1401-1404.

119. Chen F, et al. Recurrent lymphangioleiomyomatosis after living-donor lobar lung transplantation. *Transplant Proc.* 2006;38(9):3151-3153.

120. O'Brien JD, et al. Lymphangiomyomatosis recurrence in the allograft after single-lung transplantation. *Am J Respir Crit Care Med.* 1995;151(6):2033-2036.

121. Collins J, et al. Lung transplantation for lymphangioleiomyomatosis: role of imaging in the assessment of complications related to the underlying disease. *Radiology.* 1999;210(2):325-332.

122. Cook RC, et al. Recurrence of intravenous talc granulomatosis following single lung transplantation. *Can Respir J.* 1998;5(6):511-514.

123. Toyooka S, et al. Recurrent lung cancer in the mediastinum noticed after a living-donor lobar lung transplantation. *Ann Thorac Cardiovasc Surg.* 2009;15(2):119-122.

124. Garver RI Jr, et al. Recurrence of bronchioloalveolar carcinoma in transplanted lungs. *N Engl J Med.* 1999;340(14):1071-1074.

125. Baz MA, et al. Recurrence of diffuse panbronchiolitis after lung transplantation. *Am J Respir Crit Care Med.* 1995;151 (3 pt 1):895-898.

126. Assi MA, et al. Graft-vs.-host disease in lung and other solid organ transplant recipients. *Clin Transplant.* 2007;21(1):1-6.

127. Fossi A, et al. Severe acute graft versus host disease after lung transplant: report of a case successfully treated with high dose corticosteroids. *J Heart Lung Transplant.* 2009;28(5):508-510.

128. Chau EM, et al. Mediastinal irradiation for graft-versus-host disease in a heart-lung transplant recipient. *J Heart Lung Transplant.* 1997;16(9):974-979.

Interstitial Pneumonias

18

Tomonori Tanaka and Junya Fukuoka

TAKE HOME PEARLS

- The role of transbronchial biopsies in the context of interstitial pneumonia is generally limited. The primary role of transbronchial biopsies is to exclude neoplasia, sarcoidosis, and certain infections.
- Idiopathic interstitial pneumonias include usual interstitial pneumonia (UIP), nonspecific interstitial pneumonia (NSIP), acute interstitial pneumonia (AIP), and cryptogenic organizing pneumonia (COP).
- Idiopathic pulmonary fibrosis (IPF) is defined as a specific form of chronic, progressive fibrosing interstitial pneumonia of unknown etiology, occurring primarily in older adults, limited to the lungs, and associated with the histopathologic and radiologic pattern of UIP.
- UIP is characterized by a patchy pattern of fibrosis that is predominantly subpleural and lower zone, honeycomb lung and fibroblast foci.
- Idiopathic nonspecific interstitial pneumonia (NSIP) is currently defined as a specific form of chronic interstitial pneumonia of unknown etiology.
- NSIP has been identified as the most common histological pattern found in patients with collagen vascular disease.
- NSIP is histologically subdivided to cellular, cellular and fibrosing, and fibrosing NSIP, according to the amount of cellularity and fibrosis.
- AIP is a rapidly progressive interstitial pneumonia of unknown cause with pathological pattern of diffuse alveolar damage.
- The term organizing pneumonia (OP) indicates a histologic wound healing process from various

causes, such as infection, collagen vascular disease manifesting in the lung, inflammatory bowel disease, inhalational injury, hypersensitivity pneumonitis, drug toxicity, radiation therapy, and aspiration.
- COP is a specific clinicopathological form of OP without a known underlying etiology.

INTRODUCTION

The critical roles of surgical lung biopsy in interstitial pneumonias (IP) are (1) ruling out neoplastic or infectious conditions and (2) distinguishing poor prognostic patterns, such as usual interstitial pneumonia (UIP) and diffuse alveolar damage (DAD), from other interstitial pneumonias. Recognition of histological clues may also, but not always, help distinguish underlying etiologies, some of which are treatable. Histology is not always diagnostic, and the final diagnosis of IP often requires multidisciplinary discussion with experienced pulmonologists and radiologists.

APPROACH TO INTERSTITIAL PNEUMONIAS

Approach to Biopsy

The pathology of interstitial pneumonia often exhibits combinations of nonspecific findings. Characteristic proportions and combinations of inflammatory cell infiltrates, exudates, fibrosis, etc, assist with the pathological diagnosis. Correlation of clinical and radiographic findings to confirm a pathologic impression is an important, often crucial, process. For pathologists, assessment of the following clinical observations is vital for reaching a diagnosis: (1) Is the illness acute onset or chronic? (2) Does the pulmonary function test indicate restrictive change or obstructive change? (3) Does the high-resolution computed tomography (HRCT) indicate localized disease or diffuse disease? (4) Does the HRCT indicate upper lobe predominance or lung base predominance? As mentioned already, most pathologic findings in this context are rather nonspecific, and the level of confidence for a pathologic diagnosis may be low for some cases. In this setting, clinical-radiologic-pathologic correlation is vital in arriving at a diagnosis (*Figure 18-1*).

The role of transbronchial biopsies in the diagnosis of interstitial pneumonia is generally limited. The primary role of transbronchial biopsies is to exclude neoplasia, sarcoidosis, and certain infections. Some diseases such as organizing pneumonia, diffuse alveolar damage, and alveolar proteinosis can be diagnosed with appropriate clinical and radiologic correlation. A future substitute for traditional transbronchial biopsies is "cryo-biopsy" which may permit observation of a larger amount of lung tissue for diagnosis.[1]

Special Considerations of Specimen Handling

Optimal specimen handling is essential for reliable pathologic diagnosis. The specimens biopsied by video assisted thoracic surgery are deflated and stapled. The stapled surgical margin should be removed from the specimen and can potentially be used for microbiologic cultures. After the removal of stapled margin, reinflation of the specimen with fixative is very beneficial. One may use a small-gauge needle and syringe to reinflate the specimen. This reinflation may cause histologic artifacts including washing out cells or materials and overinflation of airspaces, interstitial tissue or lymphatic spaces.

Special stains

There are some special stains that are useful in the interpretation of interstitial lung diseases. The Masson trichrome stain or azan stain reveal dense collagen in a deep blue and may help identify otherwise subtle or inconspicuous chronic fibrosis. Trichrome stain is especially helpful when acute exacerbation of chronic lung disease is suspected. Elastic stains such as Verhoeff Van Giesen (VVG) stain or Movat stain demonstrate elastic fibers in blood vessels, bronchioles, pleura, and alveolar septa. VVG stains help identify the basic architecture of the lung. Elastic stains highlight subtle organizing pneumonia and vascular injury (*Figure 18-2*). When acute changes (for example, airspace fibrin and edema) are observed, stains for microorganisms such as Gomori methenamine silver (GMS) and Ziehl-Neelsen stains may be useful since infectious disease may be a cause of interstitial pneumonia.

DIFFUSE INTERSTITIAL PNEUMONIAS

Hypersensitivity Pneumonia

Clinical features of hypersensitivity pneumonia

Hypersensitivity pneumonia (HP) is a form of diffuse interstitial lung disease resulting from repeated exposure to a variety of organic dusts. Numerous

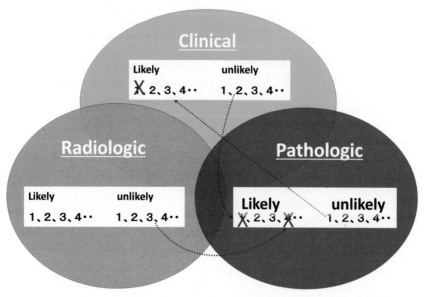

FIGURE 18-1 Clinical-radiological-pathological correlation often leads to the correct final diagnosis. Differential diagnoses may differ, though, so communication must remain active to best ensure accurate diagnosis.

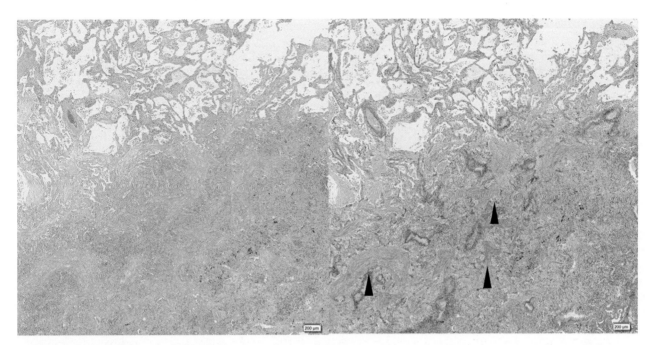

FIGURE 18-2 Consolidated eosinophilic area at the lower half (left). EVG stain highlights areas of organizing pneumonia (right, arrowheads).

responsible agents have been described, including agricultural dusts, fungi, bird proteins, and certain reactive chemicals.[2,3] The pathogenesis of HP involves both type III and type IV allergic reactions that are mediated by immune complexes and Th1 T cells. Clinically, HP can be classified into acute, subacute, and chronic forms based on the clinical presentation.[2] Acute HP follows exposure to relatively large doses of responsible antigen and almost all case are diagnosed clinically.[4] The vast majority of HP patients who undergo biopsy have either the subacute or chronic form of the disease. Untreated patients with chronic HP may develop progressive fibrosis, and in advanced stage, the disease may mimic idiopathic pulmonary fibrosis (IPF) or fibrosing nonspecific interstitial pneumonia (NSIP).[3] In both subacute and chronic forms of HP, an offending antigen is not identified in up to one-third of patients.[5] An acute exacerbation may occur both with and without further exposure to the antigen.[6-8]

The clinical diagnosis of chronic HP is challenging, relying on a combination of nonspecific findings, such as clinical symptoms and signs, characteristic radiographic features, serum precipitating antibodies against offending antigens, and a lymphocytosis on bronchoalveolar lavage.[2] Due to the absence of a diagnostic "gold standard," recognition of characteristic histological findings in surgical lung biopsies often plays an important role in diagnosis.[9]

Early recognition of the disease and avoidance of the causative antigen are crucial, since chronic HP patients may progress and die of lung fibrosis.[2]

Imaging features of hypersensitivity pneumonitis

The HRCT features of subacute HP are characterized by patchy bilateral ground glass opacities (GGO), poorly defined centrilobular nodules, lobular areas of decreased attenuation on inspiratory images, and air trapping on expiratory HRCT. GGO often involve the middle and lower lung zones. Areas of GGO and centrilobular nodules may decrease during long-term follow-up.[10] Chronic HP is characterized by the presence of intralobular reticular opacities, subpleural consolidation mainly in the upper lung fields, architectural distortion, traction bronchiolectasis, and honeycomb change. Most patients with chronic HP also show areas of GGO, poorly defined centrilobular nodules, and air trapping (*Figure 18-3*). Rarely, HRCT may show undistinguishable features from those of IPF and NSIP.[11]

Histologic features of hypersensitivity pneumonitis

Surgical lung biopsy is rarely performed for diagnosis of patients with acute HP, and almost all biopsies are for either subacute or chronic HP. If biopsied, acute HP may show cellular interstitial pneumonia and acute lung injury.[4] The triad of classic pathological features seen in subacute HP is airway-centered cellular interstitial pneumonia, chronic bronchiolitis, and nonnecrotizing granulomas[9] (*Figures 18-4* and *18-5A, B*). The nonnecrotizing granulomas are an important

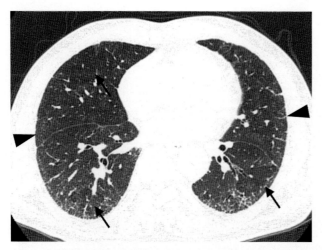

FIGURE 18-3 Hypersensitivity pneumonitis. HRCT at the level of the lower lung zone shows scattered irregular linear opacities and centrilobular nodules (arrowheads). Occasional low attenuation areas are interpreted as air trapping (arrows).

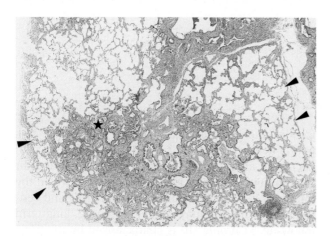

FIGURE 18-4 Hypersensitivity pneumonitis. Chronic bronchiolitis and bronchiolocentric distribution are most important characteristic features of hypersensitivity pneumonia. Note presence of peribronchiolar metaplasia (asterisk) and mucostasis along with relatively spared peripheral area (arrowheads) inside lobules.

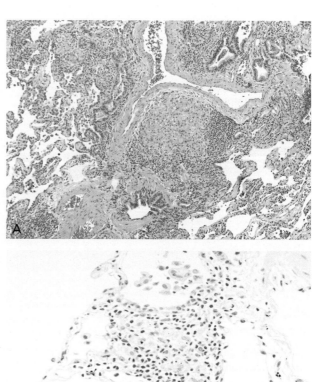

FIGURE 18-5 Hypersensitivity pneumonitis. The poorly formed nonnecrotizing granuloma is a characteristic feature for hypersensitivity pneumonitis (A). The granulomas tend to be inconspicuous and compose of a few epithelioid histiocytes (B).

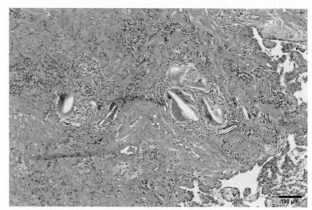

FIGURE 18-6 Hypersensitivity pneumonitis. The interstitial multinucleated giant cells with cholesterin clefts are characteristic features of hypersensitivity pneumonitis.

characteristic findings (*Figure 18-5A*). They tend to be poorly formed and composed of only a few epithelioid histiocytes (*Figure 18-5B*). Necrosis is extremely rare. If present, an infection, especially mycobacteria or fungus, should be considered.[12] Isolated interstitial multinucleated giant cells are a common finding and these often contain cholesterol clefts or Schaumann bodies[12] (*Figure 18-6*). Although these poorly formed granulomas are a characteristic finding in HP, one-third of the biopsies show no granulomas.[13] Giant cells and granulomas are known to disappear over time in HP, particularly when exposure to the antigen has ceased. One study indicated that granulomas were rarely detected in autopsies of chronic HP cases.[14]

Chronic bronchiolitis is frequent in HP, characterized by a variable infiltrate of mononuclear cells that expands the peribronchiolar interstitium, with or without accompanying fibrosis. Peribronchiolar metaplasia, representing chronic bronchiolar injury, is seen in as many as half of the surgical lung biopsies from patients with HP and is a universal finding at autopsy.[14,15] The inflammatory infiltrate is composed mainly of lymphocytes and plasma cells. Lymphoid follicles may be present around bronchioles, but are usually inconspicuous. Organizing pneumonia is also a frequent finding seen in about half of biopsies.[9]

Lung biopsies from patients with subacute HP typically show airway-centered cellular interstitial pneumonia of nonspecific interstitial pneumonia (NSIP) type. Dense fibrosis is often absent. Some cases are indistinguishable from idiopathic NSIP. Lung biopsies from patients with chronic HP shows fibrotic lung disease with more variable patterns including NSIP,[16] usual interstitial pneumonia (UIP), airway-centered interstitial fibrosis (ACIF)[17,18] and pleuroparenchymal fibroelastosis (PPFE)[19] (*Figure 18-7A, B*).

The final diagnosis of HP requires multidisciplinary discussion (MDD) with experienced clinicians and radiologists as well as clinical information of an exposure history, although, as described above, one-third of HP is diagnosed without identification of the offending antigen.

Organizing Diffuse Alveolar Damage

Clinical features of organizing diffuse alveolar damage

Organizing diffuse alveolar damage (DAD), also known as proliferative phase of DAD, is a pathologic pattern corresponding to the clinical acute respiratory distress syndrome (ARDS) or acute interstitial pneumonia (AIP) (Refer to the section on AIP below).[20-22] Organizing DAD occurs 1 to 2 weeks after the onset of symptoms. The underlying etiologies associated with organizing DAD are numerous, including infection, collagen vascular disease, drugs, inhalations, shock, sepsis, radiation, and idiopathic (AIP). The mortality rate of organizing DAD is high, up to 50% of the cases. Survivors of organizing DAD may experience recurrences and progress to chronic fibrotic lung disease.

Imaging features of organizing diffuse alveolar damage

Consolidation, traction bronchiectasis, and ground glass opacity (GGO) are the features of organizing DAD on HRCT. The areas of consolidation may regress to GGO. Patients who survive demonstrate disappearance of GGO and consolidation, and they may later show areas of hypoattenuation, cystic lesions, reticular abnormalities and associated parenchymal distortion.[23,24]

Histologic features of organizing diffuse alveolar damage

Organizing DAD is characterized by proliferation of fibroblasts/myofibroblasts admixed with scattered mononuclear inflammatory cells within the alveolar septa and airspaces (*Figure 18-8*). The alveolar fibrinous exudate, seen in the exudative phase, makes a

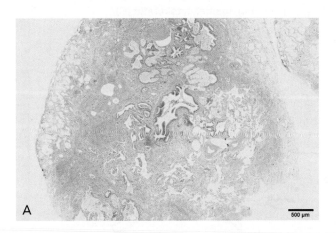

A
500 µm

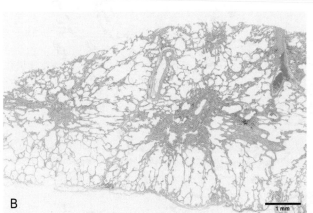

B
1 mm

FIGURE 18-7 Hypersensitivity pneumonitis. Chronic hypersensitivity pneumonitis can show patchy dense fibrosis that may be indistinguishable from usual interstitial pneumonia of idiopathic pulmonary fibrosis **(A)** or airway-centered interstitial fibrosis **(B)**.

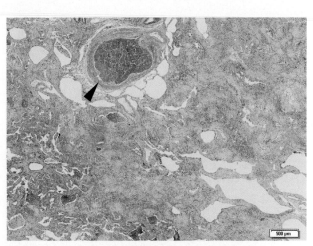

500 µm

FIGURE 18-8 Organizing DAD. Organization is seen mostly in the alveolar septa but also filling airspaces as seen in cryptogenic organizing pneumonia. Presence of fibrin thrombus in the small artery (arrowhead) is common.

transition to the organization phase with active fibrosis on the luminal surface of alveolar septa. The organization often involves collapsed alveoli and incorporates the alveolar septa. Deposition of collagen fibers may be seen but is often minimal. Pneumocyte hyperplasia develops approximately 3 to 7 days following lung injury, and is present in the organizing phase. They may demonstrate cytological atypia simulating adenocarcinoma. Detachment of pneumocytes from the interstitium is common. Intra-alveolar edema and hyaline membranes, hallmarks of exudative DAD, are often inconspicuous, and a few remnants may be identified in the thickened alveolar septa. Other characteristic findings of organizing DAD are widening of alveolar duct, squamous metaplasia, vascular injury with/without thrombus, and thickened pleura (*Figure 18-9A–C*). Squamous metaplasia is typically observed around the widened alveolar ducts. Loose intimal thickening

of the pulmonary artery along with fibrinous thrombi, evidence of vascular injury, can be found in this phase. Thickening of the pleura with slight fibrosis is a common finding as well. Some cases may resemble NSIP, especially when collapsed alveoli are incorporated and reepithelialized by proliferating pneumocytes.[25] Some cases of DAD resolve completely, but rarely, fibrosis may progress to extensive structural remodeling and honeycomb lung.

Honeycomb Lung

Clinical features of honeycomb lung

The term "honeycomb lung" was originally used to describe the macroscopic appearance of cysts in the lung regardless of background etiology.[26] Currently, honeycomb lung is limited to describe end-stage

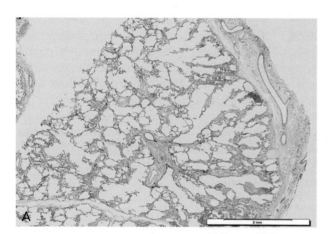

FIGURE 18-9 Organizing DAD. The widened alveolar duct due to collapse of alveolar sac (A, B). The collapsed alveolar sac can be visualized by immunostaining against cytokeratin (C).

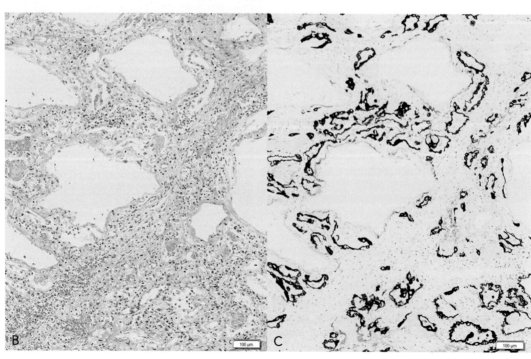

pulmonary fibrosis.[27] Idiopathic pulmonary fibrosis (IPF) is the leading cause of honeycomb lung. However, several other interstitial lung diseases have the potential to progress to honeycomb lung. These include NSIP,[28] desquamative interstitial pneumonia (DIP),[29] chronic HP and various collagen vascular diseases (CVD) manifesting in the lung.[30,31] Regardless the underlying etiology and disease, the presence of honeycomb lung is associated with a poor prognosis.[32-35]

Imaging features of honeycomb lung

The radiologic features of honeycomb lung are clustered cystic air spaces separated by well-defined thick walls, typically of diameters of 2 to 10 mm but occasionally as large as 2 cm. Honeycomb lung usually shows subpleural predominance with well-defined cyst walls and is considered a CT feature of established pulmonary fibrosis[36] (*Figure 18-10A, B*). Identification of honeycomb lung is the most important finding on HRCT for the diagnosis of IPF and current IPF guidelines state

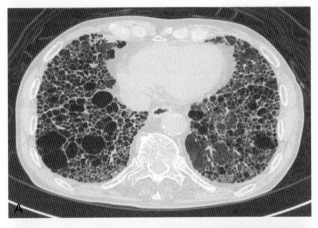
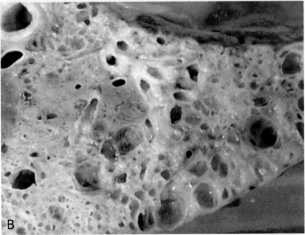

FIGURE 18-10 Honeycomb lung. Lower lung zone of the end-stage pulmonary fibrosis demonstrates multilayer of cystic lesion in CT (A). Gross appearance of honeycomb cysts is characteristically firm and rounded with little structural contents inside (B).

that identifying honeycomb cysts on the HRCT can be diagnostic of UIP without the need for a surgical lung biopsy.[37] Various lung diseases other than IPF can result in honeycomb lung. Some studies report that up to 28% of NSIP and up to 16% of DIP may progress to honeycomb lung with follow-up.[28,29,38] Although most cases of honeycomb lung are found in chronic diseases, a minority of patients with acute interstitial pneumonia or diffuse alveolar damage may develop honeycomb lung.[24,39] Traction bronchiectasis is an important condition that resembles honeycomb lung on imaging. In traction bronchiectasis there are enlarged bronchial spaces secondary to shrinkage of surrounding lung tissue. Traction bronchiectasis frequently accompanies fibrotic lung disease especially end-stage fibrotic NSIP.[40-42] Similar to honeycomb lung producing clusters of cystic spaces, confluent traction bronchiectasis and emphysematous cysts accompanied by fibrosis can present as multicystic lung, strongly mimicking honeycomb lung on imaging studies. Discriminating confluent traction bronchiectasis from honeycomb lung can be challenging even for the expert radiologist.[42]

Histologic features of honeycomb lung

The characteristic pathologic features of honeycomb lung, also recognizable by HRCT, are uniformly sized cysts ranging from 2 to 10 mm in diameter with underling dense scarring and complete destruction of normal lung architecture (*Figures 18-10* and *18-11*). The typical histologic features of honeycomb cysts are enlarged airspaces surrounded by collagen-rich scaring and metaplastic bronchiolar epithelium along the luminal surface (*Figure 18-11A, B*). Other cystic lesions that resemble honeycomb lung, but should be distinguished from it, are traction bronchiolectasia and airspace enlargement with fibrosis (AEF) (*Figure 18-12A, B*). Occasional fibroblastic foci or lymphoid aggregates may be found in the cystic walls. The term "microscopic honeycomb" applies to cystic lesions only recognizable under the microscope, although there is little consensus definition. The cysts of microscopic honeycomb are often filled with mucin or proteinaceous substances with various degrees of inflammatory cells that can prevent recognition by HRCT (*Figure 18-13*). The exact relationship between honeycomb and microscopic honeycomb is not clear. However, the high association between the two indicates that microscopic honeycomb may be a precursor of larger honeycomb cysts.

Current IPF guidelines state that when honeycomb lung is the only finding in the surgical biopsy, the biopsy falls into the diagnostic category of probable UIP.

Honeycomb lung can be an eventual end-stage of a variety of interstitial lung diseases. Therefore, it is often difficult or impossible to identify the background etiology. For this reason, the biopsy specimen should not be

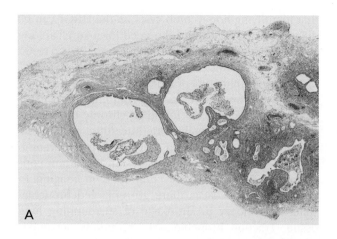

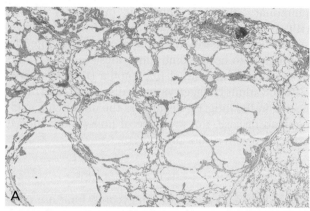

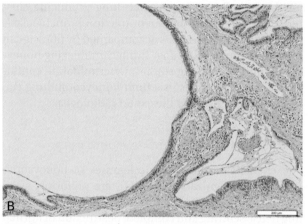

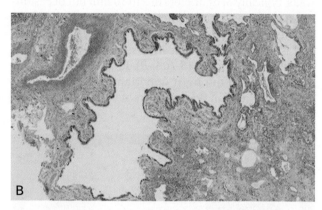

FIGURE 18-11 Honeycomb lung. The honeycomb cysts are enlarged airspaces surrounded by collagen-rich dense fibrosis (A). Cysts are often covered with ciliated bronchiolar epithelial cells with various levels of mucous production (B).

FIGURE 18-12 Other cystic lesions simulating honeycomb. Airspace enlargement with fibrosis (AEF) is an emphysematous condition associated with slight fibrosis in their walls (A). Traction bronchiolectasia can mimic honeycomb cysts. Presence of basement membrane and smooth muscle bundles adjacent to the cystic wall is a key clue of dilated bronchioles (B).

taken purely from honeycomb areas. Ideally the lung biopsy should include the full spectrum of the HRCT appearance including areas with active disease rather than end-stage honeycomb.

The exact pathogenesis of honeycomb lung remains unclear, although parenchymal collapse in the areas of lung injury is considered to be a major contributor.[43,44]

Diffuse Alveolar-Septal Amyloidosis

Clinical features of diffuse alveolar-septal amyloidosis

Amyloidosis is a rare disease characterized by the extracellular accumulation in various organs including the lungs of insoluble fibrous protein due to the formation of β-pleated sheets. These amyloid fibrils may derive from a variety of precursor proteins, frequently

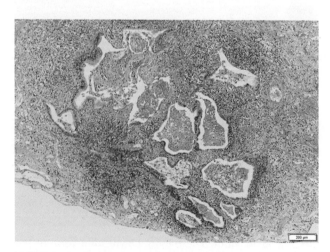

FIGURE 18-13 Honeycomb lung. Microscopic honeycomb is often filled with mucus substance or proteinous debris. Surrounding parenchyma shows various degrees of inflammatory cells.

serum amyloid A protein (AA) or monoclonal immunoglobulin light chains (AL). Amyloidosis is classified as systemic or localized, as well as primary (idiopathic) or secondary (reactive).[45,46] A diffuse alveolar-septal amyloidosis usually occurs in association with primary systemic amyloidosis or multiple myeloma.[47] Rarely, primary lung involvement with alveolar-septal amyloidosis occurs. Some cases of secondary amyloidosis are associated with diffuse lymphoid hyperplasia, hemodialysis, and collagen vascular disease, especially Sjögren syndrome.[46,48] The most common presenting symptom in patients with diffuse alveolar-septal amyloidosis is progressive dyspnea. Hemorrhagic diathesis is a known complication in amyloidosis.[48] Persistent pleural effusions are seen in 5.5% of patients and are commonly associated with cardiac amyloidosis.[45] Diffuse alveolar-septal amyloidosis usually has a poor prognosis with a median survival of only 16 months after diagnosis.[49]

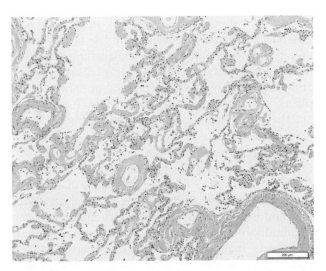

FIGURE 18-14 Diffuse alveolar septal amyloidosis. The alveolar septa show amorphous eosinophilic changes. Basic lung structures are mostly preserved.

Imaging features of diffuse alveolar-septal amyloidosis

The characteristic HRCT findings in diffuse alveolar-septal amyloidosis include abnormal reticular opacities, interlobular septal thickening, small well-defined nodules 2 to 4 mm in diameter, and confluent consolidative opacities that predominate in the subpleural regions of the middle and lower lung zones. Calcification is common in which small interstitial nodules on HRCT are characteristic findings.[50] Multiple thin-walled cysts are rarely found in the peripheral lung.[47] Diffuse alveolar-septal amyloidosis may clinically and radiologically mimic pulmonary edema or interstitial pneumonia.[45,51]

Histologic features of diffuse alveolar-septal amyloidosis

Diffuse alveolar-septal amyloidosis may be more often observed histologically at autopsy than in biopsy in patients with systemic amyloidosis. The histological features of diffuse alveolar-septal amyloidosis are acellular thickening of alveolar septa where uniform deposition of amorphous eosinophilic material along alveolar septa and within media of blood vessels is found[45] (*Figure 18-14*). The alveolar structures are usually preserved, but may be distorted. Inflammatory cell infiltrations are typically inconspicuous, and when lymphocytes and plasma cells are prominent, lymphoproliferative disorders need to be ruled out. Calcifications can be seen inside the amyloid deposits.[47] The giant cells that are frequently seen in nodular amyloidosis are not prominent in diffuse alveolar-septal amyloidosis. The diagnosis of amyloidosis requires the confirmation of amyloid deposition with special stains, such as Congo red, direct fast scarlet, crystal violet, or immunohistochemical stains for amyloid[52] (*Figure 18-15*). If special

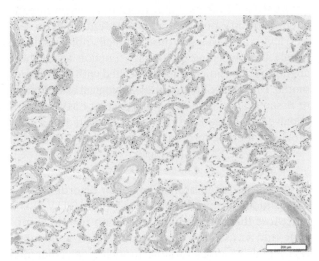

FIGURE 18-15 Diffuse alveolar septal amyloidosis. The staining of direct fast scarlet revealed diffuse deposition of amyloid in alveolar septa.

stains are negative, light chain deposition disease needs to be considered.[53] The differential diagnosis may also include fibrosing interstitial pneumonia with extensive hyalinized collagen deposition.

Infectious Interstitial Pneumonia

Clinical features of infectious interstitial pneumonia

Several virus infections are associated with specific interstitial pneumonias; however, their occurrence is rare.

Lymphoid interstitial pneumonia in HIV infection

HIV can induce interstitial pneumonia, such as lymphocytic interstitial pneumonitis (LIP) especially in children with perinatally acquired infection.[54,55] Numerous studies have shown evidence of EBV in patients with HIV infection and LIP. However, the role of EBV infection in the development of LIP remains unclear.[56] The patients demonstrate insidious onset of disease. Cough and tachypnea are the most common presenting complains.[57] The prognosis for children with LIP is variable, and the overall long-term mortality rate is high.[58]

Cytomegalovirus pneumonia

Cytomegalovirus (CMV), a member of the Herpesviridae family, is a common cause of interstitial pneumonia. Interstitial pneumonia related to cytomegalovirus (CMV) infection is often a life-threatening complication seen in immunocompromised patients. It occurs commonly after bone marrow and solid organ transplantation and in patients with acquired immunodeficiency syndrome.[59] CMV is a common copathogen in *Pneumocystis jiroveci* pneumonia (PCP). Reports of increased mortality in patients with both PCP and CMV have been reported. CMV infection may range from asymptomatic viremia to CMV pneumonia. The patients may present with low-grade fever, shortness of breath, nonproductive cough, and declining pulmonary function tests. There are no specific clinical signs associated with CMV pneumonia. Diagnosis often requires serological examination or tissue examination.[60] The presence of CMV in bronchoalveolar lavage fluid by culture is related to a poor prognosis for long-term survival.[61] Ganciclovir is used to treat or prevent CMV infection.[60]

HTLV-1–associated bronchioalveolar disorder

The human T-lymphotropic virus type I (HTLV-I) is a retrovirus that infects 10 to 20 million people worldwide and is associated with adult T-cell leukemia.[62] HTLV-1 also causes variable bronchioloalveolar disorders, such as LIP, diffuse panbronchiolitis, bronchiectasis, and miliary distribution of micronodules.[63-66] Pulmonary involvement in HTLV-1 carriers is mostly subclinical.[67]

Other viruses that can cause interstitial pneumonia include severe acute respiratory syndrome (SARS) virus, influenza virus, hepatitis C virus, herpes simplex virus, and adenovirus.[68-70]

Imaging features of infectious interstitial pneumonia

The dominant CT finding seen in HIV patients with LIP is usually diffuse ground glass opacity. Scattered thin-walled cysts can also be seen.[54] In long-term survivors of vertically acquired HIV infection, a decreased attenuation consistent with small airway disease is the most common and extensive abnormality, followed by large airway abnormalities (bronchial wall thickening, small and large airway plugging, and bronchiectasis. The natural course of HIV-related LIP remains unknown.[71]

The radiographic features of CMV pneumonia are parenchymal consolidation and multiple nodules smaller than 5 mm in diameter. The other CT findings include areas of GGO, linear opacities, nodules, or masses.[72]

HRCT findings in patients with HTLV-1 consisted mainly of miliary nodules, GGO, and thickening of the bronchovascular bundles in the peripheral lung.[73]

Histologic features of infectious interstitial pneumonia

The histologic features of infectious interstitial pneumonia are variable depending on the causative agents, severity of the disease, and time of pathological examination.

Lymphoid interstitial pneumonia in HIV infection

The most common interstitial pneumonia encountered in HIV carrier in the absence of specific infection is a lymphocytic interstitial pneumonia (LIP).[74] The LIP associated with HIV is characterized by diffuse infiltration of mature lymphocytes and a variable admixture of plasma cells in alveolar wall (*Figure 18-16A, B*).

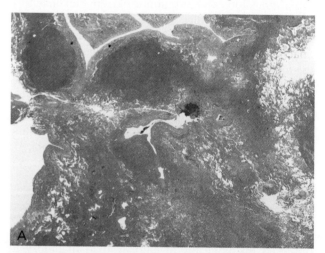

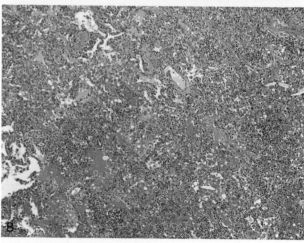

FIGURE 18-16 **LIP associated with HIV. The diffuse infiltration of mature lymphocytes is characteristic feature for LIP (A, B).**

Collagenous interstitial fibrosis is absent or inconspicuous. Occasional cystic change may be seen and surrounded by loose fibrosis with lymphocytic infiltration. Lymphoid follicle which lacks the germinal center is common. Foamy macrophages and eosinophilic exudate filling in the alveolar spaces are common in HIV patients with LIP.[75]

Cytomegalovirus pneumonia

The diagnostic histologic finding of CMV pneumonia is cellular enlargement combined with characteristic intranuclear inclusions (*Figure 18-17*). These intranuclear inclusions are round to oval and dark purple body surrounded by a clear halo, "owl's eye." (Cowdry type A inclusion) The cytoplasmic inclusions may be identified as well. CMV can infect a wide variety of cell types including epithelial cells of the airways and alveoli, fibroblasts, macrophages, histiocytes, and endothelial cells. However, the inclusions may be absent in some patients with positive viral culture. Varieties of histologic manifestations of CMV pneumonia were reported including a focal or diffuse interstitial pneumonia, miliary pattern of exudation, and DAD. Among them, DAD is the most common histological pattern. Identification of unequivocal inclusion bodies or immunohistochemical detection of viral antigen is required to confirm the diagnosis.[76] Herpes simplex virus can cause similar disease as CMV pneumonia. Herpes pneumonia shows foci of small necrosis and epithelial cells with characteristic nuclear changes which include enlarged nuclei with smudged or homogenized, ground glass, or slate-gray nuclei called Cowdry B. When difficult to distinguish, immunohistochemical techniques can help confirm the responsible virus.[77]

HTLV-1–associated bronchioalveolar disorder

The characteristic histological feature of HTLV-1–associated bronchioloalveolar disorder is micronodules less than 3 mm in diameter distributed mainly around the airways (*Figure 18-18A, B*). These nodules consist of severe lymphoid infiltration, florid tissue eosinophilia, and nonnecrotizing granulomas. The occasional small foci of necrosis may be seen inside the granuloma. It is important to rule out acid-fast bacilli infection by Ziehl-Neelsen stains as well as tissue culture. The majority of lymphocytes are T cells, and cellular atypia should not be seen. Fibrin exudates and limited amount of organizing pneumonia can be seen around the micronodular lesions. Dense fibrosis is not seen.[63,64] Other abnormality such as airway-centered pulmonary fibrosis, organizing pneumonia, and peribronchiolar inflammation simulating diffuse panbronchiolitis can be seen in a rare fashion.[78,79]

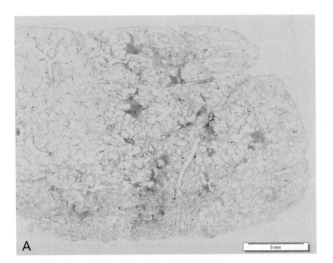

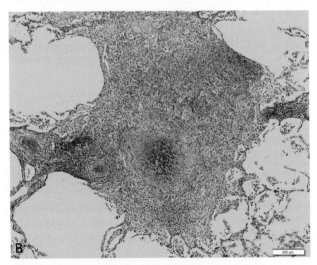

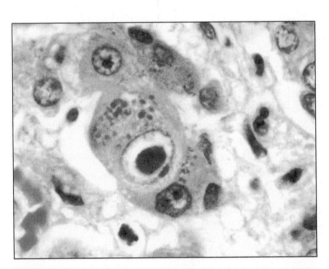

FIGURE 18-17 CMV pneumonia. The nuclear enlargement associated with owl eye appearance is characteristic feature of CMV pneumonia. The background lung often shows diffuse alveolar damage.

FIGURE 18-18 HTLV-1. The eosinophilic micronodules are randomly distributed. The micronodules are composed of poorly formed granuloma surrounded by T lymphocytes along with occasional tiny foci of necrosis (A, B).

Flock Lung

Clinical features of flock lung

The workers in flocking industry were reported to be at high risk for interstitial lung disease with unique histologic findings of lymphocytic bronchiolitis.[80,81] Flock is cut or pulverized fiber (synthetic or natural) of small diameter that produces a velvet-like coating when applied to adhesive-coated fabric or other material. On average, affected employees had a 6-year latency period until symptoms developed.[82] Although, the exact etiological agent is unknown, several studies have suggested that aerosolized flock may contain respirable-sized particles that may lead to inflammatory reactions in the lung.[81]

Most patients present with subacute or chronic symptoms including the progressive dyspnea and cough with or without sputum production. On physical examination, crackles were auscultated in all. Pulmonary function test (PFT) demonstrates a restrictive pulmonary defect with reduced diffusing capacity for carbon monoxide, although an obstructive defect may also present in some individuals. Bronchoalveolar lavage (BAL) is sometimes abnormal with eosinophilia, lymphocytosis, or neutrophilia.

Avoidance of flock exposure is the only effective therapy and is usually associated with stabilization or improvement in respiratory symptoms.[82]

Imaging features of flock lung

More than half of the exposed workers including individuals who do not develop symptoms show abnormal CT scans.[83] The most characteristic findings in FL were diffuse ground glass opacities (GGO) and micronodules.[83] Other characteristic features include bronchial wall thickening, air trapping, patchy consolidation, and peripheral honeycombing.[84] These changes often involve the entire lung and appear to be similar to hypersensitivity pneumonitis or respiratory bronchiolitis.

Histologic features of flock lung

The classic histologic feature of FL is a mixture of lymphocytic bronchiolitis, peribronchiolar inflammation, and lymphoid hyperplasia (*Figure 18-19A, B*). In most cases, lymphocytes are the predominant inflammatory cells but plasma cells are also present. Significant tissue eosinophilia can be seen in the rare occasion. Although rare, FL case may progress to pulmonary fibrosis showing usual interstitial pneumonia pattern. Alveolar macrophages were prominent within peribronchiolar alveolar space, and occasional multinucleated giant cells were reported. The pertinent negative findings for FL are the lack of granulomas, presence of fibrin, necrosis, vascular changes, and smooth muscle hyperplasia.

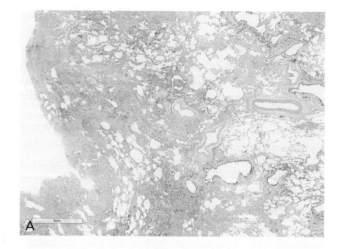

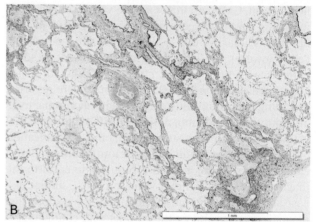

FIGURE 18-19 Flock worker's lung. Airway accentuated interstitial pneumonia. Note marked peribronchiolar inflammation and metaplasia (A, B).

Some patients may demonstrate acute to subacute lung injury and simulate organizing pneumonia or organizing diffuse alveolar damage.[85]

Hot Tub Lung

Clinical features of hot tub lung

Hot tub lung is a granulomatous lung disease caused by exposure to *Mycobacterium avium* complex (MAC) organisms contaminating hot tub water.[86,87] Initial symptom onset is usually an acute flu-like illness. The dyspnea and cough at presentation is common. Half of the patients demonstrate low-grade fever and chest tightness.[88]

For the diagnosis, MAC should be isolated from respiratory secretion, hot tub water sample, or lung tissue without other identifiable cause for the illness.[88]

Hot tub lung is more likely a form of hypersensitivity pneumonia to mycobacteria rather than a harmful infection, and treatment with antimycobacterial drugs is usually unnecessary.[88] Some patients appeared to improve with hot tub avoidance alone.[88]

Imaging features of hot tub lung

The common HRCT features in patients with hot tub lung are small nodular opacities which are usually bilateral and symmetric in most cases. The nodules demonstrate centrilobular distribution with upper lung predominance and involve more than 40% of the entire lung. Some cases can show prominent nodules. Rarely, cases may demonstrate reticular opacities with lower lung predominance. Consolidations, cysts, honeycombing, emphysema, bronchiectasis, pleural effusions, and lymph adenopathy are not the feature of hot tub lung. The air trapping is common; it may be the only abnormality on HRCT.[88,89]

Histologic features of hot tub lung

The histologic hallmark of hot tub lung is the presence of nonnecrotizing granulomas. The granulomas are distributed bronchiolocentric area mainly within alveolar spaces or around the lymphatic route (*Figure 18-20A, B*). Involvement of granuloma in the interstitial area inside

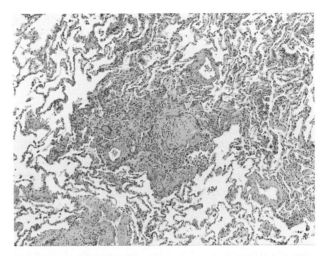

FIGURE 18-21 **Hot tub lung. Organizing pneumonia is often an accompanying feature.**

the pleura or interlobular septa is rare. The granulomas are better demarcated than those seen in hypersensitivity pneumonitis but not as well formed as those of sarcoidosis. The well-formed granulomas are typically nonnecrotizing, but may show small foci of eosinophilic central necrosis. There should be no identifiable surrounding fibrosis as seen in sarcoidosis. Special stains will demonstrate a few acid-fast bacilli within the granulomas in about one-fourth of biopsies. The cultures or polymerase chain reaction of tissue or pulmonary secretions are usually positive for MAC, but not all cases.[90] Organizing pneumonia with interstitial inflammation is often present but its extent is variable.[12] (*Figure 18-21*). Hot tub lung can be suspected solely on the basis of histologic findings. Definitive diagnosis requires a history of hot tub use or exposure to aerosolized water contaminated with mycobacterial organisms.[88]

Airway-Centered Interstitial Lung Disease

Pathogenesis of airway-centered interstitial lung disease

Several retrospective studies have described airway-centered interstitial lung disease (AC-ILD)[17,91-93] and various histologic patterns of AC-ILD have been described under different names[94] (*Table 18-1*). Some patients show positive to serum precipitins from

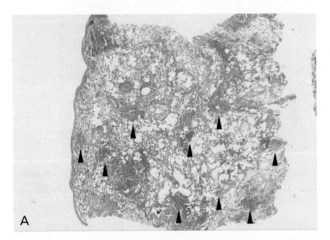

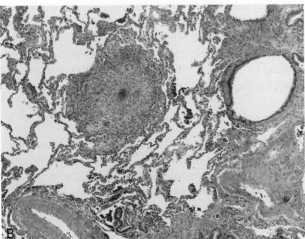

FIGURE 18-20 **Hot tub lung. The biopsy of the hot tub user showed miliary distributed granulomas (arrowheads). The culture revealed MAC infection. (A) The relatively large granuloma with giant cells is characteristic for MAC infection. (B)**

Table 18-1 Histologic Patterns of Airway-Centered Fibrotic Lung Disease

Airway-centered interstitial fibrosis
Idiopathic bronchiolocentric interstitial pneumonia
Peribronchiolar metaplasia

From Reference[94] (Allen TC. Pathology of small airways disease. *Arch Pathol Lab Med.* May 2010;134(5):702-718.)

pigeon, goose, duck, and chicken feathers indicating that part of AC-ILD are indeed chronic HP.[18] Tabaco smoking, microaspiration, and inhalation of unknown dust may be a possible cause of AC-ILD as well.

Clinical features of airway-centered fibrotic lung disease

Precise background clinical characteristics are unknown. There was a female predominance with age range of 23 to 74 years.[17,91-93,95] The presenting symptoms in patients with airway-centered fibrotic lung disease are chronic cough and slowly progressive dyspnea. Pulmonary function tests can show both obstructive and restrictive lung disease with reduced lung volumes and abnormalities of carbon monoxide diffusing capacity. One-third of patients demonstrate a mild to moderate increase of lymphocytes in bronchoalveolar lavage fluid.[17] There is a few evidence of treatment for ACC-ILD, but some reports described the efficacy of corticosteroids.[95] Reported prognoses for AC-ILD are variable. Series of Yousem et al and Churg et al showed poor prognoses where 33% to 40% of the patients had died of disease[91] On the other hand, one report indicated favorable prognosis in patients who only show peribronchiolar metaplasia.[93] Prognosis of AC-ILD may be favorable when peripheral interstitial fibrosis is not prominent morphologically.

Imaging features of airway-centered fibrotic lung disease

The characteristic features of HRCT scans in patients with ACIF are not well recognized. Reported features were peribronchovascular interstitial thickening, traction bronchiectasis, and thickened airway walls. There may be subtle abnormality indicating air trapping such as mosaic attenuation only identifiable by expiratory CT.[17] Emphysematous change may be seen in patients with extensive smoking history.

Histologic features of airway-centered fibrotic lung disease

At low magnification, the most striking feature is multiple nodular foci of airway-centered interstitial fibrosis centered on membranous and respiratory bronchioles. Variable degrees of interstitial fibrosis extended away from the affected airways (*Figure 18-22 A, B*). When levels of fibrosis become more extensive, fibrosis incorporates interlobular septa or pleura which may give pathologists a wrong impression that the fibrosis may be peripheral predominant (*Figure 18-23*). Another important caveat is that the areas adjacent to large membranous bronchiole may be a peripheral zone inside the lobule. Pathologists have to know that before entering to the pulmonary secondary lobule, bronchioles indeed run

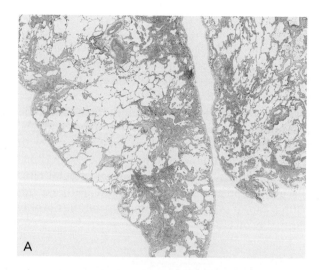

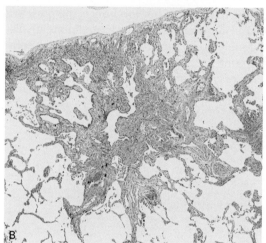

FIGURE 18-22 Airway-centered fibrotic lung disease. Interstitial fibrosis is located around the airway (A, B).

into lung parenchyma through areas outside the lobule, interlobular septa. Peribronchiolar metaplasia (PBM) is a metaplastic proliferation of bronchiolar type epithelia starting from respiratory bronchioles and a frequent finding in AC-ILD. PBM probably highlights sequels of bronchiolocentric injury.[17,91]

Differential diagnosis

AC-ILD due to causable inhalation agents always enter in the differential diagnosis. When intra-alveolar macrophage is prominent on a heavy smoking patient, respiratory bronchiolitis interstitial lung disease (RBILD) needs to be considered.[94,96] Pneumoconiosis such as mixed dust pneumoconiosis or asbestosis shows histological pattern of AC-ILD as well. The prominent dust deposition or presence of asbestos body can exclude idiopathic form of AC-ILD. Prussian blue stain is helpful for identifying the asbestos bodies and other iron-coated particles.[97]

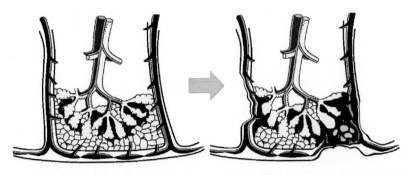

FIGURE 18-23 Airway-centered fibrotic lung disease. Initial fibrosis starts around respiratory and/or terminal bronchiole. When inhalation is the main cause, areas around recurrent branches of respiratory bronchiole are the most common place of inflammation/fibrosis (left). When disease progresses, fibrosis connects to the peripheral zone of pulmonary lobule and form scar similar to usual interstitial pneumonia (right). Blue-colored area indicates schematic image of mucin containing microscopic honeycombing (right lower corner).

IDIOPATHIC INTERSTITIAL PNEUMONIAS

Usual Interstitial Pneumonia

Pathogenesis of usual interstitial pneumonia

Idiopathic pulmonary fibrosis (IPF) is defined as a specific form of chronic, progressive fibrosing interstitial pneumonia of unknown etiology, occurring primarily in older adults, limited to the lungs, and associated with the histopathologic and radiologic pattern of usual interstitial pneumonia (UIP).[21,22,37] Although IPF is, by definition, a disease of unknown etiology, a number of potential pathogenesis has been described.

Genetic Factors

The familial forms of IPF have been reported in many researches.[98-100] The familial IPF and sporadic IPF are clinically and histologically indistinguishable, although familial forms may develop at an earlier age. The strong associations with familial IPF have been found with mutations in the surfactant protein C gene,[101] but this association has not been found in patients with the sporadic IPF.[102] Mutation of another surfactant protein A2 (SFTPA2)[103] has been identified as a responsible gene of familial IPF.[104] Recent reports have also described that genetic variants within the human telomerase reverse transcriptase (hTERT) or human telomerase RNA (hTR) components of the telomerase gene are associated with familial forms of IPF and are present in some patients with sporadic IPF. These rare mutations can be found in up to 15% of familial IPF kindred and 3% of sporadic IIP cases, and result in telomere shortening that ultimately causes apoptosis of alveolar epithelial cell.[105,106] Polymorphisms of genes encoding interleukin [IL]-1, IL-4, IL-6, IL-8, IL-10, IL-12a,[107,108] tumor necrosis factor-a,[109] angiotensin-converting enzyme,[110] transforming growth factor-β-1,[111] NOD2/CARD15, MUC5B,[112,113]

and matrix metalloproteinase-1 have been reported to have increased frequencies of IPF.[114] However, responsible driver gene mutations connecting to its pathogenesis is still unclear.

Cigarette Smoking

Cigarette smoking is strongly associated with IPF. Although not all patients with IPF are smokers, the frequency of smoking history is as high as lung cancer and COPD (eg, 60%–80%).[115-117] The odds ratio of risk to have IPF in the smoking individuals is 1.58 (95% confidence interval: 1.27–1.97).[118]

Gastroesophageal Reflux

It has been hypothesized that chronic microaspiration (ie, tracheobronchial aspiration of small amounts of gastric secretions) due to gastroesophageal reflux (GER) may cause repetitive subclinical injury to the lung leading to IPF.[119] Actually, GER can be found in some patients with IPF and is mostly clinically silent.[120] The prevalence of microaspiration in patients with IPF is not known, and it is not clear whether microaspiration represents an intrinsic risk factor or causes acute exacerbations of IPF.[121] A recent report described that the use of GER medications (PPI) improves the radiologic abnormality and patients' survival.[122]

Clinical features of usual interstitial pneumonia

Idiopathic pulmonary fibrosis is a specific form of chronic fibrosing interstitial pneumonia limited to the lung and associated with the histologic appearance of usual interstitial pneumonia (UIP) on surgical lung biopsy.[21,22,37] IPF is the most common disease in the subtype of IIPs, comprising up to 70% of the cases. IPF has an estimated prevalence of 14 to 43 per 100,000 and an estimated incidence of 7 to 16 per 100,000.[123,124] The median survival of patients with IPF after diagnosis is as poor as lung cancer being 2 to 5 years.[37] Improvement in lung physiology and radiologic abnormalities is rare.[22] The incidence of the disease increases with age for which initial presentation typically occur in the seventh decades. Patients with IPF aged less than 50 years are rare; such patients may subsequently manifest overt features of underlying conditions such as connective tissue disease that is subclinical at the time of diagnosis. Onset of symptoms is usually gradual. In most patients, symptoms have been present for more than 6 months before presentation. Ninety percent of patients have dyspnea at the time of diagnosis. Digital clubbing develops in 25% to 50% of patients, and fine end-inspiratory crackles are characteristic on chest auscultation.[37] Serum levels of Krebs von den Lungen 6 antigen (KL-6) have been reported to be elevated in IPF.[125] Connective tissue disease can present pulmonary fibrosis with UIP pattern, and ILD can be a sole clinical manifestation of these conditions.[126] Serologic testing for connective tissue disease should be performed in the evaluation of IPF.[127] Pulmonary function test shows a restrictive pattern of ventilatory defect with a decrease in DL_{co}. Pulmonary function test or chest radiographs may be normal or near normal in the early phase of IPF.[128] In smokers and exsmokers with IPF, coexistent of emphysema may result in relatively higher lung volumes compared with never-smoking patients with IPF.[117] The most common cause of death related to IPF is respiratory failure. Other causes of death include pulmonary hypertension, heart failure, lung cancer, pulmonary embolism, and infectious pneumonia.[129,130] As no therapy has been proven to be efficacious in this disease, management generally includes supportive cares (eg, supplemental oxygen, pulmonary rehabilitation), lung transplant evaluation, and identification and treatment of comorbidities.[37] New therapeutic agents including pirfenidone may show some benefit, but there is insufficient evidence to recommend their general use at this time.[131,132]

For the diagnosis of IPF, the multidisciplinary discussion between pulmonologists, radiologists, and pathologists well experienced in the diagnosis of ILD is of the utmost importance to an accurate diagnosis.

Acute Exacerbation of IPF

An acute exacerbation can occur at any course of IPF. When acute exacerbation occurs, it is often lethal. Acute respiratory worsening occurs in up to 40% of patients with IPF, and if it does, nearly half of the patients are going to death.[133] Many of these acute deteriorations are of unknown etiology and have been termed acute exacerbations of IPF.[134] The criteria for acute exacerbation of IPF have included an unexplained worsening of dyspnea within 1 month, evidence of hypoxemia as defined by worsened or severely impaired gas exchange, new radiographic alveolar infiltrates, and an absence of an alternative explanation such as infection, pulmonary embolism, pneumothorax, or heart failure.[133] Acute exacerbations of IPF can occur at any time during the course of disease,

and for some patients, may be the presenting manifestation of their disease.[135] Worsened cough, fever, and/or increased sputum have been observed.

Imaging features of usual interstitial pneumonia

High-resolution computed tomography (HRCT) imaging has a pivotal role in the diagnosis of interstitial lung diseases, particularly in the assessment of patients with suspected IPF. The chest radiograph is less useful than HRCT in evaluating patients with suspected IPF. HRCT demonstrates a characteristic pattern of subpleural, bibasilar reticular opacities, including honeycomb changes and traction bronchiectasis.[40,41,136] Honeycomb change is manifested on HRCT as clustered cystic airspaces, usually ranging from 2 to 20 mm in diameter. It is usually subpleural and is characterized by well-defined walls. Honeycomb change is a hallmark appearance of UIP; however, it is often absent in the early phase (*Figure 18-24*). When honeycomb change is absent, but the imaging features otherwise meet criteria of UIP, the imaging features are regarded as "possible UIP."[37] Ground glass opacities (GGO) are common, but usually less extensive than the reticulation. Another hallmark of UIP on HRCT is patchy distribution (temporal or spatial heterogeneity). Areas of mild and severe fibrosis and normal lung are often present in the same lobe, in the same segment, and in the same secondary lobule. The key findings of temporal or spatial heterogeneity on HRCT are various findings including normal to end-stage fibrosis locate in one secondary lobule.[136] Extensive pleural effusion, extensive GGO, profuse micronodules, diffuse mosaic attenuation, discrete cysts, consolidation, or peribronchovascular-predominant distribution suggest an alternative diagnosis.[37] In patients whose HRCT demonstrate inconsistent UIP may demonstrate UIP on histology. Such cases behave as bad as IPF and needs to be treated as IPF.[32]

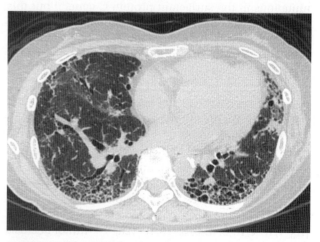

FIGURE 18-24 HRCT of UIP. Accumulation of cystic spaces directly starting from subpleural zone (honeycomb change) is characteristic and diagnostic features of UIP.

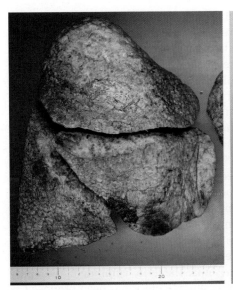
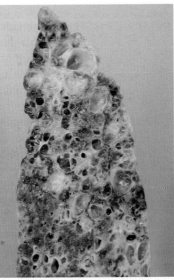

FIGURE 18-25 Macroscopic image of UIP pattern. The lung shows significant shrinkage and the pleural surface demonstrates a cobble-stoned appearance (left). The honeycomb cysts represent independent spherical space (right).

Gross features of usual interstitial pneumonia

The lung usually shows significant shrinkage, especially in the lower lobe. The pleural surface of the lungs demonstrates a cobble-stoned appearance due to the contraction of scars along the interlobular septa (*Figure 18-25*). The cut surface typically shows multiple layers of cysts, honeycomb lung, starting from subpleural area with the lower lobe predominance. Most of honeycomb cysts represent independent spherical space but often mixed

with undistinguishable spaces from traction bronchiolectasia. The upper lobe is relatively preserved.

Histologic features of usual interstitial pneumonia

UIP showed characteristic low magnification of heterogeneous appearance and patchy involvement. This patchy involvement was characterized by foci of dense fibrosis and normal lung or mild interstitial fibrosis (*Figure 18-26*).[21,37] There is an abrupt change

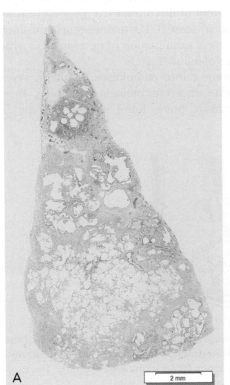
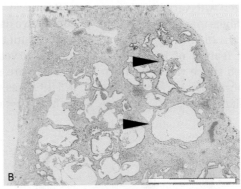
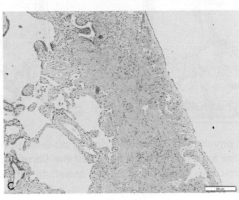

FIGURE 18-26 Usual interstitial pneumonia. The mixture of dense fibrosis and normal lung shows patchy distribution (A). Microscopic honeycombing (arrowheads) is characteristic histological feature (B). Smooth muscle hyperplasia is also frequent findings for UIP (C).

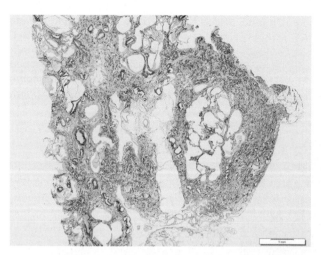

FIGURE 18-27 Usual interstitial pneumonia. Accumulation of elastic fiber mainly in the peripheral zone of the pulmonary lobule reflects the architectural destruction of UIP.

from a fibrotic area to the normal lung and little intervening transition. Involvement of peripheral areas of secondary lobules was an important feature of UIP.[137] Peripheral areas contain paraseptal regions, areas adjacent to bronchovascular bundles, and areas surrounding postcapillary venules that start inside the lobule (*Figure 18-27*). This perivenular fibrosis may progress to linear fibrotic structure simulating interlobular septa and divides the secondary lobules into smaller units (*Figure 18-28*). Another feature of low magnification is a honeycomb change described in the former section of this chapter.[27,41] The fibrotic area of UIP is composed mainly of dense hyaline collagen with variable amount of smooth muscle.[98,138] Elastic fibers may be increased in the scarred areas as well (*Figure 18-29*).[139] Fibroblastic foci are the key histological feature of UIP as well (*Figure 18-30*). They are curved shape young fibroplasia mainly composed of myofibroblasts and covered by hyperplastic type II cells. Inflammatory cells are rare

inside the fibroblastic foci, and if there are, they may be better considered as organizing pneumonia. The levels of fibroblastic foci have been reported as prognostic factor, therefore, mentioning levels of fibroblastic foci to the pulmonologist may be beneficial.[138,140-142]

Inflammatory cell infiltration is usually absent or mild. Scattered lymphoid follicles with/without germinal center may be present, but are inconspicuous.[37] When remarkable, CVD manifesting in the lung should be considered.[33,143] (*Figure 18-31*).

Current or recent exsmoker sometimes demonstrates complex histology in the cases with UIP.[144-148] Some may show the accumulation of macrophages within the alveolar spaces identical to DIP. Recognition of background UIP fibrosis is critical to distinguish DIP-like reaction from true DIP.[149] Other complex issue in this context is a coexistence of emphysema. The term "combined pulmonary fibrosis and emphysema (CPFE)" has been proposed as a possible new disease entity by Cottin et al.[117] Patients with CPFE have a significant increased risk of developing pulmonary hypertension and lung cancer.[150,151] Currently, it is not clear if CPFE represents a distinct clinical phenotype or a simply overlap of two different conditions, emphysema and interstitial pneumonia.[148]

Other histological patterns may coexist with UIP in the variable proportion, in which most common counterpart is NSIP (*Figures 18-32* and *18-33*). The term "discordant UIP" can be used for such occasions. Discordant UIP is clinically considered as a type of UIP due to the similar prognostic course with IPF; however, current IPF guidelines may classify such case into unclassifiable IIP due to mixture of multiple pathologic patterns.[152,153] Some of discordant UIP may end up to connective tissue disease (CTD) manifesting in the lung with careful clinical examination or develop CTD with months to years of follow-up.

There are some minor pathologies frequently seen in UIP cases with uncertain biological meaning. They include metaplastic bone, Kuhn hyaline in type II

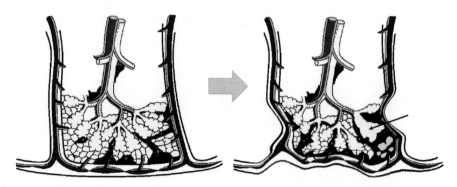

FIGURE 18-28 Usual interstitial pneumonia. Schematic view of disease progression. Fibrosis starts from margins of the pulmonary lobule and perivenular area (left). The progress of the fibrosis cause traction bronchiolectasia (arrow) and microscopic honeycombing (blue-colored zone) which often associate with mucous filling (right lower corner). The perivenular fibrosis may divide lung lobule into smaller units.

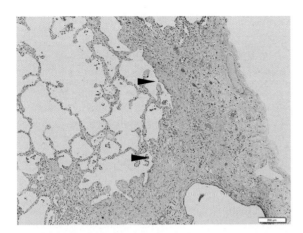

FIGURE 18-29 Usual interstitial pneumonia. Fibroblastic focus (arrowheads) is seen at the transition area from dense fibrosis to normal lung.

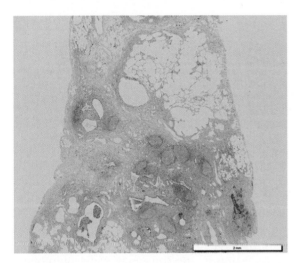

FIGURE 18-30 Usual interstitial pneumonia in patient with rheumatoid arthritis. The conspicuous lymphoid follicles with large germinal center present on the patchy fibrosis of UIP pattern.

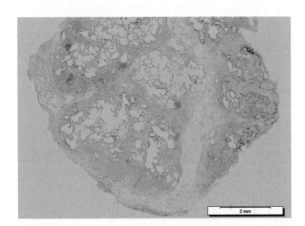

FIGURE 18-31 Difficult case of combined pulmonary fibrosis and emphysema. Part of the fibrosis shows characteristic changes of usual interstitial pneumonia although significant level of emphysema is also evident.

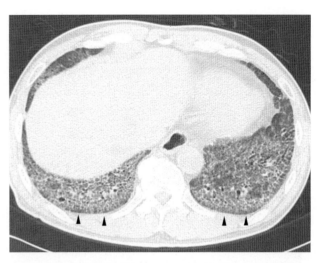

FIGURE 18-32 HRCT image of NSIP. The lower lung zone demonstrates the diffuse ground glass opacities with fine reticular shadow. The subpleural sparing is seen beneath the pleura (arrowheads).

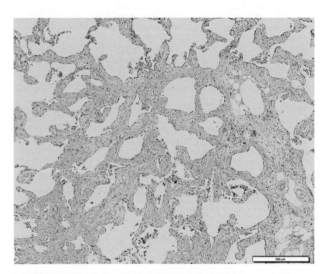

FIGURE 18-33 Fibrosing NSIP pattern. Diffuse temporally uniform fibrosis. Cellular infiltration is inconspicuous.

pneumocytes, smooth muscle hyperplasia, and subpleural fat metaplasia.[138]

IPF guidelines

The 2011 evidence-based IPF guidelines introduced the concept to describe levels of confidence for a diagnosis of UIP: definite, probable, possible, and not UIP (*Table 18-2*). Some cases do not fit well into this categorization, but it works well for the majority of cases. For the clinical trial, these guidelines should be taken into considerations to unify the diagnostic criteria.[37]

Most important criteria among them are four criteria of the UIP pattern: (1) marked fibrosis or architectural distortion with or without honeycombing in a predominantly subpleural or paraseptal distribution; (2) patchy involvement of lung parenchyma by fibrosis;

Table 18-2 Histopathological Criteria for UIP Pattern

UIP Pattern (All Four Criteria)	Probable UIP Pattern	Possible UIP Pattern (All Three Criteria)	Not UIP Pattern (Any of the Six Criteria)
• Evidence of marked fibrosis/ architectural distortion, ± honeycombing in a predominantly subpleural/ paraseptal distribution • Presence of patchy involvement of lung parenchyma by fibrosis • Presence of fibroblast foci • Absence of features against a diagnosis of UIP suggesting an alternate diagnosis (see fourth column)	• Evidence of marked fibrosis / architectural distortion, ± honeycombing • Absence of either patchy involvement or fibroblastic foci, but not both • Absence of features against a diagnosis of UIP suggesting an alternate diagnosis (see fourth column) OR • Honeycomb changes only[c]	• Patchy or diffuse involvement of lung parenchyma by fibrosis, with or without interstitial inflammation • Absence of other criteria for UIP (see the UIP Pattern column) • Absence of features against a diagnosis of UIP suggesting an alternate diagnosis (see the fourth column)	• Hyaline membranes[a] • Organizing pneumonia[a,b] • Granulomas[b] • Marked interstitial inflammatory cell infiltrate away from honeycombing • Predominant airway-centered changes • Other features suggestive of an alternate diagnosis

HRCT, high-resolution computed tomography; UIP, usual interstitial pneumonia.
[a]Can be associated with acute exacerbation of idiopathic pulmonary fibrosis.
[b]An isolated or occasional granuloma and/or a mild component of organizing pneumonia pattern may rarely be coexisting in lung biopsies with an otherwise UIP pattern.
[c]This scenario usually represents end-stage fibrotic lung disease where honeycombed segments have been sampled but where a UIP pattern might be present in other areas. Such areas are usually represented by overt honeycombing on HRCT and can be avoided by preoperative targeting of biopsy sites away from these areas using HRCT.

(3) presence of fibroblast foci; and (4) absence of features against a diagnosis of UIP suggesting an alternate diagnosis. When these four criteria are fulfilled, then pathology diagnosis becomes UIP. When the case is missing one of subpleural/paraseptal distribution, patchy involvement, or fibroblastic foci but also missing enough features to suggest alternative diagnosis, then the diagnosis becomes probable UIP. When fibrosis is the only finding, the diagnosis of possible UIP would be applied. Criteria listed in the column of "not UIP" are findings suggesting other diagnosis. Whether other diagnosis can effectively include NSIP, CVD manifesting in the lung, or chronic HP is not certain. Considering the challenge of distinguishing those conditions, simple applying of the diagnosis of "not UIP" to the case that fulfills UIP criteria otherwise is not a recommendation. Multidisciplinary discussion is strongly recommended for final diagnosis. Rarely, final diagnosis of these cases may end up to IPF eventually.

Acute exacerbation of UIP

The classic findings of acute exacerbation of UIP are acute and/or organizing diffuse alveolar damage (DAD) superimposed on the background chronic fibrosis suggestive of UIP.[134,154] Rarely, organizing pneumonia can be the major histology.[155] Any of the following findings are found: hyaline membrane, fibrinous exudate, extensive organizing pneumonia, or fibrin thrombi; possibility of acute exacerbation should be mentioned to the clinician immediately. Since the clinical course of acute exacerbation of UIP is rapid and highly lethal, the patient is better observed carefully or treated by intense corticosteroid and immune suppression therapy.[133,156,157] The extent of acute pathology may vary that is probably depending on the sampling site.

UIP pattern in collagen vascular disease

CVD manifesting in the lung may show pulmonary fibrosis highly simulating UIP pattern.[31,158] Generally, UIP pattern seen in CTD patients have fewer and smaller fibroblastic focus, more lymphoid follicles, more plasma cell infiltrations, extensive pleuritis, more vascular changes, or mixture of NSIP pathology.[33,127,143,159] When cases come with little clinical information, mentioning possibility of CVD in addition to UIP diagnosis is the recommendation. Applying UIP pattern diagnosis to the case with clear underline CVD is controversial.[160] Mentioning presence of UIP pattern may be beneficial to the pulmonologists for their therapeutic choice.

UIP pattern in chronic HP

Chronic HP may show histological features indistinguishable from UIP.[15] When causative antigen is not identified, cases showing UIP pattern and indicative pathologies for HP such as a few poorly formed granulomas or slight bronchiolocentrisity may better be diagnosed as UIP pattern along with note that the case shows suggestive features of HP in the diagnostic line. In that case, intense clinical radiological and pathological discussion is required for consensus diagnosis.[21]

Nonspecific Interstitial Pneumonia

Pathogenesis of nonspecific interstitial pneumonia

Cases with histological and radiological NSIP pattern represent heterogeneous group of disorders. Several potential pathogenesis has been reported in NSIP.[161] Idiopathic nonspecific interstitial pneumonia (NSIP) is currently defined as a specific form of chronic interstitial pneumonia of unknown etiology.

Collagen Vascular Disease

NSIP has been identified as the most common histological pattern found in patients with collagen vascular disease (CVD).[126,162] Some of the patients with NSIP develop CVDs during their follow-up.[163] It may be extremely challenging or impossible to distinguish idiopathic NSIP and interstitial pneumonia associated with CVD.[164,165] The patients with idiopathic NSIP often have positive serologic tests for collagen vascular disease. Rheumatologic studies have estimated that up to 25% of patients with features of a systemic autoimmune disease do not fulfill the criteria for CVD. There have been some conceptual proposals for such cases which include undifferentiated connective tissue disease (UCTD) and lung dominant connective tissue disease (LD-CTD). Kinder et al reported that 88% of patient classified as idiopathic NSIP met the criteria for UCTD.[25,127,166]

Organic Dust Exposure

A majority of cases with hypersensitivity pneumonia (HP) reveal NSIP pattern in which some cases lack characteristic features of HP and present indistinguishable pathology from idiopathic NSIP.[167]

Cigarette Smoking

Whether smoking tobacco really induces NSIP or not is under debate. There is one report of retrospective study based on HRCT in patients with desquamative interstitial pneumonia (DIP) suggestive of fibrotic NSIP rather than DIP. This has led to the hypothesis that a subgroup of cigarette smokers may develop a pattern of fibrotic NSIP.[168]

Clinical features of nonspecific interstitial pneumonia

The idiopathic nonspecific interstitial pneumonia (NSIP) is a second common idiopathic interstitial pneumonia (IIP) accounts for 4% to 36% of IIPs.[157] The mean age of patients at onset of NSIP is fifth to sixth decade and younger than patients with IPF. NSIP patients are more commonly female and never smokers than IPF. Onset is usually gradual; however, a minority of patients may show subacute presentation. Breathlessness,

cough, fatigue, and a history of weight loss are usual symptoms. Crackles are characteristic on chest auscultation and are initially predominantly basal but may be widespread. The NSIP patients often had positive serology for collagen vascular disease (CVD) such as antinuclear antibody, rheumatoid factor, anti-CCP antibody, anti-SS-A antibody, anti-SS-B antibody, and anti-ARS antibody. Careful attention should be paid to identify background CVD.[161,169-172] Pulmonary function testing demonstrates a restrictive ventilatory defect and a decrease DL_{co} and/or desaturation during exertion. Several reports described that the bronchoalveolar lavage (BAL) shows a higher percentage of lymphocytes in patients with NSIP compared to IPF.[173,174] Similar to patients with IPF, patients with NSIP may develop acute deterioration with an abrupt worsening of symptoms without identifiable cause. These episodes are considered as acute exacerbation of NSIP.[155] The prognosis of NSIP is favorable compared to IPF being 5 years' survival up to 80%.[161] Several studies indicate that patients with cellular NSIP have a more favorable survival than those with fibrosing NSIP.[138]

Imaging features of nonspecific interstitial pneumonia

The HRCT manifestations of NSIP consist of reticular opacities with lower lung zone predominance, associated with traction bronchiectasis and lobar volume loss. The distribution is predominantly diffuse or subpleural.[161] Although the abnormality shows peripheral predominance, different from IPF, the relative subpleural sparing of the immediate subpleural zone is characteristic.[28] Ground glass opacities (GGO) are seen in 44% to 100% of the NSIP, mostly with symmetrical appearance.[28,40,161,175] Honeycombing is usually not seen in NSIP but when present, it tends to be mild, involving less than 10% of the parenchyma.[40,161]

Histologic features of nonspecific interstitial pneumonia

The histologic features of NSIP are varying amounts of diffuse interstitial inflammation and fibrosis with a uniform appearance (*Figures 18-34A, B* and *18-35*). The NSIP is histologically subdivided into cellular, cellular and fibrosing, and fibrosing NSIP, according to the amount of cellularity and fibrosis.[25] Among them, most frequent form is a cellular and fibrotic NSIP.

Cellular NSIP demonstrates a mild to moderate interstitial chronic inflammation, containing lymphocytes and plasma cells. Fibrosis may be present to a minimum degree. Pure fibrosing NSIP is relatively rare which consist of interstitial uniform and dense fibrosis of the temporal homogeneity usually preserving the basis of alveolar architecture. Fibroblastic focus is absent or inconspicuous. Honeycomb changes are rare, but areas

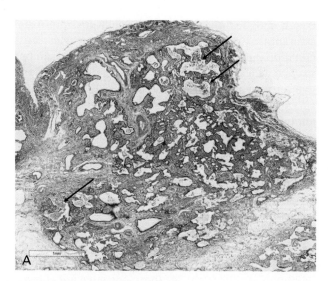
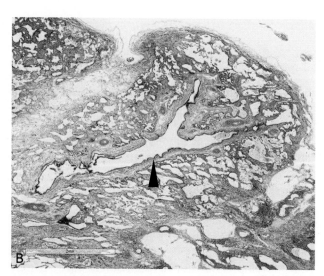

FIGURE 18-34 Fibrosing NSIP. A: The areas of interstitial fibrosis may associate enlarged airspaces simulating honeycomb cysts (arrows). B: Traction bronchiolectasia (arrowhead) is a common finding in fibrosing NSIP.

of interstitial fibrosis with enlarged airspaces are common. These enlarged spaces should be distinguished from honeycomb change, but their clear distinction is difficult for some occasion. These enlarged airspaces were more common in fibrosing NSIP than in cellular NSIP.[161]

Mixture of foci with organizing pneumonia (OP) is fairly frequent in cellular NSIP. When it is obvious, distinction between OP and NSIP may be challenging. Referring HRCT for such case is helpful for such occasion.

Differential diagnosis

Idiopathic Pulmonary Fibrosis
Distinction of NSIP from IPF is the most important clinical implications because the patients' outcome and choice of therapy are different. (See differential diagnosis of UIP.)

Collagen Vascular Disease
The most frequent subtypes of interstitial pneumonia encountered in patients with CVD are NSIP pattern.[176] Various collagen vascular diseases can associate with interstitial pneumonia similar to NSIP. Such include systemic sclerosis, polymyositis/dermatomyositis,[177] Sjögren syndrome,[178] mixed connective tissue disease,[179] anti-aminoacyl-tRNA synthetase antibodies syndrome,[171] and

rheumatoid arthritis (RA).[31] Distinction between idiopathic NSIP and NSIP associated with CVD is extremely challenging and often impossible by pathology.[164,165] Careful clinical observation and follow-up are often required for definite diagnosis.

Hypersensitivity Pneumonia
Since NSIP does not have positive diagnostic findings, distinction between NSIP and hypersensitivity pneumonia (HP) often depends on exclusion of HP. Presence of occasional poorly formed nonnecrotizing granulomas in peribronchiolar interstitium, marked bronchiolocentric accentuation, and marked peribronchiolar metaplasia should suggest HP.[93] Clinical and radiological features are critical for the distinction.

Acute Interstitial Pneumonia

Clinical features of acute interstitial pneumonia

Acute interstitial pneumonia (AIP) is a rapidly progressive interstitial pneumonia of unknown cause with pathological pattern of diffuse alveolar damage (DAD). AIP occurs over a wide age range, with a mean in sixth decades, and

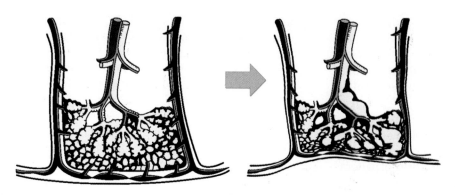

FIGURE 18-35 Nonspecific interstitial pneumonia. Schematic view of disease progression. Fibrosis starts diffusely inside whole lobule. Severity of the fibrosis may show variation inside the lobule (left). The progress of the fibrosis may cause shrinkage of the lung parenchyma resulting in traction bronchiolectasia simulating honeycombing (right).

the gender ratio is equal in most series. In most cases, it is difficult to distinguish between DAD patients with putative causes and AIP. Patients often have a prior illness suggestive of a viral upper respiratory infection with constitutional symptoms such as myalgias, arthralgias, fever, chills, and malaise. Pulmonary function tests show a restrictive disease with reduced diffusing capacity. The majority of patients has symptoms for less than 1 week before diagnosis, usually develops respiratory failure, and requires mechanical ventilation. The majority of patients fulfill the clinical criteria of ARDS. There is no established treatment, and the mortality rates are 50% or more. Most deaths occur between 1 and 2 months from the onset. Survivors of AIP may experience recurrences and develop chronic interstitial lung disease such as nonspecific interstitial pneumonia.[25] AIP needs to be distinguished from acute exacerbation of UIP, ARDS (DAD of known cause), infection, drug-induced pneumonitis, and acute eosinophilic pneumonia.[133]

Imaging features of acute interstitial pneumonia

The chest radiograph demonstrates bilateral airspace consolidation with air bronchograms in basically all patients. The distribution is usually patchy, with sparing of the costophrenic angles. Pleural effusions are uncommon. The lung volumes are usually decreased but can be normal.

The most common findings on HRCT are wide areas of ground glass opacities (GGO), traction bronchiectasis or bronchiolectasis, and architectural distortion[39] (*Figure 18-36*). The extent of the areas of GGO correlates with disease duration. Consolidation is seen in the majority of cases as well. Architectural distortion, traction bronchiolectasis, and bronchiectasis are related to poor prognosis.[39] The few patients who survive demonstrate gradual clearing of the GGO and consolidation.

Histologic features of acute interstitial pneumonia

The histological pattern of patients with AIP is the acute and/or organizing phases of diffuse alveolar

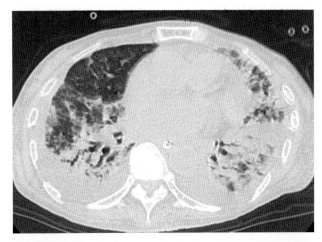

FIGURE 18-36 HRCT image of AIP. Lower lung zone shows bilateral diffuse consolidation with traction bronchiectasis.

damage (DAD) (*Figure 18-37*). The adjective "diffuse" may be confusing to general pathologists and is usually interpreted as synonymous to "widespread," and "diffuse alveolar" may be thus interpreted as all alveoli in the whole lung. However, current DAD indicates a specific type of histological reaction and may involve the lung focally.

Basically, DAD is time sequentially divided into three phases. The exudative phase of DAD is the first week following the onset of lung injury. The earliest changes of DAD may be difficult to be recognized by microscope. The type 1 pneumocytes and endothelial cells are injured, resulting in edema and exudation of plasma proteins into the alveolar spaces as a consequence of increased permeability of the alveolar-capillary barrier.[180] The type 1 pneumocytes fall into apoptosis and slough off the alveolar surface. The injury to type II cells reduces the production of surfactant, resulting in collapse of alveoli and dilatation of alveolar duct.[181] The early stage of exudative phase of DAD demonstrates interstitial and intra-alveolar edema with varying amounts of hemorrhage and fibrin exudation. Hyaline membrane is the histologic hallmark of the exudative phase and may be seen as early as 12 hours

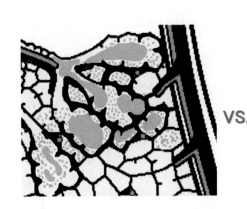
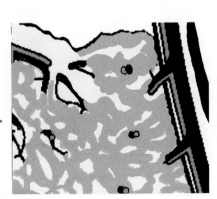

VS.

FIGURE 18-37 Acute interstitial pneumonia. Schematic view of the early exudative phase. Left image shows normal lung architecture. Right image shows initial collapse of alveolar sac and presence of inconspicuous hyaline membrane (pink colored).

following injury, but is most numerous after 3 to 5 days. The hyaline membranes are homogeneous and amorphous eosinophilic substances that are attached along the alveolar septa.[182] The infiltration of inflammatory cells such as lymphocytes, plasma cells, and macrophages is most prominent after 1 week. Fibrin thrombi are sometimes present in the pulmonary arteries. They are thought to be the result of secondary to endothelial damage. Alveolar epithelial hyperplasia develops approximately 3 to 7 days following lung injury, and is characterized by proliferation along with the alveolar septa in a hobnail fashion. Considerable atypia may be seen with nuclear enlargement, large eosinophilic nucleoli, and cellular pleomorphism. The cytoplasmic hyaline inclusions known as Kuhn hyaline, which are similar to Mallory body in liver cells, are occasionally found.[22] Detachment of the type II pneumocytes is frequent along with basal cell hyperplasia and squamous metaplasia mainly observed around the respiratory bronchioles. The organizing phase of DAD begins after 1 week of the lung injury.

Various kinds of infection, drug, and connective tissue diseases can cause DAD. Histological distinction may be difficult unless there are findings strongly suggesting each one of them. Viral inclusion, granuloma, necrosis, and abscess are strong indicator of infection. DAD from drug or connective tissue disease is mostly impossible to distinguish from AIP.

Acute Exacerbation of Chronic Interstitial Pneumonia

Acute exacerbation with background chronic interstitial pneumonia can occur at any course of the disease and can be present as an initial symptom of subclinical chronic interstitial pneumonia.[183] The key histological feature to differentiate from AIP is the existence of chronic fibrosis. The background chronic fibrosis is sometimes obscure. Elastica van Gieson, Azan, or Masson trichrome stains are helpful to identify the inconspicuous chronic fibrosis.

Cryptogenic Organizing Pneumonia

Clinical features of cryptogenic organizing pneumonia

The term organizing pneumonia (OP) indicates a histologic wound healing process from various causes, such as infection, collagen vascular disease manifesting in the lung, inflammatory bowel disease, inhalational injury, hypersensitivity pneumonitis, drug toxicity, radiation therapy and aspiration.[126] Among them, cryptogenic organizing pneumonia (COP) is a specific clinicopathological form of OP without underline etiology. The onset of COP is typically subacute. There is a similar proportion in males and females with presentation

occurring in the fifth to seventh decades.[184-186] The primary symptom includes the variable degrees of cough and dyspnea, but often begins with ones similar to upper respiratory infection, such as fever, chills, and malaise. Therefore, the COP patient often has history of receiving at least one or several courses of antibiotics. A markedly raised erythrocyte sedimentation rate (ESR), elevated C-reactive protein, and peripheral blood neutrophilia are common findings.[22] Pulmonary function tests demonstrate a restrictive disease with a moderately reduced carbon monoxide transfer factor. Bronchoalveolar lavage fluid contains increases in the total number and proportion of lymphocytes.[22] The COP patients have good prognosis with 5 years' survival of more than 80%.[187] The majority of patients recover completely with oral corticosteroids, but relapse is common. Prolonged treatment for 6 months or longer is recommended.

OP is a common histologic pattern seen in association with various conditions. A multidisciplinary discussion (MDD) is particularly important in distinguishing COP from OP related to other cause.[21,22]

Imaging features of cryptogenic organizing pneumonia

The characteristic HRCT findings of OP consist of patchy and often migratory consolidation in a subpleural, peribronchial, or band-like pattern, commonly associated with ground glass opacity (GGO) (*Figure 18-38*). Perilobular opacities and reversed halo sign may be helpful for the diagnosis. The lower lung zones are more frequently involved. Air bronchograms may be seen when consolidation is present.[22]

Areas of airspace consolidation are present on HRCT in most of patients with COP. Approximately 15% of patients with COP present with multiple nodules.[22] The

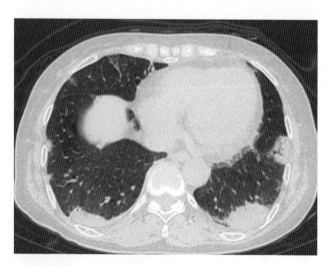

FIGURE 18-38 HRCT image of COP. The bilateral patchy consolidations are characteristic features of COP.

areas of consolidation reflect the presence of dense organizing pneumonia and filling of the alveolar duct with intraluminal plugs of granulation tissue. Mild cylindrical bronchial dilatation is commonly evident in areas of consolidation. Pleural effusions are rare.

Although the majority of patients with COP demonstrate radiographic improvement with treatment, some patients with COP show remaining disease seen on follow-up CT, and, in such cases, the lesions generally resemble a fibrotic nonspecific interstitial pneumonia pattern.[184]

Histologic features of cryptogenic organizing pneumonia

The generic term "organizing pneumonia (OP)" indicates large variations of healing process from various injuries, and can cause confusion with OP of interstitial lung disease. When OP is considered in the context of diffuse lung disease, it often indicates a patchy process characterized primarily by airspace organization involving peripheral areas of the lobules. Prototypical feature of OP is a presence of intraluminal plugs of granulation tissue (intraluminal polyps, so-called "Mason body") within alveolar ducts and surrounding alveoli. The granulation tissue is composed of fibroblasts and myofibroblasts embedded in a myxoid extracellular matrix and contains small numbers of capillaries and various amounts of inflammatory cells such as lymphocytes, macrophages, and plasma cells. The granulation tissue may be covered by reactive type II cells. Air space fibrin may be seen focally but inconspicuous.

Although transbronchial biopsy is often not useful in the diagnosis of interstitial lung diseases, it may be applicable for OP diagnosis with adequate clinical and radiological settings. Importantly, the primary role of transbronchial biopsies for such occasion is still to exclude sarcoidosis and certain infections.[22] Since OP is one of the interstitial pneumonia patterns for various etiologies, diagnosis of COP can be compelled only after the careful clinical-radiological-pathological discussion.

Differential diagnosis

Probably, most frequent and critical mistake of OP diagnosis is for fibroblastic foci of other chronic progressive disease, especially UIP. These intraluminal plugs of OP must be distinguished from a fibroblastic focus, which should be interstitial based and gradually continue to the dense chronic fibrosis. In contrast to UIP, the process of OP is temporally homogenous, and dense fibrotic scaring or honeycomb change should not be seen in the cases of OP.[22]

Another frequent mistake of OP diagnosis is for organizing DAD. Importantly, most OP cases provide patchy appearance by low magnification. If the organization diffusely involves the entire biopsy, organizing diffuse alveolar damage should be considered. The distinction between OP and organizing DAD may be extremely challenging by histology alone.

When air space fibrin is confluent, acute fibrinous and organizing pneumonia should be considered.[188] In such cases, the careful exclusion of infectious lung disease such as *Pneumocystis jirovecii* or collagen vascular disease such as granulomatosis with polyangiitis (GPA) is important.

Nonspecific interstitial pneumonia (NSIP) can associate focal OP in up to two-thirds of cases, but area of OP is considerably less than 20% of the overall biopsy specimen, and differentiation from OP is often not difficult. Occasionally, there are cases showing features of both OP and NSIP as a major histology. Such cases are often with subacute onset and frequently associated with myositis or related conditions.

REFERENCES

1. Babiak A, Hetzel J, Krishna G, et al. Transbronchial cryobiopsy: a new tool for lung biopsies. *Respiration.* 2009;78:203-208.
2. Lacasse Y, Selman M, Costabel U, et al. Clinical diagnosis of hypersensitivity pneumonitis. *Am J Respir Crit Care Med.* October 15, 2003;168(8):952-958.
3. Selman M, Pardo A, King TE Jr. Hypersensitivity pneumonitis: insights in diagnosis and pathobiology. *Am J Respir Crit Care Med.* August 15, 2012;186(4):314-324.
4. Hariri LP, Mino-Kenudson M, Shea B, et al. Distinct histopathology of acute onset or abrupt exacerbation of hypersensitivity pneumonitis. *Hum Pathol.* May 2012;43(5):660-668.
5. Sahin H, Brown KK, Curran-Everett D, et al. Chronic hypersensitivity pneumonitis: CT features comparison with pathologic evidence of fibrosis and survival. *Radiology.* August 2007;244(2):591-598.
6. Inase N, Sakashita H, Ohtani Y, et al. Chronic bird fancier's lung presenting with acute exacerbation due to use of a feather duvet. *Intern Med.* September 2004;43(9):835-837.
7. Olson AL, Huie TJ, Groshong SD, et al. Acute exacerbations of fibrotic hypersensitivity pneumonitis: a case series. *Chest.* October 2008;134(4):844-850.
8. Miyazaki Y, Tateishi T, Akashi T, Ohtani Y, Inase N, Yoshizawa Y. Clinical predictors and histologic appearance of acute exacerbations in chronic hypersensitivity pneumonitis. *Chest.* December 2008;134(6):1265-1270.
9. Myers JL. Hypersensitivity pneumonia: the role of lung biopsy in diagnosis and management. *Mod Pathol.* January 2012;25(suppl 1):S58-S67.
10. Tateishi T, Ohtani Y, Takemura T, et al. Serial high-resolution computed tomography findings of acute and chronic hypersensitivity pneumonitis induced by avian antigen. *J Comput Assist Tomogr.* March-April 2011;35(2):272-279.
11. Silva CI, Churg A, Muller NL. Hypersensitivity pneumonitis: spectrum of high-resolution CT and pathologic findings. *AJR Am J Roentgenol.* February 2007;188(2):334-344.
12. Khoor A, Leslie KO, Tazelaar HD, Helmers RA, Colby TV. Diffuse pulmonary disease caused by nontuberculous mycobacteria in immunocompetent people (hot tub lung). *Am J Clin Pathol.* May 2001;115(5):755-762.

13. Lima MS, Coletta EN, Ferreira RG, et al. Subacute and chronic hypersensitivity pneumonitis: histopathological patterns and survival. *Respir Med.* April 2009;103(4):508-515.

14. Akashi T, Takemura T, Ando N, et al. Histopathologic analysis of sixteen autopsy cases of chronic hypersensitivity pneumonitis and comparison with idiopathic pulmonary fibrosis/usual interstitial pneumonia. *Am J Clin Pathol.* March 2009;131(3):405-415.

15. Trahan S, Hanak V, Ryu JH, Myers JL. Role of surgical lung biopsy in separating chronic hypersensitivity pneumonia from usual interstitial pneumonia/idiopathic pulmonary fibrosis: analysis of 31 biopsies from 15 patients. *Chest.* July 2008;134(1):126-132.

16. Churg A, Sin DD, Everett D, Brown K, Cool C. Pathologic patterns and survival in chronic hypersensitivity pneumonitis. *Am J Surg Pathol.* December 2009;33(12):1765-1770.

17. Churg A, Myers J, Suarez T, et al. Airway-centered interstitial fibrosis: a distinct form of aggressive diffuse lung disease. *Am J Surg Pathol.* January 2004;28(1):62-68.

18. Fenton ME, Cockcroft DW, Wright JL, Churg A. Hypersensitivity pneumonitis as a cause of airway-centered interstitial fibrosis. *Ann Allergy Asthma Immunol.* November 2007;99(5):465-466.

19. Frankel SK, Cool CD, Lynch DA, Brown KK. Idiopathic pleuroparenchymal fibroelastosis: description of a novel clinicopathologic entity. *Chest.* December 2004;126(6):2007-2013.

20. Force ADT, Ranieri VM, Rubenfeld GD, et al. Acute respiratory distress syndrome: the Berlin Definition. *JAMA.* June 20 2012;307(23):2526-2533.

21. Travis WD, Costabel U, Hansell DM, et al. An official American Thoracic Society/European Respiratory Society statement: Update of the international multidisciplinary classification of the idiopathic interstitial pneumonias. *Am J Respir Crit Care Med.* September 15, 2013;188(6):733-748.

22. American Thoracic Society, European Respiratory Society. American Thoracic Society/European Respiratory Society International Multidisciplinary Consensus Classification of the Idiopathic Interstitial Pneumonias. This joint statement of the American Thoracic Society (ATS), and the European Respiratory Society (ERS) was adopted by the ATS board of directors, June 2001 and by the ERS Executive Committee, June 2001. *Am J Respir Crit Care Med.* January 15, 2002;165(2):277-304.

23. Akira M. Computed tomography and pathologic findings in fulminant forms of idiopathic interstitial pneumonia. *J Thorac Imaging.* April 1999;14(2):76-84.

24. Johkoh T, Muller NL, Taniguchi H, et al. Acute interstitial pneumonia: thin-section CT findings in 36 patients. *Radiology.* June 1999;211(3):859-863.

25. Katzenstein AL, Fiorelli RF. Nonspecific interstitial pneumonia/fibrosis. Histologic features and clinical significance. *Am J Surg Pathol.* February 1994;18(2):136-147.

26. Heppleston AG. The pathology of honeycomb lung. *Thorax.* June 1956;11(2):77-93.

27. Arakawa H, Honma K. Honeycomb lung: history and current concepts. *AJR Am J Roentgenol.* April 2011;196(4):773-782.

28. Silva CI, Muller NL, Hansell DM, Lee KS, Nicholson AG, Wells AU. Nonspecific interstitial pneumonia and idiopathic pulmonary fibrosis: changes in pattern and distribution of disease over time. *Radiology.* April 2008;247(1):251-259.

29. Kawabata Y, Takemura T, Hebisawa A, et al. Desquamative interstitial pneumonia may progress to lung fibrosis as characterized radiologically. *Respirology.* November 2012;17(8):1214-1221.

30. Ito I, Nagai S, Kitaichi M, et al. Pulmonary manifestations of primary Sjogren's syndrome: a clinical, radiologic, and pathologic study. *Am J Respir Crit Care Med.* March 15 2005;171(6):632-638.

31. Lee HK, Kim DS, Yoo B, et al. Histopathologic pattern and clinical features of rheumatoid arthritis-associated interstitial lung disease. *Chest.* June 2005;127(6):

32. Sumikawa H, Johkoh T, Colby TV, et al. Computed tomography findings in pathological 2019-2027.usual interstitial

33. Song JW, Do KH, Kim MY, Jang SJ, Colby TV, Kim DS. Pathologic and radiologic differences between idiopathic and collagen vascular disease-related usual interstitial pneumonia. *Chest.* July 2009;136(1):23-30.

34. Sumikawa H, Johkoh T, Ichikado K, et al. Nonspecific interstitial pneumonia: histologic correlation with high-resolution CT in 29 patients. *Eur J Radiol.* April 2009;70(1):35-40.

35. Sumikawa H, Johkoh T, Ichikado K, et al. Usual interstitial pneumonia and chronic idiopathic interstitial pneumonia: analysis of CT appearance in 92 patients. *Radiology.* October 2006;241(1):258-266.

36. Hansell DM, Bankier AA, MacMahon H, McLoud TC, Muller NL, Remy J. Fleischner Society: glossary of terms for thoracic imaging. *Radiology.* March 2008;246(3):697-722.

37. Raghu G, Collard HR, Egan JJ, et al. An official ATS/ERS/JRS/ALAT statement: idiopathic pulmonary fibrosis: evidence-based guidelines for diagnosis and management. *Am J Respir Crit Care Med.* March 15, 2011;183(6):788-824.

38. Kim MY, Song JW, Do KH, Jang SJ, Colby TV, Kim DS. Idiopathic nonspecific interstitial pneumonia: changes in high-resolution computed tomography on long-term follow-up. *J Comput Assist Tomogr.* March-April 2012;36(2):170-174.

39. Ichikado K, Suga M, Muller NL, et al. Acute interstitial pneumonia: comparison of high-resolution computed tomography findings between survivors and nonsurvivors. *Am J Respir Crit Care Med.* June 1, 2002;165(11):1551-1556.

40. Johkoh T, Muller NL, Colby TV, et al. Nonspecific interstitial pneumonia: correlation between thin-section CT findings and pathologic subgroups in 55 patients. *Radiology.* October 2002;225(1):199-204.

41. Watadani T, Sakai F, Johkoh T, et al. Interobserver variability in the CT assessment of honeycombing in the lungs. *Radiology.* March 2013;266(3):936-944.

42. Johkoh T, Sakai F, Noma S, et al. Honeycombing on CT; its definition, pathologic correlation, and future direction of its diagnosis. *Eur J Radiol.* January 2014;83(1):27-31.

43. Myers JL, Katzenstein AL. Epithelial necrosis and alveolar collapse in the pathogenesis of usual interstitial pneumonia. *Chest.* December 1988;94(6):1309-1311.

44. Honda T, Ota H, Arai K, et al. Three-dimensional analysis of alveolar structure in usual interstitial pneumonia. *Virchows Arch.* July 2002;441(1):47-52.

45. Sterlacci W, Veits L, Moser P, et al. Idiopathic systemic amyloidosis primarily affecting the lungs with fatal pulmonary haemorrhage due to vascular involvement. *Pathol Oncol Res.* March 2009;15(1):133-136.

46. Blancas-Mejia LM, Ramirez-Alvarado M. Systemic amyloidoses. *Annu Rev Biochem.* 2013;82:745-774.

47. Ohdama S, Akagawa S, Matsubara O, Yoshizawa Y. Primary diffuse alveolar septal amyloidosis with multiple cysts and calcification. *Eur Respir J.* July 1996;9(7):1569-1571.

48. Ogoshi T, Kawanami T, Yatera K, Mukae H. Dialysis-related amyloidosis with diffuse parenchymal lung involvement. *Intern Med.* 2012;51(23):3303-3304.

49. Utz JP, Swensen SJ, Gertz MA. Pulmonary amyloidosis. The Mayo Clinic experience from 1980 to 1993. *Ann Intern Med.* February 15, 1996;124(4):407-413.

50. Graham CM, Stern EJ, Finkbeiner WE, Webb WR. High-resolution CT appearance of diffuse alveolar septal amyloidosis. *AJR Am J Roentgenol.* February 1992;158(2):265-267.

51. Hui AN, Koss MN, Hochholzer L, Wehunt WD. Amyloidosis presenting in the lower respiratory tract. Clinicopathologic, radiologic, immunohistochemical, and histochemical studies on 48 cases. *Arch Pathol Lab Med.* March 1986;110(3):212-218.

52. Gillmore JD, Hawkins PN. Amyloidosis and the respiratory tract. *Thorax.* May 1999;54(5):444-451.

pneumonia: relationship to survival. *Am J Respir Crit Care Med.* February 15, 2008;177(4):433-439.

53. Khoor A, Myers JL, Tazelaar HD, Kurtin PJ. Amyloid-like pulmonary nodules, including localized light-chain deposition: clinicopathologic analysis of three cases. *Am J Clin Pathol*. February 2004;121(2):200-204.

54. Swigris JJ, Berry GJ, Raffin TA, Kuschner WG. Lymphoid interstitial pneumonia: a narrative review. *Chest*. December 2002;122(6):2150-2164.

55. Nielsen K, McSherry G, Petru A, et al. A descriptive survey of pediatric human immunodeficiency virus-infected long-term survivors. *Pediatrics*. April 1997;99(4):E4.

56. Joo EJ, Ha YE, Jung DS, et al. An adult case of chronic active Epstein-Barr virus infection with interstitial pneumonitis. *Korean J Intern Med*. December 2011;26(4):466-469.

57. Zar HJ. Chronic lung disease in human immunodeficiency virus (HIV) infected children. *Pediatr Pulmonol*. January 2008;43(1):1-10.

58. Simmank K, Meyers T, Galpin J, Cumin E, Kaplan A. Clinical features and T-cell subsets in HIV-infected children with and without lymphocytic interstitial pneumonitis. *Ann Trop Paediatr*. September 2001;21(3):195-201.

59. Pereyra F, Rubin RH. Prevention and treatment of cytomegalovirus infection in solid organ transplant recipients. *Curr Opin Infect Dis*. August 2004;17(4):357-361.

60. de la Hoz RE, Stephens G, Sherlock C. Diagnosis and treatment approaches of CMV infections in adult patients. *J Clin Virol*. August 2002;25(suppl 2):S1-S12.

61. Hayner CE, Baughman RP, Linnemann CC Jr, Dohn MN. The relationship between cytomegalovirus retrieved by bronchoalveolar lavage and mortality in patients with HIV. *Chest*. March 1995;107(3):735-740.

62. Cook LB, Elemans M, Rowan AG, Asquith B. HTLV-1: persistence and pathogenesis. *Virology*. January 5, 2013;435(1):131-140.

63. Fukuoka J, Tominaga M, Ichikado K, et al. Lung miliary micronodules in human T-cell leukemia virus type I carriers. *Pathol Int*. February 2013;63(2):108-112.

64. Ishii H, Kawabata Y, Amemiya Y, Ogata M, Kadota J. Multiple tiny granulomatous lesions with eosinophils in a patient with smoldering-type adult T-cell leukaemia: the possibility of a new type of bronchioloalveolopathy. *Respirology*. January 2010;15(1):182-184.

65. Einsiedel L, Fernandes L, Spelman T, Steinfort D, Gotuzzo E. Bronchiectasis is associated with human T-lymphotropic virus 1 infection in an Indigenous Australian population. *Clin Infect Dis*. January 1, 2012;54(1):43-50.

66. Matsuno O, Watanabe K, Kataoka H, Miyazaki E, Kumamoto T. A case of diffuse panbronchiolitis (DPB) in a patient positive for HTLV-1. *Scand J Infect Dis*. 2004;36(9):687-689.

67. Mori S, Mizoguchi A, Kawabata M, et al. Bronchoalveolar lymphocytosis correlates with human T lymphotropic virus type I (HTLV-I) proviral DNA load in HTLV-I carriers. *Thorax*. February 2005;60(2):138-143.

68. Bando M, Ohno S, Oshikawa K, Takahashi M, Okamoto H, Sugiyama Y. Infection of TT virus in patients with idiopathic pulmonary fibrosis. *Respir Med*. December 2001;95(12):935-942.

69. Lasithiotaki I, Antoniou KM, Vlahava VM, et al. Detection of herpes simplex virus type-1 in patients with fibrotic lung diseases. *PLoS One*. 2011;6(12):e27800.

70. Franks TJ, Chong PY, Chui P, et al. Lung pathology of severe acute respiratory syndrome (SARS): a study of 8 autopsy cases from Singapore. *Hum Pathol*. August 2003;34(8):743-748.

71. Ferrand RA, Desai SR, Hopkins C, et al. Chronic lung disease in adolescents with delayed diagnosis of vertically acquired HIV infection. *Clin Infect Dis*. July 2012;55(1):145-152.

72. Franquet T, Lee KS, Muller NL. Thin-section CT findings in 32 immunocompromised patients with cytomegalovirus pneumonia who do not have AIDS. *AJR Am J Roentgenol*. October 2003;181(4):1059-1063.

73. Okada F, Ando Y, Yoshitake S, et al. Pulmonary CT findings in 320 carriers of human T-lymphotropic virus type 1. *Radiology*. August 2006;240(2):559-564.

74. Scott GB, Hutto C, Makuch RW, et al. Survival in children with perinatally acquired human immunodeficiency virus type 1 infection. *N Engl J Med*. December 28, 1989;321(26):1791-1796.

75. Koga M, Umemoto Y, Nishikawa M, Nakashima K, Ishihara T, Furukawa S. A case of lymphoid interstitial pneumonia in a 3-month-old boy not associated with HIV infection: immunohistochemistry of lung biopsy specimens and serum transforming growth factor-beta 1 assay. *Pathol Int*. October 1997;47(10):698-702.

76. Kotton CN, Kumar D, Caliendo AM, et al. International consensus guidelines on the management of cytomegalovirus in solid organ transplantation. *Transplantation*. April 15, 2010;89(7):779-795.

77. Andrade ZR, Garippo AL, Saldiva PH, Capelozzi VL. Immunohistochemical and in situ detection of cytomegalovirus in lung autopsies of children immunocompromised by secondary interstitial pneumonia. *Pathol Res Pract*. 2004;200(1):25-32.

78. Couderc LJ, Rain B, Desgranges C. Pulmonary fibrosis in association with human T cell lymphotropic virus type 1 (HTLV-1) infection. *Respir Med*. October 2000;94(10):1010.

79. Matsuyama W, Kawabata M, Mizoguchi A, Iwami F, Wakimoto J, Osame M. Influence of human T lymphotrophic virus type I on cryptogenic fibrosing alveolitis - HTLV-I associated fibrosing alveolitis: proposal of a new clinical entity. *Clin Exp Immunol*. September 2003;133(3):397-403.

80. Kern DG, Crausman RS, Durand KT, Nayer A, Kuhn C 3rd. Flock worker's lung: chronic interstitial lung disease in the nylon flocking industry. *Ann Intern Med*. August 15, 1998;129(4):261-272.

81. Washko RM, Day B, Parker JE, Castellan RM, Kreiss K. Epidemiologic investigation of respiratory morbidity at a nylon flock plant. *Am J Ind Med*. December 2000;38(6):628-638.

82. Eschenbacher WL, Kreiss K, Lougheed MD, Pransky GS, Day B, Castellan RM. Nylon flock-associated interstitial lung disease. *Am J Respir Crit Care Med*. June 1999;159(6):2003-2008.

83. Weiland DA, Lynch DA, Jensen SP, et al. Thin-section CT findings in flock worker's lung, a work-related interstitial lung disease. *Radiology*. April 2003;227(1):222-231.

84. Atis S, Tutluoglu B, Levent E, et al. The respiratory effects of occupational polypropylene flock exposure. *Eur Respir J*. January 2005;25(1):110-117.

85. Boag AH, Colby TV, Fraire AE, et al. The pathology of interstitial lung disease in nylon flock workers. *Am J Surg Pathol*. December 1999;23(12):1539-1545.

86. Kahana LM, Kay JM, Yakrus MA, Waserman S. Mycobacterium avium complex infection in an immunocompetent young adult related to hot tub exposure. *Chest*. January 1997;111(1):242-245.

87. Embil J, Warren P, Yakrus M, et al. Pulmonary illness associated with exposure to Mycobacterium-avium complex in hot tub water. Hypersensitivity pneumonitis or infection? *Chest*. March 1997;111(3):813-816.

88. Hanak V, Kalra S, Aksamit TR, Hartman TE, Tazelaar HD, Ryu JH. Hot tub lung: presenting features and clinical course of 21 patients. *Respir Med*. April 2006;100(4):610-615.

89. Hartman TE, Jensen E, Tazelaar HD, Hanak V, Ryu JH. CT findings of granulomatous pneumonitis secondary to Mycobacterium avium-intracellulare inhalation: "hot tub lung." *AJR Am J Roentgenol*. April 2007;188(4):1050-1053.

90. Mukhopadhyay S, Gal AA. Granulomatous lung disease: an approach to the differential diagnosis. *Arch Pathol Lab Med*. May 2010;134(5):667-690.

91. Yousem SA, Dacic S. Idiopathic bronchiolocentric interstitial pneumonia. *Mod Pathol*. November 2002;15(11):1148-1153.

92. de Carvalho ME, Kairalla RA, Capelozzi VL, Deheinzelin D, do Nascimento Saldiva PH, de Carvalho CR. Centrilobular fibrosis: a novel histological pattern of idiopathic interstitial pneumonia. *Pathol Res Pract*. 2002;198(9):577-583.

93. Fukuoka J, Franks TJ, Colby TV, et al. Peribronchiolar metaplasia: a common histologic lesion in diffuse lung disease and a rare cause of interstitial lung disease: clinicopathologic features of 15 cases. *Am J Surg Pathol*. July 2005;29(7):948-954.

94. Allen TC. Pathology of small airways disease. *Arch Pathol Lab Med*. May 2010;134(5):702-718.

95. Mark EJ, Ruangchira-urai R. Bronchiolitis interstitial pneumonitis: a pathologic study of 31 lung biopsies with features intermediate between bronchiolitis obliterans organizing pneumonia and usual interstitial pneumonitis, with clinical correlation. *Ann Diagn Pathol*. June 2008;12(3):171-180.

96. Myers JL, Veal CF Jr, Shin MS, Katzenstein AL. Respiratory bronchiolitis causing interstitial lung disease. A clinicopathologic study of six cases. *Am Rev Respir Dis*. April 1987;135(4):880-884.

97. Churg A, Wright JL, Wiggs B, Pare PD, Lazar N. Small airways disease and mineral dust exposure. Prevalence, structure, and function. *Am Rev Respir Dis*. January 1985;131(1):139-143.

98. Leslie KO, Cool CD, Sporn TA, et al. Familial idiopathic interstitial pneumonia: histopathology and survival in 30 patients. *Arch Pathol Lab Med*. November 2012;136(11):1366-1376.

99. Lee HL, Ryu JH, Wittmer MH, et al. Familial idiopathic pulmonary fibrosis: clinical features and outcome. *Chest*. June 2005;127(6):2034-2041.

100. Garcia-Sancho C, Buendia-Roldan I, Fernandez-Plata MR, et al. Familial pulmonary fibrosis is the strongest risk factor for idiopathic pulmonary fibrosis. *Respir Med*. December 2011;105(12):1902-1907.

101. Chibbar R, Shih F, Baga M, et al. Nonspecific interstitial pneumonia and usual interstitial pneumonia with mutation in surfactant protein C in familial pulmonary fibrosis. *Mod Pathol*. August 2004;17(8):973-980.

102. Lawson WE, Grant SW, Ambrosini V, et al. Genetic mutations in surfactant protein C are a rare cause of sporadic cases of IPF. *Thorax*. November 2004;59(11):977-980.

103. Maitra M, Wang Y, Gerard RD, Mendelson CR, Garcia CK. Surfactant protein A2 mutations associated with pulmonary fibrosis lead to protein instability and endoplasmic reticulum stress. *J Biol Chem*. July 16, 2010;285(29):22103-22113.

104. Wang Y, Kuan PJ, Xing C, et al. Genetic defects in surfactant protein A2 are associated with pulmonary fibrosis and lung cancer. *Am J Hum Genet*. January 2009;84(1):52-59.

105. Armanios MY, Chen JJ, Cogan JD, et al. Telomerase mutations in families with idiopathic pulmonary fibrosis. *N Engl J Med*. March 29, 2007;356(13):1317-1326.

106. Tsang AR, Wyatt HD, Ting NS, Beattie TL. hTERT mutations associated with idiopathic pulmonary fibrosis affect telomerase activity, telomere length, and cell growth by distinct mechanisms. *Aging Cell*. June 2012;11(3):482-490.

107. Whyte M, Hubbard R, Meliconi R, et al. Increased risk of fibrosing alveolitis associated with interleukin-1 receptor antagonist and tumor necrosis factor-alpha gene polymorphisms. *Am J Respir Crit Care Med*. August 2000;162(2 pt 1):755-758.

108. Vasakova M, Striz I, Slavcev A, et al. Correlation of IL-1alpha and IL-4 gene polymorphisms and clinical parameters in idiopathic pulmonary fibrosis. *Scand J Immunol*. March 2007;65(3):265-270.

109. Pantelidis P, Fanning GC, Wells AU, Welsh KI, Du Bois RM. Analysis of tumor necrosis factor-alpha, lymphotoxin-alpha, tumor necrosis factor receptor II, and interleukin-6 polymorphisms in patients with idiopathic pulmonary fibrosis. *Am J Respir Crit Care Med*. May 2001;163(6):1432-1436.

110. Morrison CD, Papp AC, Hejmanowski AQ, Addis VM, Prior TW. Increased D allele frequency of the angiotensin-converting enzyme gene in pulmonary fibrosis. *Hum Pathol*. May 2001;32(5):521-528.

111. Xaubet A, Marin-Arguedas A, Lario S, et al. Transforming growth factor-beta1 gene polymorphisms are associated with disease progression in idiopathic pulmonary fibrosis. *Am J Respir Crit Care Med*. August 15, 2003;168(4):431-435.

112. Peljto AL, Zhang Y, Fingerlin TE, et al. Association between the MUC5B promoter polymorphism and survival in patients with idiopathic pulmonary fibrosis. *JAMA*. June 5, 2013;309(21):2232-2239.

113. Zhang Y, Noth I, Garcia JG, Kaminski N. A variant in the promoter of MUC5B and idiopathic pulmonary fibrosis. *N Engl J Med*. April 21, 2011;364(16):1576-1577.

114. Checa M, Ruiz V, Montano M, Velazquez-Cruz R, Selman M, Pardo A. MMP-1 polymorphisms and the risk of idiopathic pulmonary fibrosis. *Hum Genet*. December 2008;124(5):465-472.

115. Iwai K, Mori T, Yamada N, Yamaguchi M, Hosoda Y. Idiopathic pulmonary fibrosis. Epidemiologic approaches to occupational exposure. *Am J Respir Crit Care Med*. September 1994;150(3):670-675.

116. Kishaba T, Shimaoka Y, Fukuyama H, et al. A cohort study of mortality predictors and characteristics of patients with combined pulmonary fibrosis and emphysema. *BMJ Open*. 2012;2(3).

117. Cottin V, Nunes H, Brillet PY, et al. Combined pulmonary fibrosis and emphysema: a distinct underrecognised entity. *Eur Respir J*. October 2005;26(4):586-593.

118. Taskar VS, Coultas DB. Is idiopathic pulmonary fibrosis an environmental disease? *Proc Am Thorac Soc*. June 2006;3(4):293-298.

119. Tobin RW, Pope CE 2nd, Pellegrini CA, Emond MJ, Sillery J, Raghu G. Increased prevalence of gastroesophageal reflux in patients with idiopathic pulmonary fibrosis. *Am J Respir Crit Care Med*. December 1998;158(6):1804-1808.

120. Raghu G, Freudenberger TD, Yang S, et al. High prevalence of abnormal acid gastro-oesophageal reflux in idiopathic pulmonary fibrosis. *Eur Respir J*. January 2006;27(1):136-142.

121. Lee JS, Song JW, Wolters PJ, et al. Bronchoalveolar lavage pepsin in acute exacerbation of idiopathic pulmonary fibrosis. *Eur Respir J*. February 2012;39(2):352-358.

122. Lee JS, Ryu JH, Elicker BM, et al. Gastroesophageal reflux therapy is associated with longer survival in patients with idiopathic pulmonary fibrosis. *Am J Respir Crit Care Med*. December 15, 2011;184(12):1390-1394.

123. Raghu G, Weycker D, Edelsberg J, Bradford WZ, Oster G. Incidence and prevalence of idiopathic pulmonary fibrosis. *Am J Respir Crit Care Med*. October 1, 2006;174(7):810-816.

124. von Plessen C, Grinde O, Gulsvik A. Incidence and prevalence of cryptogenic fibrosing alveolitis in a Norwegian community. *Respir Med*. April 2003;97(4):428-435.

125. Ishikawa N, Hattori N, Yokoyama A, Kohno N. Utility of KL-6/MUC1 in the clinical management of interstitial lung diseases. *Respir Investig*. March 2012;50(1):3-13.

126. Tansey D, Wells AU, Colby TV, et al. Variations in histological patterns of interstitial pneumonia between connective tissue disorders and their relationship to prognosis. *Histopathology*. June 2004;44(6):585-596.

127. Fischer A, West SG, Swigris JJ, Brown KK, du Bois RM. Connective tissue disease-associated interstitial lung disease: a call for clarification. *Chest*. August 2010;138(2):251-256.

128. Kondoh Y, Taniguchi H, Ogura T, et al. Disease progression in idiopathic pulmonary fibrosis without pulmonary function impairment. *Respirology*. July 2013;18(5):820-826.

129. Panos RJ, Mortenson RL, Niccoli SA, King TE Jr. Clinical deterioration in patients with idiopathic pulmonary fibrosis: causes and assessment. *Am J Med*. April 1990;88(4):396-404.

130. Daniels CE, Yi ES, Ryu JH. Autopsy findings in 42 consecutive patients with idiopathic pulmonary fibrosis. *Eur Respir J*. July 2008;32(1):170-174.

131. Taniguchi H, Ebina M, Kondoh Y, et al. Pirfenidone in idiopathic pulmonary fibrosis. *Eur Respir J*. April 2010;35(4):821-829.

132. Noble PW, Albera C, Bradford WZ, et al. Pirfenidone in patients with idiopathic pulmonary fibrosis (CAPACITY): two randomised trials. *Lancet*. May 21, 2011;377(9779):1760-1769.

133. Collard HR, Moore BB, Flaherty KR, et al. Acute exacerbations of idiopathic pulmonary fibrosis. *Am J Respir Crit Care Med.* October 1, 2007;176(7):636-643.

134. Kondoh Y, Taniguchi H, Kawabata Y, Yokoi T, Suzuki K, Takagi K. Acute exacerbation in idiopathic pulmonary fibrosis. Analysis of clinical and pathologic findings in three cases. *Chest.* June 1993;103(6):1808-1812.

135. Sakamoto K, Taniguchi H, Kondoh Y, Ono K, Hasegawa Y, Kitaichi M. Acute exacerbation of idiopathic pulmonary fibrosis as the initial presentation of the disease. *Eur Respir Rev.* June 2009;18(112):129-132.

136. Johkoh T, Sumikawa H, Fukuoka J, et al. Do you really know precise radiologic-pathologic correlation of usual interstitial pneumonia? *Eur J Radiol.* January 24;83(1):20-26.

137. Katzenstein AL, Zisman DA, Litzky LA, Nguyen BT, Kotloff RM. Usual interstitial pneumonia: histologic study of biopsy and explant specimens. *Am J Surg Pathol.* December 2002;26(12):1567-1577.

138. Travis WD, Matsui K, Moss J, Ferrans VJ. Idiopathic nonspecific interstitial pneumonia: prognostic significance of cellular and fibrosing patterns: survival comparison with usual interstitial pneumonia and desquamative interstitial pneumonia. *Am J Surg Pathol.* January 2000;24(1):19-33.

139. Enomoto N, Suda T, Kono M, et al. Amount of elastic fibers predicts prognosis of idiopathic pulmonary fibrosis. *Respir Med.* October 2013;107(10):1608-1616.

140. Nicholson AG, Fulford LG, Colby TV, du Bois RM, Hansell DM, Wells AU. The relationship between individual histologic features and disease progression in idiopathic pulmonary fibrosis. *Am J Respir Crit Care Med.* July 15, 2002;166(2):173-177.

141. Harada T, Watanabe K, Nabeshima K, Hamasaki M, Iwasaki H. Prognostic significance of fibroblastic foci in usual interstitial pneumonia and non-specific interstitial pneumonia. *Respirology.* February 2013;18(2):278-283.

142. Enomoto N, Suda T, Kato M, et al. Quantitative analysis of fibroblastic foci in usual interstitial pneumonia. *Chest.* July 2006;130(1):22-29.

143. Cipriani NA, Strek M, Noth I, et al. Pathologic quantification of connective tissue disease-associated versus idiopathic usual interstitial pneumonia. *Arch Pathol Lab Med.* October 2012;136(10):1253-1258.

144. Kawabata Y, Hoshi E, Murai K, et al. Smoking-related changes in the background lung of specimens resected for lung cancer: a semiquantitative study with correlation to postoperative course. *Histopathology.* December 2008;53(6):707-714.

145. Kurashima K, Takayanagi N, Tsuchiya N, et al. The effect of emphysema on lung function and survival in patients with idiopathic pulmonary fibrosis. *Respirology.* July 2010;15(5):843-848.

146. Katzenstein AL. Smoking-related interstitial fibrosis (SRIF): pathologic findings and distinction from other chronic fibrosing lung diseases. *J Clin Pathol.* October 2013;66(10):882-887.

147. Katzenstein AL, Mukhopadhyay S, Zanardi C, Dexter E. Clinically occult interstitial fibrosis in smokers: classification and significance of a surprisingly common finding in lobectomy specimens. *Hum Pathol.* March 2010;41(3):316-325.

148. Wright JL, Tazelaar HD, Churg A. Fibrosis with emphysema. *Histopathology.* March 2011;58(4):517-524.

149. Fraig M, Shreesha U, Savici D, Katzenstein AL. Respiratory bronchiolitis: a clinicopathologic study in current smokers, ex-smokers, and never-smokers. *Am J Surg Pathol.* May 2002;26(5):647-653.

150. Kitaguchi Y, Fujimoto K, Hanaoka M, Kawakami S, Honda T, Kubo K. Clinical characteristics of combined pulmonary fibrosis and emphysema. *Respirology.* February 2010;15(2):265-271.

151. Cottin V. The impact of emphysema in pulmonary fibrosis. *Eur Respir Rev.* June 1, 2013;22(128):153-157.

152. Flaherty KR, Travis WD, Colby TV, et al. Histopathologic variability in usual and nonspecific interstitial pneumonias. *Am J Respir Crit Care Med.* November 1, 2001;164(9):1722-1727.

153. Monaghan H, Wells AU, Colby TV, du Bois RM, Hansell DM, Nicholson AG. Prognostic implications of histologic patterns in multiple surgical lung biopsies from patients with idiopathic interstitial pneumonias. *Chest.* February 2004;125(2):522-526.

154. Parambil JG, Myers JL, Ryu JH. Histopathologic features and outcome of patients with acute exacerbation of idiopathic pulmonary fibrosis undergoing surgical lung biopsy. *Chest.* November 2005;128(5):3310-3315.

155. Churg A, Muller NL, Silva CI, Wright JL. Acute exacerbation (acute lung injury of unknown cause) in UIP and other forms of fibrotic interstitial pneumonias. *Am J Surg Pathol.* February 2007;31(2):277-284.

156. Hyzy R, Huang S, Myers J, Flaherty K, Martinez F. Acute exacerbation of idiopathic pulmonary fibrosis. *Chest.* November 2007;132(5):1652-1658.

157. Kim DS, Collard HR, King TE Jr. Classification and natural history of the idiopathic interstitial pneumonias. *Proc Am Thorac Soc.* June 2006;3(4):285-292.

158. Park JH, Kim DS, Park IN, et al. Prognosis of fibrotic interstitial pneumonia: idiopathic versus collagen vascular disease-related subtypes. *Am J Respir Crit Care Med.* April 1, 2007;175(7):705-711.

159. Flaherty KR, Colby TV, Travis WD, et al. Fibroblastic foci in usual interstitial pneumonia: idiopathic versus collagen vascular disease. *Am J Respir Crit Care Med.* May 15 2003;167(10):1410-1415.

160. Leslie KO, Trahan S, Gruden J. Pulmonary pathology of the rheumatic diseases. *Semin Respir Crit Care Med.* August 2007;28(4):369-378.

161. Travis WD, Hunninghake G, King TE Jr, et al. Idiopathic nonspecific interstitial pneumonia: report of an American Thoracic Society project. *Am J Respir Crit Care Med.* June 15 2008;177(12):1338-1347.

162. Romagnoli M, Nannini C, Piciucchi S, et al. Idiopathic nonspecific interstitial pneumonia: an interstitial lung disease associated with autoimmune disorders? *Eur Respir J.* August 2011;38(2):384-391.

163. Park IN, Jegal Y, Kim DS, et al. Clinical course and lung function change of idiopathic nonspecific interstitial pneumonia. *Eur Respir J.* January 2009;33(1):68-76.

164. Fujita J, Ohtsuki Y, Yoshinouchi T, et al. Idiopathic non-specific interstitial pneumonia: as an "autoimmune interstitial pneumonia." *Respir Med.* February 2005;99(2):234-240.

165. Suda T, Kono M, Nakamura Y, et al. Distinct prognosis of idiopathic nonspecific interstitial pneumonia (NSIP) fulfilling criteria for undifferentiated connective tissue disease (UCTD). *Respir Med.* October 2010;104(10):1527-1534.

166. Kinder BW, Collard HR, Koth L, et al. Idiopathic nonspecific interstitial pneumonia: lung manifestation of undifferentiated connective tissue disease? *Am J Respir Crit Care Med.* October 1, 2007;176(7):691-697.

167. Vourlekis JS, Schwarz MI, Cool CD, Tuder RM, King TE, Brown KK. Nonspecific interstitial pneumonitis as the sole histologic expression of hypersensitivity pneumonitis. *Am J Med.* April 15, 2002;112(6):490-493.

168. Craig PJ, Wells AU, Doffman S, et al. Desquamative interstitial pneumonia, respiratory bronchiolitis and their relationship to smoking. *Histopathology.* September 2004;45(3):275-282.

169. Fischer A, Solomon JJ, du Bois RM, et al. Lung disease with anti-CCP antibodies but not rheumatoid arthritis or connective tissue disease. *Respir Med.* July 2012;106(7):1040-1047.

170. Koreeda Y, Higashimoto I, Yamamoto M, et al. Clinical and pathological findings of interstitial lung disease patients with anti-aminoacyl-tRNA synthetase autoantibodies. *Intern Med.* 2010;49(5):361-369.

171. Takato H, Waseda Y, Watanabe S, et al. Pulmonary manifestations of anti-ARS antibody positive interstitial pneumonia—with or without PM/DM. *Respir Med.* January 2013;107(1):128-133.

172. Kang BH, Park JK, Roh JH, et al. Clinical significance of serum autoantibodies in idiopathic interstitial pneumonia. *J Korean Med Sci.* May 2013;28(5):731-737.

173. Nagai S, Kitaichi M, Itoh H, Nishimura K, Izumi T, Colby TV. Idiopathic nonspecific interstitial pneumonia/fibrosis: comparison with idiopathic pulmonary fibrosis and BOOP. *Eur Respir J.* November 1998;12(5):1010-1019.

174. Cottin V, Donsbeck AV, Revel D, Loire R, Cordier JF. Nonspecific interstitial pneumonia. Individualization of a clinicopathologic entity in a series of 12 patients. *Am J Respir Crit Care Med.* October 1998;158(4):1286-1293.

175. Do KH, Lee JS, Colby TV, Kitaichi M, Kim DS. Nonspecific interstitial pneumonia versus usual interstitial pneumonia: differences in the density histogram of high-resolution CT. *J Comput Assist Tomogr.* July-August 2005;29(4):544-548.

176. Tzelepis GE, Toya SP, Moutsopoulos HM. Occult connective tissue diseases mimicking idiopathic interstitial pneumonias. *Eur Respir J.* January 2008;31(1):11-20.

177. Mino M, Noma S, Taguchi Y, Tomii K, Kohri Y, Oida K. Pulmonary involvement in polymyositis and dermatomyositis: sequential evaluation with CT. *AJR Am J Roentgenol.* July 1997;169(1):83-87.

178. Yamadori I, Fujita J, Bandoh S, et al. Nonspecific interstitial pneumonia as pulmonary involvement of primary Sjogren's syndrome. *Rheumatol Int.* Jul 2002;22(3):89-92.

179. Gunnarsson R, Aalokken TM, Molberg O, et al. Prevalence and severity of interstitial lung disease in mixed connective tissue disease: a nationwide, cross-sectional study. *Ann Rheum Dis.* December 2012;71(12):1966-1972.

180. Pugin J, Verghese G, Widmer MC, Matthay MA. The alveolar space is the site of intense inflammatory and profibrotic reactions in the early phase of acute respiratory distress syndrome. *Crit Care Med.* February 1999;27(2):304-312.

181. Greene KE, Wright JR, Steinberg KP, et al. Serial changes in surfactant-associated proteins in lung and serum before and after onset of ARDS. *Am J Respir Crit Care Med.* December 1999;160(6):1843-1850.

182. Ware LB, Matthay MA. The acute respiratory distress syndrome. *N Engl J Med.* May 4, 2000;342(18):1334-1349.

183. Park IN, Kim DS, Shim TS, et al. Acute exacerbation of interstitial pneumonia other than idiopathic pulmonary fibrosis. *Chest.* July 2007;132(1):214-220.

184. Lee JW, Lee KS, Lee HY, et al. Cryptogenic organizing pneumonia: serial high-resolution CT findings in 22 patients. *AJR Am J Roentgenol.* October 2010;195(4):916-922.

185. Izumi T, Kitaichi M, Nishimura K, Nagai S. Bronchiolitis obliterans organizing pneumonia. Clinical features and differential diagnosis. *Chest.* September 1992;102(3):715-719.

186. King TE, Jr., Mortenson RL. Cryptogenic organizing pneumonitis. The North American experience. *Chest.* July 1992;102(1 suppl):8S-13S.

187. Yoo JW, Song JW, Jang SJ, et al. Comparison between cryptogenic organizing pneumonia and connective tissue disease-related organizing pneumonia. *Rheumatology (Oxford).* May 2011;50(5):932-938.

188. Beasley MB, Franks TJ, Galvin JR, Gochuico B, Travis WD. Acute fibrinous and organizing pneumonia: a histological pattern of lung injury and possible variant of diffuse alveolar damage. *Arch Pathol Lab Med.* September 2002;126(9):1064-1070.

Collagen Vascular Diseases

Nahal Boroumand and Yimin Ge

TAKE HOME PEARLS

- It is important to differentiate collagen vascular disease (CVD)-ILD from idiopathic pulmonary fibrosis since they differ in treatment and prognosis.
- NSIP is the most common histopathologic pattern seen in CVD, except in rheumatoid arthritis, in which UIP is the predominant pattern.
- UIP pattern is the most common histopathologic feature associated with idiopathic pulmonary fibrosis.
- UIP pattern in an idiopathic setting has a significantly worse prognosis than fibrotic NSIP; CVD-associated UIP pattern has a favorable prognosis that is similar to NSIP.
- UIP pattern associated with rheumatoid arthritis does not have a survival advantage compared to idiopathic UIP.
- Histopathologic features that suggest an underlying CVD include:
  - Involvement of a different compartment of the lung
  - Presence of overlapping acute, subacute, and chronic lesions
  - Presence of NSIP or LIP background
  - Lymphoid follicles with germinal centers
- **Rheumatoid arthritis (RA)**
  - Pleuritis and pleural effusion are the most common pulmonary manifestation
  - Pulmonary nodules are the most specific pulmonary lesions
  - Airway involvement in RA is in the form of:

- Follicular bronchiolitis
- Obliterative bronchiolitis
- Bronchiolectasis
- Bronchiolocentric granulomatosis
- UIP pattern is the most common pattern of ILD in RA followed by NSIP
- Patients with UIP pattern have the worse prognosis
- **Systemic lupus erythematosus (SLE)**
  - Infection is the most common pulmonary complication
  - Pleuritis is the most common noninfectious pulmonary manifestation
  - Significant ILD is not a common finding in SLE
  - Acute lupus pneumonitis and cellular NSIP are the two main patterns of parenchymal lung disease in SLE
- **Progressive systemic sclerosis (PSS)**
  - Pulmonary arterial hypertension (PAH) and pulmonary interstitial fibrosis are the two most common pulmonary manifestations of scleroderma
  - ILD is more commonly associated with the diffuse cutaneous form
  - NSIP is the most common pattern of ILD in patients with sine scleroderma
  - Primary pulmonary hypertension occurs almost always in the limited cutaneous form of scleroderma
- **Polymyositis/Dermatomyositis (PM/DM)**
  - Pulmonary involvement is the most common extramuscular manifestation of disease

- Pulmonary complications include ILD, aspiration pneumonia, drug-induced lung diseases, ventilatory problems
- ILD is an important prognostic factor
- Anti-Jo 1 antibody is the strongest predictor of ILD
- NSIP is the most common pattern of ILD
- Aspiration pneumonia is a common complication of the disease
- Pleural involvement, bronchiolitis, and pulmonary hypertension are not commonly seen in these patients
- **Sjögren syndrome (SS)**
  - The most frequent pulmonary manifestations are ILD, airway diseases, and lymphoproliferative disorders.
  - ILD is the most common form of lung involvement.
  - NSIP is the most common pattern of ILD.
  - Tracheal and large airway involvement is common and results in xerotrachea and xerobronchitis.
  - Follicular bronchiolitis is common but rarely results in significant clinical problems.
- **Ankylosing spondylitis**
  - Pulmonary involvement includes apical fibrobullous disease and pneumothorax.
- **Inflammatory bowel disease (IBD)**
  - Pulmonary involvement is among the rarest extraintestinal manifestation.
  - Pulmonary manifestations in IBD are most frequently drug induced rather than the manifestation of the disease.
- **Behcet syndrome**
  - Necrotizing vasculitis involves all sizes of pulmonary arteries, veins, and capillaries.

INTRODUCTION

Pleuropulmonary involvement is a common manifestation of collagen vascular diseases (CVD) and a major source of morbidity and mortality in these patients.

Collagen vascular diseases can involve different components of the lung, including pleura, lung parenchyma, large and small airways, and vasculature. The frequency and severity of each involved component vary greatly in different collagen vascular diseases (*Table 19-1*). Pulmonary involvement can precede, coincide, or occur after the manifestations of primary collagen vascular diseases. A diagnostic dilemma arises when pulmonary manifestations, interstitial lung disease (ILD) in particular, antedate other symptoms and serologic markers. It is important to distinguish collagen vascular disease associated interstitial lung disease (CVD-ILD) from idiopathic pulmonary fibrosis (IPF), because of significant differences in prognosis and approach to treatment.

Nonspecific interstitial pneumonia (NSIP) is the most common histopathologic pattern seen in collagen vascular diseases, except in rheumatoid arthritis, in which usual interstitial pneumonia (UIP) pattern is the predominant finding. UIP pattern is also the most common histopathologic pattern in idiopathic pulmonary fibrosis (IPF) and has a significantly worse prognosis than fibrotic NSIP. However, the prognosis of NSIP and UIP in patients with collagen vascular diseases is similar and more favorable than that in idiopathic setting. The better prognosis for CVD-ILD has been attributed to higher frequency of NSIP pattern and better prognosis of UIP pattern associated CVD.[1-3] UIP pattern associated with rheumatoid arthritis is the only exception with dismal prognosis as that of UIP associated with IPF.[4] The fact that CVD associated NSIP and UIP patterns have similar survival obviates the need for surgical lung biopsy.

Histopathologic features that suggest an underlying collagen vascular disease include involvement of different compartments of the lung (especially pleura), overlapping acute, subacute, and chronic lesions, NSIP or lymphocytic interstitial pneumonia (LIP), and lymphoid follicles with germinal centers.[5] From a clinical standpoint, young age at onset, unexplained joint or cutaneous manifestations, and serologic abnormalities are suggestive of collagen vascular diseases[5] (*Table 19-2*).

Table 19-1 Pulmonary Manifestations in Collagen Vascular Diseases

	Pleura	Airway	ILD	Vasculature
RA	++	++	++	+
SLE	+++	+	+	+
SSc	−/+	−/+	+++	+++
PM/DM	−	−/+	+++	+
Sjögren syndrome	+	++	++	+

Table 19-2 Clinical and Histopathologic Features Suggestive of CVD-ILD

Clinical features	• Young age at onset • Unexplained joint or cutaneous manifestations • Serologic abnormalities
Histologic features	• Involvement of multiple lung compartments, especially pleura • Concurrent acute, subacute, and chronic lesions • NSIP or LIP background • Lymphoid follicles with germinal centers

RHEUMATOID ARTHRITIS

Rheumatoid arthritis (RA) is a systemic autoimmune disease characterized by symmetric involvement of the small peripheral joints. Pleuropulmonary involvement is an extra-articular manifestation and a major source of morbidity and mortality in these patients. It usually occurs late in the course of the disease, but it can present simultaneously or even antedate the articular manifestation in rare cases. RA may involve different components of the lung including pleura, lung parenchyma, airways, and vessels, and results in a wide variety of clinical presentations and pathologic changes (*Table 19-3*). The pulmonary manifestations

Table 19-3 Pulmonary Manifestations in Rheumatoid Arthritis

Location	Lesions
Pleura	• Pleuritis +/− effusion • Pleural fibrosis • Empyema • Interstitium • UIP > NSIP > OP = DAD • Apical fibrobullous disease • Rheumatoid nodule • Amyloidosis
Alveolus	• Diffuse hemorrhage • Eosinophilic pneumonia
Airway	• Bronchiolitis +/− fibrosis • Follicular bronchiolitis • Constrictive bronchiolitis • Bronchiectasis • Bronchocentric granulomatosis
Vasculature	• Pulmonary arterial hypertension (rare) • Vasculitis (rare)
Indirect effects	• Thoracic cage immobility

in patients with RA can also be secondary to treatment or infection.

Pleuritis and pleural effusion are the most common type of pulmonary manifestation in RA but both are nonspecific[6] (*Figure 19-1A*). Pulmonary rheumatoid nodules are the most specific pulmonary lesions that are more common in males and in patients with subcutaneous nodules. These nodules may be detected by high-resolution computed tomography (HRCT) as multiple well-defined nodules ranging in size from a few millimeters to a few centimeters. Histologically, rheumatoid nodules are necrotizing nodules surrounded by epithelioid histiocytes and giant cells that are often located subpleurally.[6] They are usually asymptomatic unless complicated by rupture, infection, hemorrhage, or bronchopleural fistula. Rupture of these nodules can result in pneumothorax or empyema. Wegener granulomatosis and infections are in the differential diagnosis of rheumatoid nodules. Necrotizing vasculitis and lack of tendency to involve the pleura help distinguish Wegener granulomatosis from rheumatoid nodules. Infectious etiologies should be excluded by appropriate cultures or special stains.

Airway involvement with airflow obstruction is a common manifestation of the disease. Airway diseases associated with RA include follicular bronchiolitis, obliterative bronchiolitis, bronchiolectasis, and bronchiolocentric granulomatosis. Follicular bronchiolitis is seen in 20% of patients and is characterized by infiltration of the bronchiolar wall by chronic inflammatory cells including lymphocytes and plasma cells, and formation of lymphoid follicles with germinal centers[6] (*Figure 19-1C*). Obliterative or constrictive bronchiolitis is an irreversible progressive form of bronchiolitis with poor prognosis. It is characterized by circumferential narrowing of the bronchiolar lumen and scarring. Patients present with dry cough and progressive dyspnea. A mosaic pattern as a result of moderate to severe air trapping may be observed on HRCT.

The reported prevalence of ILD in RA ranges widely from 4% to 68% and depends on the method of detection (HRCT, CXR, PFT) and the population studied (asymptomatic, symptomatic patients, or autopsy).[7] Approximately 14% of patients with RA have clinically significant ILD.

UIP, NSIP, organizing pneumonia (OP), LIP, respiratory bronchiolitis (RB), and desquamative interstitial pneumonia (DIP) are histopathologic patterns of ILD reported in patients with RA (*Figure 19-1D-H*). These histopathologic patterns are morphologically similar to the corresponding idiopathic forms. However, the presence of lymphoid follicles and concurrent acute, subacute, and chronic inflammatory reactions (*Figure 19-1B*) and involvement of the pleura raise the possibility of RA as an underlying cause.[5,6] UIP pattern

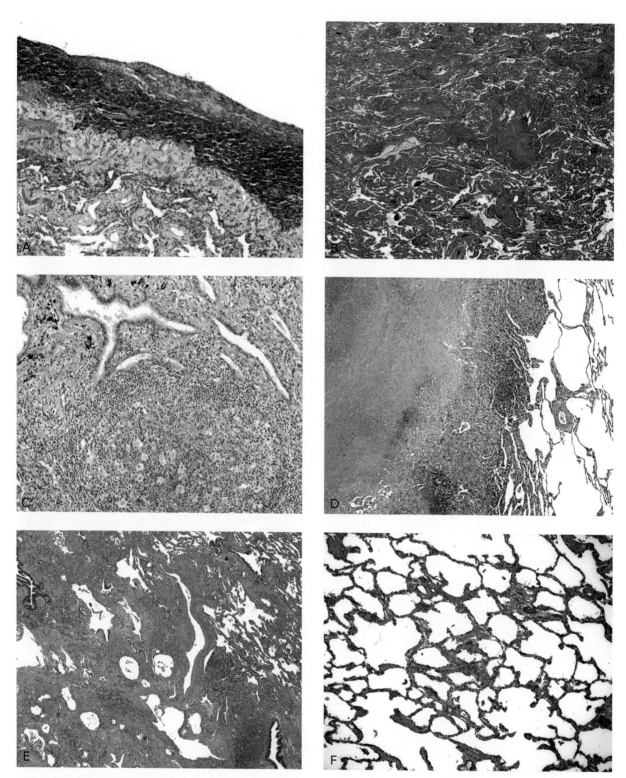

CHAPTER 19

FIGURE 19-1 Rheumatoid arthritis. A: Pleural tissue from a patient with rheumatoid arthritis (RA) lung disease shows significant pleural thickening with marked chronic inflammation and fibrosis (H&E stain). **B:** Lower power view of RA lung disease is often characterized by prominent lymphocytic infiltration with lymphoid follicles, primarily located in the alveolar septa and around the airways or blood vessels (H&E stain). **C:** Follicular bronchiolitis is a typical finding in rheumatoid arthritis (H&E stain). **D:** Rheumatoid nodule is characterized by necrotic nodule surrounded by chronic inflammation and palisading histiocytes (H&E stain). **E:** Interstitial fibrosis with usual interstitial pneumonitis (UIP)–like pattern is the most common histologic pattern of RA-related ILD (H&E stain). **F:** ILD associated with RA may also have histologic pattern simulating fibrotic nonspecific interstitial pneumonitis (NSIP) as seen in this photograph (H&E stain).

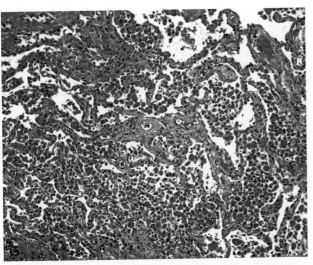 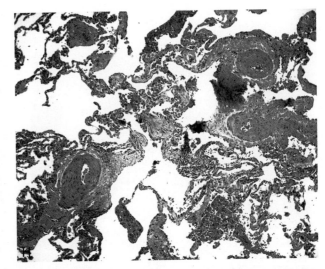

FIGURE 19-1 (Continued) G: Desquamative interstitial pneumonia (DIP)–like pattern can also be occasionally seen in ILD associated with RA with abundant lightly brown-pigmented alveolar macrophages packed in the air spaces (H&E stain). **H:** Sections of RA lung disease shows pulmonary arteries with marked intimal-medial hyperplasia resulting significant luminal stenosis, features of pulmonary arterial hypertension (PAH) (H&E stain).

is the most common pattern of ILD reported in RA followed by NSIP pattern.[7,8] Ground glass opacity and bilateral subpleural reticulation with or without honeycombing can be found in HRCT, corresponding to NSIP and UIP histopathologic patterns respectively. The patients who have ILD with UIP pattern have the worst prognosis.[4] The data are conflicting regarding whether the prognosis in patients with RA-related UIP is better than or similar to patients with idiopathic UIP.[2,4]

Acute deterioration and respiratory failure can occur in patients with ILD. Acute lung injury may presents as OP with diffuse alveolar damage (DAD).[6] Diffuse pulmonary hemorrhage is a rare complication of RA.

SYSTEMIC LUPUS ERYTHEMATOSUS

Systemic lupus erythematosus (SLE) is a systemic autoimmune disease with multiorgan involvement and a waxing and waning clinical course. It affects predominantly females between the ages of 15 and 45 years old. Pleuropulmonary involvement is seen in 20% to 90% of patients, and is more common in males and associated with higher mortality rate.

Infection is the most common pulmonary complication in SLE patients with immunosuppressive therapy. Lung biopsy is often necessary to distinguish an infectious process from underlying disease and thereby prescribe appropriate treatment.

Pleuritis is the most common noninfectious pulmonary manifestation in patients with SLE

(Figure 19-2A). Other pulmonary manifestations include parenchymal lesions, vascular diseases, diaphragmatic dysfunction, and upper airway involvement (Table 19-4).

Acute lupus pneumonitis and cellular NSIP are the two main patterns of lung parenchymal disease seen in SLE. Acute lupus pneumonitis is the most dreaded complication of SLE, occurring in 1% to 4% of the patients. Clinical manifestations include acute onset dyspnea, cough, fever, and hemoptysis. HRCT shows bilateral ground glass opacity or consolidation. The histopathologic findings are similar to diffuse alveolar damage with or without diffuse pulmonary hemorrhage[6,9] (Figure 19-2C, D).

Significant ILD is not a common finding in SLE and is only seen in 3% to 8% of the cases. NSIP is the most common pattern of ILD in these patients. Cellular NSIP is characterized by a cellular interstitial pneumonia dominated by lymphocyte and plasma cells with a varying degree of interstitial fibrosis (Figure 19-2E). Other histologic patterns include LIP (Figure 19-2B), OP, and UIP (Figure 19-2F).[1,6,9]

Pulmonary hypertension is a serious complication of SLE that may be underestimated. The pathogenesis of pulmonary hypertension in SLE includes arteriopathy with plexiform lesion and thromboembolic arteriopathy (Figure 19-2F). Rarely, pulmonary vasculitis is the cause of pulmonary hypertension[1,6,9] (Figure 19-2D).

Shrinking lung syndrome is another respiratory manifestation of SLE, characterized by unexplained dyspnea, elevation of the diaphragm, and reduced lung volume without evidence of ILD.[9]

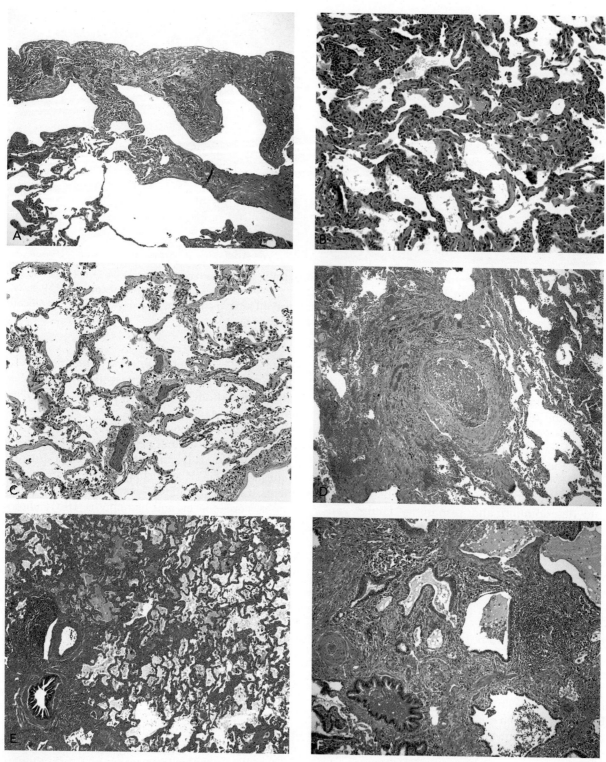

FIGURE 19-2 Systemic lupus erythematosus. **A:** Pleuritis is seen in this patient with systemic lupus erythematosus (SLE) features by pleural fibrosis and chronic inflammation (H&E stain). **B:** Acute lupus pneumonitis shows prominent interstitial inflammation with focal edema and intra-alveolar fibrin (H&E stain). **C:** Severe acute lupus pneumonitis shows alveolitis with intra-alveolar hemorrhage and hyaline membranes, features indistinguishable from diffuse alveolar damage (DAD) (H&E stain). **D:** Vasculitis with intravascular fibrin thrombus is seen in acute lupus pneumonitis with hemorrhage in the background (H&E stain). **E:** Cellular NSIP demonstrated in this picture is the most common pattern of ILD associated with SLE. Follicular bronchiolitis is also present in the left side of the picture (H&E stain). **F:** UIP pattern associated with SLE shows significant interstitial fibrosis with honeycomb change. Note the significantly thickened or occluded branches of pulmonary artery in the left lower portion of the picture, indicating SLE-included arteriopathy.

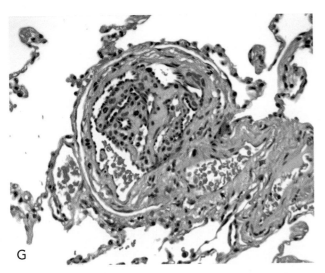

FIGURE 19-2 (Continued) G: Plexiform arteriopathy can be seen in SLE associated lung disease and may contribute to PAH.

Table 19-4 Pulmonary Manifestations in Systemic Lupus Erythematosus

Location	Lesions
Pleura	• Pleuritis +/− effusion • Pleural fibrosis
Interstitium	• Acute lupus pneumonitis • Chronic interstitial pneumonitis • NSIP > LIP = OP = UIP
Alveolus	• Diffuse alveolar hemorrhage
Vasculature	• Pulmonary arterial hypertension • Vasculitis • Thromboembolism
Airway	• Obstructive lung disease • Upper airway disease
Indirect effects	• Shrinking lung syndrome

PROGRESSIVE SYSTEMIC SCLEROSIS (PSS)

Systemic sclerosis (SSc) is a rare autoimmune connective tissue disorder that is more common in females between the ages of 45 and 64 years old. It has been classified into three groups based on the extent of skin involvement: limited cutaneous form, diffuse cutaneous form, and sine scleroderma. In the limited cutaneous form, sclerosis is limited to portions of the extremities below the elbows and knees. In the diffuse cutaneous form sclerosis extends above the elbows and the knees, and the skin is spared in sine scleroderma.

Lung involvement is a common complication of SSc and is a leading cause of morbidity and mortality in these patients. Radiologic findings include bibasilar ground glass opacity, reticulation, mild architectural distortion, and traction bronchiectasis. The subpleural lung is often spared and honeycombing fibrosis is uncommon.[6]

Pulmonary arterial hypertension (PAH) (*Figure 19-3C, D*) and pulmonary interstitial fibrosis (*Figure 19-3E*) are the two most common pulmonary manifestations of SSc.[6,10-12] PAH can be secondary to ILD or occurs in the absence of interstitial fibrosis. The primary form of PAH is almost always seen in the limited cutaneous form of scleroderma.[13]

Significant ILD is reported in 40% of patients with Ssc and is more commonly associated with the diffuse cutaneous form. NSIP is the most common pattern of ILD in patients with SSc (*Figure 19-3A, B*)[6,10,11] and is characterized by uniform paucicellular fibrosis of the interstitium. Surfactant protein D, Krebs von den Lungen-6 (KL-6), and glycoproteins secreted by type II pneumocytes have emerged as predictors of ILD.[14]

Other respiratory manifestations of the scleroderma include airway diseases (*Figure 19-3E*), pleural effusion (*Figure 19-3F*), pneumothorax, lung cancer, and recurrent aspiration with centrilobular fibrosis due to esophageal dysmotility (*Table 19-5*).[6,10,11]

POLYMYOSITIS AND DERMATOMYOSITIS

Polymyositis/dermatomyositis (PM/DM) is an idiopathic systemic autoimmune disorder with inflammation of skeletal muscles. Patients present with weakness of proximal muscles, elevated serum muscle enzymes (most commonly creatine kinase), electromyographic features of myopathy, and inflammation of muscle tissue. Polymyositis has been classified into three categories: adult and juvenile dermatomyositis and inclusion body myositis. It is a rare autoimmune disease with a female to male ratio of 2 to 1.

Pulmonary involvement is the most common extramuscular manifestation of the disease and a major cause of morbidity and mortality. Pulmonary complications occur in 40% of patients and include interstitial lung disease, aspiration pneumonia, drug-induced lung diseases, and ventilatory dysfunction (diaphragmatic and intercostal muscle weakness). Pulmonary arterial hypertension and diffuse alveolar hemorrhage with capillaritis are also reported (*Table 19-6*).

ILD may precede myositis symptoms, occur concomitantly, or present late in the course of disease.[15] Lung involvement precedes the muscle manifestation in third of the patients. The clinical course in myositis-associated ILD varies and the patients can

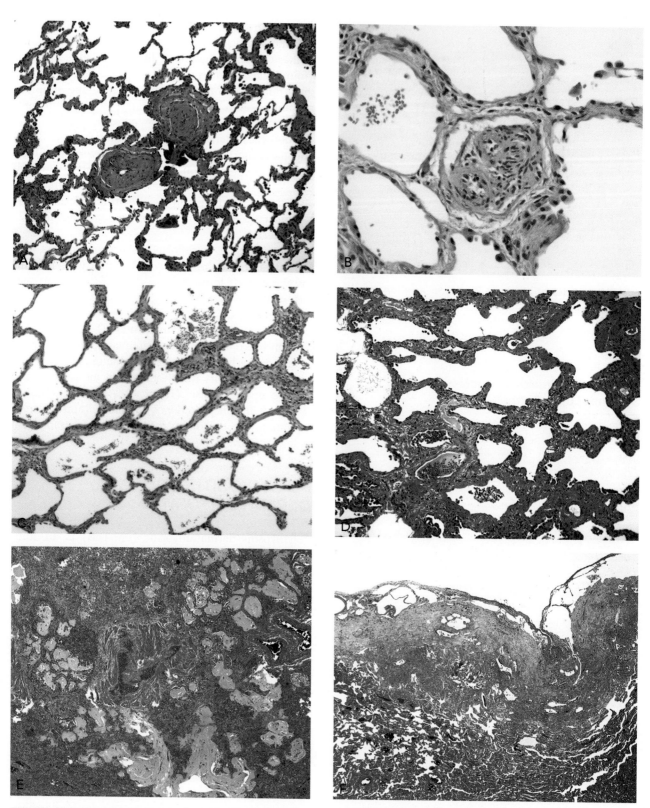

FIGURE 19-3 Progressive systemic sclerosis. A: Scleroderma-induced arteriopathy demonstrated in this picture shows marked intimal-medial proliferation with luminal stenosis and occlusion, features of PAH (H&E stain). B: A plexiform lesion is seen in a patient with PAH secondary to scleroderma (H&E stain). C and D: Fibrotic NSIP pattern is the most common ILD in patients with scleroderma, featured by paucicellular and evenly distributed fibrosis of the alveolar septa (H&E stain). E: Severe interstitial fibrosis with honeycombing can also be seen in scleroderma that simulating UIP. Note a focus of restrictive bronchiolitis in the center of the picture (H&E stain). F: Pleuritis with pleural fibrosis and chronic inflammation is seen in this patient with scleroderma, a finding less common than that in RA and SLE (H&E stain).

Table 19-5 Pulmonary Manifestations in Systemic Sclerosis

Location	Lesions
Pleura	• Pleuritis +/− effusion • Pleural fibrosis
Interstitium	• NSIP >>> UIP • DAD • COP • Aspiration pneumonia • Apical fibrobullous disease
Alveoli	• Diffuse alveolar hemorrhage
Vasculature	• Pulmonary hypertension • Vasculitis
Others	• Lung malignancy • Respiratory muscle weakness • Drug induced toxicity

Table 19-6 Pulmonary Manifestations in Polymyositis/Dermatomyositis

Location	Lesions
Pleura	• Pleuritis +/− effusion • Pleural fibrosis • Pneumothorax
Interstitium	• Interstitial lung disease (most common) • NSIP = OP > DAD > UIP • Aspiration pneumonia • Infectious pneumonia • Drug-induced interstitial lung disease
Alveoli	• Diffuse alveolar hemorrhage
Airway	• Bronchiolitis +/− fibrosis
Vasculature	• Pulmonary arterial hypertension

be asymptomatic, have a chronic course, or present acutely with progressive respiratory failure. Muscle-specific autoantibody, like anti-Jo 1, is reported in 50% to 60% of patients with ILD and is considered the strongest predictor of ILD.

HRCT shows reticular and ground glass opacities involving the lung bases and periphery that correlating with an NSIP pattern. Air space consolidation is also a common finding but honeycombing fibrosis is not common.

Histologically, the common patterns include NSIP, UIP, DAD, and OP, with NSIP being the most common.[16] These patterns are histologically similar to their idiopathic counterpart. The histologic patterns have

important prognostic value, and the best prognosis is associated with NSIP and OP, intermediate outcome with UIP pattern, and the worst prognosis with DAD.

Aspiration pneumonia is a common complication of the disease due to weakness of striated muscles of the pharynx and upper esophagus. Pleural involvement, bronchiolitis, and pulmonary hypertension are not commonly seen in patients with PM/DM.[15,16] However, pulmonary hypertension secondary to ILD and capillaritis has been reported. Patients with PM/DM are at higher risk of developing a malignancy.

SJÖGREN SYNDROME

Sjögren syndrome (SS) is a systemic autoimmune disease characterized by keratoconjunctivitis, xerostomia, and arthritis. It affects predominantly women in their 40s and 50s, with a female to male ratio of 9:1. Primary Sjögren syndrome (pSS) occurs in isolation, while secondary Sjögren syndrome (sSS) is often associated with other autoimmune disorders, especially RA. Radiologic findings are nonspecific and include a fine reticular pattern and ground glass opacity that predominantly involves the lower lobes. Architectural distortion and honeycombing are absent.

Lung involvement occurs late in the course of the disease. The most frequent pulmonary manifestations are ILD, airway diseases, and lymphoproliferative disorders. ILD is the most common form of lung involvement in Sjögren syndrome. The most common histologic pattern of ILD is NSIP (*Figure 19-4A, C*), followed by LIP, UIP, and OP (*Figure 19-4B*).[1,6,17] Involvement of trachea and large airways is common and may result in xerotrachea and xerobronchitis that manifest as nonproductive cough. The small airways are also commonly involved, with follicular bronchiolitis as a common histologic finding (*Figure 19-4D*). However, small airways involvement rarely results in significant clinical consequences (*Table 19-7*).

Patients with SS have a higher risk of developing lymphoma. The prevalence of primary pulmonary lymphoma is 1-2%,[18,19] which is usually a low-grade marginal zone B cell lymphoma.[20-22] Presence of pleural effusion and hilar and mediastinal adenopathy should raise concern for lymphoma.[23]

ANKYLOSING SPONDYLITIS

Ankylosing spondylitis (AS) is a seronegative spondyloarthritis that usually affects young males and has a strong association with HLA27. Uveitis, bowel disease, cardiac dysfunction, and pulmonary disease are the most common extra-articular manifestations of the disease.[24,25] Involvement of the lung and pleura occurs late in the

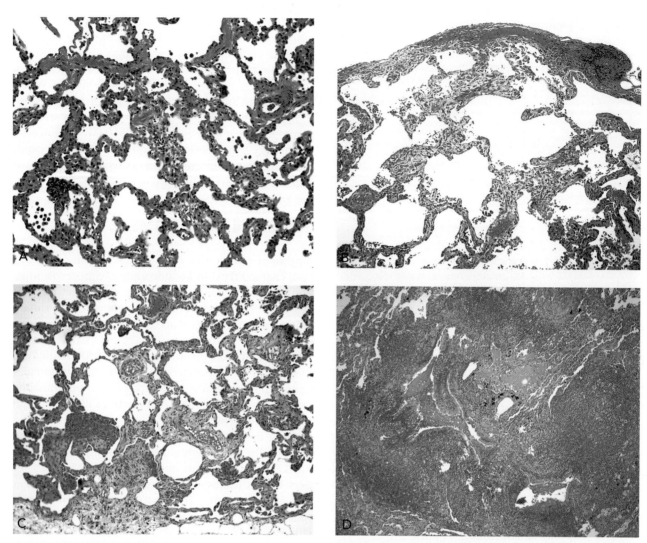

CHAPTER 19

FIGURE 19-4 Sjögren syndrome. **A:** Cellular NSIP pattern is the most common type of ILD associated with Sjögren syndrome (H&E stain). **B:** NSIP pattern with interstitial organization is often seen in ILD associated with Sjögren syndrome. Note the overlaying pleura with congestion and mild chronic inflammation, a rare finding of Sjögren syndrome compare to SLE and RA (H&E stain). **C:** Organizing pneumonia is observed in a background of NSIP in a patient with Sjögren syndrome (H&E stain). **D:** Follicular bronchiolitis is a common histologic type of small airway disease associated with Sjögren syndrome (H&E stain).

Table 19-7 Pulmonary Manifestations in Sjögren Syndrome

Location	Lesions
Pleura	• Pleuritis +/− effusion • Pleural fibrosis
Interstitium	• NSIP >LIP> OP = UIP = DAD • Amyloidosis
Airway	• Bronchiolitis +/− fibrosis • Follicular bronchiolitis • Xerotrachea
Vasculature	• Vasculitis • Pulmonary hypertension
Neoplasm	• Lymphoma

disease course and is usually asymptomatic. Pulmonary involvement consists of apical fibrobullous lesions, emphysema, bronchiectasis, and pneumothorax.[25-27]

INFLAMMATORY BOWEL DISEASE

Pulmonary diseases are among the rarest extraintestinal manifestations of inflammatory bowel disease (IBD), which may precede the intestinal manifestations in a small percentage of cases.[28] Pulmonary involvement is more common in ulcerative colitis than Crohn disease.[29,30] Airways at different levels are commonly involved and a wide spectrum of pathologic changes ranging from subglottic inflammation and fibrosis, chronic bronchitis, follicular bronchiolitis, constrictive bronchiolitis, and bronchiectasis may be seen.[31-36] NSIP, organizing pneumonia, and eosinophilic pneumonia are the patterns of ILD that may occur.[37-41] Pleuritis, pleural effusion, amyloidosis, pulmonary thromboemboli, and apical fibrosis are among other pulmonary manifestations that are seen in IBD.[42-45] It is worth noting that pulmonary manifestations in patients with IBD are most frequently drug induced.

BEHCET SYNDROME

Behcet syndrome is a systemic vasculitic syndrome characterized by uveitis and recurrent oral and genital ulcers. Pleuropulmonary involvement is reported in less than 10% of the cases and is a predictor of a poor clinical outcome.[46-48] About one-third of patients with pulmonary involvement die as a result of pulmonary complications. Necrotizing vasculitis involves all sizes of arteries, veins, and capillaries and can result in pulmonary arterial aneurysm, arterial and venous thrombosis, pulmonary infarction, and arteriobronchial fistula due to bronchial erosion by pulmonary arterial aneurysm.[49-53] Pulmonary hemorrhage and acute interstitial pneumonia are life-threatening conditions.

EHLERS-DANLOS SYNDROME

Ehlers-Danlos syndrome is a connective tissue disorder with hyperextensibility of skin and hypermobility of joints. Pulmonary manifestations in these patients include spontaneous and recurrent pneumothorax, tracheobronchomegaly, cystic changes, fibrous parenchymal scars, fibrous nodules, and pseudotumors.[54-57] The fragility of blood vessels in these patients results in pulmonary hemorrhage and hemoptysis.[58-59]

REFERENCES

1. de Lauretis A, Veeraraghavan S, Renzoni E. Connective tissue disease-associated interstitial lung disease: how does it differ from IPF? How should the clinical approach differ? *Chron Respir Dis.* 2011;8(1):53-82.
2. Park JH, Kim DS, Park I-N, et al. Prognosis of fibrotic interstitial pneumonia. Idiopathic versus collagen vascular disease-related subtypes. *Am J Respir Crit Care Med.* 2007;175(7):705-711.
3. Song JW, Do K-H, Kim M-Y, et al. Pathologic and radiologic differences between idiopathic and collagen vascular disease-related usual interstitial pneumonia. *Chest.* 2009;136(1):23-30.
4. Solomon JJ, Ryu JH, Tazelaar HD, et al. Fibrosing interstitial pneumonia predicts survival in patients with rheumatoid arthritis-associated interstitial lung disease (RA-ILD). *Respir Med.* August 2013;107(8):1247-1252.
5. Smith M, Dalurzo M, Panse P, et al. Usual interstitial pneumonia-pattern fibrosis in surgical lung biopsies. Clinical, radiological and histopathological clues to aetiology. *J Clin Pathol.* October 2013;66(10):896-903.
6. Schneider F, Gruden J, Tazlaar HD, et al. Pleuropulmonary pathology in patients with rheumatic disease. *Arch Pathol Lab Med.* 2012;136:1242-1252.
7. Kim EJ, Collard HR, King TE Jr. Rheumatoid arthritis-associated interstitial lung disease. The relevance of histopathologic and radiographic pattern. *Chest.* 2009;136(5):1397-1405.
8. Lee H-K, Kim DS, Yoo B, et al. Histopathologic pattern and clinical features of rheumatoid arthritis-associated interstitial lung disease. *Chest.* 2005;127(6):2019-2027.
9. Kamen DL, Strange C. Pulmonary manifestations of systemic lupus erythematosus. *Clin Chest Med.* 2010;31:479-488.
10. Highland KB, Garin MC, Brown KK. The spectrum of scleroderma lung disease. *Semin Respir Crit Care Med.* 2007;28:418-429.
11. Mouthon L, Berezne A, Brauner M, et al. Interstitial lung disease in systemic sclerosis. *Rev Mal Respir.* 2007;24:1035-1046.
12. Hassoun PM. Lung involvement in systemic sclerosis. *Presse Med.* January 2011;40(1 pt 2):e3-e17.
13. Hant FN, Herpel LB, Silver RM. Pulmonary manifestations of scleroderma and mixed connective tissue disease. *Clin Chest Med.* September 2010;31(3):433-449.
14. Hant FN, Silver RM. Biomarkers of scleroderma lung disease: recent progress. *Curr Rheumatol Rep.* February 2011;13(1):44-50.
15. Fathi M, Lundberg IE, Tornling G. Pulmonary complications of polymyositis and dermatomyositis. *Semin Respir Crit Care Med.* 2007;28:451-458.
16. Kalluri M, Oddis CV. Pulmonary manifestations of the idiopathic inflammatory myopathies. *Clin Chest Med.* September 2010;31(3):501-512.
17. Kokosi M, Riemer EC, Highland KB. Pulmonary involvement in Sjogren syndrome. *Clin Chest Med.* September 2010;31(3):489-500.
18. Franquet T, Gimenez A, Monill JM, et al. Primary Sjogren's syndrome and associated lung disease: CT findings in 50 patients. *AJR Am J Roentgenol.* 1997;169:655-658.
19. Hansen LA, Prakash UB, Colby TV. Pulmonary lymphoma in Sjogren's syndrome. *Mayo Clin Proc.* 1989;64:920-993.
20. Royer B, Cazals-Hatem D, Sibilia J, et al. Lymphomas in patients with Sjögren's syndrome are marginal zone B-cell neoplasms, arise in diverse extranodal and nodal sites, and are not associated with viruses. *Blood.* 1997;90:766-775.
21. Voulgarelis M, Tzioufas AG, Moutsopoulos HM. Mortality in Sjögren's syndrome. *Clin Exp Rheumatol.* 2008;26:S66-S71.
22. Kobayashi T, Muro Y, Sugiura K, Akiyama M. Pulmonary mucosa-associated lymphoid tissue lymphoma in Sjögren's syndrome without interstitial pneumonia. *Int J Rheum Dis.* 2013;16(6):780-782.
23. Kokosi M, Riemer EC, Highland KB. Pulmonary involvement in Sjogren syndrome. *Clin Chest Med.* 2010;31(3):489-500.
24. El Maghraoui A. Extra-articular manifestations of ankylosing spondylitis: prevalence, characteristics and therapeutic implications. *Eur J Intern Med.* 2011;22(6):554-560.
25. Kanathur N, Lee-Chiong T. Pulmonary manifestations of ankylosing spondylitis. *Clin Chest Med.* September 2010;31(3):547-554.
26. El Maghraoui A, Dehhaoui M. Prevalence and characteristics of lung involvement on high resolution computed tomography in patients with ankylosing spondylitis: a systematic review. *Pulm Med.* 2012;2012:965956.
27. Hasiloglu ZI, Havan N, Rezvani A, et al. Lung parenchymal changes in patients with ankylosing spondylitis. *World J Radiol.* 2012;4(5):215-219.
28. Ji XQ, Wang LX, Lu DG. Pulmonary manifestations of inflammatory bowel disease. *World J Gastroenterol.* October 7, 2014;20(37):13501-13511.
29. Loftus EV. Clinical epidemiology of inflammatory bowel disease: incidence, prevalence, and environmental influences. *Gastroenterology.* 2004;126:1504-1517.

CHAPTER 19

30. Hoffmann RM, Kruis W. Rare extraintestinal manifestations of inflammatory bowel disease. *Inflamm Bowel Dis.* 2004;10:140-147.

31. Papanikolaou I, Kagouridis K, Papiris SA. Patterns of airway involvement in inflammatory bowel diseases. *World J Gastrointest Pathophysiol.* 2014;15;5(4):560-569.

32. Mahadeva R, Walsh G, Flower CD, Shneerson JM. Clinical and radiological characteristics of lung disease in inflammatory bowel disease. *Eur Respir J.* 2000;15:41-48.

33. Butland RJ, Cole P, Citron KM, et al. Chronic bronchial suppuration and inflammatory bowel disease. *Q J Med.* 1981;50:63-75.

34. Moles KW, Varghese G, Hayes JR. Pulmonary involvement in ulcerative colitis. *Br J Dis Chest.* 1988;82:79-83.

35. Gionchetti P, Schiavina M, Campieri M, et al. Bronchopulmonary involvement in ulcerative colitis. *J Clin Gastroenterol.* 1990;12:647-650.

36. Wilcox P, Miller R, Miller G, et al. Airway involvement in ulcerative colitis. *Chest.* 1987;92:18-22.

37. Haralambou G, Teirstein AS, Gil J, et al. Bronchiolitis obliterans in a patient with ulcerative colitis receiving mesalamine. *Mt Sinai J Med.* 2001;68:384-388.

38. Heatley RV, Thomas P, Prokipchuk EJ, et al. Pulmonary function abnormalities in patients with inflammatory bowel disease. *Q J Med.* 1982;51:241-250.

39. Balestra DJ, Balestra ST, Wasson JH. Ulcerative colitis and steroid-responsive, diffuse interstitial lung disease. A trial of N = 1. *JAMA.* 1988;260:62-64.

40. Chikano S, Sawada K, Ohnishi K, Fukunaga K, Tanaka J, Shimoyama T. Interstitial pneumonia accompanying ulcerative colitis. *Intern Med.* 2001;40:883-886.

41. Hotermans G, Benard A, Guenanen H, et al. Nongranulomatous interstitial lung disease in Crohn's disease. *Eur Respir J.* 1996;9:380-382.

42. Orii S, Chiba T, Nakadate I, et al. Pleuropericarditis and disseminated intravascular coagulation in ulcerative colitis. *J Clin Gastroenterol.* 2001;32:251-254.

43. Abu-Hijleh M, Evans S, Aswad B. Pleuropericarditis in a patient with inflammatory bowel disease: a case presentation and review of the literature. *Lung.* 2010;188:505-510.

44. Smith PA, Crampton JR, Pritchard S, Li C. Pneumothorax as a presenting feature of granulomatous disease of the lung in a patient with Crohn's disease. *Eur J Gastroenterol Hepatol.* 2009;21:237-240.

45. Desai D, Patil S, Udwadia Z, Maheshwari S, Abraham P, Joshi A. Pulmonary manifestations in inflammatory bowel disease: a prospective study. *Indian J Gastroenterol.* 2011;30:225-228.

46. Chajek T, Fainaru M. Behçet's disease. Report of 41 cases and a review of the literature. *Medicine (Baltimore).* 1975;54(3):179-196.

47. Efthimiou J, Johnston C, Spiro SG, et al. Pulmonary disease in Behçet's syndrome. *Q J Med.* 1986;58(227):259-280.

48. Erkan F, Kiyan E, Tunaci A. Pulmonary complications of Behçet's disease. *Clin Chest Med.* 2002;23(2):493-503.

49. Grosso V, Boveri E, Bogliolo L, et al. Diffuse alveolar hemorrhage as a manifestation of Behçet disease. *Reumatismo.* 2013;24;65(3):138-141.

50. Kanchinadham S, Potikuri D. Multiple pulmonary arterial aneurysms in a young male patient with incomplete Behçet's syndrome. *Lung India.* 2013;30(1):76-77.

51. Jayachandran NV, Rajasekhar L, Chandrasekhara PK, et al. Multiple peripheral arterial and aortic aneurysms in Behcet's syndrome: a case report. *Clin Rheumatol.* 2008;27(2):265-267.

52. Seyahi E, Melikoglu M, Akman C, et al. Pulmonary artery involvement and associated lung disease in Behçet disease: a series of 47 patients. *Medicine (Baltimore).* 2012;91(1):35-48.

53. Uzun O, Akpolat T, Erkan L. Pulmonary vasculitis in behcet disease: a cumulative analysis. *Chest.* 2005;127(6):2243-2253.

54. Hatake K, Morimura Y, Kudo R, et al. Respiratory complications of Ehlers-Danlos syndrome type IV. *Leg Med (Tokyo).* 2013;15(1):23-27.

55. Kawabata Y, Watanabe A, Yamaguchi S, et al. Pleuropulmonary pathology of vascular Ehlers-Danlos syndrome: spontaneous laceration, haematoma and fibrous nodules. *Histopathology.* 2010;56(7):944-950.

56. Ishiguro T, Takayanagi N, Kawabata Y, et al. Ehlers-Danlos syndrome with recurrent spontaneous pneumothoraces and cavitary lesion on chest X-ray as the initial complications. *Intern Med.* 2009;48(9):717-722.

57. Dowton SB, Pincott S, Demmer L. Respiratory complications of Ehlers-Danlos syndrome type IV. *Clin Genet.* 1996; 50(6):510-514.

58. Yost BA, Vogelsang JP, Lie JT. Fatal hemoptysis in Ehlers-Danlos syndrome. Old malady with a new curse. *Chest.* 1995;107(5):1465-1467.

59. Shields LB, Rolf CM, Davis GJ, Hunsaker JC 3rd. Sudden and unexpected death in three cases of Ehlers-Danlos syndrome type IV. *J Forensic Sci.* 2010;55(6):1641-1645.

20 Asbestosis and Pneumoconiosis

Umar Nisar Sheikh and Timothy Craig Allen

TAKE HOME PEARLS

- Pneumoconiosis is due to the inhalation of inorganic dusts, and these can be fibrogenic dusts (eg, silica, asbestos), or nonfibrogenic or inert dusts (eg, carbon), or both (eg, silicates).
- The diagnosis of a specific type of pneumoconiosis should be based on reliable exposure history, relative risk of developing the disease after exposure, latency of exposure and temporal sequence with the onset of illness, and established link of exposure to a single disease.
- Clinical presentation of pneumoconiosis may vary from patients being completely asymptomatic (eg, simple coal worker's pneumoconiosis), to have mild to moderate respiratory disease (eg, asbestosis), to severe respiratory distress syndrome (eg, acute berylliosis). In many diseases, the advanced stage is manifested by increasing pulmonary dysfunction, pulmonary hypertension, and cor pulmonale.
- Radiological assessment is made by a comparison of International Labour Office (ILO) Classification System which employs standard chest radiography as diagnostic modality.
- Surgical lung biopsies obtained through thoracotomy or thoracoscopy are considered optimal specimen type for histopathological diagnosis.
- Asbestos fibers are of two main classes: the curved flexible serpentines (chrysolite is the major type) and the straight rigid amphiboles (of which amosite and crocidolite are the more important ones). The

amphiboles have a greater fibrogenic potential than the serpentines.
- Asbestos exposure is associated with asbestosis, localized pleural plaques, diffuse pleural fibrosis, recurrent pleural effusions, bronchogenic carcinoma, malignant mesotheliomas, and various extrapulmonary cancers.
- Silicosis, the most common type, is due to respirable free crystalline silica (eg, quartz). The silica dust is the most abundant and fibrogenic of all, and may contaminate virtually any other dust.
- Silica associated lung reactions includes acute silicoproteinosis, nodular silicosis (simple silicosis and complicated silicosis/progressive massive fibrosis), silicotuberculosis, rheumatoid pneumoconiosis, mixed dust fibrosis, diffuse interstitial fibrosis, and pleural silicosis. Patients with silicosis are at twice the risk for developing lung cancer.
- Coal worker's pneumoconiosis (CWP) is due to exposure of elemental carbon and various organic compounds, metals, and minerals; disease development is related to the cumulative exposure, the higher content of silica dust, the coal rank, and the specific duties of a worker. After implementation of Federal Coal Mine Health and Safety Act of 1969, the incidence has greatly reduced.
- The histopathologic findings in coal worker's pneumoconiosis include anthracosis, simple CWP, complicated CWP/progressive massive fibrosis, coal dust nodules, diffuse interstitial fibrosis, rheumatoid pneumoconiosis, and chronic/industrial bronchitis.

- Pulmonary siderosis, a relatively benign pneumoconiosis, develops due to exposure to metallic iron or iron oxides. The histologic findings include dust macules, mineral dust airways disease, and nodular fibrosis.
- Mixed-dust pneumoconiosis is due to exposure to mixed dust containing silica, silicates, and various metal particles. The histological hallmarks are macules, mixed-dust fibrotic lesions, and silicotic nodules. These mixed-dust fibrotic nodules should be significantly more in number than silicotic nodules to reliably diagnose mixed-dust pneumoconiosis.
- Silicatosis is caused by the inhalation of nonasbestos silicates, which are compounds of silica with magnesium, sodium, aluminum, among others. Sheet silicates are typically associated with parenchymal lung disease and include talc, kaolin, mica, and fuller's earth, etc. The histological lesions identified are nodules, mineral dust airway disease, granulomatous reaction, dust macules, progressive massive fibrosis, pleural fibrosis and thickening, and diffuse interstitial fibrosis.
- Berylliosis is a systemic disease caused by exposure to beryllium metal or beryllium compounds due to hypersensitivity to beryllium. Berylliosis is divided into acute and chronic forms. Acute berylliosis morphologically resembles pulmonary alveolar proteinosis. The diagnosis of chronic berylliosis is based on evidence of hypersensitivity to beryllium and identification of granulomatous inflammation with interstitial fibrosis in the lung.
- Hard metal pneumoconiosis is caused by hard metal dust that contains a mixture of tungsten carbide and cobalt, with other rare elements. The histologic hallmarks are presence of multinucleated giant cells filling the alveolar spaces and lining the alveolar walls, and identification of chronic inflammation with fibrosis centered on the bronchioles.

INTRODUCTION TO PNEUMOCONIOSIS

Parkes defined pneumoconiosis as "the non-neoplastic reaction of the lungs to inhaled mineral or organic dust… excluding asthma, bronchitis and emphysema."[1] It should be emphasized here that pneumoconiosis is not synonymous with occupational lung disease. Occupational lung disease involves a much broader concept and includes the reactions that may occur from exposure to fumes, gases, and other irritants in addition to dust.[2-4] These chemicals and other irritants depict various patterns of injury including, but not limited to, diffuse alveolar damage and hypersensitivity pneumonia which are discussed elsewhere in this book. Pneumoconiosis is primarily due to the inhalation of inorganic dusts, and the reaction of the lungs to these dusts is generally fibrosis. The histopathologic findings in these conditions can resemble those in interstitial, fibrotic, and granulomatous diseases of the lung, so it is prudent for a surgical pathologist to gain familiarity to certain diagnostic features. The principal cause of the pneumoconiosis is work-related exposure; environmental exposures have rarely given rise to these diseases.

Pneumoconiosis—Types

The primary or classic pneumoconiosis are asbestosis, silicosis, and coal workers' pneumoconiosis. Other forms of pneumoconiosis can be caused by inhaling dusts containing iron, silicates (kaolin, mica, talc), beryllium, hard metal, among other dusts. There is also a form called mixed-dust pneumoconiosis.

Pneumoconiosis—Pathogenesis

The reaction of the lung to any dust will depend on a number of independent factors which include the physical properties of dust particles (size, chemical composition, mineralogic property, immunogenicity), the length and magnitude of exposure, the individual susceptibility of host, and many other factors.[1-5] The dust particles ranging in size from 1 to 5 μm have the highest probability of deposition and retention within the respiratory tract. There is generally a latency period of years to decades between the onset of exposure and the development of clinically apparent disease.[2] Based on the intrinsic property, the classic histologic response to various dusts can be categorized into two main groups: (a) Fibrogenic dusts (eg, silica, asbestos) and (b) nonfibrogenic or inert dusts (eg, carbon, and many others). Host factors include efficiency of mucociliary clearance mechanisms and individual susceptibility due to possible other irritants, for instance concomitant tobacco smoking. Although these inorganic dust materials are the major contributory factors of the disease pathogenesis, not all patients with similar exposures develop disease. This suggests that there may be a genetic predisposition to pneumoconiosis.[6]

Finally, certain dusts types activate the inflammasomes when phagocytosed by macrophages. These innate and adaptive immune responses amplify the intensity and the duration of the local reaction. Current evidence suggests that the above-mentioned physical attributes, coupled with reactive oxygen species, macrophage-derived interleukins and cytokines, and various families of growth factors lead to lung reactions and disease propagation. These inhaled dusts are not necessarily confined to the lungs and many solutes from them may enter bloodstream and together with lung inflammation invokes systemic responses.

Cigarette smoking, as an independent prognostic factor, worsens the effects of all inhaled mineral dusts, in particular, of asbestos and silica.[1,2,7,10,24]

APPROACH TO PNEUMOCONIOSIS

The most common identifiable causes of interstitial lung diseases (ILDs) are results of occupational and environmental exposures to various inorganic or organic dusts. The diagnosis of pneumoconiosis and occupational lung disease in general is made without histologic evaluation. The diagnosis is based on a combination of clinical, epidemiological, and radiologic findings related to a history of exposure to occupational and environmental sources. The diagnosis of a specific type of pneumoconiosis should be rendered based on following information: (1) reliable exposure history; (2) relative risk of developing the disease after exposure; (3) latency of exposure and temporal sequence with the onset of illness; and (4) established link of exposure to a single disease.[7,8]

After a thorough clinical evaluation, radiological assessment of the presence, type, and severity of parenchymal and pleural abnormalities is made by comparing patient's films to the International Labour Office (ILO) Classification System. The 2011 revised edition of the guidelines supplements the preceding 2000 edition and extends the applicability of the ILO scheme to classifications of results from digital radiographic images of the chest. The standard films provide differing types (shape and size) and severity (profusion) of abnormalities seen in patients with pneumoconiosis due to asbestos, silica, and coal dust among others.[9] To date, no such standardized classification system has been proposed for computed tomography, in particular, for high-resolution computed tomography (HRCT) which is considered to be far more accurate than conventional radiography for diagnosing earlier lesions of most types of pneumoconiosis.

SPECIAL CONSIDERATIONS OF SPECIMEN HANDLING

A variety of specimens may be obtained for histologic examination in a suspected cases of nonneoplastic lung diseases. Transbronchial biopsy in general considered a suboptimal specimen to evaluate for interstitial lung diseases and pneumoconiosis. Surgical lung biopsies obtained through thoracotomy or thoracoscopy are usually desired to establish a diagnosis of diffuse interstitial lung diseases for pattern recognition owing to the large size of the specimen.[7] A standard method should be developed for handling specimens of suspected pneumoconiosis in the histopathology laboratory. If possible, a weighed portion of lung should be retained for analytic studies. A number of analytic studies can also be performed on tissue from paraffin-embedded blocks.[10] Analytic electron microscopy can be employed to identify dust particles in lung tissue.[11] The energy-dispersive form (energy dispersive x-ray analysis [EDXA]) is also a powerful technique to identify a wide range of elements with accuracy and speed.[12] Although not routinely used, mineral analysis of lung samples may prove to be a reliable technique to provide information about exposure when coupled with epidemiological and clinical information. Most of the data using mineral analysis is limited to fibrous particles such as asbestos.[12]

ASBESTOSIS

Asbestos

Asbestos is a naturally occurring hydrated silicate which is a mineral compound of silica with iron, magnesium, sodium, and other metals in varying proportions.[13] The inherent properties of these asbestiform silicates allow them to resist heat and chemical degradation and give ability to be woven with high tensile strength.[1,2,14,15] In contrast to the compact silica particles, the elongated asbestos fibers elicit a more diffuse lung reaction.[10] A detailed list of occupational and industrial settings in which asbestos exposure can occur is shown in *Table 20-1*. In general, asbestos fibers are divided into two main classes: the curved flexible serpentines (chrysolite is the major type) and the straight rigid amphiboles (of which amosite and crocidolite are the more important ones). Chrysolite fibers are the most common type used in the industry and they tend to be relatively fragile and not chemically stable under biologic conditions. Because chrysolite's fibers are relatively soluble in lung fluid, it is less likely to cause disease, and if inhaled are more readily cleared by lungs than the amphiboles. Amphibole asbestos fibers, on the other hand, are more stable and resistant, and are a culprit in a variety of reactions ranging from inflammatory and fibrosing conditions to neoplasia.[1,2,14,16,17] The ability of asbestos fibers to reach up to the terminal airways of the lung is a function of their diameter (usually length-to-diameter ratio is greater than 3; diameter less than 3 μm).[1,2,16] Although seldom clinically indicated, special techniques such as energy dispersive x-ray analysis, electron diffraction, or mass spectrometry may be used to identify specific type of asbestos fibers.[18] An increased incidence of asbestos-related cancer among household contacts of asbestos workers shows the potential hazards of very low levels of these silicates.[19-21]

Table 20-1 Work Environments and Occupations Leading to Asbestos Exposure[20]

Work Environments	
Asbestos product manufacturing (insulation and roofing)	
Automotive repair (brakes and clutches)	
Construction sites including railroads	
Mining and maritime operations	
Offshore rust removals	
Oil refineries	
Sand or abrasive manufacturers	
Shipyards/ships/shipbuilders	
Steel mills	
Occupations	
Asbestos removal workers	Demolition workers
Auto mechanics	Boilermakers
Bricklayers	Building inspectors
Carpenters	Drywallers
Electricians	Floor covering manufacturers
Furnace workers	Glazers
Grinders	Hod carriers
Insulators	Iron workers
Laborers	Longshoremen
Maintenance workers	Merchant marines
Millwrights	Operating engineers
Painters	Plasterers
Plumbers	Roofers

Diseases Associated With Asbestos Exposure

Asbestosis is defined as bilateral diffuse pulmonary interstitial fibrosis caused by the inhalation of asbestos fibers.[2,10,17,22,23] Asbestosis generally requires heavy exposure to asbestos; the severity and rate of progression of disease parallel the exposure level.[7] Diseases associated with asbestosis are listed in *Table 20-2*. Besides asbestosis, other asbestos-related disease processes in the thorax include asbestos airway disease, localized fibrous pleural plaques, diffuse pleural fibrosis, recurrent benign pleural effusions, rounded atelectasis, bronchogenic carcinoma, and mesotheliomas.[7,24] Smoking appears to facilitate the damaging effects of asbestos inhalation. The synergistic effect of tobacco smoking and asbestos exposure on the development of lung cancer is well established, with 30% to 40% of asbestosis patients developing lung cancer. Recently, asbestos has also been implicated in the development of laryngeal, ovarian, and other extrapulmonary neoplasms, including colon carcinomas, increased risk for systemic autoimmune diseases, and cardiovascular disease.[24,25]

Table 20-2 Thoracic and Extrathoracic Diseases Associated With Asbestos Exposure[2,14,24,25]

Thoracic Disease
Nonneoplastic lung and pleural disease
Asbestosis (lung parenchymal interstitial fibrosis)
Asbestos airway disease
Rounded atelectasis
Hyaline pleural plaques (most common)
Diffuse pleural fibrosis (rare)
Pleural effusions (often recurrent)
Neoplastic lung and pleural disease
Bronchogenic carcinoma
Pleural malignant mesothelioma

Extrathoracic Disease
Malignancies
Peritoneal malignant mesothelioma
Laryngeal, ovarian, and colon carcinomas
Systemic autoimmune diseases (increased risk)
Cardiovascular disease (increased risk)

Clinical Features of Asbestosis

The clinical presentation of patients with asbestosis is usually indistinguishable from idiopathic pulmonary fibrosis with progressive onset of dyspnea, worsening cough, and bibasilar inspiratory crackles with or without digital clubbing on physical examination. There is often a latency period of several years to decades from exposure to clinical manifestation. Some patients for some poorly understood mechanisms remain asymptomatic till later stages of disease. Pulmonary function tests typically show restrictive pattern, with marked reduction in diffusion capacity (DL_{co}).[1,2,7] The clinical course of asbestosis is usually one of the slow but progressive deterioration, and death is often a result of either respiratory compromise or cancer.

Imaging Features of Asbestosis

On plain chest x-ray, the typical finding in asbestosis is the presence of small, irregular opacities, usually in the midlung and lower lung zones.[26] According to ILO classification,[27] "small irregular opacities" describe irregular, linear shadows that develop in the lung parenchyma and obscure normal bronchovascular markings. The progression of asbestosis is described from a fine, reticular pattern usually at the lung bases to small, irregular opacities into a prominent interstitial pattern to the final stage of coarse interstitial pattern and honeycombing to the upper lung zones. CXR findings are rather nonspecific, however, the presence of pleural abnormalities combined with compatible clinical history increases specificity of asbestosis diagnosis. High-resolution computed tomography (HRCT) is now considered more specific and sensitive than CXR and can reliably point toward the diagnosis even in earlier stages. HRCT findings in asbestosis are consistently reproducible stage to stage for histologic findings. On HRCT, from earlier to later stages, subpleural, intralobular, small, rounded, or branching opacities correspond to peribronchiolar fibrosis (the earliest microscopic finding); thickened interlobular septa; subpleural curvilinear lines (histologically represented by combination of peribronchiolar fibrosis and atelectasis); and parenchymal bands (corresponds to fibrosis along bronchovascular sheath with architectural distortion).[28,29] With progression of disease, honeycombing is seen (histologically characterized by thick-walled, cystic spaces with a diameter of less than 1 cm).

Histologic Features of Asbestosis

Careful gross examination of the lungs and overlying pleura cannot be overemphasized in suspected cases. There is often pleural and parenchymal fibrosis typically more pronounced in the lower zones and subpleural regions in a fine, reticular pattern. Grossly, the lungs range from appearing normal to severely scarred and shrunken, and may include honeycomb change.[1,2,17,23] Bilateral parietal pleural plaques are present in the vast majority of cases and may be calcified. Although diffuse pleural fibrosis and plaques are usually footprints of an asbestos etiology of pulmonary fibrosis, diagnosis of asbestosis should not be rendered in the absence of parenchymal disease.

On histologic examination, asbestosis manifests itself in the early stages as bilateral interstitial fibrosis with or without associated visceral pleural changes and with predominantly mural or desquamative features.[2,14,17,30] The interstitial fibrosis may be patchy and subpleural especially in the earlier lesions, a feature similar to usual interstitial pneumonia (UIP). However, unlike UIP characteristic well-formed fibroblastic foci are not typically seen. Asbestos bodies, a telltale sign of asbestos exposure, are rod-like, beaded, or fusiform structures composed of asbestos fibers engulfed by macrophages and further coated by endogenous ferritin (*Figure 20-1*). The generic term ferruginous body encompasses not only asbestos particles coated with iron but also other compounds, such as aluminum silicates and glass, that may become similarly coated and instead have broad yellow or black central cores.[17,18,31] Asbestos bodies are typically found in the peribronchiolar interstitium, but, with heavy exposure, may be seen in the alveolar spaces in histologic sections, sputum samples,[32] and in thoracic lymph nodes.[33] Iron cytochemical stain may be used to highlight asbestos bodies, which impart a deep blue color. Craighead et al used discrete foci of fibrosis in the walls of bronchioles together with asbestos bodies as a minimum histologic

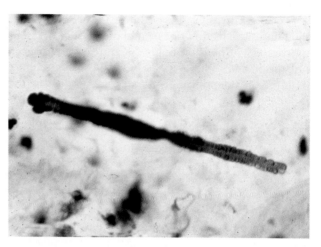

FIGURE 20-1 High-power image of an asbestos body showing a golden-brown beaded body with a clear asbestos fiber core.

criterion to diagnose asbestosis.[17] Changes associated with fibrosis include metaplastic epithelium, mild interstitial chronic inflammatory infiltrate, and mucostasis. Large honeycomb cysts, prominent smooth muscle hyperplasia, lymphoid hyperplasia, and sarcoid like granulomas, however, are exceedingly rare or unusual.[1] Hyperplastic alveolar cells may contain intracytoplasmic Mallory hyaline tissue reminiscent of that found in the cytoplasm of hepatocytes, a nonspecific finding.[34] In later stages the interstitial fibrosis becomes more diffuse and results in honeycomb lung. The involvement is more prominent in the basal segments. Based on Roggli et al,[14] the grading scheme to document severity and extent of fibrosis in asbestosis is shown in *Table 20-3*.

Table 20-3 Grading Scheme to Document the Extent and Severity of Fibrosis in Asbestosis[14]

Grade 0:	No appreciable peribronchiolar fibrosis or less than half of bronchioles affected
Grade 1:	Fibrosis confined to the walls of respiratory bronchioles with minimal involvement and involvement of more than half of the bronchioles on a slide
Grade 2:	Extension of fibrosis to involve alveolar ducts and/or ≥2 tiers of adjacent alveoli, with sparing of at least some alveoli between adjacent bronchioles
Grade 3:	Fibrotic thickening of the walls of all alveoli between ≥2 adjacent respiratory bronchioles
Grade 4:	Honeycomb changes (include microscopic honeycombing)

The change in asbestosis is often fibroelastic rather than fibrotic, a feature not seen in other types of pneumoconiosis.[35] The morphologic features are, however, not specific, and the diagnosis of asbestosis therefore requires the identification of asbestos bodies in the lesions, by conventional microscopy, electron microscopy, or incineration.[36] Digestion procedures have been developed for quantifying the content of asbestos in lung tissue. The commercial forms of asbestos (serpentines and amphiboles) may be identified in lung specimens from patients by utilizing analytic electron microscopy.[2] If asbestos bodies are not identified in routine histologic sections, specific asbestos fiber burden is typically always >2 standard deviations below the mean value when compared to histologically confirmed asbestosis cases.[37]

Pleural Plaques

Hyaline pleural plaques or pleural plaques, most common manifestation of asbestos exposure, are localized type of dense pleural fibrosis that tend to occur on the posterior inferior parietal pleura and surface of diaphragm.[1,2,17,14] It is important to diagnose correctly because it may reflect residue of healed inflammatory process unrelated to asbestos. However, it is likely related to mineral dusts exposure such as asbestos (mainly amphiboles) when the plaque is bilateral and symmetric.[2,17,38,39] The size and number of pleural plaques do not correlate with the level of exposure to asbestos or the time since exposure. The asbestos-related pleural plaques are unrelated to pleural black spots (ie, foci of accumulation of inhaled particles), suggesting that there is no pathogenetic connection between the two processes.[40] Patients are almost always asymptomatic and most cases are identified incidentally at the time of radiologic studies, autopsy, or surgery.[1,2]

On plain CXR, benign pleural plaques may be seen as focal, smooth opacities, usually less than 1 cm thick, paralleling the chest wall in profile films, or as more ill-defined opacity with irregular margins in en face images. Most asbestos-related pleural plaques are multiple, bilateral, and often symmetrical and are located in the midportion of the chest wall between the seventh and tenth ribs, following rib contours, or adjacent to the aponeurotic portion of the diaphragm and vertebral column. The prevalence of calcification in pleural plaques is reported to be 10% to 15%. The presence of bilateral, superior diaphragmatic surface calcifications with clear costophrenic angles is virtually pathognomonic for asbestos-related pleural disease.[41] HRCT scanning is reported to be 50% more sensitive in detecting pleural calcifications than conventional CXR.[42]

Grossly, the plaques are firm, discrete, slightly elevated lesions on the surface of pleura and has a shiny

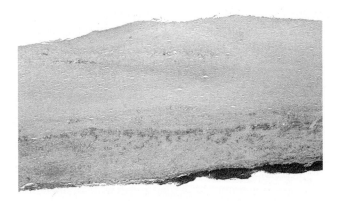

FIGURE 20-2 Low-power image of a pleural plaque showing relatively acellular fibrous pleural thickening.

surface.[1,2,14,17] Calcifications may be grossly evident.[14] Under light microscopy, pleural plaques consist of layers of dense acellular hyalinized collagen with a basket-weave pattern (*Figures 20-2* and *20-3*). There may be some fibroblastic proliferation with some nonspecific chronic inflammation around the edges of plaques, but the center is usually paucicellular. Asbestos bodies are typically not found in routine histologic stained sections of these plaques, but they have been demonstrated by the digestion-filtration techniques.[43]

Asbestos Airway Disease

Asbestos-related airway disease is usually defined by the presence of peribronchiolar and alveolar ducts thickening and fibrosis directly associated with asbestos inhalation.[2,44] The concept of asbestos airway disease is still controversial and has not gained universal agreement. It has been proposed that asbestos-induced airway may represent a precursor lesion to asbestosis.[14] Clinical findings are not well documented. Plain CXR is usually

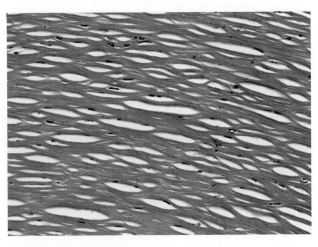

FIGURE 20-3 High-power image of a pleural plaque showing collagen bundles arranged in a basket-weave pattern.

normal; however, HRCT shows peribronchiolar fibrosis with subpleural, dot-like, branching linear opacities. Serial HRCT scan reportedly shows progression of these linear opacities to well-formed subpleural fibrosis.[28]

Histologic findings reportedly include mural thickening of respiratory bronchioles and alveolar ducts with mature fibrosis and scant to numerous asbestos bodies and dust-filled macrophages. Scant inflammatory component may also be seen.[2,44] The overall histologic appearance is reported to resemble smoking-related changes except that the amount of fibrosis is much more pronounced than caused by cigarette smoking alone. Furthermore, the fibrosis in asbestos-related airway disease is usually distal involving preferentially alveolar ducts and to some extent respiratory bronchioles, whereas it is more proximal in smoking associated changes.[44] This controversial entity requires further evidence-based studies.

Benign Asbestos Pleural Effusion

Benign asbestos-related pleural effusion is diagnosed by presence of four criteria[2,14,43] which include a reliable history of asbestos exposure, presence of pleural effusion confirmed by either radiology or thoracocentesis, absence of another disease that could cause the pleural effusion, and no malignant tumor developing within 3 years of diagnosis. Asbestos exposure rarely induces pleural effusions and estimated at 1% to 3%. It has a latency period of about 10 years from the first exposure.[1,2] The clinical presentation ranges from majority being asymptomatic to some experiencing pleuritic chest pain, cough, fever, or dyspnea. Benign, asbestos-related effusions have the same radiographic appearance as effusions due to other etiologies; the diagnosis usually is one of exclusion. Effusions are usually small, they may be unilateral or bilateral, and they tend to resolve spontaneously over 3 to 4 months, although as many as 30% recur. Some effusions are associated with pleural plaques.[28,45] Grossly, the effusions are hemorrhagic in up to 50% of cases. The fluid analysis reveal eosinophilia (25%) with normal glucose content.[43]

Rounded Atelectasis

Asbestos-related rounded atelectasis is a focal pleural-based lesion secondary to pleural and subpleural scarring which causes atelectasis of the adjacent lung, resulting in pseudotumor formation.[2,14,46] In a large series of 74 patients by Hillerdal,[46] rounded atelectasis involved predominantly lower lobes (55%) and middle lobes (39%). Patients are almost always asymptomatic and most cases are identified incidentally at the time of radiologic studies. Patients may have surgery for these rounded pseudotumor to exclude a neoplastic process.

Concomitant other asbestos-related pleural changes may also be seen.[46] On plain CXR, rounded atelectasis appears as a well-defined, rounded, or wedge-shaped mass forming an acute angle with the adjacent thickened pleura, and is usually separated from the diaphragm by interposed lung. HRCT findings include crowding of air bronchograms and the presence of a comet-tail sign, or hurricane sign, which is a curvilinear bronchovascular bundle leading into the mass.[47] Gross examination usually reveals a zone of pleural scarring and retraction associated with atelectasis of adjacent lung parenchyma producing mass effect and upon dissection, the mass usually disappears.[14,46] Routine histologic sections show marked pleural and septal fibrosis, with associated atelectatic lung parenchyma.[2,14] Lymphoid aggregates with overlying pleuritis may be seen.

Visceral Pleural Fibrosis

Visceral pleural fibrosis, also sometimes referred to as diffuse pleural fibrosis or diffuse pleural thickening, results from asbestos exposure and may coexist with pleural plaques. As the name implies, it is usually diffuse and bilateral.[1,2,14,48] About 20% of patients develop diffuse visceral fibrosis after prolonged and heavy exposure to asbestos for more than a decade.[1] Most patients are asymptomatic; those with severe disease show symptomatology of restrictive pattern of lung injury.[49] Radiologically, asbestos-related, diffuse pleural thickening is defined as a smooth, uninterrupted pleural opacity extending over at least one-quarter of the chest wall, with or without obliteration of the costophrenic angles. Pleural thickening may be difficult to diagnose using conventional chest radiographs, and differentiation between diffuse thickening and focal pleural plaques may be problematic. On HRCT scan, it is defined as an uninterrupted sheet at least 5 cm wide, 8 to 10 cm long craniocaudally, and 3 mm thick. Proliferation of extrapleural fat is a frequent finding; this presumably occurs as a response to pleural retraction.[28,50] Grossly, diffuse pleural fibrosis follows other asbestos-related diseases and is usually most severe over the lower lung zones. Rarely, in advanced cases diffuse visceral pleural fibrosis may bind the lung to the thoracic wall. Histologic findings are generally nonspecific. There is varying degree of paucicellular pleural fibrosis and thickening. Some features mimicking pleural fibrinous pleuritis may also be present. The fibrosis tends to involve the adjacent subpleural lung parenchyma in interstitial fashion for short distance. Pleural plaques, if present, show typical morphology of dense basket-weave collagenized tissue. Parenchymal changes typical of asbestosis may or may not present.[2,48] The pathologist must always keep desmoplastic malignant mesothelioma in the differential diagnosis of visceral pleural fibrosis.

Pleural fibrosis typically is acellular and lacks the storiform pattern characteristic of desmoplastic malignant mesothelioma. Furthermore, the visceral pleural fibrosis typically does not involve the lung parenchyma and lacks the independent expansile nodules, often seen in malignant mesothelioma.[2]

SILICOSIS

Silica

Silicosis is perhaps the oldest recognized occupational lung disease which had been identified in Egyptians mummies, and Hippocrates and Pliny referred to this disease.[51] Silicosis is a chronic lung disease characterized by the development of progressive parenchymal nodules and pulmonary fibrosis after the inhalation of silica.[1,2,52] On oxidation, silicon acquires oxygen radicals which upon three-dimensional networking form an average stoicheiometric formula of silicon dioxide (SiO_2).[1,2] Silica (silicon dioxide) occurs in amorphous and crystalline forms. Quartz, cristobalite, and tridymite are the three most common forms of crystalline silica, which causes silicosis. Amorphous silica is nontoxic. Silicosis occurs as a reaction to inhaled crystalline silica. Quartz is the most abundant mineral in the earth's crust and most cases of silicosis are due to quartz exposure. Occupational exposure may be direct as in stonecutting, quarry work, or sandblasting, or may be indirect when silica contaminates other dusts such as asbestos, iron, coal , etc.[65,70] A list of occupational and industrial settings in which silica exposure[53] can occur is detailed in *Table 20-4*.

Table 20-4 Occupations and Industries Leading to Respirable Crystalline Silica Exposure (1982, Bureau of Consensus)[53]

Non-mining industries
  Masonry, stonework, tile setting, and plastering
  Services to dwellings and other buildings
  Concrete , gypsum , and plaster products
  Roofing and sheet metal work
  General industrial machinery and equipment
  Medical and dental laboratories
  Combination of gas and electric and other utilities
  Miscellaneous special trade contractors
  Automotive repair shops
  Pottery and related products
Mining industries
  Oil and gas extraction
  Bituminous coal and lignite mining
  Mining and quarrying of nonmetallic minerals, except fuels
  Metal mining

Diseases Associated With Silicosis

Although recognized for decades, new cases continue to occur as shown in recent surveillance studies.[54] A number of silica associated lung reactions are identified and listed in *Table 20-5*. Patients with silicosis are at twice the risk for developing lung cancer.

Clinical Features of Silicosis

The onset of silica-induced lung diseases may be slow and insidious (classic), accelerated, or rapid (rare), depending on the intensity and duration of the silica dust exposure. A very heavy exposure of finely particulate silica dust, often in unregulated environments such as sandblasting, leads to fatal acute silicoproteinosis with a latency period of <3 years. Symptoms of cough, shortness of breath, and pleuritic pain may develop in days to several weeks, followed by weight loss and fatigue in months to years.[1,2,52] Chronic (classic or nodular) silicosis develops progressively after years of exposure to low levels of silica, with a latency period of at least 20 years. If present between 3 and 10 years, the term accelerated silicosis is sometimes used.[7] Simple silicosis patients are usually asymptomatic in earlier stages. Productive cough and dyspnea develop in more advanced stages especially with concomitant tobacco smoking owing to secondary development of chronic bronchitis. Pulmonary functions are either normal or only moderately affected early in the course, and most patients do not develop shortness of breath until progressive massive fibrosis supervenes. The disease may continue to worsen even if the patient is no longer exposed. A well-known complication of crystalline silica is to inhibit macrophage phagocytic ability against mycobacteria. This results in an increase incidence of mycobacterial (tuberculous and atypical) infections among silicotic individuals.[55] When tuberculosis sets

Table 20-5 Diseases and Lung Reactions Associated With Silica Exposure[a]

Acute silicoproteinosis
Chronic or pure nodular silicosis
  Simple silicosis (nodules less than 1 cm)
  Complicated silicosis/progressive massive fibrosis (nodules larger than 1 cm)
Conglomerate nodules
Silicotuberculosis
Rheumatoid pneumoconiosis (Caplan syndrome)
Mixed dust fibrosis
Diffuse interstitial fibrosis
Pleural silicosis
Silicotic fibrous pseudotumors
Peritoneal silicotic nodules

[a]Derived from Refs. 1, 2, 52, 75, 77.

in, fever and weight loss become chief complaints. The end-stage complications of long-term silicosis is cor pulmonale. The laboratory findings are usually non-specific and may include an elevation in sedimentation rate, presence of rheumatoid factor, antinuclear antibodies, and serum immune complexes, and a polyclonal increase in immunoglobulins especially IgG. A number of connective tissue disease (CTDs) have been linked and identified in silica exposed individuals including progressive systemic sclerosis, rheumatoid arthritis, dermatomyositis, and systemic lupus erythematosus.[56,57]

Imaging Features of Silicosis

Chest x-ray radiography in silicosis is usually positive after approximately 20 years postexposure. CXR is about 80% sensitive, and the usual findings are multiple, small (<1 cm), round and well-circumscribed, lung opacities. These opacities tend to occur in the upper and posterior regions of the lungs. These nodules are calcified in 10% to 20% of patients. With progression, the nodules may become confluent to form large opacities. This change is indicative of complicated silicosis/progressive massive fibrosis (PMF), These confluent nodules must be at least 1 cm to be classified as PMF and it occurs more frequently in silicosis than in coal worker's pneumoconiosis (discussed next in the chapter). PMF is usually symmetrical, but it may be unilateral. It appears as irregular, mass-like, or sausage-shaped opacities that are typically seen in the posterior upper lobes with associated hilar retraction.[58,59]

On HRCT, acute silicoproteinosis appears as a ground glass or alveolar pattern; no nodules are observed. The nodules of chronic silicosis on HRCT imaging are well-defined, discrete, and if present, interstitial fibrosis manifests as traction bronchiectasis, honeycombing, or large attenuations. PMF typically appears as irregular, lens-shaped, bilateral, large (>10 mm) attenuations in the posterior portions of the upper lobes in HRCT scans. These lesions are often well-circumscribed, calcified, and surrounded by cicatricial emphysema. Masses larger than 4 cm in diameter may exhibit central necrosis without cavitation. If necrosis or cavitation is seen in PMF, mycobacterial infection should always be considered. PMF can be misdiagnosed as bronchogenic carcinoma when pathognomonic characteristics, such as bilateral lens-shaped attenuations, well-defined borders, irregular calcifications, and lung nodularity, are not evident.[28,59,60]

Histologic Features of Silicosis

Acute silicoproteinosis, histologically and ultrastructurally, resembles pulmonary alveolar proteinosis. Grossly, the lung tissue is characterized by irregular zones of consolidation. Histologically, it is characterized by alveolar spaces filled with an eosinophilic, granular, PAS-positive lipoproteinaceous coagulum admixed with cell "ghosts."[61,62] Cholesterol clefts may be prominent within the intra-alveolar material. There is also a variable amount of diffuse interstitial fibrosis and irregular hyaline scars, but classic silicotic fibrous nodules are either poorly formed or absent.[1,2,52,61,62]

The gross and histologic findings of chronic nodular or pure silicosis are very similar and are characterized by the proliferation of small, discrete, hyalinized/fibrotic nodules, ranging in size from 3 to 6 mm and usually less than 1 cm, predominantly in the posterior aspects of upper lobes. The cut surfaces of these nodules are typically slate gray, firm, rounded, well demarcated, and are usually rimmed by black to brown pigmentation (anthracotic pigment) if present near or on pleural surface.[7] Bronchopulmonary lymph nodes are often involved and have nodules with similar characteristics, and often have peripheral eggshell-like calcifications.[52,56] Histologically, the earlier silicotic lesions are characterized by micronodular scars along the lymphatic network, particularly around bronchovascular bundles. In early (cellular) lesions, nodules composed of fibroblasts and histiocytes containing abundant silica particles. The developing nodules have foci of increased fibrosis with pigment-laden macrophages. The micronodules enlarge to form the discrete nodules of classic silicosis (*Figure 20-4*). The older well-formed nodules are less cellular and more like lamellated collagenized scars. Long-standing lesions may be calcified or even ossified. They may fuse to produce large masses and may undergo degenerative changes including necrosis as a result of ischemia. The edges of the nodule have a characteristic stellate shape, reminiscent of sarcoid-like naked granulomas or eosinophilic granulomas of Langerhans cell type. The arteries

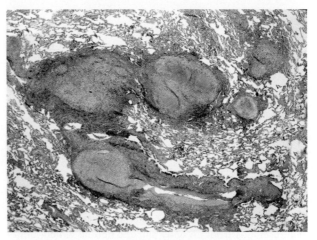

FIGURE 20-4 Low power of silicosis showing advanced silicotic nodules becoming confluent.

often show intimal and medial thickening.[1,2,7,52] The silica particles are best demonstrated under polarized light. They appear as weakly birefringent spicules with pointed ends, 5 μm or less in length, and are found both within the nodules and in the surrounding cuff of pigment-laden macrophages[63] (*Figure 20-5*). It is prudent to mention that finding only silica particles in a tissue sample does not equate to the diagnosis of silicosis. The diagnosis should be rendered when silica particles are found with characteristic collagenized or fibrous scars.[64]

Conglomerate nodules are identified in advanced stages of disease and are reflective of disease severity. They are clusters of silicotic nodules that have fused into larger (usually >1 cm in diameter) masses. The outlines of the individual silicotic nodules can still be recognized within these conglomerate nodules.[1,2,4,65,70] These should be viewed differently than complicated silicosis/progressive massive fibrosis (PMF). The defining feature of PMF is a large amorphous mass of fibrous tissue characteristically obliterates and contracts the lung parenchyma, preferentially, of upper lobe and is larger than 1 cm. PMF may also complicates other types of pneumoconiosis particularly coal worker's and asbestosis.[1,66]

Silicotuberculosis should be suspected if giant cells or granulomas are found in the capsule of silicotic nodules or PMF lesions. Larger nodules may undergo central necrosis or cavitation. If central necrosis is associated with histiocytic and granulomatous reaction in silicotic nodules, it should lower the threshold to order diagnostic workup for mycobacterial infection.[1,4,55,65]

In rheumatoid pneumoconiosis, grossly, the silicotic nodules have necrobiotic centers with light and dark laminated tissue toward the periphery. Histologic sections reveal a silicotic nodule with central necrosis surrounded by palisading histiocytes, neutrophils, fibroblasts, and collagen contributing the rheumatoid portion of the disease. Such coexistence in which rheumatoid arthritis subsumes the morphologic changes in the silicotic nodules is referred to as Caplan syndrome.[67,68]

Diffuse interstitial fibrosis, usually without typical silicotic nodules and involving significant portions of lungs, has been described in granite workers exposed to silica dust. In these patients, presence of silica dust was demonstrated by x-ray spectrometry scanning and electron microscopy. Double refractive particles which are typically found in silicotic nodes were not identified. CXR in these patients did not show typical features of pneumoconiosis.[69,70] Similarly, diffuse fibrotic lesions have been identified in foundry workers exposed to quartz admixed with cristobalite (another crystalline form of silica).[70]

Pleural silicosis, a common finding in pulmonary silicosis, manifests as dense fibrosis. Isolated pleural thickening due to silica dust may clinically and radiologically mimic malignant mesothelioma.[71] Silicotic nodules may protrude as pleural pearls. Under polarized microscopy, numerous birefringent silica particles may be seen.[72]

Silicotic fibrous pseudotumors are expansile fibrous masses in the mediastinum and peribronchial lymph nodes. They mimic sarcomas due to their infiltrative pattern of growth and local destructive behavior.[1]

Peritoneal silicotic nodules, morphologically classic silicotic nodules, have also been reported in extrathoracic sites including lymph nodes, spleen, bone marrow, liver, among others.[73] These nodules, though uncommon, almost always occur in advanced stages of pulmonary silicosis.

COAL WORKER'S PNEUMOCONIOSIS

Coal worker's pneumoconiosis (CWP) refers to progressive pulmonary reaction to inhaled coal particles and other admixed forms of dust, and the host tissue's reaction to its retention.[1,2,4,74] Coal dust is a complicated mixture of elemental carbon and various organic compounds, metals, and minerals including silicates, sulfides, carbonates, among others.[2,75] Workers of coal mines are susceptible to two types of pneumoconiosis, CWP and silicosis (discussed above). These two entities are often difficult to differentiate on conventional radiology,[76] but they show distinct histopathologic features and may have different clinical presentations as well. The likelihood of CWP development is directly related to the following: (i) the cumulative exposure to coal mine dust[2]; (ii) the higher silica dust (mainly quartz) content of the respirable dust[2,74,75]; (iii) the coal rank

FIGURE 20-5 High power of silicosis showing dust-laden macrophages from an early silicotic nodule which, under polarized light examination, show tiny silica particles with weak birefringence.

which is a measure of the geologic maturity of the coal, with different ranks having distinct physical and chemical characteristics[2,74-77]; (iv) the specific assigned duties to a worker, those who are involved in the drilling of the ceiling shafts are exposed to greater amounts of silica than those who work at the coal face.[77,78] The four major types of coal are anthracite, bituminous, subbituminous, and lignite.[2,75] The burning of coal dust produces ash, some particles of which are small enough to escape into smoke, these are termed as "fly ash." The respirable particles in fly ash consist of aluminosilicates, are angular in outline, and range in size from submicroscopic to 10 μm.[2,4] The composition of dust is another independent factor to determine the type of histologic appearance.[78] In the United States, Federal Coal Mine Health and Safety Act of 1969 placed strict controls on airborne respirable dust concentrations in underground coal mines.[79] In order to early detect and prevent of CWP, a Coal Workers' X-ray Surveillance Program (CWXSP) has been in place and administered by joint collaboration of National Institute for Occupational Safety and Health (NIOSH) with Mine Safety and Health Administration (MSHA). These combined efforts have greatly reduced the incidence of CWP and progressive massive fibrosis (PMF), the advanced form of CWP.[80]

Diseases Associated With Coal Worker's Pneumoconiosis

The disease is divided, based on radiological and histopathological features, into two main categories: simple coal worker's pneumoconiosis and complicated coal worker's pneumoconiosis/progressive massive fibrosis (PMF), depending on the extent of involvement.[1,2,74,81] The pathologic processes associated with coal dust exposure are included in *Table 20-6*.

Table 20-6 Diseases and Lung Reactions Associated With Coal Dust Exposure[a]

Anthracosis
Simple coal worker's pneumoconiosis (CWP)
Coal dust macule
Centrilobular emphysema
Complicated coal worker's pneumoconiosis/   progressive massive fibrosis
Coal nodules
Diffuse interstitial fibrosis
Rheumatoid pneumoconiosis (Caplan syndrome)
Silicotic nodules
Chronic bronchitis/industrial bronchitis

[a]Derived from Refs. 2, 4, 89.

Coal workers may also develop emphysema and chronic bronchitis independent of smoking. In contrast to silicosis, there is not enough supporting evidence that coal dust predisposes to mycobacterial infections. CWP has not been proven to independently increase lung cancer risk in the absence of tobacco smoking. Domestic indoor use of bituminous-rich coal preparations for cooking and heating is, however, associated with an increased risk of lung cancer death.[24]

Clinical Features of Coal Worker's Pneumoconiosis

Simple CWP is usually benign, causing little decrement in lung function. Patients may remain asymptomatic or have chronic productive cough. The severity of simple CWP is based on radiological extent.[81] In complicated CWP, milder forms may not affect lung function significantly. In a minority of cases (fewer than 10%), PMF develops, leading to increasing pulmonary dysfunction, pulmonary hypertension, and cor pulmonale.[81,82,83] Asymptomatic to mildly symptomatic simple CWP may progress to complicated CWP, and the presence of simple CWP also increases the risk of developing PMF.[84] If further exposure to coal dust is reduced or eliminated, it appears to halt the progression of disease to PMF in miners with simple CWP. In contrast, silicosis may still progress to PMF even after cessation of exposure.[85]

Imaging Features of Coal Worker's Pneumoconiosis

Similar to silicosis, radiographically CWP consists of multiple nodules of varying sizes. The nodules tend to be concentrated mainly in the upper lobes but they can be diffuse throughout the lungs.[86] The severity of the disease correlate well with number and sizes of the nodules; more advanced disease tend to have more and larger nodules.[87]

The chest radiograph is a relatively insensitive and nonspecific tool to identify these nodules, because both silicosis and CWP are often difficult to differentiate on conventional radiology.[76,88] In addition, CXR results may cause underestimation or overestimation of the disease extent. Moreover, normal chest radiographs do not rule out interstitial fibrosis.[88] CT scan can depict nodules that chest radiography cannot, although HRCT is best for detecting nodules smaller than 3 mm. In CWP, there is usually associated centrilobular emphysema, also best visualized on HRCT. Furthermore, CWP lesions appear as small, branching lines or ill-defined, punctate attenuations. In some cases, small areas of low attenuation with a central dot can be seen. These areas may represent either irregular fibrosis surrounding respiratory bronchioles or dust macules on dilated respiratory bronchioles. Subpleural micronodules can be seen on HRCT. These lesions can coalesce into large pseudoplaques in CWP.[28] The appearance of PMF is very similar to that of silicosis. With progression, the nodules may become confluent to form large opacities, which may also be associated with emphysema. This change is indicative of complicated CWP/progressive massive fibrosis (PMF), These confluent nodules must be at least 1 cm to be classified as PMF and it occurs more frequently in silicosis than in coal worker's pneumoconiosis (refer to imaging section in silicosis above).

Histologic Features of Coal Worker's Pneumoconiosis

Anthracosis is defined by the presence of inhaled carbon particles and is the most common lesion in coal miners' lungs. The mere presence of coal particles is not considered pathologic as it is also seen to some degree in urban dwellers and cigarette smokers. Due to the intrinsic inert nature, carbon particles, even in larger amounts, do not usually elicit any tissue reaction (ie, no fibrosis).[77] Inhaled carbon pigment reaches up to respiratory bronchioles and then engulfed by alveolar or interstitial macrophages. Histologically, it is identified as black particles/pigment, almost always, within macrophages, sometimes it may also be seen freely mixed with fibrous tissue.[7,24] These dust-filled macrophages then accumulate in the connective tissue along the bronchovascular bundles, including the pleural lymphatics, or in the lung hilus. Not uncommonly, these coal dust may get ferruginated, sometimes referred as "coal bodies." These bodies to some extent resemble asbestos bodies; however, they have a dark core in contrast to the lucent core of asbestos bodies.[1,2,81]

Coal worker's pneumoconiosis occurs when the coal dust elicits a tissue response, may be secondary to weakened host immune response. However, the lungs must be exposed for a significant amount of time to dust particles, 2 to 5 μm in diameter, in order to be retained in the alveoli.[1,2,74,75]

Simple CWP is characterized by the presence of coal dust macules with associated focal centrilobular emphysema. Grossly, these dust macules (usually 1-2 mm in diameter) are recognized by palpable, discrete, deposition of black parenchymal patches or lesions more concentrated in the upper lobes or upper portions of lower lung lobes. Pigmentation of pleural lymphatics by coal dust is one of the distinctive gross features of CWP.[1,2,89] Focal emphysematous changes may be appreciated grossly when using special barium impregnation technique (not routinely employed or needed in clinical practice).[89] These dust macules in CWP are usually more in number when compared in specimens from smokers and urban population.[90] Microscopically,

these dust macules correspond to the dust-laden alveolar macrophages and the focal emphysema is shown by dilated respiratory bronchioles surrounded by these macrophages. The macules may extend in a stellate fashion into the surrounding alveolar spaces. There is usually none to minimal fibrosis associated with these lesions.[1,2,4,89]

Complicated CWP is characterized by features of PMF with the development of large, less discrete areas of fibrosis and causing significant decline in pulmonary functions due to airway obstruction, abnormal diffusing capacity, and restrictive defects.[1,2,4,66] As mentioned above, PMF may be a feature of many different pneumoconiosis. When it occurs in CWP, grossly it is identified by large, black masses that are round, oval, or stellate in configuration and often have a central cavity obliterating large portions of the lung.[2,89] PMF nodular masses often do not respect the normal anatomic landmarks such as fissures, lobular septa, bronchi, and may traverse or destroy the vasculature.[1,2,89] Microscopically, PMF lesions consist of haphazardly arranged collagen bundles with dust particles sprinkled throughout the lesions. Endarteritis obliterans and destructive airways may be seen in the center and can be highlighted by Verhoeff elastic stain. Chronic inflammatory cells coupled with fibrosis may be seen at the periphery with vessel wall destruction leading to ischemia and subsequent central necrosis and cavitation may ensue.[89]

Coal dust nodules are nodular lesions occurring in a background of CWP, usually less than 1 cm.[1,2,89,90] Some authors advocate its presence as histologic criterion for CWP diagnosis instead of coal macules, which can also be seen in urban population, particularly with smoking habit.[90] These nodules are grossly similar to silicotic nodules, except for being black rather than slate gray. Unlike in silicosis, these coal dust nodules usually have a collarette of pigmented macrophages often surrounds the nodules, imparting a "Medusa head" appearance. These nodules are composed of coal dust admixed with fibrogenic silica dusts, leading to the formation of pigmented fibrous nodules. Hence, they are usually classified as part of mixed dust pneumoconiosis. Coal nodules are more numerous in the upper zones, but characteristically may also be found in subpleural location. These nodules may undergo degenerative changes, including calcifications and liquefactive necrosis with cholesterol clefts.

Diffuse interstitial pulmonary fibrosis has been identified in up to 16% to 20% of autopsied coal miners in some studies.[1,2,91] Grossly, the findings are similar to other diffuse fibrotic lung diseases with architectural remodeling. Histologically, there is varying degree of interstitial fibrosis, often with coal dust pigment. The end-stage cases show honeycombing.

In rheumatoid pneumoconiosis or Caplan syndrome, single or multiple well-defined nodules, often large and several centimeters in diameter, are identified on gross examination. They are preferentially situated in subpleural parenchymal tissue.[87] The cut surface usually shows concentric, lamellated dark and pale bands around the center. On histologic sectioning, they resemble classic soft tissue rheumatoid nodules with central deeply eosinophilic fibrinous necrosis surrounded by palisaded layers of fibroblasts, and macrophages with giant cells. The distinction from infectious granuloma may be challenging. The presence of giant cells and histiocytes may raise a suspicion for mycobacterial or fungal infection; however, plasma cells and palisaded fibroblasts are more characteristic of rheumatoid pneumoconiosis and rare in tuberculosis and other infections. Identification of dust rings are usually very helpful to point toward rheumatoid pneumoconiosis.[1,2,68]

Silicotic nodules may also be identified in CWP. They have less pigment and are typically densely collagenized and rounded, in contrast to the irregular contour of the coal dust nodules. The occurrence of silicotic nodules in CWP is expected due to frequent contamination of coal dust with silica particles.[2,77]

Chronic or industrial bronchitis associated with CWP is an inflammatory response in the large caliber bronchioles and main stem bronchi to the inhaled dust particles. It is histologically indistinguishable from smoker's chronic bronchitis.[4]

SIDEROSIS

Pulmonary siderosis develops as a result of exogenous iron deposition secondary to occupational exposure. The exposure is related to metallic iron or iron oxides. It is most often seen in iron workers, hematite miners, and welders (sometimes also referred to as arc-welder's lung or hematite lung), steel mills, metal alloy factories, etc.[1,2,92,93] In many instances, especially in miners and foundry workers, the exposure also contains significant amounts of silica in the workplace, resulting in a form of mixed dust fibrosis, that is, siderosilicosis, characterized by histologic features of both siderosis and silicosis (discussed later).[2,93,94]

Clinical Features of Siderosis

Pulmonary siderosis has traditionally been considered as a benign pneumoconiosis,[95] as the disease tends to be asymptomatic despite striking radiological and histopathological features.[96] Doig and McLaughlin, who first described welders siderosis in 1936, followed these cases for several years and found that about 25% of subjects demonstrated progressive radiographic reticular changes while the rest showed either no progression or had partial resolution over 9 years' time.[96,97]

They concluded that siderosis (in its pure form) was not associated with respiratory symptoms or functional impairment.

When the exposure is limited to inert metallic iron, there is minimal to absent fibrosis and patients are typically asymptomatic even with heavy exposures. When the exposure is enormous over a short period of time, the patient may depict small airway abnormalities and/or signs of emphysema. When exposed with mixed ducts, especially iron with silica, patients may become symptomatic with restrictive pulmonary pattern owing to fibrosis.[2,92,94]

Imaging Features of Siderosis

Conventional chest radiography may suggest interstitial fibrosis secondary to diffuse generalized reticular shadowing by iron pigment deposition.[92] According to Fraser et al,[98] radiographically siderosis show diffuse or micronodular opacities, more pronounced in the upper lobes, with a reticulonodular pattern.

Histologic Features of Siderosis

On gross examination, siderosis is characterized by identifying macules similar to that seen in CWP. The siderotic macules are usually red to golden brown to black due to presence of iron oxide admixed with hemosiderin particles. In severe cases, these macules may impart a striking rusty-brown gross appearance.[1,2,93] The histologic findings in siderosis include: (i) formation of macules with iron-laden macrophages in perivascular and peribronchiolar fashion; (ii) mineral dust airways disease associated with fibrosis of alveolar ducts; and (iii) nodular fibrosis.[2,99] The pigment may be found in macrophages or the interstitium, or both, with minimal to no fibrosis. The Prussian blue iron stain is helpful in identifying the iron content of the dust.[1,2,92,93] Ferruginous bodies may be observed.[100] These bodies may resemble asbestos bodies; however, they have a dark core in contrast to the lucent core of asbestos bodies. The presence of other dusts, especially silica and asbestos, may produce significant amounts of fibrosis and modify the histologic findings accordingly.

MIXED DUST PNEUMOCONIOSIS

Mixed-dust pneumoconiosis (MDP) is defined as a pneumoconiosis showing dust macules or mixed-dust fibrotic lesions with or without silicotic nodules with a history of exposure to mixed dust. The term mixed dust was coined in mid-20th century by the Europeans to describe the ferrous and nonferrous lung parenchymal lesions in foundry workers,[101-103] who were exposed to a combination of silica with nonfibrogenic silicates.[104]

Over the years, it has been realized that exposure to mixtures of dusts is a common occurrence, and in fact, most industrial exposures are mixed in nature.[7] According to Honma et al, mixed-dust fibrotic nodules should be significantly more in number than silicotic nodules in the lung to reliably diagnose MDP. Mineralogic analysis may be helpful to support the diagnosis if the exposure history is questionable.[104] Analysis typically shows the presence of silica, silicates, and various metal particles. These dust levels usually exceed the levels in general population.[12] Furthermore, MDP should be considered a diagnosis of exclusion after ruling out a specific type of pneumoconiosis. A number of occupations are associated with mixed dust exposure and diagnosis of MDP, which includes coal miners, hematite miners, quarry workers, metal miners, foundry and ceramics workers, and stonemasons.[2]

Clinical Features of Mixed Dust Pneumoconiosis

The clinical symptomatology of MDP is nonspecific and includes productive cough and dyspnea. This could be related to pneumoconiosis, smoking, or associated emphysema. Pulmonary function abnormalities are variable, and tend to be less severe than in classic pneumoconiosis.[105,106] Uncomplicated MDP follows a benign course; however, cases with diffuse interstitial fibrosis with honeycombing, may be fatal and have prognosis similar to PMF.[104]

Imaging Features of Mixed Dust Pneumoconiosis

Plain chest radiographs show a mixture of small rounded and irregular opacities as defined by the ILO standards.[10,28] In contrast, silicosis has a predominance of small rounded opacities. On HRCT, the disease is often characterized by presence of reticular, reticulolinear, or reticulonodular opacities, with areas of emphysema may be seen.[107,108]

Histologic Features of Mixed Dust Pneumoconiosis

The histological hallmark of MDP is presence of three types of lesions, to include: macules, mixed-dust fibrotic lesions, and silicotic nodules, in varying combinations.[71] Macules are usually nonpalpable lesions, similar to the macules seen in CWP, consisting of interstitial accumulations of dust-laden macrophages. They are present around bronchioles and vascular channels, with an associated delicate meshwork of reticulin fibers. Mixed-dust fibrotic lesions are palpable, irregularly contoured, stellate-shaped lesion. These fibrotic lesions resemble medusa head and have a central loosely collagenized core which is surrounded by dust-laden macrophages extending into the adjacent parenchyma like tentacles. These macules and fibrotic lesions tend to spread in a diffuse fashion into adjacent lung parenchyma, reminiscent of diffuse interstitial fibrosis pattern.[71] Silicotic nodules are rounded, firm, discrete, nodules with a whorled cut-surface. On histologic sectioning, they are usually paucicellular, fibrotic nodules with hyalinized collagen.

Under polarizing microscopy, crystalline silica shows weakly birefringent needles, whereas silicates show strongly birefringent plates.[71] The presence of crystalline silica under polarized light helps distinguish silicotic nodules from similar fibrous nodules of other etiologies. Progressive massive fibrosis or conglomerate lesions may be observed.

One of the caveats in diagnosing MDP is identifying histological hallmarks in the absence of exposure history and/or mineralogic analysis. A practical approach is to sign these cases under the diagnostic term "mixed-dust pneumoconiosis pattern."[71,104]

SILICATOSIS

Silicatosis is a type of pneumoconiosis caused by the inhalation of nonasbestos silicates. Silicates are compounds of silica with magnesium, sodium, aluminum, among others, in varying proportions.[2] The nonasbestos silicates are divided into many groups; however, only sheet silicates will be discussed. Sheet silicates are typically associated with parenchymal lung disease and include talc, kaolin, mica, and fuller's earth, etc.[2,71] The particle size significant to cause disease is usually 1 to 5 μm. Typical occupations with silicate exposure are mining and quarry work.[2] A detailed list of occupational settings where sheet silicates exposure may occur has been provided in *Table 20-7*.

Clinical Features of Silicatosis

Silicatosis usually produce mild disease. Patients are usually asymptomatic despite radiologic abnormalities. If heavy exposure occurs for prolonged periods of time, severe disease with rapidly declining pulmonary functions may occur.[1,2,109,110]

Imaging Features of Silicatosis

On various radiographic modalities, it may be very challenging to differentiate various forms of silicatosis from other pneumoconiosis. Mica and talc, for instance, are indistinguishable from asbestosis, with pleural plaques being most common finding in these exposed individuals.[99] The lung parenchymal finding in these silicates is usually characterized by a reticular pattern of interstitial

Table 20-7 Occupations and Industries Leading to Various Sheet Silicates Exposure[a]

Kaolin
Pharmaceutical industries
Ceramic factories
Plastic and rubber industries
Paper factories
Talc
Ceramic factories
Plastic and rubber industries
Paper factories
Building materials
Cosmetic industries
Pharmaceutical and insecticides manufacturing industries
Mica
Thermal and electrical insulation
Building materials
Oil-well drilling
As a filler in adhesives, cements, textures paints, enamels
Fuller's earth
Used in various industries due to its absorbent properties

[a]Derived from Ref. 2.

fibrosis, predominantly involving lower lobes. On the other hand, kaolin and fuller's earth exposure resembles silicosis, with numerous nodular opacities of varying sizes are found on imaging.[99]

Histologic Features of Silicatosis

Grossly, the lungs may appear normal, or in advanced cases may be firm due to marked fibrosis. The histological lesions identified in silicatosis are discussed below and listed in *Table 20-8*.

Nodules, one of the most common finding in silicates exposure, are gray-brown to blue in color and are usually numerous in upper and superior portion of middle lobes. While these nodules may have an appearance of medusa head nodules found in MDP and in CWP

Table 20-8 Diseases and Lung Reactions Associated With Silicates Exposure[2,111]

Nodules
Mineral dust airway disease
Granulomatous reaction
Dust macules
Progressive massive fibrosis (PMF)
Pleura fibrosis and thickening
Diffuse interstitial fibrosis

(discussed above), the degree of hyalinization and collagenization in the center correlates with the concentration of silica in the exposed dust. Some of them may have dust particles sprinkled in areas of fibrosis and giant cell granulomatous reaction. It must be emphasized here that these nodules are distinct from silicotic nodules and the nodules found in mixed dust pneumoconiosis. Under polarizing microscopy, crystalline silica shows weakly birefringent needles, whereas silicates show strongly birefringent plates.[2,71]

Dust macules are formed of dust-laden macrophages distributed in perivascular and peribronchiolar pattern, similar to the macules seen in siderosis and MDP.

Mineral dust airway disease is associated with fibrosis of alveolar ducts, with destruction of lumen may also be seen, similar to the pattern seen in siderosis. Granulomatous reaction is a unique feature seen in the workers exposed to talc, kaolin, and feldspars.[110]

Complicated silicatosis or progressive massive fibrosis have been reported in the advanced cases of talc, kaolin, mica, and feldspars exposures.[110] They are formed by the confluence of nodules with associated fibrosis, and numerous refractive particles intermixed with collagen and macrophages may be seen. Diffuse interstitial fibrosis and pleural thickening have been reported in cases of nonasbestiform silicates exposure.[2,111]

BERYLLIOSIS

Berylliosis is a systemic disease caused by exposure to beryllium metal or beryllium compounds containing dust.[1,2,112,113] Because of beryllium's characteristic physical properties, it is used in the aerospace industry for the purpose of manufacturing various equipment, ceramic parts, thermal couplings, and as a controller in nuclear reactors. Exposure may occur from these manufacturing plants as well as in the mining or extraction of beryllium.[2,113-116]

Clinical Features of Berylliosis

Berylliosis is traditionally divided into acute and chronic forms.[2,113,114] Acute berylliosis, similar to acute silicoproteinosis, develops due to massive beryllium exposure over a very short period of time. The resultant acute chemical pneumonitis is characterized by dyspnea, productive cough, chest pain, and cyanosis. Patients may clinically develop acute respiratory distress syndrome (ARDS) with a histological pattern of diffuse alveolar damage. Some patients may develop local tissue symptoms secondary to direct contact, such as conjunctivitis or nasopharyngitis, etc. The final outcome is usually complete recovery with prompt supportive therapy.[1,2,113]

Chronic berylliosis, a multiorgan disease, develops with or without documented acute disease in only about 1% of exposed workers at risk.[1,2,113] The latency of developing disease is extremely variable, ranging from few years to up to 40 years postexposure. Hypersensitivity to beryllium is thought to be the likely pathophysiologic mechanism.[1,2,114,117] To diagnose chronic berylliosis, the following criteria needs to be fulfilled: (i) evidence of hypersensitivity to beryllium by positive blood findings or bronchoalveolar lavage (BAL) beryllium lymphocyte proliferation test (BeLPT), and (ii) identification of granulomatous inflammation with interstitial fibrosis in the lung.[118-120] In chronic disease, patients may be asymptomatic or may present with insidiously progressive dyspnea and cough. Pulmonary functions show restrictive pattern, with marked reduction in diffusion capacity (DL_{co}).[1,2,113] Chronic berylliosis may have nonspecific abnormal results of blood chemistries, including hyperuricemia, hyperglycemia, hypercalcemia. Some may also show elevation of liver enzymes, angiotensin converting enzyme, and serum polyclonal immunoglobulins.

Imaging Features of Berylliosis

Acute berylliosis has the same radiographic features as of ARDS or acute chemical pneumonitis. Plain chest radiography usually shows bilateral, diffuse, hazy, ground glass opacities. Over time, these opacities may consolidate.[99,112]

Chronic berylliosis resembles sarcoidosis on imaging modalities. On plain chest radiography, chronic berylliosis shows significant hilar lymphadenopathy with associated increased interstitial markings. HRCT scan (89%) is more sensitive when compared to CXR (54%).[121,122] HRCT scans show ground glass opacities, parenchymal nodules, or thickened septal lines.[122]

Histological Features of Berylliosis

Acute berylliosis show nonspecific features of acute lung injury. A small percentage of cases with milder form of disease show interstitial edema with type II pneumocyte hyperplasia and nonspecific chronic inflammation. Most cases have severe disease, with diffuse alveolar damage with hyaline membrane formation.[2]

In chronic berylliosis, the lungs are grossly shrunken and fibrotic, with multiple nodules of varying sizes (2 cm or larger) are identified throughout the lung lobes. Only a minority of cases show extensive fibrosis or end-stage honeycombing.[2,123] Histologically, it is characterized by interstitial fibrosis often accompanied by noncaseating granulomas distributed along the lymphatic channels. The granulomas are often accompanied by chronic inflammatory infiltrate. The changes may closely mimic sarcoidosis, however, in some cases, granulomas may be poorly formed or absent.[1,2,113,114,123] Schaumann bodies and asteroid bodies within multinucleate giant cells may also be found.[2,100] With progression, these granulomas may coalesce to give rise to hyaline nodules with central necrosis; however, these are unrelated to concomitant silica exposure.[2,113] The diagnosis of chronic berylliosis can only be definitely rendered, after exclusion of sarcoidosis, by correlating the exposure history, clinical outcome, and radiographic finding. Mineralogical analysis by biochemical or physical means may be performed, but beryllium is not readily demonstrated in tissue by energy dispersive x-ray analysis.[2]

HARD METAL LUNG DISEASE

Hard metal pneumoconiosis is caused by hard metal dust that contains a mixture of tungsten carbide and cobalt, with other rare elements.[1,2,124-127] The occupational exposure to hard metal occurs in their manufacturing plants or during their use.[127] The hardness of hard metal allows its usefulness in cutting and grinding the metal tools, and most of the document cases occur in such settings. Similarly, cobalt exposure classically has been reported in diamond polishers.[128,129]

Clinical Features of Hard Metal Lung Disease

According to Churg and Green,[2] hard metal pneumoconiosis may clinically present as either IgE-mediated asthma (most common manifestation), interstitial lung disease, or syndrome resembling extrinsic allergic alveolitis. The symptomatology is according to the predominant disease, however, oftentimes the clinical findings are nonspecific. Patients usually complain of dyspnea of insidious onset and have restrictive changes with decreased lung volumes on testing. Interestingly, disease has been reported to recur after lung transplantation, even without additional exposure.[130]

Imaging Features of Hard Metal Lung Disease

Chest radiography may be normal or show nodular, reticulonodular, or reticular pattern, predominantly in cases with interstitial lung disease. Although not much data are available on HRCT findings, the typical abnormalities identified in hard metal lung disease include patchy parenchymal ground glass opacities, consolidation with centrilobular nodularity. Advanced cases may occasionally show honeycomb changes.[131]

Histologic Features of Hard Metal Lung Disease

In hard metal lung disease, the lungs are often grossly shrunken and fibrotic. The histologic hallmark is presence of multinucleated giant cells filling the terminal bronchioles and alveoli, and lining the alveolar walls. Multinucleated cells are derived both from histiocytes and hyperplastic alveolar type II pneumocytes.[12,132-134] Another distinct and helpful finding is to identify moderate amount of chronic inflammatory infiltrate and fibrosis centered on the bronchioles.[7] Lymphoid aggregates are a common finding. Due to increased numbers of macrophages, it may closely resemble DIP pattern. Uncommonly, presence of microscopic honeycomb change may mimic UIP pattern. Birefringent dust particles (cobalt, tungsten, etc) may be demonstrated within the macrophages and giant cells under polarizing light microscopy. The individual metal particles can also be identified by energy dispersive x-ray spectroscopy.[135]

REFERENCES

1. Parkes WR. *Occupational Lung Disorders.* 3rd ed. London: Butterworth-Heinemann; 1994.
2. Churg A, Green FHY. *Pathology of Occupational Lung Disease.* 2nd ed. Baltimore, MD: Williams & Wilkins; 1998.
3. Gee JBL. *Occupational Lung Disease.* New York: Churchill Livingstone; 1984.
4. Morgan WKC, Steaton A. *Occupational Lung Diseases.* 2nd ed. Philadelphia, PA: WB Saunders Co; 1984.
5. Newman L, Storey E, Kreiss K. Immunologic evaluation of occupational lung disease. *Occup Med.* 1987;2:345.
6. Yucesoy B, Luster MI. Genetic susceptibility in pneumoconiosis. *Toxicol Lett.* February 5, 2007;168(3):249-254. Epub 2006 Nov 16.
7. Travis WD, Colby TV, Koss MN, Rosado-de-Christenson ML, Müller NL, King TE Jr. Non-neoplastic Disorders of the Lower Respiratory Tract, AFIP Atlas of Nontumor Pathology, First Series, Fascicle 2, 2002.
8. American Thoracic Society; European Respiratory Society. American Thoracic Society/European Respiratory Society International Multidisciplinary Consensus Classification of the Idiopathic Interstitial Pneumonias. This joint statement of the American Thoracic Society (ATS), and the European Respiratory Society (ERS) was adopted by the ATS board of directors, June 2001 and by the ERS Executive Committee. January 15, 2002;165(2):277-304.
9. International Labour Office. Guidelines for the use of the ILO International Classification of Radiographs of Pneumoconioses, Revised edition 2011. Occupational Safety and Health Series. No. 22. Geneva: International Labour Office; 2011.
10. Katzenstein A-LA. *Katzenstein and Askin's Surgical Pathology of Non-Neoplastic Lung Disease.* (Major Prob Pathol Vol 13), 4th ed. Edinburgh, Scotland: Elsevier; 2006.
11. McDonald JW, Roggli VL, Churg A, et al. Microprobe analysis in pulmonary pathology. In: Ingram P, Shelburne J, Roggli V, et al, eds. *Biomedical Applications of Microprobe Analysis.* San Diego, CA: Academic Press; 1999:201-256.
12. Leyden DE. Energy dispersive x-ray spectrometry. *Spectroscopy.* 1986;2:28.
13. Gibbs AR, Pooley FD. Analysis and interpretation of inorganic mineral particles in "lung" tissues. *Thorax.* March 1996;51(3):327-334.
14. Roggli VL, Greenberg SD, Pratt PC, eds. *Pathology of Asbestos-Associated Disease.* Boston, MA: Little Brown; 1992.
15. Friis RH. *Praeger Handbook of Environmental Health.* Santa Barbara, CA: ABC-CLIO; 2012.
16. Churg A. Analysis of lung asbestos content. *Br J Ind Med.* October 1991;48(10):649-652.
17. Craighead JE, Abraham JL, Churg A, et al. The pathology of asbestos-associated diseases of the lungs and pleural cavities: diagnostic criteria and proposed grading schema. *Arch Pathol Lab Med.* October 8, 1982;106(11):544-596.
18. Churg A. Analysis of asbestos fibers from lung tissue: research and diagnostic uses. *Semin Respir Med.* 1986;7:281.
19. Epler GR, Fitz Gerald MX, Gaensler EA, Carrington CB. Asbestos-related disease from household exposure. *Respiration.* 1980;39(4):229-240.
20. Agency for Toxic Substances and Disease Registry. Asbestos: an overview for clinicians. http://www.atsdr.cdc.gov/asbestos/medical_community/working_with_patients/docs/overview-clin_32205_hi.pdf. Accessed November 29, 2014.
21. Schneider J, Brückel B, Fink L, Woitowitz HJ. Pulmonary fibrosis following household exposure to asbestos dust? *J Occup Med Toxicol.* November 18, 2014;9(1):39. eCollection 2014.
22. Dail DH, Hammar SP, eds. *Asbestos.* New York: Springer-Verlag; 1994.
23. Roggli, VL, Oury TD, Sporn TA, eds. *Pathology of Asbestos-Associated Diseases.* New York: Springer; 2004.
24. Vinay K, Abbas AK, Fausto N, Aster N. *Robbins & Cotran Pathologic Basis of Disease.* 9th ed. New York: Elsevier; 2013.
25. Paget-Bailly S, Cyr D, Carton M, Guida F, Stucker I, Luce D. 0234 Head and neck cancer and occupational exposure to asbestos, mineral wools and silica: results from the ICARE study. *J Occup Environ Med.* 2013;55(9):1065-1073.
26. McLoud TC. Conventional radiography in the diagnosis of asbestos-related disease. *Radiol Clin North Am.* November 1992;30(6):1177-1189.
27. International Labour Office. Guidelines for the Use of the ILO International Classification of Radiographs of Pneumoconioses. Revised Edition 2000. Occupational Safety and Health Series. No.22. Geneva: International Labour Office; 2000.
28. Akira M. High-resolution CT in the evaluation of occupational and environmental disease. *Radiol Clin North Am.* January 2002;40(1):43-59.
29. Staples CA. Computed tomography in the evaluation of benign asbestos-related disorders. *Radiol Clin North Am.* November 1992;30(6):1191-1207.
30. Hammars SP. Controversies and uncertainties concerning the pathologic features and pathologic diagnosis of asbestosis. *Semin Diagn Pathol.* 1992;9:102-109.
31. Roggli VL. *The pneumoconioses: asbestosis.* In: Saldana MJ, ed. Pathology of Pulmonary Disease. Philadelphia, PA: Lippincott; 1994:395-410.
32. Teschler H, Thompson AB, Dollenkamp R, Konietzko N, Costabel U. Relevance of asbestos bodies in sputum. *Eur Respir J.* April 1996;9(4):680-686.
33. Philippou S, Mandelartz H. [Detection of asbestos in thoracic lymph nodes in patients with asbestosis]. *Pneumologie.* June 1993;47(6):409-413.
34. Kuhn C, Kuo TT. Cytoplasmic hyalin in asbestosis: a reaction of injured alveolar epithelium. *Arch Pathol.* 1973;95:190-194.
35. Wick MR, Kendall TJ, Ritter JH. Asbestosis: demonstration of distinctive interstitial fibroelastosis. A pilot study. *Ann Diagn Pathol.* 2009;13:297-302.
36. Hyers T, Ohar J, Crim C. Clinical controversies in asbestos-induced lung diseases. *Semin Diagn Pathol.* 1992;9:97-101.

37. Schneider F, Sporn TA, Roggli VL. Asbestos fiber content of lungs with diffuse interstitial fibrosis: an analytical scanning electron microscopic analysis of 249 cases. *Arch Pathol Lab Med.* 2010;134:457-461.

38. Becklake MR. Asbestos-related diseases of the lung and other organs: their epidemiology and implications for clinical practice. *Am Rev Respir Dis.* 1976;114:187-227.

39. Churg A. Asbestos fibers and pleural plaques in a general autopsy population. *Am J Pathol.* 1982;109:88-96.

40. Mitchev K, Dumortier P, De Vuyst P. 'Black spots' and hyaline pleural plaques on the parietal pleura of 150 urban necropsy cases. *Am J Surg Pathol.* 2002;26:1198-1206.

41. Tiitola M, Kivisaari L, Zitting A. Computed tomography of asbestos-related pleural abnormalities. *Int Arch Occup Environ Health.* April 2002;75(4):224-228.

42. Majurin ML, Varpula M, Kurki T, et al. High-resolution CT of the lung in asbestos-exposed subjects. Comparison of low-dose and high-dose HRCT. *Acta Radiol.* September 1994;35(5):473-477.

43. Hillerdal G. Asbestos-related pleural disease. *Semin Respir Med.* 1987;9:65.

44. Wright JL, Churg A. Morphology of small-airway lesions in patients with asbestos exposure. *Hum Pathol.* 1984;15:68-74.

45. Bolton C, Richards A, Ebden P. Asbestos-related disease. *Hosp Med.* March 2002;63(3):148-151.

46. Hillerdal G. Rounded atelectasis. Clinical experience with 74 patients. *Chest.* 1989;95:836-141.

47. Roach HD, Davies GJ, Attanoos R. Asbestos: when the dust settles–an imaging review of asbestos- related disease. *Radiographics.* October 2002;22 Spec No:S167-S184.

48. Stephens M, Gibbs AR, Pooley FD, Wagner JC. Asbestos induced diffuse pleural fibrosis: pathology and mineralogy. *Thorax.* 1987;42:583-588.

49. Rudd RM. New developments in asbestos-related pleural disease. *Thorax.* 1996;51:210-216.

50. Tiitola M, Kivisaari L, Zitting A. Computed tomography of asbestos-related pleural abnormalities. *Int Arch Occup Environ Health.* April 2002;75(4):224-228.

51. Sherson D. Silicosis in the twenty first century. *Occup Environ Med.* November 2002;59(11):721-722.

52. Silicosis and Silicate Disease Committee. Disease associated with exposure to silica and nonfibrous silicate minerals. *Arch Pathol Lab Med.* 1988;112:673-720.

53. NIOSH hazard review. Health Effects of Occupational Exposure to Respirable Crystalline Silica. Centers for Disease Control and Prevention. National Institute for Occupational Safety and Health. April 2002. http://www.cdc.gov/niosh/docs/2002-129/pdfs/2002-129.pdf.

54. Rosenman KD, Reilly MJ, Kalinowski DJ, Watt FC. Silicosis in the 1990s. *Chest.* 1997;111:779-786.

55. Sonnenberg P, Murray J, Glynn JR, Thomas RG, Godfrey-Faussett P, Shearer S. Risk factors for pulmonary disease due to culture-positive M. tuberculosis or nontuberculous mycobacteria in South African gold miners. *Eur Respir J.* February 2000;15(2):291-296.

56. Adverse effects of crystalline silica exposure. American Thoracic Society Committee of the Scientific Assembly on Environmental and Occupational Health. *Am J Respir Crit Care Med.* February 1997;155(2):761-768.

57. Koeger AC, Lang T, Alcaix D, et al. Silica-associated connective tissue disease. A study of 24 cases. *Medicine (Baltimore).* September 1995;74(5):221-237.

58. Centers for Disease Control and Prevention. Pneumoconiosis prevalence among working coal miners examined in federal chest radiograph surveillance programs—United States, 1996-2002. *Morb Mortal Wkly Rep.* April 18 2003;52(15):336-340.

59. Kim JS, Lynch DA. Imaging of nonmalignant occupational lung disease. *J Thorac Imaging.* October 2002;17(4):238-260.

60. Ooi GC, Tsang KW, Cheung TF, et al. Silicosis in 76 men: qualitative and quantitative CT evaluation—clinical-radiologic correlation study. *Radiology.* September 2003;228(3):816-825.

61. Hoffman EO, Lamberty J, Pizzolato P, et al. The ultrastructure of acute silicosis. *Arch Pathol.* 1973;96:104.

62. Xipell JM, Ham KN, Price CG, et al. Acute silicolipoproteinosis. *Thorax.* 1977;32:104.

63. McDonald JW, Roggli VL. Detection of silica particles in lung tissue by polarizing light microscopy. *Arch Pathol Lab Med.* 1995;119:242-246.

64. Naeye RL. The anthracotic pneumoconioses. *Curr Top Pathol.* 1971;55:37-68.

65. Ziskind M, Jones RM, Weill H. Silicosis. *Am Rev Respir Dis.* 1976;113:643.

66. Leibowitz MC, Goldstein B. Some investigations into the nature and cause of massive fibrosis (MF) in the lungs of South African gold, coal, and asbestos mine workers. *Am J Ind Med.* 1987;12:129.

67. Gough J, Rivers D, Seal RME. Pathological studies of modified pneumoconiosis in coal miners with rheumatoid arthritis (Caplan's syndrome). *Thorax.* 1955;10:9-18.

68. Benedek TG. Rheumatoid pneumoconiosis. Documentation of onset and pathogenetic considerations. *Am J Ind Med.* 1973;55:515.

69. Craighead JE, Vallyathan NV. Cryptic pulmonary lesions in workers occupationally exposed to dust containing silica. *JAMA.* 1980;244(17):1939-1941.

70. Craighead JE, Kleinerman J, Abraham JL, et al. Diseases associated with exposure to silica and non-fibrous silicate minerals. *Arch Pathol Lab Med.* 1988;112:673-720.

71. Zeren E, Colby TV, Roggli VL. Silica-induced pleural disease: an unusual case mimicking malignant mesothelioma. *Chest.* 1997;112(5):1436-1438.

72. Rashid A-MH, Green FHY. Pleural pearls following silicosis. *Histopathology.* 1995,26:84-87.

73. Slavin RE, Swedo JL, Brandes D, et al. Extrapulmonary silicosis: a clinical, morphologic, and ultrastructural study. *Hum Pathol.* 1985;16:393.

74. Lapp NL, Parker JE. Coal workers' pneumoconiosis. *Clin Chest Med.* June 1992;13(2):243-252. Review. PubMed PMID: 1511552.

75. Green FH, Laqueur WA. Coal workers' pneumoconiosis. *Pathol Annu.* 1980;15(pt 2):333-410.

76. Laney AS, Petsonk EL, Attfield MD. Pneumoconiosis among underground bituminous coal miners in the United States: is silicosis becoming more frequent? *Occup Environ Med.* October 2010;67(10):652-656.

77. Davis JM, Chapman J, Collings P, et al. Variation in the histological pattern of the lesions of coal worker's pneumoconiosis in Britain and their relationship to lung dust content. *Am Rev Respir Dis.* 1983;128:118-124.

78. Laney AS, Attfield MD. Coal workers' pneumoconiosis and progressive massive fibrosis are increasingly more prevalent among workers in small underground coal mines in the United States. *Occup Environ Med.* June 2010;67(6):428-431.

79. Federal Coal Mine Health and Safety Act. Public Law no. 1969;91-173.

80. Center for Disease Control and Prevention. Pneumoconiosis prevalence among working coal miners examined in federal chest radiograph surveillance programs—United States, 1996-2002. *MMWR Morb Mortal Wkly Rep.* 2003;52:336-340.

81. Wade WA, Petsonk EL, Young B, Mogri I. Severe occupational pneumoconiosis among West Virginian coal miners: one hundred thirty-eight cases of progressive massive fibrosis compensated between 2000 and 2009. *Chest.* June 2011;139(6):1458-1462.

82. Vallyathan V, Brower PS, Green FHY, Attfield MD. Radiographic and pathologic correlation of coal workers' pneumoconiosis. *Am J Respir Crit Care Med.* 1996;154:741-748.

83. Marine WM, Gurr D, Jacobsen M. Clinically important respiratory effects of dust exposure and smoking in British coal miners. *Am Rev Respir Dis.* 1988;137:106-112.

84. Criteria for a recommended standard, Occupational exposure to respirable coal mine dust, Publication No. 95-106, National Institute for Occupational Safety and Health, US Department of Health and Human Services, NIOSH, 1995.

85. Joy GJ, Colinet JF, Landen DD. Coal workers' pneumoconiosis prevalence disparity between Australia and the United States. *Mining Engineering.* 2012;64(7):65-71.

86. Stark P, Jacobson F, Shaffer K. Standard imaging in silicosis and coal worker's pneumoconiosis. *Radiol Clin North Am.* 1992;30:1147-1154.

87. Remy-Jardin M, Remy J, Farre I, Marquette CH. Computed tomographic evaluation of silicosis and coal workers' pneumoconiosis. *Radiol Clin North Am.* November 1992;30(6):1155-1176.

88. Chong S, Lee KS, Chung MJ, Han J, Kwon OJ, Kim TS. Pneumoconiosis: comparison of imaging and pathologic findings. *Radiographics.* January-February 2006;26(1):59-77.

89. Kleinerman J, et al. Pathology standards for coal workers' pneumoconiosis. Report of the Pneumoconiosis Committee of the College of American Pathologists to the National Institute for Occupational Safety and Health. *Arch Pathol Lab Med.* July 1979;103(8):375-432.

90. Fisher ER, Watkins G, Lam NV, et al. Objective pathological diagnosis of coal worker's pneumoconiosis. *JAMA.* May 8, 1981 8;245(18):1829-1834.

91. Baum GL, Crapo JD, Celli BR. *Textbook of Pulmonary Diseases.* Vol 1. Philadelphia, PA: Lippincott-Raven; 1998:683-692.

92. Sferlazza SJ, Beckett WS. The respiratory health of welders. *Am Rev Respir Dis.* May 1991;143(5 pt 1):1134-1148.

93. Kleinfeld M, Messite J, Kooyman O, Shapiro J. Welders' siderosis. *Arch Environm Hlth.* 1969;19:70-73.

94. Funahashi A, Schlueter DP, Pintar K, Bemis EL, Siegesmund KA. Welders' pneumoconiosis: tissue elemental microanalysis by energy dispersive x ray analysis. *Br J Ind Med.* January 1988;45(1):14-18.

95. Billings CG, Howard P. Occupational siderosis and welders' lung: a review. *Monaldi Arch Chest Dis.* 1993;48:304-314.

96. Doig AT, McLaughlin AIG. Clearing of X-ray shadows in welders' siderosis. *Lancet.* 1948;1:789-791.

97. Doig AT, McLaughlin AIG. X-ray appearances of the lungs of electric arc welders. *Lancet.* 1936;1:771-775.

98. Fraser RS, Müller NL, Colman N, Pare PD, eds. Inhalation of inorganic dust (pneumoconiosis). In: *Fraser and Pares Diagnosis of Disease of the Chest.* 4th edition. Philadelphia, PA: WB Saunders Company; 1999:2386-2484.

99. Roggli VL. Rare pneumoconioses: metalloconioses. In: Saldana MJ, ed. Pathology of Pulmonary Disease. Philadelphia, PA: Lippincott; 1994:411-422.

100. Roggli VL. Asbestos bodies and non-asbestos ferruginous bodies. In: Roggli VL, Oury TD, Sporn TA, eds. Pathology of Asbestos-Associated Diseases. New York: Springer; 2004:34-37.

101. Uehlinger E. Über Mischstaubpneumokoniosen. *Schweiz Z Pathol Bakt.* 1946;9:692-700.

102. Harding HE, Gloyne RS, McLaughlin AIG. *Industrial Lung Diseases of Iron and Steel Foundry Workers.* London: HMSD; 1950:3.

103. Harding HE, McLaughlin AIG. Pulmonary fibrosis in nonferrous foundry workers. *Br J Ind Med.* 1955;12:92-99.

104. Honma K, Abraham JL, Chiyotani K, et al. Proposed criteria for mixed-dust pneumoconiosis: definition, descriptions, and guidelines for pathologic diagnosis and clinical correlation. *Hum Pathol.* December 2004;35(12):1515-1523.

105. Oxman AD, Muir DCF, Shannon HS, et al. Occupational dust exposure and chronic obstructive pulmonary disease. A systematic overview of the evidence. *Am Rev Respir Dis.* 1993; 148:38-48.

106. Bégin R, Filion R, Ostiguy G. Emphysema in silica- and asbestos-exposed workers seeking compensation. A CT scan study. *Chest.* 1995;108:647-655.

107. Shida H, Chiyotani K, Honma K, et al. Radiologic and pathologic characteristics of mixed dust pneumoconiosis. *Radiographics.* 1996;16:483-498.

108. Mester Á, Németh L, Makó E, et al. High resolution computed tomography (HRCT) of pneumoconiosis. *Cent Eur J Occup Environ Med.* 1998;4:114-129.

109. Vallyathan NV, Craighead JE. Pulmonary pathology in workers exposed to nonasbestiform talc. *Hum Pathol.* January 1981;12(1):28-35.

110. Morgan WK, Donner A, Higgins IT, Pearson MG, Rawlings W Jr. The effects of kaolin on the lung. *Am Rev Respir Dis.* October 1988;138(4):813 820.

111. Monso E, Tura JM, Marsal M, Morell F, Pujadas J, Morera J. Mineralogical microanalysis of idiopathic pulmonary fibrosis. *Arch Environ Health.* May-June 1990;45(3):185-188.

112. Meyer KC. Beryllium and lung disease. *Chest.* 1994;106:942-946.

113. Kriebel D, Brain JD, Sprince NL, Kazemi H. The pulmonary toxicity of beryllium. *Am Rev Respir Dis.* 1988;137:464-473.

114. Newman LS, Kreiss K, King TE, Seay S, Campbell PA. Pathologic and immunologic alterations in early stages of beryllium disease: re-examination of disease definition and natural history. *Am Rev Respir Dis.* 1989;139:1479-1446.

115. Kotloff RM, Richman PS, Greenacre JK, Rossman MD. Chronic beryllium disease in a dental laboratory technician. *Am Rev Respir Dis.* 1993;147:205-207.

116. Cullen MR, Kominsky JR, Rossman MD, et al. Chronic beryllium disease in a precious metal refinery. *Am Rev Respir Dis.* 1987;135:201-208.

117. Kreiss K, Mroz MM, Zhen B, Martyny JW, Newman LS. Epidemiology of beryllium sensitization and disease in nuclear workers. *Am Rev Respir Dis.* 1993;148:985-991.

118. Barna BP, Culver DA, Yen-Lieberman B, Dweik RA, Thomassen MJ. Clinical application of beryllium lymphocyte proliferation testing. *Clin Diagn Lab Immunol.* November 2003;10(6):990-994.

119. Newman LS. Significance of the blood beryllium lymphocyte proliferation test. *Environ Health Perspect.* October 1996;104(suppl 5):953-956.

120. Rossman MD, Kern JA, Elias JA, et al. Proliferative response of bronchoalveolar lymphocytes to beryllium. A test for chronic beryllium disease. *Ann Intern Med.* May 1988;108(5):687-693.

121. Saber W, Dweik RA. A 65-year-old factory worker with dyspnea on exertion and a normal chest x-ray. *Cleve Clin J Med.* November 2000;67(11):791-792, 794, 797-798, 800.

122. Newman LS, Buschman DL, Newell JD Jr, Lynch DA. Beryllium disease: assessment with CT. *Radiology.* March 1994;190(3):835-840.

123. Freiman DG, Hardy HL. Beryllium disease. The relation of pulmonary pathology to clinical course and prognosis based on a study of 130 cases from the U.S. beryllium case registry. *Hum Pathol.* March 1970;1(1):25-44.

124. Anttila S, Sutinen S, Paananen M, et al. Hard metal lung disease: a clinical, histological, ultrastructural and X-ray microanalytical study. *Eur J Respir Dis.* August 1986;69(2):83-94.

125. Davison AG, Haslam PL, Corrin B, et al. Interstitial lung disease and asthma in hard-metal workers: bronchoalveolar lavage, ultrastructural, and analytical findings and results of bronchial provocation tests. *Thorax.* February 1983;38(2):119-128.

126. Skluis-Cremer GK, Glyn Thomas R, Solomon A. Hard-metal lung disease. A report of 4 cases. *S Afr Med J.* May 2, 1987;71(9):598-600.

127. Sprince NL, Oliver LC, Eisen EA, Greene RE, Chamberlin RI. Cobalt exposure and lung disease in tungsten carbide production. A cross-sectional study of current workers. *Am Rev Respir Dis.* November 1988;138(5):1220-1226.

CHAPTER 20

128. Nemery B, Nagels J, Verbeken E, et al. Rapidly fatal progression of cobalt lung in a diamond polisher. *Am Rev Respir Dis.* 1990;141:1373-1378.

129. Nemery B, Casier P, Roosels D, et al. Survey of cobalt exposure and respiratory health in diamond polishers. *Am Rev Respir Dis.* 1992;145:610-616.

130. Frost AE, Keller CA, Brown RW, et al. Giant cell interstitial pneumonitis: disease recurrence in the transplanted lung. *Am Rev Respir Dis.* 1993;148:1401-1404.

131. Dunlop P, Müller NL, Wilson J, Flint J, Churg A. Hard metal lung disease: high resolution CT and histologic correlation of the initial findings and demonstration of interval improvement. *J Thorac Imaging.* November 2005;20(4):301-304.

132. Demedts M, Gheysens B, Nagels J, et al. Cobalt lung in diamond polishers. *Am Rev Respir Dis.* June 1984;130(1):130-135.

133. Demedts M, Gyselen A. [The cobalt lung in diamond cutters: a new disease]. *Verh K Acad Geneeskd Belg.* 1989;51(6):559-581.

134. Lison D, Lauwerys R, Demedts M, Nemery B. Experimental research into the pathogenesis of cobalt/hard metal lung disease. *Eur Respir J.* May 1996;9(5):1024-1028.

135. Stettler LE, Groth DH, Platek SF. Automated characterization of particles extracted from human lungs: three cases of tungsten carbide exposure. *Scan Electron Microsc.* 1983;I:439-448.

Acute Lung Injury

Timothy Craig Allen and Melanie C. Bois

TAKE HOME PEARLS

- Open lung biopsy in acute lung injury is the gold standard for pathologic diagnosis of patients with diffuse pulmonary infiltrates in the absence of a defined cause.
- Organizing pneumonia is characterized histologically by plugs of spindled fibroblasts and myofibroblasts. It may be associated with a known etiology, idiopathic in nature, or a component in a constellation of findings that compose a specific clinicopathologic diagnosis.
- Diffuse alveolar damage is the most common histologic finding in patients with a clinical diagnosis of acute lung injury or acute respiratory distress syndrome.
- Pulmonary edema may develop under a host of environmental and clinical conditions, including cardiogenic, noncardiogenic, during pulmonary reexpansion, or in association with high altitudes.

APPROACH TO ACUTE LUNG INJURY

The mortality in acute lung injury (ALI) is high, even with a trend toward improved survival in recent years. Forty-three percent of patients do not survive their acute pulmonary insult.[1] Acute respiratory distress syndrome (ARDS), as defined by the American European Consensus Conference (AECC) developed in 1994, include a PaO_2:$FiO_2 \leq 200$, bilateral infiltrates on chest radiograph consistent with pulmonary edema, and no evidence of cardiac failure. In patients with less profound hypoxia, a diagnosis of ALI is made when patients meet the criteria of a PaO_2:FiO_2 ratio in the range of 201 to 300, holding the remaining criteria constant. Both ALI and ARDS have acute-onset clinical presentations.[2]

The role of biopsy in ALI/ARDS is multifactorial. Patients benefit from histologic evaluation of their disease process by confirming or refuting the diagnosis, identification of infectious agents, and evaluation of the amount of fibrosis present.[3,4] The degree of fibrosis is prognostically important because patients with the worst outcomes in ALI/ARDS are those who typically develop significant pulmonary fibrosis as their lungs heal from the acute injury, rather than returning to a generally normal architecture. This irreversible, increased fibrosis leads to decreased oxygenation and pulmonary compliance, worsening patient outcome.[3]

Transbronchial biopsy may occasionally aid in the diagnosis of a patient with diffuse infiltrates. While its diagnostic yield trumps that of bronchoalveolar lavage, the majority of patients with diagnostically difficult disease require open-lung biopsy (OLB) for diagnosis.[5] In one study by Papazian and colleagues, 78% of patients with suspected acute lung injury and a negative bronchoalveolar lavage benefited from open lung biopsy, with addition of new pharmacologic agents and improved survival.[3] The safety and utility of open lung biopsy in patients with ALI/ARDS has been well documented.[6,7] OLB remains the gold standard in diagnostic evaluation of patients with diffuse infiltrates in the absence of a defined cause.[5]

SPECIAL CONSIDERATIONS OF SPECIMEN HANDLING

Evaluation of an open lung biopsy by frozen section is not uncommon. The utility of this initial evaluation will be to assess for adequacy or the need intraoperative cultures that may aid review of the permanent section.

The OLB providing the best diagnostic yield typically samples at least three lobules, correlating to an approximate size of $2.0 \times 1.0 \times 1.0$ cm, not including the stapled surgical margin. Correlation with clinical information is imperative, as patients who are immunocompromised require the histologic aid of special stains for microorganisms.[8]

While the diagnostic criteria for ARDS and ALI include diffuse pulmonary infiltrates on imaging, the possibility for sampling error still exists. Care must be taken by the surgeon to avoid areas with nonspecific fibrosis such as the apex of the upper lobes and lingula, which may interfere with diagnosis of the patient's acute process. Surgeons must also take care to sample relatively normal appearing lung parenchyma as well as the transition zone between normal-appearing and more fibrotic lung parenchyma in order to avoid sampling only nonspecific end-stage lung change. When these criteria are followed, OLB can be highly beneficial to patient care. In a study by Patel and colleagues, a diagnosis other than diffuse alveolar damage (DAD)—the histologic counterpart to the clinical diagnosis of ARDS—was made in 60% of patients receiving OLB. Common alternative diagnoses included infection, alveolar hemorrhage, and organizing pneumonia.[6]

ORGANIZING PNEUMONIA

Organization is a manifestation of lung injury to a wide range of insults. It results in a distinct histologic pattern characterized by plugs of spindled fibroblasts and myofibroblasts creating "Masson bodies." This response represents the pulmonary parenchyma's attempt at healing and has two possible outcomes: reestablishment of normal architecture or diffuse fibrosis.[9] Organizing pneumonia (OP) is a histologic finding that may been seen in three different clinical situations: (1) as its own disease entity without a known etiology, so-called "cryptogenic organizing pneumonia," or COP (2) as a nonspecific healing response after a known pulmonary insult, called "secondary organizing pneumonia," and (3) as component of a histologic pattern that confers a different, specific pathologic diagnosis.[10]

Diseases Associated With Organizing Pneumonia

Cryptogenic, or primary, organizing pneumonia is idiopathic by definition, and falls under the clinical classification of an idiopathic interstitial pneumonia.[11] COP is a diagnosis of exclusion, and the diagnosis is only rendered after other possible causative insults have been excluded.[12] The term COP has been recommended by the American Thoracic Society/European Respiratory Society since 2002, replacing the no-longer-used term for idiopathic organizing pneumonia: bronchiolitis obliterans organizing pneumonia (BOOP). This change in terminology occurred because of the similarity of the terms "bronchiolitis obliterans" and "obliterative bronchiolitis," terms that sound similar but in fact define very different clinical and pathologic entities. Unfortunately, the term BOOP still lingers in the literature in reference to the same idiopathic clinicopathologic diagnosis as COP.[12] There is marked clinical importance to the diagnosis of COP, as patients respond well to systemic corticosteroid treatment.[13]

When a specific disease association can be identified, OP is termed secondary organizing pneumonia or "organizing pneumonia associated with [underlying disease]." A large number of etiologies have been associated with pulmonary injury that is histologically arranged in an organizing pneumonia pattern (*Table 21-1*). Some of the more common entities causing secondary organizing pneumonia include prescription and illicit drug reactions, collagen vascular diseases, and immunodeficiency states. Bacterial infections, especially *Streptococcus pneumoniae*, *Legionella pneumophila*, *Mycoplasma pneumoniae*, *Nocardia asteroides*, *Chlamydia pneumoniae*, and *Staphylococcus aureus*, have been associated with the histologic features of OP.[14] Notably, no histologic criteria are able to differentiate cryptogenic organizing pneumonia from OP secondary to another cause.[9]

Organizing pneumonia itself may be histologically identified in association with other entities within the lung. For instance, nonspecific interstitial pneumonia (NSIP), respiratory bronchiolitis-associates interstitial lung disease (RBILD), and hypersensitivity pneumonitis are clinicopathologic entities in which organizing pneumonia may be seen, or may be a component (*Table 21-2*).

Clinical Features of Organizing Pneumonia

Organizing pneumonia, whether COP or secondary OP, has an insidious onset likened to a cold or flu. Characteristic symptoms of malaise, nonproductive

Table 21-1 Entities Associated With Organizing Pneumonia

Drug reactions
Common Prescription
Amiodarone, bleomycin, carbamazepine, interferon-α, -β, methotrexate
Uncommon Prescription
Acebutolol, doxorubicin, mesalamine, sulfasalazine, nitrofurantoin, sirolimus
Illicit
Cocaine

Collagen vascular diseases
Systemic lupus erythematosus
Rheumatoid arthritis
Sjögren syndrome
Ankylosing spondylitis
Polymyalgia rheumatic
Polymyositis dermatomyositis
Systemic sclerosis
Behcet disease
Mixed connective tissue disorder

Infection
Bacterial (including mycoplasma), viral, fungal, parasitic

Immunodeficiency
HIV
Common variable immunodeficiency syndrome
Organ transplantation

Malignancy
Hematologic
Solid organ

External factors
Radiation therapy
Toxic fumes
Smoke inhalation

Used with permission of Ref. 14.

Table 21-2 Organizing Pneumonia as a Component in the Diagnosis of Other Clinicopathologic Entities

Nonspecific organizing pneumonia (NSIP)

Respiratory bronchiolitis associated interstitial lung disease (RB-ILD)

Hypersensitivity pneumonitis

Granulomatosis with polyangiitis (Wegener granulomatosis)

cough, fever, and dyspnea frequently lead patients to undergo a trial of antibiotics, as physicians often interpret these patients' nondescript symptoms as a pneumonia.[14,15] Three-fourths of patients who develop COP or secondary OP are current or former smokers.[15]

Physical examination demonstrates inspiratory crackles in half to three-fourths of patients, with crackles being more common in the cases of secondary OP. Findings of chronic respiratory disease such as clubbing are extremely rare. Laboratory values often show leukocytosis, elevated erythrocyte sedimentation rate, and elevated C-reactive protein.[15]

Imaging Features of Organizing Pneumonia

Two classic imaging patterns are associated with OP. The most common pattern seen in approximately three-fourths of patients is that of changing multifocal peripheral consolidations, in which peripheral foci of consolidations vary over the time course of several weeks. The remaining 25% of patients will have a bronchocentric pattern with prominent consolidation around large bronchovascular bundles. While a host of minor patterns have also been uncommonly associated with OP, key features that narrow the differential diagnosis are that of spontaneous regression and temporal migration of opacities within the lung.[10]

There are no specific findings able to differentiate cryptogenic from secondary OP. The reverse halo sign on imaging—a central area of ground glass opacity, with peripheral consolidation— was first used to describe COP; however, it has since been shown to lack specificity for this entity.[16] Indeed, the reverse halo sign is commonly identified in not only COP and secondary organizing pneumonia, but numerous other clinicopathologic entities as well.

Histologic Features of Organizing Pneumonia

The histogenesis of OP occurs following a wide variety of acute lung insults that are of sufficient strength or intensity to result in pneumocyte injury and death. Subsequent disruption to the integrity of the basement membrane of the alveolar space leads to increased alveolar wall permeability. Plasma proteins and inflammatory cells then readily leak into alveolar spaces and are exposed to intracellular debris from dying pneumocytes, resulting in activation of the coagulation cascade and formation of abundant airspace fibrin. The inflammatory milieu in the airspaces in turn initiates the differentiation of a select population of fibroblasts into myofibroblasts.

At this stage, the histologic pattern of OP may be appreciated as loose plugs of spindled fibroblasts and myofibroblasts in bronchioles, alveolar ducts and spaces, resting in a myxoid-appearing matrix.[9] These characteristic spindled plugs termed Masson bodies, represent the lung's attempt at healing (*Figures 21-1 and 21-2*). They are generally accompanied by an interstitial inflammatory infiltrate.[17] As these plugs of fibroblasts and myofibroblasts continue to organize, the ground substance is generally resorbed, and resolution occurs with the reestablishment of normal airway architecture.[10]

Differential Diagnosis of Organizing Pneumonia

The constellation of imaging and clinical findings with an emphasis on temporal migration and spontaneous regression suggests four entities: eosinophilic pneumonia, vasculitis, alveolar hemorrhage, and OP.[10,17]

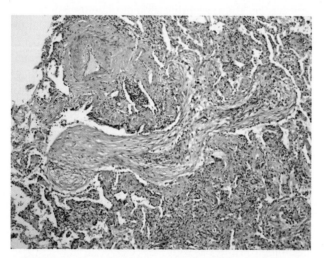

FIGURE 21-1 Organizing pneumonia presents as airspace plugs of spindled fibroblasts and myofibroblasts in a background of ground substance. These characteristic plugs are known as Masson bodies (10× hematoxylin and eosin [H&E]).

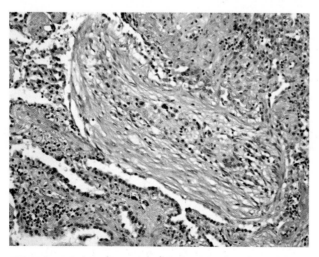

FIGURE 21-2 Higher power showing a plug of organizing pneumonia within an airspace (20× H&E).

While clinical and radiologic examination may assist in limiting the differential diagnoses, for example, the detection of autoantibodies in the patient's serum, OLB may be required for definitive diagnosis.

As noted, the presence of the histologic pattern of OP does not allow for a clinical diagnosis, and no distinguishing histologic features allow for the diagnosis COP as opposed to secondary OP caused by a preexisting insult. As such, OP must be correlated with clinical information in order that definitive and timely treatment may be provided.

DIFFUSE ALVEOLAR DAMAGE

The most common histopathologic correlate of ARDS and ALI is diffuse alveolar damage (DAD). Although ARDS does not describe a histologic finding, approximately 40% of patients with the clinical diagnosis of ARDS or ALI will demonstrate DAD on OLB.[6]

Diseases Associated With Diffuse Alveolar Damage

DAD is a nonspecific pattern of injury demonstrated by the lung in the acute setting. It is a common histologic manifestation in a wide variety of pulmonary injuries.[18] Etiologic factors that have been associated with DAD include numerous infections, including fungal, parasitic, bacterial, and viral infections, as well as exposure to environmental inhalants and ingestants, chemotherapy, drugs such as amiodarone, and systemic illnesses such as leukemic blast crisis[8] (*Table 21-3*). DAD may also occur as a idiopathic entity, for which the term "Hamman-Rich syndrome" has been historically applied.[9]

Clinical Features of Diffuse Alveolar Damage

Clinical symptoms, predominantly cough and increasing dyspnea, may be attributed to protein-rich alveolar infiltrates coupled with pulmonary surfactant dysregulation. Pulmonary edema originates from increased permeability in the microvasculature adjacent to the alveolar walls. Disruption of the microvasculature integrity leads to leakage of intravascular fluid and large plasma proteins into the interstitium and alveolar spaces. The degree of alveolar edema is dependent on coexisting damage to the alveolar epithelium.[19]

Surfactant decreases the surface tension of water, which in turn increases pulmonary compliance. Dysregulation of pulmonary surfactant results in decreased lung compliance and subsequent increased work of breathing.[19]

Table 21-3 Clinical Diagnoses Associated With Diffuse Alveolar Damage

Infection
Viral illness
Bacterial pneumonia (including legionella, mycoplasma, mycobacteria, and rickettsia)
Parasitic infection
Fungal pneumonia

Drug Reactions
Prescription
Chemotherapeutics
Amiodarone
Nitrofurantoin
Penicillamine
External beam radiation
Illicit
Heroine
Methadone

Vascular collapse
Hemorrhagic, neurogenic, cardiogenic, burns

Collagen vascular disease

Chemical inhalants and ingestants

Systemic Illness
Acute pancreatitis
Cardiopulmonary bypass
Leukemia blast crisis
Molar pregnancy
Uremia
Disseminated intravascular coagulation
Kidney and liver transplant

Pulmonary emboli (air, amniotic fluid)

Reprinted with permission from Elsevier, Castro CY. ARDS and diffuse alveolar damage: a pathologist's perspective. *Semin Thorac Cardiovasc Surg.* Spring 2006;18(1):13-19.

Imaging Features of Diffuse Alveolar Damage

Patients with DAD commonly receive mechanically ventilation as a result of their profound hypoxemia and respiratory failure. Yet imaging in DAD patients may be normal within the first 12 to 24 hours of acute onset.[5] Subsequent chest x-rays demonstrate a "white-out," or diffuse bilateral pulmonary infiltrates. CT scan shows ground glass opacities (GGO) which are heterogeneous and patchy but diffuse in distribution.[20] The GGO may be accompanied by areas of consolidation and septal thickening, most profound in the lower lung fields or dependent areas of the lung.[9,20] In a study by Chung and colleagues, patients with involvement of greater than 80% of their lung fields had statistically significant increased mortality. In addition, signs of pulmonary fibrosis on imaging, including honeycomb change and reticular opacities, portended a worse prognosis.[21]

Resolution of imaging abnormalities with patient improvement may be complete, or may result in permanent changes. Residual and sometimes debilitating fibrosis may be encountered and is generally seen in anterior and nondependent areas of the lung.[9]

Histologic Features of Diffuse Alveolar Damage

The histologic features of DAD may be subdivided into three phases that represent initial pulmonary injury, parenchymal healing, and resolution.[18,20] It is important to recognize that these phases occur in a continuum, and as such overlapping features may be present on histologic examination.

The acute phase

The acute phase may be visualized by light microscopy approximately 2 days following the inciting injury; however, electron microscopy reveals injury earlier. Ultrastructural studies demonstrate early endothelial cell swelling and widening of the endothelial cell junctions.[18] Significant damage to the alveolar basement membranes and the type I and type II pneumocytes accompany endothelial cell injury. Type I cells have been repeatedly demonstrated to be more susceptible to injury; however, necrotic type II pneumocytes may also be visualized.[18]

Histologically, alveolar and interstitial edema are evidenced by interstitial widening, and are often the first radiologic evidence of injury. Edema may be coupled with capillary congestion and variable intra-alveolar hemorrhage.[18,20] Following the influx of alveolar and interstitial edema, hyaline membranes begin to form. This histologic hallmark of the initial phase is most prominent at days 4 to 5 and may be identified by intensely eosinophilic and homogenous lining that is adherent to the alveolar ducts and spaces. The prominent eosinophilia of the hyaline membranes is attributed to the proteinaceous and nuclear debris that migrated there from the leaky capillary endothelium[20] (*Figures 21-3* and *21-4*). Injury to type II pneumocytes markedly decreases surfactant, which decreases alveolar volume and leads to partially collapsed alveolar spaces on histologic examination. Notably, an inflammatory infiltrate is generally limited during the initial phase unless it was present prior to injury due to, for example, infection.

Gross examination of the lungs in patients who die during the acute phase of DAD shows a dark bluish hue and punctate hemorrhage on the pleural surface. The lungs are heavy and firm, due to diffuse edema in both the alveolar spaces and in the interstitium.[18]

The proliferative phase

The second phase of DAD is associated with parenchymal proliferation as healing begins. Surviving type II

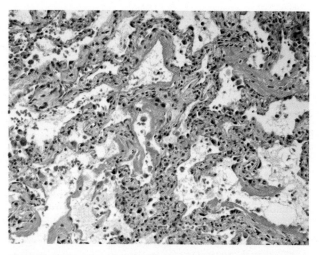

FIGURE 21-3 The acute phase of diffuse alveolar damage is characterized by eosinophilic homogenous hyaline membranes adherent to the alveolar spaces. Type II pneumocyte injury decreases surfactant and leads to partially collapsed alveolar spaces (21× H&E).

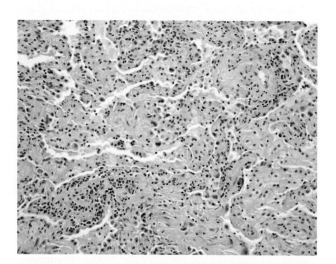

FIGURE 21-4 The proliferative phase of DAD is marked by type II pneumocyte hyperplasia with hobnailing into the alveolar spaces, and interstitial widening by a myxoid matrix. The airspaces are filled with fibroblastic population that organizes the proteinaceous debris (21× H&E).

pneumocytes become hyperplastic and extend in a hobnail pattern into the alveolar spaces as they serve as the progenitor cells for new alveolar epithelium.[19] Their activation is seen histologically by epithelial cell enlargement, vesicular chromatin, and prominent nucleoli. As interstitial fibrosis begins to form, squamous metaplasia associated with epithelial repair also becomes prominent.[18] Features of regeneration may appear concerning on open lung biopsy or cytology, so care must be taken not to overdiagnose carcinoma in the setting of robust squamous metaplasia, nuclear atypia, and mitotic activity because these features are common in the proliferative phase of DAD.

Activation of fibroblasts and myofibroblasts in the alveolar wall is evidenced by interstitial widening with a myxoid matrix and is often considered the hallmark of the proliferative phase of DAD.[8] The reparative fibroblastic population gains access to the alveolar spaces through the damaged alveolar basement membrane, wherein it begins to organize the proteinaceous debris deposited during the acute phase. The histologic appearance produced by this phenomenon may be reminiscent of organizing pneumonia, as the physiology of repair is the same.[18]

The resolution phase

Approximately 3 to 4 weeks following the initial injury, dense collagenous tissue that has been deposited in damaged parenchyma imparts a micronodular gross appearance to the pleural surface. The cut surface of the lung shows alternating areas of scarring and microcystic spaces. Histologically, reparative fibroblasts slowly replace collapsed and injured alveoli with fibrosis, resulting in fewer alveoli with enlarged air spaces and distended ducts. The interstitium and alveolar walls contain paucicellular collagenous connective tissue.[8,18]

Differential Diagnosis of Diffuse Alveolar Damage

There are a large number of causes of DAD owning to the multiple etiologies that manifest this histologic appearance (*Table 21-3*). Infections, medications and illicit drugs, inhalants, shock, external beam radiation therapy, and iatrogenic processes are a mere sample of the myriad insults that may lead to DAD. Due to the expanded differential, clinical correlation is imperative when this diagnosis is suspected.

ACUTE FIBRINOUS AND ORGANIZING PNEUMONIA

Acute fibrinous and organizing pneumonia (AFOP) is a rare pattern of acute lung injury was first identified by Beasley and colleagues in 2002.[22] It is a histologic variant that does not lend itself to classification of DAD, OP, or eosinophilic pneumonia (EP). The clinical presentation could be variable, and the pattern may be seen in patients with an acute or subacute clinical presentation.

Diseases Associated With Acute Fibrinous and Organizing Pneumonia

AFOP may be idiopathic or a sequelae of a spectrum of clinical entities. Known associations with AFOP include collagen vascular disease (specifically ankylosing spondylitis and polymyositis), infection, adverse drug reactions, and environmental exposures.

Clinical Features of Acute Fibrinous and Organizing Pneumonia

The largest study to date comprises 17 patients with a diagnosis of AFOP. The presentation of these patients was both acute and subacute, with an average of 19 days from the onset of symptoms to biopsy.[22] The clinical course has since been subdivided into two distinct presentations: an acute course with symptoms overlapping ARDS and a subacute course with favorable outcome and response to therapy.[23,24] Patient exhibited a range of clinical symptoms, including fever, cough, shortness of breath, and hemoptysis.

Imaging Features of Acute Fibrinous and Organizing Pneumonia

AFOP mimics COP on imaging studies. Patchy migratory and diffuse alveolar infiltrates tend to present predominately in the basilar and peripheral lung fields.[24] Beasley's original study quoted imaging findings that were suggestive of atypical pneumonia or pulmonary edema.[22]

Histologic Features of Acute Fibrinous and Organizing Pneumonia

Histologically, AFOP shows tight aggregates of fibrin within alveolar spaces. These fibrin "balls" distinguish themselves from the surrounding alveolar membranes by circumferential clefting. They occur in a patchy distribution within the lung parenchyma. Alveolar ducts and bronchioles peripheral to these fibrin aggregates are often filled with loose, streaming connective tissue constituting organizing pneumonia. There is a conspicuous absence of hyaline membranes associated with DAD (*Figure 21-5*).

Accompanying mild to moderate lymphoplasmacytic infiltrate is universally present in the interstitium. Rare eosinophils and neutrophils may be appreciated, but are not a predominate feature of AFOP. It should be noted that while sparse neutrophils may be appreciated in nearly every AFOP specimen, these cases fail to have the histologic criteria consistent with acute pneumonia. Similarly, cases fail to demonstrate any evidence of capillaritis.

Secondary features consistent with this diagnosis include interstitial widening due to edema and reactive type II pneumocyte hyperplasia. Notably, the presence of microorganisms or granulomatous inflammation on special stains or H&E sections excludes the diagnosis of AFOP.

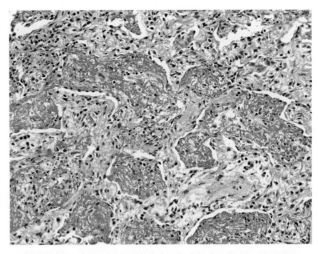

FIGURE 21-5 **Medium power of acute fibrinous and organizing pneumonia (AFOP) (H&E, 10×).**

Differential Diagnosis of Acute Fibrinous and Organizing Pneumonia

The differential diagnosis of AFOP includes DAD, OP, and EP. Beasley postulates that AFOP may in fact be the fibrous variant of DAD in light of the similar clinical course and outcomes of AFOP and DAD patients.[22] While fibrin is a constituent of the histologic diagnosis of DAD and OP, its extent and prominence in those entities is far less than in AFOP. Additionally, there is a distinct lack of hyaline membranes in AFOP, further distinguishing it as a separate entity.

PULMONARY EDEMA

Intra-alveolar fluid in the absence of acute lung injury is limited by tight epithelial junctions that prevent passive movement of fluid and solutes into the airspace. Any accumulation of fluid that circumvents this physical barrier is removed by creation of an osmotic gradient within the interstitium.

The osmotic gradient is formed by apical sodium channels on the surface of type I and type II pneumocytes. Once sodium has entered the cell, it is actively transported into the interstitium by a basolaterally located sodium-potassium ATPase. This process builds an osmotic gradient that encourages water to flow from the airspace into the interstitium via both aquaporins on the cell surface, as well as by intercellular channels. Excess interstitial edema is then removed by lymphatics, which drain the fluid back into the circulation.[25]

Limitations to this intricate design occur commonly in acute lung injury. The failure of this pathway results in intra-alveolar edema, which subsequently leads to profound hypoxia and respiratory failure.

CHAPTER 21

Noncardiogenic Edema

In contrast to cardiogenic pulmonary edema, which develops due to increased vascular pressure, noncardiogenic pulmonary edema is associated with acute lung injury and ARDS. Impaired fluid clearance from the alveolar space is not only associated with ALI/ARDS, but marked impairment is inversely correlated with survival[25,26] (*Figure 21-6*).

Several factors contribute to the accumulation of airspace fluid during lung injury. Cell death disrupts with tight epithelial junctions that provide a physical barrier against alveolar edema. The unencumbered fluid fills the airspace and is unable to be osmotically removed due to absence of the sodium-potassium pump.

Factors present as a consequence of acute pulmonary injury but in the absence of cell death also adversely affect intra-alveolar edema. Hypoxemia has been found to decrease the activity of sodium transport by 50% through a variety of mechanisms, including transcription, impairment of the apical sodium channels, impaired sodium trafficking, and endocytosis of sodium-potassium ATPases. Oxygen administration to a patient with pulmonary edema, therefore, may assist in resolution. Cytokines and oxidants associated with acute inflammation and pulmonary damage, pathogens such as viral infections, and hypercapnia also decrease the efficacy intra-alveolar fluid resolution.[25] Fluid restriction during ALI/ARDS has been shown to improve oxygenation and result in a shorter duration of mechanical ventilation.[27]

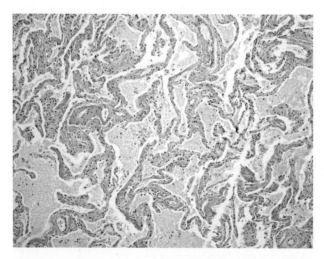

FIGURE 21-6 Edema and eosinophilic proteinaceous debris fills and expands the alveolar spaces. In the non-injured lung, a sodium-potassium ATPase pump creates an osmotic gradient, which allows water to flow from the airspace and into the interstitium. Excess fluid in the interstitium is then cleared by the lymphatics. In ALI/ARDS, this mechanism as well as tight epithelial junctions is disrupted, leading to an accumulation intra-alveolar fluid (H&E, 10×).

Reexpansion

Reexpansion pulmonary edema (RPE) occurs when a lung has been chronically collapsed for longer than 72 hours, and then is rapidly reexpanded. Clinical scenarios in which this syndrome is encountered include pneumothoraces and large volume pleural effusions. Care must be taken when expanding a chronically collapsed lung, because although the syndrome is rare (significant events occur at an incidence of approximately 1%), the mortality rate approaches 15% to 20%.[28,29]

A subset of patients is at higher risk for developing RPE. Risk factors that may predispose patients to RPE include a young age, large pneumothoraces, lung collapse for greater than 7 days, and large volume drainage of pleural effusion (>3 L).[29] The majority of patients will experience symptoms within the first 1 to 2 hours after therapeutic decompression; however, symptoms present up to 24 hours after lung expansion. Patients experience a range of symptoms including new-onset cough, dyspnea, chest pain, and frothy sputum production. Clinical hallmarks include tachypnea, tachycardia, and desaturation, as well as pulmonary crackles on auscultation.[30] Imaging assists in confirming the diagnosis with homogenous ground glass opacities, septal thickening, and consolidation throughout the reexpanded lung.[31]

Damage to pulmonary microvasculature and subsequent stress when reperfused are thought to be the driving mechanisms in RPE. Upon pulmonary collapse, the capillary endothelium and basement membrane thicken. This stiffens the pulmonary microvasculature, leaving it susceptible to damage upon reexpansion.[32]

Capillary damage occurs through both mechanical stress and inflammation. Decreased pulmonary surfactant, impaired lymphatic flow, and increased hydrostatic pressure secondary to increased venous return provide mechanical disruption to small vessels. In addition, reestablishment of perfusion in a collapsed lung elicits an inflammatory response. Reactive oxygen species produced by acute inflammation is thought to further damage the endothelium, allowing an influx of fluid into the airspace.[30]

Treatment of RPE is mainly supportive, and can range from providing supplemental oxygen in a mildly effected patient to intubation and mechanical ventilation in a severe presentation. Prevention is preferred, and is best achieved by gradual reexpansion of pulmonary parenchyma. Pleural manometry has been increasingly used to monitor intrapleural pressure during procedures.[30]

High Altitude

High-altitude pulmonary edema (HAPE) occurs in individuals ascending to a height of greater than 3000 m. Onset of symptoms occurs within 2 to 4 days of ascent and are related to the body's attempt to acclimate to a higher altitude. Early in the course of pulmonary edema, fatigue, cough, headache, and dyspnea may be encountered. As HAPE progresses, frothy sputum, occasionally with hemoptysis, desaturation, and cyanosis may be seen.[33]

HAPE occurs in both patients who live at high altitudes and are returning home from a lower-altitude trip, and to those who are newly exposed to high altitudes. The greatest risk factor for development of HAPE is a prior episode of pulmonary edema at high altitude. Patients who have experienced a prior episode have a 60% chance of recurrence upon ascension. Other important risk factors include fast ascent, cold ambient temperatures, preexisting pulmonary infection, and male gender.[33,34] Vigorous physical exercise at high altitudes is an additional risk factor, due to the increase in mean pulmonary artery pressure and pulmonary arterial wedge pressure with physical exertion.[35] Chest x-ray is significant for patchy alveolar infiltrates bilaterally that progress to confluent infiltrates in severe disease.[34]

The pathophysiology of HAPE starts with vasoconstriction of the pulmonary vasculature upon exposure to low-oxygen environment. Hypoxic pulmonary vasoconstriction is nonuniform, diverting pulmonary blood flow from areas of hyperactive vasoconstriction to regions with less constricted blood flow. Pressure increases within open pulmonary capillaries, breaking through the tight junctions in the alveolar epithelium and forcing fluid into the alveolar space.[33,34] Recall that hypoxemic environments downregulate the efficacy of the sodium potassium ATPase pump, which functions to move intra-alveolar fluid back into the interstitial space. This marked reduction in the normal mechanisms used to clear airspace fluid perpetuates the buildup of airspace edema.[34]

REFERENCES

1. Zambon M, Vincent JL. Mortality rates for patients with acute lung injury/ARDS have decreased over time. *Chest*. May 2008;133(5):1120-1127.
2. Thompson BT, Moss M. A new definition for the acute respiratory distress syndrome. *Semin Respir Crit Care Med*. August 2013;34(4):441-447.
3. Papazian L, Doddoli C, Chetaille B, et al. A contributive result of open-lung biopsy improves survival in acute respiratory distress syndrome patients. *Crit Care Med*. March 2007;35(3):755-762.
4. Donati SY, Papazian L. Role of open-lung biopsy in acute respiratory distress syndrome. *Curr Opin Crit Care*. February 2008;14(1):75-79.
5. Terminella L, Sharma G. Diagnostic studies in patients with acute respiratory distress syndrome. *Semin Thorac Cardiovasc Surg*. Spring 2006;18(1):2-7.
6. Patel SR, Karmpaliotis D, Ayas NT, et al. The role of open-lung biopsy in ARDS. *Chest*. January 2004;125(1):197-202.
7. Kao KC, Tsai YH, Wu YK, et al. Open lung biopsy in early-stage acute respiratory distress syndrome. *Crit Care*. 2006;10(4):R106.
8. Castro CY. ARDS and diffuse alveolar damage: a pathologist's perspective. *Semin Thorac Cardiovasc Surg*. Spring 2006;18(1):13-19.
9. Kligerman SJ, Franks TJ, Galvin JR. From the radiologic pathology archives: organization and fibrosis as a response to lung injury in diffuse alveolar damage, organizing pneumonia, and acute fibrinous and organizing pneumonia. *Radiographics*. November-December 2013;33(7):1951-1975.
10. Roberton BJ, Hansell DM. Organizing pneumonia: a kaleidoscope of concepts and morphologies. *Eur Radiol*. November 2011;21(11):2244-2254.
11. Larsen BT, Colby TV. Update for pathologists on idiopathic interstitial pneumonias. *Arch Pathol Lab Med*. October 2012;136(10):1234-1241.
12. Schlesinger C, Koss MN. The organizing pneumonias: an update and review. *Curr Opin Pulm Med*. September 2005;11(5):422-430.
13. Cordier JF. Cryptogenic organizing pneumonia. *Clin Chest Med*. December 2004;25(4):727-738, vi-vii.
14. Drakopanagiotakis F, Polychronopoulos V, Judson MA. Organizing pneumonia. *Am J Med Sci*. January 2008;335(1):34-39.
15. Sveinsson OA, Isaksson HJ, Sigvaldason A, Yngvason F, Aspelund T, Gudmundsson G. Clinical features in secondary and cryptogenic organising pneumonia. *Int J Tuberc Lung Dis*. June 2007;11(6):689-694.
16. Maturu VN, Agarwal R. Reversed halo sign: a systematic review. *Respir Care*. 2014;59(9):1440-1449.
17. Baque-Juston M, Pellegrin A, Leroy S, Marquette CH, Padovani B. Organizing pneumonia: What is it? A conceptual approach and pictorial review. *Diagn Interv Imaging*. 2014;95(9):771-777.
18. Tomashefski JF Jr. Pulmonary pathology of acute respiratory distress syndrome. *Clin Chest Med*. September 2000;21(3):435-466.
19. Ware LB. Pathophysiology of acute lung injury and the acute respiratory distress syndrome. *Semin Respir Crit Care Med*. August 2006;27(4):337-349.
20. Beasley MB. The pathologist's approach to acute lung injury. *Arch Pathol Lab Med*. May 2010;134(5):719-727.
21. Chung JH, Kradin RL, Greene RE, Shepard JA, Digumarthy SR. CT predictors of mortality in pathology confirmed ARDS. *Eur Radiol*. April 2011;21(4):730-737.
22. Beasley MB, Franks TJ, Galvin JR, Gochuico B, Travis WD. Acute fibrinous and organizing pneumonia: a histological pattern of lung injury and possible variant of diffuse alveolar damage. *Arch Pathol Lab Med*. September 2002;126(9):1064-1070.
23. Guimarães C, Sanches I, Ferreira C. Acute fibrinous and organising pneumonia. *BMJ Case Rep*. March 20, 2012;2012.
24. Tzouvelekis A, Koutsopoulos A, Oikonomou A, et al. Acute fibrinous and organising pneumonia: a case report and review of the literature. *J Med Case Rep*. October 12, 2009;3:74.
25. Matthay MA. Resolution of pulmonary edema. Thirty years of progress. *Am J Respir Crit Care Med*. June 1, 2014;189(11):1301-1308.
26. Ware LB, Matthay MA. Alveolar fluid clearance is impaired in the majority of patients with acute lung injury and the acute respiratory distress syndrome. *Am J Respir Crit Care Med*. May 2001;163(6):1376-1383.
27. Wiedemann HP, Wheeler AP, Bernard GR, et al. Comparison of two fluid-management strategies in acute lung injury. *N Engl J Med*. June 15, 2006;354(24):2564-2575.
28. Chakraborty PP, Chakraborty S. Reexpansion pulmonary edema. *Indian J Surg*. April 2012;74(2):174-176.
29. Echevarria C, Twomey D, Dunning J, Chanda B. Does re-expansion pulmonary oedema exist? *Interact Cardiovasc Thorac Surg*. May 2008;7(3):485-489.
30. Kasmani R, Irani F, Okoli K, Mahajan V. Re-expansion pulmonary edema following thoracentesis. *CMAJ*. December 14, 2010;182(18):2000-2002.

31. Gleeson T, Thiessen R, Müller N. Reexpansion pulmonary edema: computed tomography findings in 22 patients. *J Thorac Imaging.* February 2011;26(1):36-41.

32. Sohara Y. Reexpansion pulmonary edema. *Ann Thorac Cardiovasc Surg.* August 2008;14(4):205-209.

33. Bhagi S, Srivastava S, Singh SB. High-altitude pulmonary edema: review. *J Occup Health.* 2014;56(4):235-234.

34. Stream JO, Grissom CK. Update on high-altitude pulmonary edema: pathogenesis, prevention, and treatment. *Wilderness Environ Med.* Winter 2008;19(4):293-303.

35. Kaner RJ, Crystal RG. Pathogenesis of high altitude pulmonary edema: does alveolar epithelial lining fluid vascular endothelial growth factor exacerbate capillary leak? *High Alt Med Biol.* Winter 2004;5(4):399-409.

22 Small Airway Disease

Anatoly Urisman and Kirk D. Jones

TAKE HOME PEARLS

- The evaluation of the biopsy with airway pathology is supported by careful correlation with clinical findings (eg, obstructive physiology on pulmonary function testing) and radiologic information (eg, air trapping on CT scan).
- Clinical-radiologic-pathologic correlation can help turn a descriptive histologic diagnosis into a specific diagnosis for the patient.
- If the low-power view of a surgical lung biopsy appears nearly normal, the biopsy may show small airway disease.
- Alveolar interstitium and airspaces are often excluded from the pathologic changes of small airway disease.

INTRODUCTION

Small airway disease is an umbrella term that originally defined a group of diseases clinically associated with airway obstruction. To the pathologist, the term is more commonly used to describe pathologic changes of inflammation and fibrosis affecting the distal component of the air conducting system in the lungs (ie, the bronchioles), and is often used synonymously with bronchiolitis. This chapter will discuss the typical patterns of small airway disease and several of the specific entities associated with small airway pathology.[1-3]

APPROACH TO SMALL AIRWAY DISEASE

Pathologic evaluation of lungs for small airway disease is best performed using clinical and radiologic correlation. A wide spectrum of inflammatory and fibrotic disorders are encompassed by this term, and the pathologist may be confronted with a biopsy from a patient showing acute airflow obstruction or one with chronic progressive dyspnea and cough. In addition, these cases may show variable radiographic findings on chest computerized tomography (CT), including centrilobular nodules, "tree-in-bud" opacities, air trapping with mosaic perfusion, or may show nearly normal lungs. Several of the small airway diseases will show varying degrees of inflammation and fibrosis as they progress (eg, the evolution of inflamed necrotizing viral bronchiolitis to fibrotic constrictive bronchiolitis). The nonspecific appearance of several patterns of small airway disease combined with variable or overlapping appearance in specific diseases often makes determination of an exact etiology difficult. For pathologists, it is helpful to examine the lung biopsy to determine the histologic pattern of injury, then use this pattern as a starting point or foundation to develop a clinically useful differential diagnosis. *Figure 22-1* presents a systematic approach to evaluation of small airways disease starting with identification of the major histologic pattern followed by consideration of clinical conditions associated with that pattern.

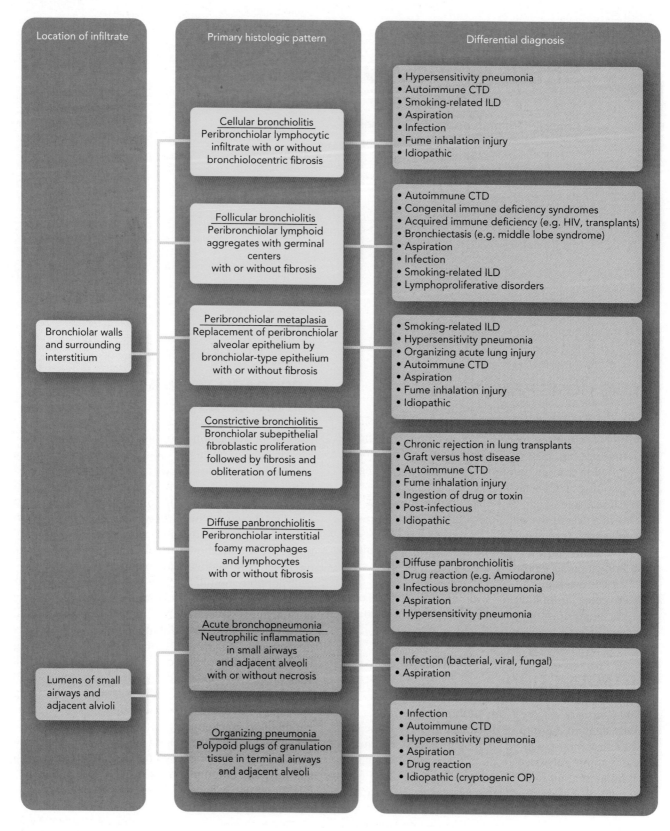

FIGURE 22-1 An algorithmic pattern-based approach to small airway disease.

SPECIAL CONSIDERATIONS OF SPECIMEN HANDLING

Handling of surgical biopsies evaluation possible small airway disease employs several principles that pathologists apply to other medical lung diseases. First, the differential diagnosis often includes infection, so it is important to verify that tissue has been sent from the operating suite for microbiologic cultures. In our practice, surgical biopsies are "inflated" by simply removing the stapled surgical margin and then vigorously shaking the specimen in a closed formalin-filled container. If injection inflation is performed, it is important to use only minimal inflation pressures in order to prevent overinflation artifacts.[4] Small airway diseases are often focal (eg, constrictive bronchiolitis), so the pathologist should be ready to obtain additional sections from tissue blocks to increase the likelihood of identifying a diagnostic lesion. Finally, use of special stains for elastic tissue (eg, Verhoeff-van Gieson) can help highlight airway and vascular structures within the pulmonary lobule.

HISTOLOGY OF SMALL AIRWAYS

Most authorities define small airways as those having lumens smaller than 2 to 3 mm. While this definition is useful for research in airflow resistance and morphometry, in clinical practice, most pathologists use a histological definition of small airways that excludes bronchi (ie, airways supported by cartilage) and includes membranous (terminal) bronchioles, respiratory bronchioles, and alveolar ducts (*Figure 22-2*). Membranous bronchioles retain a small layer of smooth muscle and adventitia and are lined

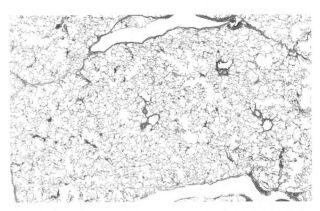

FIGURE 22-3 An overview of the pulmonary lobule shows centrally located bronchovascular bundles with paired bronchioles and pulmonary arteries, peripheral interlobular septa containing pulmonary veins, and surface pleura. This approximately 1 cm structure allows recognition and correlation of pathologic and radiologic patterns of disease.

by ciliated respiratory epithelium with occasional Clara cells. Respiratory bronchioles contain alveoli within their walls and are part of both the conducting and respiratory systems of the lung. The bronchioles extend into elongate alveolar ducts that open directly into the distal alveoli. Both alveolar ducts and alveoli are normally lined by flattened type 1 pneumocytes. The basic functional unit of the lung parenchyma, the acinus (or primary pulmonary lobule), is composed of a single respiratory bronchiole with its alveolar ducts and alveoli. Several (5-10) adjacent acini connected by membranous bronchioles and enclosed by interlobular septa containing small veins and lymphatics form the secondary pulmonary lobule (*Figure 22-3*). The secondary lobule is an important structure for histologic-radiologic correlation, as it is readily recognized on high-resolution CT (HRCT) in pathologic conditions that manifest as either centrilobular consolidations or interlobular septal thickening.[2,5]

PERIBRONCHIOLAR METAPLASIA AND BRONCHIOLOCENTRIC FIBROSIS

Histologic Features of Peribronchiolar Metaplasia

Peribronchiolar metaplasia, also known by older terms *bronchiolization of alveolar ducts* and *Lambertosis*, is characterized by replacement of the normal flat epithelium of the alveolar ducts and adjacent alveoli by bronchiolar-type cuboidal, columnar, or ciliated columnar epithelium. In most cases, peribronchiolar metaplasia is associated with bronchiolocentric fibrosis, a variable thickening of the alveolar septa by collagenous fibrosis

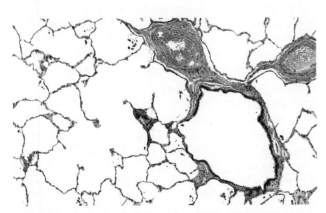

FIGURE 22-2 Normal bronchiole. This low-power view of a bronchovascular unit shows a bronchiole with a thin wall composed of smooth muscle layer, indistinct basement membrane, and surface cuboidal and columnar epithelium. The associated pulmonary artery is noted above, and the adjacent alveolar duct to the left shows thin alveolar septa.

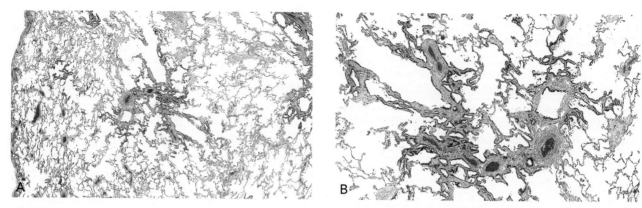

FIGURE 22-4 Peribronchiolar metaplasia and bronchiolocentric fibrosis. **A:** On low-power image, centrilobular prominence of the alveolar septa surrounding bronchovascular bundles is noted. **B:** On medium-power image, the septa in alveolar ducts and peribronchiolar alveoli are thickened by uniform fibrosis and surface proliferation of bronchiolar-type epithelium.

that imparts a reticular or lace-like prominence to the peribronchiolar alveoli when viewed at low magnification (*Figure 22-4A, B*). Peribronchiolar metaplasia as an isolated finding is rare, but it is very common in association with other injury patterns including cellular interstitial pneumonia, interstitial fibrosis (particularly bronchiolocentric), respiratory bronchiolitis and desquamative interstitial pneumonia (DIP), cellular bronchiolitis, constrictive bronchiolitis, and organizing pneumonia.[6]

Imaging Features of Peribronchiolar Metaplasia

Mosaic attenuation and air trapping appear to be the sole and nonspecific HRCT correlates of peribronchiolar metaplasia. Other radiographic findings typically reflect associated lung injury patterns such as fibrosis, emphysema, or organizing pneumonia. Interestingly, centrilobular opacities or nodules are typically not detected by CT in cases of isolated peribronchiolar metaplasia.[6]

Etiologies of Peribronchiolar Metaplasia

Peribronchiolar metaplasia and bronchiolocentric fibrosis are thought to be manifestations of subacute or chronic small airway injury. They are found in multiple conditions associated with distinctly different underlying etiologies, including chronic hypersensitivity pneumonia, autoimmune connective tissue disease (CTD), toxic fume or smoke inhalation injury, organizing acute lung injury, various pneumoconioses, and aspiration, among others. Bronchiolocentric fibrosis is also identified as a rare pathologic pattern of idiopathic interstitial lung disease. This is based on several series of cases describing airway-centered fibrosis. In these series, the prognosis was variable but many patients showed disease progression despite treatment.[7-10]

Clinical Features of Peribronchiolar Metaplasia

Given the diversity of etiologies associated with peribronchiolar metaplasia, it is not surprising that clinical manifestations are largely determined by the underlying condition. In general, however, if present in isolation, peribronchiolar metaplasia may be found in completely asymptomatic patients, while cases where there is significant associated bronchiolocentric fibrosis will typically have clinically evident interstitial lung disease.[8-10]

ACUTE BRONCHOPNEUMONIA

Histologic Features of Acute Bronchopneumonia

The primary histologic finding in acute bronchopneumonia is the accumulation of neutrophils in the terminal bronchioles, alveolar ducts, and adjacent central alveolar spaces (*Figure 22-5A, B*). This airspace consolidation is usually accompanied by accumulation of fibrin, and in severe cases epithelial cell or parenchymal necrosis is present. Alveolar macrophages may be present but are usually less numerous than neutrophils. Bacteria or fungi may be observed in some cases, often with the aid of additional histochemical staining. Bacteria are best visualized with silver impregnation stains (eg, Warthin-Starry or Steiner methods), and tissue Gram stain (eg, Brown and Brenn) may be helpful, particularly with gram-positive bacteria. Fungi may be identified with Grocott methenamine silver (GMS) stains or periodic acid-Schiff with diastase (PAS-D). It is important to remember that several important pulmonary pathogens (eg, *Histoplasma* and *Pneumocystis*) do not stain well with PAS-D. Additional correlation with microbiology cultures or ancillary molecular tests may be useful in identification of pathogenic organisms.[11]

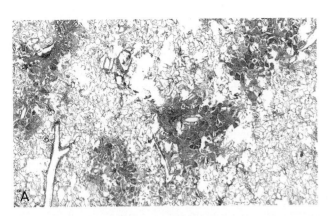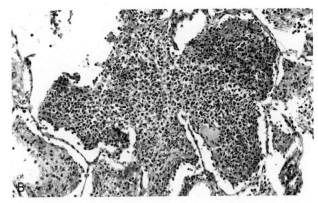

FIGURE 22-5 **Acute bronchopneumonia. A: On low-power image, multiple centrilobular regions of alveolar and bronchiolar consolidation are noted. B: On high-power image, filling of the alveolar space with neutrophils and fibrin is observed.**

Gross Features of Acute Bronchopneumonia

Gross evaluation of acute bronchopneumonia is most commonly performed in the autopsy setting. The lungs are heavier than normal and show small (<5 mm) white-tan centrilobular nodules. Larger areas of consolidation may be present, as well as areas of necrosis with or without cavitation.[11]

Imaging Features of Acute Bronchopneumonia

A spectrum of radiologic abnormalities may be observed in acute bronchopneumonia depending on timing and severity of disease. Chest CT findings may include centrilobular nodules, ground glass opacification, thickening of interlobular septa and bronchovascular bundles, and more prominent regional consolidation.[5]

Etiologies of Acute Bronchopneumonia

Acute bronchopneumonia has been described in association with a wide range of bacterial, viral, and fungal pathogens. The most common bacterial pathogens include gram-positive cocci such as *Streptococcus pneumoniae* and *Staphylococcus aureus*, gram-negative bacteria such as *Haemophilus influenzae*, *Legionella pneumophila*, and *Coxiella burnetii*, as well as "atypical" bacteria such as *Chlamydophila* species and *Mycoplasma pneumonia*.[12-14] Viral pathogens causing lower respiratory tract infections include influenza, parainfluenza, respiratory syncytial virus, adenoviruses, metapneumovirus, rhinoviruses, and coronaviruses.[15,16] Fungal pneumonias are most often secondary to opportunistic infections in immunocompromised patients. The most common fungal pathogens include *Aspergillus* species, *Mucorales* and *Rhizopus* species, *Candida* species, *Cryptococcus neoformans*, and *Pneumocystis jirovecii*.[17]

Clinical Features of Acute Bronchopneumonia

The histologic picture of acute bronchopneumonia most often correlates with the clinical diagnosis of acute pneumonia. Depending on the setting, these cases are classified as community or hospital acquired (the latter group includes ventilator-associated pneumonia). In general, hospital-acquired cases are associated with higher mortality than community-acquired cases. Pyogenic and anaerobic gram-negative bacteria, often resistant to multiple antibiotics, as well as polymicrobial infections are more frequent in hospital-acquired cases.[12,18,19]

ORGANIZING PNEUMONIA

Histologic Features of Organizing Pneumonia

Histologically, OP is characterized by consolidation of airspaces by rounded and sometimes branching polypoid plugs of granulation tissue (*Figure 22-6A, B, C*) composed predominantly of fibroblasts within a myxoid or edematous matrix. Variable numbers of intra-alveolar macrophages, foamy macrophages, lymphocytes, plasma cells, and eosinophils may also accompany the airspace organization. The plugs of organizing pneumonia are usually observed in the terminal bronchioles, alveolar ducts, and adjacent alveoli. Organizing pneumonia is a common and often nonspecific pattern of injury, which is best evaluated in the context of other histologic clues when searching for a possible etiology. Presence of fibrin or hyaline membranes in the alveoli suggests organizing acute lung injury or organizing diffuse alveolar damage. When hyaline membranes are present, a diagnosis of simple organizing pneumonia is inappropriate since the acute lung injury pattern will influence prognosis.[20] When organizing pneumonia is

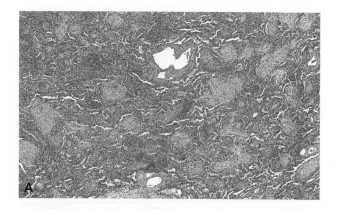

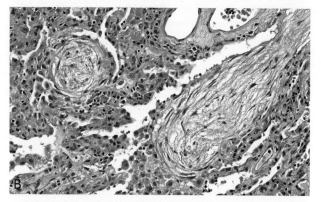

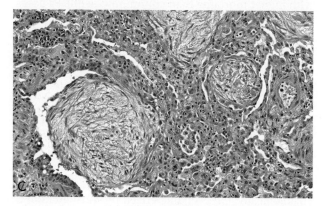

FIGURE 22-6 Organizing pneumonia. A: On low-power image, the branching rounded polypoid plugs of granulation tissue result in patchy airspace consolidation. B: On high-power image, the rounded plug of fibromyxoid tissue is noted within an airspace with surrounding pulmonary macrophages. C: A high-power view shows an intraluminal granulation tissue polyp within a bronchiole.

accompanied by prominent neutrophilia and fibrin in the airspaces, acute viral or bacterial infections should be the top consideration. Viral inclusions or other viral cytopathic changes are helpful in recognizing cases of viral pneumonia, although most such cases will have only nonspecific reactive type 2 pneumocyte hyperplasia. In cases of aspiration pneumonia, one often observes accumulation of airspace and interstitial macrophages with vacuolated cytoplasm, multinucleated

giant cells, and neutrophils. Identification of food particles or pill fragments within alveolar spaces supports the diagnosis. Organizing pneumonia is almost always accompanied by airspace filling by foamy macrophages; however, in cases with prominent macrophage accumulation, one should also consider the possibility of drug toxicity (eg, amiodarone). Focal organizing pneumonia can be found as a secondary pattern in numerous fibrosing and inflammatory conditions, including autoimmune CTD, hypersensitivity pneumonia, and in acute exacerbations of idiopathic pulmonary fibrosis. Pure involvement of airways by organizing pneumonia is exceedingly rare and should raise concern for obliterative bronchiolitis.[21-27]

Imaging Features of Organizing Pneumonia

The two main manifestations of OP on HRCT are ground glass opacities and areas of consolidation, which often have patchy distribution with lower lobe predominance and subpleural accentuation. Linear or polygonal consolidations following the outlines of the interlobular septa adjacent or surrounding normal-appearing lung (atoll sign) have high specificity for OP. Centrilobular nodules and larger areas of consolidation along the bronchovascular bundles are also frequently observed. Many cases of OP are diagnosed by imaging with compatible clinical history and do not require a lung biopsy.[23,28]

Etiologies of Organizing Pneumonia

The most common known etiologies of OP include infection, drug reaction, aspiration, and autoimmune CTD. When no etiology can be identified, the clinical diagnosis of *cryptogenic organizing pneumonia* (COP) is appropriate. It has been suggested that at least some of the cases of COP may be due to occult viral infections. OP can also be a predominant manifestation in some cases of acute hypersensitivity pneumonitis, acute rejection in lung transplants, and rarely graft versus host disease.[3]

Clinical Features of Organizing Pneumonia

COP (previously known as idiopathic bronchiolitis obliterans organizing pneumonia or BOOP) has been recognized since at least the 1980s as a distinct clinical entity with characteristic imaging findings and rapid clinical and radiological improvement upon administration of corticosteroids. Many cases of COP start as a mild flu-like illness with subsequent persistent cough and dyspnea that is not responsive to antibiotics. Over two-thirds of the patients with COP will have excellent response to prednisone therapy without relapses and overall survival of ~75%. A minority of patients develop a relapsing or chronic illness. Patients with OP secondary to autoimmune CTD have a higher frequency of relapses after the initial treatment, and a substantial number of cases will develop chronic fibrosing interstitial lung disease such as nonspecific interstitial pneumonia (NSIP).[29,30]

CONSTRICTIVE BRONCHIOLITIS

Histologic Features of Constrictive Bronchiolitis

Histologically, constrictive bronchiolitis, or obliterative bronchiolitis (OB), is characterized by bronchiolar subepithelial fibroblastic proliferation followed by fibrosis, which results in narrowing and eventual obliteration of the bronchiolar lumen (*Figure 22-7A, B*). In many cases, the lesion is not associated with significant inflammation. The findings are often subtle and focal, and multiple level sections may be necessary to visualize the diagnostic lesions. Bronchiolectasis with luminal mucus plugging or accumulation of macrophages with airspace cholesterol granuloma formation may be observed as sequelae of airway obstruction, and may be a useful clue in some cases. Elastic tissue stains, for example, Verhoeff-van Gieson (EVG), are often helpful in visualizing the presence of collapsed bronchiolar lumens with remnant smooth muscle within the scarred bronchovascular bundles.[27,31,32]

Imaging Features of Constrictive Bronchiolitis

HRCT features seen in constrictive bronchiolitis include areas of mosaic perfusion with or without reduction in the caliber of the pulmonary arteries, and air trapping on dynamic expiratory views. Variable involvement of the larger airways manifested by bronchial wall thickening and bronchiectasis is common, particularly in advanced cases.[33,34]

Etiologies of Constrictive Bronchiolitis

OB has been linked to a number of distinct etiologies. It is a well-documented complication of chronic rejection and is an important cause of mortality and morbidity in lung transplant patients.[35,36] In a similar fashion, patients status post bone marrow transplant may develop OB as a manifestation of pulmonary graft versus host disease.[37,38] Outside of the transplant population, OB is most often encountered in autoimmune CTD, particularly in rheumatoid arthritis (RA) and rarely in other CTD types.[39] OB is a rare delayed complication of viral bronchiolitis or viral pneumonia in association with several viruses, including respiratory syncytial virus (RSV), adenovirus, influenza and measles, and mycoplasma pneumonia,[40] which can result in regional hyperinflation of alveoli with decreased perfusion (eg, Swyer-James syndrome[41,42]). Many inhaled and ingested toxins have been associated with OB, including several from environmental, occupation, and therapeutic exposures (*Table 22-1*).[3]

Clinical Features of Constrictive Bronchiolitis

Symptoms of OB are nonspecific. Most patients report chronic cough and dyspnea. In lung transplant patients, OB is manifested as bronchiolitis obliterans syndrome (BOS), a subtype of chronic lung allograft dysfunction (CLAD), and is usually diagnosed without lung biopsy when there is evidence of spirometric flow obstruction not explained by other causes.[44]

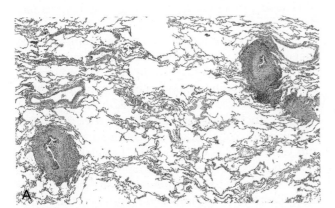
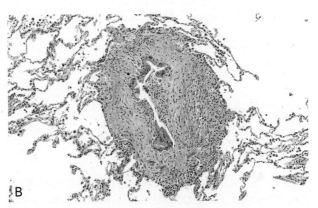

FIGURE 22-7 Constrictive bronchiolitis. **A:** On low-power image, two bronchioles show evidence of luminal narrowing by scarring. The alveolar tissue shows no pathologic alterations. **B:** On high-power image, subepithelial fibroplasia and sclerosis are noted. This mural scarring differs from the intraluminal fibromyxoid tissue observed in organizing pneumonia.

Table 22-1 Toxic Substances Associated With Small Airway Disease

Inhaled substances	Ammonia (fertilizer, production, refrigeration, explosives)
	Chlorine (bleaching, plastics, disinfectants)
	Diacetyl (food flavoring)
	Ozone (arc welding, sewage and water treatment)
	Phosgene (dye and insecticide manufacturing)
	Nitrogen dioxide (silo gas, rocket fuel, explosives, arc welding)
	Sulfur dioxide (fossil fuels, ore smelting, acid production)
Drugs and ingested substances	Amiodarone
	Busulfan
	Gold
	Lomustine
	Methotrexate
	Nitrofurantoin
	Penicillamine
	Phenytoin
	Risedronate
	Sulfasalazine
	Sauropus androgynous

Used with permission of Refs. 1 and 43.

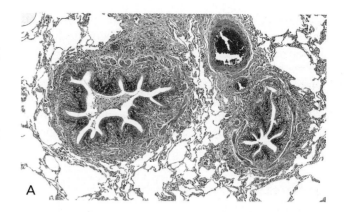

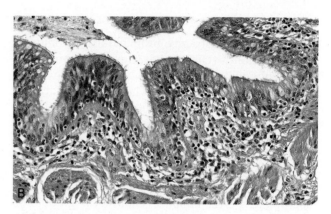

FIGURE 22-8 Cellular bronchiolitis. A: The subepithelial tissue shows a band-like infiltrate of lymphocytes with patchy extension into the surface epithelium. B: On high-power image, the lymphocytes are observed within the walls of the bronchiole.

Transbronchial biopsies of lung allografts have variable sensitivity for OB in the range of 20% to 70% and therefore are not completely reliable for diagnosis.[45,46] OB secondary to an acute environmental or occupational toxin exposure often results in an acute and sometimes life-threatening respiratory illness; however, OB may not develop for months or years following the exposure. In chronic exposures the onset may be slow. In many cases of chronic OB, there is consequent bronchiectasis. This bronchiolitis obliterans-bronchiectasis complex often results in recurrent chronic pneumonias.[40,47]

CELLULAR BRONCHIOLITIS

Histologic Features of Cellular Bronchiolitis

Cellular bronchiolitis is characterized by mononuclear inflammatory infiltrate involving bronchiolar walls and peribronchiolar interstitium (*Figure 22-8A, B*). The infiltrate is usually dominated by lymphocytes with variable numbers of plasma cells, and occasional eosinophils may be present. It is often patchy and can be present in combination with peribronchiolar metaplasia or more advanced bronchiolocentric fibrosis. These histologic features alone are not specific for a particular etiology. However, a few secondary histologic clues in combination with the primary pattern of cellular bronchiolitis, if present, may help to narrow the differential diagnosis.[48] Presence of significant numbers of interstitial foamy macrophages may suggest diffuse panbronchiolitis. Small poorly formed granulomas and giant cells in the peribronchiolar interstitium are often found in cases of hypersensitivity pneumonia. Larger granulomas, particularly with necrosis, are highly suggestive of infection, most often fungal or mycobacterial, and evaluation with AFB and GMS stains is often helpful. Cellular bronchiolitis with large numbers of eosinophils may be seen in some fungal and parasitic infections, asthma, and rare drug reactions. Superimposed respiratory bronchiolitis with accumulation of lightly pigmented (smoker's) macrophages is seen in tobacco smokers and with inhalation of other combustibles.[27,31]

Imaging Features of Cellular Bronchiolitis

Radiographic features of cellular bronchiolitis are variable. The CT scan may be normal or may show regions of hyperinflation. Centrilobular nodules with fine reticulation are noted in some cases.[49,50]

Etiologies of Cellular Bronchiolitis

As mentioned earlier, cellular bronchiolitis in the absence of other histologic clues is a nonspecific finding. It is most frequently encountered in autoimmune CTD and hypersensitivity pneumonia. Other etiologies include smoking, some airway infections, chronic aspiration, and rare drug toxicities.

Clinical Features of Cellular Bronchiolitis

Clinical manifestations are determined by the nature and severity of the underlying condition. In general, prognosis is worse in cases associated with significant fibrosis. Immunosuppressive therapy is often indicated in cases of autoimmune CTD and hypersensitivity pneumonia, and may result in significant improvement in symptoms and long-term outcomes. In cases of infection, identification of the pathogen and administration of appropriate antimicrobial therapy is the goal.

Acute bronchiolitis

Acute bronchiolitis is primarily a clinical term used to describe an acute respiratory illness in infants characterized by flu-like symptoms, wheezing, cough, and shortness of breath. Most of the cases are due to lower respiratory tract viral infection, which is classically caused by RSV.[51] However, other viruses such as adenovirus, influenza, parainfluenza, herpesviruses, coronaviruses, and metapneumovirus, as well as bacteria such as *Mycoplasma* or *Bordetella pertussis* may produce an indistinguishable clinical picture in both children and adults. Lung biopsy is not typically performed, but classic histologic changes include bronchiolar intraepithelial and subepithelial mononuclear and neutrophilic inflammation accompanied by epithelial sloughing and necrosis in severe cases[52] (*Figure 22-9A, B*). This histologic pattern is virtually never observed in isolation and is usually accompanied by features of diffuse alveolar damage (DAD), acute bronchopneumonia, or both. For this reason and to prevent confusion with the clinical meaning of this term, we avoid the use of *acute bronchiolitis* as a histologic diagnosis and instead advocate a diagnosis that specifies the primary pattern, that is, DAD or acute bronchopneumonia. In cases with significant bronchiolar necrosis and lack of prominent inflammation, noninfectious etiologies such as toxic

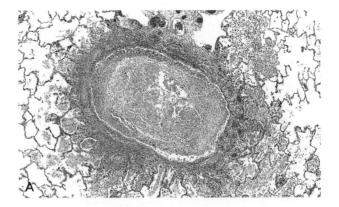

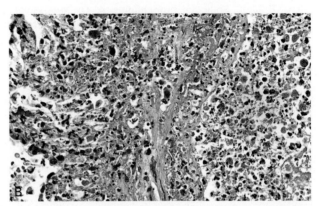

FIGURE 22-9 Necrotizing herpesvirus bronchiolitis. A: This bronchiole shows marked acute inflammation with nuclear dust, and necrosis and sloughing of the surface bronchiolar epithelium. B: On high-power image, cells with smudgy nuclear chromatin and viral inclusions are noted, consistent with herpesvirus pneumonia.

fume inhalation or drug toxicity should also be considered. Some of the patients develop constrictive bronchiolitis months or years after the initial illness.

FOLLICULAR BRONCHIOLITIS

Histologic Features of Follicular Bronchiolitis

Follicular bronchiolitis is recognized by the presence of prominent peribronchiolar and often subepithelial lymphoid aggregates with germinal center formation (*Figure 22-10A, B*). Follicular bronchiolitis often coexists with cellular bronchiolitis and thus may represent a continuum rather than two distinct patterns of injury. Evidence of luminal obstruction, mucostasis, and bronchiolectasis are also often found. Presence of significant acute inflammation should raise suspicion of airway infection. In cases where there is combined prominent lymphocytic interstitial widening of the alveolar septa with follicular bronchiolitis, a diagnosis of lymphocytic interstitial pneumonia (LIP) may be made. Nodular

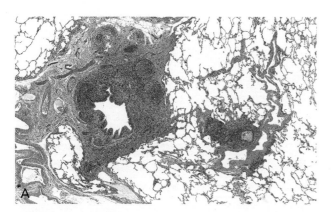 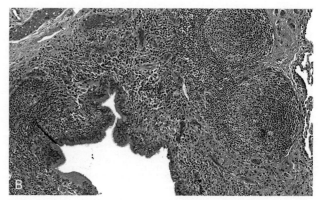

FIGURE 22-10 Follicular bronchiolitis. A: On low-power image, the bronchioles show a marked subepithelial chronic inflammatory infiltrate with rounded lymphoid follicles with germinal center formation. B: On medium-power image, the typical architecture of a germinal center is visualized.

disease or diffuse inflammatory infiltrates with parenchymal effacement should raise concern for a possible lymphoproliferative disease, and evaluation of lymphoma markers by immunohistochemistry or other ancillary methods is appropriate. Follicular bronchiolitis may also be observed distal to bronchiectasis.[53,54]

Imaging Features of Follicular Bronchiolitis

The main radiologic correlate of follicular bronchiolitis is the presence of centrilobular nodules on HRCT. Mosaic perfusion, with or without areas of segmental hyperinflation (air trapping) on expiratory views, may also be observed.[5,55]

Etiologies of Follicular Bronchiolitis

To a large extent, the etiologies associated with follicular bronchiolitis overlap significantly with those of cellular bronchiolitis. However, conditions associated with inherited and acquired immune deficiency are at the top of the differential diagnosis. These include autoimmune CTD, severe combined immunodeficiency syndrome, total or class-specific hypogammaglobulinemia, HIV/AIDS, and immunosuppression in organ transplant patients. Other etiologies include smoking, dust inhalation, and rare chronic drug reactions (eg, nitrofurantoin). Idiopathic forms have been described.[56,57] Chronic infectious pneumonias, such as in right middle lobe syndrome or cystic fibrosis, are also often associated with follicular bronchiolitis, but these cases typically show significant concurrent large airway involvement manifested by bronchiectasis and prominent acute inflammation. Lymphomas, including but not limited to extranodal marginal zone lymphoma, may mimic or have background follicular bronchiolitis.[53,58]

Clinical Features of Follicular Bronchiolitis

As in cellular bronchiolitis, clinical manifestations and treatment considerations are largely dictated by the primary etiology. Identification of an underlying immunological disorder and ruling out infection or a possible lymphoproliferative condition are the pathologist's primary concerns.

DIFFUSE PANBRONCHIOLITIS

Histologic Features of Diffuse Panbronchiolitis

Diffuse panbronchiolitis is a distinctive form of small airway disease, histologically characterized by chronic inflammation of respiratory bronchioles with interstitial accumulation of foamy macrophages, often with luminal acute and chronic inflammation (*Figure 22-11A, B*). In advanced untreated cases, associated bronchiolocentric fibrosis is also usually present. The nomenclature of the disease refers to the bilateral distribution (diffuse), and involvement of all layers of the respiratory bronchiole (pan). Special stains for microorganisms are virtually always negative; however, chronic bacterial infection often occurs in patients with advanced disease and bronchiectasis.[59,60]

Imaging Features of Diffuse Panbronchiolitis

Chest CT usually shows centrilobular nodules and branching linear densities are noted. Airway thickening and bronchiectasis with "tree-in-bud" opacities may be observed in advanced cases.[5,33]

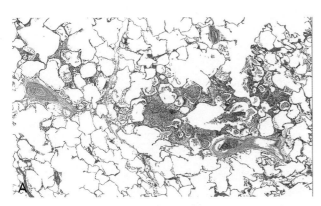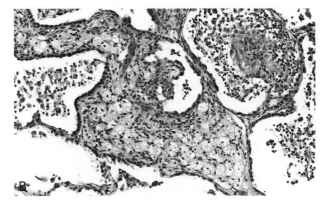

FIGURE 22-11 Diffuse panbronchiolitis. **A:** On low-power image, there is evidence of a centrilobular chronic pneumonia with surrounding normal alveolar tissue. **B:** On high-power image, the terminal bronchioles show luminal acute inflammation, mural chronic inflammation, and prominent foamy macrophage accumulation within the peribronchiolar interstitium.

Etiologies of Diffuse Panbronchiolitis

The etiology of diffuse panbronchiolitis is unknown. A familial clustering has been reported with an increase in HLA-B54.[61] The disorder is most commonly observed in Asian patients[62]; however, several cases have been reported in all races.[63,64]

Clinical Features of Diffuse Panbronchiolitis

Patients with diffuse panbronchiolitis present with a chronic cough with prominent sputum production. The majority of patients will show a long-standing chronic sinusitis. There is a male predominance, with a 2:1 male to female ratio. Most patients are between 30 and 70 years old. Recognition of the disease is paramount, as it is progressive and lethal if untreated, but may be controlled with chronic low-dose macrolide therapy with good results.[62]

OTHER BRONCHIOLITIC CONDITIONS WITH SPECIFIC ETIOLOGIES

Presence of Granulomas

Granulomas involving small airways can be found in biopsies of patients with a number of distinct etiologies. A specific etiology can be identified in a large proportion of such cases upon careful consideration of histologic features, imaging, and clinical data. Therefore, the use of the older nonspecific diagnosis *granulomatous bronchiolitis* is discouraged in such cases.

Most cases of *pulmonary sarcoidosis* have well-formed nonnecrotizing granulomas that are found within bronchovascular bundles, along interlobular septa, and in the subpleural regions. This perilymphatic (or lymphangitic) pattern of distribution is an important histologic as well as radiologic diagnostic clue [see Chapter 24]. In contrast, small poorly formed nonnecrotizing granulomas composed of loosely adherent macrophages, multinucleated giant cells with occasional cholesterol clefts, found in the peribronchiolar interstitium and adjacent airspaces should raise suspicion for *hypersensitivity pneumonia* (see Chapter 23). Necrotizing granulomas and/or significant acute inflammation are typical of *infection*, particularly fungal or mycobacterial, and should be evaluated with cultures, special stains (eg, AFB, GMS), and molecular or immunodetection tests when needed (see Chapters 12 and 13). As mentioned above, small nonnecrotizing granulomas composed of giant cells with prominent cholesterol clefts observed in dilated bronchioles, often in association with accumulation of mucus, are an important clue for possible *constrictive bronchiolitis*. Peribronchiolar granulomas have also been reported in association with inflammatory bowel disease.[65]

Mineral Dust-Related Small Airway Disease

*Mineral dust-related small airway disease*s are caused by inhalation of a variety of inorganic substances through occupational or environmental exposure, including silica, silicates, coal, asbestos, and other less common minerals. Although the exact histologic manifestations vary by the type and severity of exposure, a common set of features can be observed. Early findings include centrilobular accumulation of alveolar macrophages (respiratory bronchiolitis) containing pigmented particulates. Later, the macrophages are incorporated into the peribronchiolar interstitium resulting in formation of irregular microscopic nodules with pigment deposition (*Figure 22-12A, B*). Centriacinar emphysema is almost uniformly present. In severe cases, progressive coalescence of these

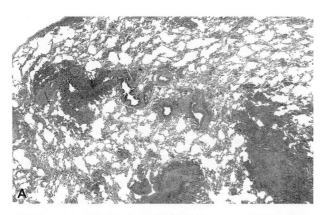
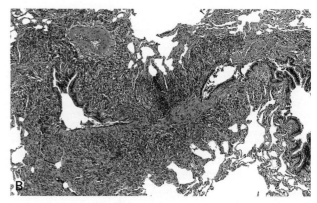

FIGURE 22-12 Dust-related bronchiolitis. A: On low-power image, a peribronchiolar nodular accumulation of macrophages containing fine particulate material is noted. B: A high-power image shows peribronchiolar histiocytes with cytoplasmic dust accumulation. In some dust-related small airway diseases, the macrophages accumulate within the peribronchiolar alveolar spaces, much like respiratory bronchiolitis of smokers.

smaller nodules leads to large areas of consolidation that are readily recognized radiologically as *progressive massive fibrosis* (PMF). Perilymphatic distribution of the nodules (ie, within bronchovascular bundles, in interlobular septa, and along the pleura) is apparent both histologically and radiographically. Upper lobes are affected more severely than the lower lobes in most inhaled dust diseases (with the exception of asbestosis). Clinical course is variable and dependent on the severity of fibrosis and emphysema. In most cases, the diagnosis is established based on exposure history and imaging findings alone, without a need for biopsy.[32] Asbestosis and other pneumoconioses are further described in Chapter 20.

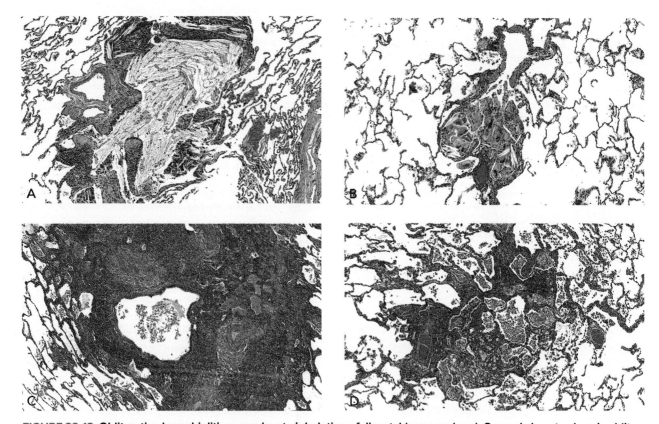

FIGURE 22-13 Obliterative bronchiolitis secondary to inhalation of diacetyl (popcorn lung). Several clues to chronic obliterative bronchiolitis are observed in this single case of a popcorn factory worker. A: Mucus plugging is noted within terminal bronchioles. B: Cholesterol granuloma formation is observed within alveolar ducts. Proximal bronchiolectasis with marked chronic inflammation is present. Numerous foamy macrophages are noted within the peribronchiolar alveolar spaces.

Small Airway Disease due to Drugs, Toxins, and Chemical Fumes

Numerous substances (*Table 22-1*), both inhaled and ingested, have been associated with interstitial lung disease and small airway injury. Acute exposures can trigger a life-threatening respiratory illness manifested histologically as DAD with parenchymal edema and bronchiolar necrosis in most severe cases. Upon withdrawal of inciting agent and administration of therapy, which may include mechanical ventilation and high-dose steroids, surviving patients often progress to an organizing stage histologically characterized by organizing pneumonia (OP). Less acute cases may have OP as the initial presentation.[66] While some patients will have full recovery, a proportion will develop chronic sequelae such as interstitial fibrosis or constrictive bronchiolitis months to years after the initial exposure. Chronic exposures may result in bronchiolocentric fibrosis with cellular or follicular bronchiolitis, as for example in nitrofurantoin or amiodarone toxicity, and may present a significant diagnostic challenge.[67,68]

Inhalation exposure to diacetyl, a flavoring agent used in manufacturing of microwave popcorn and other food products, has been linked to development of constrictive bronchiolitis in workers at popcorn manufacturing plants.[69,70] Lung biopsies from *popcorn lung* patients show a range of small airway findings, including constrictive bronchiolitis, cellular and follicular bronchiolitis, and bronchiolectasis (*Figure 22-13A–D*).

REFERENCES

1. Visscher DW, Myers JL. Bronchiolitis: the pathologist's perspective. *Proc Am Thorac Soc.* 2006;3(1):41-47.
2. Allen TC. Pathology of small airways disease. *Arch Pathol Lab Med.* May 2010;134(5):702-718.
3. Schwarz MI, King TE. *Interstitial lung disease.* 5th ed. Shelton, CT: People's Medical Publishing House-USA; 2011.
4. Churg A. An inflation procedure for open lung biopsies. *Am J Surg Pathol.* January 1983;7(1):69-71.
5. Webb WR, Müller NL, Naidich DP. *High-resolution CT of the lung.* 4th ed. Philadelphia, PA: Wolters Kluwer/Lippincott Williams & Wilkins; 2009.
6. Fukuoka J, Franks TJ, Colby TV, et al. Peribronchiolar metaplasia: a common histologic lesion in diffuse lung disease and a rare cause of interstitial lung disease: clinicopathologic features of 15 cases. *Am J Surg Pathol.* July 2005;29(7):948-954.
7. Travis WD, Costabel U, Hansell DM, et al. An official American Thoracic Society/European Respiratory Society statement: update of the international multidisciplinary classification of the idiopathic interstitial pneumonias. *Am J Respir Crit Care Med.* September 15, 2013;188(6):733-748.
8. Yousem SA, Dacic S. Idiopathic bronchiolocentric interstitial pneumonia. *Mod Pathol.* November 2002;15(11):1148-1153.
9. Churg A, Myers J, Suarez T, et al. Airway-centered interstitial fibrosis: a distinct form of aggressive diffuse lung disease. *Am J Surg Pathol.* January 2004;28(1):62-68.
10. de Carvalho ME, Kairalla RA, Capelozzi VL, Deheinzelin D, do Nascimento Saldiva PH, de Carvalho CR. Centrilobular fibrosis: a novel histological pattern of idiopathic interstitial pneumonia. *Pathol Res Pract.* 2002;198(9):577-583.
11. Delafield F. The pathology of broncho-pneumonia. *Boston Med Surg J.* November 20, 1884;111:484-487.
12. Bates JH, Campbell GD, Barron AL, et al. Microbial etiology of acute pneumonia in hospitalized patients. *Chest.* April 1992;101(4):1005-1012.
13. Ishiguro T, Takayanagi N, Yamaguchi S, et al. Etiology and factors contributing to the severity and mortality of community-acquired pneumonia. *Intern Med.* 2013;52(3):317-324.
14. Spoorenberg SM, Bos WJ, Heijligenberg R, et al. Microbial aetiology, outcomes, and costs of hospitalisation for community-acquired pneumonia; an observational analysis. *BMC Infect Dis.* 2014;14:335.
15. Pavia AT. Viral infections of the lower respiratory tract: old viruses, new viruses, and the role of diagnosis. *Clin Infect Dis.* May 2011;52(suppl 4):S284-S289.
16. Clark TW, Medina MJ, Batham S, Curran MD, Parmar S, Nicholson KG. Adults hospitalised with acute respiratory illness rarely have detectable bacteria in the absence of COPD or pneumonia; viral infection predominates in a large prospective UK sample. *J Infect.* November 2014;69(5):507-515.
17. Pound MW, Drew RH, Perfect JR. Recent advances in the epidemiology, prevention, diagnosis, and treatment of fungal pneumonia. *Curr Opin Infect Dis.* April 2002;15(2):183-194.
18. Barbier F, Andremont A, Wolff M, Bouadma L. Hospital-acquired pneumonia and ventilator-associated pneumonia: recent advances in epidemiology and management. *Curr Opin Pulm Med.* May 2013;19(3):216-228.
19. Leu HS, Kaiser DL, Mori M, Woolson RF, Wenzel RP. Hospital-acquired pneumonia. Attributable mortality and morbidity. *Am J Epidemiol.* June 1989;129(6):1258-1267.
20. Yousem SA, Lohr RH, Colby TV. Idiopathic bronchiolitis obliterans organizing pneumonia/cryptogenic organizing pneumonia with unfavorable outcome: pathologic predictors. *Mod Pathol.* September 1997;10(9):864-871.
21. Davison AG, Heard BE, McAllister WA, Turner-Warwick ME. Cryptogenic organizing pneumonitis. *Q J Med.* Summer 1983;52(207):382-394.
22. Epler GR, Colby TV, McLoud TC, Carrington CB, Gaensler EA. Bronchiolitis obliterans organizing pneumonia. *N Engl J Med.* January 17, 1985;312(3):152-158.
23. Cordier JF, Loire R, Brune J. Idiopathic bronchiolitis obliterans organizing pneumonia. Definition of characteristic clinical profiles in a series of 16 patients. *Chest.* November 1989;96(5):999-1004.
24. Bartter T, Irwin RS, Nash G, Balikian JP, Hollingsworth HH. Idiopathic bronchiolitis obliterans organizing pneumonia with peripheral infiltrates on chest roentgenogram. *Arch Intern Med.* February 1989;149(2):273-279.
25. Guerry-Force ML, Muller NL, Wright JL, et al. A comparison of bronchiolitis obliterans with organizing pneumonia, usual interstitial pneumonia, and small airways disease. *Am Rev Respir Dis.* March 1987;135(3):705-712.
26. Cordier JF. Cryptogenic organising pneumonia. *Eur Respir J.* August 2006;28(2):422-446.
27. Myers JL, Colby TV. Pathologic manifestations of bronchiolitis, constrictive bronchiolitis, cryptogenic organizing pneumonia, and diffuse panbronchiolitis. *Clin Chest Med.* December 1993;14(4):611-622.
28. Lee KS, Kullnig P, Hartman TE, Muller NL. Cryptogenic organizing pneumonia: CT findings in 43 patients. *AJR Am J Roentgenol.* March 1994;162(3):543-546.
29. Lohr RH, Boland BJ, Douglas WW, et al. Organizing pneumonia. Features and prognosis of cryptogenic, secondary, and focal variants. *Arch Intern Med.* June 23 1997;157(12):1323-1329.

30. King TE, Jr., Mortenson RL. Cryptogenic organizing pneumonitis. The North American experience. *Chest.* July 1992;102 (1 suppl):8S-13S.

31. Colby TV. Bronchiolitis. Pathologic considerations. *Am J Clin Pathol.* January 1998;109(1):101-109.

32. Wright JL, Cagle P, Churg A, Colby TV, Myers J. Diseases of the small airways. *Am Rev Respir Dis.* July 1992;146(1):240-262.

33. Hansell DM. Small airways diseases: detection and insights with computed tomography. *Eur Respir J.* June 2001;17(6):1294-1313.

34. Hansell DM. HRCT of obliterative bronchiolitis and other small airways diseases. *Semin Roentgenol.* January 2001;36(1):51-65.

35. Yousem SA, Burke CM, Billingham ME. Pathologic pulmonary alterations in long-term human heart-lung transplantation. *Hum Pathol.* September 1985;16(9):911-923.

36. Burke CM, Theodore J, Dawkins KD, et al. Post-transplant obliterative bronchiolitis and other late lung sequelae in human heart-lung transplantation. *Chest.* December 1984;86(6):824-829.

37. Yousem SA. The histological spectrum of pulmonary graft-versus-host disease in bone marrow transplant recipients. *Hum Pathol.* June 1995;26(6):668-675.

38. Yokoi T, Hirabayashi N, Ito M, et al. Broncho-bronchiolitis obliterans as a complication of bone marrow transplantation: a clinicopathological study of eight autopsy cases. Nagoya BMT Group. *Virchows Arch.* October 1997;431(4):275-282.

39. Urisman A, Jones KD. Pulmonary pathology in connective tissue disease. *Semin Respir Crit Care Med.* April 2014;35(2):201-212.

40. Schlesinger C, Meyer CA, Veeraraghavan S, Koss MN. Constrictive (obliterative) bronchiolitis: diagnosis, etiology, and a critical review of the literature. *Ann Diagn Pathol.* October 1998;2(5):321-334.

41. Parambil JG, Yi ES, Ryu JH. Obstructive bronchiolar disease identified by CT in the non-transplant population: analysis of 29 consecutive cases. *Respirology.* April 2009;14(3):443-448.

42. Epler GR. Diagnosis and treatment of constrictive bronchiolitis. *F1000 Med Rep.* 2010;2:32.

43. Rosenow EC 3rd, Myers JL, Swensen SJ, Pisani RJ. Drug-induced pulmonary disease. An update. *Chest.* July 1992;102(1):239-250.

44. Verleden GM, Raghu G, Meyer KC, Glanville AR, Corris P. A new classification system for chronic lung allograft dysfunction. *J Heart Lung Transplant.* February 2014;33(2):127-133.

45. Kramer MR, Stoehr C, Whang JL, et al. The diagnosis of obliterative bronchiolitis after heart-lung and lung transplantation: low yield of transbronchial lung biopsy. *J Heart Lung Transplant.* July-August 1993;12(4):675-681.

46. Cagle PT, Brown RW, Frost A, Kellar C, Yousem SA. Diagnosis of chronic lung transplant rejection by transbronchial biopsy. *Mod Pathol.* February 1995;8(2):137-142.

47. Lynch JP, 3rd, Weigt SS, DerHovanessian A, Fishbein MC, Gutierrez A, Belperio JA. Obliterative (constrictive) bronchiolitis. *Semin Respir Crit Care Med.* October 2012;33(5):509-532.

48. Jones KD, Urisman A. Histopathologic approach to the surgical lung biopsy in interstitial lung disease. *Clin Chest Med.* March 2012;33(1):27-40.

49. Gruden JF, Webb WR, Warnock M. Centrilobular opacities in the lung on high-resolution CT: diagnostic considerations and pathologic correlation. *AJR Am J Roentgenol.* March 1994;162(3):569-574.

50. Muller NL, Miller RR. Diseases of the bronchioles: CT and histopathologic findings. *Radiology.* July 1995;196(1):3-12.

51. Aherne W, Bird T, Court SD, Gardner PS, McQuillin J. Pathological changes in virus infections of the lower respiratory tract in children. *J Clin Pathol.* February 1970;23(1):7-18.

52. Kindt GC, Weiland JE, Davis WB, Gadek JE, Dorinsky PM. Bronchiolitis in adults. A reversible cause of airway obstruction associated with airway neutrophils and neutrophil products. *Am Rev Respir Dis.* August 1989;140(2):483-492.

53. Yousem SA, Colby TV, Carrington CB. Follicular bronchitis/bronchiolitis. *Hum Pathol.* July 1985;16(7):700-706.

54. Nicholson AG, Wotherspoon AC, Diss TC, et al. Reactive pulmonary lymphoid disorders. *Histopathology.* May 1995;26(5):405-412.

55. Howling SJ, Hansell DM, Wells AU, Nicholson AG, Flint JD, Muller NL. Follicular bronchiolitis: thin-section CT and histologic findings. *Radiology.* September 1999;212(3):637-642.

56. Romero S, Barroso E, Gil J, Aranda I, Alonso S, Garcia-Pachon E. Follicular bronchiolitis: clinical and pathologic findings in six patients. *Lung.* November-December 2003;181(6):309-319.

57. Aerni MR, Vassallo R, Myers JL, Lindell RM, Ryu JH. Follicular bronchiolitis in surgical lung biopsies: clinical implications in 12 patients. *Respir Med.* February 2008;102(2):307-312.

58. Fortoul TI, Cano-Valle F, Oliva E, Barrios R. Follicular bronchiolitis in association with connective tissue diseases. *Lung.* 1985;163(5):305-314.

59. Poletti V, Chilosi M, Casoni G, Colby TV. Diffuse panbronchiolitis. *Sarcoidosis Vasc Diffuse Lung Dis.* June 2004;21(2):94-104.

60. Iwata M, Colby TV, Kitaichi M. Diffuse panbronchiolitis: diagnosis and distinction from various pulmonary diseases with centrilobular interstitial foam cell accumulations. *Hum Pathol.* April 1994;25(4):357-363.

61. Chen Y, Kang J, Wu M, Azuma A, Zhao L. Differential association between HLA and diffuse panbronchiolitis in Northern and Southern Chinese. *Intern Med.* 2012;51(3):271-276.

62. Kudoh S, Keicho N. Diffuse panbronchiolitis. *Clin Chest Med.* June 2012;33(2):297-305.

63. Fitzgerald JE, King TE Jr, Lynch DA, Tuder RM, Schwarz MI. Diffuse panbronchiolitis in the United States. *Am J Respir Crit Care Med.* August 1996;154(2 Pt 1):497-503.

64. Baz MA, Kussin PS, Van Trigt P, Davis RD, Roggli VL, Tapson VF. Recurrence of diffuse panbronchiolitis after lung transplantation. *Am J Respir Crit Care Med.* March 1995;151(3 pt 1):895-898.

65. Camus P, Colby TV. The lung in inflammatory bowel disease. *Eur Respir J.* January 2000;15(1):5-10.

66. Churg A, Green FHY. *Pathology of Occupational Lung Disease.* 2nd ed. Baltimore, MD: Williams & Wilkins; 1998.

67. Rosenow EC 3rd, DeRemee RA, Dines DE. Chronic nitrofurantoin pulmonary reaction. Report of 5 cases. *N Engl J Med.* December 5, 1968;279(23):1258-1262.

68. Larsen BT, Vaszar LT, Colby TV, Tazelaar HD. Lymphoid hyperplasia and eosinophilic pneumonia as histologic manifestations of amiodarone-induced lung toxicity. *Am J Surg Pathol.* April 2012;36(4):509-516.

69. Parmet AJ, Von Essen S. Rapidly progressive, fixed airway obstructive disease in popcorn workers: a new occupational pulmonary illness? *J Occup Environ Med.* March 2002;44(3):216-218.

70. Kreiss K, Gomaa A, Kullman G, Fedan K, Simoes EJ, Enright PL. Clinical bronchiolitis obliterans in workers at a microwave-popcorn plant. *N Engl J Med.* August 1, 2002;347(5):330-338.

23 Hypersensitivity Pneumonitis

Roberto Barrios and Miguel O. Gaxiola

TAKE HOME PEARLS

- Hypersensitivity pneumonitis is an entity with common clinical and histopathological features due to a large number of environmental agents.
- The pathologist may identify an acute, subacute, or chronic form but most likely biopsies obtained show a subacute and a chronic change.
- The triad of interstitial pneumonitis, ill-formed airway-centered granulomas, and bronchiolitis is strongly suggestive of the entity, but they are not specific and some well-documented cases of HP may lack the three components.
- The final diagnosis is made with clinical and radiological findings and a careful history but it is seldom dependent solely on the biopsy findings.

INTRODUCTION

Hypersensitivity pneumonitis (HPS), also known as extrinsic allergic alveolitis, is a clinicopathological entity characterized by an interstitial and small airway inflammatory response to a large number of possible environmental antigens.[1]

Hypersensitivity pneumonitis (HP), also known as extrinsic allergic alveolitis, to the pathologist represents an interstitial granulomatous pneumonitis. To the clinician HP is a group of interstitial lung diseases caused by the repeated inhalation of antigenic organic particles in susceptible individuals. The disease may present as an acute, subacute, or chronic illness. Since the acute form resembles a "flu-like illness," it is rarely seen by the clinician or the pathologist and therefore, most of the information described in the literature is based on observations from patients with the subacute or chronic forms. It usually presents as repeated episodes of respiratory symptoms that subside after cessation of the antigen exposure. If the patient continues exposure to the causal antigen HP may be irreversible and progress to diffuse interstitial fibrosis.

PREVALENCE

It is difficult to establish with certainty the prevalence of HP since it varies depending on geographic and seasonal factors.[2-5] The presence of local occupational settings such as manufacturing plants and other occupational-related factors also has to be considered in the geographic variation reported in the literature. Some studies have estimated the prevalence of farmer's lung, one of the most common forms of hypersensitivity pneumonitis, at approximately 9% in the humid zones of Scotland and 2.3% in the drier zones of East Lothian. Other reports estimate a prevalence of farmer's lung to be between 11.5 and 193 per 100,000 individuals in different regions of England. The prevalence of another form of HP, pigeon breeder's disease, may be between 10% and 20% in individuals regularly exposed to pigeon antigens although some reports mention lower figures (1.4 per 1000 and 1 per 5000).[4]

Table 23-1 Some Examples of Hypersensitivity Pneumonitis

Disease	Antigen Source	Probable Antigen
Plant products		
Farmer's lung	Moldy hay	Thermophilic actinomycetes *Saccharopolyspora rectivirgula* (formerly known as *Micropolyspora faeni*) *Thermoactinomyces vulgaris* *Aspergillus* species *Penicillium* species *Candida* species *Fusarium* species
Bagassosis	Moldy pressed sugar cane (bagasse)	Thermophilic actinomyces *T sacchari* *T vulgaris*
Mushroom worker's disease	Moldy compost and mushrooms	Thermophilic actinomyces *S rectivirgula* *T vulgaris* *Aspergillus* species Mushroom spores
Suberosis	Moldy cork	*Penicillium* species

Used with permission of Ref. 3.

ETIOLOGY

A wide variety of organic antigens derived from various microorganisms including bacteria, fungi, protozoa, and various plant or animal proteins are known causes of hypersensitivity pneumonitis and the name for each form of HP is derived from the setting in which it occurs (*Table 23-1*).[5-10] Exposure to causal antigens can occur in occupational, home, or hobby settings. A form of HP that probably deserves special attention in some geographic areas is the so-called "hot tube disease" which is caused by nontuberculous mycobacteria.[16] It has been described in immunocompetent healthy individuals with a history of hot tub exposure who developed a clinical picture of HP. Examination of lung biopsies from these patients reveals nonnecrotizing granulomas, and *Mycobacterium avium-intracellulare* complex has been demonstrated by culture. Although it is controversial whether these cases can be considered mycobacterial infections or HP, hot tub disease is now considered by many authors a form of HP.

New forms of hypersensitivity pneumonitis are continuously reported in the literature such as mollusk shell hypersensitivity pneumonitis from inhalation of dust produced during the manufacture of nacre buttons from sea-snail shells and summer pneumonitis, a type of extrinsic allergic alveolitis described in Japan caused by *Trichosporon cutaneum*.[8]

CLINICAL FEATURES

In the acute form of the disease the symptoms begin 4 to 6 hours after inhalation of the antigen and starts with influenza-like symptoms: fever, malaise, chills, dyspnea, and cough. The severity varies from a mild flu-like illness to an acute attack of pulmonary edema. The symptoms usually reach a peak 18 to 24 hours after exposure and, if further exposure to the antigen is prevented, the clinical condition resolves without treatment. This disease is frequently mistaken clinically as influenza.

In the chronic form of the disease in which there is repeated inhalation of the responsible antigen, patients frequently present with chronic fatigue, dyspnea, anorexia, and occasionally weight loss. This stage is often progressive and may result in progressive respiratory failure. Physical examination in both forms of the disease is usually nonspecific, and rales are heard in most patients.

PATHOGENESIS

The pathogenesis of HP is complex and some aspects of the disease, such as individual susceptibility, are poorly understood. HP probably results from a combination of an immune complex mediated mechanism at the beginning of the disease and a delayed cellular component due to Th1 T cells during the subacute and chronic stages. The subacute and chronic forms of the disease are characterized by an alveolitis sustained by CD8+ cytotoxic T lymphocytes, granuloma formation, and fibrosis. A number of proinflammatory cytokines and chemokines play an important role since they can activate alveolar macrophages, induce migration of CD8+ lymphocytes into the pulmonary parenchyma, and promote the development of the granulomatous reaction in the interstitial compartment. Macrophages are also critical in the development of the lesion with upregulation of L-selectin, chemokines. An important consideration is that only a minority of individuals exposed to the same antigens that cause HP develop the disease and the reasons for that are not clear but there appears to be a genetic predisposition linked to the major histocompatibility complex (MHC). The results of some of these studies suggest the presence of several alleles and haplotypes that increase the susceptibility to develop the disease.[9-20]

HISTOPATHOLOGIC FEATURES

Acute Stage

The histologic features of the acute stage of HP are not well known because it is very uncommon to see biopsies from these patients during acute episodes since at the beginning of the disease the diagnosis may not be suspected. In addition, it is highly unlikely that a patient would undergo a lung biopsy at this stage of the disease. The few reports of acute HP that have been published describe a neutrophilic infiltrate in the alveoli and respiratory bronchioles (acute bronchiolitis) and occasionally a pattern of diffuse alveolar damage and even small vessel vasculitis.[6]

Subacute Stage

HP in the subacute stage has been well described in the literature and is characterized by an interstitial pneumonitis formed predominantly by lymphocytes, loose granulomas characterized by occasional multinucleated giant cells admixed with lymphocytes (*Figure 23-1*). These granulomas are poorly circumscribed and occasionally contain cholesterol clefts[26] (*Figure 23-2*). Schaumann bodies may be present. In addition, foci of organizing pneumonia and fibrosis are also seen. The disease is predominantly airway centered (*Figure 23-3*) and the inflammatory infiltrate consists mostly of lymphocytes

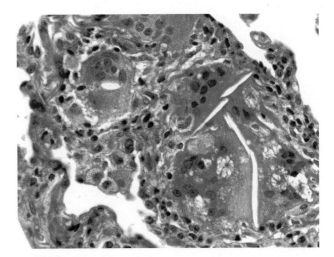

FIGURE 23-2 Granuloma with cholesterol clefts and asteroid bodies (400×).

and some plasma cells. In approximately 50% of clinically proven HP giant cells are absent; it is important to keep this in mind since absence of giant cells does not rule out HP. Furthermore, the presence of giant cells is suggestive of HP but not specific. In some biopsies, especially those from pigeon breeder's disease, foamy macrophages may be seen in small groups in a pattern resembling small foci of endogenous lipid pneumonia.[14,19] Whether these foamy macrophages represent foci of postobstructive endogenous lipid pneumonia or macrophages containing inhaled particles is not clear. Although the term used as a synonym for this disease: "extrinsic allergic alveolitis" may suggest that eosinophils, seen associated with allergic diseases are seen in HP; however, in HP eosinophils are scant or absent in most cases. The so-called intraluminal budding fibrosis consists of polypoid plugs of loose, organizing connective tissue that protrudes into the lumens of alveolar ducts and bronchioles

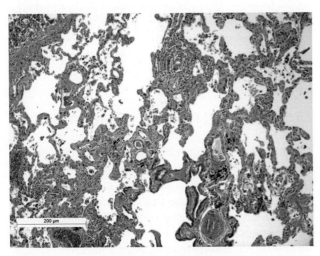

FIGURE 23-1 Interstitial lymphocytic infiltrate with an ill-defined granuloma and metaplastic changes in the vicinity of an airway (40×).

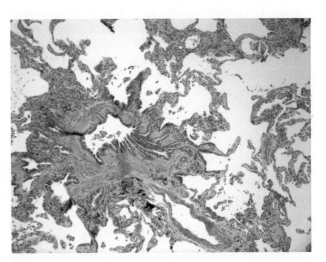

FIGURE 23-3 Airway-centered fibrosis on chronic HP. There is fibrosis of a membranous bronchiole and residual inflammation at the periphery (100×).

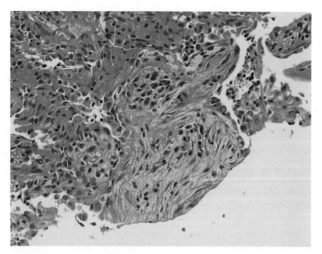

FIGURE 23-4 Fibroblastic "plugs" characteristic or organizing pneumonia in a case of HP (400×).

(a BOOP-like pattern) is seen in approximately two-thirds of cases (*Figure 23-4*).[3] As HP progresses diffuse interstitial fibrosis develops and it may result in a nonspecific pattern of end-stage fibrosis although frequently this fibrosis is airway centered. Although vasculitis has been mentioned as a component of acute HP, it is not seen in biopsies from subacute and chronic forms of the disease. Vascular lesions, when present, probably reflect secondary hypertensive vascular disease and consist of medial hypertrophy of arteries and muscularization of arterioles as well as fibrous intimal thickening of arteries.

Chronic Stage

Chronic cases of HP have been difficult to study but in a series of clinical history, radiology, and pathology of 13 confirmed cases of chronic HSP three histologic patterns were described: NSIP-like, which was relatively homogenous with linear fibrosis, UIP-like in which peripheral fibrosis, patchy distribution, and architectural distortion were present, and mixed which had irregular, predominately peribronchiolar fibrosis. [21-25] Poorly formed granulomas were found in all patterns and this may be a clue to the pathologist although the granulomas ranged from recognizable granulomas to scattered giant cells in the interstitium. In some cases Schaumann bodies were the only sign of possible granulomas.[16] The described changes may be seen in combination with changes due to other causes, such as individuals with HP who live at high altitude.[27]

DIFFERENTIAL HISTOLOGIC DIAGNOSIS

HP must be separated histologically from a number of conditions that may share similar histopathological findings[28] such as lymphoid interstitial pneumonia

(LIP), sarcoidosis, berylliosis, infection, nonspecific interstitial pneumonia (NSIP), and usual interstitial pneumonia (UIP). Nowadays the diagnosis of lymphoid interstitial pneumonia is uncommon but an interstitial lymphoid infiltrate is much more prominent in LIP than HP, and extensively involves alveolar septa. Granulomas and intraluminal budding fibrosis are more common in HP than LIP. In most cases the separation of sarcoidosis and HP is straightforward, but occasionally it may be difficult. The granulomas of HP, as mentioned previously, are "poorly formed" or "ill defined," they are loose and tend to show bronchiolocentric predilection while the granulomas of sarcoidosis tend to be tightly packed, well defined, and distributed along bronchovascular bundles and the pleura. Since infectious etiology can produce the histologic picture of HP, special stains should be performed to rule out the presence of acid-fast bacilli, fungi, and *Pneumocystis carinii*.

The nonspecific interstitial pneumonia (NSIP) pattern can considerably overlap with the HP pattern. In fact, an NSIP pattern has been described in clinically well-documented cases of HP. An exposure history helps distinguish between the two. The fibrotic phase of HP can occasionally be confused with UIP. Temporal heterogeneity with dense may even be seen in HP. The presence of granulomas is helpful in such cases. The same constellation of histologic features seen in HP, including peribronchiolar inflammation, scattered poorly formed granulomas, and intraluminal fibrosis, may be seen in collagen vascular disease, drug reactions, and infection. While lung biopsy findings are suggestive, the ultimate diagnosis of HP requires correlation with clinical findings to identify the offending antigen. Clinical and serologic information is required to exclude a collagen vascular disease and drug reaction.[29]

In summary, the histologic findings previously described are not specific. The lung has limited forms of tissue response to various environmental and endogenous injuries. The final diagnosis of HP should not be based on the pathology alone, but should be done with careful radiological and clinical information to document antigen exposure and an association between symptomatology and antigen exposure.

MANAGEMENT AND PROGNOSIS

Elimination of exposure to the antigen from the patient's environment is the first step in treatment. Pharmacologic therapy may be needed in severe cases: Prednisone, typically beginning at 60 mg/day, plus supplemental oxygen for hypoxemia and other appropriate supportive measures are needed in patients who present with significant respiratory insufficiency. Prednisone usually is continued until there is significant symptomatic and functional improvement. There are conflicting results with the administration of corticosteroids on the long-term course of various forms of HP. In a study of pigeon breeders with HP, there were no significant clinical outcome differences between cases who were treated with steroids and those who were not.[30]

In acute HP, symptoms of fever, chills, and cough disappear within days after exposure ceases. There is usually improvement in the first 2 weeks after an acute attack, but mild abnormalities in pulmonary function may persist for several months. Acute episodes are self-limited and do not require treatment other than avoidance of repeated exposure. The subacute and chronic forms of HP are recognized later in the course of illness and have a poorer prognosis than a single acute episode. As expected, patients with fibrotic HP have a significantly worse prognosis when compared with those with nonfibrotic chronic HP.

REFERENCES

1. Fink JN. Hypersensitivity pneumonitis. *Clin Chest Med.* 1992; 13(2):303-309.

2. Patel AM, Ryu JH, Reed CE. Hypersensitivity pneumonitis: current concepts and future questions. *J Allergy Clin Immunol.* 2001;108(5):661-670.

3. Yi ES. Hypersensitivity pneumonitis. *Crit Rev Clin Lab Sci.* 2002;39(6):581-629.

4. Grant IW, Blyth W, Wardrop VE, Gordon RM, Pearson JC, Mair A. Prevalence of farmer's lung in Scotland: a pilot survey. *Br Med J.* 1972;1(799):530.

5. Christensen LT, Schmidt CD, Robbins L. Pigeon breeders' disease—a prevalence study and review. *Clin Allergy.* 1975;5(4):417-430.

6. Staines FH. A survey of farmer's lung. *J Coll Gen Pract.* 1961;4:351-356.

7. Halpin DM, Graneek BJ, Turner-Warwick M, Newman Taylor AJ. Extrinsic allergic alveolitis and asthma in a sawmill worker: case report and review of the literature. *Occup Environ Med.* 1994 Mar;51(3):160-164.

8. Yoo CG, Kim YW, Han SK, et al. Summer-type hypersensitivity pneumonitis outside Japan: a case report and the state of the art. *Respirology.* 1997;2(1):75-77.

9. Ando M. [Allergic pneumonia. Pathogenesis of summer hypersensitivity pneumonitis]. *Arerugi.* 1994;43(9):1151-1155.

10. Flaherty DK, Braun SR, Marx JJ, Blank JL, Emanuel DA, Rankin J. Serologically detectable HLA-A, B, and C loci antigens in farmer's lung disease. *Am Rev Respir Dis.* 1980;122(3):437-443.

11. Rittner C, Sennekamp J, Mollenhauer E, et al. Pigeon breeder's lung: association with HLA-DR 3. *Tissue Antigens.* 1983;21(5): 374-379.

12. Selman M, Teran L, Mendoza A, et al. Increase of HLA-DR7 in pigeon breeder's lung in a Mexican population. *Clin Immunol Immunopathol.* 1987;44(1):63-70.

13. Ando M, Hirayama K, Soda K, Okubo R, Araki S, Sasazuki T. HLA-DQw3 in Japanese summer-type hypersensitivity pneumonitis induced by Trichosporon cutaneum. *Am Rev Respir Dis.* 1989; 140(4):948-950.

14. Camarena A, Juarez A, Mejia M, et al. Major histocompatibility complex and tumor necrosis factor-alpha polymorphisms in pigeon breeder's disease. *Am J Respir Crit Care Med.* 2001;163(7):1528-1533.

15. Orriols R, Aliaga JL, Anto JM, et al. High prevalence of mollusk shell hypersensitivity pneumonitis in nacre factory workers. *Eur Respir J.* 1997;10(4):780-786.

16. Khoor A, Leslie KO, Tazelaar HD, Helmers RA, Colby TV. Diffuse pulmonary disease caused by nontuberculous mycobacteria in immunocompetent people (hot tub lung). *Am J Clin Pathol.* 2001;115(5):755-762.

17. Agostini C, Trentin L, Facco M, Semenzato G. New aspects of hypersensitivity pneumonitis. *Curr Opin Pulm Med.* 2004;10(5): 378-382.

18. Barrios R, Selman M, Franco R, Chapela R, Lopez JS, Fortoul TI. Subpopulations of T cells in lung biopsies from patients with pigeon breeder's disease. *Lung.* 1987;165(3):181-187.

19. Coleman A, Colby TV. Histologic diagnosis of extrinsic allergic alveolitis. *Am J Surg Pathol.* 1988;12(7):514-518.

20. Schuyler M. Hypersensitivity pneumonitis. In: Crapo JD, Glassroth J, Karlinsky J, King T, eds. *Baum's Textbook of Pulmonary Disease.* 7th ed. Philadelphia, PA. Lippincott Williams & Wilkins; 2004.

21. Agostini C, Calabrese F, Poletti V, et al. CXCR3/CXCL10 interactions in the development of hypersensitivity pneumonitis. *Respir Res.* 2005;6(1):20.

22. Churg A, Muller NL, Flint J, et al. Chronic hypersensitivity pneumonitis. *Am J Surg Pathol.* 2006;30:201-208.

23. Ryu JH, Myers JL, Swensen SJ. Bronchiolar disorders. *Am J Respir Crit Care Med.* 2003;168(11):1277-1292.

24. Perez-Padilla R, Gaxiola M, Salas J, Mejia M, Ramos C, Selman M. Bronchiolitis in chronic pigeon breeder's disease. Morphologic evidence of a spectrum of small airway lesions in hypersensitivity pneumonitis induced by avian antigens. *Chest.* 1996;110(2):371-377.

25. Reyes CN, Wenzel FJ, Lawton BR, Emanuel DA. The pulmonary pathology of farmer's lung disease. *Chest.* 1982;81(2):142-146.

26. Kawanami O, Basset F, Barrios R, Lacronique JG, Ferrans VJ, Crystal RG. Hypersensitivity pneumonitis in man. Light- and electron-microscopic studies of 18 lung biopsies. *Am J Pathol.* 1983;110(3):275-289.

27. Lupi-Herrera E, Sandoval J, Bialostozky D, et al. Extrinsic allergic alveolitis caused by pigeon breeding at a high altitude (2,240 meters). Hemodynamic behavior of pulmonary circulation. *Am Rev Respir Dis.* 1981;124(5):602-607.

28. Grunes D, Beasley, MB. Hypersensitivity pneumonitis: a review and update of histologic findings. *J Clin Pathol.* 2013;66: 888-895.

29. Sahin H, Brown KK, Curran-Everett D, et al. Chronic hypersensitivity pneumonitis: CT features comparison with pathologic evidence of fibrosis and survival. *Radiology.* 2007;244:591-598.

30. de Gracia J, Morell F, Bofill JM, et al. Time of exposure as a prognostic factor in avian hypersensitivity pneumonitis. *Respir Med.* 1989; 83:139-143.

CHAPTER 23

24 Pulmonary Sarcoidosis

Roberto Barrios and Alfredo Valero Gómez

TAKE HOME PEARLS

- Sarcoidosis is a multisystem granulomatous disease of unknown etiology with lung involvement in 90% of the cases.
- The diagnostic histopathologic feature, although not specific, is the presence of noncaseating granulomas in various tissues composed of epithelioid histiocytes and multinucleated giant cells sharply circumscribed from surrounding normal lung.
- Most of the granulomas follow a lymphangitic and bronchovascular distribution in contrast to other granulomatous diseases.
- The presence of bronchial subepithelial granulomas results in high yield on transbronchial biopsies.
- The sarcoidal granuloma is well circumscribed and over time develops peripheral fibrosis and hyalinization.
- Up to 40% of the granulomas contain inclusions (asteroid bodies, Schaumann bodies, calcium oxalate crystals); these inclusions are not specific and can be seen in other granulomatous diseases.

INTRODUCTION

Sarcoidosis is a multisystem granulomatous disease of unknown cause, characterized by a variable clinical presentation and course. More than 90% of patients exhibit thoracic involvement with mediastinal and hilar lymph node enlargement or parenchymal lung disease, but any organ may be involved.[1]

EPIDEMIOLOGY

Sarcoidosis occurs worldwide with the highest incidence occurring in the United States (among African Americans) and Sweden. The incidence is lower in the Asian population and very rare in some Latin-American countries like Mexico. It frequently presents in individuals in their 20s and affects more females than males.[1]

ETIOLOGY

The etiology of sarcoidosis remains unknown but most authors agree that the disease is seen in genetically predisposed individuals exposed to some environmental agents. Infectious agents, specifically mycobacteria, have been proposed as possible agents playing a role in the development of the lesions.[2,3]

PATHOGENESIS

The development and accumulation of granulomas represent the basic pathologic abnormality in sarcoidosis. Sarcoidal granulomas are tightly organized collections of macrophages and macrophage-derived epithelioid cells encircled by lymphocytes. Fused epithelioid cells, which over time become multinucleated giant cells, are often found scattered throughout the granuloma.[4] Accumulation and activation of inflammatory/effector cells, in addition to the proliferation of immune cells, lead to the formation of the typical sarcoid granulomas, that is, compact structures made by a central core of epithelioid and multinucleated phagocyte cells surrounded by T cells, especially CD4 T cells, but also rare CD8 T lymphocytes and B cells. Sarcoidosis is characterized by a compartmentalization of CD4+ T helper 1 (Th1) lymphocytes and activated monocyte/macrophages in involved organs, including the lung, lymph nodes, and skin.[5,6] In approximately 60% of patients the disease spontaneously resolves, but in some subjects the persistence of the antigenic stimulus favors a chronic inflammatory state, granuloma lung formation, and, in some cases, an evolution toward fibrosis.[7,8] A complex network of cytokines and chemokines play a crucial role in the pathogenesis of sarcoidosis: early phases are characterized by a local overproduction of Th1 cytokines,[9,10] such as interleukin 2 (IL-2) and interferon γ (IFN-γ), associated with the high expression of macrophage-derived molecules such as IL-15, CXCL10, CXCL16, CCL5, and CCL20. Th17, a new CD4+ effector T-cell population, has been recently described. Initially identified for its ability to produce IL-17A, IL-17F, and IL-22, Th17 cells develop in response to IL-23 and IL-1β. These cells express CD4, CD45RO, CCR6 (receptor of the chemokine CCL20), CCR4, and the subunit IL-23R (the specific receptor for the p19 chain of IL-23). In addition, Th17 lymphocytes express a specific master transcription factor known as retinoic acid–related orphan receptor (ROR)γt and release an array of cytokines, including proinflammatory molecules such as tumor necrosis factor α (TNF-α) and IL-6.[12] Recent studies have highlighted the effector role of Th17 cells in a number of pathological conditions, including autoimmunity and inflammation. In particular, the Th17 subset has been linked to Th1 chronic inflammatory diseases, such as psoriasis and inflammatory bowel diseases, and also lung fibrosis. Fibrosis has been associated with a shift in the involved lymphocytes from the TH1 (IL-2 and IFN-γ) to the TH2 phenotype (IL-4, -10, and -13). This fibrotic process irreversibly alters organ architecture and function. Increased 1-α-hydroxylase activity in macrophages within granulomas and the alveoli converts 25-hydroxyvitamin D to the biologically active form 1,25-dihydroxyvitamin D (calcitriol), thereby resulting in increased intestinal absorption of calcium. Although sarcoidosis is predominantly a T-cell-driven disease, the presence of polyclonal hyperglobulinemia indicates that B lymphocytes may also play a role.[11,12]

The diagnosis is usually of exclusion and is established when clinicoradiological findings are supported by histologic evidence of noncaseating epithelioid cell granulomas. Granulomatous inflammation of known causes and local sarcoid-like reactions must be excluded. Parameters used to assess sarcoidosis disease expression include chest radiographic staging (CXR), lung function, organ involvement, and, more recently, dyspnea and fatigue scales.[13] Cell infiltration of activated Th1 cells represents the immunological hallmark of sarcoidosis.[14]

CLINICAL FINDINGS

Up to 90% of patients with sarcoidosis have pulmonary involvement.[1] Symptomatic individuals commonly experience fatigue, night sweats, and weight loss. Pulmonary function tests show a restrictive pattern, more often than an obstructive pattern, owing to fibrosis. Obstruction may be caused by endobronchial disease, bronchial stenosis, distortion of airways, or increased airway reactivity. Pulmonary sarcoid is staged by radiographic findings.[15,16] Histologic diagnosis is made either by the presence of nonnecrotizing granulomas on transbronchial biopsy or by on a biopsy of mediastinal lymph nodes. The latter can be accomplished by mediastinoscopy or by transbronchial needle aspiration (TBNA). The yield of TBNA is increased if it is done by endobronchial ultrasound guidance.[17] The rate of positive biopsy results of transbronchial biopsy is 40% (higher with restrictive disease) and much higher (near 90%) with TBNA of enlarged lymph nodes.

Up to 35% of cases of sarcoidosis are a part of Löfgren syndrome.[18] Löfgren syndrome differs from other types of sarcoidosis, however, in important ways. Löfgren syndrome, an acute form of the disease, consists of erythema nodosum, arthritis, and bilateral hilar adenopathy. Fever and uveitis may also accompany Löfgren syndrome. Erythema nodosum occurs predominantly in women, whereas arthritis predominates in men. It is more common in young white women from Scandinavia and Ireland, and is uncommon in blacks.[1]

The most common radiographic finding is intrathoracic lymph node enlargement with or without parenchymal lung involvement. Mediastinal lymphadenopathy without hilar adenopathy is extremely rare. Hilar lymph node enlargement is usually symmetrical, and less than 3% of patients have unilateral enlargement.

Endobronchial sarcoidosis may lead to bronchial stenosis and recurrent obstructive pneumonias. Pleural effusions on plain radiography are uncommon (1%-3% of patients). Pulmonary hypertension may complicate sarcoidosis, particularly when pulmonary fibrosis is present.

GROSS FINDINGS

The gross appearance of pulmonary sarcoidosis depends on the stage of the disease. In early phases the lung may look normal or show small pleural tan nodules. Over time the nodules are more conspicuous in the interlobular septa. In advanced stages there is interstitial fibrosis and honeycombing. In less than 5% of the cases sarcoidosis can present as solitary nodules (so-called nodular sarcoidosis). Pulmonary fibrosis can be seen but although it has been mentioned in the literature as a frequent cause of honeycomb lung, this finding is unusual. Bilateral lymph node involvement is common with enlarged intrapulmonary and Hilar lymph nodes. The lymphangitic distribution of the sarcoidal lesions can be seen as prominent wide interlobular septa on cut surface of the lung.

HISTOLOGICAL CHARACTERISTICS

The characteristic lesion in sarcoid is the nonnecrotizing granuloma. Typically the granulomas are nonnecrotizing; however, it is well known that up to 40% of granulomas may contain small central areas of necrosis or fibrinoid change but necrosis is usually not prominent and the presence of abundant necrosis is unlikely and more suggestive of a different etiology such as infection. Sarcoidal granulomas are well-circumscribed aggregates of epithelioid cells with lymphocytes and fibroblast at the periphery of the lesion and sharply circumscribed from surrounding normal lung (*Figure 24-1*). Multinucleated giant cells are usually present in florid lesions. Over time the granulomas are surrounded by concentric fibrosis that surrounds the cellular portion of the granulomatous inflammation.[19] Long-standing lesions may show predominantly partially hyalinized fibrosis (*Figure 24-2*). The various cellular and noncellular components of the sarcoidal granulomas and not specific and can be seen in other granulomatous diseases but in most cases

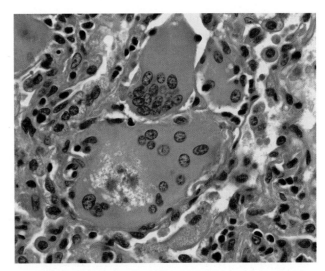

FIGURE 24-2 **Asteroid bodies. Multinucleated giant cell containing asteroid bodies showing a central core, rays, and vacuoles (400×).**

it is possible to find the previously mentioned epithelioid histiocytes admixed with multinucleated giant cells. These cells may exhibit a number of inclusions including asteroid bodies, calcium oxalate crystals, and Schaumann (conchoidal) bodies. Asteroid bodies are cytoskeletal structures found in the cytoplasm and consist of a speculated star-shaped structure varying from 3 to 30 μm with several "rays" in a radiated configuration (*Figure 24-3*). Since these bodies are found in granulomas of different etiologies, they are nonspecific and should not be mistaken for inhaled environmental or infectious agents. Laminated concretions composed of calcium and proteins known as Schaumann bodies (*Figure 24-3*) are found within giant cells in

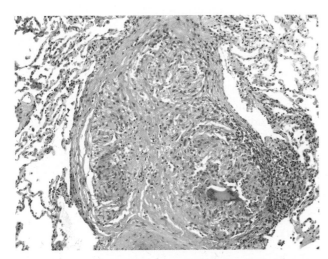

FIGURE 24-1 **Sarcoidal-type granulomas. They are well circumscribed, composed of epithelioid and multinucleated giant cells and a lymphocytic component. Early fibrosis and hyalinization can be seen at the periphery (200×).**

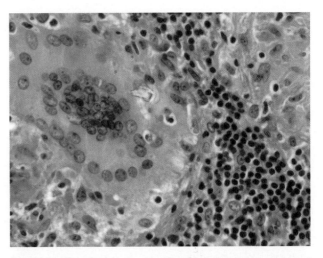

FIGURE 24-3 **Schaumann body formed by inclusions of calcium and protein inside of multinucleated giant cells (400×).**

approximately 60% of the granulomas. Schaumann bodies are usually intracytoplasmic; however, if large enough, they may extrude into the extracellular space. Though characteristic, these microscopic features are not pathognomonic of sarcoidosis, because asteroid and Schaumann bodies may be encountered in other diseases with granulomatous inflammation. Calcium oxalate crystals are also found in granulomas; they are birefringent under polarized light and are frequently mistaken by inhaled environmental agents.

The relatively high frequency of granulomas in the bronchial submucosa accounts for the high diagnostic yield of bronchoscopic biopsies (*Figure 24-4*). Vasculitis seen in over half of cases and involvement of adventitia and media of arteries and veins may cause pulmonary hypertension (*Figure 24-5*).

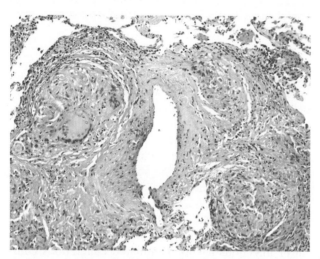

FIGURE 24-4 Granulomas involving bronchovascular sheaths. Vascular involvement can lead to pulmonary hypertension (200×).

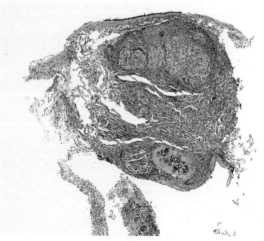

FIGURE 24-5 Granulomas in bronchial mucosa. A partially denuded bronchial epithelium can be seen in this transbronchial biopsy that contains nonnecrotizing granulomas (40×).

DIFFERENTIAL DIAGNOSIS

Although, as previously mentioned, the diagnosis of sarcoidosis is a diagnosis of exclusion, there are some distinguishing features in the histopathology of sarcoidosis that, although not specific, may help suggest the diagnosis over other granulomatous diseases, and these features are (1) lack or minimal necrosis as discussed before. (2) The morphology of the granulomas: Sarcoidal granulomas are well defined, well circumscribed, and in contrast to other pulmonary granulomatous diseases, it usually does not spread or involve adjacent lung parenchyma. (3) The distribution of the granulomas in sarcoidosis is typically lymphangitic following interlobular septa, bronchovascular septa, and visceral pleura. (4) Involvement of bronchi which frequently allows the pathologist to make the diagnosis by transbronchial biopsies since the granulomas can be found in a subepithelial location. Differential diagnosis should include infection, especially fungi and mycobacteria, hypersensitivity pneumonitis, collagen vascular disease, drug reaction, Crohn disease, metals reaction. Berylliosis can be indistinguishable from sarcoidosis and elemental analysis and careful clinical history help in the diagnosis. Advanced disease with prominent interstitial fibrosis can mimic usual interstitial pneumonia (UIP); however, the distribution of the fibrosis in UIP is predominantly subpleural and basal whereas in sarcoidosis it tends to be more central.[20] Sarcoidosis is a disease that recurs in transplanted patients although the disease is usually not as severe as what is seen in the patient's native lungs.[21]

TREATMENT

The natural history of the disease is variable. While some patients recover, others progress or have relapses. Oral corticosteroids remain the first line of therapy in most cases but they are aimed at reduction of symptoms. The American Thoracic Society recommends a starting dose of 20 to 40 mg of prednisone daily or on alternate days. The use of other immunosuppressive agents is reserved for those patients who do not improve on steroids. Methotrexate, cyclosporin A, azathioprine are agents that have been used with various degrees of success. Patients with severe progressive pulmonary disease may be candidates for lung transplantation but the possibility of recurrence should be kept in mind.[21]

REFERENCES

1. Iannuzzi MC, Rybicki BA, Teirstein AS. Sarcoidosis. *N Engl J Med.* 2007;357:2153-2165.
2. Gupta D, Agarwal R, Aggarwak AN, et al. Molecular evidence for the role of mycobacteria in sarcoidosis: a meta-analysis. *Eur Respir J.* 2007;30:508-516.

3. Drake WP, Dhason R, Hajizadeh R, et al. Cellular recognition of Mycobacterium ESAT-6 and katG peptides in systemic sarcoidosis. *Infect Immunol.* 2007;75:527-530.

4. Rosen Y. Pathology of sarcoidosis. *Semin Respir Crit Care Med.* 2007;28(1):36-52.

5. Agostini C, Facco M, Chilosi M, Semenzato G. Alveolar macrophage-T cell interactions during Th1-type sarcoid inflammation. *Microsc Res Tech.* 2001;53:278-287.

6. Agostini C, Meneghin A, Semenzato G. T-lymphocytes and cytokines in sarcoidosis. *Curr Opin Pulm Med.* 2002;8:435-440.

7. Baughman RP, Culver DA, Judson MA. A concise review of pulmonary sarcoidosis. *Am J Respir Crit Care Med.* 2011;183: 573 Y581.

8. Ma Y, Gal A, Koss MN. The pathology of pulmonary sarcoidosis: update. *Semin Diagn Pathol.* 2007;24:150-161.

9. Baughman RP, Culver DA, Judson MA, et al. A concise review of pulmonary sarcoidosis. *Am J Respir Crit Care Med.* 2011;183(5):573-581.

10. Prasse A, et al. Th1 cytokine pattern in sarcoidosis is expressed by bronchoalveolar CD4+ and CD8+ T cells. *Clin Exp Immunol.* 2000;122(2): 241–248.

11. Gerke AK, Hunninghake G. The immunology of sarcoidosis. *Clin Chest Med.* 2008;29:379-390.

12. Facco M, Baesso I, Miorin M, et al. Expression and role of CCR6/CCL20 chemokine axis in pulmonary sarcoidosis. *J Leukoc Biol.* October 2007;82(4):946-955.

13. Baughman RP, Teirstein AS, Judson MA, et al. A Case Control Etiologic Study of Sarcoidosis (ACCESS) research group. Clinical characteristics of patients in a case control study of sarcoidosis. *Am J Respir Crit Care Med.* 2001;164:1885-18893.

14. The ACCESS Research Group. Design of a case control etiologic study of sarcoidosis (ACCESS). *J Clin Epidemiol.* 1999;52(12):1173-1186.

15. Prabhakar HB, Rabinowitz CB, Gibbons FK, et al. Imaging features of sarcoidosis on MDCT, FDG PET, and PET/CT. *AJR Am J Roentgenol.* 2008;190(3 suppl):S1-S6 18287458.

16. Kieszko R, Krawczyk P, Michnar M, et al. The yield of endobronchial biopsy in pulmonary sarcoidosis: connection between spirometric impairment and lymphocyte subpopulations in bronchoalveolar lavage fluid. *Respiration.* 2004;71:72-76.

17. de Boer S, Milne DG, Zeng I, Wilsher ML. Does CT scanning predict the likelihood of a positive transbronchial biopsy in sarcoidosis? *Thorax.* 2009;64:436-439.

18. Mana J, Gómez-Vaquero C, Montero A, et al. Löfgren's syndrome revisited: a study of 186 patients. *Am J Med.* 1999;107:240-245.

19. Gall AA, Koss MB. The pathology of sarcoidosis. *Curr Opin Pulm Med.* 2002;8:445-451.

20. Xu L, Kligerman S, Burke A. End-stage sarcoid lung disease is distinct from usual interstitial pneumonia. *American J Surg Path.* April 2013;37(4):593-600.

21. Xu L, Kligerman S, Todd N, Burke A. Pulmonary sarcoidosis: necrotizing granulomas on explant, with recurrence on surveillance biopsies. *Pathol Case Rev.* May/June 2013;18(3):138-143.

25 Smoking-Related Lung Diseases

Nahal Boroumand and Yimin Ge

TAKE HOME PEARLS

- RB is usually an incidental histologic finding in smokers who are otherwise asymptomatic.
- RB-ILD is histologically and radiologically indistinguishable from RB, and can only be determined based on pulmonary function test.
- Histologically, RB and RB-ILD are characterized by accumulation of lightly pigmented macrophages in distal air spaces and mild bronchiolar and peribronchiolar fibrosis.
- Patients with RB-ILD have good prognosis and improve with cessation of smoking.
- DIP is associated with smoking in majority of cases but it has been reported in pneumoconiosis, rheumatological diseases, and drug reaction.
- RB-ILD and DIP have significant morphological overlap and represent a spectrum of lesions with RB-ILD being the mildest form and DIP being the most severe form.
- Patients with DIP may develop acute exacerbation with a mortality rate of 6% to 30%, whereas no acute exacerbation or mortality reported in patients with RB-ILD.
- The relationship between DIP and fibrosing NSIP is unclear. Although they have morphological overlap, prognosis in DIP is significantly better than fibrotic NSIP.
- PLCH has strong association with smoking and often affects upper and middle zones of the lung.
- PLCH is characterized by bilateral diffuse bronchiolocentric nodules with or without cavitation or cystic changes.

- The nodules are typically in stellate shape and are composed of Langerhans cell histiocytes, lymphocytes, plasma cells, and eosinophils, and become fibrotic in late stages.
- Emphysema is defined as permanent abnormal enlargement of air spaces distal to terminal bronchioles by destruction of the alveolar septa with little or no fibrosis.
- Centriacinar emphysema is the most common type of emphysema and has a strong association with smoking
- Combined pulmonary fibrosis and emphysema (CPFE) is defined as combination of emphysema and diffuse interstitial lung disease with increased risk of developing pulmonary hypertension, acute lung injury, and lung cancer.

INTRODUCTION

In addition to cancer and chronic obstructive pulmonary disease (COPD), tobacco smoking is known to have a causal relationship with certain diffuse interstitial and bronchiolar lung diseases, including respiratory bronchiolitis interstitial lung disease (RB-ILD), desquamative interstitial pneumonia (DIP), and pulmonary Langerhans cell histiocytosis (PLCH). Smoking is also considered a risk factor for developing idiopathic pulmonary fibrosis (IPF) and rheumatoid arthritis–associated interstitial lung disease (RA-ILD). Some cases of acute eosinophilic pneumonia and pulmonary hemorrhage syndromes have also been attributed to smoking (*Table 25-1*). On the other hand, some

TABLE 25-1 Classification of Smoking-Related Interstitial Lung Diseases

Chronic interstitial lung diseases
- Respiratory bronchiolitis interstitial lung disease (RB-ILD)
- Desquamative interstitial pneumonia (DIP)
- Pulmonary Langerhans cell histiocytosis

Acute interstitial lung diseases (possibly caused by smoking)
- Acute eosinophilic pneumonia
- Pulmonary hemorrhage syndromes

Interstitial lung diseases (more common in smokers)
- Usual interstitial pneumonia/idiopathic pulmonary fibrosis
- Rheumatoid arthritis–associated interstitial lung disease

interstitial lung diseases such as hypersensitivity pneumonitis and sarcoidosis are less prevalent in smokers than nonsmokers; it is believed that smoking protects against the development of these diseases.[1,2]

The term smoking-related interstitial lung disease has been proposed to encompass RB-ILD, DIP, and PLCH. This classification is supported by the fact that an overwhelming majority of these patients have a history of smoking, the coexistence of these diseases in smokers, improvement of disease upon smoking cessation, and recurrence with resumption of smoking.[2]

RESPIRATORY BRONCHIOLITIS INTERSTITIAL LUNG DISEASE (RB-ILD)

RB was first described by Niewoehner et al in 1974, as a ubiquitous histopathological finding in the lung of young cigarette smokers.[3] It is characterized by aggregation of lightly brown-pigmented macrophages in the respiratory bronchioles, alveolar duct, and adjacent alveoli (*Figure 25-1A*). Mild inflammation and fibrosis might be present in bronchiolar wall and adjacent alveolar septa (*Figure 25-1B, Table 25-2*). RB can be an incidental finding in smokers who are otherwise asymptomatic.

RB-ILD is a mild form of pulmonary interstitial disease that histopathologically and radiologically is indistinguishable from RB. It was originally described by Myers et al in 1985 to explain clinical interstitial lung disease in six cigarette smoking patients who had restrictive pattern on pulmonary function test and/or interstitial marking on plain chest x-ray (CXR). The patients did not have any histopathologic findings other than RB in their surgical lung biopsy.[4] The authors suggested that fibrosis and inflammation of

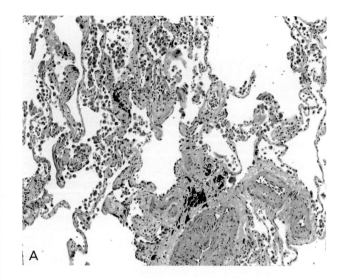

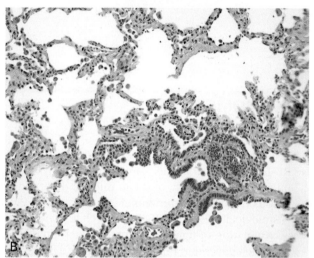

FIGURE 25-1 A: Lower magnification view of RB/RB-ILD shows abundant brown pigmented macrophages in the alveolar spaces adjacent to respiratory bronchiole (H&E stain). B: Medium magnification depictures lightly brown-pigmented macrophages in the respiratory bronchiole and alveoli with minimal to mild inflammation and fibrosis in peribronchiolar tissue and adjacent alveolar septa (H&E stain).

TABLE 25-2 Histologic Features of Respiratory Bronchiolitis

- Pigmented macrophages in membranous and respiratory bronchioles, alveolar ducts, and adjacent alveoli
- Mild bronchiolitis (fibrosis chronic inflammation)

bronchiolar wall and extension into the adjacent alveolar septa distinguish RB-ILD from RB. However, studies done by Fraig et al[5] and Yousem et al[6] concluded that there is no histopathologic feature that can separate RB from RB-ILD.

TABLE 25-3 Differential Diagnosis of Smoking-Related Interstitial Lung Diseases

	Clinical	HRCT	Pathology
RB-ILD	Chronic cough and dyspnea	Bronchiolocentric nodules; ground glass opacities	Pigmented macrophages in membranous and respiratory bronchioles, alveolar ducts, and adjacent alveoli
DIP	Chronic cough and dyspnea	Ground glass opacities; reticular opacities	Pigmented macrophages fill alveolar spaces diffusely
PLCH	Chronic cough and dyspnea, occasional pneumothorax	Cysts, bronchiolocentric nodules with or without cavitation	Stellate or medusa head nodules around bronchioles variable cellularity with Langerhans cells and eosinophils; older nodules increasingly less cellular and more fibrotic

Clinical Features

RB-ILD is almost exclusively seen in young adult smokers and has an equal sex distribution. Patients usually present with cough and mild dyspnea. Pulmonary function test (PFT) shows a mix of obstructive and restrictive pattern and mild decrease in carbon monoxide diffusing capacity (DL_{CO}). Physical examination reveals inspiratory crackles in approximately half of the patients, but digital clubbing is uncommon. This diagnosis can only be established in the presence of RB and absence of other interstitial lung diseases.[7]

Radiologic Findings

Radiologic findings in patients with RB-ILD include diffuse reticulonodular opacity in CXR and centrilobular nodules with ground glass opacity in high-resolution computed tomography (HRCT). It predominantly affects the upper lobe. Similar radiologic findings are reported in asymptomatic smokers.[8,9]

Histologic Findings

Pathologic findings in RB-ILD are indistinguishable from RB and also include the presence of lightly pigmented macrophages in the small bronchioles, alveolar ducts, and adjacent alveolar spaces with mild bronchiolar and peribronchiolar fibrosis (*Figure 25-1A, B*).

Differential Diagnosis

The differential diagnoses include DIP, PLCH, and asbestosis. RB and RB-ILD are histologically indistinguishable. RB-ILD can be distinguished from DIP by the extent of accumulation of pigmented macrophages in the alveolar spaces, which in RB-ILD is peribronchiolar and in DIP is diffuse. In addition, thickening of the alveolar septa by fibrosis and inflammation may be present in DIP. In some cases, the distinction between RB-ILD

and DIP is difficult because of significant morphological overlap. PLCH is another smoker's lung disease characterized by a bronchiolocentric fibrotic or cellular stellate lesion with Langerhans cell histiocytes in addition to the presence of smoker's macrophages in the peribronchiolar alveolar spaces. Identifying the stellate-shape bronchiolocentric lesions helps differentiate these two entities (*Table 25-3*). History of occupational exposure to asbestos and identification of asbestos bodies in H&E- and iron-stained biopsy specimens help differentiate asbestos-related bronchiolar fibrosis from RB-ILD.

Treatment and Prognosis

Patients with RB-ILD have a favorable clinical course and good prognosis. They usually improve with cessation of smoking, thus it is important to differentiate RB-ILD from other interstitial lung diseases.

DESQUAMATIVE INTERSTITIAL PNEUMONIA (DIP)

DIP is one of the rarest idiopathic interstitial pneumonias, comprising less than 10% of the cases. It was first described by Liebow et al in 1965, and was believed to be a diffuse lung disease resulting from desquamation of pneumocytes.[10] Later it became clear that the cells in alveoli are alveolar macrophages rather than pneumocytes. The majority of DIP cases are associated with smoking; however, DIP has been reported in pneumoconiosis, rheumatological diseases, and some drug reactions.[11] DIP has a close relationship with RB-ILD. Both have strong association with smoking and they can have significant morphological overlap. Therefore, it is postulated that DIP and RB-ILD represent different points along the spectrum of smoking-related interstitial lung disease. The relationship between DIP and fibrosing nonspecific interstitial pneumonia (NSIP) is

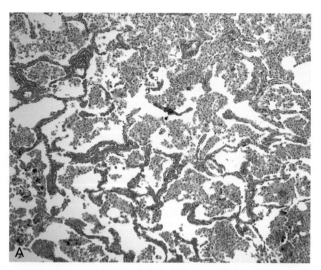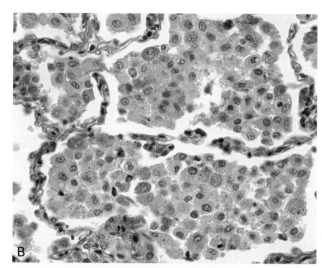

FIGURE 25-2 **A:** Microscopic examination of DIP at low magnification is featured by diffuse involvement of the lung parenchyma with abundant intra-alveolar macrophages and mild thickening of the alveolar septa (H&E stain). **B:** High magnification view of DIP shows alveolar spaces impacted with abundant lightly brown-pigmented macrophages (H&E stain).

not clear. Although they can have morphological overlap, the prognosis in DIP is significantly better than fibrotic NSIP. DIP in children is a different disease and at least in some of them is manifestation of surfactant dysfunction.[11]

Clinical Features

Patients with DIP usually present in the fourth to fifth decade of life. It is more common in men with a male to female ratio of 2 to 1. Patients present with a persistent cough and progressive shortness of breath. Systemic symptoms like fever, fatigue, and weight loss may exist. Physical examination shows bilateral basal inspiratory crackles. PFT shows mild restrictive disease with significant decrease in DL_{CO}.

Radiologic Findings

CXR findings are variable and nonspecific, ranging from normal to predominantly reticulonodular or ground glass opacity. HRCT shows widespread bilateral patchy ground glass opacity. These findings are more prominent in lower and peripheral zones of lung. Irregular linear opacity and limited reticular pattern are frequently seen in the subpleural area and lower lung zone, which represent fibrosis.[2]

Pathologic Findings

DIP is a diffuse process characterized by the presence of an excessive number of lightly brown-pigmented macrophages in the alveolar spaces throughout the lung

parenchyma with variable degree of interstitial inflammation and fibrosis (*Figure 25-2A, B*). Lymphoid follicles and scattered eosinophils are often present. There is no scarring fibrosis or remodeling of the lung parenchyma (*Table 25-4*).

A finely granular hemosiderin pigment can be detected by Prussian blue stain for iron. DIP is closely related to RB-ILD with significant overlapping features. They likely represent the two extremes of a disease spectrum, with RB-ILD being the mildest form and DIP being the most severe. The overlapping histologic features can make the distinction difficult. However, it is still preferred to keep these two entities separate because of significant difference in prognosis. DIP patients may develop acute exacerbation in their course and they have a mortality rate of 6% to 30%, whereas no mortality or acute exacerbation has been reported in patients with RB-ILD.[11] Evidence also shows that RB-ILD often progresses to centrilobular

TABLE 25-4 Histologic Features of Desquamative Interstitial Pneumonia

- Diffuse filling of alveolar spaces by abundant pigmented macrophages
- Mild to moderate interstitial fibrosis and chronic inflammation
- No significant architectural alterations (eg, honeycombing fibrosis)
- Absence of eosinophilic microabscesses
- Absence of inorganic dusts (eg, asbestos)
- Absence of granulomas

emphysema, whereas DIP does not. On the other hand, the relationship between DIP and fibrotic NSIP is not clear. Although there are some overlapping morphologic features, the prognosis for DIP is considerably better than that of fibrotic NSIP.[11]

Differential Diagnosis

RB-ILD and fibrotic NSIP are in the differential diagnosis with DIP. Bronchiolocentric distribution of pigmented macrophages without interstitial pneumonia or lymphoid follicles helps distinguish RB-ILD from DIP. Lack of pigmented macrophages in the air spaces and presence of organizing pneumonia distinguish fibrotic NSIP from DIP.[11]

Histiocyte-rich infections, chronic eosinophilic pneumonia treated with steroids, and chronic hemorrhage with hemosiderosis are among the conditions that need to be considered in the differential diagnosis.

Treatment and Prognosis

Overall prognosis is good in patients with DIP. The majority of patients with DIP respond to smoking cessation and steroid therapy, although some progress to end-stage fibrosis.

PULMONARY LANGERHANS CELL HISTIOCYTOSIS (PLCH)

PLCH is a rare disease comprising less than 5% of diffuse lung disease. It is a chronic progressive disorder characterized by bilateral diffuse bronchiolocentric stellate nodules. PLCH is mostly an isolated process but it can be part of a systemic disorder. Approximately 15% of adults with PLCH have extrapulmonary manifestations. The pathogenesis is poorly understood but is strongly associated with smoking. More than 90% of the patients are current or former smokers. It is likely that smoke constituents activate epithelial cells and other cell types in the airways to produce cytokines that subsequently promote recruitment, activation, and retention of Langerhans cells in the subepithelial regions of the airways. The disease can resolve after cessation of smoking or it can progress. Recurrent PLCH has been reported in transplanted lung.

Clinical Findings

PLCH tends to affect young adults usually in the third to fifth decades of life, and it seems to affect both sexes equally. Patients usually present with nonspecific symptoms including cough, shortness of breath, and chest pain, sometimes accompanied by systemic symptoms

TABLE 25-5 Clinical Features of Pulmonary Langerhans Cell Histiocytosis

- Patients range typically from 20 to 50 years old
- Over 90% of patients are current or former smokers
- Approximately one-third of patients are asymptomatic at the time of diagnosis
- Spontaneous pneumothorax occurs in 10% to 15%
- Extrapulmonary findings in 15% of adult patients
- Pulmonary hypertension is a common complication with poor prognosis

such as fever and weight loss. About a third of patients are asymptomatic when the disease is discovered. About 10% to 15% of patients present with spontaneous pneumothorax which can be recurrent. Pulmonary hypertension is a common complication of PLCH and is associated with poor prognosis (*Table 25-5*). The physical examination is usually normal. PFT shows markedly reduced DL_{CO}, but the total lung capacity and expiratory flow rate is preserved.

Radiologic Findings

CXR shows a bilateral reticulonodular pattern with sparing of the lung bases. In advanced stage of the disease cystic changes and hyperinflation can be seen. HRCT shows bronchiolocentric nodules with or without cavitation, and cystic spaces with variable wall thickness and an occasional highly irregular outline. These lesions are mostly distributed in the upper and middle zone of the lungs. The costophrenic angle is spared.

Pathologic Findings

In the early stage of the disease there is an interstitial infiltrate around small airways. As disease progresses, the infiltrate becomes nodular (*Figure 25-3A*). The inflammatory infiltrate is composed of Langerhans histiocytes, lymphocytes, plasma cells, and eosinophils (*Figure 25-3B*). Langerhans cells can be identified by visualization of Birbeck granules by electron microscopy or positive immunostaining for S100, CD1a (*Figure 25-3C*), and Langerin. Cavitation is a well-recognized feature of PLCH and may ultimately progress to cystic changes that are responsible for pneumothorax (*Figure 25-3A*). In the advanced stage, the nodules become less cellular and more fibrotic (*Figure 25-3D*). The typical nodules of PLCH are roughly symmetric stellate lesions with central fibrosis. Pigmented macrophages are present in surrounding alveolar spaces (*Figure 25-3D*). The nodules show temporal heterogenicity with variations in cellularity and fibrosis, representing different stages of the disease[1,2,12] (*Table 25-6*).

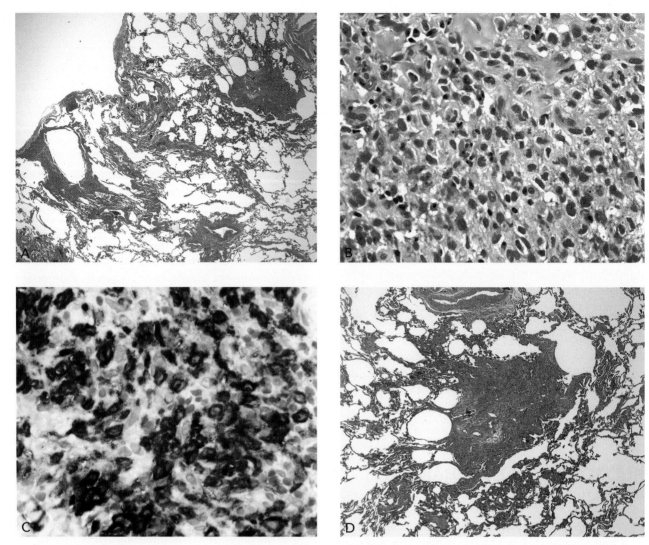

FIGURE 25-3 A: Microscopic view of PLCH shows a bronchiolocentric distribution of stellate shape nodules in this low-magnification view. Cystic change or cavitation is a well-recognized feature and can be seen in the subpleural nodule on the left side of the picture (H&E stain). **B:** High magnification view of an early stage PLCH demonstrates a cellular infiltrate composed of Langerhans cell histiocytes, lymphocytes, plasma cells, and eosinophils. The Langerhans cell histiocytes are featured by pale basophilic nuclei, nuclear groves, and indistinct cell borders (H&E stain). **C:** Immunostain for CD1a highlights Langerhans cell histiocytes in PLCH nodule (immunohistochemical stain). **D:** In advanced stage, the PLCH nodule becomes hypocellular and fibrotic with typical symmetrical stellate shape (H&E stain).

TABLE 25-6 Histologic Features of Pulmonary Langerhans Cell Histiocytosis

- Bilateral bronchiolocentric nodules mainly affect the upper and middle lobes
- Nodules are roughly symmetrical, stellate or medusa-head, and often cavitate
- Nodules vary in cellularity progressing from highly cellular to fibrotic as they age
- Cellular nodules in early stages consist of Langerhans cells with variable numbers of eosinophils; lymphocytes and plasma cells also present
- Langerhans cells are immunopositive for S100, CD1a, and Langerin, and contain Birbeck granules on electron microscopy

Differential Diagnosis

The differential diagnosis includes RB, chronic eosinophilic pneumonia, and usual interstitial pneumonia (UIP). RB lacks the bronchiolocentric, cellular, or fibrotic stellate lesions that are seen in PLCH. The inflammatory infiltrate in chronic eosinophilic pneumonia is present in alveolar spaces, whereas in PLCH it is interstitial. The fibrotic scar in PLCH is bronchiolocentric, stellate shaped, and lacks the patchy pattern of UIP.

Prognosis and Treatment

The natural history of PLCH in adults varies and is unpredictable. Most of the cases remain stable and some cases may regress. There are some patients who may progress despite smoking cessation. In patients with mild disease, smoking cessation might be the only necessary treatment. Corticosteroids and chemotherapeutic agents have been used to treat progressive cases with occasional favorable responses. Pulmonary hypertension is a common complication of the disease and portends poor prognosis. Patients with PLCH have an increased incidence of lung cancer, lymphoma, and myeloproliferative disorders.

EMPHYSEMA

Emphysema is defined as permanent abnormal enlargement of air spaces distal to the terminal bronchioles with destruction of the alveolar septa with little or no fibrosis.

It is classified to proximal acinar (centriacinar), panacinar, distal acinar, and irregular based on the affected part of the acinus.

Centriacinar Emphysema

Centriacinar emphysema is the most common type of emphysema, accounting for approximately 85% of cases. It has a strong association with smoking and mostly involves the upper lobes and posterior part of the lungs. Gross examination of emphysematous lung usually discovers enlarged airspaces (*Figure 25-4B*) that may become significant large air pockets named blebs or bullae (*Figure 25-4A*). Histologically, centriacinar emphysema involves the respiratory bronchioles and adjacent alveoli, hence the term centriacinar (*Figure 25-4C, D*).

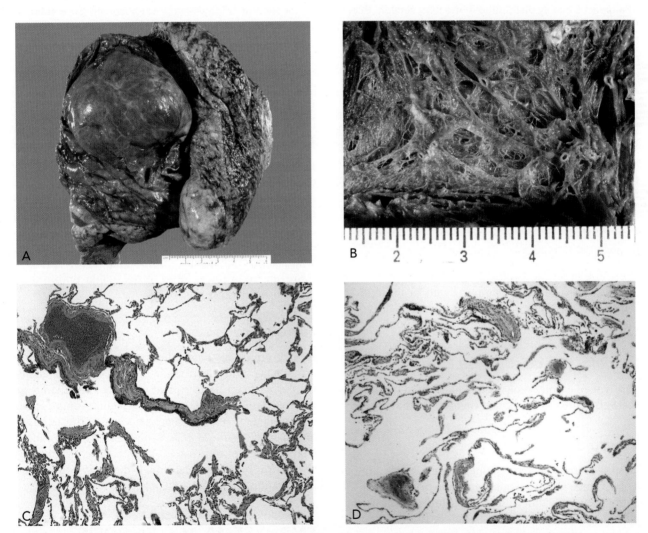

FIGURE 25-4 A: An explanted lung from a long-term smoker shows a giant subpleural air collection (bulla), a common complication of emphysema. **B:** Gross appearance of emphysematous lung shows severe destruction of normal lung parenchyma resulting in markedly enlarged air spaces. **C:** Microscopic examination of centriacinar emphysema shows enlarged air spaces located around a respiratory bronchiole (H&E stain). **D:** Floating pieces of destructed alveolar septa are observed in enlarged air spaces. Presence of a small artery adjacent to the enlarged air space indicates the centriacinar location of emphysema (H&E stain).

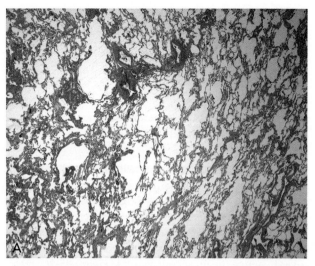 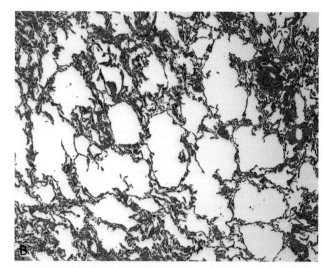

FIGURE 25-5 A: Section of explanted lung from a patient with α₁-antitrypsin deficiency depictures a diffuse enlargement of airspaces evenly distributed in the lung section. Bcentriacinar location of emphysema is not observed (H&E stain). **B:** High magnification of panacinar emphysema shows emphysematous change involves the entire acinus with floating pieces of alveolar septa in enlarged airspaces (H&E stain).

Panacinar Emphysema

Panacinar emphysema comprises 5% of cases. It involves the entire acinus and is diffusely distributed throughout the lungs (*Figure 25-5A, B*), although the lower lobes are more severely involved. This type of emphysema is seen in patients with α₁-antitrypsin deficiency.

Distal Acinar (Localized) Emphysema

Distal acinar emphysema accounts for approximately 5% of the cases, and it involves the distal part of the acinus. It is focal and mainly located in the apex of the lungs. This type of emphysema is seen in young people and often results in spontaneous pneumothorax.

Irregular (Paracicatricial) Emphysema

This type of emphysema occurs adjacent to pulmonary scars and constitutes approximately 5% of the cases.

Clinical Findings

Dyspnea is the main complaint in patients with emphysema. Cough may exist but is not a major symptom. The patient is usually thin with a barrel chest and appears to be in respiratory distress. Respiratory sounds are faint and far in auscultation, and the chest is hyperresonant in percussion.

PFT shows increased volume of the lung (TLC), air flow obstruction with increased residual volume, decreased FEV_1 due to the lack of elastic recoil and collapse of the bronchiole, and decreased diffusion capacity (DL_{CO}) due to the loss of alveolar surface.

Gross Findings

Lungs are enlarged and overinflated. Enlargement of the airspaces may result in formation of bullae (enlarged air spaces more than 1 cm in size) and blebs (dissection of the visceral pleura by air). The distribution varies depending on the type of emphysema. In centriacinar emphysema, upper lobes are more severely involved, whereas in panacinar emphysema, involvement is more severe in lower lobes; distal acinar emphysema commonly involves the apex.

Histologic Findings

Emphysema is histologically characterized by enlarged air spaces and destruction of the alveolar septa, which are seen as free floating pieces in dilated air spaces (*Figure 25-4D*). In centriacinar emphysema a small artery is often seen adjacent to the enlarged air space (*Figure 25-4C*), while the emphysematous change involves entire acini in panacinar emphysema (*Figure 25-5A, B*). Emphysema is diagnosed by clinical information, PFT, CXR, and particularly HRCT.

EMPHYSEMA AND FIBROSIS

Emphysema is defined by the National Institutes of Health (NIH) as abnormal permanent enlargement of airspaces distal to terminal bronchioles, associated

CHAPTER 25

with destruction of the alveolar walls and without obvious gross fibrosis. In recent years, however, coexistence of emphysema and fibrosis has been described in two different settings:

1. Emphysema associated with a diffuse fibrosing interstitial lung disease, most commonly UIP. The condition is called combined pulmonary fibrosis and emphysema syndrome and is of clinical significance since it affects the pulmonary function and causes pulmonary hypertension.
2. Emphysema associated with localized fibrosis, which is a part of either emphysema or respiratory bronchiolitis or both, and is only occasionally associated with physiological or radiological changes of an interstitial lung disease. This condition is called smoking-related interstitial fibrosis or clinically occult interstitial fibrosis in smokers. It is important to know that this condition is not a diffuse fibrosing interstitial pneumonia and does not imply a poor prognosis.

COMBINED PULMONARY FIBROSIS AND EMPHYSEMA (CPFE) SYNDROME

CPFE syndrome is the simultaneous presence of emphysema and diffuse interstitial lung disease. CPFE occurs mostly in current or previous smokers, but it can also be seen in patients with some occupational exposure or collagen vascular diseases, especially rheumatoid arthritis and systemic sclerosis.[13-15] It is more common in males, with a male/female ratio of 9 to 1.

Clinical Findings

Patients with CPFE present with severe dyspnea, despite relatively normal spirometry and lung volumes. DL_{CO} is significantly reduced. There is increased risk of pulmonary hypertension, acute lung injury, and lung cancer in these patients.

Radiologic Findings

HRCT shows bibasilar reticular abnormalities with basal and subpleural predominance, traction bronchiectasis, and honeycombing.

Pathologic Findings

Emphysema predominantly involves the upper lobe and is frequently paraseptal, while interstitial fibrosis predominantly involves the lower lobe. The interstitial fibrosis mostly has an UIP pattern but can also simulate NSIP, DIP, or RB-ILD[13,14] (*Table 25-7*).

TABLE 25-7 Features of Combined Pulmonary Fibrosis and Emphysema (CPFE)

- Emphysema and diffuse interstitial fibrosis coexist in the same patient
- Mostly current or former smokers
- Male predominant (male:female = 9:1)
- Severe dyspnea associated with near-normal pulmonary function tests
- Emphysema is upper lobe predominant and interstitial fibrosis is lower lobe predominant
- Usual interstitial pneumonia pattern is most common fibrotic pattern
- Patients have increased risk of pulmonary hypertension, acute lung injury, and lung cancer
- Prognosis related to pulmonary hypertension

Prognosis

The natural history of CPFE is different from emphysema or interstitial lung disease alone. The prognosis in CPFE is determined by pulmonary hypertension.[13,14]

SMOKING-RELATED INTERSTITIAL FIBROSIS (SRIF)

SRIF is a distinct form of chronic interstitial fibrosis. It is usually an incidental finding in smokers or exsmokers and is found in nonneoplastic areas of the lungs that are removed due to cancer. Patients are usually asymptomatic or mildly symptomatic and disease has a stable course.

Histologically, it is characterized by marked thickening of the alveolar septa with hyalinized fibrosis associated with respiratory bronchiolitis and emphysema. The dense fibrosis surrounds the emphysematous spaces underneath the pleura that can mimic the honeycombing lung in UIP.[16,17] It is important to distinguish SRIF from UIP and other idiopathic interstitial pneumonias.

REFERENCES

1. Vassallo R. Diffuse lung diseases in cigarette smokers. *Semin Respir Crit Care Med.* 2012;33(5):533-542.
2. Vassallo R, Ryu JH. Smoking-related interstitial lung diseases. *Clin Chest Med.* 2012;33(1):165-178.
3. Niewoehner DE, Kleinerman J, Rice DB. Pathologic changes in the peripheral airways of young cigarette smokers. *N Engl J Med.* 1974;291(15):755-758.
4. Myers JL, Veal CF Jr, Shin MS, et al. Respiratory bronchiolitis causing interstitial lung disease: a clinicopathologic study of six cases. *Am Rev Respir Dis.* 1987;135(4):880-884.
5. Fraig M, Shreesha U, Savici D, et al. Respiratory bronchiolitis: a clinicopathologic study in current smokers, ex-smokers, and never smokers. *Am J Surg Path.* 2002;26(5):647-653.

6. Yousem SA, Colby TV, Gaensler EA. Respiratory bronchiolitis-associated interstitial lung disease and its relationship to desquamative interstitial pneumonia. *Mayo Clin Proc.* 1989;64(11):1373-1380.

7. Churg A, Muller NL, Wright JL. Respiratory bronchiolitis/interstitial lung disease. *Arch Pathol Lab Med.* 2010;134(1):27-32.

8. Desai SR, Ryan SM, Colby TV. Smoking related interstitial lung diseases: histopathological and imaging perspectives. *Clin Radiol.* 2003;58:259-268.

9. Galvin JR, Franks TJ. Smoking-related lung disease. *J Thorac Imaging.* 2009;24:274-284.

10. Liebow AA, Steer A, Billingsley JG. Desquamative interstitial pneumonia. *Am J Med.* 1965;39:369-404.

11. Tazelaar HD, Wright JL, Churg A. Desquamative interstitial pneumonia: *Histopathology.* 2011;58(4):509-516.

12. Suri HS, Yi ES, Nowakowski GS, et al. Pulmonary Langerhans cell histiocytosis. *Orphanet J Rare Dis.* 2012;33(5):533-542.

13. Cottin V, Cordier JF. Combined pulmonary fibrosis and emphysema in connective tissue disease. *Curr Opin Pulm Med.* September 2012;18(5):418-427.

14. Wright JL, Tazelaar HD, Churg A. Fibrosis with emphysema. *Histopathology.* 2011;58(4):517-524.

15. Jankowich MD, Rounds SI. Combined pulmonary fibrosis and emphysema syndrome. *Chest.* 2012;141(1):222-231.

16. Katzenstein AL. Smoking-related interstitial fibrosis (SRIF): pathologic findings and distinction from other chronic fibrosing lung disease. *J Clin Pathol.* 2013;66(10):882-887.

17. Katzenstein AL, Mukhopadhyay S, Zanardi C, et al. Clinically occult interstitial fibrosis in smokers: classification and significance of a surprisingly common finding in lobectomy specimens. *Human Pathol.* March 2010;41(3):316-325.

Alveolar Infiltrates

Alberto M. Marchevsky

TAKE HOME PEARLS

- The lung reacts acutely to infections, drugs, toxins, and other pathogens with various clinical and pathologic manifestations of the acute lung injury syndrome (ALI). Among the pathologic manifestations are pulmonary edema and diffuse alveolar damage.
- The clinicopathologic patterns of injury in pulmonary infectious processes include lobar or segmental pneumonia, bronchopneumonia, acute interstitial pneumonia, and mixed pneumonic patterns.
- Acute alveolitis is most frequent in patients with bacterial pneumonias, although it can be seen as a result of fungal or viral infections. It is characterized by the presence of numerous neutrophils in intra-alveolar spaces, admixed with eosinophilic fibrin, debris, and variable number of red blood cells.
- Pneumonias secondary to viral infections, M pneumoniae, Chlamydia sp, Pneumocystis jiroveci, and other organisms usually present with interstitial infiltrates rather than acute alveolitis.
- Approximately 5% to 15% of community-acquired pneumonias in the United States result from aspiration.
- Necrotizing pneumonia is an infrequent complication of bacterial and viral pneumonias characterized by the development of pulmonary necrosis, lung abscess formation, empyema, bronchopleural fistula, diffuse alveolar damage, and/or sepsis.
- Pulmonary abscess is an acute or subacute pneumonia that destroys the lung parenchyma, creating one or more intrapulmonary cavities.

- Organizing pneumonia is a condition defined pathologically by the presence of granulation tissue, and myofibroblastic proliferation with early fibrosis in alveolar ducts and sacs. It can also extend into respiratory bronchioles, resulting in bronchiolitis obliterans. It is a pathological pattern rather than a specific clinicopathologic entity.
- Acute fibrinous and organizing pneumonia (AFOP) is a recently described histologic pattern of acute or subacute lung injury The most characteristic histopathologic feature of AFOP is the presence of extensive intra-alveolar fibrin in the form of fibrin "balls" with scanty or absent neutrophils.
- Lipoid pneumonia is a condition characterized by the accumulation of lipid containing macrophages in the lung. It can be classified as exogenous and endogenous lipoid pneumonia.
- Pulmonary conditions associated with eosinophilia include asthma, acute and chronic eosinophilic pneumonia, pulmonary Langerhans cell histiocytosis, some cases of hypersensitivity pneumonitis (extrinsic allergic alveolitis), viral and other infectious pneumonia, drug reaction, allergic bronchopulmonary aspergillosis, bronchocentric granulomatosis, radiation pneumonitis, lung cancer, Churg-Strauss syndrome, acute cellular rejection, and other conditions.
- Acute eosinophilic pneumonia typically presents with a severe acute illness of a few days duration and presence of >25% of eosinophils on bronchoalveolar lavage fluid and/or tissue eosinophilia.
- Lung tissues in patients with acute eosinophilic pneumonia show a large number of interstitial

eosinophils and a smaller number of intra-alveolar eosinophils associated with changes of the exudative and/or proliferative phases of DAD.

- Lung tissues in patients with chronic eosinophilic pneumonia show extensive intra-alveolar accumulation of macrophages admixed with variable numbers of eosinophils, edema fluid, and a proteinaceous exudate that can appear as "colloid like."
- The histopathological changes of chronic eosinophilic pneumonia can be associated with foci of organizing pneumonia, bronchiolitis obliterans, eosinophilic microabscesses, small number of epithelioid granulomas, and focal necrosis.
- Desquamative interstitial pneumonia–like pattern is characterized by the presence of numerous pigmented macrophages within alveoli in a diffuse distribution throughout the lung parenchyma.
- Pulmonary alveolar proteinosis is a rare condition characterized by the presence of abundant granular, eosinophilic, acellular material within the alveolar spaces resulting from the intra-alveolar accumulation of lipoproteinaceous surfactant material as a consequence of alveolar macrophage abnormalities.

ACUTE LUNG INJURY

The lung reacts acutely to infections, drugs, toxins, and other pathogens with various clinical and pathologic manifestations of the acute lung injury syndrome (ALI).[1] The pathologic findings in acute lung injury include pulmonary edema, diffuse alveolar damage, and several conditions characterized by the presence of cellular alveolar infiltrates that are generally diagnosed as acute pneumonias (*Table 26-1*).[2]

Pulmonary Edema

Pulmonary edema is a form of acute lung injury characterized by the transudation of fluid from the capillary space into the pulmonary interstitium and intra-alveolar

Table 26-1 Pathologic Findings in Acute Lung Injury

Pulmonary edema
Diffuse alveolar damage
    Exudative phase
    Proliferative phase
Pneumonias
    Acute alveolitis
        Lobar pneumonia
        Segmental pneumonia
        Bronchopneumonia
    Acute interstitial pneumonia

spaces.[3] It can result from *increase in capillary hydrostatic pressure* (eg, secondary to mitral stenosis and other causes of left ventricular failure), *increased capillary permeability* (eg, secondary to inhaled toxins, oxygen toxicity, and others), *lymphatic insufficiency* (eg, secondary to metastatic carcinoma with lymphangitic spread, silicosis, others), *decreased colloid osmotic pressure* (eg, secondary to hypoproteinemia), *decreased interstitial pressure* (eg, secondary to hyperinflation, rapid removal of pleural fluid, others), or *unknown mechanisms* (eg, high altitude, heroin, neurogenic events, others).[3-8]

Clinical features of pulmonary edema

Depending on the severity of the pulmonary edema patients present with various degrees of shortness of breath ranging from dyspnea on exertion, paroxysmal nocturnal dyspnea, and/or orthopnea to severe dyspnea at rest.[4,5] Patients with severe pulmonary edema also develop frothy, blood tinged sputum. Physical examination reveals decreased breath sounds, fine inspiratory crepitation, rales, crackles, and/or rhonchi that are more prominent at the lung bases.

Imaging features of pulmonary edema

Chest radiographs show an enlarged heart in patients with cardiogenic pulmonary edema.[4] The chest radiographs of patients with early pulmonary edema show the presence of Kerley B lines seen as short, linear, horizontal markings that are most prominent near the pleural surfaces of the lower lobes.[8] Imaging findings in patients with more advanced pulmonary edema include the presence of bilateral densities that radiate from the hilar regions with a "butterfly appearance."

Gross features of pulmonary edema

Edematous lungs are heavy, congested, firm, pink-red (*Figure 26-1*) and exhibit the presence of frothy fluid in airways on section.[2] Measurements of lung weights are very useful to detect the presence of pulmonary edema at autopsy in patients who lack the presence of pneumonia or other pathology. Adult lungs weighing over 500 g in the absence of other pathology are considered severely edematous at our hospital.

Histologic features of pulmonary edema

Pulmonary edema is characterized histopathologically by the presence of intra-alveolar slightly eosinophilic exudates that are usually finely granular (*Figure 26-2*).[2] Marked vascular and capillary congestion is also present, particularly in patients with cardiogenic pulmonary edema. Patients with chronic cardiogenic pulmonary edema secondary to mitral stenosis or other conditions can also exhibit the presence of hemosiderosis with

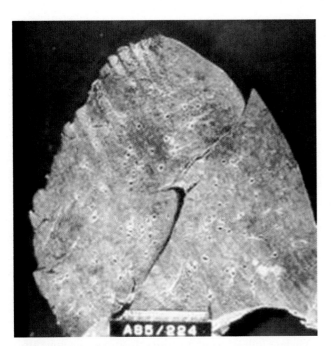

FIGURE 26-1 Acute lung injury. Lung at autopsy is heavy, congested, and diffusely congested.

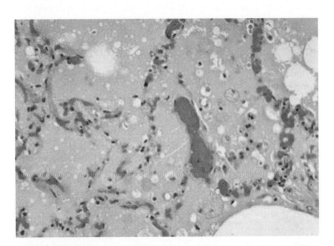

FIGURE 26-2 Intra-alveolar edema. The alveoli are filled with eosinophilic, slightly bubbly intra-alveolar exudate. Capillary congestion is also present (hematoxylin and eosin).

numerous intrapulmonary iron laden macrophages, vascular changes of secondary pulmonary hypertension such as vascular wall medial hypertrophy, and intimal thickening in pulmonary arterioles and pulmonary veins. Foci of microscopic osseous metaplasia can also be seen in patients with chronic cardiogenic pulmonary edema.

Diffuse Alveolar Damage

Diffuse alveolar damage (DAD) is the pathologic manifestation of the acute respiratory distress syndrome (ARDS), a catastrophic form of ALI characterized by

Table 26-2 Conditions Associated With Diffuse Alveolar Damage

Idiopathic
  Acute interstitial pneumonia (AIP)
Direct acute lung injury
  Infectious pneumonias
  Gastric contents aspiration
  Smoke inhalation
  Ammonia inhalation
  Drug reactions
  Fat embolization
  Drowning
  radiation injury
  Others
Indirect acute lung injury
  Gram-negative sepsis
  Major trauma
  Acute pancreatitis
  Opiate and barbiturate overdose
  Transfusion-related acute lung injury (TRALI)
  Disseminated intravascular coagulation (DIC)
  Paraquat poisoning
  Eclampsia
  Others

acute onset, bilateral pulmonary infiltrates visible on chest roentgenograms, severely impaired oxygenation, absence of pulmonary hypertension, and high mortality rate.[2] ALI and ARDS can develop as a result of direct or indirect lung injury secondary to a wide variety of pathogens (*Table 26-2*).[9-15]

Clinical features of diffuse alveolar damage

Patients with ARDS present with acute onset shortness of breath, rapid development of bilateral pulmonary infiltrates, hypoxia with $PaO_2:FiO_2$ ratio ≤ 300 mm Hg, and absence of pulmonary hypertension with pulmonary arterial wedge pressure ≤ 18 mm Hg. ARDS patients require hospitalization in intensive care units and intubation.[13] The syndrome can develop a variety of acute complications such as pneumothorax and pneumomediastinum (3%-20%), nosocomial pneumonia (>35%), multiorgan dysfunction (>80%) and is associated with high mortality (approximately 40%). Patients with ALI that survive the acute phase of ARDS can develop long-term complications such as mild to severe impairment in pulmonary function, neuromuscular weakness, and posttraumatic stress syndrome.

Imaging features of diffuse alveolar damage

Chest roentgenograms of ARDS patients show bilateral pulmonary infiltrates that may develop a few hours after hypoxemia.[13,15] The infiltrates are generally seen as densities that radiate from the hilar regions, giving a butterfly appearance.[16,17] These findings are not specific and can be seen in other patients with ALI secondary to pulmonary edema or pneumonia. Chest CT of ARDS patients shows homogeneous, bilateral densities that are more prominent in gravitationally dependent areas of the lung. The opacifications can be associated with ground glass changes, microcystic bullae, pneumothorax, and/or pneumomediastinum.

Gross features of diffuse alveolar damage

Grossly, the lungs of patients with the early phases of DAD are heavy, congested with diffuse pink-red, firm consolidation (*Figure 26-1*).[2] These gross changes are grossly indistinguishable from those seen in pulmonary edema or early bronchopneumonia. The lungs of patients with the later phases of DAD are also heavy but develop a red-gray cut surface with grossly visible, regularly distributed, airspaces. In normal lungs the alveoli are invisible to the naked eye as they are smaller than the resolution power of the human eye and have soft, pliable walls. In contrast, airspaces in DAD become grossly visible as a diffuse and regularly distributed fine honeycomb resulting from airspace enlargement and slightly firm and thickened edematous alveolar walls.

DAD can develop secondarily to patients with chronic lung diseases, particularly those with usual interstitial pneumonia (UIP) and other chronic lung diseases, resulting in acute exacerbation of the disease.[12] In these cases the gross features described above are superimposed on the chronic lung changes of UIP.

Histologic features of diffuse alveolar damage

The pathologic manifestations of DAD are usually divided into those of an early "exudative" phase and those of a subsequent "proliferative" phase.[10,11,14] These changes can develop in a heterogenous manner in different parts of the lung, with some areas exhibiting exudative microscopic features and others more advanced proliferative changes.

The earliest pathologic changes of the exudative phase of DAD result from injury and necrosis of endothelial cells and type I and II pneumocytes.[2,10] The initial changes can be seen under electron microscopy and include edema and disruption of the basement membrane between the capillary space and the adjacent alveolar space, papillary processes on the surface of pneumocytes type I, and electron lucent densities in the cytoplasm of endothelial cells. Within hours of the acute injury the lungs develop abnormalities that are visible under light microscopy, including congestion, increased number and margination of neutrophils in alveolar capillaries, and fibrin thrombi. Approximately 1

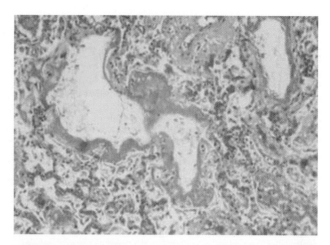

FIGURE 26-3 **Diffuse alveolar damage exudative phase. The alveoli exhibit characteristic eosinophilic hyaline membranes at the periphery of alveolar spaces (hematoxylin and eosin).**

to 3 days following acute injury the lungs develop intra-alveolar edema secondary to leaky capillaries and hyaline membranes (*Figure 26-3*). The latter are diagnostic of the exudative phase of DAD and appear as intensely eosinophilic band-like exudates that characteristically line alveolar airspaces and ducts and are composed of fibrin admixed with necrotic cellular debris. A small number of neutrophils can also be seen adjacent to the hyaline membranes, but their presence in great numbers in DAD patients usually suggests the possibility of a secondary infectious pneumonia.

The proliferative phase of DAD starts developing 5 to 7 days after the acute injury.[10,11] The alveoli adjacent to the hyaline membranes show reactive type II pneumocytes with enlarged nuclei, prominent eosinophilic nucleoli, and a hobnail appearance (*Figure 26-4*). Myofibroblasts appear later on in exudative areas and proliferate within alveoli and ducts to form granulation tissue polyps composed of spindle cell admixed with a myxoid stroma (*Figure 26-5*). These myxoid fibroblastic tissue proliferations are also present within alveolar walls, a characteristic finding in DAD. Foci of squamous metaplasia are focally present in lung tissues with the proliferative phase of DAD and are not diagnostic of a viral pneumonia.

In approximately half of ARDS patients the intra-alveolar fibrosis becomes progressively diffuse and extensive during the proliferative phase of DAD, resulting in pulmonary failure and death within days or weeks of the acute injury.[10,15] In other patients, the early fibroproliferative changes of DAD resolve with clearance of the immature intra-alveolar fibroblastic exudates, apoptosis of myofibroblasts, and phagocytosis of the debris by alveolar macrophages. Patients with a more protracted course of DAD often develop variable established lung fibrosis and vascular changes with vascular

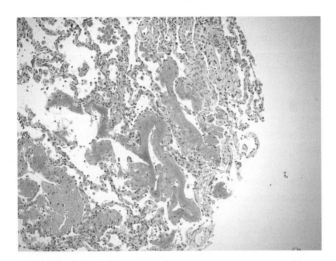

FIGURE 26-4 **Diffuse alveolar damage exudative phase. As the alveolar damage progresses the lung exhibits, in addition to hyaline membranes, the presence of reactive pneumocyte type II with cuboidal cytoplasm, round nuclei, and focally prominent nucleoli (hematoxylin and eosin).**

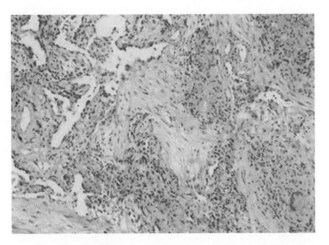

FIGURE 26-5 **Diffuse alveolar damage proliferative phase. The alveolar spaces are diffusely fibrotic and filled with myofibroblastic foci admixed with a myxoid stroma (hematoxylin and eosin).**

remodeling, medial hypertrophy of pulmonary arteries, intimal fibrosis of arteries and veins, and arterialization of pulmonary arterioles. These pathologic changes often result in chronic loss of pulmonary function and/or secondary pulmonary hypertension.

ACUTE PNEUMONIA: PNEUMONIA VERSUS PNEUMONITIS

Pneumonia is the term generally used to describe inflammatory lung conditions secondary to infections, such as bacterial pneumonias, viral pneumonias, and other organisms.[18-20] In contrast, the term pneumonitis is generally used to describe noninfectious inflammatory lung conditions, such as those associated with drugs, hypersensitivity, environmental and other factors.[21,22] However, this terminology is not used consistently in the literature, resulting in some confusion. For example, the most important idiopathic diffuse lung diseases with interstitial fibrosis such as UIP, nonspecific interstitial pneumonia (NSIP), and others include the word "pneumonia" in their nomenclature although none of these conditions are, by definition, postinfectious.[23] There is a similar problem with the designation of acute pneumonias, as the idiopathic form of ALI showing pathologic changes of DAD is designated as "acute interstitial pneumonia" (AIP), although it is not caused by an infection.[23] AIP is discussed under the general topic of interstitial lung diseases.

Acute Infections Pneumonias

Lobar pneumonia, bronchopneumonia, and acute interstitial pneumonias

A wide variety of microorganisms can cause acute infections pneumonias in immunocompetent and immunosuppressed hosts.[24] Infectious organisms can reach the lungs and cause acute infectious pneumonias through various routes, including the airways, the pulmonary vasculature or direct extension from the chest wall, thoracic spine, esophagus, and other mediastinal structures; the aerogenous route is the most common pathway of pulmonary infection. Hospital-acquired pneumonias or nosocomial pneumonias are most often caused by *Staphylococcus aureus* and gram-negative organisms such as Acinetobacter sp, Pseudomonas aeruginosa, and others (*Table 26-3*). Common infectious

Table 26-3 Most Frequent Causes of Community-Acquired Pneumonia

Streptococcus pneumonia
Haemophilus influenza
Legionella sp
Staphylococcus aureus
Pseudomonas aeruginosa
Escherichia coli
Klebsiella pneumonia
Proteus mirabilis
Mycoplasma pneumonia
Chlamydophila pneumonia
Chlamydophila psittaci
Chlamydophila burnetii
Influenza A and B viruses
Mixed
Other

agents causing pneumonias in immunocompromised hosts include Pneumocystis jiroveci, cytomegalovirus, herpes virus, Candida sp, Aspergillus sp, and other organisms.[24,25]

The clinicopathologic patterns of injury in pulmonary infectious processes include lobar or segmental pneumonia, bronchopneumonia, acute interstitial pneumonia, and mixed pneumonic patterns. A detailed discussed of the pathology of acute pneumonias caused by particular infections agents and a description of acute and/or chronic granulomatous pneumonias caused by mycobacteria, fungi, and other organisms is beyond the scope of this chapter.

Clinical features of acute pneumonia

Acute infectious pneumonias can affect anyone but are more frequent in infants and children younger than 2 years, people older than 65 years old, patients with chronic diseases such as asthma, chronic obstructive pulmonary disease, chronic interstitial lung disease, and heart disease, and individuals with immunosuppression secondary to HIV/AIDS, chemotherapy for cancer, long-term corticosteroid use, or organ transplantation.[24] Cigarette smoking, hospitalization, and ventilator therapy are also risks for pneumonia. More than 6 million cases of pneumonia are diagnosed yearly in the United States and the disease is listed as the sixth most frequent cause of death.

Patients with infectious pneumonias present with acute onset cough, production of sputum that may be green or blood tinged, fever $\geq 102°F$, shortness of breath, shaking chills, chest pain, tachycardia, weakness, headaches, nausea, vomiting, and/or diarrhea. Symptoms can vary from mild to severe.[19,24,25] Patients with viral pneumonias usually but not always develop these symptoms more slowly and in a more insidious manner than those with bacterial pneumonia, with predominance of weakness and respiratory symptoms. Older patients and immunosuppressed individuals may develop minimal or absent fever and mild respiratory symptoms in the presence of significant abnormalities on chest imaging studies and/or sudden changes in mental awareness.

Physical examination of the chest in patients with acute pneumonia reveals the presence of rhonchi, dullness due to lack of aeration, rales, abnormal bubbling and/or crackling sounds. Pulse oximetry shows variable degrees of hypoxia. Blood counts usually show the presence of leukocytosis in patients with bacterial pneumonias and lymphocytosis in those with viral infections. Serologic tests are particularly helpful for the diagnosis of viral and other nonbacterial pneumonias.

Cultures of sputum, nasal swabs are generally sufficient for an etiological diagnosis of mild community-acquired pneumonias. Patients with more severe pneumonias who require hospitalization and show negative

sputum cultures often undergo bronchoscopy with cultures of bronchioloalveolar (BAL) fluids. Patients with negative BAL cultures and progressive respiratory problems often undergo video-assisted thoracoscopic surgery (VATS) with wedge lung biopsies and cultures of lung tissues obtained under sterile conditions in the operating room.[26]

Patients with bacterial pneumonia usually respond within days to antibiotic therapy but can develop progressive respiratory failure, resulting in admissions to intensive care units (ICU) for intubation and mechanical ventilation.[25] They can also develop complications such as bacteremia, sepsis, pleural effusion, empyema, lung abscess, and others. Patients with viral pneumonias usually improve within 1 to 3 weeks of diagnosis but may develop secondary bacterial pneumonias and/or some of the complications listed above.

Imaging features of acute pneumonia

The imaging findings of a patient with acute pneumonia need to be interpreted in correlation with the clinical manifestations as they resemble those seen in pulmonary edema, ARDS, drug-induced pulmonary disease, acute eosinophilic pneumonia, cryptogenic organizing pneumonia (COP), pulmonary vasculitis, intra-alveolar hemorrhage, and other conditions.[27]

Chest radiography and CT are the most useful imaging modalities for the evaluation of patients with suspected acute pneumonia. Pneumonias present on chest x-rays as localized pulmonary disease with a lobar or segmental distribution or as bilateral generalized abnormalities. Lobar pneumonias are usually secondary to bacterial infections and appear as subpleural alveolar filling defects or densities that spread toward the core portions of the lung until an entire lobe is involved by a homogenous consolidation usually associated with air bronchograms. Similar densities can involve only segmental portions of a lung in segmental pneumonias. Lobar or segmental pneumonias can also appear on chest roentgenograms as round infiltrates, particularly in children.

Bilateral generalized pulmonary abnormalities can be seen on the chest x-rays of patients with bacterial and viral pneumonias. Bacterial infections causing bronchopneumonia present with multiple, bilateral poorly defined nodular infiltrates with or without cavitation or with bilateral lung consolidation. Viral infections and pneumonias secondary to Mycoplasma pneumoniae usually present with diffuse bilateral interstitial or mixed interstitial and confluent alveolar opacities.[18]

Lobar, segmental, and generalized pulmonary infiltrates can also be associated with pleural effusion, cavitation, pneumothorax, and other manifestations on chest roentgenograms.

Chest CT is a useful adjunct to roentgenograms in selected cases with pneumonia as it provides cross-sectional images that show the pattern and distribution pattern of pulmonary processes in much more detail than conventional chest x-rays.[18,27] Patients with acute bronchopneumonia can show multifocal or lobar homogeneous opacities, acinar nodules, ground glass opacities, and/or air bronchograms. Patients with interstitial acute pneumonias usually show septal thickening, bronchovascular bundle thickening, ground glass opacities, and variable alveolar opacities. High-resolution CT scan is occasionally used for the diagnosis of patients with unusual pneumonias, such as fungal pneumonias and those seen in immunocompromised individuals.

Gross features of acute pneumonia

Acute pneumonia exhibits various gross features that involve an entire lobe or segment(s) in instances of lobar or segmental pneumonias and almost an entire lung or both lungs in a multifocal manner in others.[28] Early pneumonias exhibit a congested, red, edematous lung parenchyma resulting from the presence of congestion and edema as manifestations of early acute inflammation. Pneumonias that are 2 to 3 days old show the presence of yellow-gray, firm infiltrates admixed with red areas. These yellow-gray areas represent cellular infiltration and become progressively more prominent from days 3 to 7. These findings involve an entire lobe in lobar pneumonias or present as ill-defined multifocal and bilateral areas in patients with bronchopneumonia (*Figure 26-6*). Gross changes in lobar pneumonia tend to be homogeneous while those in bronchopneumonia are more heterogenous, as the inflammatory infiltrates in the various ill-defined nodules of the disease progress

at different times. Patients with bronchopneumonia also have a higher tendency to develop cavitation, particularly in those infected with *S. aureus* or *Klebsiella sp.*

Patients with diffuse acute interstitial pneumonias tend to show gross features similar to those of DAD.[29]

Lobar and segmental pneumonias and bronchopneumonia tend to regress after approximately 1 week on antibiotic therapy with progressive regression of the yellow-gray infiltrates and areas of congestion. They can progress to necrotizing pneumonia, lung abscess, or organizing pneumonia, pathologic processes that are described later on in this chapter. Patients with diffuse acute interstitial pneumonias tend to have a more protracted clinical course that can last for 2 to 3 weeks prior to regression.[18,27,29] Rarely viral pneumonias can progress to diffuse fibrosis of the lung, similar to the fibroproliferative response seen in DAD.

The pleura of patients with pneumonia frequently shows localized or diffuse pleuritis and appear congested, dull, and/or covered by a yellow loosely adherent fibrinous exudate. Pleural effusion and empyema, characterized by the presence of yellow or yellow-green pus within the pleural cavity, can be seen grossly as a complication of acute pneumonia.

Histologic features of acute pneumonia

Patients with lobar pneumonia, segmental pneumonia, and bronchopneumonia usually exhibit variable degrees of acute alveolitis while those with diffuse acute interstitial pneumonia show a cellular interstitial pneumonia with infiltration of alveolar septa, ducts, and interstitium by round cell infiltrates (*Figure 26-7*).[28,29]

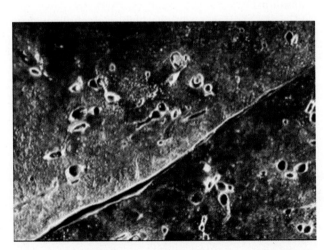

FIGURE 26-6 Bronchopneumonia. Lung at autopsy is heavy, congested with ill-defined yellow-gray infiltrates distributed in a multifocal pattern.

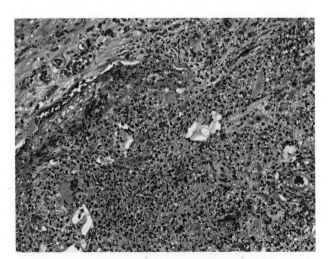

FIGURE 26-7 Acute alveolitis, usually associated with bacterial pneumonia or bronchopneumonia. The alveolar spaces are filled with neutrophils. Marked congestion and intra-alveolar exudates are also present (hematoxylin and eosin).

CHAPTER 26

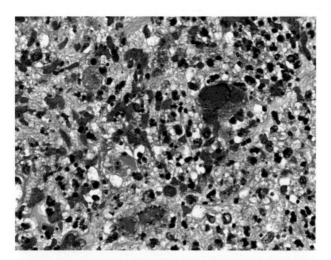

FIGURE 26-8 Acute alveolitis caused by viral infection. Certain viruses like adenovirus, herpes virus, and others can cause acute alveolitis. Notice the presence of large cells with "smudged nuclei" suggestive of viral changes (hematoxylin and eosin).

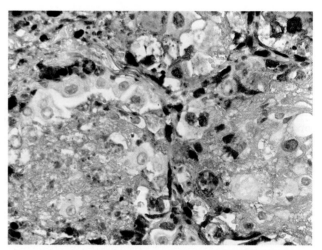

FIGURE 26-9 In situ hybridization showing reactivity for herpes virus in a biopsy with viral pneumonia (ISH).

Acute alveolitis is most frequent in patients with bacterial pneumonias, although it can be seen as a result of fungal or viral infections (*Figure 26-8*). It is characterized by the presence of numerous neutrophils in intra-alveolar spaces, admixed with eosinophilic fibrin, debris, and variable number of red blood cells. Acute alveolitis is diffuse within an entire lobe in patients with lobar pneumonia and patchy and multifocal in those with bronchopneumonia. The intra-alveolar infiltrates usually appear approximately 2 days after onset of the acute pneumonia and become more prominent during the following few days. Acute alveolitis is frequently associated with acute inflammation of bronchial and bronchiolar epithelium. In patients successfully treated with antibiotics, the infiltrates rapidly decrease and are replaced by numerous alveolar macrophages that engulf debris until the inflammatory progress subsides. The pleura in these conditions frequently show variable acute inflammation and eosinophilic fibrinous exudates in areas adjacent to the pneumonic process.

Pneumonias secondary to viral infections, M pneumoniae, Chlamydia sp, Pneumocystis jiroveci, and other organisms usually present with interstitial infiltrates rather than acute alveolitis.[29] The interstitial infiltrates are composed mostly of lymphocytes with variable number of monocytes and plasma cells. They can be associated with hyaline membranes and other changes of DAD, acute bronchitis and bronchiolitis, and rarely vasculitis. Viral inclusions can be seen in pneumonias secondary to adenovirus, herpes virus, and cytomegalovirus. Adenovirus shows the presence of "smudge nuclei" (*Figure 26-8*); herpes virus shows the presence of basophilic intranuclear inclusions and multinucleated cells while cytomegalovirus infection

induces the formation of large cells with both intranuclear and intracytoplasmic inclusions. The presence of viral changes can be confirmed by immunostains (*Figure 26-9*).

Not all patients with viral pneumonias present with diffuse interstitial infiltrates and the pathologic changes in these conditions can include pulmonary edema, DAD, and/or acute bronchitis/bronchiolitis.

Aspiration Pneumonia

Aspiration pneumonias result from the inhalation of oropharyngeal or gastric contents into the lower airways.[30,31] Aspirated materials can be gastric contents, food contents, bacteria, and oil (eg, mineral oil or vegetable oil). Approximately 5% to 15% of community-acquired pneumonias in the United States result from aspiration.

Certain clinical conditions such as alcoholism, drug overdose, seizures, stroke and other neurological disorders, head trauma, general anesthesia, nasogastric tube insertion, bronchoscopy and other procedures, esophageal strictures and neoplasms, and other conditions predispose to aspiration pneumonia. Aspiration of oropharyngeal or gastric contents can result in a chemical pneumonitis, Mendelson syndrome, and bacterial pneumonia.

Aspiration of a foreign body may cause a respiratory emergency due to airway obstruction; it can also be followed by a subsequent bacterial pneumonia.

Clinical features of aspiration pneumonia

Chemical pneumonitis or Mendelson syndrome usually occurs in patients with altered levels of consciousness secondary to seizures, cerebrovascular accident, and other neurological problems and in those with a history of drug overdose.[30,31] Patients develop acute onset of dyspnea and rapid breathing, wheezing, cough, and production of pink and/or frothy sputum, clinical findings resembling the acute lung injury syndrome. The chemical pneumonitis is frequently complicated by secondary bacterial pneumonias manifested with fever and leukocytosis.

Bacterial pneumonias secondary to aspiration usually occur in patients with chronic impairment of airway defense mechanisms such as cough, gag reflex, and immune mechanisms, such as alcoholics, persons with poor dentition, esophageal strictures, and other conditions.[28] Patients develop fever, cough, tachypnea, tachycardia, decreased breath sounds, pleural friction rub, altered mental status, leukocytosis, hypoxemia, normal or low CO_2 levels with respiratory alkalosis, and hypotension in patients who develop septic shock. Sputum and other cultures usually yield *Streptococcus pneumoniae, Staphylococcus aureus, Haemophilus influenza, Enterobacteriaceae, Pseudomonas aeruginosa,* and methicillin-resistant *Staphylococcus aureus* (MRSA) as the most common pathogens. Blood cultures are needed to exclude the possibility of bacteremia.

Bronchoscopy is often performed in patients with aspiration pneumonia, particularly when aspiration of a foreign body is suspected.[31] It allows for collection of materials with protected brush or bronchoalveolar lavage to culture for pathogens and help guide antibiotic therapy. Patients with secondary pleural effusion or empyema usually undergo thoracentesis. Intubation and mechanical ventilation may be required in patients with severe aspiration pneumonia, particularly those that progress to ARDS. Patients with anaerobic bacteria, MRSA, or other pathogens who do not readily respond to antibiotic therapy may require surgical treatment for wedge biopsy, closed tube drainage of an empyema, decortication or lung resection in rare patients with complications such as severe pulmonary bleeding.[26]

Patients with severe aspiration chemical pneumonitis have a high mortality rate that can be up to 70%. Aspiration bacterial pneumonias are also associated with a high mortality rate. For example, patients with nosocomial aspiration pneumonia have approximately 30% 30-day mortality due to the high incidence of bacteria that are resistant to antibiotic therapy and complications.

Imaging features of aspiration pneumonia

The location of the pulmonary infiltrates in aspiration pneumonias depend on the position of the patient when the episode of aspiration developed, but in general they are more common in the right middle lobe and the lower lobes.[31] Patients who aspirate while standing tend to develop bilateral lower lobe opacities. Patients lying down in the left lateral decubitus position are more likely to develop left-sided opacities. Alcoholics tend to develop right upper lobe infiltrates.

Patients with chemical pneumonitis show roentgenographic changes similar to those seen in pulmonary edema, with the development of ill-defined, poorly circumscribed opacities that are more prominent in perihilar areas and involve one or both lower lobes. Patients with bacterial pneumonia develop poorly circumscribed opacities in a lobar, segmental, or bronchopneumonic distribution, sometimes associated with air bronchograms. Bacterial pneumonias secondary to aspiration often progress to a lung abscess with development of lucencies and/or air fluid levels within the pulmonary infiltrates. Pleural effusions with blunting of the costophrenic angles are frequent findings in patients with aspiration pneumonia.

Chest CT scans are not generally needed in patients with aspiration pneumonia but can be helpful to demonstrate the presence of cavitation or empyema in selected patients, as it provides better definition of the pulmonary opacities than the plain radiographs.

Gross features of aspiration pneumonia

The lungs of patients with chemical pneumonitis show at autopsy gross findings of acute lung injury.[1,13] They are heavy, congested with diffuse consolidation of the pulmonary parenchyma by edema fluid. The airways are frequently filled with frothy, pink fluid.

Patients with bacterial pneumonias show similar findings to those of lobar pneumonia or bronchopneumonia.[28] Patients who progress to the development of lung abscess show cavities filled with yellow-green pus and lined by irregular yellow-gray tissue. Only rarely foreign matter such as food contents can be grossly identified within pneumonia areas. The pleura overlying the areas of pneumonia show fibrinous pleuritis, with a yellow-gray dull surface focally covered by loosely adherent exudates. Patients with secondary empyema show the presence of bloody or yellow-green-gray fluid in a pleural cavity that is lined by congested, thickened pleura.

Histologic features of aspiration pneumonia

The airways in patients with chemical pneumonitis are frequently edematous, congested with areas of recent hemorrhage.[30,31] The pulmonary parenchyma is congested, with intra-alveolar edema, hyaline membranes, reactive type II pneumocytes, intra-alveolar myofibroblastic proliferation, and other changes related to DAD.

Patients with aspiration bacterial pneumonias show acute alveolitis in a diffuse or patchy distribution associated with marked congestion, intra-alveolar edema, and reactive type II pneumocytes. Gram-positive bacteria can be visualized with Gram stains. Lung specimens with necrotizing pneumonia and cavitation also exhibit necrotic alveolar structures and accumulation of neutrophils, necrotic debris, and amorphous eosinophilic material within the abscess cavity.

The pleura shows reactive fibrinous pleuritis with deposition of amorphous eosinophilic material on its surface, reactive mesothelial cells exhibiting polygonal cytoplasm, round nuclei and prominent nucleoli, and granulation tissue proliferation with developing of branching capillaries that are generally distributed at 90° angle to the pleural surface.

Necrotizing Pneumonia

Necrotizing pneumonia is an infrequent complication of bacterial and viral pneumonias characterized by the development of pulmonary necrosis, lung abscess formation, empyema, bronchopleural fistula, DAD, and/or sepsis.[20] In immunocompetent individuals, necrotizing pneumonias are due to very virulent microorganisms, antibiotic resistant bacteria, and/or bacterial pneumonias superimposed on viral pneumonias such as those reported recently for pandemic H1N1 influenza.[19,20,32] *Staphylococcus aureus* strains that produce Panton-Valentine leukocidin account for a significant proportion of necrotizing pneumonias in immunocompetent patients.[25] Other frequent pathogens include *Streptococcus pneumoniae, Klebsiella pneumoniae,* and anaerobic bacteria such as *Clostridium perfringens, Clostridium septicum,* and others.[20,25,33]

Necrotizing pneumonia in immunosuppressed individuals is usually caused by bacterial infections associated with fungal infections such as invasive candidiasis, invasive aspergillosis, and others and/or viral infections such as herpes virus and cytomegalovirus.[29]

Clinical features of necrotizing pneumonia

Patients develop signs and symptoms of a severe infection with high fever, productive cough, hemoptysis, tachypnea, tachycardia, decreased breath sounds, pleural friction rub, altered mental status, leukocytosis, hypoxemia, respiratory alkalosis, hypotension, and frequent septic shock.[20,25,33] Hypoxemia and respiratory alkalosis are frequently severe, requiring admission to an ICU and mechanical ventilation.

Patients with lung cavities can develop massive hemoptysis that requires surgical resection.[26] Pleural effusion, empyema, and bronchopulmonary fistula that require chest tube placement and/or decortication are also frequent.

Imaging features of necrotizing pneumonia

Patients with necrotizing pneumonia show chest x-ray findings similar to those described above for lobar pneumonia or bronchopneumonia with cavitation.[18,27] Pleural effusion with air fluid levels secondary to bronchopleural fistula is frequent. Imaging findings usually progress rapidly to diffuse bilateral pulmonary infiltrates, as seen in DAD.

Gross features of necrotizing pneumonia

The lungs of necrotizing pneumonia are frequently consolidated with a red, firm, hemorrhagic surface.[28] On section they exhibit red parenchyma with patchy yellow-gray infiltrates and frequent cavitation. The cavities contain hemorrhagic material and are lined by irregular yellow-gray walls. Airways are markedly congested with mucosal hemorrhage. The pleural surface shows gross findings of acute fibrinous pleuritis or empyema, as described above.

Histologic features of necrotizing pneumonia

Depending on the etiology of necrotizing pneumonia, the lungs show histopathologic findings of acute alveolitis admixed with areas of DAD and/or interstitial infiltrates by lymphoid cells.[29] Bacterial necrotizing pneumonias show severe acute alveolitis, with foci of hemorrhagic necrosis of the pulmonary parenchyma, acute bronchitis and bronchiolitis, and cavitation.[28] Gram stains frequently show clumps of gram-positive or -negative organisms.

Patients with influenza or other viral necrotizing pneumonia show pulmonary edema, hyaline membranes and other findings of DAD, variable interstitial infiltrates by lymphoid cells, and patchy areas of acute alveolitis. Hemorrhagic necrosis, cavitation, and pleural changes as described above are also frequent.

Immunosuppressed patients with necrotizing pneumonia secondary to Pneumocystis jiroveci show interstitial infiltrates by lymphoplasmacytic cells, extensive characteristic foamy alveolar casts, and necrosis of alveolar septa.[34,35] The cysts of the organisms can be readily identified with GMS stains. Immunosuppressed patients with aspergillosis and other vasoinvasive fungi show extensive intra-alveolar hemorrhage, patchy areas of acute alveolitis, hyaline membranes and other findings of DAD, and intra-alveolar or intravascular fungal aggregates. The fungal organisms are often easily visible on H&E-stained sections and are better shown on GMS and PAS stains.

Pulmonary Abscess

Pulmonary abscess is an acute or subacute pneumonia that destroys the lung parenchyma, creating one or more intrapulmonary cavities.[36-38] Its frequency has decreased in patients with community-acquired pneumonia as a result of effective antibiotic therapy. It is more frequent in patients with oral disease such as periodontal disease or gingivitis, aspiration pneumonia, local lesions such as lung cancer, altered consciousness secondary to alcoholism, coma, drug abuse, anesthesia, or seizures, esophageal diseases such as achalasia, stricture, and others. Pulmonary abscess can also develop in patients with sepsis or immunocompromised hosts as a result of HIV infection, steroid therapy, chemotherapy, malnutrition, and severe trauma.

Clinical features of pulmonary abscess

Pulmonary abscess can develop acutely or subacutely from infections by anaerobic bacteria such as Clostridium sp and Clostridium putridum, gram-negative organisms such as Bacteroides sp, Fusobacterium sp, Proteus sp, Aerobacter sp, Escherichia Coli, gram-positive organisms such as Peptostreptococcus sp, Microaerophilic streptococcus, and Actinomyces sp, and opportunistic organisms such as Candida sp, Legionella sp, Mycobacteria, and others.[36-38] Rarely pulmonary abscesses can be caused by Entamoeba histolytica.

Most adult patients with pulmonary abscesses have symptoms for at least 2 weeks prior to diagnosis, including intermittent fever, productive cough, hemoptysis, general malaise, night sweats, and weight loss.[37] Sputum is putrid, particularly in patients with large cavities caused by anaerobic bacteria. Physical examination reveals absent breath sounds, coarse bronchi, pleural rubbing.

Children can develop multiple lung abscesses secondary to Staphylococcus pneumonia infection.[38] These infections are frequently hematogenous and tend to result in a more acute clinical course than adults, with high fever, chills, tachypnea, and production of putrid sputum.

Pulmonary abscesses caused by anaerobic bacteria such Clostridium sp usually present as complications of lobar or segmental pneumonias or lung infarcts and can progress to involve an entire lung or both lungs.[33]

Cultures of sputum, bronchoalveolar lavage fluid, protected bronchial brush samples, transtracheal aspirates, transthoracic aspirates, and/or wedge lung biopsies are needed for the etiological diagnosis of a lung abscess and selection of proper antibiotic therapy.[36] Bronchoscopy and percutaneous drainage can be used for evacuation of the cavitary contents of pulmonary abscesses. Selected patients with pulmonary abscesses that do not respond to antibiotic therapy or develop severe hemoptysis are treated with surgical resection.

Approximately 1/3 of patients with pulmonary abscesses develop empyema. They are drained with chest tubes and often undergo decortication.

The prognosis of patients with pulmonary abscesses depends on the underlying condition. The presence of necrotizing pneumonia, large size (>6 cm), immunocompromised, tumors associated with bronchial obstruction, and young or old age are poor prognostic features.[28] Patients with pulmonary abscess caused by anaerobic bacteria are usually very ill and frequently develop sepsis with high mortality.

Imaging features of pulmonary abscess

Chest roentgenograms show the presence of ill-defined opacities with a lobar, segmental, or bronchopneumonic distribution associated with single or multiple lucencies.[36-38] Air fluid levels are seen in patients where the pulmonary abscess opens to the airways or the pleura, resulting in pneumopyothorax. Chest x-rays may need to be taken in the lateral decubitus position to demonstrate cavities in patients with pulmonary abscess associated with a neoplasm, atelectasis, pneumothorax, extensive pleural effusion, or pleural thickening. Chest CT scans are very useful to demonstrate the presence of cavitation within lung opacities that do not show visible lucencies or air fluid levels on chest roentgenograms.

Gross features of pulmonary abscess

Pulmonary abscesses show a cavity surrounded by consolidated areas of pneumonia. The peripheral pneumonic areas show a red to yellow-gray, firm, consolidated surface.[28] The cavities can be single or multiple, particularly in children, contain hemorrhagic material and are lined by irregular yellow-gray walls.[38] Airways are markedly congested with mucosal hemorrhage. The pleural surface shows findings of acute fibrinous pleuritis or empyema, as described above.

Histologic features of pulmonary abscess

Pulmonary abscesses show histopathologic findings of acute alveolitis and/or organizing pneumonia with variable amounts of intra-alveolar fibromyxoid proliferation.[28] The areas adjacent to the cavity show destruction of the pulmonary parenchyma with acute on chronic inflammation, hemorrhage, and/or variable amounts of fibrosis. In contrast to lung cavities secondary to granulomatous pneumonia, epithelioid granulomas are absent. Foreign body granulomas can be seen, particularly in patients with aspiration pneumonia.

The lumen of lung abscesses shows necrotic debris, red blood cells, amorphous eosinophilic material, neutrophils, and alveolar macrophages. Gram stains can show clumps of gram-positive or -negative organisms, particularly in patients who do not respond to antibiotic therapy. Patients with empyema show the pleural changes described above.

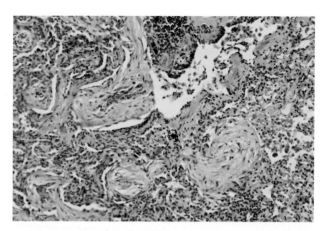

FIGURE 26-10 Organizing pneumonia showing the presence of intra-alveolar young fibrotic tissue composed of myofibroblasts in a myxoid background (hematoxylin and eosin).

Organizing Pneumonia

Organizing pneumonia is a condition defined pathologically by the presence of granulation tissue, and myofibroblastic proliferation with early fibrosis in alveolar ducts and sacs (*Figure 26-10*).[39] It can also extend into respiratory bronchioles, resulting in bronchiolitis obliterans (*Figure 26-11*). It is a pathological pattern rather than a specific clinicopathologic entity.

Organizing pneumonia can develop as a complication of infectious pneumonia, lung abscess, empyema, lung neoplasms, aspiration pneumonia, granulomatous pneumonia, drug reaction, radiation therapy, collagen vascular disease, pulmonary infarction, middle lobe syndrome, and other conditions listed in *Table 26-4*.[39] Idiopathic organizing pneumonia with or cryptogenic bronchiolitis obliterans is currently designated

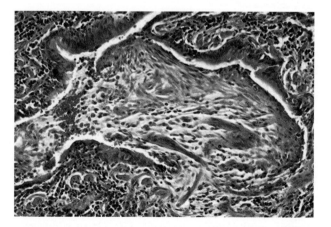

FIGURE 26-11 Presence of bronchiolitis obliterans in a lung biopsy from a patient with cryptogenic organizing pneumonia. The lumen of a respiratory bronchiole if filled by young fibrotic tissue composed of myofibroblasts in a myxoid background (hematoxylin and eosin).

Table 26-4 Conditions Associated With Organizing Pneumonia

Idiopathic
  Cryptogenic organizing pneumonia (COP)
Infectious pneumonia
  Chlamydia pneumoniae
  Coxiella pneumophila
  Legionella pneumophila
  Mycoplasma Pneumonia
  Nocardia asteroids
  Pseudomonas aeruginosa
  Serratia marcescens
  Staphylococcus aureus
  Streptococcus group B
  Herpes virus
  Human immunodeficiency virus (HIV)
  Influenza virus
  Parainfluenza virus
  Cryptococcus neoformans
  Pneumocystis jiroveci
  Other organisms.
Drug reaction
  Amiodarone
  Bleomycin
  Tacrolimus
  Interferon alfa
  Cocaine
  Others
Collagen vascular diseases
  Rheumatoid arthritis
  Sjögren syndrome
Other conditions
  Sweet's syndrome
  Ulcerative colitis
  Crohn's disease
  Polymyalgia rheumatica
  Autoimmune thyroiditis

as cryptogenic organizing pneumonia (COP), an entity that is discussed with interstitial lung diseases.[40]

Clinical features of organizing pneumonia

The clinical manifestations of organizing pneumonia are variable and depend on the underlying condition associated with this pathologic pattern.[39] Patients with postinfectious organizing pneumonia usually exhibit subacute fever, malaise, shortness of breath, and weight loss. They can also develop hemoptysis, arthralgias, chest pain, and other symptoms. Physical examination is variable and can show areas of dullness on auscultation, rales, wheezing, and other nonspecific findings. Blood counts and chemistries do not show characteristic findings.

The diagnosis of organizing pneumonia can be suspected clinically but is usually established pathologically.

The histopathological pattern can be seen on transbronchial biopsies but often require wedge lung biopsies for diagnoses. Treatment is variable, depending on the underlying condition associated with organizing pneumonia and often includes corticosteroid therapy.

Imaging features of organizing pneumonia

The imaging features of organizing pneumonia are heterogenous and depend on the underlying condition associated with this pathologic pattern.[39] Patients usually exhibit on chest x-ray and/or chest CT scans single or multiple patchy, ill-circumscribed alveolar opacities.[40] These opacities can be unilateral or bilateral in distribution. Chest CT scans can also show ground glass consolidation, nodular infiltrates with a predominant bronchocentric distribution, and air bronchograms (*Figure 26-12*).

Solitary infiltrates secondary to organizing pneumonia can appear as localized nodules or masses on chest x-rays and CT scans and simulate lung cancer or metastatic lesions. Patients with COP, drug reaction, and connective tissue disorders can also show interstitial and small alveolar opacities on CT scan.

Gross features of organizing pneumonia

The gross features of organizing pneumonia are variable and depend on the underlying conditions associated with this pathologic pattern.[39,40] In general, areas of organizing pneumonia appear as ill-defined, single or multiple, soft to firm gray areas of consolidation.

Histologic features of organizing pneumonia

Organizing pneumonia is a distinct type of repair to lung injury that reflects a form of pulmonary "wound healing". Early stages of organizing pneumonia show type I pneumocyte necrosis, visible only by electron microscopy; proliferation of type II pneumocytes showing repair changes such as enlarged size, prominent nucleoli, and anisocytosis; and accumulation of intraalveolar fibrin with focal hyaline membranes.[39,40] Later stages of organizing pneumonia show characteristic Masson bodies resulting from the intra-alveolar proliferation of spindle myofibroblastic cells (*Figure 26-13*). These areas of intra-alveolar organization appear as branching buds that fill the lumina of alveolar sacs and ducts. They are composed of spindle myofibroblastic cells admixed with a somewhat basophilic, loose, myxoid connective tissue matrix. More advanced stages of organizing pneumonia show collagenization of the intra-alveolar fibrotic areas, with development of a more eosinophilic connective tissue matrix. Similar pathologic findings can be seen in respiratory bronchioles, resulting in focal or multifocal bronchiolitis obliterans.

The histopathologic features of organizing pneumonia are similar to those seen in the proliferative phase of DAD but usually show different distribution in both conditions. They are diffuse in DAD and patchy or multifocal in COP or secondary organizing pneumonias. As it is often difficult to determine on a transbronchial or wedge lung biopsy whether the process is diffuse or patchy as a result of sampling issues, a microscopic finding of organizing pneumonia needs to be correlated with the clinical findings to interpret the pathological findings in proper context. For example, if the organizing pneumonia histopathological pattern is seen in a patient with a subacute or chronic clinical condition, the biopsy changes can be interpreted as COP or secondary organizing pneumonia. If the patient has a clinical syndrome suggesting ARDS, the findings are more likely the result of the proliferative phase of DAD.

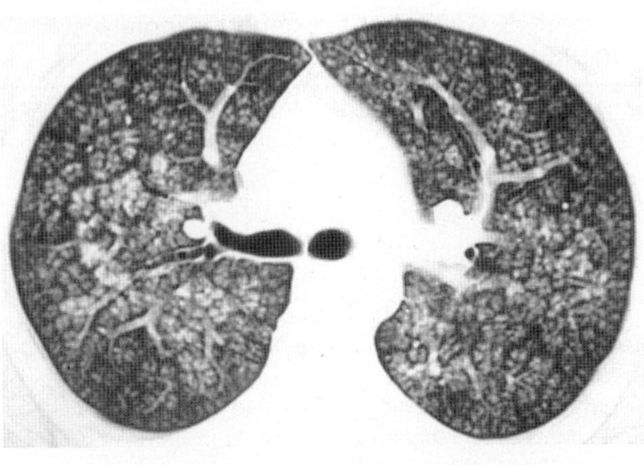

FIGURE 26-12 Chest computerized tomogram of a patient with cryptogenic organizing pneumonia showing characteristic bilateral nodular intra-alveolar densities.

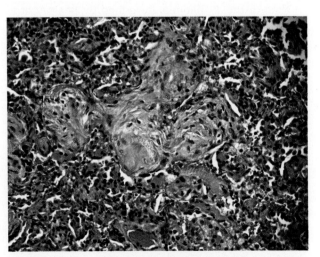

FIGURE 26-13 Organizing pneumonia showing "Masson bodies" characterized by the presence of intra-alveolar fibromyxoid infiltrates (hematoxylin and eosin).

Correlation of the microscopic findings of organizing pneumonia with the imaging findings is also important. Patients with ARDS usually have diffuse and bilateral lung opacities, as described above. Individuals with COP or secondary organizing pneumonia usually have patchy, unilateral, or bilateral infiltrates and other changes described above.

Acute Fibrinous and Organizing Pneumonia

Acute fibrinous and organizing pneumonia (AFOP) is a recently described histologic pattern of lung injury described by Beasley et al in a study of 17 open lung biopsy specimens and autopsy specimens from patients with a clinical picture of acute or subacute lung injury evaluated at the Armed Forces Institute of Pathology.[9] This histologic pattern is different than those typically seen in DAD, COP, and eosinophilic pneumonia and is characterized by the presence of extensive intra-alveolar fibrin admixed with areas of organizing pneumonia.

Clinical features of acute fibrinous and organizing pneumonia

Patients with AFOP present with an acute or subacute illness with spiking fever, cough, shortness of breath, malaise, weakness, chest, pleural, or abdominal pain, and/or hemoptysis.[9] Associated conditions included collagen vascular disease such as polymyositis and ankylosing spondylitis, hairspray use, lymphoma, corticosteroid therapy, and others. Sputum cultures show bacteria such as Haemophilus influenza and Acinetobacter baumannii in a few patients. Treatment is variable, with some patients being treated with steroids, antibiotics or both, in addition to mechanical ventilation.

Nine of the 17 patients described by Beasley et al had a clinical course similar to patients with DAD and died of the disease, suggesting that AFP may represent a fibrinous variant of DAD.

Imaging features of acute fibrinous and organizing pneumonia

The most common radiographic features in patients with AFOP include bilateral basilar infiltrates, bilateral airspace disease, bilateral reticular nodular infiltrates, and diffuse patchy infiltrates.[9]

Gross features of acute fibrinous and organizing pneumonia

The gross features of AFOP have not been described in detail as the majority of the patients had been diagnosed by lung biopsy.

Histologic features of acute fibrinous and organizing pneumonia

The most characteristic histopathologic feature of AFOP is the presence of extensive intra-alveolar fibrin in the form of fibrin "balls" with scanty or absent neutrophils.[9] The fibrin is found in a patchy distribution and can involve 25% to 90% of the alveolar spaces. The fibrin "balls" are associated with patchy areas of organizing pneumonia showing intra-alveolar loose connective tissue formation. A mild to moderate interstitial lymphoplasmacytic infiltrate, mild type 2 pneumocyte hyperplasia, and focal, mild fibroblastic proliferation with myxoid stroma within alveolar walls are also present.

Hyaline membranes, eosinophils, areas of acute alveolitis and/or bronchopneumonia, pulmonary abscess, and granulomatous inflammation are absent in AFOP.

Stains for microorganisms, such as Grocott methenamine silver, Ziehl-Neelsen, Brown-Brenn, or Brown-Hopps, are negative.

Lipoid Pneumonia

Lipoid pneumonia is a condition characterized by the accumulation of lipid containing macrophages in the lung.[30] It can be classified as exogenous and endogenous lipoid pneumonia. Exogenous lipoid pneumonia is an uncommon condition resulting from the aspiration or inhalation of lipid materials such as mineral oil and others listed in *Table 26-5*. It is more frequent in children and adults older than 50 years old and in patients with neurological or gastrointestinal disorders that affect swallowing or cough reflex.

Endogenous lipoid pneumonia is an obstructive pneumonitis secondary to tumors or other pathologic processes that occlude or compress large or small airways. It can also be seen adjacent to necrotic neoplasms, granulomas, and other chronic pathologic processes.

Table 26-5 Causes of Exogenous Lipoid Pneumonia

Aspiration of mineral oil
Laxatives
Lip balm
Flavored lip gloss
Accidental aspiration of petroleum-based products in children
Aspiration secondary to gastroesophageal reflux (GERD)
Aspiration of liquid hydrocarbons
Fire eaters
Workers exposed to oil-containing industrial products
Machinery lubrication
Spraying of pesticides or paints.
Mineral oil embolization
Use of rectal or subcutaneous products

Clinical features of lipoid pneumonia

Patients with lipoid pneumonia are often asymptomatic and are diagnosed because of abnormal chest roentgenograms.[30] They can also present with fever, cough, dyspnea, and other symptoms simulating a bacterial pneumonia. Patients with chronic lipoid pneumonia can present with chest pain, hemoptysis, weight loss, intermittent fevers, and wheezing.

Physical examination of the chest can be normal in patients with lipoid pneumonia or show dullness on percussion, crackles, wheezes, or rhonchi. Routine blood tests are unremarkable, although they can show leukocytosis. Pulmonary function tests can show a restrictive pattern.

Imaging features of lipoid pneumonia

The chest x-rays and CT scans of patients with lipoid pneumonia can exhibit a variety of findings that depend to some extent on the etiology of the syndrome.[30,41-47] They include localized or multifocal opacities often associated with air bronchograms, a fine "spun-glass" appearance, occasional cavitation, interstitial markings, single or multiple nodules and/or masses that can simulate a primary or metastatic lung malignancy and ground glass opacities associated with interlobular septal thickening (crazy-paving pattern) with a basilar predominance. Rare patients develop atelectasis secondary to bronchial narrowing by granulation tissue or oil.

Magnetic resonance imaging (MRI) can be particularly helpful for the diagnosis of lipoid pneumonia as it can show findings that are characteristic for fat or blood, such as high intensity signal on T1-weighted images with a slow decrease of signal on T2-weighted images.

Endogenous lipoid pneumonia secondary to bronchial obstruction typically show on chest roentgenograms or CT scans parenchymal opacities that are localized to areas distal to the obstructed airway.

Gross features of lipoid pneumonia

Lipoid pneumonia typically appears as yellow-gray areas of consolidation in the pulmonary parenchyma, so-called golden pneumonia.[48] Patients with chronic exogenous lipoid pneumonia can show single or multiple firm, gray, fibrotic nodules that closely simulate the gross appearance of a neoplasm.

Histologic features of lipoid pneumonia

Cytological samples such as bronchoalveolar lavage and bronchial wash fluid show the presence of numerous macrophages with a vacuolated cytoplasm in patients with lipoid pneumonia (*Figure 26-14*).[30,41-47] The vacuoles tend to be larger in cases of exogenous lipoid pneumonia (*Figure 26-15*). Stains with oil red O

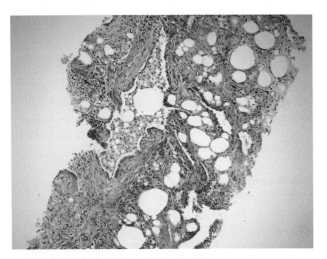

FIGURE 26-14 Transbronchial biopsy from a patient with exogenous lipoid pneumonia showing numerous intra-alveolar macrophages with foamy cytoplasm (hematoxylin and eosin).

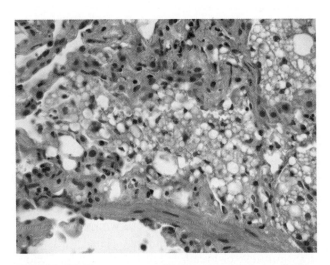

FIGURE 26-15 Exogenous lipoid pneumonia at higher power showing the presence of large intracytoplasmic vacuoles within the cytoplasm of alveolar macrophages (hematoxylin and eosin).

of cytological samples not fixed in alcohol confirm the lipid nature of these vacuoles.

Vegetable oils, such as those in sesame seed, poppy seed, and olive oil, cause little reaction and are seldom seen in biopsies. Animal and mineral oils elicit an inflammatory reaction with accumulation in alveolar spaces and interstitium of lipid-laden macrophages with a vacuolated cytoplasm. Multinucleated giant cells, chronic inflammatory cells, cholesterol clefts, lipoid granulomas, and variable fibrosis are also present.

Most of the oil material is removed from the lung by airways but some material is removed through the pulmonary lymphatics to the regional lymph nodes. Therefore, foamy macrophages, multinucleated giant cells, and lipoid granulomas can be seen along the lymphatic routes of the lung, such as in perivascular/peribronchiolar spaces, septa and the pleura.

Oil red O staining of lung sections that have not been processed in alcohol is useful to confirm a diagnosis of lipoid pneumonia. Fixation in osmium is also a sensitive method to demonstrate the presence of oil droplets within the lung and black intracytoplasmic deposits in lipid-laden macrophages.

Endogenous lipoid pneumonia shows accumulation of lipid-laden macrophages within alveoli associated with the deposition of amorphous eosinophilic proteinaceous material resulting from degenerating cells, including surfactant from type II pneumocytes. The cytoplasmic vacuoles within macrophages tend to be smaller and less distinct than those seen in patients with exogenous lipoid pneumonia.

Eosinophilic Pneumonia

Pulmonary conditions associated with eosinophilia include asthma, acute and chronic eosinophilic pneumonia, pulmonary Langerhans cell histiocytosis, some cases of hypersensitivity pneumonitis (extrinsic allergic alveolitis), viral and other infectious pneumonia, drug reaction, allergic bronchopulmonary aspergillosis, bronchocentric granulomatosis, radiation pneumonitis, lung cancer, Churg-Strauss syndrome, acute cellular rejection, and other conditions.[49-57]

Clinical features of eosinophilic pneumonia

Acute eosinophilic pneumonia is an unusual form of acute lung injury that affects patients of both genders and all ages.[57] They typically present with a severe acute illness of a few days' duration associated with myalgia, shortness of breath, pleuritic chest pain, hypoxemia, no evidence of infection and presence of >25% of eosinophils on bronchoalveolar lavage fluid, and/or tissue eosinophilia. Physical examination shows high fever, respiratory distress, and bibasilar or diffuse crackles. Peripheral blood eosinophilia is unusual at presentation but becomes more apparent during the course of the disease. Patients often develop respiratory failure requiring intubation and mechanical ventilation. Diagnosis requires bronchoalveolar lavage. Transbronchial and/or wedge lung biopsies can also be helpful to confirm the diagnosis and exclude the possibility of an infection prior to corticosteroid therapy. Acute eosinophilic pneumonia usually responds promptly to corticosteroid therapy.

Chronic eosinophilic pneumonia is a subacute or chronic condition that is more prevalent in women than men (2:1).[52-55] Patients present with cough, fever, dyspnea, and weight loss and/or symptoms of asthma. Symptoms are insidious and can last from a minimum of 2 weeks to several months prior to diagnoses. Physical examination shows nonspecific findings such as rales, wheezes, and dullness to percussion and/or decrease in breath sounds. Bronchoalveolar lavage shows eosinophilia. Peripheral blood eosinophilia is present in approximately half of the patients.

Some patients with chronic eosinophilic pneumonia have spontaneous resolution of their illness, but most individuals required corticosteroid therapy that often results in dramatic improvement within 1 to 2 days of treatment. Relapses are frequent, particularly in patients are treated for less than 6 months with corticosteroids. Rare patients with chronic eosinophilic pneumonia develop a superimposed acute illness that resembles acute eosinophilic pneumonia.

Imaging features of eosinophilic pneumonia

The chest x-rays of patients with acute eosinophilic pneumonia usually show extensive alveolar and interstitial infiltrates involving all lobes and small, usually bilateral, pleural effusions.[51,56]

The chest x-rays of patients with chronic eosinophilic pneumonia usually show localized or bilateral peripheral densities that involved the outer 2/3 of the lung perihilar regions, sparing the perihilar regions. The pattern of bilateral peripheral densities that spare perihilar areas is virtually diagnostic of chronic eosinophilic pneumonia and has been compared to the "photographic negative" of pulmonary edema. Some patients with chronic eosinophilic pneumonia show atypical imaging findings such as nodular infiltrates, lower lobe infiltrates and cavitation.

Chest CT scan shows similar findings as described above and frequently document the presence of associated mediastinal adenopathy.

Gross features of eosinophilic pneumonia

The lungs of patients with acute eosinophilic pneumonia shows similar findings to those described for acute lung injury.[49,50] They are heavy, pin-red, congested, and edematous.

Chronic eosinophilic pneumonia appears grossly as areas of ill-circumscribed gray pulmonary consolidation without any distinctive growth features from other forms of pneumonia. Rare cases can show cavitation.[53]

Histologic features of eosinophilic pneumonia

Lung tissues in patients with acute eosinophilic pneumonia show a large number of interstitial eosinophils (*Figure 26-16*) and a smaller number of intra-alveolar eosinophils associated with changes of the exudative and/or proliferative phases of DAD, such as hyaline membranes, reactive type II pneumocytes, and

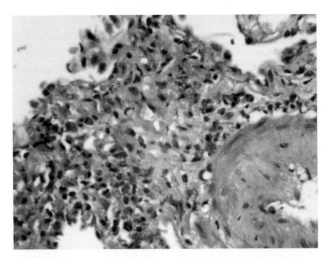

FIGURE 26-16 Transbronchial biopsy from a patient with acute eosinophilic pneumonia. The patient presented with severe dyspnea and other clinical findings of acute lung injury. The biopsy shows the presence of numerous interstitial eosinophils (hematoxylin and eosin).

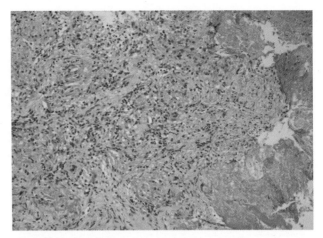

FIGURE 26-18 Wedge lung biopsy from patient with chronic eosinophilic pneumonia. The alveoli are filled with eosinophils, macrophages, and fibroblasts (hematoxylin and eosin).

intra-alveolar myofibroblastic proliferation with myxoid stroma (*Figure 26-17*).[2,50,57] Perivascular inflammation with eosinophils, focal thrombi, and acute fibrinous pleuritis are also usually present. No vasculitis or granulomas are seen.

Lung tissues in patients with chronic eosinophilic pneumonia show extensive intra-alveolar accumulation of macrophages admixed with variable numbers of eosinophils (*Figure 26-18*), edema fluid, and a proteinaceous exudate that can appear as "colloid like."[53-55] Tissue eosinophilia is variable in different microscopic fields and there is no minimum eosinophil count threshold necessary for diagnosis other than the presence of a large number of eosinophils in at least some microscopic fields. Small numbers of intra-alveolar or interstitial lymphocytes and plasma cells can also be present. Alveolar septa can be slightly thickened with type II pneumocyte hyperplasia, but alveolar walls are generally difficult to identify with certainty in the presence of dense intra-alveolar exudates. Multinucleated giant cells and Charcot-Leyden crystals can also be occasionally be identified.

The histopathological changes of chronic eosinophilic pneumonia can be associated with foci of organizing pneumonia (*Figure 26-19*), bronchiolitis obliterans, eosinophilic microabscesses, small number of epithelioid granulomas, and focal necrosis. True vasculitis is rare in chronic eosinophilic pneumonia

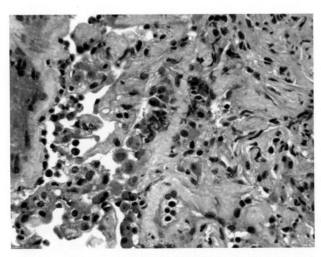

FIGURE 26-17 The biopsy from the same patient with acute eosinophilic pneumonia also shows the presence of reactive pneumocytes and intra-alveolar fibrin (hematoxylin and eosin).

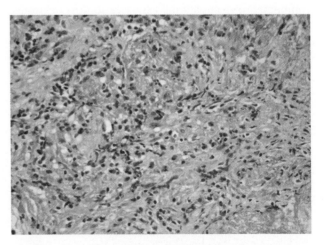

FIGURE 26-19 Chronic eosinophilic pneumonia showing, in addition to a prominent number of eosinophils, the presence of intra-alveolar fibrin and fibrosis, features usually seen in the early organizing pattern of injury (hematoxylin and eosin).

and the presence of vasculitis, tissue eosinophilia, and asthma should suggest the possibility of the Churg-Strauss syndrome.

It is important to exclude in lung biopsies from patients with acute or chronic eosinophilic pneumonia the presence of viral changes (eg, herpes virus, cytomegalovirus, others), fungi such as Cryptococcus sp, Coccidioides sp, and Histoplasma sp, and other infections that can be associated with tissue eosinophilia.[29]

Desquamative Interstitial Pneumonia–Like Pattern

Desquamative interstitial pneumonia (DIP) is a syndrome described by Liebow et al in 1965 and characterized by the diffuse intra-alveolar accumulation of slightly pigmented macrophages.[58-64] Liebow et al described DIP as a form of idiopathic interstitial lung disease to be distinguished from usual interstitial pneumonia (UIP) and assumed that these cells were desquamated pneumocytes.[65] Subsequent studies with electron microscopy demonstrated that the intra-alveolar cells were macrophages rather than epithelial cells but the term DIP was preserved for historical reasons.

DIP as described by Liebow et al is a rare condition usually associated with heavy cigarette smoking and characterized by clinicopathologic features that overlap with those of respiratory bronchiolitis interstitial lung disease (RB-ILD).[62] The latter is characterized by the presence of a patchy DIP-like reaction centered on respiratory bronchioles while the infiltrates by intra-alveolar macrophages are diffuse and bilateral in DIP.

DIP-like patterns with patchy or diffuse intra-alveolar infiltration by alveolar macrophages and without the classical clinical and imaging findings of DIP are seen more frequently in nonsmokers in patients with environmental or occupational exposure to dust or fumes, resolving viral pneumonia, collagen vascular disease, and drug reaction.[58-64] For example, DIP-like reactions have been reported in patients exposed to fire-extinguisher powder, diesel and welding fumes, beryllium and copper dust, tungsten carbide production and in textile factories manufacturing upholstery fabric by gluing finely chopped nylon filaments ("flock") to cotton or other fabrics using latex adhesive.[62] DIP-like reactions have also been reported in association with rheumatoid arthritis, drugs such as sirolimus, viral infection, and marijuana users.

Clinical features of desquamative interstitial pneumonia–like pattern

Patients with DIP-like reactions are usually adults between 40 and 60 years of age, with male predominance (2:1).[58-65] They can be asymptomatic but usually present with shortness of breath on exertion and persistent cough. Some patients also develop chest pain, systemic symptoms such as weight loss and fatigue, and rarely hemoptysis. Most patients with DIP-like reactions present with insidious clinical findings but rare individuals develop acute, fulminant clinical symptoms.

Physical examination reveals bibasilar end-inspiratory crackles, variable cyanosis, and occasional clubbing. Pulmonary function tests show impaired diffusion, particularly during exercise. Blood counts, routine chemistries, and immunological analysis are generally negative. Bronchoalveolar lavage findings are nonspecific but show the presence of numerous alveolar macrophages with finely pigmented cytoplasm.

Patients are treated with cessation of smoking and/or occupational exposures and long-term corticosteroid therapy and usually remain stable or improve. Complete recovery is possible in some patients. Untreated patients usually deteriorate with progression into interstitial fibrosis.

Imaging features of desquamative interstitial pneumonia–like pattern

Chest radiographs are often normal but can show a variety of somewhat nonspecific findings such as widespread or patchy ground glass opacities with lower lung zone or peripheral predilection, and granular or nodular opacities.[59,61,63,64] High-resolution chest CT scans shows bilateral ground glass attenuation with lower lung zone or peripheral distribution in the majority of cases. Linear opacities and reticular patterns are also frequent, usually confined to lower lung zones. Traction bronchiectasis and small peripheral cysts have also been described in patients with DIP-like reactions. Patients with chronic disease can develop peripheral and limited honeycomb changes.

Gross features of desquamative interstitial pneumonia–like pattern

The lungs can appear as slightly indurated in patients with mild DIP-like pattern or firm, indurated, and somewhat nodular in cases with more advanced disease.[63] Patients with chronic disease can exhibit focal subpleural fine honeycombing and mild, diffuse interstitial fibrosis.

Histologic features of desquamative interstitial pneumonia–like pattern

DIP-like pattern is characterized by the presence of numerous macrophages within alveoli in a diffuse distribution throughout the lung parenchyma (*Figure 26-20*).[59,61,63,64] The macrophages have abundant amphophilic cytoplasm and often contain a finely granular light-brown pigment (*Figure 26-21*). Few

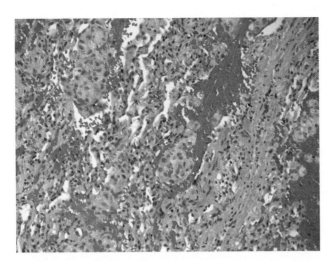

FIGURE 26-20 Desquamative interstitial pneumonia–like pattern. Alveolar spaces are filled with numerous macrophages (hematoxylin and eosin).

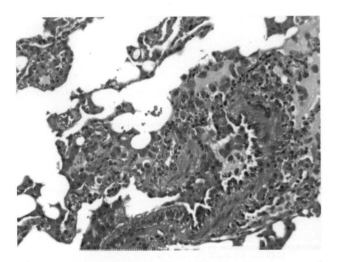

FIGURE 26-21 Respiratory bronchiolitis. The lumen of a respiratory bronchiole and the adjacent alveoli show numerous macrophages with intracytoplasmic finely granular brown pigment (hematoxylin and eosin).

multinucleated giant cells are also present within alveolar spaces. The alveolar architecture is preserved, with focal infiltration of the interstitium by lymphoid cells and/or a moderate number of eosinophils. Lymphoid aggregates can be present. Interstitial fibrosis is usually absent or mild, except in subpleural areas. Patients with long-standing DIP-like pattern may show focally moderate to severe subpleural fibrosis with distortion of the architecture and cyst formation.

The intracytoplasmic granules seen in the intra-alveolar macrophages characteristic of DIP-like pattern stain finely with Pearl iron and D-PAS stains. Their cell origin can be confirmed with immunostains for CD68 or CD163.[63] Immunostains for CD1a and S100 are negative.

The findings of DIP-like reactions can be seen on transbronchial biopsies but this diagnosis often requires

examination of wedge lung biopsies. Correlation of the clinicopathologic findings with the occupational or environmental history is important to triage biopsies from selected patients for scanning electron microscopy with energy-dispersive x-ray analysis for the detection of inorganic particles.[58-65]

Pulmonary Alveolar Proteinosis

Pulmonary alveolar proteinosis is a rare condition characterized by the presence of abundant granular, eosinophilic, acellular material within the alveolar spaces resulting from the intra-alveolar accumulation of lipoproteinaceous surfactant material as a consequence of alveolar macrophage abnormalities (*Figure 26-22*).[66-78]

Pulmonary alveolar proteinosis is idiopathic in approximately 90% of patients and is probably an autoimmune disease in which granulocyte-macrophage colony-stimulating factor (GM-CSF), a lymphokine that promotes macrophage differentiation and maturation, is blocked by autoantibodies, resulting in poor macrophage function and impaired surfactant clearance.[68,71,74]

Rare cases of congenital pulmonary alveolar proteinosis developing as a result of disorders of surfactant metabolism have been described. Multiple protein mutations involving surfactant or surfactant-associated proteins have been described in these children as a result of autosomal dominant and recessive patterns of inheritance.

Pulmonary alveolar proteinosis can also be secondary to hematological malignancy, infections by HIV and other viruses, Nocardia, Pneumocystis jiroveci, fungi and other organisms, drug reaction, acute silicosis, exposure to aluminum and kaolin.[69,76,78] Pulmonary alveolar proteinosis treated with allogeneic bone marrow transplant has also been described.[79,80]

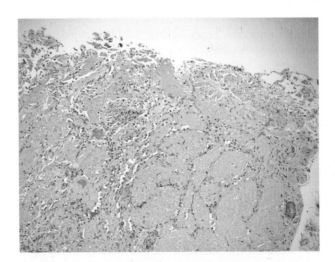

FIGURE 26-22 Transbronchial biopsy from patient with alveolar proteinosis showing the presence of densely eosinophilic intra-alveolar exudate (hematoxylin and eosin).

Clinical features of pulmonary alveolar proteinosis

Pulmonary alveolar proteinosis is more frequent in smokers and in males and it is usually seen in patients in their third to fifth decade of age.[76,77] Patients can be asymptomatic or present with shortness of breath and cough. Some patients can also develop fever, hemoptysis, chest pain, and fatigue. Physical examination may reveal no abnormalities or the presence of mild inspiratory rales. Blood counts and chemistries are usually normal. Pulmonary function tests show impaired diffusion and a restrictive pattern in some patients. Bronchoalveolar lavage is usually very helpful to suspect the diagnosis of pulmonary alveolar proteinosis, as the fluid has a characteristic white appearance resembling milk and shows abundant granular amorphous casts that exhibit strong PAS positivity. Eosinophils can also be seen in cases secondary to drug reaction. Rarely, the presence of silica particles is seen in BAL fluid, raising a suspicion for environmental exposure. The presence of anti-GM-CSF antibodies can be detected in the serum or BAL fluid.

Patients with idiopathic pulmonary alveolar proteinosis are usually treated successfully with whole lung lavage to remove the intra-alveolar material and autoantibodies and GM-CSF injections.[77] The treatment of secondary pulmonary alveolar proteinosis depends on the underlying associated condition. The prognosis of children with congenital pulmonary alveolar proteinosis is poor.[81,82]

Imaging features of pulmonary alveolar proteinosis

Chest radiographs usually show variable densities distributed in a perihilar location.[66,67,76] High-resolution CT scans show ground glass attenuation with perihilar distribution and thickening of the interlobular septa resulting in the "crazy-paving' pattern. Patients with pulmonary alveolar proteinosis often show prominent imaging abnormalities that are somewhat out of proportion to mild symptoms and clinical findings.

Gross features of pulmonary alveolar proteinosis

The lungs show patchy, firm yellow, firm areas of consolidation that can exude milky fluid on section.

Histologic features of pulmonary alveolar proteinosis

The lung shows patchy or diffuse intra-alveolar accumulation of granular, deeply eosinophilic material, some cholesterol clefts, focal, mild type II pneumocyte hyperplasia, and no significant interstitial fibrosis or

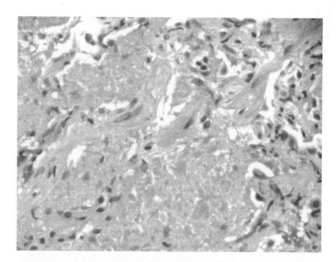

FIGURE 26-23 The eosinophilic exudate of alveolar proteinosis is finely granular. Note the absence of significant inflammation or fibrosis in alveolar septa (hematoxylin and eosin).

distortion of the alveolar architecture (*Figure 26-23*). The eosinophilic material stains strongly with D-PAS stain.[66-77,79,81,82]

The diagnosis of pulmonary alveolar proteinosis can be rendered on transbronchial biopsies or less frequently on wedge lung biopsies. In patients with secondary pulmonary alveolar proteinosis, examination of the biopsies with polarized light can show the presence of numerous silica-like crystals. GMS and Gram stains can show the presence of Pneumocystis jiroveci, fungi, Nocardia, or other infectious organisms.[69]

REFERENCES

1. Ware LB, Herridge M. Acute lung injury. *Semin Respir Crit Care Med*. 2013;34:439-440.
2. Beasley MB. The pathologist's approach to acute lung injury. *Arch Pathol Lab Med*. 2010;134:719-727.
3. Murray JF. Pulmonary edema: pathophysiology and diagnosis. *Int J Tuberc Lung Dis*. 2011;15:155-60, i.
4. Alwi I. Diagnosis and management of cardiogenic pulmonary edema. *Acta Med Indones*. 2010;42:176-184.
5. Bachmann M, Waldrop JE. Noncardiogenic pulmonary edema. *Compend Contin Educ Vet*. 2012;34:E1.
6. Eisenhut M. The pathophysiology of pulmonary edema caused by inflammation. *Int J Tuberc Lung Dis*. 2011;15:1135-1136.
7. Jaworski K, Maslanka K, Kosior DA. Transfusion-related acute lung injury: a dangerous and underdiagnosed noncardiogenic pulmonary edema. *Cardiol J*. 2013;20:337-344.
8. Martindale JL, Noble VE, Liteplo A. Diagnosing pulmonary edema: lung ultrasound versus chest radiography. *Eur J Emerg Med*. 2013;20:356-360.
9. Beasley MB, Franks TJ, Galvin JR, et al. Acute fibrinous and organizing pneumonia: a histological pattern of lung injury and possible variant of diffuse alveolar damage. *Arch Pathol Lab Med*. 2002;126:1064-1070.
10. Castro CY. ARDS and diffuse alveolar damage: a pathologist's perspective. *Semin Thorac Cardiovasc Surg*. 2006;18:13-19.

11. Fukuda Y, Ishizaki M, Masuda Y, et al. The role of intraalveolar fibrosis in the process of pulmonary structural remodeling in patients with diffuse alveolar damage. *Am J Pathol.* 1987;126:171-182.

12. Kaarteenaho R, Kinnula VL. Diffuse alveolar damage: a common phenomenon in progressive interstitial lung disorders. *Pulm Med.* 2011;2011:531302.

13. Poletti V, Casoni GL, Cancellieri A, et al. Diffuse alveolar damage. *Pathologica.* 2010;102:453-463.

14. Sugiyama K, Kawai T. Diffuse alveolar damage and acute interstitial pneumonitis: histochemical evaluation with lectins and monoclonal antibodies against surfactant apoprotein and collagen type IV. *Mod Pathol.* 1993;6:242-248.

15. Thompson BT, Matthay MA. The Berlin definition of ARDS versus pathological evidence of diffuse alveolar damage. *Am J Respir Crit Care Med.* 2013;187:675-677.

16. Kobayashi H, Itoh T, Sasaki Y, et al. Diagnostic imaging of idiopathic adult respiratory distress syndrome (ARDS)/diffuse alveolar damage (DAD) histopathological correlation with radiological imaging. *Clin Imaging.* 1996;20:1-7.

17. Miniati M, Pistolesi M. Imaging strategies in the detection and evaluation of ARDS. *Schweiz Med Wochenschr.* 1993;123:464-472.

18. Franquet T. Imaging of pulmonary viral pneumonia. *Radiology.* 2011;260:18-39.

19. Hidron AI, Low CE, Honig EG, et al. Emergence of community-acquired meticillin-resistant Staphylococcus aureus strain USA300 as a cause of necrotizing community-onset pneumonia. *Lancet Infect Dis.* 2009;9:384-392.

20. Yazer J, Giacomantonio M, Macdonald N, et al. Severe necrotizing pneumonia in a child with pandemic (H1N1) influenza. *CMAJ.* 2011;183:215-219.

21. Cruz P, Torres M, Higuera O, et al. Taxane-induced Pneumonitis: our clinical experience. *Arch Bronconeumol.* 2014;50(1):45.

22. Griese M, Haug M, Hartl D, et al. Hypersensitivity pneumonitis: lessons for diagnosis and treatment of a rare entity in children. *Orphanet J Rare Dis.* 2013;8:121.

23. Travis WD, Costabel U, Hansell DM, et al. An official American Thoracic Society/European Respiratory Society statement: update of the international multidisciplinary classification of the idiopathic interstitial pneumonias. *Am J Respir Crit Care Med.* 2013;188:733-748.

24. Ho ED. Community-acquired pneumonia in adults and children. *Prim Care.* 2013;40:655-669.

25. Kreienbuehl L, Charbonney E, Eggimann P. Community-acquired necrotizing pneumonia due to methicillin-sensitive Staphylococcus aureus secreting Panton-Valentine leukocidin: a review of case reports. *Ann Intensive Care.* 2011;1:52.

26. Reimel BA, Krishnadasen B, Cuschieri J, et al. Surgical management of acute necrotizing lung infections. *Can Respir J.* 2006;13:369-373.

27. Franquet T. Imaging of pneumonia: trends and algorithms. *Eur Respir J.* 2001;18:196-208.

28. Woodhead M, Klassen-Fischer M, Neafie R, et al. Pulmonary bacterial infections. In: Hasleton P, Flieder D, eds. *Spencer's Pathology of the Lung.* Cambridge: Cambridge University Press; 2013.

29. Kradin R, Fishman J. Pulmonary viral infections. In: Hasleton P, Flieder D, eds. *Spencer's Pulmonary Pathology.* Cambridge: Cambridge University Press; 2013.

30. Betancourt SL, Martinez-Jimenez S, Rossi SE, et al. Lipoid pneumonia: spectrum of clinical and radiologic manifestations. *AJR Am J Roentgenol.* 2010;194:103-109.

31. Franquet T, Gimenez A, Roson N, et al. Aspiration diseases: findings, pitfalls, and differential diagnosis. *Radiographics.* 2000;20:673-685.

32. Sawicki GS, Lu FL, Valim C, et al. Necrotising pneumonia is an increasingly detected complication of pneumonia in children. *Eur Respir J.* 2008;31:1285-1291.

33. Palmacci C, Antocicco M, Bonomo L, et al. Necrotizing pneumonia and sepsis due to Clostridium perfringens: a case report. *Cases J.* 2009;2:50.

34. Miller RF, Huang L, Walzer PD. Pneumocystis pneumonia associated with human immunodeficiency virus. *Clin Chest Med.* 2013;34:229-241.

35. Baumann S, Reinwald M, Haghi D, et al. Coinfection of Pneumocystis jirovecii and invasive pulmonary aspergillosis in an immunocompromised patient: a diagnostic challenge. *Onkologie.* 2013;36:582-584.

36. Puligandla PS, Laberge JM. Respiratory infections: pneumonia, lung abscess, and empyema. *Semin Pediatr Surg.* 2008;17:42-52.

37. Magalhaes L, Valadares D, Oliveira JR, et al. Lung abscesses: review of 60 cases. *Rev Port Pneumol.* 2009;15:165-178.

38. Patradoon-Ho P, Fitzgerald DA. Lung abscess in children. *Paediatr Respir Rev.* 2007;8:77-84.

39. Cordier JF. Organising pneumonia. *Thorax.* 2000;55:318-328.

40. Cordier JF. Cryptogenic organising pneumonia. *Eur Respir J.* 2006;28:422-446.

41. Seaton A. Lipoid pneumonia in a fire breather. *Occup Med (Lond).* 2010;60:406.

42. Marchiori E, Zanetti G, Mano CM, et al. Lipoid pneumonia in 53 patients after aspiration of mineral oil: comparison of high-resolution computed tomography findings in adults and children. *J Comput Assist Tomogr.* 2010;34:9-12.

43. Khilnani GC, Hadda V. Lipoid pneumonia: an uncommon entity. *Indian J Med Sci.* 2009;63:474-480.

44. Hadda V, Khilnani GC. Lipoid pneumonia: an overview. *Expert Rev Respir Med.* 2010;4:799-807.

45. Harris K, Chalhoub M, Maroun R, et al. Lipoid pneumonia: a challenging diagnosis. *Heart Lung.* 2011;40:580-584.

46. Papla B, Urbanczyk K, Gil T, et al. Exogenous lipoid pneumonia (oil granulomas of the lung). *Pol J Pathol.* 2011;62:269-273.

47. Ishimatsu K, Kamitani T, Matsuo Y, et al. Exogenous lipoid pneumonia induced by aspiration of insecticide. *J Thorac Imaging.* 2012;27:W18-W20.

48. Weill H, Ferrans VJ, Gay RM, et al. Early lipoid pneumonia. roentgenologic, anatomic and physiologic characteristics. *Am J Med.* 1964;36:370-376.

49. Marchand E, Cordier JF. Idiopathic chronic eosinophilic pneumonia. *Orphanet J Rare Dis.* 2006;1:11.

50. Liu KT, Wu MH, Chiu CH, et al. Idiopathic acute eosinophilic pneumonia. *J Chin Med Assoc.* 2006;69:330-333.

51. Furuiye M, Yoshimura N, Kobayashi A, et al. Churg-Strauss syndrome versus chronic eosinophilic pneumonia on high-resolution computed tomographic findings. *J Comput Assist Tomogr.* 2010;34:19-22.

52. Kumasawa F, Kobayashi T, Noda A, et al. Chronic eosinophilic pneumonia presenting with acute onset. *Asian Pac J Allergy Immunol.* 2012;30:321-325.

53. Alam M, Burki NK. Chronic eosinophilic pneumonia: a review. *South Med J.* 2007;100:49-53.

54. Sano S, Yamagami K, Yoshioka K. Chronic eosinophilic pneumonia: a case report and review of the literature. *Cases J.* 2009;2:7735.

55. Frank RE, Jr. Chronic eosinophilic pneumonia. *J Insur Med.* 2007;39:199-204.

56. Daimon T, Johkoh T, Sumikawa H, et al. Acute eosinophilic pneumonia: thin-section CT findings in 29 patients. *Eur J Radiol.* 2008;65:462-467.

57. Sohn JW. Acute eosinophilic pneumonia. *Tuberc Respir Dis.* 2013;74:51-55.

58. Heyneman LE, Ward S, Lynch DA, et al. Respiratory bronchiolitis, respiratory bronchiolitis-associated interstitial lung disease, and desquamative interstitial pneumonia: different entities or part of the spectrum of the same disease process? *AJR Am J Roentgenol.* 1999;173:1617-1622.

59. Craig PJ, Wells AU, Doffman S, et al. Desquamative interstitial pneumonia, respiratory bronchiolitis and their relationship to smoking. *Histopathology.* 2004;45:275-282.

60. Ischander M, Fan LL, Farahmand V, et al. Desquamative interstitial pneumonia in a child related to cigarette smoke. *Pediatr Pulmonol.* 2014;49(3):E56-E58.

61. Elkin SL, Nicholson AG, du Bois RM. Desquamative interstitial pneumonia and respiratory bronchiolitis-associated interstitial lung disease. *Semin Respir Crit Care Med.* 2001;22:387-398.

62. Godbert B, Wissler MP, Vignaud JM. Desquamative interstitial pneumonia: an analytic review with an emphasis on aetiology. *Eur Respir Rev.* 2013;22:117-123.

63. Tazelaar HD, Wright JL, Churg A. Desquamative interstitial pneumonia. *Histopathology.* 2011;58:509-516.

64. Chaudhary PK, Jain SK, Jain KP, et al. Desquamative interstitial pneumonia. *J Assoc Physicians India.* 1993;41:303-305.

65. Liebow AA, Steer A, Billingsley JG. Desquamative interstitial pneumonia. *Am J Med.* 1965;39:369-404.

66. Huizar I, Kavuru MS. Alveolar proteinosis syndrome: pathogenesis, diagnosis, and management. *Curr Opin Pulm Med.* 2009;15:491-498.

67. Campo I, Mariani F, Rodi G, et al. Assessment and management of pulmonary alveolar proteinosis in a reference center. *Orphanet J Rare Dis.* 2013;8:40.

68. Carey B, Trapnell BC. The molecular basis of pulmonary alveolar proteinosis. *Clin Immunol.* 2010;135:223-235.

69. Punatar AD, Kusne S, Blair JE, et al. Opportunistic infections in patients with pulmonary alveolar proteinosis. *J Infect.* 2012;65:173-179.

70. Khan AR, Sulaman A, Abbasi MA, et al. Primary alveolar proteinosis. *J Ayub Med Coll Abbottabad.* 2012;24:120-122.

71. Sarac S, Milic R, Zolotarevski L, et al. Primary pulmonary alveolar proteinosis. *Vojnosanit Pregl.* 2012;69:1005-1008.

72. Wang T, Lazar CA, Fishbein MC, et al. Pulmonary alveolar proteinosis. *Semin Respir Crit Care Med.* 2012;33:498-508.

73. Patel SM, Sekiguchi H, Reynolds JP, et al. Pulmonary alveolar proteinosis. *Can Respir J.* 2012;19:243-245.

74. Shattuck TM, Bean SM. Pulmonary alveolar proteinosis. *Diagn Cytopathol.* 2013;41:620-622.

75. Borie R, Danel C, Debray MP, et al. Pulmonary alveolar proteinosis. *Eur Respir Rev.* 2011;20:98-107.

76. Das M, Salzman GA. Pulmonary alveolar proteinosis: an overview for internists and hospital physicians. *Hosp Pract (1995).* 2010;38:43-49.

77. Campo I, Kadija Z, Mariani F, et al. Pulmonary alveolar proteinosis: diagnostic and therapeutic challenges. *Multidiscip Respir Med.* 2012;7:4.

78. McDonnell MJ, Reynolds C, Tormey V, et al. Pulmonary alveolar proteinosis: report of two cases in the West of Ireland with review of current literature. *Ir J Med Sci.* 2014;183(1):123-127.

79. Pidala J, Khalil F, Fernandez H. Pulmonary alveolar proteinosis following allogeneic hematopoietic cell transplantation. *Bone Marrow Transplant.* 2011;46:1480-1483.

80. Tabata S, Shimoji S, Murase K, et al. Successful allogeneic bone marrow transplantation for myelodysplastic syndrome complicated by severe pulmonary alveolar proteinosis. *Int J Hematol.* 2009;90:407-412.

81. de Blic J. Pulmonary alveolar proteinosis in children. *Paediatr Respir Rev.* 2004;5:316-322.

82. McCook TA, Kirks DR, Merten DF, et al. Pulmonary alveolar proteinosis in children. *AJR Am J Roentgenol.* 1981;137:1023-1027.

27 Drug Reactions and Radiation-Induced Lung Injury

Fumi Kawakami and Hidehiro Takei

TAKE HOME PEARLS

- Drug-induced pulmonary toxicity can be caused by any of more than 700 drugs.
- There are two major roles for pathologists in the interpretation of a biopsy from an individual with a suspected drug reaction: (1) elimination of other conditions, especially infection and malignancy, and (2) recognition of the histological pattern of lung injury.
- Drug-induced bronchospasms have frequently been reported with the use of nonsteroidal anti-inflammatory drugs, anti-infective agents, and cardiovascular drugs such as angiotensin-converting enzyme inhibitor, amiodarone, and β-blockers.
- A number of drugs have been documented to cause noncardiogenic pulmonary edema, including hydrochlorothiazide, ethchlorvynol, opiates, tocolytics, protamine, and salicylates.
- Typical agents that cause diffuse pulmonary hemorrhage include anticoagulants, amphotericin B, high-dose cyclophosphamide, mitomycin C, cytarabine (ara-C), and d-penicillamine.
- Cytotoxic drugs, such as bleomycin, busulfan, carmustine (BCNU), cyclophosphamide, melphalan, and mitomycin, are most commonly associated with diffuse alveolar damage.
- Bleomycin, cyclophosphamide, and methotrexate are the most common drugs causing organizing pneumonia, and less often it is caused by amiodarone, nitrofurantoin, penicillamine, and sulfasalazine.
- All forms of idiopathic interstitial pneumonia have been reported as manifestations of pulmonary drug toxicity, most commonly nonspecific interstitial pneumonia, particularly with amiodarone, methotrexate, and carmustine.
- Drug-induced eosinophilic pneumonia is seen with a number of drugs, particularly acetylsalicylic acid, amiodarone, bleomycin, carbamazepine, captopril, phenytoin, hydrochlorothiazide, mesalamine, minocycline, nitrofurantoin, penicillamine, sulfasalazine, and sulfonamides.
- Drug-induced lymphoid hyperplasia (LH), including diffuse LH, follicular bronchiolitis, lymphoid interstitial pneumonia, and lymphocytic perivascular cuffing, has been reported as one of the manifestations of amiodarone-related lung toxicity.
- Sarcoidosis-like changes have been reported as systemic adverse effects of interferon-α and interferon-β administration.
- Etanercept, leflunomide, mesalamine, sirolimus, and methotrexate may cause a hypersensitivity pneumonia type reaction.
- Drug-induced pulmonary alveolar proteinosis has been described with amiodarone, cyclophosphamide, busulfan, bleomycin, mitomycin C, etoposide, chlorambucil, leflunomide, and sirolimus, and more recently, fentanyl and other inhaled drugs.
- Approximately 10% of cases of lupus erythematosus are believed to be induced by drugs and more than 100 different drugs have been reported to cause lupus syndrome, with the most common being hydralazine, procainamide, quinidine, isoniazid, diltiazem, and minocycline.
- Drug-induced pulmonary veno-occlusive disease is known to occur in association with the use of

oral contraceptives and various chemotherapeutic agents, such as bleomycin, busulfan, carmustine, lomustine, and nitrosoureas.

- Anorectic drugs, such as aminorex and phentermine/fenfluramine (phen-fen), and illicit drugs, such as cocaine and methamphetamine, can induce pulmonary hypertension.
- Pleural disease may be caused by cardiovascular agents (practolol, amiodarone, and minoxidil), ergoline drugs (methysergide and bromocriptine), sclerotherapy agents (sodium morrhuate and absolute alcohol), and chemotherapeutic agents (bleomycin, mitomycin, procarbazine, methotrexate, and cyclophosphamide).
- Radiation-induced lung injury is an adverse effect of thoracic irradiation, which is usually employed for treatment of carcinomas of the lung, esophagus, thyroid, and breast, as well as for hematologic malignancies.

OVERVIEW OF DRUG TOXICITY

Awareness of drug-induced lung toxicity is increasing rapidly. In the 1970s, only 19 drugs had been reported to have the potential to cause pulmonary disease.[1] In the 1990s, at least 150 such agents were recognized,[2,3] and to date, over 700 have been identified.[4] This means that drug-induced pulmonary toxicity can occur in patients receiving any medication, including some that are marketed as health foods. Usually, agents administered intravenously or orally are more likely to cause drug-induced lung toxicity, but ocular and topical medications may also produce this adverse effect.[5] Thus, it is important to consider the possibility of drug-induced lung disease when diagnosing any clinical condition affecting the lung. This diagnosis may be largely based on exclusion of other potential causes of the symptoms observed, because there are no specific symptoms, signs, radiologic findings, or laboratory findings indicating that the pathology is drug induced.[6] For this reason, drug-induced lung toxicity is one of the most challenging fields in diagnostic pulmonary pathology.

The role of pathological examination in the diagnosis and management of drug-induced lung toxicity is rather limited. Invasive biopsies are not usually performed because the clinical symptoms of drug-induced lung toxicity are often mild, and clinicians therefore tend to recommend cessation of the causative drug as a first-line therapy. When the clinical presentation is unusual or other conditions cannot be excluded clinically, lung biopsy may be performed. There are two major roles for pathologists in the interpretation of a biopsy from an individual with a suspected drug reaction: (1) elimination of other conditions, especially infection

and malignancy and (2) recognition of the histological pattern of lung injury.

The pathogenesis of drug-induced lung toxicity is poorly understood. The condition seems to be multi-factorial and underlying mechanisms may vary with each causative agent. However, in general, direct and indirect injury to the pneumocytes and capillary endothelial cells owing to cytokine cascades and free radicals may play important roles. Interestingly, the mechanisms of molecular target drugs-induced lung toxicity are unique and reflect the fundamental biological mechanisms of action of the causative drugs. For instance, gefitinib, a selective epidermal growth factor receptor (EGFR) tyrosine kinase inhibitor, increases lung tissue vulnerability to damage through inhibition of alveolar repair.[6-8]

This chapter reviews the characteristic clinical, radiographic, and pathologic features of drug-induced lung toxicity. Several representative drugs, and the characteristic pathophysiological states caused by drug-induced lung toxicity, are described.

Differential Diagnosis of Drug Toxicity

The proposed criteria for the definitive diagnosis of a drug reaction are listed below.[9,10]

1. The timing of drug administration should be consistent with an adverse reaction occurring after a latent period.
2. Other possible causes (eg, infection, malignancy, and progression of the underlying disease) must be completely excluded.
3. The adverse reaction resolves following discontinuation of the suspect drug, and recurs with rechallenge.
4. The patient was exposed to only one drug and there was no comorbid state that could be related to the adverse reaction observed.
5. The pattern of adverse reaction (clinical, radiological, and/or histological) is consistent with the drug administered.

Because these criteria are quite rigorous and some requirements may be ethically contraindicated, very few cases fulfill them completely. Thus, most pulmonary drug reactions remain unproven. The degree of relationship between a drug and a potential adverse effect on the lungs can be classified as (1) causative, (2) probable, (3) possible, (4) coincidental, or (5) negative (unrelated).[1] Because diagnosis of drug-induced lung toxicity is often based on exclusion, adequate clinical and radiological information is essential to initiate its pathologic investigation. On occasion, a typical histologic pattern can be identified from biopsy and cytology specimens.

Clinical and Radiologic Patterns of Lung Injury

Clinical diagnosis of drug toxicity requires a constant awareness that the drug may be the cause, because the manifesting symptoms are nonspecific and overlap with those of numerous other pulmonary diseases, including infections, pulmonary manifestations of primary systemic diseases, progression of the underlying malignancy, and incidental comorbid idiopathic lung diseases. Drug toxicity may manifest as an acute or subacute reaction, chronic fibrosing pneumonitis, and/or pulmonary vascular disease.[11] Interestingly, drug-induced lung toxicity can present as an acute manifestation in patients who have been administered the causative drug for years,[6,12] or even become clinically evident years after drug discontinuation. Carmustine is a representative drug and is associated with late-onset pulmonary adverse effects, with a latency of as long as 8 to 20 years.[13-15]

Cessation of the drug is an essential and sufficient "treatment" for drug-induced lung toxicity and most patients have a good prognosis. However, some cases may need corticosteroid administration. Unfortunately, no treatment can reverse pulmonary fibrosis once it has developed.

High-resolution computed tomography (HRCT) is currently the best noninvasive method for assessing changes associated with drug-induced lung toxicity. Several radiologic patterns of drug-induced respiratory disease have been identified, including the nonspecific interstitial pneumonia (NSIP) pattern, usual interstitial pneumonia (UIP)–like pattern, hypersensitivity pneumonia (HP)–like pattern, pulmonary edema with or without diffuse alveolar damage (DAD), bronchiolitis obliterans (BO), and diffuse alveolar hemorrhage.[16] However, one report indicated that HRCT had an accuracy of only 45% for predicting the specific histology of drug-induced lung toxicity.[17] Despite its limited ability to predict these histological patterns, HRCT is a valuable tool for monitoring time-dependent changes and treatment response.

Specific serum markers for drug-induced lung injury have not been established. Levels of KL-6, a well-known marker for interstitial lung disease, increase in some cases of drug-induced lung toxicity such as DAD and chronic fibrosing interstitial pneumonia, but not in organizing pneumonia or HP.[18] Surfactant proteins SP-A and SP-D have been reported as reliable markers of pulmonary fibrosis, but are not specific for drug-induced damage.[19] Increased levels of serum ADAM8 have been reported in drug-induced eosinophilic lung inflammation.[20]

Pathology-Based Classifications

Since drug-induced lung toxicity does not have any specific histologic patterns and can display as many different patterns as lung injuries due to other causes, its diagnostic pathology is one of the most challenging fields in thoracic pathology. In addition, a single agent may produce a variety of nonspecific histologic patterns with a range of clinical courses, while a variety of agents may produce similar histologic patterns. Histological recognition of various different patterns within the lesion may be helpful for appropriate classification of the lesion. In general, concomitant acute and chronic changes may be a key feature suggestive of drug-induced lung toxicity.[21]

These factors can limit the pathologist's role in the diagnosis of drug-induced lung toxicity, emphasizing the importance of careful exclusion of other potential causes when examining the specimens.[22]

In this chapter, histological patterns often seen in drug-induced lung toxicity will be discussed, along with clinical and radiological characteristics.

Drug-induced airway changes

Several drugs can adversely affect the upper respiratory tracts and cause alterations in airway function. Clinical manifestations of drug-induced airway change include asthma-associated bronchospasms, laryngeal edema (*Figure 27-1*), and cough. A bronchospasm may present as an isolated event or as part of a drug-induced anaphylaxis. Drug-induced bronchospasms have frequently been reported with the use of nonsteroidal anti-inflammatory drugs (NSAIDs), anti-infective agents, and cardiovascular drugs such as angiotensin converting enzyme (ACE) inhibitor, amiodarone, and β-blockers.[23] ACE inhibitors provide a representative example of agents that cause cough. These inhibit the degradation of kinins, as well as the conversion of angiotensin I to angiotensin II.

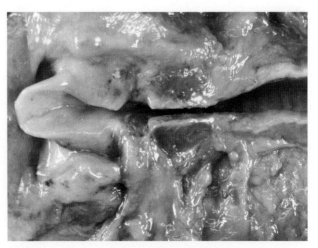

FIGURE 27-1 Drug-induced airway change: laryngeal and epiglottal edema.

CHAPTER 27

Increased levels of kinins irritate the airways, resulting in cough.[24] Inhaled medications are also likely to act as airway irritants.

Since drug-induced airway changes are usually functional and reversible, pathological examination is not generally required.

Drug-induced pulmonary edema

Noncardiogenic pulmonary edema is a syndrome characterized by severe hypoxemia and detection of bilateral diffuse infiltrates on chest radiography, without evidence of heart failure. The known causes include infections, trauma, disseminated intravascular coagulation, and drugs. A number of drugs have been documented to cause noncardiogenic pulmonary edema, including hydrochlorothiazide, ethchlorvynol, opiates, tocolytics, protamine, and salicylates.[21,25-27] Although ethchlorvynol, opiates, and salicylates induce pulmonary edema at levels associated with acute or chronic overdose, hydrochlorothiazide can cause it at levels within the therapeutic range.[27-29] The pathophysiology of drug-induced pulmonary edema is not fully understood, and multiple causative mechanisms have been proposed. Several drugs can act as potential antigens or haptens, initiating an immune cascade that can lead to lung toxicity associated with immune-mediated hypersensitivity, resulting in pulmonary edema.[30] Chest radiographs typically show bilateral interstitial and alveolar infiltrates, usually without cardiomegaly. Although drug-induced pulmonary edema is a potentially life-threatening adverse drug reaction, it can usually be diagnosed and managed without pathological examination. Histological evaluation may be performed at autopsy (*Figure 27-2*).

Drug-induced pulmonary hemorrhage

Although diffuse pulmonary hemorrhage is an uncommon complication of drug therapy, a large number of drugs have been implicated as a cause of hemorrhage through a variety of mechanisms. Patients on anticoagulants and drugs that affect coagulation pathways can develop pulmonary hemorrhage. Drug-induced vasculitis and DAD are known to increase the risk for pulmonary hemorrhage. Early-phase DAD, if severe enough, can cause pulmonary hemorrhage (*Figure 27-3A*). Drug-related lupus syndrome and Churg-Strauss syndrome (CSS), affecting the lung microvasculature (ie, small vessel vasculitis and capillaritis), can also cause drug-induced pulmonary hemorrhage.[31] Drug-induced medium to large-vessel vasculitis is infrequent. Typical agents that cause diffuse pulmonary hemorrhage include anticoagulants, amphotericin B, high-dose

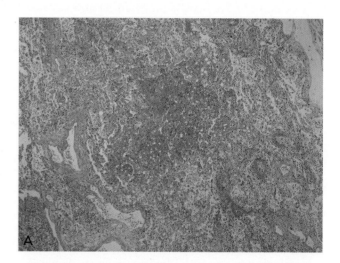

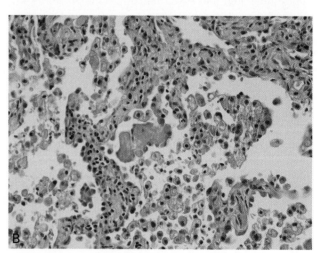

FIGURE 27-3 Drug-induced intra-alveolar hemorrhage. A: Acute hemorrhage with subsequent diffuse alveolar damage. B: In the chronic phase, hemosiderin-laden macrophages and fibrin deposits are observed in the alveolar spaces.

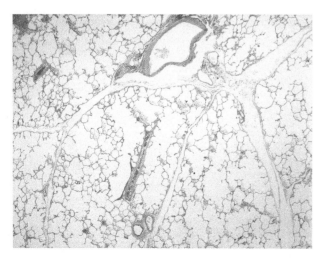

FIGURE 27-2 Drug-induced pulmonary edema: prominent septal thickening is observed. The pulmonary architecture is well preserved.

cyclophosphamide, mitomycin C, cytarabine (ara-C), and D-penicillamine.[21,32,33]

Once it develops, pulmonary hemorrhage can be associated with significant morbidity and mortality. Affected patients can present with acute respiratory distress and hemoptysis may occur, although this is uncommon.

Chest radiographs typically show bilateral heterogeneous and homogenous opacities. Focal consolidation is a less common finding. HRCT usually shows bilateral, scattered, or diffuse areas of ground glass opacity.[34]

Histological examination is rarely attempted in cases of drug-induced pulmonary hemorrhage. In cases of pulmonary hemorrhage associated with drug-related vasculitis, skin biopsy is a more common and preferable method used to assess the presence of leukocytoclastic vasculitis.[35] The presence of hemosiderin-laden macrophages in the alveolar spaces and pulmonary parenchyma can suggest prior episodes of pulmonary hemorrhage, in the appropriate context (*Figure 27-3B*).

Drug-induced diffuse alveolar damage

DAD is a common manifestation of drug-induced lung toxicity. Cytotoxic drugs, such as bleomycin, busulfan, carmustine (BCNU), cyclophosphamide, melphalan, and mitomycin, are most commonly associated with DAD.[21,36]

Affected patients present with dyspnea, cough, and occasionally, fever. The symptoms progress rapidly, resulting in life-threatening respiratory failure.

Chest radiographs show bilateral heterogeneous or homogeneous opacities, often with a mid and lower lung distribution pattern, that commonly progress to diffuse opacification. HRCT in early DAD typically shows scattered or diffuse areas of ground glass opacity.[34] Fibrosis typically develops within 1 week, but may not be evident initially on chest radiographs. With progressive fibrosis, however, marked architectural distortion and honeycomb change can occur.[21]

The mechanism of drug-induced DAD is largely understood to involve drug-related necrosis of type II pneumocytes and alveolar capillary endothelial cells.[21] Histological findings in drug-induced DAD are similar to those of DAD due to other causes. The early phase is mainly associated with acute exudative changes and characterized by alveolar and interstitial edema and hyaline membranes, and is most prominent within a week of the initiation of lung injury[21,32,36] (*Figure 27-4A*). Gradual changes, including repair and proliferation of type II pneumocytes and interstitial organization, are seen in the late phase, which typically occurs after 1 or 2 weeks[21,32,35-38] (*Figure 27-4B*). Distinctive atypia of type II pneumocytes is common in certain types of cytotoxic drug-induced DAD, and is known to be prominent among patients who are administered busulfan,

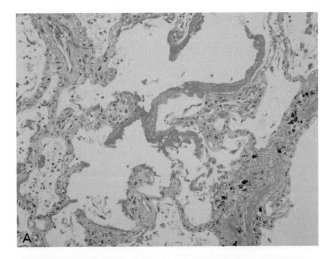

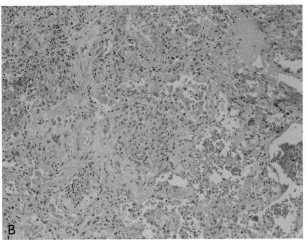

FIGURE 27-4 Drug-induced diffuse alveolar damage. A: In the early exudative phase, prominent hyaline membrane formation and interstitial edema are characteristic findings. B: Late phase methotrexate-induced organizing diffuse alveolar damage. Interstitial fibrosis and lymphocytic infiltration with prominent histiocytic accumulation in the alveolar spaces are seen (used with permission of Drs Tomonori Tanaka and Junya Fukuoka, Nagasaki University, Japan).

bleomycin, and carmustine.[36,39] If the injury is severe, progressive and irreversible fibrosis may occur.[21]

Drug-induced organizing pneumonia

OP, previously referred to as bronchiolitis-obliterans organizing pneumonia (BOOP), is a fairly common manifestation of pulmonary drug toxicity.[40] Bleomycin, cyclophosphamide, and methotrexate are the most common drugs causing this form of lung injury.[21,32,33] In comparison, OP induced by amiodarone, nitrofurantoin, penicillamine, and sulfasalazine is less common, but may still occur.[33]

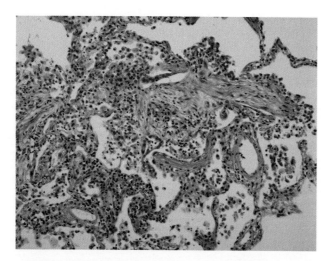

FIGURE 27-5 Amiodarone-induced organizing pneumonia. Alveolar ducts are filled with young fibroblastic polypoid lesions. Lymphoplasmacytic infiltrates in the alveolar septa and abundant intra-alveolar macrophages are present.

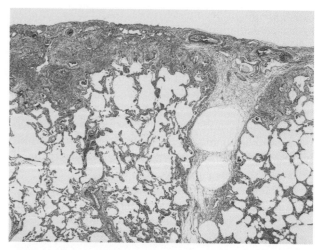

FIGURE 27-6 Drug-induced interstitial fibrosis: mesalazine-induced chronic fibrosing pneumonia showing an NSIP pattern. Subpleural interstitial fibrosis is present (used with permission of Drs Tomonori Tanaka and Junya Fukuoka, Nagasaki University, Japan).

Affected patients present with a subacute onset of progressive dyspnea, dry cough, and fever. Drug-induced OP is typically resolved by drug cessation, but the patient may also require corticosteroid therapy.

Chest radiographs show bilateral scattered heterogeneous and homogeneous ground glass opacities.[34] These areas are typically peripheral in distribution and are equally distributed between the upper and lower lobes.[41] HRCT often shows associated poorly defined nodular areas of consolidation and bronchial dilatation. Nodules distributed in a centrilobular pattern and branching linear opacities show "tree-in-bud" opacities.[41,42] A large nodule, resembling a metastatic disease radiologically, has been reported in association with bleomycin administration.[43-45]

Histologically, OP is characterized by patchy involvement of the lung parenchyma, with immature fibroblastic plugs (Masson bodies) found within the respiratory bronchioles, alveolar ducts, and adjacent alveolar spaces (*Figure 27-5*). Lymphocytic infiltration has also been noted.[21,38,41,42]

Drug-induced interstitial inflammation and fibrosis

All forms of idiopathic interstitial pneumonia have been reported as manifestations of pulmonary drug toxicity, and considerable overlap of two or more histological patterns may be seen.[46] The most commonly encountered form is an NSIP pattern, with cases fulfilling the diagnostic criteria for UIP or desquamative interstitial pneumonia (DIP) being less common.[6,10,46] A number of drugs cause pulmonary toxicity with an NSIP pattern, for example, amiodarone, methotrexate, and carmustine.[14,21,32,35,36,47,48]

Affected patients present with an insidious onset of dyspnea and dry cough, usually within several months of initiating therapy, while pulmonary fibrosis may occur many years following drug exposure. Low-grade fever and malaise are common.[49] When considering drug-related interstitial pneumonia, it is important to consider and exclude lung involvement in the primary disease, especially in patients with autoimmune disorders in which various interstitial pneumonias may develop.[6]

Chest radiographs usually show diffuse heterogeneous opacities.[21,48,49] In the early phase, HRCT scans may only show scattered or diffuse areas of ground glass opacity.[41,48] In the advanced fibrosing phase, traction bronchiectasis and honeycombing are found, predominantly at the base of the lung.[34]

Histologically, NSIP is characterized by relatively uniform parenchymal involvement with mild diffuse fibrosis and mild-to-moderate lymphocytic infiltrates (*Figure 27-6*). Interstitial inflammation is typically more homogeneous and more cellular than that associated with UIP. Reactive hyperplastic type II pneumocytes may be predominant.[32]

Drug-induced eosinophilia

Drug-induced eosinophilic pneumonia is one of the most important conditions to be considered in differential diagnosis in patients whose bronchoalveolar lavage (BAL) or lung tissue samples show eosinophilia. Other potential causes are acute and chronic idiopathic eosinophilic pneumonia, parasitic and fungal infections, and allergic bronchopulmonary aspergillosis (ABPA). A number of drugs can cause this condition, particularly acetylsalicylic acid, amiodarone, bleomycin, carbamazepine, captopril, phenytoin, hydrochlorothiazide, mesalamine, minocycline, nitrofurantoin, penicillamine, sulfasalazine, and sulfonamides.[4]

Based on the clinical pattern of the disease, eosinophilic pneumonia (drug-induced and idiopathic) is classified into the following four types: (1) simple pulmonary eosinophilia, (2) eosinophilic pneumonia, (3) chronic fibrosing pneumonitis with eosinophilia, and (4) CSS.[50] Patients may present with febrile illness, respiratory failure, and dry cough, with BAL showing greater than 25% eosinophils, or eosinophilic pneumonia at lung biopsy.[51,52] Notably, most of the patients do not show peripheral blood eosinophilia. In contrast, chronic toxicity is usually accompanied by peripheral blood eosinophilia and is associated with an indolent clinical course.[5]. Drug-induced CSS can be triggered by asthma medications such as leukotriene inhibitors (eg, zafirlukast, montelukast, and pranlukast).[50,53,54] The clinical presentation of drug-induced CSS cannot be distinguished from that of idiopathic CSS. Patients initially present with symptoms of asthma and allergic rhinitis, followed by peripheral blood eosinophilia and systemic vasculitis. Although drug-induced eosinophilic pneumonia usually responds well to drug cessation, administration of corticosteroids may be required, especially for CSS, which usually requires treatment with long-term corticosteroids and cytotoxic medications.[50]

Chest radiographs show foci of air-space consolidation and focal ground glass opacities.[55] Cavitation is rare in drugs causing eosinophilic pneumonia, except in cases with CSS, but it is common in ABPA and parasitic and fungal infections.

The histology of drug-induced eosinophilic pneumonia is characterized by the accumulation of eosinophils and macrophages in the alveoli. Alveolar septa are thickened and infiltrated by eosinophils, lymphocytes, and plasma cells.[36] In acute cases, hyaline membranes are often present. Cases of chronic fibrosing pneumonitis show a fibrosing NSIP or UIP pattern with interstitial eosinophils, and progress to irreversible pulmonary fibrosis and honeycombing.[56] Although pulmonary vasculitis or capillaritis with eosinophilia in lung biopsy specimens are indicative of drug-induced CSS, in practice, biopsy from other organs, such as the skin, may be preferred. Drug-induced eosinophilic pneumonia demonstrates a variable degree of overlapping of the histologic patterns described above and may therefore be difficult to categorize histologically[6,57] (*Figure 27-7*). In addition, making a histological diagnosis of eosinophilic pneumonia in patients after corticosteroid administration is challenging, because eosinophils disappear rapidly from pulmonary tissue after therapy. Eosinophilic pneumonia with therapeutic modulation should be considered in patients in whom eosinophilic pneumonia is highly suspected, even if tissue eosinophilia is not prominent.[58-60]

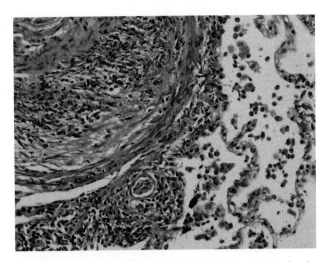

FIGURE 27-7 Drug-induced eosinophilic pneumonia: In acute eosinophilic pneumonia, the alveolar spaces are filled with eosinophils. In this particular case, intra- and perivascular eosinophilic infiltrate is notable.

Drug-induced lymphocytic infiltrates

Drug-induced lymphocytic infiltrates may exhibit a pattern of cellular or fibrosing NSIP or of lymphoid hyperplasia (LH).[10,57,61,62]

An NSIP pattern is the most common manifestation of drug-induced lung toxicity.[6] A number of drugs produce this effect, such as amiodarone, various cytotoxic agents, and gefitinib. This pattern is histologically characterized by relatively uniform parenchymal involvement, with diffuse fibrosis and/or lymphocytic aggregation[63,64] (*Figures 27-8A and B*).

Drug-induced LH, including diffuse LH, follicular bronchiolitis, lymphoid interstitial pneumonia, and lymphocytic perivascular cuffing, has been reported as one of the manifestations of amiodarone-related lung toxicity.[62] Given the particular histological pattern, the differential diagnosis includes autoimmune/connective tissue diseases, immunodeficiency syndromes, and low-grade lymphoproliferative disorders, particularly bronchus-associated lymphoid tissue lymphoma.[65] In cases showing features of diffuse micronodular LH, LIP, or perivascular lymphoid cuffing, Epstein-Barr virus or mycoplasma infections, cellular NSIP, and HP can be added to the differential diagnosis.[65,66] Distinguishing drug-induced LIP from lymphoproliferative disorders may require evaluation of the clonality of infiltrating lymphocytes by flow cytometry, immunohistochemistry, or in situ hybridization.

Drug-induced granulomatous inflammation

Sarcoidosis-like changes have been reported as systemic adverse effects of interferon-α and interferon-β administration.[6,10,46,67-69] Although the skin and lungs are

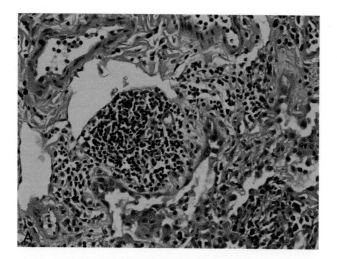

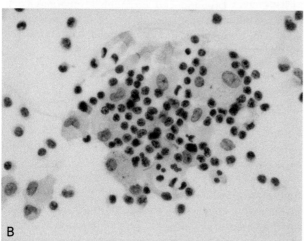

FIGURE 27-8 Drug-induced lymphocytic interstitial pneumonia. A: Methotrexate-induced interstitial pneumonia with lymphoid aggregates in the alveolar septa. B: In the same case, the BAL specimen contained alveolar macrophages and a large number of small lymphocytes.

most commonly affected, many other organs can also be involved, including the nervous system, eye, kidney, heart, liver, salivary glands, and joints.[68] Usually, dyspnea, cough, and production of sputum develop several months after drug administration.

Chest radiographs and HRCT often show lymphadenopathy, and parenchymal abnormalities (eg, diffuse nodularity and reticulonodular infiltrates) may also be seen.[69]

The presence of granulomas (*Figure 27-9*) should always raise the possibility of infectious etiologies. Special stains for fungi and acid-fast microorganisms, and culture, are crucial to exclude these infectious agents.

In contrast to sarcoidosis-like granulomatous reaction, drug-induced granulomatous inflammation usually exhibits an HP-like pattern and may show a pattern of extrinsic allergic alveolitis (EAA).[70] Etanercept, leflunomide, mesalamine, sirolimus, and methotrexate are representative causative drugs[6,10,46]

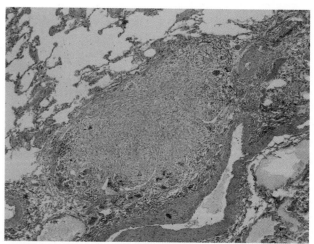

FIGURE 27-9 Drug-induced sarcoidosis-like pulmonary change: Nonnecrotizing sarcoidal granuloma is present, adjacent to the bronchovascular bundle.

HP is an inflammatory interstitial lung disease related to exposure and sensitization to a particular antigen.[71] The pathogenesis of HP involves both type III and type IV hypersensitivity reactions. Drug-induced HP typically shows a subacute onset of dyspnea, dry cough, fever, skin rash, and headache.[6] Peripheral blood eosinophilia is present in approximately 40% of patients. Chest radiographs often show diffuse acinar infiltrates, and pleural effusions may also be present (*Figure 27-10A*). Histologically, poorly formed nonnecrotizing granulomas in the alveolar spaces, instead of along lymphatic routes, are typical features of HP (*Figure 27-10B*). However, the changes detected in biopsies vary widely, from active inflammation to chronic fibrosis, depending on the stage and causative antigens.[72,73] Necrotizing granulomas are rare. They can result from administration of sirolimus, although an infectious etiology should always be considered.[74-76]

Drug-induced pulmonary alveolar proteinosis

Pulmonary alveolar proteinosis (PAP) is a rare condition characterized by the accumulation of lipoproteinaceous surfactant material in the alveolar spaces[77] (*Figure 27-11*). Ninety percent of PAP cases are primary and 10% occur due to a variety of causes, including dust inhalation, malignancy (especially hematolymphoid malignancies), and, less commonly, drug exposure.[4,77] Drug-induced PAP has been described with amiodarone, cyclophosphamide, busulfan, bleomycin, mitomycin C, etoposide, chlorambucil, leflunomide, and sirolimus, and more recently, fentanyl and other inhaled drugs have been linked with PAP.[4,10,78] Although most cases of drug-induced PAP

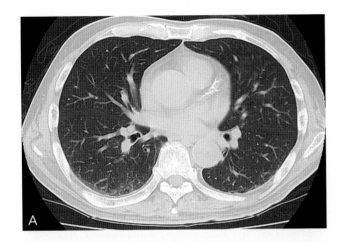

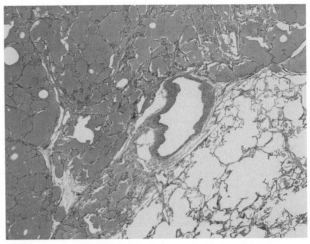

FIGURE 27-11 Drug-induced alveolar proteinosis: Eosinophilic proteinaceous material fills the alveolar spaces. This patient had a long history of traditional Chinese medicine use.

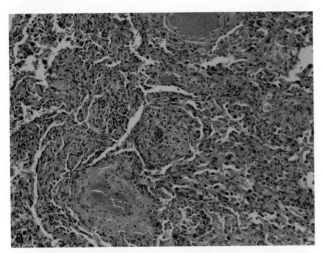

FIGURE 27-10 Drug-induced hypersensitivity pneumonia-like pulmonary change. A: Computed tomography of methotrexate-induced lung injury. Diffuse increases in the alveolar density and focal reticular opacity are noted. B: Diffuse interstitial lymphocytic infiltrate with small non-necrotizing granuloma.

are diagnosed from incidental microscopic findings, in some cases a long-standing progressive exertional dyspnea and minimally productive cough, fatigue, weight loss, chest pain, and low-grade fever are seen.[79] The mean age of presentation is around 40 years, two-thirds of the patients are male, and three-quarters are smokers.[77]

Radiologically, PAP usually shows a "crazy paving" pattern (ie, diffuse ground glass opacities with super-imposed interlobular septal thickening) on HRCT.[80]

Drug-induced lupus syndrome

Approximately 10% of cases of lupus erythematosus are believed to be induced by drugs. Diagnosis of drug-induced lupus syndrome requires: (1) a positive antinuclear antibody (ANA) test; (2) exposure to an offending drug; and (3) one clinical feature of lupus in a patient without a known history of lupus.[81] More than

100 different drugs have been reported to cause lupus syndrome, with the most common being hydralazine, procainamide, quinidine, isoniazid, diltiazem, and minocycline.[82] More recently, antitumor necrosis factor (TNF)-α antibodies and type I interferon have been added to this list.

The symptoms are similar to those of systemic lupus erythematosus (SLE); however, pleuropulmonary involvement is seen more frequently (50% of the cases)[83] and the central nervous system, kidney, and skin are less affected than in SLE. Because drug-specific T cells or antibodies are absent, drug-induced lupus syndrome does not seem to be a typical drug hypersensitivity reaction. Typically, a long exposure history and administration of a high-dose increases risk for drug-induced lupus syndrome.[84] This disease develops several months after initiation of the medication and tends to resolve rapidly after drug withdrawal. However, it can also cause life-threatening pulmonary renal syndrome and fatal alveolar hemorrhage. Immunologically, patients present with a positive ANA test and antihistone antibodies, but rarely test positive for either anti-dsDNA or anti-Sm/U1-RNP antibodies. In addition, antineutrophil cytoplasmic antibody (ANCA)/myeloperoxidase (MPO) reactivity, cardiolipin, and dsDNA targeting are seen in cases of drug-induced lupus with life-threatening pulmonary-renal syndrome, and hydralazine, propylthiouracil, penicillamine, anti-TNF blockers, and type I interferons are reportedly linked to this condition.[85]

Although histologic evaluation of drug-induced lupus syndrome is seldom attempted, transbronchial biopsy and cytologic examination may be performed to exclude other causes of lung disease, such as infections and malignancies. Acute lung injury and pulmonary hemorrhage are commonly seen in cases of lupus syndrome (*Figure 27-12*).

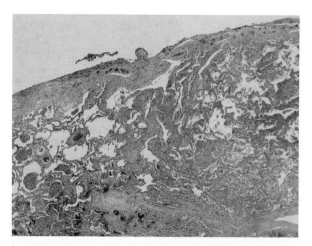

FIGURE 27-12 Drug-induced lupus syndrome: In the acute phase, active alveolitis and capillaritis, resulting in alveolar hemorrhage, are characteristic findings.

Drug-induced pulmonary veno-occlusive disease

Pulmonary veno-occlusive disease (PVOD) is characterized by the obstruction of small pulmonary veins, as well as evidence of pulmonary arterial hypertension and occlusive changes in pulmonary arteries. Drug-induced PVOD is known to occur in association with the use of oral contraceptives and various chemotherapeutic agents, such as bleomycin, busulfan, carmustine, lomustine, and nitrosoureas.[86-92]

Drug-induced PVOD occurs within 1 year of initiation of the causative drug. This is a fatal condition, and its clinical course from the onset, to death by respiratory failure, is generally short.

It is important to recognize occlusive lesions in small pulmonary venules histologically in biopsy specimens (*Figure 27-13*). However, small veno-occlusive lesions

may mimic mild pulmonary interstitial fibrosis and are thus easily missed. Elastic stain is helpful for the detection PVOD in this setting.[89]

Drug-induced pulmonary hypertension

Pulmonary hypertension is a rare and potentially life-threatening disease. Its incidence increased 10-fold in the 1960s, and it has become apparent that a range of drugs can cause pulmonary hypertension.[93-95] These include anorectic drugs, such as aminorex and phentermine/fenfluramine (phen-fen), and illicit drugs, such as cocaine and methamphetamine.[96]

Histologically, drug-induced pulmonary hypertension is generally indistinguishable from idiopathic disease[94,95] (*Figures 27-14A* and *B*).

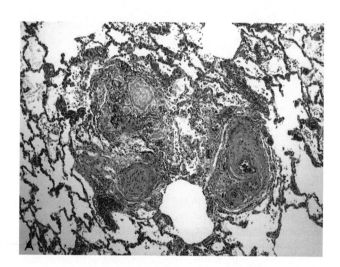

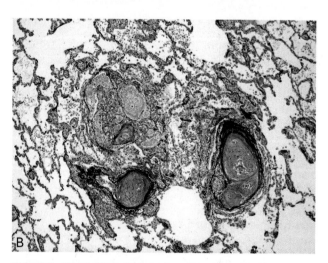

FIGURE 27-14 Drug-induced pulmonary hypertension. A: Marked myointimal thickening of small pulmonary arteries, resulting in luminal obstruction, is evident. B: Elastic stain highlighting the lesions (used with permission of Dr Toshiaki Morito, Kagawa Rosai Hospital, Japan).

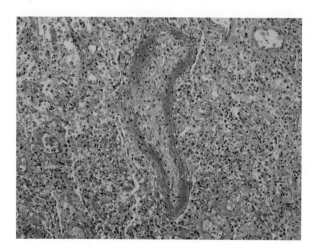

FIGURE 27-13 Drug-induced pulmonary veno-occlusive disease: Small pulmonary vein is completely occluded by intimal fibrosis.

Drug-induced pleural changes

Drug-induced pleural disease is less common than drug-induced lung disease.[97] Pleural disease may be caused by cardiovascular agents (practolol, amiodarone, and minoxidil), ergoline drugs (methysergide and bromocriptine), sclerotherapy agents (sodium morrhuate and absolute alcohol), and chemotherapeutic agents (bleomycin, mitomycin, procarbazine, methotrexate, and cyclophosphamide).[83] Although most drugs that affect the pleura simultaneously involve the lung parenchyma, some cytotoxic agents, such as methotrexate and bleomycin, may have pleura-specific effects.

The manifestations of drug-induced pleural disease are as follows: (1) asymptomatic pleural effusion, (2) acute pleuritis, and (3) symptomatic pleural thickening. Although these might hold clues to this disease, these features are generally nonspecific. Pleural fluid eosinophilia is also seen in drug-induced pleural disease, and known causative agents include valproic acid, propylthiouracil, isotretinoin, nitrofurantoin, bromocriptine, dantrolene, gliclazide, and mesalamine.[98] The mechanism of this disease is still under debate; however, hypersensitivity reactions and direct or indirect toxic effects of the causative drugs may contribute to the pathogenesis.[99]

Histologic features of the affected pleura are nonspecific (*Figure 27-15*). Pathological examination is usually not performed for this diagnosis and therapeutic decision making.

Specific Drugs

Cyclophosphamide

Cyclophosphamide is an alkylating agent widely used as a chemotherapeutic drug for the treatment of various malignancies, and as an immune suppressor for

the treatment of autoimmune disorders, inflammatory disorders, and posttransplant maintenance.[39] Cyclophosphamide is metabolically activated in the liver by the cytochrome P450 2B6 (CYP2B6) enzyme to form phosphoramide mustard and then induces cellular death by forming irreversible DNA adducts, in particular, interstrand DNA crosslinks at guanine N-7 positions.[100] Cyclophosphamide-induced lung toxicity reportedly affected less than 1% of patients; however, the true incidence may be difficult to estimate given the presence of multiple confounding variables, such as concomitant use of other cytotoxic drugs, opportunistic infections, coexistent pulmonary diseases, radiation pneumonitis, and oxygen toxicity.[101]

There are two types of cyclophosphamide-induced lung toxicity: early onset and late onset.[48,102] The early-onset type occurs weeks to months after initiation of cyclophosphamide. It is essentially reversible by cessation of cyclophosphamide, and/or corticosteroid treatment. The major pathologic feature of this type is reported to be interstitial infiltration of inflammatory cells. In contrast, the late-onset type occurs years after initiation of cyclophosphamide. It may develop over 10 years after initiation and even months to years after discontinuation. Despite corticosteroid therapy, the late-onset type usually has an unfavorable prognosis, with a mortality rate of over 60%. Histologically, the late-onset type is reported to show interstitial collagen deposition, proliferation of type II pneumocytes (*Figure 27-16*), and interstitial inflammatory infiltrate, resulting in various patterns of interstitial changes similar to DAD, NSIP, OP, and progressive interstitial fibrosis.[35,102,103] Pleural thickening is one of the characteristic features of the late-onset type.[104] However, these histologic findings are similar to those seen in lung toxicity caused by busulfan and other cytotoxic agents.

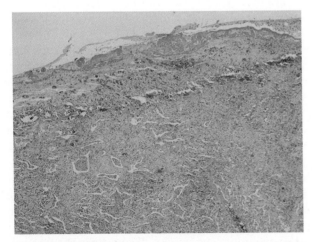

FIGURE 27-15 Drug-induced pleural change: methotrexate-induced diffuse alveolar damage with severe fibrinous pleuritis (used with permission of Drs Tomonori Tanaka and Junya Fukuoka, Nagasaki University, Japan).

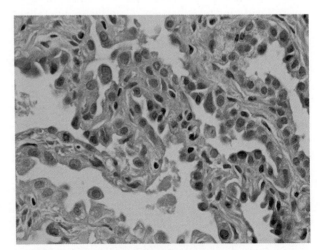

FIGURE 27-16 Cyclophosphamide-induced pulmonary toxicity: marked type II pneumocyte proliferation and atypia (used with permission of Drs Tomonori Tanaka and Junya Fukuoka, Nagasaki University, Japan).

Phen-fen

Coadministration of phentermine and fenfluramine (phen-fen) increases extracellular levels of dopamine and serotonin in experimental models, respectively, and provide effective treatment for obesity and substance abuse disorders.[105,106] Fenfluramine and its active *d*-isomer (*d*-fenfluramine) are reportedly linked to primary pulmonary hypertension and valvular heart disease.[107] No association of phentermine with pulmonary hypertension has been reported to date. The mechanism of fenfluramine-related pulmonary hypertension is unknown, but elevated serum serotonin level might cause a chronic increase in pulmonary arterial pressure and induce growth of arterial smooth muscle cells, resulting in pulmonary hypertension.[108] Another hypothesis is that fenfluramine may block K^+ channels in pulmonary artery smooth muscle cells and increase perfusion pressure in the lung.[109] Cardiopulmonary side effects occur in approximately 10% of patients treated with diet pills containing fenfluramine, and it is often fatal.[110] The risk increases with an exposure duration of longer than 3 months, and peaks after 1-year exposure.[107]

Histological findings in phen-fen-induced lung toxicity are identical to those of pulmonary hypertension resulting from other causes.[94,95] The findings range from intimal and medial thickening, to plexiform lesions.

Bleomycin

Bleomycin is an antitumor antibiotic produced by *Streptomyces verticillus* and is used in the chemotherapeutic regimen for various malignant neoplasms. Lung toxicity is the most serious complication of this therapy. The mean incidence of bleomycin-induced lung toxicity is 6% to 10% but some reports have indicated that up to 46% of patients were affected.[111] The risk of bleomycin-induced lung toxicity is correlated with age (above 40 years), smoking, renal-function impairment, and a cumulative dose >400 mg, and it has also been suggested that bleomycin increases sensitivity to oxygen toxicity.[11,112]

Bleomycin-induced lung toxicity may show acute fulminate, subacute, or indolent features.[5,46] Common presenting clinical features are cough, dyspnea, and occasional fever. In addition to drug withdrawal, the treatment usually requires corticosteroid administration. A clinical response usually occurs within weeks, rather than days, and is most often seen in those with a significant inflammatory component. Bleomycin-induced pneumonitis is thought to resolve in the majority of patients over time.[113]

Radiological features are variable, with the typical pattern including bilateral basal subpleural opacification with loss of volume. Later, progressive consolidation and honeycombing is seen. HRCT typically shows ground glass opacification in the mid and lower zones.

Distinctive nodular densities may be observed, that mimic metastatic tumors.[45]

Although DAD is the most common histological manifestation of bleomycin-induced lung toxicity,[21] various histological patterns have been reported, including NSIP, OP, PVOD, eosinophilic pneumonia, and pleuritis.[21,39,40,83] In long-term cases, pulmonary fibrosis can eventually be observed.

Amiodarone

Amiodarone is an antiarrhythmic agent that is used to treat supraventricular and ventricular tachycardia. The incidence of pulmonary toxicity is estimated as 5% to 10% and it typically occurs several months after starting the medication.[114-116] The risk is directly related to the dose and duration of administration.[117,118] Advanced age, underlying pulmonary disease, oxygen therapy, and surgery are also proposed to increase the risk for amiodarone-induced pulmonary toxicity.[114,119]

The clinical manifestation of amiodarone-induced lung toxicity usually includes subacute onset of dyspnea, dry cough, and diffuse pulmonary infiltration.[114-116] As febrile episodes are common, it can sometimes be difficult to distinguish from infectious disease.[49,116] It can be reversed following cessation of medication (and corticosteroid treatment) in most cases.

Amiodarone-induced lung toxicity shows variable manifestations on chest radiographs and HRCT, including diffuse or localized, well-defined or ill-defined interstitial, alveolar, or mixed ground glass opacities that might not be bilateral[34,49] (*Figure 27-17A*). As a rare manifestation, discrete mass forming lesions have also been reported.[120] In cases with long-term administration, increased CT signal attenuation in the liver or spleen, reflecting deposition of amiodarone metabolites, was also observed.

Variable histological findings have also been reported in amiodarone-induced lung toxicity. In addition to the classical features of OP,[49,121] acute or organizing DAD,[121,122] chronic interstitial pneumonitis with fibrosis, pulmonary hemorrhage,[123] lymphoid hyperplasia, eosinophilic pneumonia,[62] or nodular collections of foamy macrophages with central necrosis[120] have been reported. Although not highly specific, accumulation of intra-alveolar foamy macrophages is the most characteristic of these findings, and the observation of vacuolated pneumocytes also helps identify this condition[49] (*Figures 27-17B* and *C*). Ultrastructurally, intra-alveolar macrophages and pulmonary parenchyma contain whorled, lamellar, membrane-bound, electron dense inclusions.[35,116,121,122,124] Numerous intra-alveolar foamy macrophages are also diagnostic in the BAL cellular profile. BAL fluid from patients with this disease usually shows an increased total cell count, with abundant foamy macrophages in a background of mixed

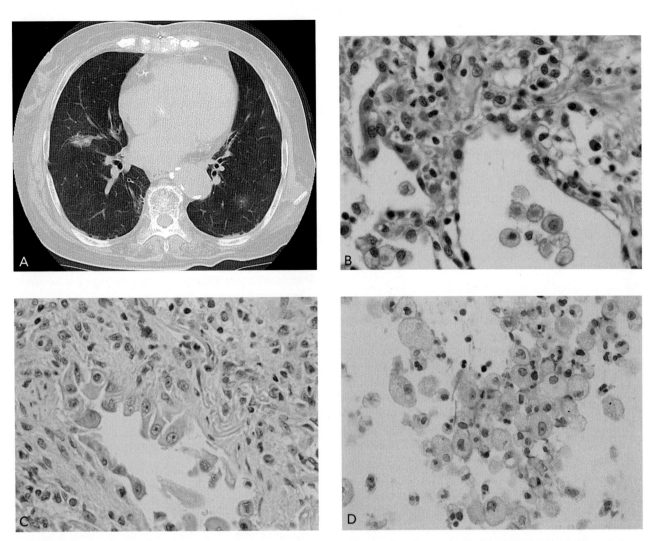

FIGURE 27-17 Amiodarone-induced pulmonary toxicity. **A:** Computed tomography of amiodarone-induced lung injury, indicating patchy ground glass opacity. **B:** Interstitial fibrosis with lymphocytic and eosinophilic infiltration is observed. Intra-alveolar macrophages show characteristic cytoplasmic vacuolation. **C:** Type II pneumocytes show nuclear enlargement, prominent nucleoli, and cytoplasmic vacuolar change. **D:** A BAL specimen containing a large number of macrophages with vacuolated cytoplasm (used with permission of Drs Tomonori Tanaka and Junya Fukuoka, Nagasaki University, Japan).

inflammatory cells (*Figure 27-17D*). Amiodarone-induced pleural effusions may also contain foamy macrophages.[125]

Carmustine (BCNU)

Carmustine or bis-chloroethyl nitrosourea (BCNU) is a nitrosourea compound categorized as an alkylating agent. It is used as a chemotherapeutic drug for the treatment of several types of malignant brain tumor and breast cancer. It is also used as part of the chemotherapeutic preconditioning protocol for bone marrow transplantation.[39] Carmustine is able to form interstrand crosslinks in DNA and exerts its tumoricidal effects via chloromethylation of DNA at the O^6 position of guanine, resulting in prevention of DNA replication and

transcription.[126] Because carmustine is almost always used with other chemotherapeutic drugs and radiation therapy, the frequency of carmustine-related lung toxicity is hard to estimate. However, up to 58% of patients treated with high-dose chemotherapy regimens including carmustine show some degree of pulmonary toxicity,[127] and its frequency of pulmonary complication is the highest among nitrosoureas.[39,128-131]

The high frequency of carmustine-induced lung toxicity may be due to delayed pulmonary repair. Several situations are recognized as risk factors for carmustine-related lung toxicity: high-dose administration, preexisting lung disease, lung function abnormality, thoracic irradiation (usually given for carcinomas of the lung, esophagus, thyroid, and breast), and concomitant use of cyclophosphamide.[132]

Carmustine-induced lung toxicity shows two distinct forms of clinical presentation: acute and chronic. The acute form occurs weeks after administration, and DAD is the most common manifestation.[133] The chronic form is less common, and usually occurs months to years following therapy. Irreversible pulmonary interstitial fibrosis may occur within 40 days after a single course of carmustine.[134] On the other hand, survivors of brain tumors can develop carmustine-induced lung fibrosis with characteristic subpleural pulmonary fibrosis involving the upper lobes over 10 years after treatment.[13-15] Histologically, the chronic form generally shows an NSIP pattern.[14] Fibrosing pleuritis and PVOD have also been reported following carmustine administration.[21]

Nitrofurantoin

Nitrofurantoin is an antibiotic agent used in the treatment of urinary tract infections. Although nitrofurantoin-induced lung toxicity occurs infrequently, given the widespread use of this drug, it is one of the most common causes of drug-induced lung toxicity.[97,135]

Acute and chronic nitrofurantoin-induced lung toxicities have been described. The acute manifestation is more common, occurs within 2 weeks of administration of nitrofurantoin,[136] and is thought to result from a hypersensitivity reaction to the drug. Clinical findings include fever, dyspnea, cough, and peripheral eosinophilia,[21] with radiologic findings of diffuse bilateral, predominantly basal heterogeneous opacities.[137] The prognosis is favorable and most patients recover after cessation. In one study, the acute manifestation improved within 15 days, with approximately 50% of the patients becoming asymptomatic within 24 hours, and 88% within 72 hours.[138] Although pathological examination is rarely attempted, acute nitrofurantoin-induced lung toxicity has been reported to show histological features of the early stages of DAD, diffuse alveolar hemorrhage, OP, hypersensitivity pneumonitis, and cellular NSIP.[40,139]

Chronic lung toxicity is less common and usually occurs months or years after nitrofurantoin administration. It presents as insidious onset dyspnea on exertion and cough. Treatment involved drug cessation and the patient may require corticosteroid therapy. Chronic toxicity is associated with a poorer prognosis that acute toxicity. Recovery from chronic toxicity may take from months to a year, and mortality may reach 10%.[46,140-142] Chronic fibrosing interstitial pneumonia with features of UIP and NSIP is a common histopathologic manifestation of chronic toxicity, and OP, DIP, granulomatous/giant cell interstitial pneumonia, and pleuritis have also been reported.[21,35,83,143]

Mitomycin C

Mitomycin C is a chemotherapeutic agent derived from *Streptomyces caespitosus*. It has antitumor and antibiotic activity, and is widely used in the treatment of various carcinomas. An estimated 5% to 10% of patients receiving systemic mitomycin C develop drug-induced lung toxicity.[144] This adverse effect is generally recognized to occur in a dose-dependent manner.[145] However, even intravesical instillations for bladder cancer carry some degree of risk for fetal pulmonary adverse effects, despite the low rate of systemic mitomycin C absorption.[146]

Clinically, two forms of mitomycin C-induced lung toxicity are known: the acute type, which usually occurs as pulmonary manifestations of hemolytic uremic syndrome (HUS),[147,148] and the subacute type. HUS develops shortly after the administration of mitomycin C. Noncardiogenic acute pulmonary edema due to increased permeability occurs in addition to microangiopathic hemolytic anemia, thrombocytopenia, fever, and renal failure.[149] Subacute onset mitomycin C-induced lung toxicity typically occurs 3 to 12 months after administration[128] with progressive dyspnea, dry cough, fever, and hypoxemia.[150] The pathological features are characterized by DAD, OP, pulmonary fibrosis, and pleuritis.[21,35,83,150-152]

RADIATION-INDUCED LUNG INJURY

Radiation-induced lung injury (RILI) is an adverse effect of thoracic irradiation, which is usually employed for treatment of carcinomas of the lung, esophagus, thyroid, and breast, as well as for hematologic malignancies.[153-155] The beneficial effects of radiotherapy for thoracic malignancies may be offset by RILI.[156] Approximately 5% to 10% of patients develop RILI as a consequence of therapeutic radiation, and this incidence is 13% to 37% in patients with lung cancer.[157]

Although the precise mechanisms of RILI are still unknown, it has been proposed that radiation pneumonitis and the ensuing pulmonary fibrosis may be associated with a cytokine cascade that is triggered by irradiation, resulting in direct and indirect cellular injury.[128,158] Type I pneumocytes are the first target to incur damage and undergo apoptosis. The capillary endothelium is also directly affected.[159-161] Radiation-induced oxidative stress and free radical generation may indirectly damage DNA in all lung cells.[128,153,159-161]

Clinical Features of Radiation-Induced Lung Injury

RILI is usually divided into two stages, namely, acute radiation pneumonitis and chronic fibrosis. Although chronic fibrosis may develop in the absence of clinically apparent acute disease, the processes of acute pneumonitis and chronic fibrosis are generally assumed to be tightly connected via the cytokine cascade.[159]

The dose schedule and intensity of radiotherapy influences the risk of RILI. The most consistent predictor

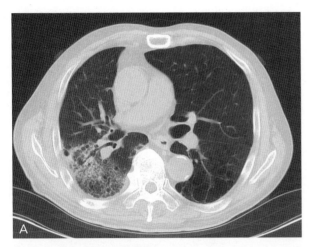
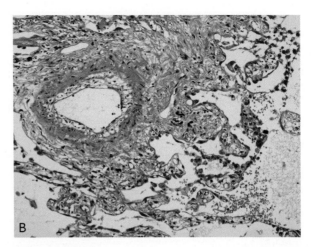

FIGURE 27-18 Acute radiation-induced pneumonitis. **A:** Computed tomography axial view of the lungs, 2 months after radiation therapy for stage IIIb squamous cell carcinoma. Reticular pattern and consolidation are confined to the radiation field. **B:** Histologically, prominent type II pneumocyte hyperplasia with interstitial edema is observed. Vascular degeneration is commonly seen in cases of acute radiation pneumonia.

of pneumonitis is the cumulative dose of radiotherapy that has been administered to normal lung tissue.[162,163] Increased risk has also been associated with preexisting underlying lung disease and patient age.[164-168] The patient's history of prior irradiation, the type of radiotherapy employed, and the presence of concomitant chemotherapeutic agents also influence risk.[153-155] Although no reliable prophylaxis for RILI has been proposed, immunomodulators, interferons, and corticosteroids may be administered as premedications.[128,160]

Clinically, acute radiation pneumonitis typically presents 2 or 3 months after radiotherapy with nonspecific symptoms (eg, shortness of the breath and cough, with or without mild fever).[10,160,161] It may be erroneously attributed to another cardiovascular or respiratory disorders, including pulmonary infection, tumor metastasis, or tumor recurrence. Radiographic findings are varied and include ground glass changes, localized consolidation, and ill-defined nodules, typically limited to the irradiated field[10,153,160] (*Figure 27-18A*) corresponding to the histologic findings of acute pneumonitis (*Figure 27-18B*). Radiographic changes may precede the onset of acute radiation pneumonitis or be present in asymptomatic patients.[46]

Chronic fibrosis is permanent scarring of lung tissue that occurs more gradually typically beginning after 6 months and generally stabilizing after 2 years, resulting in a permanent impairment of oxygen transfer.[10] Although radiologic findings may spread beyond the irradiated field and may even also involve the contralateral lung[128,153 155,160] (*Figure 27-19A*), corresponding to a widespread area of histologic chronic fibrosis

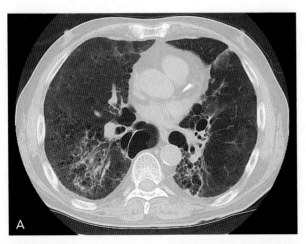
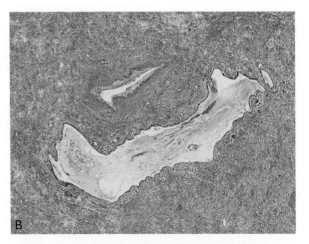

FIGURE 27-19 Chronic radiation fibrosis of lungs. **A:** Computed tomography axial view of the lungs, 6 months after radiation therapy for stage IIIb squamous cell carcinoma. Dense fibrosis is observed in the irradiated paramediastinal regions. In addition, consolidation and honeycombing with cystic spaces are bilaterally and diffusely observed. **B:** Alveolar spaces are completely replaced by dense fibrosis with lymphocytic infiltration. Degeneration of the pulmonary artery with intimal thickening is noted.

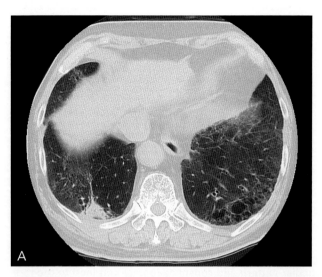

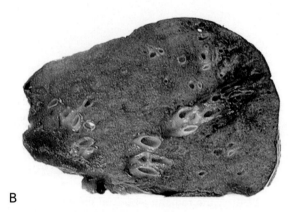

FIGURE 27-20 Chronic radiation fibrosis of lungs due to heavy particle radiation therapy. **A:** Computed tomography axial view of the lungs, 4 years after the initial therapy for stage Ib squamous cell carcinoma. Localized dense fibrosis is seen. **B:** Macroscopically, localized scar-like fibrosis with anthracosis is observed.

(*Figure 27-19B*), it is usually confined to the irradiated field on radiographs (*Figures 27-20A* and *B*).

Although most cases of acute radiation pneumonia do not require further treatment, the mortality rate associated with severe radiation pneumonitis may approach 50%.[156] Consequently, it has been reported that 2.3% of all patients who received thoracic radiotherapy or chemoradiation therapy for advanced cancer died of RILI.[169] The initial treatment for RILI is corticosteroid administration, but this does not reverse the fibrotic phase.[170]

Histologic Features of Radiation-Induced Lung Injury

Acute pneumonitis

The pathological changes caused by lung irradiation can be divided into several phases.[171] During the first latency, which occurs immediately and up to 3 months after irradiation, there is an acute inflammatory infiltrate with associated type I pneumocyte depletion in the alveolar surfaces. Hyaline membranes may be prominent and the histology mimics the DAD exudative phase.[10,160,161,172] This exudative phase is followed by an organizing phase, with marked type II pneumocyte proliferation. Cellular atypia of type II pneumocytes, atypical stromal cells (ie, radiation fibroblasts), and degeneration of the blood vessels are common and often prominent findings[46] (*Figure 27-18B*).

Chronic fibrosis

As a consequence of DAD, the fibrotic process gradually progresses. Approximately 6 months after irradiation,

active collagen production by the fibroblasts is seen, resulting in fibrosis, scarring, and destruction of the normal architecture, processes that can progress for months to years.[10] Fibrosis is most prominent in the lung parenchyma, especially in the perivascular regions.[161,172] Blood vessels and airways are surrounded by scar-like dense fibrosis. Vascular changes, including myointimal proliferation, intramural hyalinization, and elastosis, are more evident (compared to acute radiation pneumonitis) and arteries tend to be more severely affected than veins[161] (*Figure 27-19B*). Various epithelial metaplastic changes are often present. Pleural adhesions and fibrous thickening are common findings in chronic radiation fibrosis.[46] Subpleural honeycomb fibrosis is sometimes observed, although this is rare.

REFERENCES

1. Rosenow EC. The spectrum of drug-induced pulmonary disease. *Ann Intern Med.* 1972;77:977-991.
2. Fraser RS, Müller NL, Colman N, Pare PD. Pulmonary disease caused by toxins, drugs, and irradiation. In: Fraser RS, Müller NL, Colman N, Pare PD, eds. *Diagnosis of Diseases of the Chest.* 4th ed. Philadelphia, PA: WB Saunders; 1999:2517-2592.
3. Rosenow EC. Drug-induced pulmonary disease. *Dis Mon.* 1994;40:253-310.
4. Pneumotox Web site. http://www.pneumotox.com. Accessed January 2014.
5. Beasley MB, Rudner GA. Drug-and therapy-induced lung injury. In: Hasleton P, Flieder DB, eds. *Spencer's Pathology of the Lung.* 6th ed. Cambridge: Cambridge University Press; 2013:585-604.
6. Camus P, Bonniaud P, Fanton A, Camus C, Baudaun N, Foucher P. Drug-induced and iatrogenic infiltrative lung disease. *Clin Chest Med.* 2004;25:479-519.
7. Delaunois LM. Mechanisms in pulmonary toxicology. *Clin Chest Med.* 2004;25:1-14.

8. Vahid B, Marik PE. Pulmonary complications of novel antineo-plastic agents for solid tumors. *Chest*. 2008;133:528-538.
9. Irey NS. Teaching monograph. Tissue reactions to drugs. *Am J Surg Pathol*. 1976;82:613-647.
10. Travis WD, Colby TV, Koss MN, Rosado-de-Christenson ML, Müller NL, King TE. Drug and radiation reactions. In: Travis, WD. *Atlas of Non-tumor Pathology: Non-neoplastic Disorders of the Lower Respiratory Tract*. Washington, DC: AFIP Press; 2002:321-350.
11. Ozkan M, Dweik RA, Ahmad M. Drug-induced lung disease. *Cleve Clin J Med*. 2001;68:782-785.
12. Camus P, Rosenow EC 3rd. Iatrogenic lung disease. *Clin Chest Med*. 2004;25:XIII-XIX.
13. Durant JR, Norgard MJ, Murad TM, Bartolucci AA, Langford KH. Pulmonary toxicity associated with bischloroethyl nitrosourea (BCNU). *Ann Intern Med*. 1979;90:191-194.
14. Holoye PY, Jenkins DE, Greenberg SD. Pulmonary toxicity in long-term administration of BCNU. *Cancer Treat Rep*. 1976;60:1691-1694.
15. O'Driscoll BR, Hasleton PS, Taylor PM, Poulter LW, Gattameneni HR, Woodcock AA. Active lung fibrosis up to 17 years after chemotherapy with carmustine (BCNU) in childhood. *N Eng J Med*. 1990;323:378-382.
16. Lindell RM, Hartman TE. Chest imaging in iatrogenic respiratory disease. *Clin Chest Med*. 2004;25:15-24.
17. Cleverley JR, Screaton NJ, Hiorns MP, Flint JD, Müller NL. Drug-induced lung disease: high-resolution CT and histological findings. *Clin Radiol*. 2002;57:292-299.
18. Ohnishi H, Yokoyama A, Yasuhara Y, et al. Circulating KL-6 levels in patients with drug induced pneumonitis. *Thorax*. 2003;58:872-875.
19. Takahashi H, Fujishima T, Koba H, et al. Serum surfactant proteins A and D as prognostic factors in idiopathic pulmonary fibrosis and their relationship to disease extent. *Am J Respir Crit Care Med*. 2000;162:1109-1114.
20. Matsuno O, Ono E, Ueno T, et al. Increased serum ADAM8 concentration in patients with drug-induced eosinophilic pneumonia -ADAM8 expression depends on the allergen route of entry. *Respir Med*. 2010;104:34-39.
21. Myers JL. Pathology of drug-induced lung disease. In: Katzenstein ALA, ed. *Katzenstein and Askin's Surgical Pathology of Non-neoplastic Lung Disease*. 3rd ed. Philadelphia, PA: WB Saunders; 1997:81-111.
22. Zitnik RJ, Matthay RA. Drug-induced lung disease. In: Schwartz MI, King TE, eds. *Interstitial Lung Disease*. London: BC Decker; 1998:423-449.
23. Leuppi JD, Schnyder P, Hartmann K, Reinhart WH, Kuhn M. Drug-induced bronchospasm: analysis of 187 spontaneously reported cases. *Respiration*. 2001;68:345-351.
24. Fuller RW, Dixon CM, Cuss FM, Barnes PJ. Bradykinin-induced bronchoconstriction in humans. Mode of action. *Am Rev Respir Dis*. 1987;135:176-180.
25. Reed C, Glauser F. Drug-induced noncardiogenic pulmonary edema. *Chest*. 1991;100:1120-1124.
26. Lock BJ, Eggert M, Cooper JA Jr. Infiltrative lung disease due to noncytotoxic agents. *Clin Chest Med*. 2004;25:47-52.
27. Lee-Chiong T Jr, Matthay RA. Drug-induced pulmonary edema and acute respiratory distress syndrome. *Clin Chest Med*. 2004;25:95-104.
28. Heffner JE, Sahn SA. Salicylate-induced pulmonary edema. Clinical features and prognosis. *Ann Intern Med*. 1981;95:405-409.
29. Knowles SR, Wong GA, Rahim SA, Binkley K, Phillips EJ, Shear NH. Hydrochlorothiazide-induced noncardiogenic pulmonary edema: an underrecognized yet serious adverse drug reaction. *Pharmacotherapy*. 2005;25:1258-1265.
30. Kaarteenaho R, Kinnula VL. Diffuse alveolar damage: a common phenomenon in progressive interstitial lung disorders. *Pulm Med*. 2011;2011:531302.
31. Nathani N, Little MA, Kunst H, Wilson D, Thickett DR. Churg-Strauss syndrome and leukotriene antagonist use: a respiratory perspective. *Thorax*. 2008;63:883-888.
32. Kay JM. Drug-induced lung disease. In: Hasleton PS, ed. *Spencer's Pathology of the Lung*. 5th ed. New York: McGraw-Hill; 1996:551-595.
33. Rosenow EC, Myers JL, Swensen SJ, Pisani RJ. Drug-induced pulmonary disease: an update. *Chest*. 1992;102:239-250.
34. Rossi SE, Erasmus JJ, McAdams HP, Sporn TA, Goodman PC. Pulmonary drug toxicity: radiologic and pathologic manifestations. *Radiographics*. 2000;20:1245-1259.
35. Smith GWJ. The histopathology of pulmonary reactions to drugs. *Clin Chest Med*. 1990;11:95-117.
36. Pietra GG. Pathologic mechanisms of drug-induced lung disorders. *J Thorac Imaging*. 1991;6:1-7.
37. Tomashefski JF Jr. Pulmonary pathology of acute respiratory distress syndrome. *Clin Chest Med*. 2000;21:435-466.
38. American Thoracic Society; European Respiratory Society. American Thoracic Society/European Respiratory Society International Multidisciplinary Consensus Classification of the Idiopathic Interstitial Pneumonias. This joint statement of the American Thoracic Society (ATS), and the European Respiratory Society (ERS) was adopted by the ATS board of directors, June 2001 and by the ERS Executive Committee, June 2001. *Am J Respir Crit Care Med*. 2002;15:165:277-304.
39. Limper AH. Chemotherapy-induced lung disease. *Clin Chest Med*. 2004;25:53-64.
40. Epler GR. Drug-induced bronchiolitis obliterans organizing pneumonia. *Clin Chest Med*. 2004;25:89-94.
41. McAdams HP, Rosado-de-Christenson ML, Wehunt WD, Fishback NF. The alphabet soup revisited: the chronic interstitial pneumonias in the 1990s. *Radiographics*. 1996;16:1009-1033.
42. Epler GR, Colby TV, McLoud TC, Carington CB, Gaensler EA. Bronchiolitis obliterans organizing pneumonia. *N Engl J Med*. 1985;312:152-158.
43. Cohen MB, Austin JH, Smith-Vaniz A, Lutzky J, Grimes MM. Nodular bleomycin toxicity. *Am J Clin Pathol*. 1989;92:101-104.
44. McCrea ES, Diaconis JN, Wade JC, Johnston CA. Bleomycin toxicity simulating metastatic nodules to the lungs. *Cancer*. 1981;48:1096-1100.
45. Santrach PJ, Askin FB, Wells RJ, Azizkhan RG, Merten DF. Nodular form of bleomycin-related pulmonary injury in patients with osteogenic sarcoma. *Cancer*. 1989;64:806-811.
46. Gal AA. Drug and radiation toxicity. In: Tomashefski JF Jr, Cagle PT, Farver CF, Fraire AE, eds. *Dail and Hammar's Pulmonary Pathology: Volume I: Nonneoplastic Lung Disease*. 3rd ed. New York: Springer; 2008:807-830.
47. Kuhlman JE, Teigen C, Ren H, Hurban RH, Hutchins GM, Fishman EK. Amiodarone pulmonary toxicity: CT findings in symptomatic patients. *Radiology*. 1990;177:121-125.
48. Cooper JA Jr, White DA, Matthay RA. Drug-induced pulmonary disease. 1. Cytotoxic drugs. *Am Rev Resp Dis*. 1986;133:321-340.
49. Kennedy J, Myers J, Plumb V, Fulmer J. Amiodarone pulmonary toxicity: clinical, radiologic, and pathologic correlations. *Arch Intern Med*. 1987;147:50-55.
50. Allen JN. Drug-induced eosinophilic lung disease. *Clin Chest Med*. 2004;25:77-88.
51. Philit F, Etienne-Mastroianni B, Parrot A, Guerin C, Robert D, Cordier JF. Idiopathic acute eosinophilic pneumonia: a study of 22 patients. *Am J Respir Crit Care Med*. 2002;166:1235-1239.
52. Solomon J, Schwarz M. Drug-, toxin-, and radiation therapy-induced eosinophilic pneumonia. *Semin Respir Crit Care Med*. 2006;27:192-197.
53. Wechsler ME, Garpestad E, Flier SR, et al. Pulmonary infiltrates, eosinophilia, and cardiomyopathy following corticosteroid withdrawal in patients with asthma receiving zafirlukast. *JAMA*. 1998;279:455-457.

54. Weller PF, Plaut M, Taggart V, Trontell A. The relationship of asthma therapy and Churg-Strauss syndrome: NIH workshop summary report. *J Allergy Clin Immunol.* 2001;108:175-183.

55. Johkoh T, Müller NL, Akira M, et al. Eosinophilic lung diseases: diagnostic accuracy of thin-section CT in 111 patients. *Radiology.* 2000;216:773-780.

56. Yousem SA. Eosinophilic pneumonia-like areas in idiopathic usual interstitial pneumonia. *Mod Pathol.* 2000;13:1280-1284.

57. Flieder DB, Travis WD. Pathologic characteristics of drug-induced lung disease. *Clin Chest Med.* 2004;25:37-45.

58. Carrington CB, Addington WW, Goff AM, et al. Chronic eosinophilic pneumonia. *N Eng J Med.* 1969;280:787-798.

59. Pope-Harman AL, Davis WB, Allen ED, Christoforidis AJ, Allen JN. Acute eosinophilic pneumonia. A summary of 15 cases and review of the literature. *Medicine (Baltimore).* 1996;75:334-342.

60. Tazelaar HD, Linz LJ, Colby TV, Myers JL, Limper AH. Acute eosinophilic pneumonia: histopathologic findings in nine patients. *Am J Respir Crit Care Med.* 1997;155:296-302.

61. Lombard CM. Drug-induced pulmonary disease. In: Saldana MJ ed. *Pathology of Pulmonary Disease.* Philadelphia, PA: JB Lippincott; 1994:149-157.

62. Larsen BT, Vaszar LT, Colby TV, Tazelaar HD. Lymphoid hyperplasia and eosinophilic pneumonia as histologic manifestations of amiodarone-induced lung toxicity. *Am J Surg Pathol.* 2012;36:509-516.

63. Travis WD, Matsui K, Moss J, Ferrans VJ. Idiopathic nonspecific interstitial pneumonia: prognostic significance of cellular and fibrosing patterns: survival comparison with usual interstitial pneumonia and desquamative interstitial pneumonia. *Am J Surg Pathol.* 2000;24:19-33.

64. Travis WD, Hunninghake G, King TE Jr, et al. Idiopathic nonspecific interstitial pneumonia: report of an American Thoracic Society project. *Am J Respir Crit Care Med.* 2008;177:1338-1347.

65. Guinee DG Jr. Update on nonneoplastic pulmonary lymphoproliferative disorders and related entities. *Arch Pathol Lab Med.* 2010;134:691-701.

66. Swigris JJ, Berry GJ, Raffin TA, Kuschner WG. Lymphoid interstitial pneumonia: a narrative review. *Chest.* 2002;122:2150-2164.

67. Butnor KJ. Pulmonary sarcoidosis induced by interferon-alpha therapy. *Am J Surg Pathol.* 2005;29:976-979.

68. Goldberg HJ, Fiedler D, Webb A, Jagirdar J, Hoyumpa AM, Peters J. Sarcoidosis after treatment with interferon-alpha: a case series and review of the literature. *Respir Med.* 2006;100:2063-2068.

69. Rosen Y. Interferon-alpha and Sarcoidosis. *Am J Surg Pathol.* 2005;29:1544.

70. Coleman A, Colby TV. Histologic diagnosis of extrinsic allergic alveolitis. *Am J Surg Pathol.* 1988;12:514-518.

71. Agostini C, Trentin L, Facco M, Semenzato G. New aspects of hypersensitivity pneumonitis. *Curr Opin Pulm Med.* 2004;10:378-382.

72. Foucher P, Biour M, Blayac JP, et al. Drugs that may injure the respiratory system. *Eur Respir J.* 1997;10:265-279.

73. Camus P, Foucher P, Bonniaud P, Ash K. Drug-induced infiltrative lung disease. *Eur Respir J Suppl.* 2001;32:93s-100s.

74. Chhajed PN, Dickenmann M, Bubendorf L, Mayr M, Steiger J, Tamm M. Patterns of pulmonary complications associated with sirolimus. *Respiration.* 2006;73:367-374.

75. Pham PT, Pham PC, Danovitch GM, et al. Sirolimus-associated pulmonary toxicity. *Transplantation.* 2004;77:1215-1220.

76. Weiner SM, Sellin L, Vonend O, et al. Pneumonitis associated with sirolimus: clinical characteristics, risk factors and outcome—a single-centre experience and review of the literature. *Nephrol Dial Transplant.* 2007;22:3631-3637.

77. Seymour JF, Presneill JJ. Pulmonary alveolar proteinosis: progress in the first 44 years. *Am J Respir Crit Care Med.* 2002;166:215-235.

78. Chapman E, Leipsic J, Satkunam N, Churg A. Pulmonary alveolar proteinosis as a reaction to fentanyl patch smoke. *Chest.* 2012;141:1321-1323.

79. Frazier AA, Franks TJ, Cooke EO, Mohammed TL, Pugatch RD, Galvin JR. From the archives of the AFIP: pulmonary alveolar proteinosis. *Radiographics.* 2008;28:883-899.

80. Holbert JM, Costello P, Li W, Hoffman RM, Rogers RM. CT features of pulmonary alveolar proteinosis. *AJR Am J Roentgenol.* 2001;176:1287-1294.

81. Hess E. Drug-related lupus. *N Engl J Med.* 1988;318:1460-1462.

82. Lenert P, Icardi M, Dahmoush L. ANA (+) ANCA (+) systemic vasculitis associated with the use of minocycline: case-based review. *Clin Rheumatol.* 2013;32:1099-1106.

83. Huggins JT, Sahn SA. Drug-induced pleural disease. *Clin Chest Med.* 2004;25:141-153.

84. Cameron HA, Ramsay LE. The lupus syndrome induced by hydralazine: a common complication with low dose treatment. *Br Med J.* 1984;289:410-412.

85. Merkel PA. Drugs associated with vasculitis. *Curr Opin Rheumatol.* 1998;10:45-50.

86. Ellis DA, Capewell SJ. Pulmonary veno-occlusive disease after chemotherapy. *Thorax.* 1986;41:415-416.

87. Joselson R, Warnock M. Pulmonary veno-occlusive disease after chemotherapy. *Hum Pathol.* 1983;14:88-91.

88. Knight BK, Rose AG. Pulmonary veno-occlusive disease after chemotherapy. *Thorax.* 1985;40:874-875.

89. Lombard CM, Churg A, Winokur S. Pulmonary veno-occlusive disease following therapy for malignant neoplasms. *Chest.* 1987;92:871-876.

90. Montani D, Achouh L, Dorfmüller P, et al. Pulmonary veno-occlusive disease: clinical, functional, radiologic, and hemodynamic characteristics and outcome of 24 cases confirmed by histology. *Medicine (Baltimore).* 2008;87:220-233.

91. Rose AG. Pulmonary veno-occlusive disease due to bleomycin therapy for lymphoma. Case reports. *S Afr Med J.* 1983;64:636-638.

92. Doll DC, Yarbro JW. Vascular toxicity associated with antineoplastic agents. *Semin Oncol.* 1992;19:580-596.

93. Gurtner HP. Pulmonary hypertension, "plexogenic pulmonary arteriopathy" and the appetite depressant drug aminorex: post or propter? *Bull Eur Physiopathol Respir.* 1979;15:897-923.

94. Higenbottam T, Laude L, Emery C, Essener M. Pulmonary hypertension as a result of drug therapy. *Clin Chest Med.* 2004;25:123-131.

95. Kramer MS, Lane DA. Aminorex, dexfenfluramine, and primary pulmonary hypertension. *J Clin Epidemiol.* 1998;51:361-364.

96. Tomashefski JF Jr, Hirsch CS. The pulmonary vascular lesions of intravenous drug abuse. *Hum Pathol.* 1980;11:133-145.

97. Cooper JA Jr, White DA, Matthay RA. Drug-induced pulmonary disease. Part 2: Noncytotoxic drugs. *Am Rev Respir Dis.* 1986;133:488-505.

98. Morelock SY, Sahn SA. Drugs and the pleura. *Chest.* 1999;116:212-221.

99. Antony VB. Drug-induced pleural disease. *Clin Chest Med.* 1998;19:331-340.

100. Johnson LA, Malayappan B, Tretyakova N, et al. Formation of cyclophosphamide specific DNA adducts in hematological diseases. *Pediatr Blood Cancer.* 2012;58:708-714.

101. Spector JI, Zimbler H, Ross JS. Early-onset cyclophosphamide-induced interstitial pneumonitis. *JAMA.* 1979;242:2852-2854.

102. Malik SW, Myers JL, DeRemee RA, Specks U. Lung toxicity associated with cyclophosphamide use. Two distinct patterns. *Am J Respir Crit Care Med.* 1996;154:1851-1856.

103. Segura A, Yuste A, Cercos A, et al. Pulmonary fibrosis induced by cyclophosphamide. *Ann Pharmacother.* 2001;35:894-897.

104. Abdel Karim FW, Ayash RE, Allam C, Salem PA. Pulmonary fibrosis after prolonged treatment with low-dose cyclophosphamide. A case report. *Oncology*. 1983;40:174-176.

105. Weintraub M. Long-term weight control study: conclusions. *Clin Pharmacol Ther*. 1992;51:642-646.

106. Baumann MH, Ayestas MA, Dersch CM, Brockington A, Rice KC, Rothman RB. Effects of phentermine and fenfluramine on extracellular dopamine and serotonin in rat nucleus accumbens: therapeutic implications. *Synapse*. 2000;36:102-113.

107. Abenhaim L, Moride Y, Brenot F, et al. Appetite-suppressant drugs and the risk of primary pulmonary hypertension. International Primary Pulmonary Hypertension Study Group. *N Engl J Med*. 1996;335:609-616.

108. Hervé P, Launay JM, Scrobohaci ML, et al. Increased plasma serotonin in primary pulmonary hypertension. *Am J Med*. 1995;99:249-254.

109. Weir EK, Reeve HL, Huang JM, et al. Anorexic agents aminorex, fenfluramine, and dexfenfluramine inhibit potassium current in rat pulmonary vascular smooth muscle and cause pulmonary vasoconstriction. *Circulation*. 1996;94:2216-2220.

110. Sachdev M, Miller WC, Ryan T, Jollis JG. Effect of fenfluramine-derivative diet pills on cardiac valves: a meta-analysis of observational studies. *Am Heart J*. 2002;144:1065-1073.

111. Sleijfer S. Bleomycin-induced pneumonitis. *Chest*. 2001; 120:617-624.

112. Gilson AJ, Sahn SA. Reactivation of bleomycin lung toxicity following oxygen administration. A second response to corticosteroids. *Chest*. 1985;88:304-306.

113. Jensen JL, Goel R, Venner PM. The effect of corticosteroid administration on bleomycin lung toxicity. *Cancer*. 1990;65:1291-1297.

114. Martin WJ 2nd, Rosenow EC 3rd. Amiodarone pulmonary toxicity. Recognition and pathogenesis (Part 2). *Chest*. 1988;93:1242-1248.

115. Kennedy JI Jr. Clinical aspects of amiodarone pulmonary toxicity. *Clin Chest Med*. 1990;11:119-129.

116. Fraire AE, Guntupalli KK, Greenberg SD, Cartwright J Jr, Chasen MH. Amiodarone pulmonary toxicity: a multidisciplinary review of current status. *South Med J*. 1993;86:67-77.

117. Martin WJ 2nd, Rosenow EC 3rd. Amiodarone pulmonary toxicity. Recognition and pathogenesis (Part I). *Chest*. 1988;93:1067-1075.

118. Yamada Y, Shiga T, Matsuda N, et al. Incidence and predictors of pulmonary toxicity in Japanese patients receiving low-dose amiodarone. *Circ J*. 2007;71:1610-1616.

119. Camus P, Martin WJ 2nd, Rosenow EC 3rd. Amiodarone pulmonary toxicity. *Clin Chest Med*. 2004;25:65-75.

120. Ruangchira-Urai R, Colby TV, Klein J, Nielsen GP, Kradin RL, Mark EJ. Nodular amiodarone lung disease. *Am J Surg Pathol*. 2008;32:1654-1660.

121. Myers JL, Kennedy JI, Plumb VJ. Amiodarone lung: pathologic findings in clinically toxic patients. *Hum Pathol*. 1987;18:349-354.

122. Dean PJ, Groshart KD, Porterfield JG, Iansmith DH, Golden EB Jr. Amiodarone-associated pulmonary toxicity. A clinical and pathologic study of eleven cases. *Am J Clin Pathol*. 1987;87:7-13.

123. Camus P, Colby TV, Rosenow EC 3rd. Amiodarone pulmonary toxicity. In: Camus P, Rosenow EC 3rd. eds. *Drug-Induced and Iatrogenic Respiratory Disease*. London: Hodder Arnold; 2010:240-259.

124. Colgan T, Simon GT, Kay JM, Pugsley SO, Eydt J. Amiodarone pulmonary toxicity. *Ultrastruct Pathol*. 1984;6:199-207.

125. Stein B, Zaatari GS, Pine JR. Amiodarone pulmonary toxicity. Clinical, cytologic and ultrastructural findings. *Acta Cytol*. 1987;31:357-361.

126. Pegg AE. Mammalian O6-alkylguanine-DNA alkyltransferase: regulation and importance in response to alkylating carcinogenic and therapeutic agents. *Cancer Res*. 1990;50:6119-6129.

127. Chap L, Shpiner R, Levine M, Norton L, Lill M, Glaspy J. Pulmonary toxicity of high-dose chemotherapy for breast cancer: a non-invasive approach to diagnosis and treatment. *Bone marrow Transplant*. 1997;20:1063-1067.

128. Abid SH, Malhotra V, Perry MC. Radiation-induced and chemotherapy-induced pulmonary injury. *Curr Opin Oncol*. 2001;13:242-248.

129. Weiss RB, Poster DS, Penta JS. The nitrosoureas and pulmonary toxicity. *Cancer Treat Rev*. 1981;8:111-125.

130. Smith AC, et al. The pulmonary toxicity of nitrosoureas. *Pharmacol Ther*. 1989;41:443-460.

131. Massin F, Coudert B, Foucher P, et al. Nitrosourea-induced lung diseases. *Rev Mal Respir*. 1992;9:575-582.

132. Twohig KJ, Matthay RA. Pulmonary effects of cytotoxic agents other than bleomycin. *Clin Chest Med*. 1990;11:31-54.

133. Litam JP, Dail DH, Spitzer G, et al. Early pulmonary toxicity after administration of high-dose BCNU. *Cancer Treat Rep*. 1981;65:39-44.

134. Lieberman A, Ruoff M, Estey E, Seidman I, Lieberman I, Wise A. Irreversible pulmonary toxicity after single course of BCNU. *Am J Med Sci*. 1980;279:53-56.

135. Hallas J, Gram LF, Grodum E, et al. Drug related admissions to medical wards: a population based survey. *Br J Clin Pharmacol*. 1992;33:61-68.

136. Boggess KA, Benedetti TJ, Raghu G. Nitrofurantoin- induced pulmonary toxicity during pregnancy: a report of a case and review of the literature. *Obstet Gynecol Surv*. 1996; 51:367-370.

137. Morrison DA, Goldman AL. Radiologic patterns of drug-induced lung disease. *Radiology*. 1979;131:299-304.

138. Holmberg L, Boman G, Bottiger LE, Eriksson B, Spross R, Wessling A. Adverse reactions to nitrofurantoin. Analysis of 921 reports. *Am J Med*. 1980;69:733-738.

139. Geller M, Dickie HA, Kass DA, Hafez GR, Gillespie JJ. The histopathology of acute nitrofurantoin-associated pneumonitis. *Ann Allergy*. 1976;37:275-279.

140. Mendez JL, Nadrous HF, Hartman TE, Ryu JH. Chronic nitrofurantoin-induced lung disease. *Mayo Clin Proc*. 2005;80:1298-1302.

141. Rosenow EC 3rd, DeRemee RA, Dines DE. Chronic nitrofurantoin pulmonary reaction. Report of 5 cases. *N Engl J Med*. 1968;279:1258-1262.

142. Sheehan RE, Wells AU, Milne DG, Hansell DM. Nitrofurantoin-induced lung disease: two cases demonstrating resolution of apparently irreversible CT abnormalities. *J Comput Assist Tomogr*. 2000;24:259-261.

143. Padley SP, Adler B, Hansell DM, Müller NL. High-resolution computed tomography of drug-induced lung disease. *Clin Radiol*. 1992;46:232-236.

144. Okuno SH, Frytak S. Mitomycin lung toxicity: acute and chronic phases. *Am J Clin Oncol*. 1997;20:282-284.

145. Verweij J, van Zanten T, Souren T, Golding R, Pinedo HM. Prospective study on the dose relationship of mitomycin C-induced interstitial pneumonitis. *Cancer*. 1987;60:756-761.

146. Wada H, Nakano Y, Yamada H, Saiga T, Yamanaka A, Sakai N. Intravesical mitomycin-C-induced interstitial pneumonia. *Respiration*. 2010;80:256-259.

147. Jolivet J, Giroux L, Laurin S, Gruber J, Bettez P, Band PR. Microangiopathic hemolytic anemia, renal failure, and noncardiogenic pulmonary edema: a chemotherapy-induced syndrome. *Cancer Treat Rep*. 1983;67:429-434.

148. Chang-Poon VY, Hwang WS, Wong A, Berry J, Klassen J, Poon MC. Pulmonary angiomatoid vascular changes in mitomycin C-associated hemolytic-uremic syndrome. *Arch Pathol Lab Med*. 1985;109:877-878.

149. Sheldon R, Slaughter D. A syndrome of microangiopathic hemolytic anemia, renal impairment, and pulmonary edema in

chemotherapy-treated patients with adenocarcinoma. *Cancer.* 1986;58:1428-1436.

150. Gunstream SR, Seidenfeld JJ, Sobonya RE, McMahon LJ. Mitomycin-associated lung disease. *Cancer Treat Rep.* 1983; 67:301-304.

151. Buzdar AU, Legha SS, Luna MA, Tashima CK, Hortobagyi GN, Blumenschein GR. Pulmonary toxicity of mitomycin. *Cancer.* 1980;45:236-244.

152. Orwoll ES, Kiessling PJ, Patterson JR. Interstitial pneumonia from mitomycin. *Ann Intern Med.* 1978;89:352-355.

153. Abratt RP, Morgan GW, Silvestri G, Willcox P. Pulmonary complications of radiation therapy. *Clin Chest Med.* 2004;25:167-177.

154. Abratt RP, Morgan GW. Lung toxicity following chest irradiation in patients with lung cancer. *Lung Cancer.* 2002;35:103-109.

155. Rosiello RA, Merrill WW. Radiation-induced lung injury. *Clin Chest Med.* 1990;11:65-71.

156. Wang JY, Chen KY, Wang JT, et al. Outcome and prognostic factors for patients with non-small-cell lung cancer and severe radiation pneumonitis. *Int J Radiat Oncol Biol Phys.* 2002;54:735-741.

157. Rodrigues G, Lock M, D'Souza D, Yu E, Van Dyk J. Prediction of radiation pneumonitis by dose-volume histogram parameters in lung cancer-a systematic review. *Radiother Oncol.* 2004;71:127-138.

158. Rubin P, Johnston CJ, Williams JP, McDonald S, Finkelstein JN. A perpetual cascade of cytokines postirradiation leads to pulmonary fibrosis. *Int J Radiat Oncol Biol Phys.* 1995;33:99-109.

159. Tsoutsou P, Koukorakis M. Radiation pneumonitis and fibrosis: mechanisms underlying its pathogenesis and implications for future research. *Int J Radiat Oncol Biol Phys.* 2006;66:1281-1293.

160. Movsas B, Raffin TA, Epstein AH, Link CJ Jr. Pulmonary radiation injury. *Chest.* 1997;111:1061-1076.

161. Fajardo LF, Berthrong M, Anderson RE, eds. Lung. In: *Radiation Pathology.* Oxford: Oxford University Press; 2001:198-207.

162. Armstrong JG, Zelefsky MJ, Leibel SA, et al. Strategy for dose escalation using 3-dimensional conformal radiation therapy for lung cancer. *Ann Oncol.* 1995;6:693-697.

163. Graham MV, Purdy JA, Emami B, et al. Clinical dose-volume histogram analysis for pneumonitis after 3D treatment for non-small cell lung cancer (NSCLC). *Int J Radiat Oncol Biol Phys.* 1999;45:323-329.

164. Claude L, Pérol D, Ginestet C, et al. A prospective study on radiation pneumonitis following conformal radiation therapy in non–small-cell lung cancer: clinical and dosimetric factors analysis. *Radiother Oncol.* 2004;71:175-181.

165. Schild SE, Stella PJ, Geyer SM, et al. The outcome of combined-modality therapy for stage III non–small-cell lung cancer in the elderly. *J Clin Oncol.* 2003;21:3201-3206.

166. Rancati T, Ceresoli GL, Gagliardi G, Schipani S, Cattaneo GM. Factors predicting radiation pneumonitis in lung cancer patients: a retrospective study. *Radiother Oncol.* 2003;67:275-283.

167. Monson JM, Stark P, Reilly JJ, et al. Clinical radiation pneumonitis and radiographic changes after thoracic radiation therapy for lung carcinoma. *Cancer.* 1998;82:842-850.

168. Inoue A, Kunitoh H, Sekine I, Sumi M, Tokuuye K, Saijo N. Radiation pneumonitis in lung cancer patients: a retrospective study of risk factors and the long-term prognosis. *Int J Radiat Oncol Biol Phys.* 2001;49:649-655.

169. Ohe Y. Treatment-related death from chemotherapy and thoracic radiotherapy for advanced cancer. *Panminerva Med.* 2002;44:205-212.

170. Sekine I, Sumi M, Ito Y, et al. Retrospective analysis of steroid therapy for radiation-induced lung injury in lung cancer patients. *Radiother Oncol.* 2006;80:93-97.

171. Kong FM, Ten Haken R, Eisbruch A, Lawrence TS. Non-small-cell lung cancer therapy-related pulmonary toxicity: an update on radiation pneumonitis and fibrosis. *Semin Oncol.* 2005;32(suppl 3):S42-S54.

172. Tomashefski JF Jr. Iatrogenic diffuse alveolar damage: oxygen toxicity and radiation-induced injury. In: Saldana MJ, ed. *Pathology of Pulmonary Disease.* Philadelphia, PA: JB Lippincott; 1994:143-147.

28

Storage Diseases

Hidehiro Takei and Fumi Kawakami

TAKE HOME PEARLS

- Lysosomal storage diseases (LSDs) are a group of approximately 50 unique, genetically distinct, inherited metabolic disorders that result from lysosomal dysfunction.
- Gaucher disease is the most common and Fabry disease is the second most common of the LSDs.
- In Niemann-Pick disease, the lungs show diffuse endogenous lipid pneumonia with an accumulation of lipid-laden macrophages, called Niemann-Pick cells, within the alveolar spaces.
- Glycosphingolipid accumulation causes airway obstruction in Fabry disease.
- Infiltration of pulmonary interstitium, alveolar spaces and capillaries by Gaucher cells filled with glucocerebroside is characteristic of Gaucher disease.
- Intracytoplasmic accumulation of cholesterol ester in multiple types of pulmonary cells occurs in cholesteryl ester storage disease.
- Pulmonary fibrosis is the most serious complication and the major cause of death for patients with Hermansky-Pudlak syndrome.

INTRODUCTION

Lysosomal storage diseases (LSDs) are a group of approximately 50 unique, genetically distinct, inherited metabolic disorders that result from lysosomal dysfunction. The estimated combined incidence is reportedly 1 in approximately 7000 to 8000 live births.[1,2] Gaucher disease is the most common and Fabry disease is the

second most common of the LSDs. LSDs affect mostly children (ie, infantile and juvenile forms) although adult-onset diseases are well known. Most LSDs occur secondary to genetic defects that cause total deficiency or reduced activity of specific native enzymes within the lysosomes. All of them are characterized by progressive intralysosomal accumulation of specific macromolecular compounds, which are normally enzymatically catabolized, in a variety of tissues and organs, causing progressive damage that can become life threatening. It is well known that the central nervous and reticuloendothelial systems are most frequently involved, and these organ systems have been extensively studied. Respiratory system involvement can also be observed although little attention has been paid to the lung. A lung biopsy is usually not taken since the diagnosis is made on the basis of extrapulmonary diseases. Given a significant cause of morbidity and mortality in patients with LSDs, awareness and histopathologic recognition of the respiratory system involvement is important. Lung involvement in LSD patients should be included in the differential diagnosis of interstitial lung diseases.

NIEMANN-PICK DISEASE

Niemann-Pick disease (NPD) is a clinically and biochemically heterogeneous disorder that affects lipid metabolism. This disease is inherited in an autosomal recessive pattern. Based on the clinical presentation and the genetic cause, six variants (types A-F) of NPD have been described.[3] Of these variants, types A-C are well characterized clinically. The main symptoms include

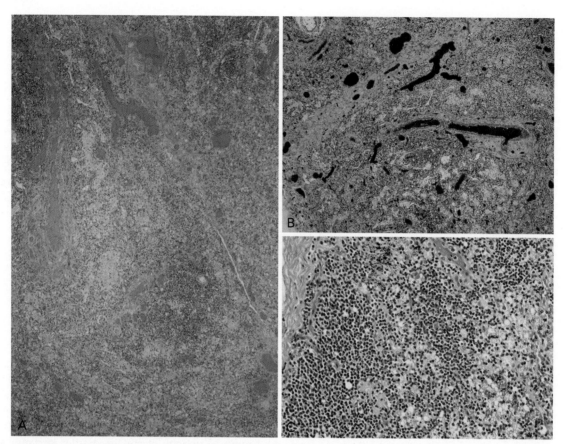

FIGURE 28-1 Niemann-Pick disease type C. A: Low-power image showing congested autopsied lung with mild interstitial fibrosis and diffuse endogenous lipid pneumonia and focal aggregates of lymphocytes (H&E). B: Low-power image showing mild peribronchial and interlobular septal fibrosis (trichrome stain). C: Intermediate-power image showing lymphocytic aggregate admixed with lipid-laden macrophages (H&E).

hepatosplenomegaly, failure to thrive/growth retardation, and progressive deterioration of the nervous system. Types A and B are caused by an absence or deficiency of acid sphingomyelinase due to the *SMPD1* gene mutations, with abnormal intracellular accumulation of sphingomyelin in various organs. Clinically, these diseases appear to represent opposite ends of a phenotypic continuum. Type A, also referred to as the neurological type, is the most devastating form with nervous system involvement, resulting in early childhood death. Type B shows heterogeneous clinical manifestations with chronic visceral involvement, which are usually slower in progression than type A. Given that the nervous system is not generally involved (ie, nonneurological type), patients with Type B disease usually survive into adulthood. Type C is biochemically, genetically, and clinically distinct from types A and B, and is caused by defective intracellular processing and transport of low-density, lipoprotein-derived cholesterol resulting in the intracellular accumulation of excessive amounts of cholesterol and other lipids (*Figure 28-1*). Genetically, it consists of defining two different genetic complementation groups, NPC1 (95% of cases) and NPC2, with causative mutations in the *NPC1* or *NPC2* gene, respectively.[4] Type C is

typically a chronic neurodegenerative disorder involving both the viscera and the central nervous system. This disease is characterized by extremely heterogeneous clinical presentation and variable life expectancy.

Clinical Features of Lung Involvement

Pulmonary involvement was reported in NPD types A-C, although it is difficult to determine its exact incidence in NPD since the literature mostly consists of isolated single reports or small patient series. Of all variants, lung involvement has been most commonly described in Type B disease. Respiratory symptoms at diagnosis include isolated dyspnea, chronic cough, recurrent lung infections, asthma, and respiratory failure.[5-7] The most common symptom in patients with type A disease is (recurrent) pulmonary infections, leading to respiratory insufficiency. In contrast, in type B disease two most frequent symptoms are recurrent lung infections and dyspnea, with a variable course ranging from stable chronic obstructive pulmonary disease to chronic respiratory insufficiency that requires oxygen therapy.[6] Asymptomatic patients or patients with mild respiratory system complaints are not uncommon in type B,

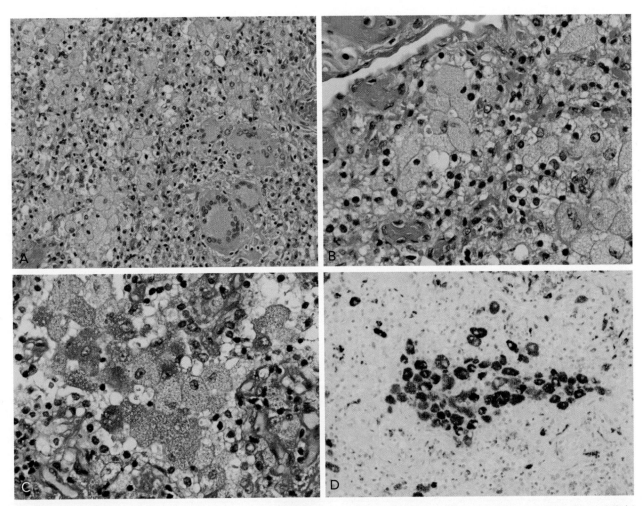

FIGURE 28-2 Niemann-Pick disease type C. A: High-power image showing an intra-alveolar accumulation of lipid-laden macrophages (ie, Niemann-Pick cells) and a few multinucleated giant histiocytes (H&E). **B:** High-power image showing Niemann-Pick cells characterized by rounded or polygonal histiocytes with abundant foamy cytoplasm (H&E). **C:** High-power image showing Niemann-Pick cells with numerous PAS-positive droplets filling the cytoplasm (PAS stain). **D:** Intermediate-power image showing Niemann-Pick cells highlighted with CD68 immunohistochemical stain.

while severe and fatal lung disease is also reported. Asymptomatic patients at diagnosis develop at least some respiratory symptoms during follow-up.[6,7] In type C disease, some patients are asymptomatic, while others develop recurrent lung infections and fatal acute/chronic respiratory failure.[5-7] Alterations of the immune response are more abundant in type C compared to other types, although recurrent lung infections are commonly seen for all the NPD types.[8] Pulmonary alveolar lipoproteinosis has rarely been reported in association with NPC2.[9,10]

Imaging Features

The vast majority of radiological features reported in the literature are those of type B disease. Mendelson et al reported that chest radiography and thin-section CT revealed interstitial lung disease in 90% and 98% of 52 patients with type B disease examined, respectively,

which indicated that pulmonary involvement was a common manifestation of the disease in patients of all ages.[11] Of note is that abnormal imaging findings do not necessarily correlate with the results of pulmonary function tests in these patients.

Chest CT imaging features are nonspecific for this disease and include ground-glass opacities, thickened interlobular septa, and intralobular lines.[5-7,11] On occasion, the combination of these patterns results in the "crazy-paving" sign seen on CT.[11] Atelectasis can be seen.

Pathologic Features

Histologically, the lungs of type B disease show predominantly diffuse endogenous lipid pneumonia with an accumulation of lipid-laden macrophages, called Niemann-Pick cells, within the alveolar spaces. Areas of interstitial foamy macrophages and variable interstitial fibrosis are also seen. Niemann-Pick cells are characterized by generally enlarged histiocytes with abundant finely vacuolated cytoplasm and eccentrically located nuclei. These cells show CD68 immunoreactivity. In type C disease, the histologic features are similar to those of type B (*Figure 28-2*). Nicholson et al reported that vacuolated cytoplasmic changes in type 2 pneumocytes were seen in type C disease, not type B disease, and that those in airway ciliated epithelial cells were noted in type B disease, not type C disease.[5]

Ultrastructurally, the macrophages contain numerous enlarged lysosomes packed with concentric lamellar myelin-like inclusions.

Treatment by whole bronchoalveolar lavage (BAL) using flexible bronchoscopy has been described. Cytological examination of BAL fluid reveals characteristic foamy macrophages with a distended cytoplasm and small eccentrically located nuclei, which account for more than 90% of total number of alveolar macrophages.[6] Eosinophils are not found.

Diagnostic Laboratory Tests

NPD types A and B are diagnosed by measuring the acid sphingomyelinase activity in white blood cells. This enzyme test cannot reliably detect carries of the condition. Molecular genetic (DNA) testing is also available for diagnostic confirmation. DNA tests can be done to diagnose carriers.

NPD type C is diagnosed by assaying cultured fibroblasts for cholesterol esterification and staining for unesterified cholesterol with filipin (ie, filipin test).[12] The diagnosis is confirmed by DNA mutation tests for *NPC1* and *NPC2* genes.

FABRY DISEASE

Fabry disease (FD) is an X-linked recessive, inherited LSD caused by absent or deficient activity of alfa-galactosidase A (α-GAL) due to mutations in the *GLA* gene. This results

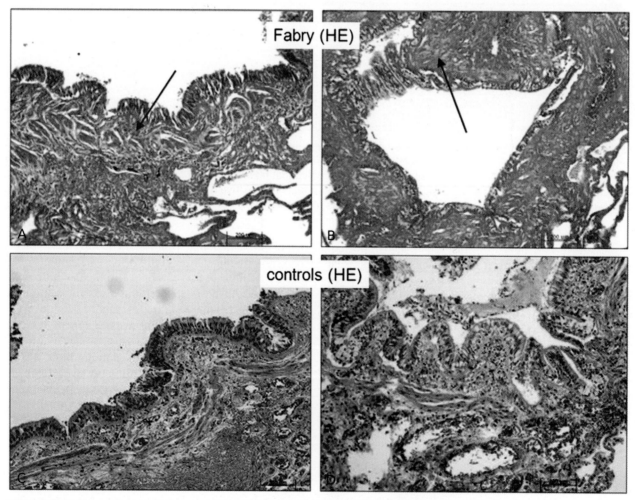

FIGURE 28-3 Fabry disease. Pronounced hypertrophy/hyperplasia of the bronchial smooth muscle cells (arrow, A and B) compared to an age-matched control (C and D) (H&E) (Reprinted with permission from Elsevier, used with permission of Franzen D et al. Pulmonary involvement in Fabry disease: overview and perspectives. *Eur J Intern Med* 2013;24:707-713).

in a progressive abnormal accumulation of glycosphingolipids, particularly globotriaosylceramide (GL-3), in a variety of cell types including vascular endothelial cells, and renal, cardiac and nerve cells, leading to organ dysfunction. The estimated prevalence of this disorder is 1/117,000 in the general population.[13] The characteristic clinical features include acroparesthesias/pain crisis, cutaneous angiokeratomas, hypohidrosis/anhidrosis, corneal opacity, gastrointestinal symptoms, heat and cold intolerance, and hearing loss and tinnitus. Most severe complications include renal insufficiency and cardiovascular and cerebrovascular diseases, which can be lethal. The disease predominantly affects males (hemizygotes); however, most female heterozygotes develop symptoms and sings of FD via yet unknown mechanisms, and later on, a high percentage of women develop vital organ damage.[14] The recombinant human α-GAL is now available for patients with FD as an enzyme replacement therapy and is becoming the treatment of choice for FD.

Clinical Features of Lung Involvement

Pulmonary involvement, manifesting clinically as cough, wheeze, or dyspnea, is frequent in patients with FD,[15] although it is generally underappreciated compared with other organ involvement. Chronic obstructive lung disease, specifically involving the small airways, is much more prevalent in patients with FD than would be expected in the general population. The prevalence of airway obstruction, assessed by a clinically significant reduction in spirometric parameters, was reportedly 26% of women and 61% of men.[16] A significant age- and gender-dependent progression of pulmonary involvement was shown on the basis of the serial follow-up data.[16] Enzyme replacement therapy may alleviate pulmonary dysfunction in patients with FD.[17,18]

Imaging Features

Chest x-ray is frequently normal.[15] CT features were reportedly heterogeneous, ranging from ground-glass opacities to marked pulmonary fibrosis (rare).[19]

Pathologic Features

Histologically, hyperplasia/hypertrophy of the bronchial smooth muscle cells is seen (*Figure 28-3*).[20] This is considered to be secondary to glycosphingolipid accumulation within these cells and results in small airway disease. There is no evidence for involvement of the pulmonary interstitium in this disease. Ultrastructurally, diagnostic lamellar inclusion bodies can be identified in type II pneumocytes and bronchial epithelial cells, which are generally found in transbronchial biopsy specimens.[21] Cytologic

specimens of induced sputum were reported to show these inclusions within the ciliated bronchial epithelial cells, using electron microscopy.[22]

Diagnostic Laboratory Tests

The diagnosis of FD in male patients is made by measuring the level of alfa-galactosidase A activity in a blood sample. The diagnosis is confirmed by mutational analysis of *GLA* gene. In female, only mutational analysis can reliably identify female carriers.

GAUCHER DISEASE

Gaucher disease (GD) is the most prevalent lysosomal storage disease and is inherited in an autosomal recessive manner. GD is caused by deficient activity of beta-glucocerebrosidase due to mutations in *GBA* gene, resulting in accumulation of glucocerebroside within cells primarily of mononuclear phagocyte system. The hallmark of GD is the presence of lipid-laden macrophages (Gaucher cells) in a variety of tissues, primarily in the spleen, liver, bone marrow, lymph nodes, and the central nervous system. The overall incidence of GD is approximately 1:40,000 individuals.[23] The frequency and distribution of *GBA* mutations varies among different ethnic groups and races, and the frequency is known to be the highest in the Ashkenazi Jewish heritage with the carrier frequency of 1 in 18.[24]

CD has a continuum of clinical manifestations from a perinatal lethal form to an asymptomatic form. There are three major clinical types (1, 2, and 3). GD is characterized clinically by hepatosplenomegaly, anemia and thrombocytopenia, bone lesions, and pulmonary lesions, with (neuronopathic type; types 2 and 3) or without (nonneuronopathic type; type 1) primary central nervous system involvement. GD type 1 is the most common form of this disorder, and may appear early in life or adulthood. GD type 2 usually causes life-threatening medical problems beginning in infancy, while GD type 3 tends to progress more slowly than type 2. Enzyme replacement therapy is available.

Clinical Features of Lung Involvement

Lung involvement is a well-known complication described in all types of GD, although not common at presentation. It varies in symptomatology from asymptomatic to severe dyspnea. Severe pulmonary disease seems to occur mainly in children with a more severe course of GD (ie, types 2 and 3).[25] Pulmonary disease is associated with high mortality in these patients. Kerem et al reported in their prospective study that >2/3 of patients (children and adults) with GD type I have some pulmonary function abnormality although

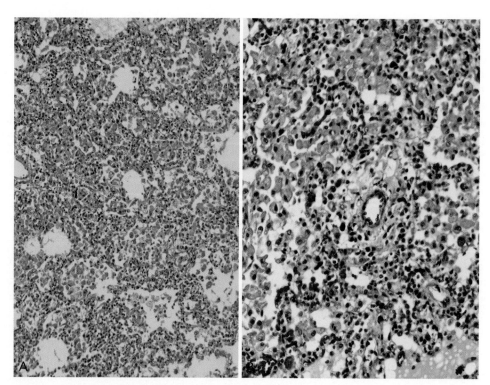

FIGURE 28-4 Gaucher disease. A: low-power image showing edematous autopsied lung with alveolar spaces filled with foamy macrophages (ie, Gaucher cells) (H&E). B: Intermediate-power image showing edema and inconspicuous fibrosis (trichrome stain).

many show no clinical manifestations.[26] For genotype-phenotype correlations, Santamaria et al suggested that GD patients with L444P homozygous mutation might have an increased risk for developing primary lung disease.[27] Pulmonary arterial hypertension and hepatopulmonary syndrome (HPS) are rare pulmonary vascular complications seen in GD type 1 patients with long-standing liver disease.[28] Intrapulmonary (micro)vascular dilatation probably due to failure of the damaged liver to clear circulating pulmonary vasodilators and to inhibition of circulating vasoconstrictors by the damaged liver is the defining pathological feature of HPS, which leads to severe hypoxemia.[29] Enzyme replacement therapy is reported to be marginally effective in contrast to the dramatic reduction in organomegaly.[30,31]

Imaging Features

Chest x-ray and CT scans are not specific for the diagnosis of lung involvement of GD. Chest x-ray may be normal. Radiological pulmonary findings are more frequent and more severe in GD type 2 and type 3 than in GD type 1. High-resolution CT (HRCT) demonstrates interstitial lung disease or a mixed interstitial and alveolar pattern. HRCT findings include thickening of the interlobular and intralobular septa and ground glass opacities.

Pathologic Features

The pathologic hallmark of GD is the presence of Gaucher cells (GCs) in organs (*Figure 28-4*). The following histological patterns are described in pulmonary involvement of GD:[32-34] (i) interstitial infiltration of GCs in the perivascular, peribronchial, and septal region with fibrosis, (ii) alveolar spaces filled with GCs, (iii) capillary plugging with GCs. Pattern (iii) with subsequent occlusion may be associated with pulmonary hypertension that is seen in GD.

GCs are filled with glucocerebroside to an extreme level and are morphologically characterized by eccentrically located nuclei and abundant cytoplasm with the characteristic "wrinkled tissue paper" appearance (*Figure 28-5*). Periodic acid-Schiff stain highlights GCs with strongly positive granular or fibrillar material in the cytoplasm. Immunohistochemically, GCs express CD68; however, they usually exhibit relatively light CD68 immunoreactivity in contrast to alveolar macrophages.[35]

GCs are identified in the bronchoalveolar lavage specimens by cytologic examination.[36]

Diagnostic Laboratory Tests

Enzymatic assay to evaluate beta-glucosidase (glucocerebrosidase) activity in leukocytes or cultured fibroblasts

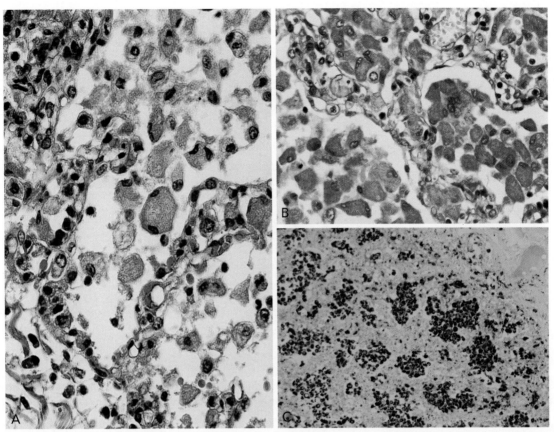

FIGURE 28-5 Gaucher disease. **A:** High-power view showing an intra-alveolar accumulation of Gaucher cells. They are characterized by voluminous cytoplasm with a "wrinkled tissue paper" appearance and the nuclei that are pushed off to the periphery (H&E). **B:** High-power view showing intra-alveolar Gaucher cells with **PAS** positive, finely granular cytoplasm containing glucocerebroside (PAS stain). **C:** Low-power view showing Gaucher cells with high intracellular immunohistochemical expression of CD68.

combined with molecular analysis of *GBA* is now the gold standard. However, the enzyme activity test is unreliable for carrier detection. Target mutation analysis of four known mutations in *GBA* is useful for Ashkenazi Jewish population since these mutations account for approximately 90% of the disease-causing alleles.[24]

Bone marrow examination reveals the presence of Gaucher cells. However, this examination is not a reliable diagnostic test given that this finding is nonspecific.[24]

CHOLESTERYL ESTER STORAGE DISEASE

Lysosomal acid lipase (LAL) deficiency due to mutations in the lysosomal acid lipase gene (*LIPA*) causes an autosomal recessive lipid storage disorder. There are two major clinical phenotypes: infantile-onset Wolman disease (WD) and later-onset cholesteryl ester storage disease (CESD). WD is a fulminant subtype with absent or less than 1% of normal LAL activity, while

CESD is an often unrecognized, later-onset subtype and can present in infancy, childhood, or adulthood, depending on the residual LAL activity.[37] Deficiency of LAL activity results in lysosomal accumulation of cholesteryl ester and to a lesser extent, triglycerides, predominantly in the liver, spleen, and macrophages throughout the body.

Clinical manifestations of CESD include chronic liver disease (diffuse microvesicular steatosis progressing to cirrhosis), hepatosplenomegaly, elevated serum transaminases, and type IIb hyperlipoproteinemia (ie, elevated serum LDL-cholesterol and triglycerides, with normal to low HDL-cholesterol concentrations). Premature demise is mostly due to liver failure. Cardiovascular complications related to accelerated atherosclerosis secondary to chronic hyperlipidemia are major causes of morbidity.[37,38] There is no specific treatment at present, but enzyme replacement therapy has shown encouraging results.[37] Liver transplantation can be effective for patients with end-stage liver disease.[39]

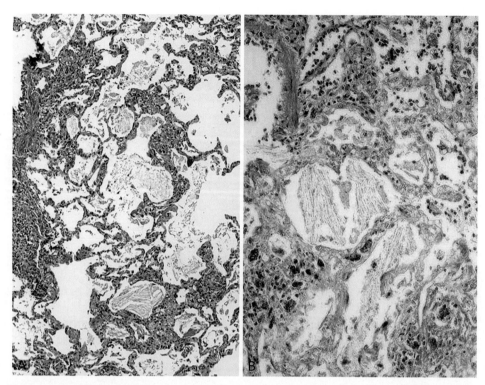

FIGURE 28-6 Cholesteryl ester storage disease. **A:** low-power and **B:** intermediate-power images showing intracellular (ie, within alveolar macrophages) and extracellular accumulation of elliptical cholesterol ester clefts within the alveolar spaces, and thickened alveolar septa (H&E).

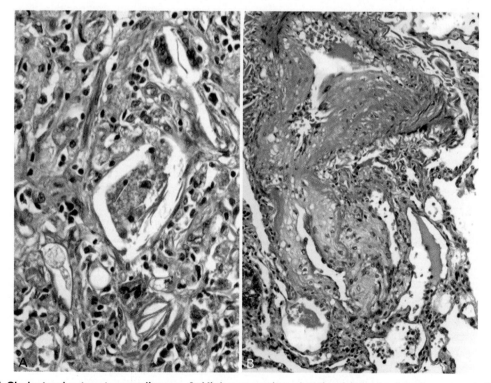

FIGURE 28-7 Cholesteryl ester storage disease. **A:** High-power view showing intracytoplasmic accumulation of cholesterol esters within alveolar macrophages and pulmonary interstitial cells. Multinucleated histiocytes are also seen (H&E). **B:** Intermediate-power view showing focal fibrous intimal thickening and intracellular accumulation of cholesterol ester within fibroblasts and medial smooth muscle cells (H&E).

Clinical Features of Lung Involvement

Pulmonary manifestations are extremely rare. No specific clinical features are reported. Pulmonary hypertension due to accelerated atherosclerosis may be seen.[40,41]

Imaging Features

No specific/characteristic radiological features are reported.

Pathologic Features

Intracytoplasmic accumulation of cholesterol ester is seen within different cells in lung, including pulmonary interstitial cells, alveolar macrophages, and fibroblasts (*Figures 28-6 and 28-7*). Focal concentric intimal deposition of foam cells and extracellular lipid may be seen in pulmonary arteries.[40,41]

Diagnostic Laboratory Tests

Biochemical assay for LAL enzyme activity is performed. After the enzyme test has shown deficiency, DNA mutation analysis of the *LIPA* gene can be done as a confirmatory test. Immunoreactivity for LAMP1, LAMP2, or cathepsin D, or demonstration of pathognomonic cholesteryl ester crystals or their remnant clefts by electron microscopy in liver biopsies can be used to establish the diagnosis.[37]

HERMANSKY-PUDLAK SYNDROME

Hermansky-Pudlak syndrome (HPS) is a rare, autosomal recessive, multisystem disorder characterized by a classic triad of oculocutaneous albinism, bleeding diathesis due to platelet dysfunction (platelet storage pool defect), and lysosomal accumulation of ceroid lipofuscin in a variety of tissue. Other clinical manifestations include pulmonary fibrosis, kidney disease, neutropenia, visual impairment, and granulomatous colitis. These clinical features are thought to occur as a consequence of defective formation, trafficking, or function of intracellular lysosome-related organelles, most importantly, melanosomes in skin melanocytes and retinal pigment epithelial cells, platelet dense granules, and lamellar bodies in alveolar type II epithelial cells.[42,43] Although worldwide it is an extremely rare disorder and is estimated to affect 1 in 500,000 to 1 in 1,000,000,[44] HPS is most common in northwest Puerto Rico, where the frequency is approximately 1 in 1800.[45] The following nine genetic loci have been associated with different distinct HPS subtypes in humans: *HPS-1*, *AP3B1* (causing HPS-2), *HPS-3*, *HPS-4*, *HPS-5*, *HPS-6*, *DTNBP1* (causing HPS-7), *BLOC1S3* (causing HPS-8), and *BLOC1S6* (causing HPS-9).[46] HPS-1 is the most

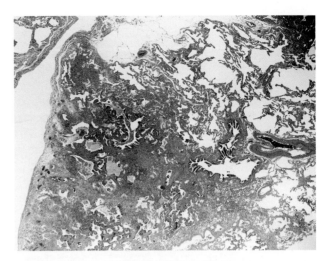

FIGURE 28-8 Hermansky-Pudlak syndrome. Low-power view showing a UIP-like pattern characterized by a subpleural area of fibrosis with honeycombing and patchy inflammatory infiltrates as well as areas of alveolated parenchyma without fibrosis (H&E). (Used with permission of Mary Beth Beasley, MD, Mount Sinai Hospital, NY).

common subtype in both Puerto Rican and non-Puerto Rican populations, and is also the most severe subtype clinically.[47] There is no known cure for HPS. Patients with HPS die of causes directly related to the syndrome, with an average survival age of 30 to 50 years.

Clinical Features of Lung Involvement

Pulmonary fibrosis (PF) is the most serious complication and the major cause of death for patients with HPS. Of the subtypes, PF is seen only in HPS-1, HPS-2, and HPS-4. In one series, pulmonary symptoms developed in 61% of patients with HPS1, the most common subtype, with onset at a mean age of 35 years.[48] HPS interstitial pneumonia shares the same aggressive course of lung fibrosis with usual interstitial pneumonitis (UIP), resulting in progressive dyspnea, reduced exercise capacity, loss of life quality, and eventual death.[49] PF typically manifests in the third and fourth decades of life and can progress to death within a decade.[49] Lung transplantation is the potentially life-extending therapy for severe PF. Steroid therapy is not effective.

Imaging Features

Routine chest x-ray findings include reticulonodular pattern, perihilar fibrosis, pleural thickening, and interstitial infiltrates, while high-resolution CT (HRCT) scan shows septal thickening, ground-glass opacities, reticulation, subpleural cysts, bronchiectasis, pleural thickening, and peribronchovascular thickening.[50] These interstitial abnormalities are distributed diffusely in all lobes, with a peripheral predominant involvement especially in early stage.[50] Pulmonary functional deficits

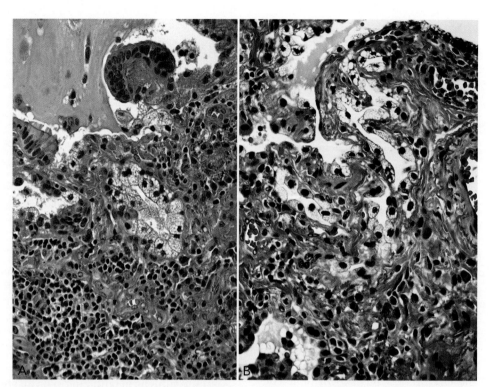

FIGURE 28-9 Hermansky-Pudlak syndrome. A, B: High-power view showing prominent vacuolated pneumocytes lining alveolar spaces. Interstitial fibrosis with lymphoplasmacytic infiltrate is noted (H&E) (Used with permission of Mary Beth Beasley, MD, Mount Sinai Hospital, NY).

assessed by pulmonary function tests correlate with HRCT scan evidence of progression/severity of interstitial lung disease.[49,50]

Pathologic Features

Grossly, PF in HPS is characteristically uneven in distribution without specific localization, in contrast to usual interstitial pneumonitis (UIP), which is characterized by subpleural and basal predominant fibrosis.[51]

Histologically, a UIP-like pattern or a nonspecific interstitial pneumonia-like pattern of fibrosis is seen in the lung (*Figures 28-8 and 28-9*).[35] A diffuse interstitial lymphocytic infiltrate is recognized. Active fibroblastic foci seen in UIP are generally not present in HPS.[51,52] Prominent vacuolated pneumocytes lining alveoli and individual and clusters of histiocytes containing fine and course brown pigments (ie, ceroid) that stained with periodic acid-Schiff are seen in fibrotic areas. On ultrastructural examination, these cells contain giant lamellar bodies within the cytoplasm, which represent vesicles of abnormal lysosomes.[52] Although pathogenesis underlying the PF of HPS is unknown, there is a speculation that intracellular disruption of type II pneumocytes due to accumulation of ceroid triggers a cascade of inflammation, cytokine production, and fibroblastic proliferation, ultimately resulting in PF.[47] Cytological examination of bronchoalveolar lavage can show alveolar macrophages with foamy accumulation of ceroid.[50]

Diagnostic Laboratory Tests

The reliable method of diagnosing HPS is by a deficiency of dense bodies observed by whole mount electron microscopy of platelets. Prolongation of the bleeding time despite normal platelet counts and impaired secondary aggregation response in platelet aggregation studies is noted.

Molecular genetic testing (sequencing) is clinically available for all known genes involved in this disease.[46] Since prognosis and treatment varies among the subtypes of HPS with respect to the occurrence of pulmonary fibrosis, molecular genetic typing for accurate diagnosis of HPS subtype is important.

In Puerto Rican, the *HPS-1* founder mutation, a 16-bp duplication in exon 15, is most common (comprising approximately 75% of patients) and can be tested with target mutation analysis.[46] Severely affected individuals with pulmonary dysfunction can be tested for *HPS1* and *HPS4* mutations initially.

REFERENCES

1. Meikle PJ, Hopwood JJ, Clague AE, Carey WF. Prevalence of lysosomal storage disorders. *JAMA*. 1999;281:249-254.
2. Poupetova H, Ledvinova J, Berna L, Dvorakova L, Kozich V, Elleder M. The birth prevalence of lysosomal storage disorders in the Czech Republic: comparison with date in different populations. *J Inherit Metab Dis*. 2010;33:387-396.

3. Minai OA, Sullivan EJ, Stoller JK. Pulmonary involvement in Niemann-Pick disease: case report and literature review. *Respir Med.* 2000;94:1241-1251.

4. Millat G, Chikh K, Naureckiene S, et al. Niemann-Pick disease type C: spectrum of HE1 mutations and genotype/ phenotype correlations in the NPC2 group. *Am J Hum Genet.* 2001;69:1013-1021.

5. Nicholson AG, Florio R, Hansell DM, et al. Pulmonary involvement by Niemann-Pick disease. A report of six cases. *Histopathology.* 2006;48:596-603.

6. Guillemot N, Troadec C, de Villemeur TB, Clement A, Fauroux B. Lung disease in Niemann-Pick disease. *Pediatr Pulmonol.* 2007;42:1207-1214.

7. Gulhan B, Ozcelik U, Gurakan F, et al. Different features of lung involvement in Niemann-Pick disease and Gaucher disease. *Respir Med.* 2012;106:1278-1285.

8. Castenada JA, Lim MJ, Cooper JD, Pearce DA. Immune system irregularities in lysosomal storage disorders. *Acta Neuropathol.* 2008;115:159-174.

9. Bjurulf B, Spetalen S, Erichsen A, Vanier MT, Strom EH, Stromme P. Niemann-Pick disease type C2 presenting as fatal pulmonary alveolar lipoproteinosis: morphological findings in lung and nervous tissue. *Med Sci Monit.* 2008;14:CS71-75.

10. Griese M, Brasch F, Aldana VR, et al. Respiratory disease in Niemann-Pick type C2 is caused by pulmonary alveolar proteinosis. *Clin Genet.* 2010;77:119-130.

11. Mendelson S, Wasestin MP, Dnik R, et al. Type B Niemann-Pick disease findings at chest radiography, thin-section CT, and pulmonary function testing. *Radiology.* 2006;238:339-345.

12. Wraith JE, Baumgartner MR, Bembi B, et al. Recommendations on the diagnosis and management of Niemann-Pick disease type C. *Mol Genet Metab.* 2009;98:152-165.

13. Meikle PJ, Hopwood JJ, Clague AE, Carey WF. Prevalence of lysosomal storage disorders. *JAMA.* 1999;281:249-254.

14. Wilcox WR, Oliveira JP, Hopkin RJ, et al. Females with Fabry disease frequently have major organ involvement: lesions from the Fabry registry. *Mol Genet Metab.* 2008;93:112-128.

15. Brown LK, Miller A, Bhuptani A, et al. Pulmonary involvement in Fabry disease. *Am J Respir Crit Care Med.* 1997;155:1004-1010.

16. Magage S, Lubanda JC, Susa Z, et al. Natural history of the respiratory involvement in Anderson-Fabry disease. *J Inherit Metab Dis.* 2007;30:790-799.

17. Kim W, Pyeritz RE, Bernhardt BA, Casey M, Litt HI. Pulmonary manifestations of Fabry disease and positive response to enzyme replacement therapy. *Am J Med Gen part A.* 2007;143A:377-381.

18. Wang RY, Abe JT, Cohen AH, Wilcox WR. Enzyme replacement therapy stabilizes obstructive pulmonary Fabry disease associated with respiratory globotriaosylceramide storage. *J Inherit Metab Dis.* 2008;31(suppl 2):S369-S374.

19. Koskenvuo JW, Kantola IM, Nuutila P, et al. Cardiopulmonary involvement in Fabry's disease. *Acta Cardiol.* 2010;65:185-192.

20. Franzen D, Krayenbuehl PA, Lidove O, Aubert JD, Barbey F. Pulmonary involvement in Fabry disease: overview and perspective. *Eur J Intern Med.* 2013.

21. Gaggl M, Kain R, Jaksch P, et al. *A single lung transplant in a patient with Fabry disease: Causality or far-fetched? A case report. Case Rep Transplant.* 2013;2013:905743.

22. Kelly MM, Leigh R, McKenzie R, Kamada D, Ramsdale EH, Hargreave FE. Induced sputum examination: diagnosis of pulmonary involvement in Fabry's disease. *Thorax.* 2000;55:720-721.

23. Mehta A. Epidemiology and natural history of Gaucher's disease. *Eur J Intern Med.* 2006;17:S2-S5.

24. Pastores GM, Hughes DA. Gaucher disease. July 27, 2000 [Updated July 21, 2011]. In: Pagon RA, Adam MP, Bird TD, et al. eds. *GeneReviews*™ [Internet]. Seattle (WA): University of Washington, Seattle; 1993-2013.

25. Goitein O, Elstein D, Abrahamov A, et al. Lung involvement and enzyme replacement therapy in Gaucher's disease. *Q J Med.* 2001;94(8):407-415.

26. Kerem E, Elstein D, Abrahamov A. Pulmonary function abnormalities in type I Gaucher disease. *Eur Respir J.* 1996;9:164-166.

27. Santamaria F, Parenti G, Guidi G, et al. Pulmonary manifestations of Gaucher disease. An increased risk for L444P homozygotes? *Am J Respir Crit Care Med.* 1998;157:985-989.

28. Lo SM, Liu J, Chen F, et al. Pulmonary vascular disease in Gaucher disease: clinical spectrum, determinants of phenotype and long-term outcomes of therapy. *J Inherit Metab Dis.* 2011;34:643-650.

29. Kim JH, Park CH, Pai MS, Hahn MH, Kim HJ. Hepatopulmonary syndrome in Gaucher disease with right-to-left shunt: evaluation and measurement using Tc-99m MAA. *Clin Nucl Med.* 1999;24:164e6.

30. Goitein O, Elstein D, Abrahamov A, et al. Lung involvement and enzyme replacement therapy in Gaucher's disease. *QJ Med.* 2001;94:407-415.

31. Lee SY, Mak AW, Huen KF, Lam ST, Chow CB. Gaucher disease with pulmonary involvement in a 6-year-old girl: report of resolution of radiographic abnormalities on increasing dose of imiglucerase. *J Pediatr.* 2001;139:862-864.

32. Banjar H, Tulbah A, Ozand P. Pediatric pulmonary Gaucher disease: two patterns of lung involvement. *Ann Saudi Med.* 1997;17:464-467.

33. Amir G, Ron N. Pulmonary pathology in Gaucher's disease. *Hum Pathol.* 1999;30:666-670.

34. Miller A, Brown LK, Pastores GM, Desnick RJ. Pulmonary involvement in type 1 Gaucher disease: functional and exercise findings in patients with and without clinical interstitial lung disease. *Clin Genet.* 2003;63:368-376.

35. Allen TC. Pulmonary Langerhans cell histiocytosis and other pulmonary histiocytic diseases: a review. *Arch Pathol Lab Med.* 2008;132:1171-1181.

36. Djordjević M, Minic P, Sarajlija A, Djuricic SM, Djokic D, Markovic O. Pulmonary involvement in siblings with Gaucher disease type III. *Vojnosanit Pregl.* 2011;68:1071-1074.

37. Bernstein DL, Hulkova H, Bialer MG, Desnick RJ. Cholesteryl ester storage disease: review of the findings in 135 reported patients with an underdiagnosed disease. *J Hepatol.* 2013;58:1230-1243.

38. Elleder M, Chlumska A, Hyanek J, et al. Subclinical course of cholesteryl ester storage disease in an adult with hypercholesterolemia, accelerated atherosclerosis, and liver cancer. *J Hepatol.* 2000;32:528-534.

39. Ambler GK, Hoare M, Brais R, et al. Orthotopic liver transplantation in an adult with cholesterol ester storage disease. *JIMD Rep.* 2013;8:41-46.

40. Michels VV, Driscoll DJ, Ferry GD, Duff DF, Beaudet AL. Pulmonary vascular obstruction associated with cholesteryl ester storage disease. *J Pediatr.* 1979;94:621-623.

41. Cagle PT, Ferry GD, Beaudet AL, Hawkins EP. Clinicopathologic conference: pulmonary hypertension in an 18-year-old girl with cholesteryl ester storage disease (CESD). *Am J Med Genet.* 1986;24:711-722.

42. Boissy RE, Richmond B, Huizing M, et al. Melanocyte-specific proteins are aberrantly trafficked in melanocytes of Hermansky-Pudlak syndrome-type 3. *Am J Pathol.* 2005;166:231-240.

43. Huizing M, Gahl WA. Disorders of vesicles of lysosomal lineage: the Hermansky-Pudlak syndromes. *Curr Mol Med.* 2002;2:451-467.

44. Izquierdo NJ, Royuela MA, Maumenee IH. Possible origins of the gene of Hermansky-Pudlak in Puerto Rico. *PR Health Sci J.* 1993;12:147-148.

45. Witkop CJ, Nunez Babcock M, Rao GH, et al. Albinism and Hermansky-Pudlak syndrome in Puerto Rico. *Bol Asoc Med PR.* 1990;82:333-339.

46. Gahl WA, Huizing M. Hermansky-Pudlak syndrome. July 24, 2000 Jul 24 [Updated February 28, 2013]. In: Pagon RA, Adam MP, Bird TD, et al. eds. *GeneReviews*™ [Internet]. Seattle (WA): University of Washington, Seattle; 1993-2013. Available from: http://www.ncbi.nlm.nih.gov/books/NBK1287/.

CHAPTER 28

47. Pierson DM, Ionescu D, Qing G, et al. Pulmonary fibrosis in Hermansky-Pudlak syndrome. *Respiration.* 2006;7:382-395.

48. Brantly M, Avila NA, Shortelersuk V, Lucero C, Huizing M, Gahl WA. Pulmonary function and high-resolution CT findings in patients with an inherited form of pulmonary fibrosis, Hermansky-Pudlak syndrome, due to mutations in HPS-1. *Chest.* 2000;117:129-136.

49. Mahavadi P, Guenther A, Gochuico BR. Hermansky-Pudlak syndrome interstitial pneumonia. It's the epithelium, stupid! *Am J Respir Crit Care Med.* 2012;186:939-940.

50. Avila NA, Brantly M, Premkumar A, Huizing M, Dwyer A, Gahl WA. Hermansky-Pudlak syndrome: radiography and CT of the chest compared with pulmonary function tests and genetic studies. *AJR.* 2002;179:887-892.

51. Tager AM, Sharma A, Mark EJ. Case 32-2009: a 27-year-old man with progressive dyspnea. *N Engl J Med.* 2009;361:1585-1593.

52. Nakatani Y, Nakamura N, Sano J, et al. Interstitial pneumonia in Hermansky-Pudlak syndrome: significance of florid foamy swelling/degeneration (giant lamellar body degeneration) of type-2 pneumocytes. *Virchows Arch.* 2000;437:304-313.

29 Large Airway Diseases

Michael P. Sedrak, Jason T. Koshy and Timothy Craig Allen

TAKE HOME PEARLS

- Smoking is the most common cause of chronic bronchitis.
- Common histologic findings include chronic subepithelial bronchial inflammation and bronchial gland hyperplasia and hypertrophy.
- Cystic fibrosis is caused by a mutation of the *CFTR* gene located on chromosome 7.
- There are over 900 known mutations of *CFTR*, the most common being the delta 508.
- The major bacterial pathogen in cystic fibrosis is *Pseudomonas aeruginosa*.
- Tracheobronchopathia osteochondroplastica is defined as the abnormal deposition of bone or cartilage in the tracheobronchial tree.
- It is present on the anterior and lateral aspects of the large airways.
- The exact etiology of tracheobronchopathia osteochondroplastica is unknown.

CHRONIC BRONCHITIS

Etiologies of Chronic Bronchitis

The most common cause of chronic bronchitis (CB) is cigarette smoking.[1] Smoking impairs respiratory ciliary movement and macrophage activity and also causes hypertrophy and hyperplasia of mucus secreting glands.[2] The net effect of these events is the buildup of mucus facilitation of pathogen growth. Most (70%-80%) acute exacerbations of CB are estimated to be due to viral and bacterial respiratory infections.[3] Common bacterial causes of these acute exacerbations include *Haemophilus influenza, Moraxella catarrhalis*, and *Streptococcus pneumoniae*; and viral causes include adenovirus, influenza, and parainfluenza. Repeated infections cause persistent inflammation and further damage to lung parenchyma. Less common causes of CB include air pollution and occupational exposures such as silica dust.

Clinical Features of Chronic Bronchitis

Chronic bronchitis has no sex predilection, and affected patients typically share the same clinical history of long-term smoking. CB is clinically defined as a productive cough of at least 3 months duration for two consecutive years with other causes of the cough being ruled out. Because CB is part of the COPD spectrum, patients tend to take a longer time exhaling than inhaling. Worsening dyspnea and wheezing may be signs of an acute exacerbation of CB. Fluoroquinolones such as moxifloxacin have been shown to be effective in treating bacteria-caused exacerbations of CB.[4] As with most chronic lung diseases, cardiac function may be affected in some patients presenting with cor pulmonale. This is typically due to pulmonary hypertension caused by chronic hypoxia and tissue destruction secondary to CB.

Imaging Features of Chronic Bronchitis

Chest radiograph of patients with CB are often unremarkable.[5] Nonspecific findings include bronchial wall

611

thickening and increased lung markings.[6] Pulmonary hyperexpansion is another common x-ray finding. In high-resolution CT scan, small pits can often be detected along the inner surfaces of large bronchi and when multiple, causing an "accordion-like" appearance.[7]

Histologic Features of Chronic Bronchitis

Chronic subepithelial bronchial inflammation is typically seen histologically in patients with CB. When directly caused by a respiratory infection, necrosis of the mucosa can be seen.[8] Bronchial gland hypertrophy and hyperplasia is also present. The Reid index, defined as the ratio of the gland thickness to the bronchial wall thickness measured from the epithelial basement membrane to the perichondrium, is often used to make a diagnosis of chronic bronchitis postmortem.[9] A normal Reid index is less than 0.4 while a greater value is indicative of CB. Anthracotic pigment deposition is characteristic, as virtually all CB patients are or have been smokers. Other CB findings include squamous metaplasia of the bronchial epithelium and smooth muscle hypertrophy. However, these findings are nonspecific as they are often present secondary to any chronic lung injury.

CYSTIC FIBROSIS

Etiologies of Cystic Fibrosis

Cystic fibrosis (CF) is an autosomal recessive disease caused by a mutation in the *CFTR* gene which encodes for a transmembrane conductance regulator. Normally the protein regulates the conductance of negatively charged ions such as chloride out of the cell. If the *CFTR* gene is mutated chloride cannot be properly removed from the cell and as a result, chloride and sodium ions accumulate within cells, thereby drawing fluid into the cells and causing dehydration of the mucus that normally coats these surfaces.[10] The result is the buildup of thick extracellular mucus, causing the well-known pulmonary manifestations of CF. There are over 900 known mutations of the *CFTR* gene, located on chromosome 7, associated with clinical disease.[11] These mutations can cause defective protein synthesis, defective maturation, blocked activation, reduced channel conductance, decreased abundance, or impaired regulation. The most common mutation is the delta 508, a three nucleotide deletion resulting in the loss of the amino acid phenylalanine.[12] Because of the autosomal recessive nature of its transmission, mutations in both the paternal and maternal alleles are required for disease presentation.[13]

Clinical Manifestations of Cystic Fibrosis

The clinical presentation of CF is variable due to its multiorgan distribution. *CFTR* is normally expressed in the epithelium of the skin, lungs, pancreas, liver, and gastrointestinal tract. In the lung, infection is currently recognized as the major cause of mortality in patients with CF. Excessive mucus builds up, causing airway obstruction that leads to respiratory symptoms such as chronic cough, wheezing, shortness of breath, and sputum production. This excessive mucoid environment also facilitates bacterial growth. The major bacterial pathogen in CF is *Pseudomonas aeruginosa* while other common bacteria seen include *Staphylococcus aureus, Haemophilus influenzae, Stenotrophomonas maltophilia, Achromobacter xylosoxidans,* and *Burkholderia* species.[14] Bronchiectasis, part of the chronic obstructive pulmonary disorder spectrum, is another complication of CF. This occurs when excessive mucus in the airways causes chronic infection and inflammation. The excessive inflammation causes bronchiolar smooth muscle to break down leading to abnormal dilation of the airways. As with other chronic lung injury processes, cardiac complications such as cor pulmonale are common in patients with CF.

Imaging Features of Cystic Fibrosis

No radiologic finding is considered diagnostic of CF but there are characteristic features. On chest x-ray lung hyperinflation with flattening of the diaphragm is frequently seen and thought to be an early finding in CF. Atelectasis is seen when mucus plugging is extensive. Bronchiectasis is the most common finding seen on CT scan and is also secondary to mucus buildup. Consolidation due to bacterial pneumonia is often seen. Cystic lung changes are a sign of later stage disease.

Gross Features of Cystic Fibrosis

Grossly CF lungs are enlarged and edematous. The cut surface reveals consolidation of lung parenchyma. Large and small airways are dilated and frequently filled with mucus plugs. Cysts and parenchymal fibrosis are often seen in severe cases.

Histologic Features of Cystic Fibrosis

Microscopically, CF lungs show correlation with the classic gross findings. Extensive infiltration of intra-alveolar neutrophils, cellular debris, and fluid draw a parallel with the gross findings of consolidation. Microabscess formation and mucin filled airways with muciphages are classic findings. In areas of chronic disease, fibrosis and cyst formation can predominate.

TRACHEOBRONCHOPATHIA OSTEOCHONDROPLASTICA

Etiologies of Tracheobronchopathia Osteochondroplastica

Tracheobronchopathia osteochondroplastica (TO) is a rare disease of unknown etiology characterized by bony or cartilaginous submucosal nodules that project into the tracheobronchial lumen.[15] Though a direct relationship has yet to be proven, malignancy, familial inheritance, chronic inflammation, metabolic disorders, and amyloidosis are thought to correlate with presence of TO.[16] There are two theories to the pathogenesis of this disease. The first, by Virchow, posits the formation of enchondromas which undergo calcification and ossification leading to nodule formation.[17] The second, by Aschoff-Freiburg, posits the ossification of elastic connective tissue.[18]

Clinical Features of Tracheobronchopathia Osteochondroplastica

Approximately 300 cases of TO have been reported since it was first described in 1857.[19] Symptoms of disease include shortness of breath, chronic cough, sputum production, and chest tightness.[20] However, many patients are asymptomatic and accordingly the incidence of TO is likely underreported. Patients are typically middle age and there is a male predilection. The treatment of TO is symptomatic, with some patients showing improvement with inhaled corticosteroids. Complete removal of this lesion is not thought to be necessary.

Imaging Features of Tracheobronchopathia Osteochondroplastica

Using fiberoptic bronchoscopy, the submucosal nodules in TO can be easily visualized and biopsied. Chest x-ray can be normal; however, CT scan often shows the characteristic pattern of calcification of the anterior and lateral aspects of the large airway wall. The posterior aspect of the trachea is always spared as it lacks cartilage.

Gross Features of Tracheobronchopathia Osteochondroplastica

TO is limited to the large airways and does not involve lung parenchyma or other organs.[21] It is most commonly observed in the distal two-thirds of the trachea and proximal bronchi but it can be seen anywhere from the larynx to the peripheral bronchi.[22] The distinguishing gross feature of TO is the presence of multiple smooth white submucosal nodules on the anterior and/or lateral aspects of the large airways giving rise to a "cobblestone" like appearance to the lumen.

Histologic Features of Tracheobronchopathia Osteochondroplastica

The pathology of TO is found in the submucosa, with islands of benign cartilage, calcification and bone expanding the submucosa and creating grossly identifiable lumen-narrowing nodules. The bronchial mucosa may contain chronic inflammation with varying degrees of squamous metaplasia. Ulceration of the mucosa is uncommon but may occasionally occur in symptomatic patients.

BRONCHIECTASIS

Bronchiectasis is defined as abnormal permanent dilation of the cartilaginous airways (bronchi) and often has an associated acute or chronic inflammatory infiltrate.[23,24] There is a broad spectrum of pathologic findings and severity that can be seen in bronchiectasis. Mild cases have subtle dilation that may only be noted microscopically by comparing adjacent bronchial artery, which is normally of similar size. Severe cases may exhibit striking, grossly observable dilatation with dilated airways extending almost to the pleural surface. There are numerous causes of bronchiectasis, some of which predominantly affect the lung while others are systemic disorders (Table 29-1).[25,26]

Clinical Features of Bronchiectasis

All ages and both sexes can be affected by bronchiectasis. Patients may be asymptomatic or symptomatic with the former identified radiographically and only symptomatic during disease exacerbation. Frequent symptoms include purulent sputum, cough, dyspnea, fever, and hemoptysis. Patients may also have coexisting sinusitis. Acute exacerbations are identified by increased cough, breathlessness, sputum production, and pleuritic chest pain. Physical examination of the chest in patients with bronchiectasis reveals the presence of crackles, squeaks/rhonchi, and rarely clubbing.[27,28]

Sputum microscopy, culture, and cytology are often useful. A variety of organisms may infect individuals with bronchiectasis and management requires cultures with appropriate sensitivity studies or serologic tests for the diagnosis of viral and other nonbacterial pneumonias.

TABLE 29-1 Associations and Causes of Bronchiectasis

Systemic Disorders
Collagen vascular diseases
  Sjögren syndrome
  Rheumatoid arthritis
  Ankylosing spondylitis
  Systemic lupus erythematosus

Celiac disease
Inflammatory bowel disease
Sarcoidosis
Human immunodeficiency virus (HIV) infection
Amyloidosis

Conditions Predominantly Affecting the Lung
Postinfectious bronchial damage
  Bacteria (Pseudomonas, Haemophilus)
  Virus (influenza virus, adenovirus)
  Fungi (Aspergillus species)

Abnormal host defense
  Primary
    Hypogammaglobulinemia
    Complement deficiency

  Secondary
    Malignancy (chronic lymphocytic leukemia),
      immune modulation following transplantation,
      chemotherapy

Mechanical bronchial obstruction
  Intrinsic: foreign body, viscid secretions, tumor
  Extrinsic: tumor, adenopathy

Congenital
  Cystic fibrosis
  Pulmonary sequestration
  Miscellaneous anomalies (T:E fistula, bronchomalacia,
    ectopic bronchi, bronchial cysts)
  α_1-Antitrypsin deficiency
  Ciliary dysfunction (Kartagener syndrome,
    immotile cilia)
  Marfan syndrome

Asthma
Middle lobe syndrome
Noninfectious postinflammatory pneumonitis
  Aspiration
  Inhalation of toxins

Idiopathic pulmonary fibrosis
Idiopathic

Imaging Features of Bronchiectasis

The sensitivity of chest radiographs is low, and many patients have no or nonspecific abnormalities. Plain films may show parallel linear opacities in a "tram track" appearance that correspond to thickened bronchial walls. Tubular opacities may be seen and correspond to mucus-filled bronchi. Cystic spaces with air fluid levels may also be seen.

High-resolution CT can readily diagnose bronchiectasis with high sensitivity and specificity.[29] Radiologic diagnosis can be rendered with one or more of the following findings: internal bronchial diameter greater than that of the adjacent pulmonary artery; visualization of bronchi abutting the mediastinal pleura; lack of bronchial narrowing in which the bronchus maintains the same diameter before, and for more than 2 cm after, branching. The appearance of ectatic bronchi on HRCT depends on the type of bronchiectasis (cylindrical, cystic, or varicose) and on the orientation of the bronchi. In cylindrical bronchiectasis with a horizontal course appears as parallel lines (tram tracks) while a vertical course creates a "signet-ring" appearance with the internal bronchial diameter larger than the supplying pulmonary artery. Cystic bronchiectasis results in a cluster of thin-walled cystic spaces with air-fluid levels. Varicose bronchiectasis is characterized by nonuniform bronchial dilatation.[30-32]

Gross Features of Bronchiectasis

The gross findings of bronchiectasis are well described from autopsy studies. Fewer than half of cases of bronchiectasis are bilateral. The lower lobes are more frequently involved. Fully developed cases of bronchiectasis have a dramatic appearance with dilated bronchi that may be filled with tenacious mucopurulent secretions. The clinical significance, if any, of the gross classification of the forms of bronchiectasis, noted above, has yet to be determined. Transverse ridging by hypertrophied circular smooth muscle bundles may be seen. Mild bronchiectasis may be difficult to appreciate in collapsed lobes (*Figure 29-1*).

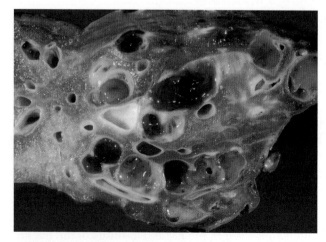

FIGURE 29-1 Gross image of bronchiectasis, showing dilated bronchi filled with mucopurulent secretions.

Histologic Features of Bronchiectasis

There is a wide range of histologic findings in bronchiectasis. Some cases have mild histologic changes which correlate with a lack of signs and symptoms, while severe, symptomatic cases can have florid acute and chronic inflammation with fibrosis. The bronchial wall often exhibits chronic inflammation with ulcerated or metaplastic mucosa. The lumen may be filled with acute inflammation and mucopurulent or necrotic debris (*Figure 29-2*). On bronchoscopic biopsy, necrotic debris associated with bronchiectasis may suggest an underlying neoplastic process with necrosis, but a broad differential diagnosis and strict adherence to diagnostic criteria provide the best approach to avoid confusion. Severe cases may show transmural destruction of the bronchial wall including the mucosa, submucosa, muscularis propria, and cartilage. These changes are not restricted to bronchi and may be seen in distal bronchioles as well. Occasionally, neuroendocrine cell hyperplasia may arise along small bronchi and bronchioles.

Secondary alveolar changes may occur, particularly if there is associated pneumonia. Specific changes depend on the chronicity of pneumonia and include acute bronchopneumonia, organizing bronchopneumonia, organizing pneumonia with septal fibrosis, and intra-alveolar macrophages. Pleural fibrosis and lymphoid hyperplasia may be seen, the latter may raise the concern for a lymphoproliferative disorder in transbronchial biopsy specimens. Zones of atelectasis alternating with zones of emphysema may be seen. Finally, fibrotic zones of lung tissue may have all the features of honeycomb change with mucus pooling and metaplastic epithelium and may raise the possibility of primary pulmonary interstitial fibrosing diseases such as usual interstitial fibrosis.

MIDDLE LOBE SYNDROME

Middle lobe syndrome is a disease of chronic airway obstruction and fixed atelectasis of the right middle lobe. The syndrome includes other downstream effects of obstruction such as bronchitis and bronchiolitis-associated parenchymal changes.

Etiologies of Middle Lobe Syndrome

The position and relatively long and narrow bronchus of the right middle lobe and lingula are thought to be predisposed to obstruction. Early studies highlighted cases in children and proposed compression of the bronchial tree in the right middle lobe and lingula by lymphoid hyperplasia.[33] Later studies demonstrated more common occurrence in adults due to obstruction from a variety of etiologies and associations summarized in *Table 29-2*, while some cases have no recognizable cause for obstruction.[34,35]

Clinical Features of Middle Lobe Syndrome

Middle lobe syndrome can be seen in a wide age range and can affect males and females. The most common presentation is a middle-aged or elderly woman (so-called Lady Windemere syndrome) presenting with chronic cough, hemoptysis, chest pain, dyspnea, or

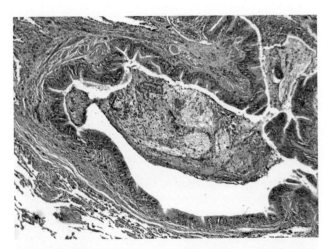

FIGURE 29-2 Medium power image of bronchiectasis showing dilated bronchial lumen containing mucopurulent debris.

TABLE 29-2 Associations and Causes of Middle Lobe Syndrome

Nonneoplastic Associations and Causes
Intrinsic bronchial obstruction
Foreign body aspiration
Edema of bronchial mucosa
Submucosal fibrosis/scarring
Granulation tissue
Reactive lymph node hyperplasia
Broncholithiasis
Extrinsic bronchial obstruction
Calcification/lymphadenopathy
Esophageal traction diverticula
Granulomatous infection (tuberculosis, histoplasmosis)
Neoplastic Causes
Benign or malignant; primary or metastatic
Result in obstruction by endobronchial mass or extrinsic bronchial compression

fever—all symptoms that are typical of chronic recurrent atelectasis. Severe asthma complicated by mucus plugging of the bronchus may manifest as middle lobe syndrome.[36] Occasionally, patients may be asymptomatic but have abnormal radiographs.

Imaging Features of Middle Lobe Syndrome

Radiography demonstrates consolidation of the right middle lobe or lingula accompanied by bronchiectasis and consolidation of the lung parenchyma. Patchy infiltrates, broncholithiasis, and pleural effusions are less commonly seen.[37]

Gross Features of Middle Lobe Syndrome

There is a wide range of gross features that can be observed in middle lobe syndrome depending on the activity and chronicity of the process. Bronchiectasis with or without foreign body material or mucus plugging may be seen causing bronchial obstruction and downstream atelectasis.

Histologic Features of Middle Lobe Syndrome

The most common findings in middle lobe syndrome are bronchiectasis, follicular bronchiolitis, and organizing pneumonia. Atelectasis, necrotizing and nonnecrotizing granulomatous inflammation and abscesses also frequently occur. In cases with granulomatous inflammation, acid-fast stain may highlight mycobacterial organisms. Often *Mycobacterium avium-intracellulare* or *Mycobacterium fortuitum* can be identified. Hemosiderosis and interstitial fibrosis with honeycomb change may also be seen. Although these findings are nonspecific, the diagnosis of middle lobe syndrome is appropriate when the disease is restricted to the right noddle lobe and/or lingula.

MUCOID IMPACTION

Mucoid impaction is a distinct clinicopathologic syndrome with mucus plugs in dilated segmental and/or subsegmental bronchi. The mucus characteristically has the appearance of so-called "allergic mucin."[38-40]

Clinical Features of Mucoid Impaction

Many patients with mucoid impaction have an underlying allergic disease, often asthma or allergic bronchopulmonary aspergillosis and, less frequently, chronic bronchitis or cystic fibrosis. Patients may have symptoms related to the underlying condition, obstructive pneumonia beyond the impaction, or may be asymptomatic with characteristic radiologic findings.

Imaging Features of Mucoid Impaction

The radiographic findings in patients with mucoid impaction of the bronchi are characteristic with branching or band-like densities arranged in a bronchial distribution. They tend to involve the upper lobes. The opacities have a "gloved finger sign" or "inverted V or Y" appearance. Upon removal of the inspissated mucus, residual bronchial dilatation may be the only finding. Occasionally, a solitary nodule may be observed.[41,42]

Gross Features of Mucoid Impaction

Gross examination reveals dilated, firm bronchi that contain brownish to green tenacious mucus (*Figure 29-3*).

Histologic Features of Mucoid Impaction

Mucoid impaction is characterized histologically by bronchi distended by mucus with a laminated appearance. It must be present before the diagnosis is invoked because mucus plugging can occur in a number of airway diseases. The layers are composed of eosinophils, fibrin, neutrophils, mucus, eosinophil cytoplasmic granular debris, and Charcot-Leyden crystals. The crystals are elongated and hexagonal brightly eosinophilic structures that range in size from several microns to nearly 100 μm.

Changes seen in asthma including goblet cell hyperplasia and thickened basement membrane may accompany changes that result from compression by the impaction.[43] Compression changes include mural

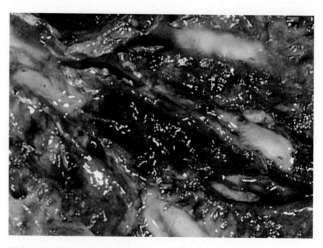

FIGURE 29-3 Gross image of mucoid impaction showing dilated, firm bronchi containing tenacious mucus.

thinning, cartilaginous atrophy, and epithelial metaplasia including squamous metaplasia. It is prudent to perform fungal stains whenever "allergic mucin" is found. Staining may highlight fungal hyphae in cases of allergic bronchopulmonary fungal disease, which may manifest as mucoid impaction.

BRONCHOCENTRIC GRANULOMATOSIS

Bronchocentric granulomatosis is granulomatous and necrotizing destruction of bronchial mucous membrane lining with palisaded histiocytes.

Etiologies of Bronchocentric Granulomatosis

Bronchocentric granulomatosis is a pathologic reaction pattern that can have noninfectious and infectious etiologies. Noninfectious etiologies include rheumatoid arthritis, Wegener granulomatosis, and allergic bronchopulmonary fungal disease. Infectious causes include mycobacterial infections, most commonly tuberculosis and mycobacterium avium intracellulare. Fungal infections have also been linked to bronchocentric granulomatosis, most commonly histoplasmosis, blastomycosis, and coccidiomycosis. Rarely, echinococcosis has produced this pattern of injury.[44]

Clinical Features of Bronchocentric Granulomatosis

Most commonly bronchocentric granulomatosis is identified in the setting of a hypersensitivity reaction, often chronic asthma or allergic bronchopulmonary aspergillosis. Patients typically present with cough, wheezing, fever, and peripheral eosinophilia.

Imaging Features of Bronchocentric Granulomatosis

Bronchocentric granulomatosis often has radiographic findings similar to mucoid impaction, which may be associated. These include band-like or branching opacities in a bronchial distribution and subsequent parenchymal consolidation. In patients without an underlying hypersensitivity, speculated nodules may be seen measuring up to 5 cm.[45]

Gross Features of Bronchocentric Granulomatosis

Gross examination of bronchocentric granulomatosis shows bronchi and large bronchioles replaced by necrotic "cheesy" material. Cases associated with hypersensitivity, either asthma or allergic bronchopulmonary aspergillosis, have tenacious green mucus distending the bronchi, typical of mucoid impaction.

Histologic Features of Bronchocentric Granulomatosis

Microscopic examination demonstrates granulomas with central necrosis and an outward rim of plump palisaded histiocytes where one would expect bronchi, specifically adjacent to pulmonary arteries. Elastin stain may be used to visualize the remnant of the single elastic membrane of the bronchial walls amidst the necrosis and acute and chronic inflammation, often including eosinophils. Densely aggregated eosinophilic granules can induce a foreign body–like giant cell reaction.

Foci of residual bronchi with only partial replacement by necrotizing granulomas may be seen, with the lumina filled with necrotic debris. Hypersensitivity-associated bronchocentric granulomatosis may also have mucoid impaction of the proximal airway with allergic mucin and downstream lung parenchyma containing a mixed inflammatory infiltrate typical of obstructive pneumonia. Special stains for mycobacterial and fungal organisms should routinely be performed to exclude infectious etiologies; fungal stain may also be useful in identifying degenerating organisms in allergic bronchopulmonary aspergillosis.

BRONCHOLITHIASIS

Broncholiths are calcified material in the airways, most commonly representing calcified lymph nodes that have partially or completely eroded through the bronchial wall. Broncholithiasis may also be complicated by bronchial obstruction or severe distortion of the tracheobronchial tree.[46-48]

Etiologies of Broncholithiasis

Tuberculosis and histoplasmosis are two of the most common causes of old calcified granulomas involving regional lymph nodes that compress and erode adjacent bronchi, resulting in broncholithiasis.

Clinical Features of Broncholithiasis

Broncholithiasis affects men and women equally, most often in the sixth decade, although there is a broad age range. Symptoms include hemoptysis, cough, fever, chills, wheezing, and distinctly, albeit rarely, expectorating calcified material (lithoptysis).

Imaging Features of Broncholithiasis

Key radiographic features include calcified peribronchial or endobronchial lymph nodes with associated bronchial distortion and, depending on the degree of bronchial compression, atelectasis, bronchiectasis, and air trapping.[49]

Gross Features of Broncholithiasis

Calcified lymph nodes are identified distorting or eroding into the airways with a connecting sinus tract. Additional complications of broncholithiasis may be seen including hemorrhage and downstream effects including parenchymal consolidation.

Histologic Features of Broncholithiasis

Microscopically, a lymph node with old calcified granulomas and surrounding chronic inflammation and fibrosis are characteristic features. Fungal stains may be performed to help identify organisms within the granulomas. Acute inflammation often accompanies erosion into the bronchial lumen. Secondary complications such as bronchiectasis and/or obstructive pneumonia may be seen.

ASTHMA

Etiologies of Asthma

Asthma is extremely common, involving up to 15 million people in the United States. It is mostly a disease of childhood, often associated with atopy; however, adults of any age can become asthmatics. Childhood atopy occurs via a genetic susceptibility to the development of hypersensitivity type I reactions to antigens such as fungi, pollen, and dust mites, with the production of IgE antibodies.[50] African Americans acquire asthma more frequently than Caucasians, and also exhibit a higher disease-related mortality. Adult-onset asthma is typically nonatopic, often termed "intrinsic asthma," and is induced nonallergenically by a variety of things such as cold, exercise, or viruses.[47]

Clinical Features of Asthma

Asthma is a disease characterized by acute, paroxysmal, generally reversible airway narrowing causing wheezing, dyspnea, and cough. It frequently exhibits airway hyperresponsiveness, intense bronchoconstriction due to various stimuli, resulting in dyspnea and wheezing. Asthma also characteristically exhibits airflow obstruction, caused by structural airway changes related to airway remodeling, edema, and mucus

plugging. The clinical diagnosis is generally based on the patient's symptoms, with or without measurement of airway hyperresponsiveness. Diagnosis in patients who have a greater than 10 pack-year history of smoking may require additional pulmonary function testing.

Imaging Features of Asthma

X-ray changes with asthma are nonspecific. Bronchial wall thickening and hyperinflation are common findings; however, many patients with asthma do not demonstrate hyperinflation. CT scan is typically not a part of the workup of a typical asthma patient; however, CT scan may be used for examining patients with ill-defined disease to exclude other etiologies such as hypersensitivity pneumonitis, or to evaluate for complications such as allergic bronchopulmonary aspergillosis.[51]

Gross Features of Asthma

Grossly, asthmatic lungs are overexpanded with areas of atelectasis. Predominantly in the upper lobes, bronchiectasis and mucus plugging may be widespread.

Histologic Features of Asthma

Biopsy is generally unnecessary for the diagnosis of asthma. Asthma is characterized histologically by marked goblet cell hyperplasia, bronchial and bronchiolar smooth muscle hyperplasia, basement membrane thickening, prominent mucus plugging, and a bronchiolocentric mixed inflammatory cell infiltrate, typically containing a prominent eosinophilic component, extending through the airway wall (*Figures 29-4* and *29-5*). Mast cells may be identified, some of which show degranulation. There may be some seromucinous

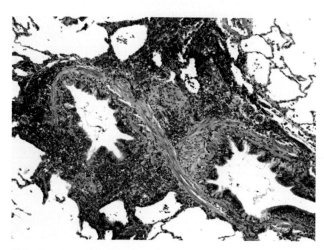

FIGURE 29-4 Medium power image of asthma showing smooth muscle hyperplasia and a bronchiolocentric mixed inflammatory cell infiltrate.

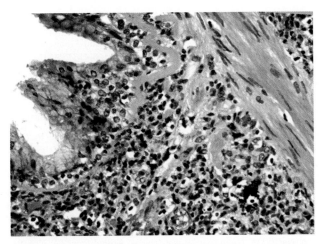

FIGURE 29-5 High-power image of asthma showing an abundance of eosinophils within the mixed inflammatory cell infiltrate.

gland hyperplasia, but the Reid index is not increased as it typically is in patients with chronic bronchitis. Curschmann spirals may be identified on sputum examination.[52,53]

ALLERGIC BRONCHOPULMONARY ASPERGILLOSIS

Clinical Features of Allergic Bronchopulmonary Aspergillosis

Allergic bronchopulmonary aspergillosis (ABPA) is a lung disease arising in approximately 15% of patients with asthma and cystic fibrosis, which is related to a hypersensitivity reaction to chronic Aspergillus airway colonization. It may occur at any age, and is clinically characterized by wheezing, fever, pulmonary infiltrates on chest x-ray, and increased sputum production. Increased spore counts during summer and autumn seasons may cause disease exacerbations in ABPA patients. Patients may develop acute disease, with pulmonary infiltrates, airway obstruction due to mucus plugging, and transient eosinophilia, and progress to chronic ABPA with increasing dyspnea due to progressive bronchiectasis and pulmonary fibrosis.[54]

Imaging Features of Allergic Bronchopulmonary Aspergillosis

Chest x-ray often shows transient bilateral upper lobe infiltrates in acute ABPA. As disease advances, CT scan exhibits increasing central bronchiectasis with mucus plugging and progressive pulmonary fibrosis, generally within the upper lobes.[55]

Gross Features of Allergic Bronchopulmonary Aspergillosis

Grossly, lungs show predominantly upper lobe involvement with mucus plugging, bronchiectasis, and variable amounts of end-stage lung fibrosis.

Histologic Features of Allergic Bronchopulmonary Aspergillosis

ABPA is not typically biopsied for diagnosis. Histologically, it exhibits mucus plugging and bronchiectasis with associated eosinophilic pneumonia and/or bronchocentric granulomatosis. Diagnosis rests on correlation of clinical, radiologic, and laboratory findings including peripheral blood eosinophilia, elevated total serum IgE, sputum eosinophilia, precipitating IgG antibodies to *Aspergillus*, and a positive skin prick test for *Aspergillus fumigatus* antigen. Treatment with steroids may alter the laboratory findings.[56]

REFERENCES

1. Decramer M, Janssens W, Miravitlles M. Chronic obstructive pulmonary disease. *Lancet*. April 2012;379(9823):1341-1351.
2. Jazeela F, Olade RB, Lessnau KD. Bronchitis. Medscape. March 2014. http://emedicine.medscape.com/article/297108-overview#aw2aab6b2b3aa.
3. Sethi S, Murphy TF. Infection in the pathogenesis and course of chronic obstructive pulmonary disease. *N Engl J Med*. November 2008;359(22):2355-2365.
4. Liu KX, Xu B, Wang J, et al. Efficacy and safety of moxifloxacin in acute exacerbations of chronic bronchitis and COPD: a systematic review and meta-analysis. *J Thorac Dis*. March 2014;6(3):221-229.
5. Takasugi J, Godwin J. Radiology of chronic obstructive pulmonary disease. *Radiol Clin North Am*. 1998;36:29-55.
6. Webb WR. Radiology of obstructive pulmonary disease. *Am J Roentgenal*. 1997;169:637-647.
7. Zompatori M, Zverzelatti N, Gentile T, Spagiarri L, Laporta T, Fecci L. Imaging of the patient with chronic bronchitis: an overview of old and new signs. *Radiol Med*. 2006;111:634-639.
8. Leslie KO, Wick MR. Pathology of the large and small airways. *Practical Pulmonary Pathology*. 2005;8:263; Elsevier.
9. Reid L. Pathology of chronic bronchitis. *Lancet*. 1954;1:275-278.
10. Cystic fibrosis (CF). *Encyclopædia Britannica. Encyclopædia Britannica Online*. Encyclopædia Britannica Inc, 2014. http://www.britannica.com/science/cystic-fibrosis.
11. Noone PG, Pue CA, Zhou Z, et al. Lung disease associated with the IVS8 5T allele of the CFTR gene. *Am J Respir Crit Care Med*. 2000;(162):1919-1924.
12. Loo TW, Bartlett MC, Clarke DM. Introduction of the most common cystic fibrosis mutation (ΔF508) into human P-glycoprotein disrupts packing of the transmembrane segments. *J Biol Chem*. 2002;277:27585-27588.
13. Warwick G, Elston C. Improving outcomes in patients with cystic fibrosis. *Practitioner*. 2011;255(1742):29-32, 3.
14. *Cystic Fibrosis Foundation Patient Registry 2009 Annual Data Report*. Bethesda, MD: Cystic Fibrosis Foundation; 2010.
15. Prakash UBS. Tracheobronchopathia osteochondroplastica. *Semin Respir Crit Care Med*. 2002;23(2);167-176.

620 Lung and Pleural Pathology

16. Zhang XB, Zeng HQ, Cai XY, Zhang YJ. Tracheobronchopathia osteochondroplastica: a case report and literature review. *J Thoracic Dis*. 2013;5(5):E182-E184.

17. Virchow R. *Die krankhaften Geschwülste*. Vol 1. Berlin: Hirschwald; 1863:442-443.

18. Aschoff-Freiburg L. Ueber Tracheopathia Osteoplastica. *Verh Dtsch Gesch Pathol*. 1910;14:125-127.

19. Laine M, Elfihri S, Kettani F, Bourkadi JE. Tracheobronchopathia osteochondroplastica associated with skin cancer: a case report and review of the literature. *BMC Res Notes*. 2014;7(1):637.

20. Zhu Y, Wu N, Huang HD, et al. A clinical study of tracheobronchopathia osteochondroplastica: findings from a large chinese cohort. *PLoS one*. 2014;9(7):e102068.

21. Abu-Hijleh M, Lee D, Braman SS. Tracheobronchopathia osteochondroplastica: a rare large airway disorder. *Lung*. 2008;186:353-359.

22. Jindal S, Nath A, Neyaz Z, Jaiswal S. Tracheobronchopathia osteochondroplastica—a rare or overlooked entity. *J Radiol Case Rep*. March 2013;7(3):16-25.

23. Heard BE, Khatchatourov V, Otto H, Putov NV, Sobin L. The morphology of emphysema, chronic bronchitis, and bronchiectasis: definition, nomenclature, and classification. *J Clin Pathol*. September 1979;32(9):882-892.

24. Whitwell F. A study of the pathology and pathogenesis of bronchiectasis. *Thorax*. September 1952;7(3):213-239.

25. Hansell DM. Bronchiectasis. *Radiol Clin North Am*. January 1998;36(1):107-128.

26. Barker AF. Bronchiectasis. *N Engl J Med*. May 2, 2002;346(18):1383-1393.

27. Nicotra MB, Rivera M, Dale AM, Shepherd R, Carter R. Clinical, pathophysiologic, and microbiologic characterization of bronchiectasis in an aging cohort. *Chest*. October 1995;108(4):955-961.

28. Sheikh S, Madiraju K, Steiner P, Rao M. Bronchiectasis in pediatric AIDS. *Chest*. November 5, 1997;112(5):1202-1207.

29. Kang EY, Miller RR, Müller NL. Bronchiectasis: comparison of preoperative thin-section CT and pathologic findings in resected specimens. *Radiology*. June 1995;195(3):649-654.

30. Grenier P, Maurice F, Musset D, Menu Y, Nahum H. Bronchiectasis: assessment by thin-section CT. *Radiology*. October 1986;161(1):95-99.

31. Young K, Aspestrand F, Kolbenstvedt A. High resolution CT and bronchography in the assessment of bronchiectasis. *Acta Radiol*. November 1991;32(6):439-441.

32. Kim JS1, Müller NL, Park CS, Grenier P, Herold CJ. Cylindrical bronchiectasis: diagnostic findings on thin-section CT. *AJR Am J Roentgenol*. March 1997;168(3):751-754.

33. Dees SC, Spock A. Right middle lobe syndrome in children. *JAMA*. July 4, 1966;197(1):8-14.

34. Eskenasy A, Eană-Iorgulescu L. Pathology of the middle lobe syndromes. A histopathological and pathogenetic analysis of sixty surgically-cured cases. *Med Interne*. January-March 1982;20(1):73-80.

35. Kwon KY, Myers JL, Swensen SJ, Colby TV. Middle lobe syndrome: a clinicopathological study of 21 patients. *Hum Pathol*. March 1995;26(3):302-307.

36. Nuhoğlu Y, Bahçeciler N, Yüksel M, et al. Thorax high resolution computerized tomography findings in asthmatic children with unusual clinical manifestations. *Ann Allergy Asthma Immunol*. March 1999;82(3):311-314.

37. Byrd R Jr, Payne JL, Roy TM. Lingular and middle lobe infiltrates in an elderly woman. *Chest*. October 1995;108(4):1156-1157.

38. Hutcheson JB, Shaw RR, Paulson DL, Kee JL Jr. Mucoid impaction of the bronchi. *Am J Clin Pathol*. May 1960;33:427-432.

39. Katzenstein AL, Liebow AA, Friedman PJ. Bronchocentric granulomatosis, mucoid impaction, and hypersensitivity reactions to fungi. *Am Rev Respir Dis*. April 1975;111(4):497-537.

40. Jelihovsky T. The structure of bronchial plugs in mucoid impaction, bronchocentric granulomatosis and asthma. *Histopathology*. March 1983;7(2):153-167.

41. Angus RM, Davies ML, Cowan MD, McSharry C, Thomson NC. Computed tomographic scanning of the lung in patients with allergic bronchopulmonary aspergillosis and in asthmatic patients with a positive skin test to Aspergillus fumigatus. *Thorax*. June 1994;49(6):586-589.

42. Neeld DA, Goodman LR, Gurney JW, Greenberger PA, Fink JN. Computerized tomography in the evaluation of allergic bronchopulmonary aspergillosis. *Am Rev Respir Dis*. November 1990;142(5):1200-1205.

43. Hogg JC. The pathology of asthma. *Clin Chest Med*. December 1984;5(4):567-571.

44. Bosken CH, Myers JL, Greenberger PA, Katzenstein AL. Pathologic features of allergic bronchopulmonary aspergillosis. *Am J Surg Pathol*. March 1988;12(3):216-222.

45. Ward S, Heyneman LE, Flint JD, Leung AN, Kazerooni EA, Müller NL. Bronchocentric granulomatosis: computed tomographic findings in five patients. *Clin Radiol*. April 2000;55(4):296-300.

46. Arrigoni MG, Bernatz PE, Donoghue FE. Broncholithiasis. *J Thorac Cardiovasc Surg*. August 1971;62(2):231-237.

47. Schmidt HW, Clagett OT, Mcdonald JR. Broncholithiasis. *J Thorac Surg*. February 1950;19(2):226-245.

48. Seo JB, Song KS, Lee JS, et al. Broncholithiasis: review of the causes with radiologic-pathologic correlation. *Radiographics*. October 2002;22 Spec No:S199-S213.

49. Conces DJ Jr, Tarver RD, Vix VA. Broncholithiasis: CT features in 15 patients. *AJR Am J Roentgenol*. August 1991;157(2):249-253.

50. Wardlaw AJ, Brightling CE, Green R, Woltmann G, Bradding P, Pavord ID. New insights into the relationship between airway inflammation and asthma. *Clin Sci (Lond)*. 2002;103:201-211.

51. Woods AQ, Lynch DA. Asthma: an imaging update. *Radiol Clin N Am*. 2009;317-329.

52. Beasley R, Burgess C, Crane J, Pearce N, Roche W. Pathology of asthma and its clinical implications. *J Allergy Clin Immunol*. 1993;92:148-154.

53. Kay AB. Pathology of mild, severe, and fatal asthma. *Am J Respir Crit Care Med*. 1996;154:S66-S69.

54. Franquet T, Muller Gimenez A, Guembe P, de la Torre J, Bague S. Spectrum of pulmonary aspergillosis: histologic, clinical, and radiologic findings. *Radiographics*. 2001;21:825-837.

55. Khan AN, Jones C, Macdonald S. Bronchopulmonary aspergillosis: a review. *Curr Probl Diagn Radiol*. 2003;32:156-168.

56. Levy MB. Allergic bronchopulmonary aspergillosis and cystic fibrosis. *Front Biosci*. 2003;8:s579-s583.

Molecular Diagnostics of Pulmonary Neoplasia

Sanja Dacic

TAKE HOME PEARLS

- Diagnostic samples from lung cancer patients may be used for molecular analyses.
- Type of tissue fixatives, fixation time, processing protocols, and storage conditions can affect the quality and quantity of DNA, RNA, and proteins in the specimens.
- Recent studies using more sensitive techniques, including next generation sequencing, have demonstrated homogeneity of driver mutations between primary tumors and metastases.
- Recently published CAP/IASLC/AMP guidelines for molecular testing in lung carcinoma recommend EGFR and *ALK* testing for adenocarcinomas and mixed lung cancers with an adenocarcinoma component.
- Assessment of the specimen adequacy for molecular analysis should be determined by each laboratory performing molecular testing.
- Selection of lung cancers for molecular testing is based on the diagnosis provided by the pathologist.

TUMOR TISSUE SAMPLE

The most common diagnostic specimens from lung cancer patients include sputum cytology, thoracentesis, transthoracic fine-needle aspirate, bronchoscopy including bronchoalveolar lavage, bronchial brush and wash, endobronchial and transbronchial biopsy, transbronchial needle aspiration (TBNA) and endobronchial ultrasound-needle aspiration (EBUS), endoscopic ultrasound-needle aspiration (EUS), and resection specimens. Diagnostic samples from lung cancer patients may be used for molecular analyses. Larger tumor samples, such as resection specimens, are preferred for any type of molecular analysis although that may not be always feasible. Cytology specimens (FNAs, or brushings) and needle core biopsies are frequently seen in diagnostic practice, but many older studies indicated that small samples may be insufficient for molecular analysis. They are more likely to fail the mutational analysis by direct Sanger sequencing or are frequently exhausted after diagnostic workup. However, in daily clinical practice, molecular assays should be able to utilize cytology specimens, otherwise many patients will be left without the benefit of molecular testing. Many recent studies have shown that molecular analysis can be successfully performed on cytology specimens particularly if cell blocks are available.[1-4] It has also been shown that smear preparations can be used for mutation assays, but may not be suitable for FISH analysis which requires nonoverlapping tumor cells.

TISSUE PROCESSING

Type of tissue fixatives, fixation time, processing protocols, and storage conditions can affect the quality and quantity of DNA, RNA, and proteins in the specimens.

PCR and FISH assays can be performed on fresh, frozen, formalin-fixed paraffin-embedded (FFPE), or alcohol-fixed specimens. The most commonly used fixative in pathology is 10% neutral-buffered formalin (NBF). The second most common fixative is alcohol (70% ethanol) particularly for cytology specimens. It is known that alcohol is equally good as10% NBF for DNA-based molecular assays.[5-7] Most molecular assays are inhibited by heavy metal fixatives (eg, Zenker, B5, B plus, acid zinc formalin (AZF)), due to competition between the metals in the fixative and the Mg needed as a cofactor for most DNA polymerases and other enzymes involved in molecular assays. Acidic solutions (eg, Bouin solution, bone decalcifying solutions) fragment DNA extensively.[6,7] Bone metastases are usually decalcified in acidic solutions, which makes molecular analysis very difficult. The use of nonacidic chelating decalcifying solutions may better preserve DNA for molecular testing. Specimens processed with heavy metal fixatives and acidic solutions should not be used for PCR or FISH assays. Fixation time can significantly impact quality and feasibility of molecular assays. Unfortunately, fixation time, except for HER2, is not standardized.[8-10] The most recent consensus was to adopt recommendations for HER2 testing which include fixation times of 6 to 12 hours for small biopsy samples and 8 to 18 hours for larger surgical specimens. According to the CAP Laboratory Accreditation Program Checklist, information about fixation times should be included in the pathology report.

SPECIMEN TYPE

Morphologic and molecular heterogeneity of lung adenocarcinoma has been extensively discussed in the literature.[8] Many older studies using different molecular methods and interpretation criteria reported molecular heterogeneity between different areas of the same tumor, as well as between primary tumors and metastases/recurrences.[9] However, more recent studies using more sensitive techniques, including next-generation sequencing, have demonstrated homogeneity of driver mutations between primary tumors and metastases.[10,11] These observations provide strong support for recommending that primary tumors or metastatic lesions are equally suitable for testing.[12-14] In cases with synchronous multiple primary tumors, molecular testing should be performed on each tumor. The choice of which sample to test should be based primarily on the specimen qualities themselves (tumor content and preservation), rather than whether they are primary or metastatic lesions. Patients should not be subjected to a procedure to obtain tissue from a metastasis prior to initiation of TKI therapy if a prior metastatic or primary lesion is available and is suitable for analysis. This is in contrast to patients who develop acquired resistance after an initially successful response to TKI who should be subjected to repeat tissue procurement for analysis of the mechanism of resistance.

To date, guidelines have not recommended gene amplification as a major selection criterion for targeted therapies. An argument can be made that gene amplification, unlike driver mutations, is a relatively late event in the progression of lung carcinoma, and therefore metastases may be a more suitable specimen for assessment of gene amplification rather than the primary tumor. This has to be further investigated in clinical trials that correlate gene amplification with patient response to targeted therapy.

TUMOR TYPE AND MOLECULAR TESTING

Adenocarcinoma and Mixed Adenocarcinoma

Recently published CAP/IASLC/AMP guidelines for molecular testing in lung carcinoma recommend EGFR and *ALK* testing for adenocarcinomas and mixed lung cancers with an adenocarcinoma component (eg, pleomorphic carcinoma, carcinosarcoma, adenosquamous). EGFR and *ALK* testing are not recommended for squamous cell carcinoma, small cell carcinoma, or large cell neuroendocrine carcinoma. Testing can be done in cases when an adenocarcinoma component cannot be excluded in a small sample or in cases with unusual clinical characteristics such as squamous cell carcinoma occurring in a never smoker. Recently, the proposed IASLC/ATS/ERS classification for lung adenocarcinoma emphasized associations between subtype of lung adenocarcinoma and genotype. However, the guidelines for molecular testing recommend that adenocarcinoma subtype should not be used as a selection criterion for molecular testing. Large cell carcinomas with adenocarcinoma immunophenotype should also be subjected to the recommended molecular testing for lung adenocarcinomas.

Squamous Cell Carcinoma

A spectrum of targetable or potentially targetable driver mutations and copy number changes in squamous cell carcinoma has been recently published.[15] Currently, there is no guideline for routine clinical molecular testing in squamous cell carcinoma outside of clinical trials.

ADEQUACY OF SPECIMEN FOR MOLECULAR TESTING

Assessment of the specimen adequacy for molecular analysis should be determined by each laboratory performing molecular testing. Only adequately processed specimens as discussed above should be considered for molecular analysis. It is important that a pathologist assess the tumor content in the specimen. A representative H&E slide should have a high proportion of tumor cells. Selected slides should have no or a minimal amount of admixed nonneoplastic cells (eg, lymphocytes, nonneoplastic lung). Similarly, necrotic tissue and abundant mucin should be avoided. The minimum percent of tumor cells required for molecular analysis is determined by the methodology used. For example, for unmodified Sanger sequencing, a minimum mutated allele frequency of 25% is required. That corresponds to a minimum cancer cell content of approximately 50% for heterozygous mutations with no polysomy or amplification. More sensitive mutation detection techniques have sensitivities in the range of 1% to 10%. These are general recommendations, and each laboratory must determine the minimum amount of tumor cells for each specimen type that will be accepted by the laboratory. Our laboratory requires an absolute minimum number of viable tumor cells per specimen for each test. For example, at least 300 viable tumor cells are required from a formalin-fixed paraffin embedded specimen submitted for unmodified Sangers sequencing. For FISH assays, at least 100 nonoverlapping, viable tumor cells are needed. Cases that do not meet these criteria are rejected as insufficient/inadequate for molecular studies. The tumor DNA content per specimen may be enriched by either manual or laser capture microdissection. A pathologist should review the representative H&E tumor slide and mark the area for microdissection. It is known that PCR- based assays in cases with a low copy number DNA template can generate sequence artifacts, mainly guanine to adenine transitions.

Selection of Tests

Molecular alterations and tumor histology are summarized in *Table 30-1*. The CAP/IASLC/AMP guideline for molecular testing of lung cancer provides guidelines for *EGFR* and *ALK* testing.[15-17] However, demand is increasing for more comprehensive testing of a larger number of potentially targetable genes. The underlying genetic alteration determines the type of molecular assay. Although numerous assays for the assessment of mutations are commercially available, laboratories may use any validated method with sufficient performance characteristics. In contrast, different methods for assessment of *ALK* rearrangement with similar diagnostic performance have been reported.[16-19] The Food and Drug Administration approved the *ALK* Break Apart FISH Probe Kit (Abbott Molecular, Des Plaines, IL) as a companion diagnostic for targeted therapy with crizotinib in lung cancers.

TABLE 30-1 Targetable Genetic Abnormalities in Main Histologic Subtypes of Non-Small-Cell Lung Carcinoma

Genetic abnormality	Adenocarcinoma (%)	Squamous Cell Carcinoma (%)
EGFR mutations	10-50	<1
KRAS mutations	10-30	6
ALK rearrangements	5	<1
BRAF mutations	2	2
PIK3CA		
Mutations	2	2
Amplification	6	30
MET amplification	3	10
HER2		
Mutation	4	<1
Amplification	6	2

Mutation Assays

A large number of mutational assays have been developed, and direct DNA sequencing was the method used in the initial trials that established EGFR mutations as predictors of response to EGFR-TKI (*Table 30-2*). There is no consensus agreement on which is the best assay, because each assay has certain advantages and disadvantages. The major advantage of DNA sequencing is that it can detect all mutations, including novel variants, and it identifies the exact mutation. In contrast, other mutational methods (eg, single-strand conformation polymorphism (SSCP), denaturing high performance liquid chromatography (DHPLC), amplification refractory mutation system [ARMS]) may miss mutations that are not assayed, but are more sensitive, requiring fewer tumor cells and less time than DNA sequencing. Laboratories may use any mutational method with clinically acceptable specificity and sensitivity for mutation detection. Since Sangers sequencing was, until recently, the most common method used in clinical practice, it is recommended that any other mutation method must be at least as sensitive as the Sanger sequencing technique. Turnaround time and spectrum of mutations detected are important and should be taken into consideration. It is believed that the ideal test should be able to detect mutations in specimens with 10% tumor cells. Interpretation of ultrasensitive tests should be made with caution as they may have a higher percentage of false-positive results. False-positive results can be a result of mispriming or low cross-contamination. High sensitivity methods may also detect small mutated subclones, which may not correlate well

TABLE 30-2 DNA Mutation Assays[42]

Method	Advantages	Disadvantages
Sanger-chain termination method	• Gold standard • Complete sequence	• Very time consuming • Cannot detect deletions, translocations, or copy number changes
Pyrosequencing—sequencing by synthesis method	• More sensitive than Sanger. Provides percentage of mutated versus wild-type DNA • Works well with fragmented DNA from FFPET samples	• Short read length limits technique to hot spots • Limited accuracy at detecting changes in homopolymer runs
Allele-specific RT-PCR	• Very high sensitivity • Widely used for clinical testing for oncogene mutations	• Scalability constraints limit application to hot spots
RT-PCR melting curve analysis	• High sensitivity • Provides percentage of mutated versus wild-type DNA	• Often difficult to resolve differences in melt curves • Difficult to standardize • Multiplex capability is limited
MS-based mutations analysis (MALDI-TOF)	• High sensitivity • High resolution of DNA fragments • Detects frame shift mutations and germline SNPs	• MS resolution window balanced with PCR amplicon design requirements combine to limit scalability

with the response to targeted therapy and may possibly represent artifactual mutations. Similarly, formalin fixation causes DNA damage that can result in sequence artifacts. It is known that one artificial mutation per 500 bases may be observed in the analysis of formalin-fixed tissue with low DNA content. The frequency of errors depends on the damage and cross linking of DNA by formalin. The accuracy of results can be ensured by duplicate amplifications of FFPE samples. For direct DNA sequencing, mutational artifacts should be distinguished from true mutations by bidirectional sequencing and by confirmatory sequencing of independent PCR products. Furthermore, whole genome amplification should be used to increase the amount of template DNA in insufficient specimens which are also run in duplicate.

Sangers sequencing detects all mutations in the sequenced exons, but mutation-specific methods are designed to test only for selected mutations. Therefore, a very common question is which mutations should be selected for testing when using a mutation-specific method. It is felt that clinical mutation testing should be able to detect all individual mutations that have been reported in at least 1% of mutated tumors. A summary of hot-spot mutations in *EGFR* lung adenocarcinoma is shown in *Table 30-3*.

Fluorescence In Situ Hybridization (FISH)

FISH assays have been developed to detect a wide variety of genomic alterations important in diagnostic pathology, including amplifications, chromosomal translocations, and gains and losses of either entire chromosomes or specific chromosomal regions. The current CAP/IASLC/AMP guideline for molecular testing only recommends FISH for *ALK* rearrangement testing. However, many laboratories perform additional FISH testing for targetable genes such as *ROS1* and *RET*. FISH for *MET* amplification in cases of resistance to *EGFR*-TKI or as a primary target for MET inhibitors is also very common. Standardization of FISH methodology should be relatively simple since many of the clinical laboratories are following similar procedure protocols using commercially available probes. Specimen requirements in respect to specimen type, fixation, and tissue processing are the same as for mutational analysis. There is an increasing need for simultaneous analysis of multiple chromosomal regions using differentially labeled probes.

Assays for gene amplification use a probe specific for the target gene of interest, often together with a differentially labeled probe for the corresponding centromere (*Figure 30-1*). Samples positive for amplification show multiple target gene signals. The ratio of target gene signals to centromere signal defines amplification. The ratio value that is considered positive for amplification depends on the gene and should correlate with a positive response to therapy. Amplifications, including low level, can be distinguished from polysomy for the entire chromosome (*Figure 30-2*).

Two types of FISH probes have been designed to detect chromosomal translocations: fusion probes and

TABLE 30-3 *EGFR* Mutations Accounting Individually for At Least 1% of All *EGFR* Mutations[12,14]

EGFR Exon	EGFR Codon	Mutations (Amino Acid)	Nucleotide Substitutions	Approximate % of All *EGFR* Mutations
18	E709	E709K E709A E709G E709V E709D E709Q	c.2125G>A c.2126A>C c.2126A>G c.2126A>T c.2127A>C, c.2127A>T c.2125G>C	1%
	G719	G719S G719A G719C G719D	c.2155G>A c.2156G>C c.2155G>T c.2156G>A	2%-5%
19	K739 I740 P741 V742 A743 I744	Insertions 18 bp ins		1%
	E746 L747 R748 E749 A750 T751 S752 P753	Deletions 15bp del 18bp del 9 bp del 24bp del 12bp del		45%
20	S768 V769 D770 N771 P772 H773 V774	Insertions		4%-10%
	S768	S768I	c.2303G>T	1%-2%
	T790	T790M	c.2369C>T	2%[b]
21	L858	L858R L858M	c.2573T>G c.2572C>A (rare)	40%
	L861	L861Q L861R	c.2582T>A, c.2582T>G	2%-5%

break-apart probes. Fusion probe sets consist of differentially labeled probes to two distinct loci that are not normally in close proximity to each other (one probe is typically labeled with a green signal and the other with a red signal). In a normal cell, one will identify two red and two green signals. In the presence of a translocation between these loci, one red and one green signal (corresponding to the normal chromosomes) and one yellow fusion signal (corresponding to one of the derivative chromosomes) will be identified (*Figure 30-3*). False-positive signals may occur in cells where the two probes are in close proximity to each other, producing a yellow fusion signal. It is important for each laboratory to test negative control cases and develop their own cutoff criteria for the percentage of nuclei containing a fusion pattern in order for the test to be interpreted as positive. The second most common strategy for translocation detection uses "break-apart" probes. The "break-apart" assay consists of two differentially labeled probes that hybridize to the same gene and are specific for regions that lie on opposite sides of the translocation breakpoint. Cells without a translocation show two yellow fusion signals. In the presence of a translocation involving the target gene, one set of probes is split, resulting

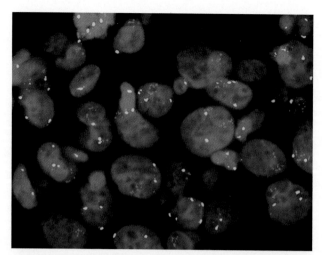

FIGURE 30-1 Lung adenocarcinoma positive for MET amplification with multiple target gene signals (red signals).

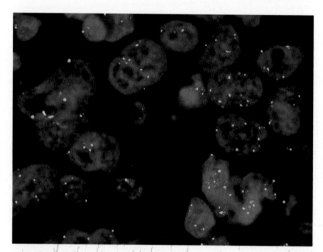

FIGURE 30-2 Lung adenocarcinoma with chromosome 7 polysomy showing multiple centromeric signals (green signal).

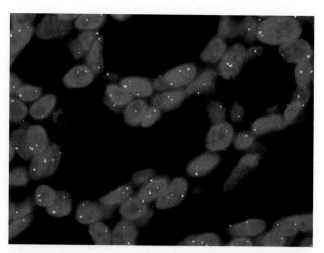

FIGURE 30-3 Fusion probe sets consist of differentially labeled probes to two distinct loci that are not normally in close proximity to each other. An example of KIF5B-RET translocation with one red and one green signal (corresponding to the normal chromosomes) and one yellow fusion signal (corresponding to one of the derivative chromosomes).

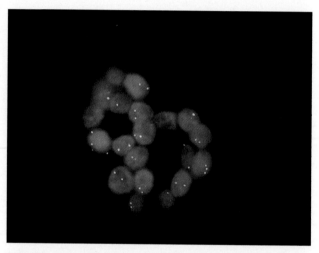

FIGURE 30-4 "Break-apart" FISH assay consists of two differentially labeled probes that hybridize to the same gene, on opposite sides of the translocation breakpoint. Cells without a translocation show two yellow fusion signals. An example of *ALK* translocation with one red and one green signal (corresponding to the two derivative chromosomes) and one yellow fusion signal (the normal chromosome).

in one red and one green signal (corresponding to the two derivative chromosomes) in addition to one yellow fusion signal (the normal chromosome) (*Figure 30-4*). This break-apart strategy is especially valuable for detecting translocations involving so-called "promiscuous" genes, where translocations may occur with multiple partner genes.

FISH assays are most frequently performed on the whole paraffin section usually 5 μm thick. Increased nuclear truncation is usually seen on thinner sections, while thicker sections show greater nuclear overlap and are more difficult to deparaffinize, leading to suboptimal hybridization. The unstained tissue sections should be prepared without tissue folding, which could also lead to greater nuclear overlap. Areas of crushed tissue also show significant nuclear overlap and should be avoided.

ALK-*FISH Assay*

The FISH break-apart assay was used in the initial studies that demonstrated significant clinical response of patients with *ALK*-rearranged tumors to treatment with the *ALK*-TKI crizotinib.[20] As noted previously, the US Food and Drug Administration has approved a commercial assay (Abbott Molecular Probes) as a "companion diagnostic" to select patients for treatment with crizo-tinib. The assay contains a SpectrumOrange-labeled 300 kb probe on the telomeric 3' side of *ALK* and a SpectrumGreen-labeled 442 kb probe on the centro-meric 5' side. Cells without translocation show a fused yellow signal, while *ALK* rearrangement is seen as distinct and separated orange and green signals. Clinical laboratories performing this test should show reproducible performance with normal controls, and with known abnormal patient specimens and cell lines. Outside of the USA, laboratories may choose to use laboratory-developed *ALK* probes for FISH. It is desirable that validation studies show comparable or superior performance to the commercial "companion diagnostic" assay. It is very important to pay attention to possible variability in clone growth, reagents, and DNA-labeling enzymes. Laboratories may follow their standard operating procedures that have been successful for FISH on FFPE tissue sections. Size of tissue, tissue preservation, and the duration and type of fixation may require modifications in the protease digestion protocol. Overdigestion should be avoided, because chromatin may show artifactual "split signals" that may result in false-positive interpretations. Although this additional step prolongs turnaround time, it is more important to modify the digestion than to reject the specimen for analysis. Similarly, hybridization and washing steps should be standardized. Although this could be done manually, use of an automated tissue processor and standardized commercial tissue digestion kits improves consistency.

A pathologist should identify areas for analysis and interpretation. Areas of interest should be marked on the H&E-stained slide adjacent to the section used for FISH analysis. Interpretation should be performed in areas of the slide with good signal, minimal background, and at least 50% of analyzable nuclei. Scoring should be performed by either a pathologist or an experienced cytotechnologist who has knowledge of solid tumor morphology. Scoring can be performed with one scorer in cases with clearly negative or positive results (>50% of cells). More complex and difficult cases should be independently scored by two interpreters.

The typical signal pattern for *ALK* rearranged adenocarcinoma is a "split signal pattern" with an orange/green fusion signal, one separate orange and one separate green signal (*Figure 30-4*). The *ALK* gene is considered rearranged if a gap between separated green and red signals is larger than two signal diameters and if this pattern is observed in ≥15% of analyzed nuclei. The identification of a two diameter gap requires experience with interpretation of FISH assays, and inclusion of well-characterized positive control sections is an essential part of the assay. *ALK*-FISH can be very heterogenous and other patterns can be observed including extra isolated 3'*ALK* signal, additional fusion signals from polysomy, and more complex *ALK* rearrangements.

ROS1-*FISH Assay*

Chromosomal rearrangements involving the *ROS1* gene were originally described in glioblastomas, where *ROS1* (chromosome 6q22) is fused to the *FIG* gene (chromosome 6q22 immediately adjacent to *ROS1*). *ROS1* fusions are identified in approximately 2% of lung adenocarcinoma.[21] ROS1 gene fusion partners in lung adenocarcinoma include CD74, SLC34A2, and SDC4. Currently there are several commercially available FISH break-apart probes. The presence of an ROS1 rearrangement leads to a split signal and the ROS1 gene is considered rearranged if a gap between separated green and red signals is larger than two signal diameters. Studies suggest that the *ALK/MET* inhibitor crizotinib may effectively inhibit the growth of *ROS1*-positive tumors.[22-24] Currently there are several commercially available FISH probes as well as an antibody for immunohistochemistry.[25] Because of potential response to an FDA-approved drug, there is an increasing demand for detection of *ROS1* rearrangements.

KIF5B-RET-*FISH Assay*

Approximately 2% of lung adenocarcinomas are reported to harbor a novel gene fusion involving the *RET* tyrosine kinase gene partnered with either *KIF5B* or *CCDC6*.[26-28] *RET* is a receptor tyrosine kinase and somatic and germline mutations in the *RET* gene are associated with multiple endocrine neoplasia type 2 syndrome and sporadic medullary thyroid cancer. The somatic *RET* fusion genes, mostly recognized as *CCDC6-RET* (PTC1) and *NCOA4-RET* (PTC3), are associated with sporadic and radiation-induced papillary thyroid cancer. Our group recently observed increased frequency of *RET* rearrangement in patients with a history of therapeutic radiation for breast carcinoma or mediastinal Hodgkin lymphoma, and suggested that *RET* chromosomal rearrangement may represent a genetic mechanism of radiation-induced lung cancer. The FISH interpretation criteria are not standardized. Based on our internal validation studies, tumors with ≥12.8% of cells displaying *RET* rearrangement are considered to be FISH positive.

MET *Amplification*

Amplification of *MET* is documented in 4.1% of lung adenocarcinomas, but *MET* overexpression is probably more common. Mutations in *MET* occur rarely in lung carcinoma. A number of recent clinical trials have demonstrated strong activity of *MET* inhibitors in patients with a variety of advanced or metastatic tumors, including non-small-cell lung cancer (NSCLC), breast, prostate, liver, and renal cancer.[29] *MET* inhibitors have also displayed clinical benefits in patients with NSCLC and patients with breast cancer who had developed resistance to *EGFR* therapy.[30,31] These recent data clearly indicate that HGF/SF-MET therapeutics may have potential in several groups of cancer patients either alone or in combination with inhibitors of other signaling pathways. *MET* is likely a targetable gene, and the companion diagnostics at this point is uncertain. A randomized phase II trial with MetMAb (Hoffmann-La Roche, Mississauga, ON), an anti-Met monoclonal antibody, suggested that protein expression may be more reliable than amplification in predicting MetMAb benefit.[32-34] The FISH *MET* assay is relatively easy to interpret. Different laboratories use different interpretation criteria for amplification. A recent study indicated that SISH shows a good correlation with *MET* immunohistochemistry and FISH results.[35]

Other Assays for Targeted Therapies

Many clinical laboratories lack technical expertise for molecular assays. Furthermore, molecular assays are expensive compared to other standard assays such as immunohistochemistry which is performed and readily interpreted by most surgical pathologists. Sensitivity and specificity of antibodies potentially used as a selection criterion for targeted therapies should be determined before they can be adopted for clinical work. Although not recommended as a screening method for gene mutations or gene rearrangements, immunohistochemistry may be considered in cases with insufficient tumor tissue for molecular assays or in cases with technically suboptimal molecular assays. Performance characteristics of commercially available mutation-specific antibodies are summarized in *Table 30-4*.

Immunohistochemistry

EGFR

Although mutation-specific EGFR antibodies are commercially available, their use for *EGFR* testing in lung cancers is not recommended.[11-13] Mutation-specific rabbit monoclonal antibodies detects two most common *EGFR* mutations (exon 19 deletions and exon 21 L858 mutation).[36-39] The reported specificity is 100%; however, the reported sensitivity ranges from 50% to 99%. Reduced sensitivity was mostly reported for exon 19 deletions other than 15bp.[32] Another confounding factor is the potential inter- and intraobserver interpretation variability that should always be taken into account. Furthermore, it is very difficult to control preanalytical and analytical variables. Staining heterogeneity and false-positive results have been reported with both antibodies.

There are two other types of EGFR IHC including IHC for total EGFR and phosphorylated EGFR. IHC for total EGFR is not an acceptable test for the selection of EGFR TKI therapy because it does not correlate with the presence of *EGFR* mutations. There is a lack of experience with IHC for phosphorylated EGFR in clinically processed pathology specimens, and therefore it should not be used in the clinical practice.

TABLE 30-4 Immunohistochemistry of Targetable Genomic Alterations in Lung Carcinoma

Target	Clone	Provider	Specificity (%)	Sensitivity (%)
EGFR	Exon 19 (E746-A750) Rabbit monoclonal	Cell Signaling Technology, Danvers, MA	85.3-100	40-100
	Exon 21 (L858R) Rabbit monoclonal	Cell Signaling Technology, Danvers, MA	91-98.5	36-95.2
ALK	D5F3 Rabbit monoclonal	Cell Signaling Technology, Danvers, MA	75-99	91-100
	5A4 Rabbit monoclonal	Novocastra, New Castle, UK	87.5-98	100
	ALK1 M7195 Mouse monoclonal	Dako, Carpinteria, CA	91-99	64-100
BRAF	V600 Clone VE1 Mouse monoclonal	Ventana, Tucson, AZ	100%	90.5
ROS	D4D6 Rabbit monoclonal	Cell Signaling Technology, Danvers, MA	92	100

TABLE 30-5 Most Commonly Used Next-Generation Sequencing Platforms in Clinical Laboratories

Parameter	Life Technologies	Ilumina	Illumina
	Ion Torrent PGM	**MiSeq**	**HiSeq**
Method of sequencing	Semiconductor sequencing technology	Sequencing by synthesis (SBS)	Sequencing by synthesis (SBS)
Clinical NGS application	Targeted sequencing for genes or gene panels	Targeted sequencing for genes or gene panels	Whole genome, exome, transcriptome, targeted sequencing for large gene panels
Time/run	4-5 hours	24 hours	3-10 days
Length of reads (base pairs)	100-200 bp	150-200 bp	150-300 bp
Minimal DNA input	10 ng	50-250 ng	250 ng-1 µg
Advantages	Low amount of DNA allows to perform NGS on small biopsies and FNA samples, fastest sequencing time	Fast, high accuracy	Allows to perform broadest number of NGS applications, discovery tool
Disadvantages	Errors in homopolymer regions	Cost of reagents, higher amount of starting DNA	Cost of reagents, higher amount of starting DNA, complex bioinformatics analysis

Used with permission of Dacic S, Nikiforova MN. Present and future molecular testing in lung carcinoma, *Adv Anatom Pathol* (submitted).

ALK

Immunohistochemistry for *ALK* protein expression is readily available, and the antibodies used in lymphomas (mouse monoclonal antihuman CD246, clone *ALK*1; Dako, Carpinteria, CA) are suboptimal for detection of protein expression in *ALK*-rearranged lung cancers. Several recent studies using a mouse monoclonal, clone 5A4 (Novocastra, Newcastle, United Kingdom), and a rabbit monoclonal anti-human CD246 (clones D5F3 and D9E4) from Cell Signaling Technology (Danvers, MA) demonstrate excellent correlation with FISH results.[16,17,40,41] Even though FISH is recommended as the standard method, *ALK* immunohistochemistry may be considered for initial *ALK* screening and positive immunostaining results can be confirmed by the FDA-approved FISH assay. This approach would reduce costs of unnecessary FISH testing. Also it could be used as a backup method in cases technically suboptimal for FISH analysis.

ROS1

A ROS1 IHC antibody (D4D6, Cell SignalingTechnology [CST], Danvers, MA) has recently been described, which appears to specifically detect ROS1-fusion proteins in NSCLC.[25] A recent report indicates excellent correlation with ROS1 rearrangements by FISH with 100% sensitivity and 92% specificity.

Next-Generation Sequencing

Next-generation sequencing (NGS) or massively parallel sequencing technology provides a more rapid and lower cost analysis of multiple gene alterations in one assay. The most commonly used technologies currently are summarized in *Table 30-5*.[42] The overall cost per test is lower by Sangers sequencing, but when the cost per base is taken into consideration, Sangers sequencing is actually more expensive than NGS. The main challenge for clinical implementation of NGS is the expertise, particularly in computational biology which is essential for meaningful data interpretation. Furthermore, small sample size seems to be even a greater challenge for these new approaches. Data on the accuracy, sensitivity, specificity, and clinical validity of these assays are very limited.

OTHER CONSIDERATIONS IN MOLECULAR TESTING

Role of the Pathologist

Selection of lung cancers for molecular testing is based on the diagnosis provided by the pathologist. The distinction between adenocarcinoma and squamous cell carcinoma is critical in the management of the lung carcinoma patient and the diagnosis of NSCLC in surgical pathology reports should be avoided as much as possible. If a diagnosis cannot be made based on morphologic criteria alone, immunoperoxidase studies may provide the diagnosis. Pathology reports may include the type of fixative that was used and time of fixation since that may influence the assay performance and interpretation. If mutational testing will be performed on FFPE tissue, the pathologist should select a paraffin block with most cellular areas containing >50% of the viable tumor cells.

Practical Considerations for Molecular Testing in Lung Carcinomas

Molecular workup represents an additional step in the workup of available tumor tissue, and therefore turnaround time becomes very important. An important question is whether molecular testing should be performed as a reflex test or should be performed only at the request of the treating physician. A turnaround time of 10 working days from the diagnostic procedure to the final report has been suggested. Achieving that goal is very challenging if samples are submitted to a reference laboratory. Testing by outside laboratories makes integration of all available data about the tumor (eg, histology, stage, mutational profile) in one report and in the patient's medical records potentially more difficult. This may be less of a problem if the testing is performed at the same institution. Reflex testing significantly reduces the turnaround time for molecular testing. It is important to precisely define criteria for testing such as tumor type, tumor stage, and specimen type to avoid unnecessary testing that would result in increased workload and overall cost. It is essential to test only patients who are candidates for TKI therapy.

REFERENCES

1. Aisner DL, Deshpande C, Baloch Z, et al. Evaluation of EGFR mutation status in cytology specimens: an institutional experience. *Diagn Cytopathol*. 2013;41:316-323.
2. Bozzetti C, Naldi N, Nizzoli R, et al. Reliability of EGFR and KRAS mutation analysis on fine-needle aspiration washing in non-small cell lung cancer. *Lung Cancer*. 2013;80:35-38.
3. Cai G, Wong R, Chhieng D, et al. Identification of EGFR mutation, KRAS mutation, and *ALK* gene rearrangement in cytological specimens of primary and metastatic lung adenocarcinoma. *Cancer Cytopathol*. 2013;121:500-507.
4. Dejmek A, Zendehrokh N, Tomaszewska M, Edsjo A. Preparation of DNA from cytological material: effects of fixation, staining, and mounting medium on DNA yield and quality. *Cancer Cytopathol*. 2013;121:344-353.
5. Gillespie JW, Best CJ, Bichsel VE, et al. Evaluation of non-formalin tissue fixation for molecular profiling studies. *Am J Pathol*. 2002;160:449-457.
6. Baloglu G, Haholu A, Kucukodaci Z, Yilmaz I, Yildirim S, Baloglu H. The effects of tissue fixation alternatives on DNA content: a study on normal colon tissue. *Appl Immunohistochem Mol Morphol*. 2008;16:485-492.
7. Moore JL, Aros M, Steudel KG, Cheng KC. Fixation and decalcification of adult zebrafish for histological, immunocytochemical, and genotypic analysis. *Biotechniques*. 2002;32:296-298.
8. Travis WD, Brambilla E, Noguchi M, et al. International Association for the Study of Lung Cancer/American Thoracic Society/European Respiratory Society: international multidisciplinary classification of lung adenocarcinoma. *J Thorac Oncol*. 2011;6:244-285.
9. Monaco SE, Nikiforova MN, Cieply K, Teot LA, Khalbuss WE, Dacic S. A comparison of EGFR and KRAS status in primary lung carcinoma and matched metastases. *Hum Pathol*. 2010;41:94-102.
10. Vignot S, Frampton GM, Soria JC, et al. Next-generation sequencing reveals high concordance of recurrent somatic alterations between primary tumor and metastases from patients with non-small-cell lung cancer. *J Clin Oncol*. 2013;31:2167-72.
11. Yatabe Y, Matsuo K, Mitsudomi T. Heterogeneous distribution of EGFR mutations is extremely rare in lung adenocarcinoma. *J Clin Oncol*. 2011;29:2972-2977.
12. Lindeman NI, Cagle PT, Beasley MB, et al. Molecular testing guideline for selection of lung cancer patients for EGFR and *ALK* tyrosine kinase inhibitors: guideline from the College of American Pathologists, International Association for the Study of Lung Cancer, and Association for Molecular Pathology. *J Mol Diagn*. 2013;15:415-453.
13. Lindeman NI, Cagle PT, Beasley MB, et al. Molecular testing guideline for selection of lung cancer patients for EGFR and *ALK* tyrosine kinase inhibitors: guideline from the College of American Pathologists, International Association for the Study of Lung Cancer, and Association for Molecular Pathology. *J Thorac Oncol*. 2013;8:823-859.
14. Lindeman NI, Cagle PT, Beasley MB, et al. Molecular testing guideline for selection of lung cancer patients for EGFR and *ALK* tyrosine kinase inhibitors: guideline from the College of American Pathologists, International Association for the Study of Lung Cancer, and Association for Molecular Pathology. *Arch Pathol Lab Med*. 2013;137:828-60.
15. Perez-Moreno P, Brambilla E, Thomas R, Soria JC. Squamous cell carcinoma of the lung: molecular subtypes and therapeutic opportunities. *Clin Cancer Res*. 2012;18:2443-51.
16. Sholl LM, Weremowicz S, Gray SW, et al. Combined use of *ALK* immunohistochemistry and FISH for optimal detection of *ALK*-rearranged lung adenocarcinomas. *J Thorac Oncol*. 2013;8:322-328.
17. Mino-Kenudson M, Chirieac LR, Law K, et al. A novel, highly sensitive antibody allows for the routine detection of *ALK*-rearranged lung adenocarcinomas by standard immunohistochemistry. *Clin Cancer Res*. 2010;16:1561-1571.
18. Rodig SJ, Mino-Kenudson M, Dacic S, et al. Unique clinicopathologic features characterize *ALK*-rearranged lung adenocarcinoma in the western population. *Clin Cancer Res*. 2009;15:5216-5223.
19. Soda M, Choi YL, Enomoto M, et al. Identification of the transforming EML4-*ALK* fusion gene in non-small-cell lung cancer. *Nature*. 2007;448:561-566.
20. Kwak EL, Bang YJ, Camidge DR, et al. Anaplastic lymphoma kinase inhibition in non-small-cell lung cancer. *N Engl J Med*. 2010;363:1693-1703.
21. Bergethon K, Shaw AT, Ou SH, et al. ROS1 rearrangements define a unique molecular class of lung cancers. *J Clin Oncol*. 2012;30:863-870.
22. Komiya T, Thomas A, Khozin S, Rajan A, Wang Y, Giaccone G. Response to crizotinib in ROS1-rearranged non-small-cell lung cancer. *J Clin Oncol*. 2012;30:3425-3426; author reply 6.
23. Sequist LV. ROS1-targeted therapy in non-small cell lung cancer. *Clin Adv Hematol Oncol*. 2012;10:827-828.

24. Takeuchi K, Soda M, Togashi Y, et al. RET, ROS1 and *ALK* fusions in lung cancer. *Nat Med*. 2012;18:378-381.

25. Sholl LM, Sun H, Butaney M, et al. ROS1 immunohistochemistry for detection of ROS1-rearranged lung adenocarcinomas. *Am J Surg Pathol*. 2013;37:1441-1449.

26. Kohno T, Ichikawa H, Totoki Y, et al. KIF5B-RET fusions in lung adenocarcinoma. *Nat Med*. 2012;18:375-377.

27. Kohno T, Tsuta K, Tsuchihara K, Nakaoku T, Yoh K, Goto K. RET fusion gene: Translation to personalized lung cancer therapy. *Cancer Sci*. 2013;104(11):1396-1400.

28. Yokota K, Sasaki H, Okuda K, et al. KIF5B/RET fusion gene in surgically-treated adenocarcinoma of the lung. *Oncol Rep*. 2012;28:1187-1192.

29. Landi L, Minuti G, D'Incecco A, Cappuzzo F. Targeting c-MET in the battle against advanced nonsmall-cell lung cancer. *Curr Opin Oncol*. 2013;25:130-136.

30. Bean J, Brennan C, Shih JY, et al. MET amplification occurs with or without T790M mutations in EGFR mutant lung tumors with acquired resistance to gefitinib or erlotinib. *Proc Natl Acad Sci U S A*. 2007;104:20932-20937.

31. Engelman JA, Zejnullahu K, Mitsudomi T, et al. MET amplification leads to gefitinib resistance in lung cancer by activating ERBB3 signaling. *Science*. 2007;316:1039-1043.

32. Sattler M, Reddy MM, Hasina R, Gangadhar T, Salgia R. The role of the c-Met pathway in lung cancer and the potential for targeted therapy. *Ther Adv Med Oncol*. 2011;3:171-184.

33. Surati M, Patel P, Peterson A, Salgia R. Role of MetMAb (OA-5D5) in c-MET active lung malignancies. *Expert Opin Biol Ther*. 2011;11:1655-1662.

34. Penuel E, Li C, Parab V, et al. HGF as a circulating biomarker of onartuzumab treatment in patients with advanced solid tumors. *Mol Cancer Ther*. 2013;12:1122-1130.

35. Dziadziuszko R, Wynes MW, Singh S, et al. Correlation between MET gene copy number by silver in situ hybridization and protein expression by immunohistochemistry in non-small cell lung cancer. *J Thorac Oncol*. 2012;7:340-347.

36. Cooper WA, Yu B, Yip PY, et al. EGFR mutant-specific immunohistochemistry has high specificity and sensitivity for detecting targeted activating EGFR mutations in lung adenocarcinoma. *J Clin Pathol*. 2013;66:744-748.

37. Jiang G, Fan C, Zhang X, et al. Ascertaining an appropriate diagnostic algorithm using EGFR mutation-specific antibodies to detect EGFR status in non-small-cell lung cancer. *PLoS One*. 2013;8:e59183.

38. Brevet M, Arcila M, Ladanyi M. Assessment of EGFR mutation status in lung adenocarcinoma by immunohistochemistry using antibodies specific to the two major forms of mutant EGFR. *J Mol Diagn*. 2010;12:169-176.

39. Kitamura A, Hosoda W, Sasaki E, Mitsudomi T, Yatabe Y. Immunohistochemical detection of EGFR mutation using mutation-specific antibodies in lung cancer. *Clin Cancer Res*. 2010;16:3349-3355.

40. Han XH, Zhang NN, Ma L, et al. Immunohistochemistry reliably detects *ALK* rearrangements in patients with advanced non-small-cell lung cancer. *Virchows Arch*. 2013;463:583-591.

41. Conklin CM, Craddock KJ, Have C, Laskin J, Couture C, Ionescu DN. Immunohistochemistry is a reliable screening tool for identification of *ALK* rearrangement in non-small-cell lung carcinoma and is antibody dependent. *J Thorac Oncol*. 2013;8:45-51.

42. Cronin M, Ross JS. Comprehensive next-generation cancer genome sequencing in the era of targeted therapy and personalized oncology. *Biomark Med*. 2011;5:293-305.

Index

Page references followed by *f* indicate figures; page references followed by *t* indicate tables.